Evidence-Based Practice Manual

EVIDENCE-BASED PRACTICE MANUAL

Research and Outcome Measures

in Health and Human Services

Edited by

Albert R. Roberts

Kenneth Yeager

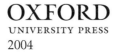
OXFORD
UNIVERSITY PRESS
2004

OXFORD
UNIVERSITY PRESS

Oxford   New York
Auckland   Bangkok   Buenos Aires   Cape Town   Chennai
Dar es Salaam   Delhi   Hong Kong   Istanbul   Karachi   Kolkata
Kuala Lumpur   Madrid   Melbourne   Mexico City   Mumbai   Nairobi
São Paulo   Shanghai   Taipei   Tokyo   Toronto

Published by Oxford University Press, Inc.
198 Madison Avenue, New York, New York 10016

www.oup.com

Oxford is a registered trademark of Oxford University Press

Library of Congress Cataloging-in-Publication Data
Evidence-based pratice manual: Research and outcome measures in health and human
services / edited by Albert R. Roberts, Kenneth Yeager.
p. cm.
Includes bibliographical references and index.
ISBN 13 978-0-19-516500-5
ISBN 0-19-516500-4
1. Medicine—Practice—Handbooks, manuals, etc.   2. Evidence-based
medicine—Handbooks, manuals, etc.   3. Human
services—Research—Methodology—Handbooks, manuals, etc.   I. Roberts,
Albert R.   II. Yeager, Kenneth.
R728   .D47   2004
362.1—dc22   2003066653

3 5 7 9 8 6 4

Printed in the United States of America
on acid-free paper

PREFACE

Evidence-based practice (EBP) is the most challenging and critical practice area of health care and human services. EBP has the potential, when systematically implemented, to prevent numerous avoidable deaths and injuries, while improving the quality of life for millions of individuals. The *Evidence-Based Practice Manual* was developed as an all-inclusive and comprehensive, practical desktop reference. It includes 104 original chapters specially written by the most prominent and experienced medical, public health, psychology, social work, criminal justice, and public policy practitioners, researchers and professors in the United States and Canada.

There has been widespread interest in finding the most up-to-date information on evidence-based assessment measures, treatment protocols, and interventions in health care and human service settings. This interdisciplinary, major reference book has systematically integrated the latest methods of locating and taking action based on evidence-based practice.

Six key features of the book are as follows:

1. The first interdisciplinary volume on locating and applying evidence-based assessment measures, treatment plans, and interventions;
2. Emphasis on practical, user-friendly, step-by-step methods for conducting evidence-based practice as well as practice-based research;
3. Emphasis on concise summaries of the substantive evidence gained from methodologically rigorous quantitative and qualitative research;
4. Identification and discussion of each essential stage of program evaluation, quantitative research, qualitative studies, quality and operational improvement, research grant applications, validating measurement tools, and utilizing statistical procedures;
5. Illustration and summary of key issues, concepts, outcome measures, how-to approaches, practice-based research guidelines, and evidence-based mental health treatment applications;
6. A comprehensive glossary with almost 500 concise definitions of every facet of evidence-based practice, research designs, epidemiological research, research grants, program evaluation, outcome measurement, assessment tools, research ethics, and quality assurance measures.

The chapter authors were invited to prepare a concise, readable, state-of-the art and practical chapter in their area of practice-based research and/or evidence-based practice. Each chapter provides sufficient basic and advanced knowledge so that all readers will be able to quickly grasp the essence and useful evidence and tools in each chapter. This Desk Reference will provide health care and human service administrators, policymakers, practitioners, and researchers and program evaluators with ready access to the knowledge base and substantive empirical evidence to make timely and critical decisions.

During the past decade there has been growing recognition and reliance on evidence-based practice in the professions of medicine, public health, psychology, social work, and criminal justice. Evidence-based practice is based on systematic reviews of a body of research and evaluation studies on a particular treatment or intervention practice. Hand-in-hand with the movement toward evidence-based practice has been a search for methodologically rigorous practice-based research and empirical evidence resulting from the studies. Therefore, this volume was developed based on the following three objectives.

1. To identify and discuss the latest protocols and methods of evidence-based practice;
2. To identify experts in the field to prepare original chapters that include systematic reviews of previous research on the effectiveness of particular assessment measures or treatment protocols for specific physical or mental health disorders.
3. To select experts who have completed scientific, methodologically rigorous medical, public health, or social science research and invite them to prepare specially designed chapters sharing their key findings and substantive empirical evidence.

Health care and human service professionals are confronted by tumultuous times. Demands for services and upon care providers are greater than ever. Previously accepted practice priorities are being rapidly revised by accreditation bodies so the newest priorities are patient safety, applying the highest standards of care, and documentation of patient progress. The changes occur due to (1) technological innovations that have resulted in greater time pressure on managers and individual practitioners; (2) increased demand for service in a managed care environment that requires cost containment; and (3) increasing difficulties in physicians' obtaining malpractice insurance and the litigation that ensues following an adverse medical outcome, which has reinforced the necessity for documenting the best practices and evidence-based applications in health care and human services. Advances in health care and human services do not come without a price. Possibly the greatest cost is that of time constraints on the individual practitioner. Professionals involved in the complex tasks of today's health care and human services arena are confronted on a daily basis with issues of time management. Currently, the application of technological advances rather than reducing the practitioner's time is in many cases increasing the amount of time and effort required to handle major tasks.

With that in mind, the *Evidence-Based Practice Manual* provides 104 concise, quickly referenced, originally prepared chapters to assist direct care practitioners and administrators in identifying and applying cutting-edge protocols and evidence-based practice within their agencies and practice environment. It is our hope that the information contained within this volume will serve as a fingertip reference on evidence-based practice and practice-based research by providing step-by-step application models for direct care practitioners working in health care and human services. Our ultimate goal is for this new Desk Reference to act as a springboard to further applications of evidence-based practice throughout all health care and human services settings. It is our contention that evidence-based practice is never complete; there is always room for updating and expansion. We consider ourselves lifelong learners, and as a result we compiled and edited this original volume to provide the foundation knowledge base, skills, and guidelines on evidence-based practice. It is our hope that future editions will build on this solid foundation, and readers will contact us with suggestions for additions in the important years ahead.

This is the first all-inclusive major reference book to include the latest information on

I.   Critical Issues in Evidence-Based Practice such as protocols for identifying evidence-based practices, implementing evidence-based and practice-based studies, establishing standardized measures in health care and mental health, and applying technological advances.
II. Research Ethics and Step-by-Step Research Grant Guidelines, including methodological approaches to writing grants; ethical and practical challenges in research grants; step-by-step grant application processes; refinement of grantsmanship skill building; and conducting cost-benefit analysis to fulfill a state contract.
III. Evidence-Based Practice Guidelines for Diagnosis and Intervention, including specific evidence-based practice guidelines; procedures for implementing and applying practice guidelines; measurement and critical reasoning skills in evidence-based practice; and facilitating practitioner use of evidence-based practice in areas such as
     • Treatment with children and adolescents
     • Culturally specific applications
     • Crisis assessment and intervention
     • Suicide assessment and prevention
     • Conduct disorder
     • Depression
     • Domestic Violence
     • Anxiety

- Obsessive-Compulsive Disorder
- Post-Traumatic Stress Disorder
- Couples Therapy
- Family Treatment

IV. Epidemiological and Public Health Research, including basic and advanced methodology skills; disease surveillance methods; randomized research processes; and disease prevention models.

V. An Emphasis on Clinical Practice Measurement, including issues of validity and reliability; risk-adjusted health and mental health outcomes; statistical methodology; measurement through computer technology; and consumer-based outcomes.

VI. Discussion of Assessment Tools and Measures, including locating the best available measurement tools and scales for children, adults, couples, and families; constructing and validating these assessment tools; how to use brief assessment tools and computer assisted scales; and how to develop scales and measurement instruments.

VII. An Emphasis on Program Evaluation Skill Development, including empowerment evaluation; evaluation strategies; process vs. outcome measurement; international service evaluation; step-by-step needs assessment; budgeting and fiscal management; logic models; system change evaluation; and quality measurement.

VIII. Qualitative Research Methods and Exemplars in direct care settings, cancer prevention, intensive care units, and mental health settings, and with families of the mentally ill, domestic violence victims, African American women with breast cancer, and homeless family members.

IX. Quantitative Research Exemplars, including experimental, correlational, logistic regression, meta-analysis, and secondary data analysis with mental health, health care, and law enforcement service consumers, and antisocial children in St. Louis, Missouri, public schools, victims of theft at Atlantic City casinos, elderly homicide victims in New York City, convicted felons in treatment programs developed by drug courts in the Southwest, and caregivers of the mentally ill in NAMI-based programs (National Alliance for the Mentally Ill).

X. Discussion of an Array of Quality and Operational Improvement Frameworks and Applications, including quality management in risk reduction; balanced scorecards; measurement of client perception; disease management; benchmarking; and strategic planning.

Two final features of this volume that readers should find very helpful are the comprehensive listing of over 120 Internet resources and websites and a glossary of nearly 500 terms at the end of the book. The thorough listing and description of evidence-based practice (EBP) websites is interdisciplinary, including criminology, education, medicine, nursing, psychology, public health, social work, and university library and medical library association websites. The detailed glossary allows readers to quickly look up key terms.

ACKNOWLEDGMENTS

First and foremost, we express our gratitude to our three esteemed consulting editors who recommended topics and chapter authors, and who also systematically completed peer reviews of many of the draft chapters. Without the dedication, diligence, and commitment of Professors Kevin Corcoran, Cheryl Regehr, and Phyllis Solomon, we would never have been able to keep to the tight contractual schedule and deadlines. Equally important was our team of prolific chapter authors who wrote the 104 original chapters in line with our guidelines and specifications. We are also particularly grateful to three esteemed chapter authors who exceeded our high expectations by each contributing three original chapters to this volume—Dr. Edward J. Mullen, Professor of Social Work at Columbia University; Dr. David L. Streiner, Professor of Psychiatry at the University of Toronto; and Dr. Harris Chaiklin, Professor Emeritus, University of Maryland at Baltimore. We feel most fortunate to have recruited over 100 of the leading research and clinical authorities to write specially designed chapters. Special thanks also go to a group of 22 dedicated and diligent peer reviewers for their timely reviews and technical assistance:

Gunner Almgren, Ph.D.
Beverley J. Antle, Ph.D.
Gary L. Bowen, Ph.D.
Natasha Bowen, Ph.D.
Michael J. Camasso, Ph.D.
Richard Caputo, Ph.D.
Harris Chaiklin, Ph.D.
Cynthia Franklin, Ph.D.

Leon Ginsburg, Ph.D.
Karen S. Knox, Ph.D.
Gordon MacNeil, Ph.D.
Leonard A. Marowitz, M.S.
C. Aaron McNeece, Ph.D.
Edward J. Mullen, D.S.W.
Scott Okamoto, Ph.D.
Nathaniel J. Pallone, Ph.D.
Carrie J. Petrucci, Ph.D.
Frederic G. Reamer, Ph.D.
Michael J. Smith, D.S.W.
David W. Springer, Ph.D.
David L. Streiner, Ph.D.
Vikki L. Vandiver, D.P.H.

We have been blessed with an exceptional editor, Joan H Bossert, to whom we give special acknowledgment for very useful guidance and insights, while being the significant sounding board in helping us process new ideas in the development of this book. Assistant editor Maura Roessner deserves our appreciation for completing numerous forms, producing total page estimates, and processing copyright releases, especially during the final transmittal stage of overseeing the manuscript as it left the New York editorial office to production. We are particularly thankful to Jessica Ryan, production manager and production editor for her diligence in keeping this large volume on schedule through all of the complex production stages such as copyediting, proofreading, and indexing. We express our appreciation to Evelyn Roberts Levine for writing glossary terms and definitions as well as compiling, organizing, and editing the multiple glossary terms and definitions submitted by the 104 lead chapter authors.

Special thanks for encouragement and support go to our respective universities. At Rutgers University, Dr. Arnold Hyndman, Dean and Professor of Cell Biology; and at Ohio State University Medical Center, Dr. Kadu Saveanu, Chairperson, Department of Psychiatry. Finally, we both thank our wives, Beverly J. Roberts and Donna Yeager, for their understanding during the numerous weekends and evenings over the past two years when they lost our companionship while we devoted ourselves to completing this book.

Albert R. Roberts, Ph.D.
Piscataway, New Jersey
Kenneth R. Yeager, Ph.D.
Columbus, Ohio

CONTENTS

SECTION IX: PRACTICE BASED QUANTITATIVE RESEARCH EXEMPLARS

SECTION X: ESTABLISHING, MONITORING, AND MAINTAINING QUALITY AND OPERATIONAL IMPROVEMENT

EPILOGUE

CONTRIBUTORS

ALBERT R. ROBERTS, Ph.D., B.C.E.T.S., D.A.C.F.E., is Professor of Criminal Justice and Social Work (former Chairperson), and Director of Faculty and Curriculum Development, Administration of Justice and Interdisciplinary Criminal Justice Programs in the Faculty of Arts and Sciences, Livingston College Campus at Rutgers, the State University of New Jersey in Piscataway. He has been a tenured professor at Rutgers University since 1989, prior to which he taught at Indiana University, Seton Hall University, Brooklyn College of CUNY, and the University of New Haven. Dr. Roberts has 30 years full-time university teaching experience including 15 years of administrative experience (ten years as Chair, and five years as a Program Director). Dr. Roberts received his M.A. degree in Sociology from the Graduate Faculty of Long Island University, and a D.S.W. in 1978 and a Ph.D. in 1981 from the School of Social Work and Community Planning at the University of Maryland in Baltimore. In addition, his doctoral studies at the University of Maryland included a double specialization in research methods and criminology. In 2002, Professor Roberts was the recipient of The Richard W. Laity Academic Leadership Award of the Rutgers Council of AAUP (American Association of University Professors) Chapters. Dr. Roberts is the founding Editor-in-Chief of the *Brief Treatment and Crisis Intervention* journal (Oxford University Press). He currently serves on the Editorial Boards of six professional journals. In January 2002, Dr. Roberts edited a special issue of the *Brief Treatment and Crisis Intervention* journal on Stress, Crisis, and Trauma Intervention Strategies in the Aftermath of the September 11th Terrorism Attacks (see Dr. Roberts website for further details *www.crisisinterventionnetwork.com.*)

Dr. Roberts is a member of The Board of Scientific and Professional Advisors, and a Board Certified Expert in Traumatic Stress for The American Academy of Experts in Traumatic Stress. He is also a Diplomate of the American College of Forensic Examiners. Dr. Roberts is the founding and current editor of the 41-volume Springer Series on Social Work (1980 to present), and the 8-volume Springer Family Violence Series. He is the author, co-author, or editor of approximately 160 scholarly publications, including numerous peer-reviewed journal articles and book chapters, and 25 books. His recent books include: *Handbook of Domestic Violence Intervention Strategies,* Oxford University Press (2002); *Social Workers' Desk Reference* (includes 146 chapters and is co-edited by Gilbert J. Greene, Oxford University Press, 2002), *Crisis Intervention Handbook: Assessment, Treatment and Research,* 2d ed. Oxford University Press, 2000), *Juvenile Justice Sourcebook* (in press, Oxford University Press), and *Battered Women and their Families: Intervention Strategies and Treatment Approaches,* 2d ed. (1998).

Dr. Roberts recent current projects include: continuing to teach courses on crisis intervention, domestic violence, introduction to criminal justice, research methods, program evaluation, victimology and victim assistance, special topics, and juvenile justice at Rutgers University; directing the 18-credit *Certificate Program in Criminal Justice Policies and Practices* at Livingston College of Rutgers University; training crisis intervention workers and clinical supervisors in crisis assessment and crisis intervention strategies; and training police officers and administrators in domestic violence policies and crisis intervention. He is a lifetime member of the Academy of Criminal Justice Sciences (ACJS), has been a member of the National Association of Social Workers (NASW) since 1974, and for many years has been listed in *Who's Who in America*, *Who's Who in Medicine and Health-care*, and *Who's Who Among Human Service Professionals*. Dr. Roberts was the recipient of the Teaching Excellence Award by Sigma Alpha Kappa Chapter of the National Criminal Justice Honor Society in both 1997 and 1998, and is a Charter Member of the Gamma Epsilon Chapter of Alpha Delta Mu National Social Work Honor Society at Indiana University (1985–present).

KENNETH R. YEAGER, Ph.D., LISW, is the Director of Quality and Operational Improvement for Ohio State University Harding Behavioral Healthcare and Medicine and Director of OSU and Harding Behavioral Healthcare and Medicine Outpatient Psychiatric Clinics. For the past eight years Dr. Yeager has served as adjunct professor in the Ohio State University College of Social Work. He is also Clinical Assistant Professor of Psychiatry in the Department of Psychiatry of The Ohio State University. Dr. Yeager completed his doctoral degree at The Ohio State University, College of Social Work. Dr. Yeager has greater than fifteen years experience in mental health and substance dependence treatment as both administrator and clinician. Currently, Dr. Yeager is a Treating Clinician for the National Football League Program for Substances of Abuse. Areas of research interest include: development of quality metrics, implementation of quality improvement processes within medical and psychiatric healthcare settings, impact of co-morbid diagnosis on rehospitalization rates, substance dependence with mentally ill chemical abusers, and processes of addiction and recovery with resistant populations. Dr. Yeager is an active member of the editorial board for the Brief Treatment and Crisis Intervention journal.

KEVIN CORCORAN, Ph.D., J.D., is Professor, Graduate School of Social Work, Portland State University in Oregon. He holds a B.A. in English from Colorado State University, an M.A. in Counseling from the University of Colorado, M.S.W., Ph.D. from University of Pittsburgh School of Social Work, and a J.D. from the University of Houston. Dr. Corcoran's research specializations are measurement in clinical practice, rapid assessment instruments, evidence-based social work practice, and legal issues of social work. He has authored or edited eight books including *Measures for Clinical Practice* (200, with Joel Fischer), *Maneuvering the Maze of Managed Care* (1996, with Vikki Vandiver), and most recently *Social Work Practice* (2001, with Harold Briggs). He has also written nearly eighty articles and book chapters and has served on eight editorial boards. He is a former board member of the Society of Social Work and Research. Dr. Corcoran is a founding board member of Oxford University Press's journal, *Brief Treatment and Crisis Intervention*. He also practices commercial and community mediation in Portland, Oregon.

CHERYL REGEHR, Ph.D., RSW, is an Associate Professor of Social Work at University of Toronto. She is also the Director of the Centre for Applied Social Research at the University of Toronto, and a faculty member in the Faculty of Law and the Institute for Health Sciences. Her practice background includes direct service in mental health, sexual assault recovery programs, and sex offender treatment programs and in administration of community and emergency mental health programs and sexual assault care centers. She was the Clinical Director of the Critical Incident Stress Team at Pearson International Airport for 10 years and remains involved with trauma interventions in organizations. Dr. Regehr's program of research involves examining aspects of recovery from trauma in such diverse populations as victims of rape, firefighters, police, and ambulance workers witnessing traumatic events, families of emergency responders, and child welfare workers. Her most recent research entitled Retribution, Restoration, and Victim Healing examines the impact of various public and court processes on victims of assault. Other research investigates means of evaluating professional competence. These research projects are primarily funded by the Social Sciences and Humanities Research Council of Canada. Her publications address both issues of trauma and the interface between the law and mental health. She has a forthcoming book with Oxford University Press, which is entitled "In the Line of Fire: Trauma in the Emergency Services."

Dr. Regehr has been a member of committees adjudicating grants for the Social Sciences and Humanities Research Council of Canada and a committee focusing on evaluation of professional competence in the health professions for the Canadian Institute for Health Research. She was recently awarded the Sandra Rotman Chair for her research and teaching in social work practice and was awarded Teacher of the Year by students in the Faculty of Social Work for the third consecutive year. She is a member of the editorial board and Research Commentaries Editor for the *Brief Treatment and Crisis Intervention* journal and *Currents—The Journal of New Scholarship*. She reviews manuscripts for 10 journals in psychiatry, psychology, and social work and grant applications for three public research councils.

PHYLLIS SOLOMON, Ph.D., is a Professor in the School of Social Work, University of Pennsylvania who teaches in the area of research. She has a secondary appointment in the Department of Psychiatry, School of Medicine, University of Pennsylvania. She earned her B.A. in sociology from Russell Sage College, M.A. in sociology, and Ph.D. in social welfare both from Case Western Reserve University. She has over 30 years of research, planning, and administrative experience. She has worked in the state psychiatric system and in a community research and planning agency where she conducted research and evaluations and designed service interventions. Prior to her current position, she was a Professor in the Department of Psychiatry at Hahnemann University. Dr. Solomon has served on numerous federal research and service review panels. Much of her research has been funded by the National Institute of Mental Health, Substance Abuse Mental Health Services Administration, state departments of mental health. She has extensively published and presented on issues concerning adults with serious mental illness and their families. She has co-edited two books on psychiatric rehabilitation, *Psychiatric Rehabilitation in Practice* and *New Developments in Psychiatric Rehabilitation*, and coauthored *Community Services to Discharged Psychiatric Patients*. She is Director of an NIMH Social Work Research Development Center that focuses on service interventions for adults with severe mental illness and their families. In 1997, her article with others on the results of a family education intervention that appeared in *Schizophrenia Bulletin* received first place by the Society for Social Work and Research. She was the 1999 recipient of the Armin Loeb Award from International Association of Psychosocial Rehabilitation Services for her research in psychosocial rehabilitation; and in 2002 she received the Outstanding Non-psychiatrist Award from the American Association of Community Psychiatrists for her extraordinary contribution to community mental health. She is listed in numerous directories, including a number of editions of *Who's Who in America, Who's Who in Medicine and Healthcare, 500 Notable Women, Outstanding Scholars of the 20th Century*, to name a few.

Jonathan S. Abramowitz, Ph.D.
Mayo Clinic
Rochester, MN

Sara Ackerman, MPH
Doctoral Candidate
Department of Anthropology
University of North Carolina
Chapel Hill, NC

Gunnar Almgren, Ph.D.
Associate Professor
School of Social Work
University of Washington
Former Director, Social Work Department
University of Washington Medical Center
Seattle, WA

Beverly J. Antle, Ph.D., R.S.W.
Academic and Clinical Specialist, Social Work
Director of PKU Program, Division of Clinical
    and Metabolic Genetics
The Hospital for Sick Children
Toronto, ON

Charles Auerbach, Ph.D.
Professor
Wurzweiler School of Social Work
Yeshiva University
New York, NY

William Bacon, Ph.D.
Research Associate, Columbia University
School of Social Work and Consultant
Owen Consulting Inc.
Brooklyn, NY

Ahmed M. Bayoumi, M.D., M.S.
Assistant Professor, Associate SGS Member
Department of Health Policy Management and
    Evaluation
University of Toronto
St Michaels Hospital
Inner City Research Unit
Toronto, ON

Ciomara Beninca, Ph.D.
Hospital Psychologist
University Faculty
City General Hospital
Passo Fundo, Brazil

Jacquelin Berman, Ph.D.
Director of Research
New York City
Department of Aging
New York, NY

Bernard Bloom, Ph.D.
Professor Emeritus
Department of Psychology
University of Colorado
Boulder, CO

Patrick Bordnick, MPH, Ph.D.
Assistant Professor
University of Georgia
School of Social Work
Athens, GA

Gary L. Bowen, Ph.D.
William R. Kenan, Jr. Distinguished Professor
School of Social Work
University of North Carolina at Chapel Hill
Chapel Hill, NC

Natasha K. Bowen, Ph.D.
Assistant Professor
School of Social Work
University of North Carolina at Chapel Hill
Chapel Hill, NC

Patricia Brownell, Ph.D.
Assistant Professor
Graduate School of Social Service
Fordham University at Lincoln Center
New York, NY

Michael J. Camasso, Ph.D.
Rutgers University
Associate Professor of Public Policy
Livingston Campus
New Brunswick, NJ

Richard K. Caputo, Ph.D.
Professor
Wurzweiler School of Social Work
Yeshiva University
New York, NY

Colleen Carpenter, MA, MPH
Program Coordinator for Nigeria, Ipas
Chapel Hill, NC

Mary Anne Casey, Ph.D.
Consultant
Minneapolis, MN

Harris Chaiklin, Ph.D.
Professor Emeritus
University of Maryland
School of Social Work
Columbia, MD

Thomas J. Chapel, MA, MBA
Senior Health Scientist
Centers for Disease Control and Prevention
Office of the Director/Office of Program
   Planning and Evaluation
Atlanta, GA

Nancy Claiborne, Ph.D., ACSW
Assistant Professor
School of Social Welfare
University at Albany, SUNY
Albany, NY

Patricia A. Cody, M.S.W.
Research Associate
University of Texas, Austin
Austin, TX

Marc Corbière, Ph.D.
Research Associate
Department of Psychiatry
University of British Columbia
Vancouver, B.C.

Jacqueline Corcoran, Ph.D.
School of Social Work
Northern Virginia Campus
Virginia Commonwealth University
Alexandria, VA

Kevin Corcoran, Ph.D., J.D.
Professor
Graduate School of Social Work
Portland State University
Portland, OR

Cindy Crusto, Ph.D.
Associate Research Scientist
Yale University School of Medicine
New Haven, CT

Gary L. Dick, Ph.D.
Assistant Professor
School of Social Work
University of Cincinnati
Cincinnati, OH

Jeffrey Draine, Ph.D.
Assistant Professor
University of Pennsylvania
School of Social Work
Philadelphia, PA

Sophia F. Dziegielewski, Ph.D.
Professor
School of Social Work
University of Central Florida
Orlando, FL

Jo Anne Earp, ScD
Professor
Department of Health Behavior and Health
    Education
School of Public Health
University of North Carolina at Chapel Hill
Chapel Hill, NC

Eugenia Eng, MPH, DrPH
Professor
Department of Health Behavior and Health
    Education
School of Public Health
University of North Carolina at Chapel Hill
Chapel Hill, NC

Hattie Ellis, M.Ed.
Counselor
Beddington High School
STEP Project Community Advisor
Step County, NC

Anna Faul, Ph.D.
Associate Dean Academic Affairs
Kent School of Social Work
Louisville, KY

Ronald Feldman, Ph.D.
Ruth Harris Ottman Centennial Professor
Director, Center for the Study of Social Work
    Practice
Columbia University
School of Social Work
New York, NY

David Fetterman, Ph.D.
Professor and Director
M.A. Program in Evaluation and Public Policy
Stanford University
School of Education
Stanford, CA

Prudence Fisher, Ph.D.
NIMH-DISC Training Center at Columbia
    University
New York State Psychiatric Institute
New York, NY

Anne E. Fortune, Ph.D.
Professor
School of Social Welfare
University at Albany
State University of New York
Albany, NY

Cynthia G.S. Franklin, Ph.D.
Professor
University of Texas at Austin
School of Social Work
Austin, TX

Eileen D. Gambrill, Ph.D.
Professor
U.C. Berkley
School of Social Welfare
Berkley, CA

Dr. Jacques Gardon
Unité d'Epidémiologie
Institut Pasteur de la Guyane
Paris, France

Margaret M. Geehan, MS
Doctoral student in Educational Theory and
    Practice
State University of New York at Albany
Albany, NY

Catherine Grenier Sennelier, MD, MBA
Assistant Professor
Public Health Department
Dochin Hospital
(Assistance Publique—Hôpitaux de Paris).
Paris, France

Leonard Gibbs, Ph.D.
Professor
Department of Social Work
University of Wisconsin
Eau Claire, WI

Leon Ginsberg, Ph.D.
Interim Dean and
Carolina Distinguished Professor
University of South Carolina
School of Social Work
Columbia, SC
Former Commissioner of Higher Education
State of South Carolina

Graham Glancy, M.D.
Associate Professor
Department of Psychiatry
Faculty of Medicine
University of Toronto
Toronto, Cannada

D. Gohdes
Principal Researcher
Montana Department of Public Health and
    Human Services
Helena, MT

William Gomes, Ph.D.
Professor of Psychology
Universidade Federal do Rio Grande do Sul
Porto Alegre Rio Grande Do Sul, Brazil

Ellen Goldstein, M.A.
Center for AIDS Prevention Studies
University of California
San Francisco, CA

Ken Graap, M.Ed.
Doctoral Student
Department of Psychology
Emory University
Atlanta, GA

Diana P. Hackbarth, RN, Ph.D., FAAN
School of Nursing
Loyola University Chicago
Chicago, IL

Hildi Hagedorn, Ph.D., LP
Minneapolis Veterans Affairs Medical Center
Staff Psychologist
Minneapolis VA Medical Center
Minneapolis, MN

Helen P. Hartnett, Ph.D.
Assistant Professor
The University of Kansas
School of Social Welfare
Lawrence, KS

Mary Beth Harris, Ph.D., LMSW-ACP
Director, New Mexico Highlands University
School of Social Work at Rio Rancho
Albuquerque, NM

Carol Harvey, Ph.D.
Associate Director
Center for State Health Policy
Institute for Health, Healthcare Policy and
    Aging Research
Rutgers University
New Brunswick, NJ

Todd Harwell, M.P.H.
Coordinator Montana DPHSS Chronic Disease
    and Health Promotion
Montana Department of Public Health and
    Human Services
Helena, MT

Robert Hayward, MD, MPH, FRCPC
Director, Centre for Health Evidence
Associate Professor, Departments of Medicine
    and Public Health Sciences
University of Alberta
Edmonton, Alberta

Heidi Heft La Porte, D.S.W
Assistant Professor
Wurzweiler School of Social Work
Yeshiva University
New York, NY

S. D. Helgerson
Department of Community Medicine
University of North Dakota
School of Medicine and Health Sciences and
Montana Department of Public Health and
    Human Services
Grand Forks, ND

Michael Hendryx, Ph.D.
Assistant Director of Mental Health Services
    Research

The Washington Institute for Mental Illness
  Research and Training (WIMIRT)
Department of Psychology WSU
Spokane, WA

James J. Hennessy, Ph.D.
Professor
Fordham University at Lincoln Center
Department of Educational Psychology
New York, NY

Lori Holleran, Ph.D.
Assistant Professor
The University of Texas at Austin
School of Social Work
Austin, TX

Gregory S. Holzman, MD, MPH
Associate Professor
University of North Dakota School of
  Medicine and Health Sciences
Department of Community Medicine
Department of Family Medicine
Grand Forks, ND

Dr. Ronald J. Hunsicker
President/CEO
National Association of Addiction Treatment
  Providers
Lancaster, PA

Donna E. Hurdle, Ph.D.
Assistant Professor
School of Social Work
Arizona State University
Tempe, AZ

Stephen W. Hwang, MD, MPH
Inner City Health Research Unit
St. Michael's Hospital
Toronto, Ontario

Radha Jagannathan, Ph.D.
Assistant Professor
Edward J. Bloustein School of Planning and
  Public Policy
Rutgers University
New Brunswick, NJ

Eric D. Johnson, Ph.D.
Assistant Professor
Couple and Family Therapy Graduate Program
Drexel University
Philadelphia, PA

Catheleen Jordan, Ph.D.
Professor
School of Social Work
University of Texas Arlington
Arlington, TX

Stephen A. Kapp, Ph.D.
Associate Professor
The University of Kansas
School of Social Welfare
Lawrence, KS

David Katz, MA
Loyola University of Chicago
Chicago, IL

Elizabeth King Keenan, Ph.D., LCSW
Assistant Professor
Department of Social Work
Southern Connecticut State University
New Haven, CT

Stuart A. Kirk, DSW, Professor
Department of Social Welfare
University of California, Los Angeles (UCLA)
Los Angeles, CA

Karen Knox, Ph.D.
Associate Professor and
Director of Field Instruction
School of Social Work
Southwest Texas State University
Austin, TX

Dawn Koontz, Ph.D.
Psychologist
Anxiety Disorder Clinic
St. Louis Medical Center
St. Louis, MO

Richard Krueger, Ph.D.
Professor
Graduate School of Education
University of Minnesota
Minneapolis, MN

Michel Landry, Ph.D.
Director of Professional Services and Research
Dollard-Cormier Rehabilitation Center
Adjunct Professor
Department of Psychology
University of Montreal
Montreal, Canada

Gerald LaSalle, M.A.
Doctoral Candidate
City University of New York Graduate Center
John Jay College of Criminal Justice
New York, NY
Adjunct Lecturer in Criminal Justice
Rutgers University

Doug Leigh, Ph.D.
Assistant Professor of Education
Pepperdine University
Graduate School of Education and Psychology
Culver City, CA

Sarah J. Lewis, Ph.D.
Associate Professor
School of Social Work
Barry University
Miami, FL

Marc Lipton, Ph.D.
Clinical Social Worker in Private Practice
Former Commissioner, Baltimore City
    Department of Mental Health
Towson, MD

Paul J. Longo, Ph.D.
Institute for Local Government Administration
    and Rural Development
Ohio University
Athens, OH

Christopher Lucas, M.D.
Columbia Psychiatric Institute and
Department of Psychiatry
Columbia Presbyterian Medical Center
New York, NY

Rochelle E. Martin, M.Sc.
Research Associate
Inner City Health Research Unit
St. Michael's Hospital
Toronto, Ontario

Sherri McCarthy, Ph.D.
Professor of Psychology
Northern Arizona University
Yuma, AZ

Charles McClintock, Ph.D.
HOD Dean
Fielding Graduate Institute
Santa Barbara, CA

C. Aaron McNeece, Ph.D.
Walter Hudson Research Professor
School of Social Work
Florida State University
Tallahassee, FL
Former Director, Institute of Health and
    Human Services Research
Florida State University

Céline Mercier, Ph.D.
Professor
Department of Preventive and Social Medecine
University of Montreal
Associate Professor
Department of Psychiatry
McGill University
Director of the Research and Information
    Technologies Department at the Lisette-
    Dupras
and West Montreal Rehabilitation Centers
Montreal, Quebec

Etienne Minvielle, MD, Ph.D.,
Chargé de Recherche CNRS
Chief Researcher
Center for Health Economics and
    Administration Research
Paris, France

Faye Mishna, Ph.D.
Assistant Professor
Faculty of Social Work
University of Toronto
Toronto, Canada

Gary Mitchell, M.S.W.
Assistant Director
Anxiety Disorder Clinic
St. Louis University Medical Center
St. Louis, MO

Carol T. Mowbray, Ph.D.
Professor
School of Social Work
University of Michigan
Ann Arbor, MI

Edward J. Mullen, Ph.D.
Distinguished Professor and Director
NIMH Mental Health Services Research
    Doctoral Training Program
Columbia University
Graduate School of Social Work
New York, NY

Carlton E. Munson, Ph.D.
Professor
University of Maryland
School of Social Work
Baltimore, MD

Peter E. Nathan, Ph.D.
University of Iowa Foundation
Distinguished Professor of Psychology
Department of Psychology
College of Liberal arts and Sciences, and
Department of Community and Behavioral
    Health
College of Public Health
University of Iowa
Iowa City, Iowa

Dianna L. Newman, Ph.D.
Evaluation Consortium
University at Albany/SUNY
Albany, NY

William R. Nugent, Ph.D.
Director, Doctoral Program
Professor of Social Work
The University of Tennessee
Knoxville, TN

Scott Okomoto, Ph.D.
Assistant Professor
School of Social Work
Arizona State University
Tempe, AZ

Julianne S. Oktay, Ph.D.
Professor and Director of the Doctoral Program
University of Maryland
School of Social Work
Baltimore, MD

Dennis K. Orthner, Ph.D.
Distinguished Professor
School of Social Work
University of North Carolina at Chapel Hill
Chapel Hill, NC

Nathaniel J. Pallone, Ph.D.
University Professor of Psychology
Center of Alcohol Studies
Rutgers University, Busch Campus
Piscataway, N.J.
Co-Editor, *Current Psychology* journal and
Editor-in-Chief, *Offender Rehabilitation and
    Counseling*

Natalia Pane, Ph.D.
Senior Analyst, Planning and Evaluation
    Team
American Institutes for Research
Washington, DC

Ms. Eunice Y. Park-Lee, MSW
Doctoral Candidate
University of Maryland Baltimore
School of Social Work
Baltimore, MD

Heather Parris, MSSW
University of Tennessee
College of Social Work
Kingsport, TN

Michel Perreault, Ph.D.
Researcher
Douglas Hospital in Montreal
Associate Professor
Department of Psychiatry
McGill University

Carrie J. Petrucci, Ph.D.
Assistant Professor, Social Work Department
California State University at Long Beach
Long Beach, CA
Former Research Associate, California
    Governor's Commission on
Criminal Justice
Sacramento, CA

Laurent Polidori, Ph.D.
Remote Sensing Specialist
Head, Laboratoire Régional de Télédétection
Institut de Recherche pour le Développement
    Guyane
Cayenne, French Guiana

Enola K. Proctor, Ph.D.
Frank J. Bruno Professor of Social Work
    Research
Dean for Research
George Warren Brown School of Social Work
Washington University
St. Louis, MO

Charles Ray, M.Ed.
President and Chief Executive Officer
National Council for Community Behavioral
    Healthcare
Rockville, MD

Frederic G. Reamer, Ph.D.
Professor
School of Social Work
Rhode Island College
Providence, RI

Cheryl Regehr, Ph.D.
Associate Professor
Faculty of Social Work
Director, Centre for Applied Social Research
University of Toronto
Toronto, Ontario

William J. Reid, DSW
Distinguished Professor
School of Social Welfare
The University at Albany
State University of New York
Albany, NY

Albert R. Roberts, Ph.D.
Professor of Criminal Justice and Social Work
Director of Faculty Development
Faculty of Arts and Sciences
Rutgers University
Livingston College Campus
Piscataway, N.J.
Editor-in-Chief, Brief Treatment and Crisis
    Intervention journal

Gina Pisano Robertiello, Ph.D.
Assistant Professor
Department of Criminal Justice
Seaton Hall University
South Orange, NJ

Aaron Rosen, Ph.D.
Barbara A. Bailey Professor Emeritus of Social
    Work
Washington University St. Louis
St. Louis, MO

Richard N. Rosenthal, M.D.
Professor of Clinical Psychiatry
Columbia University College of Physicians and
    Surgeons
Chairman, Department of Psychiatry
St. Luke's Roosevelt Hospital Center
New York, NY

Howard A. Savin, Ph.D.
Senior Vice President and Chief Clinical
    Officer
Devereux Foundation
Villanova, PA

Dr. Ian Shaw
Professor of Social Work
Department of Social Policy and Social Work
University of York
Heslington, York
Editor-in-Chief, Qualitative Research
    journal

Daniel Schnopp-Wyatt, M.A., Ph.D.
Professor
Pikeville College
Pikeville, KY

Stephanie A. Schwartz, Ph.D.
Post Doctoral Fellow
Mayo Clinic
Rochester, NY

Tazuko Shibusawa, Ph.D.
Associate Professor
Columbia University
School of Social Work
New York, NY

Diana Silimperi, M.D.,
Deputy Project, Technical Director
Quality Assurance Project
Center for Human Services
Bethesda, MD

Jennifer A. Smith, B.A.
Doctoral Student, Psychology
University at Albany
State University New York
Albany, NY

Michael J. Smith, D.S.W.
Professor
Hunter College School of Social Work
City University of New York
New York, NY

Carol A. Snively, Ph.D.
Assistant Professor
University of Missouri
School of Social Work
Columbia, MO

Phyllis Solomon, Ph.D.
Professor
University of Pennsylvania
School of Social Work
Philadelphia, PA

David W. Springer, LMSW-ACP, Ph.D.
Associate Professor and Associate Dean of
    Academic Affairs
The University of Texas at Austin
School of Social Work
Austin, TX

David L. Streiner, Ph.D., C.Psych.
Assistant V. P., Research
Director, Kunin-Lunenfeld Applied Research
    Unit
Baycrest Centre for Geriatric Care
Professor, Department of Psychiatry
University of Toronto
Toronto, Ontario
Co-Editor, Evidence-Based Mental Health
    journal

Gregory Teague, Ph.D.
Associate Professor
Department of Mental Health Law and Policy
Lou la Parte Florida Mental Health Institute
University of South Florida
Tampa, FL

Annelise Tran
Doctoral Candidate
Engineer in Remote Sensing
Laboratoire Regional de Teledetection
Institut de Recherche pour le Developpement
Cayenne, French Guiana

James C. Thomas, MPH, Ph.D.
Associate Professor of Epidemiology
Director of the Program in Public Health
    Ethics
School of Public Health
University of North Carolina
Charlotte, NC

Kirtley Thornton, Ph.D.
Clinical Psychologist
Director, Center for Health Psychology
South Plainfield, NJ

Tom Trabin, Ph.D., M.S.M.
Vice President
The Partnership for Behavioral Healthcare
    Central Link
Lead Consultant, Carter Forum Initiative
Tiburon, CA

Charles L. Usher, Ph.D.
Wallace H. Kuralt, Sr., Professor of Public
    Welfare Policy

School of Social Work
The University of North Carolina at Chapel
    Hill
Chapel Hill, NC

Henry Vandenburgh, Ph.D.
Assistant Professor
School of Management
SUNY Institute of Technology
New York, NY

Vikki L. Vandiver, Dr.P.H.
Associate Professor
Graduate School of Social Work
Portland State University
Portland, OR
Book Review Editor, Community Mental
    Health Journal

Michael A. van Zyl, Ph.D.
Associate Dean for Research
Kent School of Social Work
University of Louisville
Louisville, KY

Tisna Veldhuyzen van Zanten
Quality Assurance Project
Center for Human Services
Bethesda, MD

Gail Viamonte, Ed.D.
Professor
University of Maryland
College Park, MD

Lynda F. Voigt, Ph.D.
Fred Hutchinson Cancer Research Center,
    Seattle, WA
Department of Epidemiology
School of Public Health and Community
    Medicine
University of Washington
Seattle, WA

M. Elizabeth Vonk, Ph.D.
Associate Professor and Director
Part-time M.S.W. Program
University of Georgia
School of Social Work
Athens, GA

Joseph Walsh, Ph.D.
Associate Professor
School of Social Work

Virginia Commonwealth University
Richmond, VA

Abraham Wandersman, Ph.D.
Professor
Department of Psychology
University of South Carolina
Columbia, SC

Thomas Franklin Waters, Ph.D.
Associate Professor of Criminal Justice
Northern Arizona University-Yuma
Yuma, AZ

Marjorie Weishaar, Ph.D.
Clinical Professor
Department of Psychiatry and Human
   Behavior
Brown University Medical School
Providence, RI

Mark Willenbring, MD
Director of the Addictive Disorders Section
Minneapolis VA Medical Center
Professor of Psychiatry
University of Minnesota
Minneapolis, MN

Michael E. Woolley
Doctoral Student
School of Social Work
University of North Carolina at Chapel Hill
Chapel Hill, NC

Mona Williams-Hayes Ph.D.
Visiting Professor
School of Social Work
The University of Tennessee
Knoxville, TN

Craig Winston LeCroy
Professor
Arizona State University
School of Social Work
Tempe, AZ

John S. Wodarski, Ph.D.
Director of Research and
Professor of Social Work
The University of Tennessee
Knoxville, TN
Editor-in-Chief, *Human Behavior in the Social
   Environment* journal

Kenneth R. Yeager, Ph.D.
Director, Quality and Operational
   Improvement and Outpatient Clinic
OSU and Harding Behavioral Healthcare and
   Medicine
The Ohio State University Medical Center
Columbus, OH

Maryanne Yoshioka, Ph.D.
Associate Professor
School of Social Work
Columbia University
New York, NY

SECTION I
Overview and Critical Issues

SYSTEMATIC REVIEWS OF EVIDENCE-BASED STUDIES AND PRACTICE-BASED RESEARCH: HOW TO SEARCH FOR, DEVELOP, AND USE THEM

1

Albert R. Roberts & Kenneth Yeager

We live in a scientific age in which new medical and social science advances are reported almost daily, and the pace of change is breathtaking. In the midst of this, health and social services consumers are bombarded with information about medications, surgeries, alternative health care approaches, and psychosocial interventions that are "guaranteed" to ease their burden and enhance their lives each time they open their e-mail, turn on the TV, or go to the mailbox. Individuals are faced with choices of herbal remedies, gadgets, intrusive physical interventions, and intriguingly named psychological treatments, for example, eye movement desensitization and reprocessing (EMDR), to manage everything from life-threatening illness to unappealing aspects of their appearance. While some view this as the age of the educated consumer, few individuals have the ability to sift through the available data and make informed decisions. Rather, many of those seeking and requiring treatment turn to health care and mental health professionals with the expectation that these professionals will have the knowledge base to determine which treatment methodology is going to result in the most positive outcome with the least cost in terms of suffering, time, and money. As a result of the trust placed in

them, health care and mental health professionals have a fiduciary duty to acquire the knowledge required to answer the question "What do you recommend?" based on the best available scientific information.

The overriding objective of this volume is to bridge and augment health and human services practices with scientific research inquiry. Toward the end of the 20th century, there was a consistent trend toward bridging practice and research. In the early 21st century, evidence-based practice is beginning to proliferate worldwide in major universities, medical centers, mental health centers, schools, and family treatment centers. From empirical and evidence-based outcome studies conducted within these centers and in the community, best practice guidelines and treatment protocols are emerging that allow practitioners to provide the optimal treatment or intervention to any individual, family, or group seeking assistance. This book attempts to consolidate state-of-the-art evidence-based knowledge so that graduate students and practitioners in the medical and human services professions have all of the latest research and evaluation guidelines, research exemplars, and evidence-based protocols available in one volume.

Our primary goal in compiling and editing

the *Evidence-Based Practice Manual* is to make the latest evidence-based protocols, practice-based research designs and exemplars, evaluation research, and assessment tools and measures accessible to all education, medical, public health, psychology, public policy, and social work professionals. The secondary goal in developing this volume is to provide clinical research and program evaluation models to facilitate agency and consumer accountability on the part of health and human service professionals. The editors firmly believe that medical and psychosocial diagnosis, treatment plans, and service delivery need to be based on a scientific epistemology. Specifically, all professionals need to have easy access to the latest evidence-based research findings on medical and psychosocial treatment effectiveness, longitudinal follow-up of behavior change and medical remission following intervention, research evaluation of health and social work programs, and cost-benefit studies.

This volume contains 11 parts. The first part, consisting of 11 chapters, provides an overview of best practices, expert consensus models, evidence-based practices, and critical issues and methods of developing and disseminating practice-based research knowledge in the medical, epidemiology, mental health, public health, psychotherapy, criminology, statistical and quantitative, and qualitative research areas. The six chapters in the second part examine ethical issues while providing step-by-step grant guidelines for the accountable professional. The third part, consisting of 19 chapters, examines the latest evidence-based practices in health and human service settings. The six chapters in the fourth part focus on epidemiological basics and different types of public health research. The fifth part of this volume, also consisting of six chapters, focuses on conceptualization, operationalization, and measurement in research and evaluation studies. The 13 chapters in the sixth part of this book all focus on assessment tools and measures. The sixth part underscores the importance of monitoring and maintaining quality and operational improvement. The 13 chapters in the seventh part all focus on program evaluation strategies, approaches, issues, and models. The 21 chapters in the eighth and ninth parts of this book identify and discuss qualitative and quantitative practice-based research exemplars. The tenth section of this volume, containing 8 chapters, focuses on the establishment, application, and institutionalization of quality assurance,

quality management, and operational improvement through program monitoring and outcome measures. The final section contains the epilogue, which distinguishes efficacy from effectiveness studies and bridges the present to the future with a discussion of the clinical utility of intervention research.

This overview chapter will systematically introduce and integrate the different operational definitions of evidence-based practice, practice-based research, assessment tools and measures, and evaluation research. The 104 chapters of this volume methodically examine the following:

1. The steps in formulating a problem and selecting the research question
2. The process of determining the appropriate research method
3. Specific methodological issues such as randomization, reliability and validity, and outcome measurement
4. The steps in obtaining research funding
5. The process of conducting program and service evaluations and determining performance indicators
6. Technological issues such as use of computer technology, statistical analysis, and electronic medical records
7. Standards and guidelines for evidence-based practice or best practice

DEFINING EVIDENCE-BASED PRACTICE

It is important to begin with a common understanding of the similarities and differences between evidence-based practice and practice-based research. We asked three esteemed professors to identify and discuss their definitions and the similarities and differences between evidence-based practice (EBP) and practice-based research (PBR).

According to Dr. Edward J. Mullen, professor and director of the National Institute of Mental Health (NIMH) Mental Health Services Research Doctoral Training Program at Columbia University Graduate School of Social Work:

Evidence-based practice (EBP) and practice-based research (PBR) have similarities and differences in meaning. Both phrases refer to the relationship between research and practice. EBP places emphasis on the practitioner's use of scientifically validated assessment, intervention, and evaluation procedures, as well as the practitioner's use of critical thinking when making practice decisions that matter to service recipients. However, a frequently heard criticism of EBP is that there is little relevant research available regarding most questions that a practitioner asks. Further, it is often said that much of the research that is available is of little use because so many scientific studies are conducted in contexts that have little resemblance to realistic practice situations.

Accordingly, many are now calling for finding new ways to bridge this gap between practice and research by supporting efforts to conduct research that will be of direct relevance to practitioners and which will be usable in service systems. Such applied practice-based research can take at least two forms. On the one hand, translational research is looked to since this is a form of research that seeks to take basic research findings from one field or from highly controlled contexts and adapt the findings to realistic practice contexts. Alternatively, another approach is to foster researcher and practitioner partnerships in the conduct of practice research so as to enhance relevance. This is a two-way street in which one can move from research findings to practice contexts or, alternatively, begin with realistic practice problems as the stimulus for research. The phrase *practice-based research* can be used to signify efforts to bridge this gap between practice and research. In turn, findings from such efforts can be used to support EBP.

According to Dr. David L. Streiner, professor of psychiatry at the University of Toronto Medical Center and assistant vice-president and research director for Kunin-Lunenfeld Applied Research Unit at Baycrest Centre for Geriatric Care:

The link between practice and research is a two-way street. Good clinical practice must be informed by the best available evidence regarding treatment and diagnosis (evidence-based practice). However, in order for this research to be clinically relevant and useful, it must be both well executed and informed by actual clinical practice (practice-based research). This may consist of carefully done case histories, documentation of symptom clusters, or, ideally, N of 1 studies. The clinician cannot be divorced from what is being found in labs and studies with patients, nor can the researcher be isolated from what problems patients are presenting with, and how they are currently being treated.

An example of the usefulness of careful clinical observation of a small number of cases was recently, and unfortunately, provided by the outbreak of sudden acute respiratory syndrome (SARS) in Toronto. After "only" two deaths, it was possible to both identify this new syndrome and to trace all of the other cases to close contact with these two people, resulting in measures (e.g., screening all hospital visitors, quarantines, protective clothing, and mandatory hand washing of all people entering hospitals) that quickly broke the cycle of infections.

According to Dr. Phyllis Solomon, Professor of Social Work and affiliated Professor of Medicine at the University of Pennsylvania:

Evidence-based practice has two components. One component is basing practice decisions on empirically based evidence as to the interventions or intervention strategies that are likely to produce the desired outcomes. In other words, employing interventions that have empirically been determined to be effective for the particular problem being targeted, including the findings being applicable to the characteristics of the client or client system to be served. The second aspect is to evaluate the implementation of these interventions to ensure that they are being implemented as intended and that the intended outcomes are achieved, with no unintended negative consequences. Whereas practice-based research is scientifically investigating issues related to practice, which may or may not specifically address questions of practice effectiveness. There is clearly some overlap between these two areas, for engaging in evidence-based practice means that practice-based research is being undertaken. The caveat here is that evaluation research must be considered within the domain of research. The arena of practice-based research includes a host of research questions beyond questions of effectiveness of interventions, but still retains the expectation that knowledge gained from this research will result in more effective practice. It is important to note that both evidence-based practice and practice-based research contribute to the development of empirically-based practice knowledge.

EBP has been defined as the conscientious, explicit, and judicious use of the best available scientific evidence in professional decision making (Sackett, Richardson, Rosenberg, & Haynes, 1997). More simply defined, it is the use of treatments for which there is sufficiently persuasive evidence to support their effectiveness in attaining the desired outcomes (Rosen & Proctor, 2002). In chapter 18 of this book, Rosen and Proctor suggest that evidence-based practice is comprised of three assertions: (a) intervention decisions based on empirical, research-based support; (b) critical assessment of empirically supported interventions to determine their fit to and appropriateness for the practice situation at hand; and (c) regular monitoring and revision of the course of treatment based on outcome evaluation.

In general, decision making using evidence-based methods is achieved in a series of steps (Gibbs & Gambrill, 2002; Hayward, Wilson, Tunis, & Bass, 1995). The first step is to evaluate the problem to be addressed and formulate answerable questions. These questions can include: What is the best way of assisting an individual with these characteristics who suffers from depression? or Which group treatment method is most effective in reducing recidivism among batterers?

The next step is to gather and critically evaluate the evidence available. Evidence is generally ranked hierarchically according to its scientific strength. It is understood that various types of intervention will have been evaluated more frequently and rigorously by virtue of the length of time they have been used and the settings in which they are used. Thus, for newer treatments, only Level 4 evidence may be available (see Table 1.1). In such cases, practitioners should use the method with caution, continue to search for evidence of its efficacy, and be prepared to evaluate the method's efficacy in their own practice. The final steps involve applying the results of the assessment to practice or policy and then continuously monitoring the outcome.

While the concepts of evidence-based practice are reasonably consistent throughout the health and social science disciplines, individualized definitions are useful.

Evidence-Based Medicine

Evidence-based medicine is the conscientious, explicit, and judicious use of current best evidence in making decisions about the care of individual patients. The practice of evidence-based medicine means integrating individual clinical expertise with the best available external clinical evidence from systematic research. By best available external clinical evidence we mean clinically relevant research, often from the basic sciences of medicine, but especially from patient centered clinical research into the accuracy and precision of diagnostic tests (including the clinical examination), the power of prognostic markers, and the efficacy and safety of therapeutic, rehabilitative, and preventive regimens. External clinical evidence both invalidates previously accepted diagnostic tests and treatments and replaces them with new ones that are more powerful, more accurate, more efficacious, and safer. (Sackett et al., 1997, pp. 71–72)

Evidence-Based Clinical Practice

"Evidence-based clinical practice is an approach to decision making in which the clinician uses the best evidence available, in consultation with the patient, to decide upon the option which suits that patient best" (Muir Gray, 1997, p. 102).

Evidence-Based Practice in Health Care

Evidence-based health care "takes place when decisions that affect the care of patients are taken with due weight accorded to all valid, relevant information" (Hicks, 1997, p. 8).

TABLE 1.1 Levels of Evidence

Level	Description
1	Meta-analysis or replicated randomized controlled trials (RCT) that include a placebo condition/control trial or are from well-designed cohort or case control analytic study, preferably from more than one center or research group, or national consensus panel recommendations based on controlled, randomized studies, which are systematically reviewed.
2	At least one RCT with placebo or active comparison condition, evidence obtained from multiple time series with or without intervention, or national consensus panel recommendations based on uncontrolled studies with positive outcomes or based on studies showing dramatic effects of interventions.
3	Uncontrolled trial or observational study with 10 or more subjects, opinions of respected authorities, based on clinical experiences, descriptive studies, or reports of expert consensus.
4	Anecdotal case reports, unsystematic clinical observation, descriptive reports, case studies, and/or single-subject designs.

Evidence-based practice (EBP) is an approach to health care wherein health professionals use the best evidence possible, i.e. the most appropriate information available, to make clinical decisions for individual patients. EBP values, enhances and builds on clinical expertise, knowledge of disease mechanisms, and pathophysiology. It involves complex and conscientious decision-making based not only on the available evidence but also on patient characteristics, situations, and preferences. It recognizes that health care is individualized and ever changing and involves uncertainties and probabilities. Ultimately EBP is the formalization of the care process that the best clinicians have practiced for generations." (McKibbon, 1998, p. 396)

Evidence-Based Nursing

The conduct of research is of little value unless findings are used in practice to improve patient care. Contributions of nursing to improve patient outcomes can be optimized by the use of evidence-based practice guidelines and research-based nursing treatments. . . . It is the professional responsibility of all nurses to use the most recent scientific evidence in their practice. Additionally, it is the responsibility of nurse leaders to create practice environments that foster critical thinking, questioning of current practice, and systems to support and encourage nurses to access and implement research evidence in delivery of care. (Kleiber & Titler, 1998, p. 21)

Evidence-Based Social Work

Evidence-based [social work] dictates that professional judgments and behaviors should be guided by two distinct but interdependent principles. First, whenever possible, practice should be grounded on prior findings that demonstrate empirically that certain actions performed with a particular type of client or client system are likely to produce predictable, beneficial, and effective results. . . . Secondly, every client system, over time, should be individually evaluated to determine the extent to which the predicted results have been attained as a direct consequence of the practitioner's actions. (Cournoyer & Powers, 2002, p. 799)

MEDICINE AND EVIDENCE-BASED PRACTICE

A catalyst to the expansion and increased utilization of Evidence-Based Medicine seems to be both the Users' Guides series of articles published in the *Journal of the American Medical Association* (JAMA) between 1993 and 2000,

and the outstanding edited book based on 33 articles compiled by Doctors Gordon H. Guyatt and Drummond Rennie (2002). The strength of Guyatt and Rennie's (2002) *Users' Guides to the Medical Literature* is that it is compact and in paperback format, with a CD-rom included. The primary objective of this handbook is to improve clinical decision-making through an awareness, systematic literature search, and critical evaluation of the evidence, and its application to particular patient problems.

The leading discipline in the application of evidence-based practice is the field of medicine. This may be in part due to the critical and sometimes lifesaving nature of decision-making processes within the medical field. There may be additional contributing factors such as the quantitative nature of medical science lending itself well to the application of evidence-based treatment.

The practice of evidence-based medicine begins with a comprehensive systematic review of the literature. The next step is an open-minded and rigorous evaluation of evidence presented. Physicians are challenged to examine three elements critical to the successful implementation of evidence-based medicine. First, the evidence must connect to the treatment and to the ideal overall health outcomes. Second, there must be a control group. Third, the research design must account for any possible confounding factors that could affect the outcomes independently of the treatment. Once the evidence has been evaluated (see table 1.1), the physician's next task is to determine if the evidence demonstrates the effectiveness, benefit, and value of the treatment for its stated application. When the evidence has been thoroughly reviewed by the physicians and review groups with full understanding of the analysis, a set of recommendations should be made based on the efficacy of the procedure found within the literature. For example:

1. It is advised that this be done in a periodic health examination *or* a diagnostic procedure should be done, *or* treatment of a medical problem should be given. There is good evidence (Level 1) to support the recommendation.
2. This may be done in periodic health examination, *or* a diagnostic procedure may be done, *or* treatment of a medical problem may be given.
3. It should be done in most cases. There is

fair evidence (Level 2) to support the recommendation.

4. It should not be done in most cases. There is poor evidence (Level 3) regarding the recommendation, which may be made on other grounds.

5. It is advised that this not be done in a periodic examination, *or* a diagnostic procedure should not be done, *or* treatment of a medical problem should not be given. There is good evidence (Level 1) to support the recommendation that this not be done.

There are numerous ways in which physicians can participate in the practice of evidence-based medicine. All begin with the realization and appreciation that medicine has become far too complicated for physicians to make treatment decisions without a systematic review of evidence. Therefore, many physicians rely on practice guidelines and additional decision-making support tools that are based on principles of evidence to assist with their decision-making process. Nevertheless, we fully appreciate the fact that the decision to follow practice guidelines requires a delicate balance of reviewing the weight of evidence for a particular intervention and the individualized needs of the patient. Medical care in the real world is different from the type of medicine practiced in clinical trials. In the real world populations served are often older than those in clinical trials, with multiple diagnoses requiring multiple integrated treatments, while those in controlled studies suffer only from the condition under investigation. Clinical trials will tell us what treatments are effective but will not provide information regarding which patients should receive them. Therefore, it must be accepted that clinical guidelines and evidence-based medicine provide only guidelines for care, that medical practice and other forms of human care must be inclusive of opinion and collaborative decision making and must always be tailored to meet the individualized need of the patient combined with the treatment team's best judgment in order to obtain the best outcome.

PSYCHOLOGY AND EVIDENCE-BASED PRACTICE

Evidence-based psychotherapy emerged in the early 1990s, and by 1993 the concept of evidence-based psychotherapy had grown sufficiently in scope to warrant the American Psychological Association's publication of established empirically validated treatments (Chambless, 1993; Chambless, 1996a; Chambless, 1996b; Chambless et al., 1996). However, publication of the guidelines was not met with universal enthusiasm, and in the ensuing debates the term *empirically validated* was softened to *empirically supported* treatments. The semantic change alone did not end the controversy, which led to longstanding divisions among American psychologists. Many argued that the publication of such a list was unhelpful and scientifically unjustified because the criteria for evidence-based practice excluded clinical judgment from the scientific assessment of effectiveness. Additionally it was believed that the listing of empirically supported treatments failed to take into account evidence supporting rival hypotheses of factors that influenced the outcome of treatment, including the strong evidence for the centrality of the therapeutic alliance.

In the United Kingdom an alternative strategy for achieving evidence-based practice was implemented that permitted psychotherapists to further develop innovative approaches that built on practice wisdom. From this foundation, psychotherapeutic processes were then formally evaluated through a process of random controlled studies. This process facilitated a balance between research evidence and clinical consciousness that would support and expand clinical practice through the establishment of clinical practice guidelines.

Psychologists have developed evidence-based guidelines for specific populations within multidisciplinary organizations. One example is the *Practice Guidelines* from the International Society for Traumatic Stress Studies, edited by Foa, Keane, and Friedman (2000), that reviews the evidence and suggests guidelines for working with various populations suffering from posttraumatic stress disorder (PTSD). In addition, by virtue of their methodological rigor, psychologists have contributed significantly to the conduct of research on practice efficacy through the development of research methods and specific tools for measuring characteristics and change. David Streiner, for example, has provided an invaluable service to medical, psychology, and social work colleagues through his series of books, book chapters, and articles describing research and statistical methods and identifying their application to practice situations (see chapters 14, 37, and 50, this volume).

Although these efforts in both North America and the United Kingdom have had a substantial impact on the development of evidence-based practice within the practice of psychotherapy, this progress seems to have been relatively slow in comparison to the progress made within the field of medicine. Within the fields of psychotherapy, psychology, and many other disciplines there has been a fundamental distrust of practice guidelines and evidence-based practice. This distrust stems from professional training and skill formulation of practitioners who have been taught to emphasize the uniqueness of individuals and who frequently reject the medical metaphor of a prescriptive approach to psychotherapy.

If the tension between the prescriptive nature of practice guidelines and the traditionally more individualized practice of psychotherapy is not sufficient to slow the establishment of evidence-based practice, there are additional concerns for many therapists that the research evidence is incomplete, misleading, unfairly biased, and detrimental to the highly individualized practice of psychology. Nevertheless, examination of evidence within the field of psychology continues to progress, practice guidelines are established, and practitioners are moving forward with an awareness of the problems and limitations that may be presented through the application of evidence-based practice. This has been fostered in no small part through the development of national guidelines issued by the National Institutes of Health and National Institute of Mental Health in combination with evidence-based sources such as the Campbell and Cochrane collaborations, providing resources for practitioners. The Campbell collaboration is an international organization designed to prepare and disseminate systematic reviews of high-quality controlled studies on the effectiveness of educational criminology and social practices and policies. The Cochrane collaboration and the Cochrane library in Oxford, England, have produced databases summarizing the best and most current evidence available through controlled studies of interventions and treatment protocols for health care and human services.

SOCIAL WORK AND EVIDENCE-BASED PRACTICE

The social work field has experienced similar tensions regarding evidence-based practice. On one hand there is a push primarily by those in academic settings to evaluate practice and establish practice guidelines and on the other hand a reticence by practitioners to read and integrate research into their practices. Supporting this reluctance is another group of academics who criticize evidence-based approaches as reductionistic and mindless empiricism.

Social work has a history related to evidence-based practice dating back to the 1970s and the work of Mullen and Dumpson (1972), Fischer (1973), and Jayaratne and Levy (1979).

The point of departure is Mullen and Dumpson's classic book *Evaluation of Social Intervention* (1972). This book examines 16 field experiments testing the effects of social work interventions including social casework, social group work, and community organization. The volume included all of the known field experiments conducted through 1971 that examined social work interventions. Fifteen internationally recognized social work experts critically assessed these findings and discussed implications for social work practice and education. At the time, Edward Mullen was the director of research and evaluation at the Community Service Society of New York and an associate professor at Fordham University. James R. Dumpson was the dean of the Fordham University Graduate School of Social Service. Contributing authors included Werner Boehm, Edgar Borgatta, James Breedlove, Donald Feldstein, Ludwig Geismar, Wyatt Jones, Harold Lewis, Carol Meyer, Helen Harris Perlman, Simon Slavin, John Turner, Walter Walker, and Gene Webb. The editors convened a national conference to discuss the studies and the book chapters. This conference was attended by 125 representatives of most of the U.S. graduate schools of social work and was held at Fordham University in 1971. This was the first major call for a move toward evidence-based practice in social work.

In his classic article, "Is Casework Effective?: A Review," Joel Fischer (1973) underscored the critical importance of carefully conducted research in order to determine whether or not casework was effective. Fischer reviewed the serious limitations of 11 studies that were supposed to determine the effectiveness of casework services. His book led to a strident debate on the role of research in social work practice. The debate has continued for more than 30 years, and the profession of social work has slowly come to realize the importance of research in measuring treatment effectiveness.

Jayaratne and Levy provided a description of

"empirical clinical practice" in their 1979 text. In this text, the authors advocated for practitioners to seek evidence, measure client progress, and document treatment outcome in order to provide objective rather than subjective data to guide clinical practice.

The debate over establishing practice guidelines became most heated in 1997 with an article written by Myers and Thyer that raised the question "Should social work clients have the right to effective treatment?" In this article, they asserted that social work codes of ethics should include the clients' right to effective treatment and social workers' obligation to be educated about and provide such treatments. In the ensuing war of letters, critics countered that such a suggestion ignores the complexity of individual problems, ignores clinical expertise, is merely a cost-cutting measure, and is impossible (see Gibbs & Gambrill, 2002). Nevertheless, many social work researchers, educators, and practitioners have continued to strive toward evidence-based practice. The premise that social work practice must be based on empirically tested and verified knowledge is now widely accepted and endorsed by leaders and social work organizations (Rosen, Proctor, & Staudt, 2003). Concern still exists, however, that research evidence is not easily accessed by practitioners and is not readily translated into practice (Gambrill, 2000; Howard, McMillen, & Pollio, 2003). Thus, considerable time and effort is being directed toward the establishment of practice guidelines (Rosen et al., 2003) and in determining methods for teaching best practices based on empirical evidence to trainees in the field (Howard et al., 2003).

However, it is the scope of social work practice—which spans a multitude of service areas and treatment modalities including behavioral therapy, supportive counseling, marital or family treatment, family and children services, mental illness treatment, health care, gerontology, and many more—that has led to difficulties in defining contemporary evidence-based treatment in social work. It is also social work's unique contribution to the holistic care approach to the individual that has led the profession to an appreciation of the need for evidence-based practice. Within the past decade social workers have been given increased responsibilities in the form of care management, interdisciplinary communication, treatment planning, and resource management, all within the context of a managed care environment. These trends have high-lighted the need for social workers to practice intervention with manualized treatment protocols and strategic plans that effectively meet the needs of individuals, families, groups, programs, and organizations.

For those disciplines embracing evidence-based care, social work has become an integrated component, synthesizing and analyzing evidence currently available in the literature and working to establish clinical care pathways and practice guidelines within many care delivery systems. In addition, social workers have a history of gathering data and monitoring the outcome of the population served. It is the goal of agencies such as the National Center for Social Work Research, the National Association of Social Workers, and the Society for Social Work and Research to continue to establish and develop evidence-based practice through the application of ongoing quantitative and qualitative evaluation of outcomes. The social work profession in conjunction with other professional disciplines represents a remarkable resource of scientific measurement and practitioner's talent able to contribute greatly in the area of practice-based research, thus moving forward the goals of evidence-based practice. Evidence of social work's involvement in evidence-based practice is found in this volume in the chapters by Proctor and Rosen, Gibbs and Gambrill, and Mullen and Bacon, which outline the processes by which evidence can be translated into practice. In addition, social work scholars have contributed multiple submissions on measures for evaluating practice and creating new evidence for the assessment of others.

Social work professor Eileen D. Gambrill (2003) at the University of California at Berkeley incisively underscores the potential of EBP:

"Professionals have an obligation to inform clients about services found to be effective and to avoid harm. Concerns that practitioners were continuing to use methods found to be harmful was a key reason for the development of EBP. . . . EBP calls for candid descriptions of limitations of research studies and use of research methods that critically test questions addressed. . . . (The critical question is): How effective have we been in maximizing the flow of knowledge that contributes to helping clients and minimizing the flow of misleading, inaccurate material that diminishes opportunities to help clients and may result in harm" (Gambrill, 2003, pp. 5, 6 and 18).

OPERATIONALIZING AND INTEGRATING PRACTICE-BASED RESEARCH WITH EVIDENCE-BASED PRACTICE

The concept of integrated evidence-based practice is not new. This concept has a very long history dating to the early 1900s in the writings of Joseph Rowntree, who discussed rigor in the assessment of problems and the development of solutions. Mary Richmond in 1917 and Richard Cabot in 1933 followed this work. Evidence-based medicine has a longstanding tradition. In the broadest sense this includes the scientific tradition that has brought medicine to its current status of practice. Narrowing the scope somewhat, evidence-based medicine involves aspects of medicine requiring the burden of proof. This includes the use of hypothesis testing and calculation of statistical significance to interpret clinical research. An example is the Food and Drug Administration's criteria for new drug approval, which includes providing acceptable evidence of effectiveness and safety factors associated with the drug being tested.

As the concept of evidence-based medicine has expanded so has the idea of evidence-based practices. Areas of recent focus have included pharamacological and psychosocial treatment of mental illness, neurocognitive disorders, and substance dependence (Brink, 2003). However, to date, there has been a lack of integration regarding the application of evidence-based practice both within disciplines and across disciplines. Variation in practice-based research approaches, bottlenecks in communication of emerging best practice methods, and the failure to embrace research methodologies that harness the potential of collaborative user interfaces slow the advancement of evidence-based care. The purpose of this chapter is to explore and elaborate on the potential for multidisciplinary collaborations within the application of evidence-based practice.

So what exactly is the difference between practice-based research and evidence-based practice? Naturally, there are overlaps, but generally speaking practice-based research serves as the springboard for the development of evidence-based practice. Practice-based research:

- includes the application of rigorous, systematic, and objective procedures to obtain reliable and valid knowledge relevant to direct clinical practice, education, activities, and programs.

- involves research that employs systematic, empirical methods demonstrating valid and reliable measurement across evaluators, practitioners, and observers among multiple studies by the same or different investigators yielding replicated results, while maintaining awareness of individualized variance in response to interventions and care plans.
- analyzes and evaluates data through experimental or quasi-experimental methods, examining individuals, entities, programs, and interventions within a variety of settings across a variety of conditions with appropriate controls to evaluate the effects of the condition of interest. Controlled and randomized studies are preferable.
- provides sufficient detail and clarity to permit replication or at minimum the opportunity to build systematically on previous study findings.
- is published in peer-reviewed journals or approved by panels of independent experts through a process of rigorous and objective scientific review.

What then is the basis for variance present within the understanding and operational definitions of evidence-based practice?

- First, there are differences both within and between disciplines when addressing various approaches to similar problems with evidence-based care.
- Second, source data contributing to the evidence-based practice foundation does not currently lend itself to the infusion of new knowledge gained from practice settings.

Practice-based research in fact is the foundation for evidence-based care. Therefore, the goal of this book is to present an integrated model showing examples of practice-based research that will serve as a tool for practitioners to bridge the gap between practice, research, and emergent best practices within evidence-based practice. Multidisciplinary or interdisciplinary teams are essential to the integration and development of practice-based research. According to Dziegielewski (2003) in the multidisciplinary team professionals from multiple disciplines work together, each having clear roles and responsibilities designed to assist the client. Within the interdisciplinary team, however, although these professionals from different disciplines continue to work together, they often share roles and responsibilities, often completing tasks not considered traditional for their particular fields. For example, the social worker is expected to know about medications and the effects they can have on intervention outcomes, even though social workers have traditionally not been specifically trained in this area.

Therefore, in health care, whether services are provided through multidisciplinary or interdisciplinary teams, evidence-based practice has come to be equated with practice effectiveness. The examples presented in the chapters of this book are designed to equip practitioners with additional strategies for dealing with the rapidly changing environment where the acquisition of new knowledge and innovative practice is an essential ingredient for innovation in caregiving. We believe when research-based practice principles are appropriately applied, practice-based research will result—thereby fueling the establishment, refinement, and integration of evidence-based practice.

IMPLEMENTATION OF AN INTEGRATED MODEL OF EVIDENCE-BASED PRACTICE AND PRACTICE-BASED RESEARCH

Adoption of practice-based research and evidence-based practice requires utilization of the inherent knowledge of multidisciplinary or interdisciplinary teams. The basis for this is taking the understanding and experience of each individual practitioner and joining it with that of the research-practitioner to better assist the populations to be served. The knowledge acquired by these practitioners has become a part of a growing "toolbox" of practice-based strategies to be further explored, invented, or refined through more traditional approaches to research. When this knowledge is mixed with the skills of the practitioner-researcher, evidence-based research evolves. In essence, this combination approach capitalizes on and creates an entirely logical progression of informal research questions and methods for answering these questions, testing practice methods, and measuring outcomes as applied to issues of direct relevance to the field of interest. (See figure 2.1 for EBP resources.)

Establishment of practice-based research requires practitioners to make use of their inherent knowledge, understanding, and experiences with the population served through their inter-

actions and informal research processes. The emphasis is on descriptive, historical, and naturalistic approaches. This process information is then available for scrutiny through the rigors of scientific or social science methodology conducted by persons whose professional training has prepared them to conduct such analysis. This method, which utilizes the combination of skill and professional energy, serves to recognize how important it is for practice not to be conducted in a laboratory but rather within the practice setting, providing a necessary feedback loop for further exploration. Thus, practice-based research will accomplish the following important collaborative goals:

- Providing equal representation from all disciplines.
- Providing access for input from a variety of practitioners' groups and users of research generated.
- Promotion of new and innovative approaches to high-risk populations.
- Keeping pace with rapidly changing population needs.
- Addressing questions of importance to the discipline and the population served.
- Capitalizing on the synergistic effectiveness of collaborative approaches.
- Continually improving the quality of care provided.
- Working to minimize bias in research.
- Establishing communication for dissemination of information/knowledge gained.
- Ensuring an atmosphere of growth recognizing parallel application of practice within similar or same populations.

Currently, practitioners are challenged with unprecedented choices in theoretical approaches, community options, medications, and practice approaches. At the same time the challenge exists of providing services and treatment in the most cost-effective manner. The relevance of Senge's ideas (1995) and a growing number of others including those affiliated with the Institute of Medicine is reflective of the need for organizations to invoke their own research strategies and evidence-based practice approaches as a basis for advancing scientific knowledge-building in health care.

Today more than ever it is important for practitioners to be aware of the rapidly changing environment in which care is provided as well as the increasing number of new treatment approaches, processes, and technological advancements available. Practice-based research provides a powerful tool based on the principle that the experience, wisdom, and insight of the practitioner form the structure that can facilitate identification and framing of research questions that are relevant to practice and can improve practice methods. In turn, the research results should be ones that are in theory more easily assimilated into everyday practice. Essential skills necessary for the development of practice-based research include but are not limited to the following:

• Experience in raising research questions from practice.
• Developing or adapting appropriate research methodologies to address practice-based research questions.
• Application of the research methodology within a practice context.
• Development of methods for the generation, evaluation, and application of relevant professional knowledge in practice settings.
• Flexibility in development of methodology to facilitate maximizing input of multidisciplinary team members in the care design/clinical pathway or algorithm of best practice.

In refining practice-based research skills, teams attempt to provide a sense of how this approach can be applied within a multitude of professional settings and visualize what promise this can bring to the complex human interactions faced within the practice environment. The basis of practice-based research is that of the team coming from a "need-to-know" stance. This will require reframing of the hierarchical system approach generally adopted by our (Western) science.

The concept of practice-based research is inclusive in part of the concept of "organizational sensemaking" contained in the work of Weick (1996) on the understanding of organizational science. In a learning, researching multidisciplinary team all members are actively involved in identifying, analyzing, and solving problems, enabling the discipline to further advance and improve its capabilities, knowledge base, and understanding of the impact of multiple systems involved. Within such a learning/research environment there is no preconceived model for knowing. However, there is an overarching philosophy or attitude about the nature of practice.

In establishing such an environment the learning and adaptive capability of the entire discipline is greatly enhanced. The group will find that it is able to adapt more rapidly and to manage issues in a more efficient manner, embracing change in a progressively evolving, scientific, medical, and social approach.

One resource that can help the practitioner find the best available evidence is a series of secondary journals: *Evidence-Based Mental Health* (*EBMH*), *Evidence-Based Nursing*, and *Evidence-Based Medicine* (*EBM*). The oldest, *EBM*, has been around for about 10 years and the youngest, *EBMH*, for five. For each of the journals an experienced team scans up to 200 journals, applying rules to select only those articles that meet rigorous methodological standards for both quantitative and qualitative research. They then prepare a summary of the article, which takes up about two-thirds of a page. The remainder of the page is taken up by a commentary, written by a research-oriented clinician, that places the article in the context of previous research and current clinical practice. In this way the reader gets the bottom line for the best current articles about treatments, diagnosis, etiology, and natural history.

CONCLUSION

This volume provides direction to health, mental health, and human service professionals based on collective wisdom emanating from the practice experience and empirical research of the multidisciplinary contributors. It is intended to inspire professionals to take up the challenges of evidence-based practice and practice-based research in the form of systematic program evaluations, outcome studies of manualized treatment protocols, randomized controlled studies, epidemiological studies, survey research, consumer satisfaction studies, and cost-effectiveness studies. It is also intended to provide practical guidance to those embarking on this process both in terms of steps to achieve the outcomes and tools required in the journey. We are confident that practitioners, when provided with the necessary skills and tools, will produce compelling evidence that will direct the continued development of effective treatment and intervention approaches. In the next edition of this book we look forward to publishing an increasing number of chapters containing the research and practice guidelines produced by frontline practice researchers, epidemiologists, clinicians, and university professors.

References

Brink, L. (2003). Integrating evidence based practice with quality management (Special report: Evidence-based practices). *Behavioral Healthcare Tomorrow, 12,* 17–21.

Chambless, D. L. (1993). Task force on promotion and dissemination of psychological procedures. A report adopted by the Division 12 Board, October 1993. Washington, DC: American Psychological Association.

Chambless, D. L. (1996a). Identification of empirically supported psychological interventions. *Clinician's Research Digest,* (Suppl. 14), 1–2.

Chambless, D. L. (1996b). In defense of dissemination of empirically supported psychological interventions. *Clinical Psychology, 3,* 230–235.

Chambless, D. L., Sanderson, W. C., Shoham, V., Bennett Johnson, S., Pope, K. S., Crits-Christoph, P., Baker, M., Johnson, B., Woody, S. R., Sue, S., Beutler, L., Williams, D. A., & McCurry, S. (1996). An update on empirically validated therapies. *The Clinical Psychologist, 49,* 5–18.

Cournoyer, B., & Powers, G. (2002). Evidence-based social work: The quiet revolution continues. In A. R. Roberts & G. J. Greene (Eds.), *Social Workers' Desk Reference* (pp. 798–807). New York: Oxford University Press.

Dziegielewski, S. F. (2003). The changing face of health care practice: Professional practice in managed behavioral health care (2nd ed.). New York: Springer.

Fischer, J. (1973). Is casework effective?: A review. *Social Work, 28,* 5–30.

Foa, E., Keane, T., & Friedman, M. (2000). *Effective Treatments for PTSD: Practice Guidelines for the International Society for Traumatic Stress Studies.* New York: Guilford Press.

Gambrill, E. (2000). Evidence-based practice: An alternative to authority-based practice. *Families in Society, 80*(4), 341–350.

Gambrill, E. (2003). Editorial: Evidence-based practice: Sea change or the Emeror's new clothes? *Journal of Social Work Education, 39*(1), 1–18.

Gibbs, L., & Gambrill, E. (2002). Evidence based practice: Counterarguments to objections. *Research on Social Work Practice, 12*(3), 452–476.

Guyatt, G., & Rennie, D. (2002). *Users' guide to the medical literature: Essentials of evidence-based clinical practice.* Chicago, IL: American Medical Association Press.

Hayward, R., Wilson, M., Tunis, S., & Bass, E. (1995). User guides to evidence based medicine. *Journal of the American Medical Association, 274*(20), 1630.

Hicks, N. (1997). Evidence based healthcare. *Bandolier, 4*(39), 8.

Howard, M., McMillen, C., & Pollio, D. (2003). Teaching evidence-based practice: Toward a new paradigm for social work education. *Research on Social Work Practice, 13*(2), 234–259.

Jayaratne, S., & Levy, R. L. (1979). *Empirical Clinical Practice.* New York: Columbia University.

Kleiber, C., & Titler, M. G. (1998). *Journal of Nursing Quality Assurance, 2*(1), 21–27.

McKibbon, K. A. (1998). Evidence based practice. *Bulletin of the Medical Library Association, 86*(3), 396–401.

Muir Gray, J. A. (1997). *Evidence-based healthcare: How to make health policy and management decisions.* London: Churchill Livingstone.

Mullen, E. J., & Dumpson, J. R. (Eds.). (1972). *Evaluation of social intervention* (1st ed.). San Francisco: Jossey-Bass.

Myers, L., & Thyer, B. (1997). Should social work clients have the right to effective treatment? *Social Work, 42*(3), 288–298.

Rosen, A., & Proctor, E. (2002). Standards for evidence-based social work practice. In A. R. Roberts & G. J. Greene (Eds.), *Social Workers' Desk Reference* (pp. 743–747). New York: Oxford University Press.

Rosen, A., Proctor, E., & Staudt, M. (2003). Targets of change and interventions in social work: An empirically based prototype for developing practice guidelines. *Research on Social Work Practice, 13*(2), 208–233.

Sackett, D., Richardson, W., Rosenberg, W., & Haynes, R. (1997). *Evidence-based medicine: How to practice and the EBM.* New York: Churchill Livingstone.

Senge, P. (1995). Building learning organizations. In N. O. Graham (Ed.), *Quality in healthcare: Theory, application and evolution.* Gaithersberg, MD: Aspen.

Weick, K. E. (1996). Speaking to practice. *Journal of Management Inquiry, 5,* 251–258.

2 IMPLEMENTING BEST PRACTICE AND EXPERT CONSENSUS PROCEDURES

Kevin Corcoran & Vikki L. Vandiver

EVIDENCE-BASED PRACTICE AND THE EMERGENCE OF SCIENTIFIC THOUGHT

Evidence-based practice (EBP) reflects the continuum in the development of the scientific revolution. Prior to the scientific revolution, methods of answering questions were paramount to the accuracy of the answer (Dear, 2001). The scientific revolution, in contrast, improved the soundness of the methods in order to increase the likelihood of more accurate observations. Improved methods tended to provide more persuasive evidence.

Evidence-based practice is generally this same scientific revolution. It is a process of utilizing a variety of databases to find an appropriate guide to an intervention for a particular diagnostic condition (Vandiver, 2002; Vandiver & Corcoran, 2002). The goal is to select the most accurate, valid if you will, information derived from the best available methods. This may, as is often the case for theory development, be an in-depth description of a single case or a few cases, for example, Piaget's small children, J. B. Watson's Baby Albert, Skinner's few pigeons and only daughter, and, yes, even Freud's cases. While the accuracy of these examples varies considerably, what is common to them all is that social scientists have used more rigorous methods to test, support, refute, and revise these and other areas of case assessment in the behavioral and social sciences.

WHAT IS EVIDENCE-BASED PRACTICE?

Evidence-based practice is a way for clinicians to select from the corpus of the available evidence the most useful information to apply to a particular client who has sought services. Utilizing evidence-based practice approaches is currently considered the industry standard in many helping disciplines, from medicine to managed mental health care. It is as if we had just gotten comfortable with the notion of *best practices* and now use a more contemporary term. As a consequence, the very definition of evidence-based practice has become more illusive, if not ambiguous. Some restrict the term to systematic reviews using meta-analytic procedures. Others use a wider scope in determining evidence-based practice that may include less rigorous studies and influential cases studies. Additionally, there is the evidence delineated by a group of experts in an area or intervention, who in turn produce guidelines (i.e., expert consensus guidelines). These guidelines possess varying degrees of accuracy. This source of evidence-based practice may—by design—have less restrictive inclusion criteria in order to be a broader source of information. Presumably, the experts will have incorporated the same sources considered in the systematic reviews resulting in the same breadth of studies and use of quantitative synthesis.

KEY SOURCES OF EBP

For the practitioner who routinely sees clients several times a day and who frequently faces an unfamiliar and challenging case, it is useful to consider three sources of information on how to deliver the best intervention available that is also the most useful. The three general sources are (a) systematic reviews, (b) practice guidelines, and (c) expert consensus guidelines (see Figure 2.1).

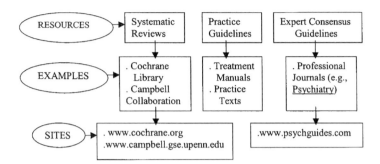

FIGURE 2.1 Resources for Implementing Evidence-Based Practice
Approaches

Systematic Reviews

For the typical practitioner the critical concern is
not simply the best intervention available, but
also the one that is most useful for the client's
circumstances. This is reflected in Gibbs and
Gambrill's (2002) review of evidence-based practice, which asserts that "evidence applies to the
client(s) at hand" in the context of "the values
and expectations of the clients" (p. 453).

The chief source of systematic reviews is the
Cochrane Library, which contains more than
1,500 systematic reviews of medical, nursing,
and health procedures. In the behavioral and social sciences the Campbell Collaboration provides systematic reviews in the areas of crime
and delinquency, education, and social welfare.
Reviews are also frequently available through
professional journals. This is nicely illustrated
by Wilson, Lipsey, and Soydan (2003), who published a systematic review of juvenile justice
with minority youth the very week this chapter
was written. Additionally, many journals such
as *Brief Treatment and Crisis Intervention, Evidence-Based Mental Health, Journal of Clinical
Psychology,* and *Research on Social Work Practice* are committed to publishing systematic reviews.

Other critical sources of such evidence are the
cutting-edge articles published first in a leading
peer-reviewed journal. These articles are not
only the most up-to-date information available,
but also will eventually be incorporated into future systematic reviews. Staying abreast of the
best research in the field still means the well-
read practitioner is likely to stay ahead in the
field.

As may be suggested from the number of
sources of systematic reviews, the quality of the
review itself may vary. In fact, the reviews will
vary in quality and thoroughness. Additionally,
the quantitative methods of data synthesis are
not without controversy (Fischer, 1990), and this
controversy is not terribly new (Glass & Miller,
1978). Inevitably, resulting uncertainties regarding data synthesis methods give rise to the same
concern in applying *any* evidence on which to
build a practice, namely, the veracity of the data.
Is the evidence persuasive for this particular client whose problem is similar in some ways and
different in many others? What would the reasonable and prudent practitioner in the same situation do with this evidence?

Practice Guidelines

Another source for evidence-based practice is the
use of practice guidelines. These are also known
as treatment manuals and include expert consensus guidelines. These sources are distinguishable
from systematic reviews not only by the method
of integrating the available evidence, but also by
the fact that the practice guidelines are reflective of earlier times when practice was guided by
authority (Gambrill, 1999). Practice guidelines
and expert consensus guidelines are readily
available to a wide audience of practitioners in a
variety of disciplines. Additionally, many guidelines and manuals are very practical and direct
in facilitating session-to-session therapeutic activities.

Practice guidelines also refer to statements
and recommendations for conducting an intervention. Terms associated with practice guidelines include *treatment protocols, standards, options, parameters, preferred practice,* and *best
practice.* There are, of course, important distinctions such as standards that are considered a pre-
requisite to all competent practice, guidelines
that are more like suggestions, and options that

are other approaches to consider when appropriate (Havinghurst, 1991).

A valuable source of this form of evidence-based practice is practice texts (e.g., Corcoran, 2000), handbooks (e.g., Roberts & Greene, 2002), and manuals (e.g., LeCroy, 1994; Steketee, 1999). Roberts and Greene's *Desk Reference* (2002) has no less than 33 chapters that are relevant to some definition of evidence-based practice. Most textbooks in production and under contract are likely to delineate evidence-based practice while others may find the need for an updated edition. What is striking about these sources is their variety. Some publishers are committed to producing treatment manuals, such as New Harbinger Publications, which has eight diagnosis-specific manuals in production. Texts such as Corcoran's (2000) may focus more on intervention while others are more diagnostic related (Roth & Foragny, 1996), age specific, (Simpson, 1998), or setting specific, such as juvenile justice (e.g., Roberts, 2004). Thus, we see that the clinician attempting to integrate evidence-based practice must inevitably consider the value of that evidence as it relates to the client. Again, judging the veracity of the evidence is a crucial task.

Expert Consensus Guidelines

Expert consensus guidelines are distinguishable from practice guidelines in that they are typically developed by a broad-based panel of experts. For example, McEvoy, Scheifler, and Thomas's *Practice Guidelines for Schizophrenia* (1999) surveyed more than 300 experts from a variety of disciplines and family and advocacy groups. Despite the wide scope of experts that potentially strengthens expert consensus guidelines, these guidelines are limited and rarely consider cultural differences. Frequently, consensus guidelines are marketed by professional organizations. Professional journals such as *Psychiatry* and the *Journal of Clinical Psychology* frequently publish expert consensus guidelines. A useful Web site for guidelines on a number of psychiatric conditions is *www.psychguides.com*.

ELEMENTS OF EVIDENCE-BASED TREATMENT PLANS

Evidenced-based treatment plans reflect an intervention selected from the best available information appropriate to the values and preferences of a particular client. An evidence-based treatment plan should include seven elements or steps: (a) a biopsychosocial assessment using standardized instruments; (b) an accurate and up-to-date diagnosis using all five axes of the DSM; (c) valid behavioral descriptions of the identified problems or focus of treatment; (d) relevant goals and observable description of the planned target of change; (e) selection of a diagnostic, specific, evidence-based guideline derived from systematic reviews, practice guidelines, or expert consensus guidelines and delineation of a particular/specific treatment plan; (f) repeated administration of outcome measures of the problem, the goals of treatment, or both; and (g) monitoring of client change over the course of treatment and critical evaluation of the treatment outcome. The most critical component of the treatment plan is that the intervention is guided by evidence and delineated in a systematic manner for targeted and observable outcomes.

In the previous section, we discussed the three kinds of resources that the practitioner can draw from to develop an evidence-based treatment plan. Using the seven elements or steps of a treatment plan, the Figure 2.2 illustrates where EBP resources are most often used. There are four main elements or steps where EBP resources are utilized: diagnosis, problem identification, intervention, and outcome.

GUIDELINES FOR IMPLEMENTING EBP

When thoughtfully applied, evidence-based practice will likely strengthen a treatment plan and, in turn, will increase the likelihood of client change and goal attainment. In other words, an intervention derived from evidence-based practice is likely to enhance treatment effectiveness. Vandiver (2002) suggests four summary guidelines for implementing evidence-based knowledge into practice settings: (a) let the assessment be the guide to selecting the appropriate diagnosis, practice guideline, and intervention; (b) use information from all three sources (i.e., systematic reviews, expert consensus guidelines, and practice guidelines) as a guide for determining the most appropriate interventions; (c) if no guideline is available for a particular diagnostic category (e.g., schizoaffective disorder), a review of the professional literature for cutting-edge research or prac-

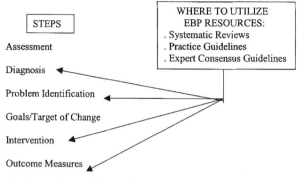

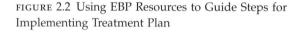

FIGURE 2.2 Using EBP Resources to Guide Steps for Implementing Treatment Plan

tice articles is in order; and (d) practice guidelines are guides, supplements if you will, and will never substitute for sound clinical and professional judgment.

CAVEATS FOR IMPLEMENTING EBP

Applying evidence-based practice is the end stage of the search for a practice approach to guide a particular intervention with a unique client. It is never as easy as the article suggests or the manual directs, including the suggestions from this chapter. The results of a search for evidence-based procedures will likely provide several to select and adapt to one's client. Thus, the clinician must sift through more information than less in developing a treatment intervention for the actual client. One's own client (the one who may be late or overly hostile or affected by the weather or the traffic) is seemingly never as uniform as those in the systematic reviews or the description by experts. Such is the variability of clinical practice. It is more difficult than we want to admit. We believe that one of the first steps in applying evidence-based practice is whether the clinician has carefully considered the credibility of the evidence that will guide the procedures.

As summarized by Vandiver (2002), much more successful work has been done on developing evidence-based interventions than has occurred in disseminating guidelines and protocols or seeing that they are easily available and integrated into routine practice. Advances in using evidence-based interventions have had limited success in some managed mental health care settings. For evidence-based practice to be successful it must first be accessible and then applied. This is greatly facilitated by those interventions that are manualized (e.g., LeCroy, 1994), are structured in a step-by-step format (Steketee, 1990), or contain treatment protocols such as those from the Cochrane Library that provide practical steps and procedures for facilitating client change. All too often, however, evidence-based practice requires that the practitioner structure the intervention into a workable treatment plan, which means that the session-by-session planning is unique and appropriate for the particular client condition.

CONCLUSION

In summary, what we consider a predictable continuum in the scientific revolution has, we believe, a Janus face. One side is designed to disseminate the best available knowledge to guide practice while the other side is marked by the lack of centralized and readily available information that is easily applied. This reflects the problem noted above—that there has been more success in developing evidence-based practice information than in dissemination. The challenges of using evidence-based practice are increased because the information that is available itself has variability in accuracy and utility and therefore must be weighed by the practitioner to determine its application. Add to all of this the fact that the field of available information that is, in fact, evidence for practice is growing so rapidly that keeping up is a formidable task even for the most committed practitioner who sees clients daily, whether in an independent practice, a clinic, hospital, or community setting. In the end, isn't improvement in treatments and procedures one of the targets and benefits of the scientific revolution in the first place?

For a detailed discussion of evidence-based practice concepts, databases to guide treatments, and the 5 steps to EBP clinical decisions in medical settings, see chapter 3 in this book.

References

Corcoran, J. (2000). *Evidence-based social work practice with families.* New York: Springer.

Dear, P. (2001). *Revolutionizing the sciences: European knowledge and its ambitions, 1500–1700.* Princeton, NJ: Princeton University Press.

Fenley, M. A., Gaiter, J. L., Hummett, M., Liburd, L. C., Mercy, J. A., O'Carroll, P. W., Onwuachi-Saunders, C., Powell, K. E., & Thornton, T. N. (1993). *The prevention of youth violence: A framework for community action.* Atlanta, GA: Center for Disease Control and Prevention.

Fischer, J. (1990). Problems and issues in meta-analysis. In L. Videka-Sherman & W. Reid (Eds.), *Advances in clinical social work research* (pp. 297–325). Silver Spring, MD: National Association of Social Workers.

Gambrill, E. (1999). Evidence-based practice: An alternative to authority-based practice. *Families in Society, 80,* 341–350.

Gibbs, L., & Gambrill, E. (2002). Evidence-based practice: Counterarguments to objections. *Research on Social Work Practice, 12,* 452–476.

LeCroy, C. W. (1994). *Handbook of children and adolescent treatment manuals.* New York: Lexington.

Roberts, A. R. (Ed.) (2004). *Juvenile justice sourcebook: Past, present, and future.* New York: Oxford University Press.

Roberts, A. R., & Greene, G. J. (Eds.) (2002). *Social workers' desk reference.* New York: Oxford University Press.

Roth, A., & Fonagy, P. (1996). *What works for whom? A critical review of psychotherapy research.* New York: Guilford Press.

Simpson, J. S., Koroloff, N., Friesen, B. J., Gac, J. (Vol. Eds.) (1999). *Promising practices in family-provider collaboration: Vol. 2. Systems of care: Promising practices in children's mental health, 1998 series.* Washington, DC: Center for Effective Collaboration and Practice, American Institutes for Research.

Steketee, G. (1999). *Overcoming obsessive-compulsive disorder: A behavioral and cognitive protocol for the treatment of OCD.* Oakland, CA: New Harbinger Publications.

Vandiver, V. L. (2002). Step-by-step practice guidelines for using evidence-based practice and expert consensus in mental health settings. In A. R. Roberts & G. J. Greene (Eds.), *Social workers' desk reference.* New York: Oxford University Press.

Vandiver, V. L., & Corcoran, K. (2002). Guidelines for establishing effective treatment goals and treatment plans with axis I disorders. In A. R. Roberts & G. J. Greene (Eds.), *Social workers' desk reference.* New York: Oxford University Press.

Wilson, S. J., Lipsey, M. W., & Soydan, H. (2003). Are mainstream programs for juvenile delinquency less effective with minority youth than majority youth? A meta-analysis of outcomes research. *Research on Social Work Practice, 13,* 3–26.

3 OVERVIEW OF EVIDENCE-BASED PRACTICE

Richard N. Rosenthal

INTRODUCTION AND OPERATIONALLY DEFINING EVIDENCE-BASED PRACTICE

In the good old days clinicians defined best practices from the guild's platform, and then the public tacitly accepted them. When the doctor ordered something, it was accepted as correct; if a specialist offered it, it was implicitly accepted as the best approach (Kramer & Glazer, 2001). Without detracting from the role of clinical experience and mentoring for the honing of clinical judgement in trainees, today's Dr. Welby is faced with the unlikely proposition of having to read an estimated 19 articles a day in his or her field just to keep up with the advances in clinical research. As such, without higher-level strategies to organize and evaluate qualitatively the increasing torrent of information, the knowledge base of any clinician is likely to drift away from the center or be doomed to become ever more specialized and restricted over time. Although there is a clear place for individual expertise, it has become apparent that expert intuitions and opinions are not necessarily correspondent with the results of systematic reviews of high quality research. Even the most experienced clinicians need help from reliable studies and other sources of statistical data in order to complement their clinical experience with accurate estimates of benefit and harm (Donald, 2002). Given the rapid pace with which practice is evolving, "without current best evidence, practice risks becoming rapidly out of date, to the detriment of patients" (Sackett, Rosenberg, Gray, Haynes, & Richardson, 1996).

Evidence-based practice (EBP) in behavioral health means the use of clinical interventions for a specific problem that has been (a) evaluated by well-designed clinical research studies, (b) published in peer-reviewed journals, and (c) consistently found to be effective or efficacious upon consensus review. The intention is to improve the process and outcome of care. Evidence-based practice has its roots in evidence-based medicine (EBM), the philosophic underpinnings of which emanate from 19th century France and which, more recently, Cochrane (1972) proposed as the set of methods needed to understand the effectiveness and efficiency of specific clinical interventions. The term *evidence-based medicine* was coined in the 1980s as a term for the clinical learning strategy developed at McMaster Medical School in Canada in the 1970s (Rosenberg & Donald, 1995). In order to clarify the nature of EBP, which is essentially an extension of EBM to disciplines beyond medicine, I will first describe the underlying process of EBM. According to Sackett and colleagues (1996), EBM is the conscientious explicit and judicious use of current best evidence in making decisions about the care of individual patients. This is done by asking questions, finding and appraising relevant data, and harnessing that information in the form of reliable estimates of benefit and harm for everyday clinical practice (Rosenberg & Donald, 1995). This approach to clinical problem solving requires integrating individual clinical expertise with the best available clinical evidence from systematic research.

EBM is the process of systematically finding, appraising, and using contemporaneous research findings as the basis for clinical decisions. This process is generally described as having five well-defined steps (Rosenberg & Donald, 1995; Sackett et al., 1996):

1. Format a structured, clear, and answerable clinical question from a patient's problem or information need.

2. Search the literature for relevant clinical articles that might answer the question.
3. Conduct a critical appraisal on the selected research articles and rank the evidence for its validity and usefulness (clinical applicability).
4. Formulate and apply a clinical intervention based on the useful findings, or "best evidence."
5. Conduct clinical audits to determine if the protocol was implemented properly (identify issues/problems).

Format a Structured, Clear, and Answerable Clinical Question

Evidence-based medicine can be initiated by questions related to diagnosis, prognosis, treatment, iatrogenic harm, quality of care, or health economics (Rosenberg & Donald, 1995). However, most of the time it pertains to finding the best treatment of a particular problem in the context of conditions that obscure the best clinical decision, that is, where the proper clinical intervention is not easily intuited but where making one choice or another will have significant meaning and consequence to the patient (Donald, 2003). Refining the question to one, which will yield a robust set of studies from the literature, takes some practice.

Search the Literature for Relevant Clinical Articles

Armed with a well-formed question, the clinician must construct a search for studies among electronic databases that is broad enough to include all relevant articles but not so broad that there is too much information to process. Another way to frame this is that high sensitivity of searching methodology will tend to reduce the specificity of the product, thus including many clearly unrelated articles in the search result. The specific detail of conducting searches is provided in chapters 1, 2, and 20 in this book.

Conduct a Critical Appraisal and Rank the Evidence for Validity and Usefulness

Conducting a critical appraisal requires specifying which outcome variables will be examined, the inclusion criteria to be used (e.g., random-

ized clinical trial), finding studies that meet these criteria, determining effect sizes for each of the outcome variables in the selected studies, and combining effect sizes across the selected studies and subjecting the result to tests for bias (Ziguras, Stuart, & Jackson, 2002). Clinical decision making is a complex process. Apart from evidence from research, clinical decisions are based on the context of a patient's current situation and his or her desires and values, as well as the values and clinical experience of the clinician. Having selected the studies with the most valid evidence, one must then weigh benefits and risks of applying the best practice versus the costs and inconveniences of alternatives in the context of the patient's values (Guyatt et al., 2000). A treatment's effectiveness and the clinician's decision to use that treatment must not automatically be determined solely by efficacy but rather by a decision as to the appropriateness of the intervention. A patient with a terminal illness and severely restricted quality of life may reasonably choose to reject cardiopulmonary resuscitation in the event of cardiac arrest, even though that intervention may be effective in restoring a heartbeat.

Formulate and Apply a Clinical Intervention Based on the Useful Findings, or "Best Evidence"

Having determined the relative benefits and harms of a specific intervention, established its suitability for the identified patient, and decided that the system of care can properly support the intervention, the clinician implements the protocol.

Conduct Clinical Audits to Determine If the Protocol was Implemented Properly

Generating information about intervention process and outcome in the context of care delivery is the domain of practice-based research, which will be discussed in later sections of this book. The intention supported by this step is to provide feedback both to the practitioner and, if he or she works within a network, to the network in the form of positive reinforcement if the intervention was effective for the patient or information from which to derive corrective action if it wasn't. This can be done either as a quality improvement protocol or can be generated by practitioners or delivery systems as a formal research study.

Part of the evolving art in EBP revolves around how one accesses studies and systematic reviews and determines the highest quality evidence in order to answer the clinical questions. The next section of this chapter examines two domains that affect that process. The first area is that of the key concepts such as methodological quality and related levels of evidence that must guide any process of critical appraisal or systematic review. The second domain is the concept of the hierarchy of information resources, which allows one to interact with research-based information at ever higher levels of extraction.

KEY CONCEPTS AND DATABASES TO GUIDE TREATMENTS THAT FACILITATE POSITIVE CLIENT CHANGE

Key Concepts 1: Levels of Evidence, Methodological Quality

In the United States, levels of evidence are a well-known concept in the legal system, where the potential impact on the defendant dictates the standard level of evidence required. These levels move from the "preponderance of evidence" in deciding simple civil cases to a standard of "clear and convincing" evidence, and finally to requiring evidence based on certitude "beyond a reasonable doubt" in criminal cases. The development of a systematic approach to evaluating the strength of scientific evidence is a more recent development. EBM and EBP rest on an underlying postulate about a hierarchy of evidence to guide clinical decision making; thus, the evidence-based practitioner must be able to assess the quality of evidence in research studies, systematic reviews, and practice guidelines (Guyatt et al., 2000).

Methodological quality answers the question of how well are systematic bias, nonsystematic bias, and inferential error protected against in the design, conduct, and analysis of any study (Lohr & Carey, 1999). That is, how valid overall is the evidence? Validity has two main domains with respect to its use in evaluating the results of clinical studies. Internal validity is the extent to which outcome differences between compari-

son groups in the study are truly attributable to the clinical intervention (i.e., how correct are the results?). External validity is the extent to which the results can be generalized to populations outside the particular group studied (i.e., how will this intervention work for my patient?).

Randomization of subjects into studies tends to reduce allocation bias, that is, it lowers the risk of confounding variables in comparison groups and increases internal validity. However, the gain in internal validity is often at the expense of external validity, which is reduced when potential subjects are not included in the research, whether through narrow inclusion criteria, local unavailability of the research study, or patient decisions not to participate. For example, in testing psychotropic medications in randomized controlled trials (RCTs) for new drug applications to the Food and Drug Administration (FDA), the pharmaceutical industry has tended to conduct efficacy trials on narrowly defined samples of patients in order to maximize the differential benefit (effect size) in treated subjects as compared to controls. However, the broader the mix of subjects with problem x included in a study, the more likely a true positive result of the study intervention will be of benefit for any other person in the population with problem x. Compared to efficacy research that typically has highly restricted inclusion criteria and subjects with homogeneous characteristics, this is the focus of effectiveness research in behavioral health. As such, one can augment external validity by broadening inclusion criteria, offering the study at multiple sites, and supporting patient participation (McKee et al., 1999).

In order to evaluate the clinical literature for the best evidence to be used in constructing an EBP, one must understand that the strength of evidence presented in a study can be rated according to established standards. Guyatt and colleagues (2000) suggest that evidence in clinical studies can be broadly defined as any empirical observation about the apparent relationship between events. Early attempts by the Canadian Task Force on the Periodic Health Examination (1979) to identify and assess studies according to methodological quality have evolved into several hierarchically based systems developed to rate the strength of scientific evidence in clinical studies. Although there has been continuing differentiation and digression in the levels of evidence in recent years (e.g., see http://www.cebm.net/toolbox.asp), the main demarcations have remained explicit and stable, having been driven mostly by differences in internal validity among the study designs. Fortunately, most hierarchically based systems follow a similar pattern of ranking strength of evidence, starting with the highest level of evidence in multipatient studies:

1. Systematic reviews or meta-analysis of multiple, well-designed controlled studies
2. Well-designed individual experimental studies (randomized, controlled)
3. Well-designed quasi experimental studies (nonrandomized, controlled)
4. Well-designed nonexperimental studies (nonrandomized, uncontrolled)
5. Case series and clinical examples, expert committee reports with critical appraisal
6. Opinions of respected authorities, based on clinical experience

A simpler "A-B-C" system, based on the rating system used by the Agency for Healthcare Research and Quality (AHRQ, formerly AHCPR [Agency for Healthcare Policy and Research]) in developing its depression guidelines (Depression Guideline Panel, 1993), is the consensus panel decision process used by the guidelines development work group at the Texas Medication Algorithm Project (Gilbert et al., 1998). The A-B-C system fits evidence from a broad range of sources into three categories and may be somewhat reductionistic as compared to the levels of evidence from the Center for Evidence-Based Medicine at Oxford University (2001). However, this formal system is an active attempt to form consensus based on the strength of evidence from scientific studies, as opposed to relying on expert opinion or clinical consensus (Suppes et al., 2002). This system rates as A-level evidence to support a recommendation as that evidence which comes from randomized, placebo-controlled studies with raters blinded to study hypotheses and subjects' group membership. Obviously, high-grade evidence from systematic reviews and meta-analyses of randomized, controlled trials also fall into the A category. The B-level data are those from either very large case studies or unblinded controlled studies. This level therefore includes both well-designed quasi-experimental (not randomized) and nonexperimental (neither controlled nor randomized) studies. The C level of evidence is generated from pilot studies, case series, and case reports.

A well-designed individual RCT can provide strong evidence, particularly if there is a large sample size and the target population is diverse and geographically distributed, as in a multisite clinical trial. Observational studies such as cohort studies offer less reliable evidence than RCTs because they cannot plainly control for confounding variables between the groups studied, increasing the risk of selection bias. In addition, observational or nonexperimental studies have been described as tending to overestimate or underestimate treatment effects in an idiosyncratic fashion, making them less valid than RCTs; however, there has been some recent dispute about this (Benson & Hartz, 2000; Concato, Shah, & Horwitz, 2000; McKee et al., 1999). In addition, there are conditions where nonrandomized, uncontrolled studies can provide powerful evidence—for example, when an intervention yields the obvious, consistent, and dramatic result that the introduction of penicillin treatment did in the 1940s (Concato, Shah, & Horwitz, 2000). Generally, unsystematic clinical observations provide the weakest level of evidence from studies because they are typically made in a small number of patients, and there are no safeguards against scientific bias. Without a control group against which to compare outcomes, case studies have low internal validity. Because of small numbers of participants, these studies tend to have low external validity. For those wanting a short primer to help in understanding the different types of research methods, the EBM tutorial website at the State University of New York (SUNY) Health Sciences Center at Brooklyn gives a brief and lucid set of descriptions (http://servers.medlib.hscbklyn.edu/ebm/toc.html).

Key Concepts 2: Hierarchy of Information Resources

Clearly, it is more time-efficient and preferable for clinicians to read one systematic review about a topic than to spend many hours searching for and reading all of the primary literature (Williamson, German, Weiss, Skinner, & Bowes, 1989). Searching, appraising, and selecting from the primary literature is usually beyond the scope of busy individual practitioners. Still, the evidence-based practitioner must have core skills in interpreting statistical results and levels of evidence as well as access to evidence-based resources (Donald, 2002). In dealing with the problem of time limitations on busy clinicians for conducting evidence-based practice, Guyatt and colleagues (2000) offer the mnemonic 4S to describe the hierarchy of information resources available to clinicians. This hierarchy of information preprocessing offers increasing efficiencies in finding an evidence base for treating specific disorders in specific patients: (a) primary *Studies*, where the process is the methodical selection of only well-designed, highly relevant studies; (b) *Summaries* or systematic reviews; (c) *Synopses* of studies or systematic reviews; and (d) *Systems* of information.

Systematic reviews provide an overview of all available evidence pertaining to a specific clinical question. Evidence is located, evaluated, and synthesized using a strict scientific design that must also be reported in the review. Systematic reviews, as compared to traditional narrative reviews, attempt to reduce bias through the inclusiveness and reproducibility of the search process as well as the selection process for studies that are included (AHRQ, 2002). In addition, systematic reviews apply a rigorous critical appraisal compared to narrative reviews and are typically generated in answer to a narrow clinical question (Cook, Mulrow, & Haynes, 1997). As such, the results can be used with more confidence than narrative reviews for decision making about delivery of health care. A meta-analysis is a particular type of systematic review that uses statistical methods to combine and summarize the results of several primary studies, but it can only be done properly with RCT as the study design (Cook, Mulrow & Haynes, 1997). Systematic reviews derived from broad and comprehensive searches also provide another strength—they can reveal what is not known at a particular level of evidence. Compared to systematic reviews, the risk of relying on narrative reviews is that the selection of studies may be idiosyncratic, incomplete, or inaccurate, such that outdated or ineffective clinical directions may continue to be promoted whereas new and effective ones may not be recommended (Antman, Lau, Kupelnick, Mosteller, & Chalmers, 1992).

Synopses provide a further extraction of key methods and results of individual studies or systematic reviews for use in clinical decision making. The typical format of an evidence-based synopsis is the structured abstract, which is specifically designed to quickly reveal information

about the validity of results and about applying these results to practice. These abstracts are often found in the newer secondary journals, which select papers from other journals based on whether the studies are of high methodological quality. Systems of information provide a linkage of related high-grade summaries that expands the narrow orientation of evidence-based practice from specific clinical problems into broader approaches to disease management. These may appear as practice guidelines, treatment algorithms, or decision-support software (Guyatt et al., 2000). An important caveat, however, is that systems for rating the strength of a body of evidence are currently much less uniform than those for rating the quality of a given study (AHRQ, 2001).

Rating scales and checklists have been generated that offer a standard approach to rating the strength of evidence in an individual study or a whole body of evidence. In particular, the best scales take into account the design of the study being examined. For example, the main risk for an invalid conclusion from observational studies is the presence of confounding variables between groups in addition to the variable being tested. Therefore, appropriate scales for rating observational studies ask explicit questions about how much information is available to assure the suitability of the comparison groups in addition to rating the quality of the exposure or intervention, the measurement of outcomes, and the statistical analysis (AHRQ, 2002; Goodman, Berlin, Fletcher, & Fletcher, 1994). A good source for finding various scales and checklists that can be used to assess the strength of scientific evidence in systematic reviews, RCTs, and observational studies is the AHRQ Evidence Report number 47, "Systems to Rate the Strength of Scientific Evidence" (2002), which can be found at www.ahrq.gov/clinic/epcix.htm.

Because EBM involves routine use of research evidence, it was not possible prior to the introduction of large electronic research databases in the early 1990s (Donald, 2002). The years following have produced an increasing torrent of information. The types of clinical questions that EBM is best suited to answer are questions about treatment, risk factors, diagnostic tests, and epidemiology (Donald, 2003). Where there is much research, the search can be limited to RCTs. If observational studies (cohort, retrospective, cross-sectional, or nonrandomized) are going to be used, one should probably only include those that at least incorporate a control group (Benson & Hartz, 2000). Conference proceedings, technical reports, and discussion papers (known as *gray literature*) are not typically indexed on the main databases, yet they should be accessed when possible from specialist libraries and databases in order to reduce publication bias. However, the validity of results reported in conference proceedings should be assessed before including them in the review.

LIMITATIONS

Limitations in Determinations of Quality

The concept of research quality measurement is relatively straightforward; however, the actual quality determined may vary depending on the instrument used to measure it. In behavioral health there is neither consensus about the most valid process measures, such as proper dosage of medications or psychotherapy sessions, nor about the most valid outcomes metrics, such as quality of life or change in symptoms (Kramer & Glazer, 2001).

Limitations in EBP Approaches

EBM and EBP have theoretical and practical limits. EBM addresses questions about the probabilities of benefit or harm to people rather than answering questions about underlying mechanisms of pathology or cure. As such, the domain of EBM/EBP is constrained to a subset of questions in clinical practice and policy that can assist the clinician in choosing whether to treat with a certain intervention or not, but EBM/EBP will not answer questions about what is actually wrong with the depressed patient's mood or dopamine receptors (Donald, 2002). Like any machine, EBP methods can only accomplish what they are designed to do. A related limitation is that even with a well-formed question the best evidence for a particular problem will be of questionable value if the problem has not been framed correctly or the diagnosis is wrong. This is why increasing diagnostic validity through a best-efforts approach to diagnosis or problem identification is so important.

The EBM approach will inevitably expose the gaps in the evidence, especially in mental health where there are many disorders with a scanty empirical research base. However, evidence alone is not sufficient to appropriately treat patients; neither is it likely that externally derived evidence will become a substitute for clinical judgment. Both individual clinical expertise and the best available external evidence are necessary for good clinical practice. "Without clinical expertise, practice risks becoming tyrannized by evidence, for even excellent external evidence may be inapplicable to or inappropriate for an individual patient" (Sackett et al., 1996). Clinicians must always weigh the risks and benefits of a particular intervention in a specific patient, regardless of the evidence base supporting that intervention, because patients may have characteristics related to compliance, age, comorbidity, and so on, that affect the estimates of benefit and risk that come from critical appraisals of the literature. If EBM is applied in an uncritical or non-patient-centered way, the results may be harmful (Naylor, 1995). As such, the issue of relevance is as important as the strength of evidence when attempting to apply results.

The critical appraisal process will generate different outcomes depending on the problem being solved, which limits its generalizability (Rosenberg & Donald, 1995). Because individual answers to clinical questions can be idiosyncratic, there should be some opportunity to generate a higher-level set of approaches that are more generic, that have greater external validity. As such, this rationale becomes one's motivation to discover the best practices, which are really about effectiveness, or how well a treatment works when given to a heterogeneous community sample of persons with a particular disorder.

Another practical limit in implementing EBP is external to the query and search process. Rather, it is located in systems of care as the lack of support structures needed for sustained evidence-based decision making. Furthermore, feasibility of evidence-based practice is constrained by lack of institutional commitment to EBP principles and insufficient skills for interpreting evidence-based information (Donald, 2002).

Limitations in Hierarchies of Evidence

Although empiricism serves as the philosophical foundation of evidence-based science, there is criticism that being overly dependent on empiricism will unnecessarily constrain the conceptual framework of psychiatry (Harari, 2001). Because processes used during the conduct of randomized controlled trials are the best at reducing confounding variables and other sources of bias, the RCT method, originally developed from bench models of empirical science, generates the most reliable evidence with the highest internal validity. However, this paradigm has essentially created a tyranny of this form of evidence in psychiatry and behavioral health. The AHRQ suggests separating out magnitude of effect from the quality of evidence, as the effect size and its positive (benefit) or negative (harm) impact is a different matter from the quality of the data. Evans (2003), in a critique of relying solely on efficacy as the indicator of the evidence quality, proposes a hierarchy of evidence that adds two independent dimensions of appropriateness and feasibility to the formal evaluation. Appropriateness does not rest solely with providers or provider systems because patient acceptance has a key role in whether or not an intervention will be useful. For example, naltrexone is highly efficacious at blocking opioid receptors, but its use in opioid dependent persons to treat addiction without other psychosocial interventions is severely limited by nonadherence with the medication regimen.

Limitations in Implementation

Feasibility can and should be evaluated in a systematic fashion, and results generated through systematic reviews and multicenter studies offer the best evidence for evaluating an intervention's feasibility (Evans, 2003). Simply because a particular intervention is effective does not mean it will be broadly implemented. Stakeholders in programmatic approaches that are not evidence-based tend not to cease providing that type of treatment simply because other evidence-based formats have been discovered. Their resistance to adoption of newer, evidence-based practices is typically composed of intellectual, economic, social, and philosophical components working in concert (Corrigan, Steiner, McCracken, Balser, & Barr, 2001). Action research is a strategy that uses a variety of quantitative and qualitative scientific methods to elucidate and address in situ problems in the care environment (Meyer, 2000). As such, action research that explores the relationships between attitudes and aspects of care or barriers to implementation of new practices can provide good quality evidence about an intervention's feasibility (Evans, 2003).

MOVEMENT TOWARD THE DEVELOPMENT OF PRACTICE GUIDELINES AND EXPERT CONSENSUS GUIDELINES

Best Practices

EBM and EBP are bottom-up approaches, starting with a specific question that derives from the problems in setting effective and appropriate treatment for a specific patient. In contrast, best practice is a top-down approach defined as the measurement, benchmarking, and identification of processes that result in better outcomes (Kramer & Glazer, 2001). Whereas the traditional point of view about mental health practice has been the individual clinician or individual clinic, the perspective of best practice requires an organizational approach to assessing variations in practice from the individual level up through groups such as hospitals and provider agencies and through regions (Glazer, 1998). The components necessary to establish best practices are data collection systems, systemic quality improvement processes, and systems of health care providers. Much of what has recently served as the basis of best practices has been gleaned from analysis and benchmarking of pooled provider data, which is often of low quality (e.g., low-resolution clinical information from hospital financial encounter data and billing records). More recently agencies such as AHRQ and the Joint Commission on Accreditation of Healthcare Organizations have created quality indicators that are driving health care provider systems toward the acquisition of better-quality clinical data for their performance improvement initiatives. When a provider organization is given feedback against benchmarks, it tends to drive the quality process. This is not only true at the macrolevel but also on the individual level, for example, when subjecting research papers to peer review (Goodman et al., 1994). However, over and above the specific contributions to individual treatment decisions made through EBM, EBM provides professional bodies with fair and scientifically rigorous means to make best-practice decisions and develop guidelines and standards (Donald, 2002). This point is important because most clinical guidelines have

TABLE 3.1 Evidence-Based Resources

Tool kit sites

New York Academy of Medicine: *http://www.ebmny.org/teach.html*
Oxford University: *http://cebm.jr2.ox.ac.uk/docs/toolbox.html*
University of Alberta: *http://www.med.ualberta.ca/ebm/ebm.htm*
University of Toronto Centre for Evidence-Based Medicine, Canada: *http://www.cebm.utoronto.ca/teach/*
Health Information Research Unit (HIRU), McMaster University, Canada: *http://hiru.mcmaster.ca/*

Systematic reviews of the literature

National Health Society Centre for Reviews and Dissemination: *http://www.york.ac.uk/inst/crd/centre.htm*
Centre for Evidence-Based Medicine, Oxford: *http://cebm.jr2.ox.ac.uk/docs/prospect.html*
Swedish Council on Technology Assessment in Health Care (SBU): *http://www.sbu.se/sbu-info.html*
Cochrane Collaboration database of systematic reviews: *http://cochrane.mcmaster.ca/*
Health Services/Technology Assessment Text (HSTAT), U.S. National Library of Medicine: *http://hstat.nlm.nih.gov/hq/Hquest/screen/HquestHome/s/49321*
Abstracts of SBU reports:*http://www.sbu.se/abstracts/abstracts.html*
The *Bandolier* newsletter on evidence-based health care

For an expanded list of Evidence-Based Resources see Appendix 2.

not been constructed using high-grade evidence (Shaneyfelt, Mayo-Smith, & Rothwangl, 1999). This may be especially true of behavioral health guidelines, where issues of practice have traditionally been viewed from the perspective of the individual practitioner (Glazer, 1998).

Guidelines Development

Though originally developed through the integration of expert clinical judgment (consensus guidelines), practice guidelines as currently defined are clinical decision rules that have been systematically developed with critical assessment and evaluation of the existing literature using the best available evidence (evidence-based guidelines). This shift from expert consensus to evidence-based consensus is partly due to the increasing recognition, using critical appraisal and systematic review, that expert opinion has relatively low validity as scientific evidence when compared to meta-analyses or systematic reviews. A practical application of evidence-based approaches to clinical guidelines development is the Texas Medication Algorithm Project (TMAP). Medication treatment algorithms have been suggested as a strategy to provide uniform care at predictable costs. TMAP is a three-phase study designed to provide solid data on the use-

fulness of medication algorithms. In the initial phase, medication algorithms for the treatment of several severe mental disorders were developed. Then a feasibility study of these algorithms was conducted in the next phase. Finally, having demonstrated the feasibility of using these algorithms, a validation phase was implemented. This study compared the outcome and costs of using a combination of an algorithm matched to a specific disorder in one group to another group using treatment as usual including a mismatched algorithm, then to a third group using typical treatment and no use of algorithms to drive treatment (Shon et al., 1999).

CONCLUSION

EBP is a powerful technology-based methodology that can support clinical decisional process, but it must start with a valid diagnosis or problem properly framed into a specific question. The well-described and standardized process entails grading studies on the strength of evidence, necessitating in those conducting EBP a working knowledge of the general standards of the hierarchies of evidence. Once a critical appraisal of the broadly screened literature results in the best evidence for action, the intervention must be weighed in context of its acceptability to the patient's desires and values and the system's capacity to successfully implement it. Limitations intrinsic to the process are that EBP is necessary but not sufficient to drive proper clinical decision making for specific patients. The patient's clinical state and values render an evidence-based intervention suitable or not suitable. Limitations to EBP found within care systems tend to be at the level of diminished implementation due to poor conceptual buy-in, deficient knowledge, or systemic inertia.

References

Agency for Healthcare Research and Quality (AHRQ). (2002). *Systems to rate the strength of scientific evidence: Summary.* (Evidence Report/Technology Assessment No. 47, AHRQ Pub. No. 02-E015). Washington, DC: U.S. Department of Health and Human Services, Public Health Service. Retrieved February 13, 2003, from www.ahrq.gov/clinic/epcix.htm.

Agency for Healthcare Research and Quality (AHRQ). (2001). *Current methods of the U.S. preventive services task force: A review of the process.* Retrieved February 13, 2003, from www.ahcpr.gov/clinic/ajpmsuppl/harris/1.htm.

Antman, E. M., Lau, J., Kupelnick, B., Mosteller, F., & Chalmers, T. C. (1992). A comparison of results of meta-analyses of randomized control trials and recommendations of clinical experts: Treatments for myocardial infarction. *Journal of the American Medical Association, 268,* 240–248.

Benson, K., & Hartz, A. J. (2000). A comparison of observational studies and randomized, controlled trials. *New England Journal of Medicine, 342,* 1878–1886.

Canadian Task Force on the Periodic Health Examination. (1979). The periodic health examination. *Canadian Medical Association Journal, 121,* 1193–1254.

Center for Evidence-Based Medicine at Oxford University. (2001). *Levels of Evidence.* Retrieved January 2, 2003, from http://www.cebm.net/toolbox.asp.

Cochrane, A. L. (1972). *Effectiveness and efficiency: Random reflections on health services.* London: Nuffield Provincial Hospitals Trust.

Concato, J., Shah, N., & Horwitz, R. I. (2000). Randomized, controlled trials, observational studies and the hierarchy of research designs. *New England Journal of Medicine, 342,* 1887–1892.

Cook, D. J., Mulrow, C. D., & Haynes, R. B. (1997). Systematic reviews: Synthesis of best evidence for clinical decisions. *Annals of Internal Medicine, 126,* 376–380.

Corrigan, P. W., Steiner, L., McCracken, S. G., Balser, B., & Barr, M. (2001). Strategies for disseminating evidence-based practices to staff who treat people with serious mental illness. *Psychiatric Services, 52,* 1598–1606.

Depression Guideline Panel. (1993). *Depression in primary care: Vol 1. Detection and diagnosis* (Clinical Practice Guideline No. 5, AHCPR Pub. No. 93-0550). Rockville, MD: U.S. Department of Health and Human Services, Agency for Health Care Policy and Research.

Donald, A. (2002). Evidence-based medicine: Key concepts. *Medscape General Medicine, 4*(2) http://www.medscape.com/viewpublication/122_index.

Donald, A. (2003). How to practice evidence-based medicine. *Medscape General Medicine, 5*(1), http://www.medscape.com/viewpublication/122_index.

Evans, D. (2003). Hierarchy of evidence: A framework for ranking evidence evaluating healthcare interventions. *Journal of Clinical Nursing, 12,* 77–84.

Gilbert, D. A., Altshuler, K. Z., Rago, W. V., Shon, S. P., Crismon, M. L., Toprac, M. G., et al. (1998). Texas Medication Algorithm Project: Definitions, rationale, and methods to develop medication algorithms. *Journal of Clinical Psychiatry, 59*(7), 345–351.

Glazer, W. M. (1988). Defining best practices: A prescription for greater autonomy. *Psychiatric Services, 49,* 1013–1016.

Goodman, S. N., Berlin, J., Fletcher, S. W., & Fletcher, R. H. (1994). Manuscript quality before and after peer review and editing at *Annals of Internal Medicine. Annals of Internal Medicine, 121,* 11–21.

Guyatt, G. H., Haynes, R. B., Jaeschke, R. Z., Cook, D. J., Green, L., Naylor, C. D., et al. (2000). Users guide to the medical literature XXV. Evidence-based medicine: Principles for applying the users guides to patient care. *Journal of the American Medical Association, 284,* 1290–1296.

Harari, E. (2001). Whose evidence? Lessons from the philosophy of science and the epistemology of medicine. *Australia and New Zealand Journal of Psychiatry, 35,* 724–730.

Kramer, T. L., & Glazer, W. N. (2001). Our quest for excellence in behavioral health care. *Psychiatric Services, 52,* 157–159.

Lohr, H. N., & Carey, T. S. (1999). Assessing "best evidence": Issues in grading the quality of studies for systematic reviews. *Joint Commission Journal on Quality Improvement, 25,* 470–479.

McKee, M., Britton, A., Black, N., McPherson, K., Sanderson, C., & Bain, C. (1999). Interpreting the evidence: Choosing between randomised and non-randomised studies. *British Medical Journal, 319,* 312–315.

Meyer, J. (2000). Using qualitative methods in health related action research. *British Medical Journal, 320,* 178–181.

Naylor, C. D. (1995). Grey zones of clinical practice:

Some limits to evidence-based medicine. *Lancet, 345*, 840–842.

Raine, R., Haines, A., Sensky, T., Hutchings, A., Larkin, K., & Black, N. (2002). Systematic review of mental health interventions for patients with common somatic symptoms: Can research evidence from secondary care be extrapolated to primary care? *British Medical Journal, 325*, 1082–1093.

Rosenberg, W., & Donald, A. (1995). Evidence based medicine: An approach to clinical problem solving. *British Medical Journal, 310*, 1122–1126.

Sackett, D. L., Rosenberg, W. M. C., Gray, J. A. M., Haynes, R. B., & Richardson, W. S. (1996). Evidence based medicine: What it is and what it isn't. *British Medical Journal, 312*, 71–72.

Shaneyfelt, T. M., Mayo-Smith, M. F., & Rothwangl, J. (1999). Are guidelines following guidelines? The methodological quality of clinical practice guidelines in the peer-reviewed medical literature. *Journal of the American Medical Association, 281*, 1900–1905.

Shon, S. P., Crismon, M. L., Toprac, M. G., Trivedi, M., Miller, A. L., Suppes, T., et al. (1999). Mental health care from the public perspective: The Texas Medication Algorithm Project. *Journal of Clinical Psychiatry, 60*(Suppl. 3), 16–20; discussion, 21.

Suppes, T., Dennehy, E. B., Swann, A. C., Bowden, C. L., Calabrese, J. R., Hirschfeld, R. M., et al. (2002). Report of the Texas Consensus Conference Panel on medication treatment of bipolar disorder 2000. *Journal of Clinical Psychiatry, 63*(4), 288–299.

Williamson, J. W., German, P. S., Weiss, R., Skinner, E. A., & Bowes, F., III. (1989). Health science information management and continuing education of physicians: A survey of U.S. primary care practitioners and their opinion leaders. *Annals of Internal Medicine, 110*, 151–160.

Ziguras, S. J., Stuart, G. W., & Jackson, A. C. (2002). Assessing the evidence on case management. *British Journal of Psychiatry, 181*, 17–21.

INFORMING HEALTH CHOICES

4

Reflections on Knowledge Integration Strategies for Electronic Health Records

Robert Hayward

This chapter explores the informational requirements of informed decision making, illustrates how changes in information tools can affect health care practice, and highlights possible implications for a new culture of knowledge integration. The chapter begins with a brief examination of how information systems can support the kinds of health care choices most likely to improve patient safety, satisfaction, and outcomes. The next section explores the information needs of health care decision makers, defines evidence-based practice and policy making, and considers information behaviors implicit in evidence-based decision making. Evidence-based informatics is described as an approach to highlighting the validity, importance, and applicability of information supporting decisions within day-to-day health care practice. Third is a discussion and classification of information tools now proliferating in the health care workplace. The importance of information convenience, discrimination, and integration is highlighted. The fourth section considers how improving information technology and methods can affect the information culture of health care organizations. Each section suggests implications for future health care management and education and the potential impact on the quality of future medical care.

OVERVIEW

A health policy agenda is emerging that is preoccupied with evidence. From national agencies to regional health authorities and from subspecialist clinics to primary health centers, every participant in the health care endeavor is aware of evidence: the need for it, the lack of it, the various definitions of it. How is it that physician practices vary so much and that solid information takes so long to find its way to practice? That the best evidence should always buttress health choices is blindingly obvious to most lay people.

A health informatics agenda is emerging that is preoccupied with technology. After years of under-investment in information systems, the Canadian National Forum on Health placed evidence-based information systems on a par with women's health as a key deliverable for the next decade of health reform (National Forum on Health, 1997). Major financial commitments—including Canada's InfoWay—fuel the expectation that "better information" will beget "better health" (Advisory Council on Health Infostructure, 1999; Alberta wellnet, 2003. These strategic information initiatives often assert that improvements will occur because better information will affect the choices of patients, practitioners, and policy makers.

In reality, more information may worsen the plight of busy decision makers. They experience information hunger in the midst of plenty. The content of health knowledge is so volatile and expansive that physicians increasingly must manage, not contain, information (Harris, Salasche, & Harris, 2001). In order for better information to yield better health, at least three things must happen. First, health care decision makers must discern better from worse infor-

mation. Second, changes in knowledge must trigger changes in health practices. Finally, improved outcomes must result from altered practices. In short, better information begets better health through the medium of better choice. For patients, practitioners and policy makers to make more informed choices, they need to

- know what to do (because best information supporting best practices is readily available at the point of decision making),
- do what is known (with aids to problem recognition, question formulation, resource selection, information acquisition, and use), and
- understand what is done (because information use is monitored and managed).

Informed choice is facilitated when information about health is connected with information about how to improve health. To attract clinician attention a health information system must be ubiquitous, accessible, dependable, and credible. It must present all information—patient reported, clinician observed, and research derived—in a way that highlights its validity, importance, and applicability for individual patients. To retain clinician attention a health information system must complement, not conflict with, the predominantly oral culture of information exchange in health care. The information tools must make it easier for decision makers to find and use high quality information when reflecting with colleagues, consultants, and clients. Most importantly, information tools must decrease the clinician's total informational burden while easing communications with colleagues and participation in virtual learning and decision-making communities. Clinicians' work should be supported by an information culture that rewards explicit approaches to uncertainty and acceptance of just-in-time knowledge.

INFORMATION NEEDS

Individual patients hope that health practitioners will identify health problems, articulate relevant options for managing each problem, assemble the best available information about the outcomes associated with each treatment option, solicit patient preferences for each outcome, and promote practices that win compliance and achieve valued results. Groups of patients hope that practitioners will work to prevent, detect, and treat health problems in a way that is fiscally responsible and that maximizes all patients' opportunity to avail themselves of high-quality health care. To meet patients' expectations, individually and in aggregate, clinicians face forbidding information management tasks.

Capable information managers discern uncertainty, craft answerable questions, map questions to different types of knowledge, seek valid evidence from appropriate sources, and prudently apply knowledge in patient care. Over the last decade Internet advances have removed technical barriers to just-in-time knowledge. We are left struggling with how best to facilitate the better application of knowledge to practice, and how to know which information behaviors are most effective.

Evidence-Based Practice

Evidence-based practice (EBP) is a particular conceptualization about what it means to enable informed choice. EBP tries to bridge the gap between evidence and practice. Knowing that there is premature adoption of incompletely tested ideas on the one hand and failure of adoption of proven knowledge on the other, scientists suggest that there is a faulty connection at the point where evidence and practice meet (Haynes et al., 1995). It is distressing to those who produce and summarize evidence that so much strong evidence remains unheeded in day-to-day practice. For the producers of evidence the starting point for EBP is the meritorious clinical trial.

Potential consumers of evidence, however, are distressed by the huge backlog of common and important clinical problems for which evidence is unavailable, and may never become available, or exists but is confusing, conflicting, or, because of mismatches to clinical circumstances, inapplicable. For the consumers of evidence, the starting point is a specific clinical problem.

From the clinician's point of view, health care depends on many types of information and there are many disconnects between information and practice. Even when good, pertinent evidence is readily available clinicians must apply it in a fuzzy context that implicitly or explicitly includes consideration of costs, patient preferences, comorbidity, and a broad range of health outcomes, many of which do not figure in clinical experiments. It is little wonder, then, that busy clinicians often are intimidated by the call to EBP. They protest that it is difficult, time-consuming, and impractical. It devalues expertise and it forebodes Hamlet-like indecision. In response, the proponents of EBP ask clinicians to focus on being more aware of the type and strength of any link between what we do and why we do it. The evidence-based decision maker should greet any information source with questions about the following:

- Validity: Is the information likely to be true?
- Importance: If true, will the information make a difference that patients will care about?
- Applicability: Can the information be used?

Promoting EBP is, at its core, an approach to information management. It holds that informational support for informed decision making must make explicit the following implicit attributes of clinical problem solving:

- recognition of patient or population health problems,
- exposing of uncertainty in how we manage those problems,
- articulating questions that must be answered to resolve the uncertainty,
- selecting appropriate sources of knowledge to answer the questions,
- finding information from those sources,
- sifting believable and relevant information from distracting information, and
- determining if and how any new information can be used.

These tasks are not restricted to the use of clinical trial results. They pertain as much to books, papers, and expert opinion as to primary research reports.

Evidence-Based Policy

EBP heralds a major change in the philosophy driving health care decisions as well as a shift in sources, types, and applications of health information. In *Creating a Culture of Evidence-Based Decision Making in Health*, the National Forum on Health defined evidence-based decision making as "the *systematic* [italics added] application of the *best available* [italics added] evidence to the evaluation of options and to decision making in clinical, management and policy settings" (National Forum on Health, 1998). Evidence-based decision making's adoption as a new mode of addressing health policy has pivotal implications for those who generate and those who use health information. Evidence-based health care expresses commitment to

- improve the transparency of reasoning behind policies.
- increase accountability by justifying decisions on the basis of valid information that can stand up to scrutiny.
- gauge uncertainty by making explicit the strength of evidence supporting policy.
- make policy decisions driven by the best outcomes for the health care dollar.

The nature of health care accountability has changed significantly within a generation. Consumers are better educated, more informed, and more skeptical than ever before. The public has access to information previously only available to professionals. In addition to consumer demands, every health profession is being challenged to demonstrate that it is making a positive impact on the health of its patients. Evidence of interventions' effectiveness and impact on health outcomes is being demanded from all health care providers.

Evidence-Based Informatics

More evidence does not make evidence-based practice. Indeed, by removing technical and operational barriers to information access we have exposed a more fundamental problem: busy physicians have difficulty applying new knowledge to patient care (Guyatt & Rennie, 2002). The last thing clinicians need is knowledge dumped at the bedside while they are ill equipped to discern the relevant details. What they do need are highly refined distillates of valid, important, and applicable patient-reported, clinician-observed, and research-derived evidence—all presented in a way that is easy to understand, readily available, and tightly linked to patient priorities.

Evidence-based informatics (EBI) accepts this challenge. It is the study of how knowledge-aware systems can improve the application of best evidence about the effects of health care practices: coupling what is known to what is done. EBI makes at least two important contributions. It helps decision makers

- know how to know by helping them voice meaningful questions, direct the questions to the right type of knowledge source, and then search, select, and synthesize information; and
- use what is known by highlighting the settings, patients, and practitioners to which the knowledge pertains.

Evidence-based health information systems are a subset of knowledge-based systems. They answer questions of validity with links to evidence supporting recommendations, answer questions of importance with presentations of information in clinically meaningful terms, and answer questions of applicability with details about the patients and circumstances to which the information applies.

EBI promotes timely access to accurate synopses of clinical data together with digests of relevant evidence about the meaning of the data. Tapping the efficiency and overwhelming power of computerized information systems, EBI links knowledge with practice with technologies that can put information at the bedside.

Implications

EBP portends a change in what it means to be a clinician. Proficiency with just-in-time knowledge requires more than good information retrieval skills. Rapid access must be paired with rapid assessment. The core assumption of EBP is that the *way* one knows is as important as *what* one knows. The imperative for EBP is a given, as is the rapid shift from static paper-based information resources to dynamic electronic resources. What remains is for professionals and professional associations to determine how they will bring themselves in line with an approach to health care that emphasizes competency in informed decision making. A health care environment driven by evidence-based practice will require

- stakeholders to make practical changes in the way health information is managed and presented.
- continuing change management paired to clinical information systems deployment, highlighting the fact that continuing professional development is inseparable from continuing clinical practice.

- a renewed understanding of how considerations of validity, importance, and applicability affect ways of knowing in a particular health discipline.

Most medical education institutions have an inadequate "infostructure" (hardware, software, and networks supporting electronic information exchange) across the continuum of teaching. Standards for health informatics teaching are not uniform, and few schools have facilities that support experiential learning with the types of information systems that clinicians encounter in practice. There are few if any links between educators and the information systems infrastructure of the health regions in which universities reside. Stakeholders wishing to improve their profile in the area of evidence-based informatics will need to define the types of health information that matter most, how such evidence is being generated, where it resides, and how it might be accessed by learners.

Informatics initiatives need to be seen as allies by practitioners and policy makers in their efforts to choose wisely and knowledgeably. These groups already feel overwhelmed by information overload. They want to be making the right decisions: right for patients, right scientifically, right for society's demands for cost control. Health education communities have a huge opportunity to facilitate the transition that practitioners feel they must make. This can be done by addressing the barriers to EBP, using experiential learning approaches to teach practical ways to overcome them, and working with health regions to make evidence training available at the point of care (Lau et al., 1999).

INFORMATION TOOLS

These are times of great expectation for health informatics. In a world frenzied by an information revolution, many anticipate knowledge beamed to the bedside in service of a new, better, health system. These are also times of great challenge for health institutions. As hospitals reorganize, regionalize, and downsize, their patients, practitioners, and funders demand better application of what is known to what is done:

- Patients want reassurance that they are receiving quality care.

- Practitioners want fast access to data and knowledge that is easy to find, easy to read, and easy to apply.
- Policy makers want new approaches to disseminating information and managing its impact on care.

That information technologies continue to grow in quantity, quality, and sophistication is encouraging. That health institutions must compensate for years of deferred maintenance and under-investment in information systems is discouraging. Although costs-per-computing-event are decreasing, user appetite for information services is growing faster than ever before. The gap between demand and capacity for information management is growing.

This section examines some of the immediate information problems of health institutions and the emerging strategies that can be used to meet those needs. New information systems must be deployed to serve

- information convenience (the right information presented the right way at the right time for the right person),
- information discrimination (valid and important information discerned from misleading and distracting information), and
- information integration (meaningful relationships between information from different sources are highlighted).

Information Needs

The emergence of a knowledge-based health economy is changing the information behaviors of hospitals, community practices, libraries, and the general public. The needs listed in Table 4.1 are made all the more urgent by a growing conviction that less-than-optimal information services are a threat to patient safety (Leape et al., 1998).

Information Technology

Computers have become so commonplace that changes in the health care workplace are now coupled to changes in computing technology. An organization's infostructure is determined by how computers are deployed to support its mission-critical functions. The health care infostructure is undergoing profound change now

TABLE 4.1 Information Needs and Their Implications

Need	Implication
As health systems are regionalized, with different care specialities concentrated at different locations, **health information networks** are being developed to facilitate reliable access to **multiple information resources at multiple locations**. Multitasking personal computers have become popular but are potentially **costly to support.**	Different practitioners have **different information needs**. Information systems need to allow for these differences by customizing how information is presented for each user type. The computer industry produces hugely powerful workstations and computer operating systems, but health practitioners need ways to focus them for individualized clusters of information tasks.
High **quality knowledge software** is now widely available. Electronic textbooks, drug information databases, decision support systems, practice guidelines, and medical education programs are available and affordable. New software appears daily and changes frequently.	Demand for **knowledge-integration services** increases because the experience, skills, and tools required to manage knowledge-based software are rare.
Most practitioners, patients, and policy makers are too busy to attend computer courses.	Users need **on-line training** opportunities and simple aids for **selecting appropriate software** for a particular clinical question.
The Internet has become a powerful and popular source of health information. Recognized for its power by nurses and physicians, who want access, it is still not provided in many health institutions because of concerns about security.	Health institutions are looking for ways to provide controlled **Internet access** without risking exposure to computer viruses and inappropriate use of the World Wide Web.
Software vendors frequently demand reimbursement based on the number of users or uses. New confidentiality laws mandate that health institutions monitor who accesses information found in clinical systems.	Health institutions need information about **who uses software, when, and for what purpose.**
Hospitals and practitioners have come under intense pressure to **control costs**. Many use practice guidelines, care maps, clinical pathways, and other information tools to try to influence practitioner behavior.	Health organizations need to monitor information behaviors and usage patterns and track who has interacted with the information tools and with what results. They need to survey staff about new information policies and practices.
The knowledge and skills concentrated in **libraries** make them the best candidates for meeting the knowledge management needs of offices, hospitals, and regions.	Libraries need to be integrated into regional information networks, and they need to be equipped with systems and skills for **wide-area knowledge management**. In the past practitioners were urged to go to libraries. Now the libraries must use the Internet to go to practitioners. Better still, librarians should use the Internet to offer a virtual presence to clinicians.

Need	Implication
As society shifts from passive multimedia information dissemination (e.g., television) to active multimedia dissemination (e.g., Internet) **patients are becoming avid health information consumers. Indeed, many patients enjoy better access to health knowledge databases than the health practitioners they go to for help.**	Patients need help to recognize better quality sources of information and to understand the relevance and applicability of information to their unique circumstances. Physicians need to hone new skills in rapid assessment of Internet resources and new approaches to patient education.

that multiple information products (multisource) can be delivered at the same time (multitasking) to multiple hardware platforms (multiplatform) using multiple communications media (multimedia).

Multisource

A WORLDWIDE HEALTH INFORMATION COMMUNITY By making virtually unlimited numbers and types of health information resources available in a consistent, compatible format, Internet communication and markup protocols remove barriers to information exchange, promote access to and use of knowledge, and fundamentally change the role of health care libraries.

Perhaps the most far-reaching change in clinical computing relates to the creation of a worldwide health care information community, on the Internet, in which all health care practitioners and institutions can participate. No longer are personal computers limited to local software. In the age of interpersonal computing, the Internet provides a robust medium for intercomputer communication, universal standards for document and database exchange, and opportunities for decentralized health care data and knowledge management.

The Internet is defined by a protocol (TCP/IP) that governs how messages are sent from one computer to another. Layered on top of this protocol are methods for creating secure communication channels between multiple computers at the same institution or between institutions. The Internet can and has been used to create multi-institutional networks and regional health information systems.

Internet communications protocols also facilitate software-to-software communication. Functions such as electronic mail, discussion lists, file transfer, and software updates are available under a common interface available to all Internet-aware software applications. Documents and databases can be stored in forms that will display on any computer with direct links to these communications tools. The user need only "click" on an item or link of interest to download or display information, send a message to the author, check a reference, or place an order for a reprint. One information resource can query another resource using standardized protocols for sending information requests from one place to another. Indeed, computing resources from around the world become indistinguishable from those stored on the local computer. Place is immaterial on the Internet. The advent of XML (extensible markup language) has brought features of databases and documents together in ways that are easy for nonexperts to manipulate and customize.

UBIQUITOUS HEALTH PUBLISHING Now that popular word processors can produce, save, and publish information in an Internet-ready form, anyone can share information on the Internet. Although this removes barriers to the exchange of health knowledge, it encourages informational anarchy because there are few controls on the quality, authenticity, or durability of Internet-based information.

INTELLECTUAL PROPERTY In general, Internet developers can create links to a wide range of independent information resources on the Internet. Health practice recommendations can be seamlessly linked to supporting evidence. In this way a new domain of intellectual property has been created. Over and above the content of a document, there is value in the relationships that have been created between that document and other information resources.

JUST-IN-TIME KNOWLEDGE Health care knowledge is highly volatile, changing at an ever-increasing rate. The Internet makes it possible to view large public databases the instant they are updated, to subscribe to "channels" broadcasting the most recent changes in databases, and to provide instant feedback to database authors concerning problems in the content of health knowledge resources. The best electronic journals include alert services that automatically send practitioners updates about new information in their fields of interest.

VIRTUAL LIBRARIES As journals, textbooks, government databases, and other resources proliferate on the Internet, this distributed network is starting to replace the library as the preferred source of health knowledge. Most Canadian health libraries have shifted from paper to electronic journal subscriptions. A new generation of librarians is emerging, who are focused on managing Internet-based information resources and virtual collections assembled from multiple databases at multiple locations.

Multitasking

Today's personal computers exceed the power of decade-old mainframes with phenomenal increases in speed, storage capacity, and display capabilities. This greatly extends the scalability of health information systems and brings previously esoteric capabilities of artificial intelligence, expert guidance, and decision support within reach of everyday health care workers. Such opportunity highlights a need for investment, for understanding of the best uses of these new tools, and for relatively greater attention to software than hardware in health institution spending.

TERMINAL–MAINFRAME DYAD Computer networks of the 1970s and 1980s commonly enslaved computer terminals to one or more mainframe computers. The terminals could display only one type of information at a time. Even systems allowing access to knowledge-based resources such as pharmacopoeia required the user to exit from one application, connect to the database, then navigate a number of keyboard-driven menus to get the desired information. Another set of menus had to be negotiated to get back to the clinical information that prompted a search for evidence.

CLIENT–SERVER MYAD In the 1990s computers were liberated from the terminal–mainframe hierarchy. Modern operating systems support multitasking so that more than one software application can be available on the same computer at the same time. The user can quickly switch from a laboratory test result display, for example, to one or more databases that help the user decide how to use and apply the test result in practice. In this way multiple software programs can access multiple mainframe computers. With the emergence of secure Internet connections those computers can be anywhere in the world. Indeed, now that the best information resources tend to be most current in their Internet iterations, the modern computer workstation again resembles a terminal—a multitasking terminal.

Multithreading

Modern computer systems also support "multithreading," where multiple software applications can perform multiple functions simultaneously on one or more computer processors at one or more locations. The increasing power of computer workstations and the increasing capacity, or bandwidth, of computer networks have enabled the development of decentralized computer networks: client–server communities with no fixed hierarchy. They are dynamic and can accommodate hardware and software changes more easily, support freer communications, and collaboratively tackle complex computational tasks. Moreover, remote desktop access protocols allow Internet devices to be used to control more powerful computers and software applications from remote and mobile locations—in effect nesting computers within computers within other computers.

Multiplatform

DIVERSIFICATION OF HARDWARE The reach of computers has been greatly extended through miniaturization, mobilization, and modularization. Classical computers, with keyboards and display screens, are giving way to a great diversity of personal computing "appliances." Digital telephones can send and receive electronic mail, televisions can browse the Internet, and bedside technologies (e.g., automated vital signs monitors) are integrated with computer networks. Indeed, a number of hospitals are installing wireless drug dispensing systems, where medication carts are network devices that continuously communicate with a central database about which drugs are needed and received by patients.

The diversification of computing technology is changing health practices at the point of care and helping to streamline health data collection. However, most health sciences curricula do not attend to these developments and do not equip students with the tools they need to decide how best to integrate these systems into their practice and continuing education. Students are rarely taught about the information properties of data collected and stored in these systems and how the data can be used to measure their performance.

Miniaturization. It is now possible to pack the power of a sophisticated multimedia workstation into a portable device the size of a notebook, and the power of a professional productivity workstation into a palm-sized device the size of a pack of cards. Some portable computers dispense with keyboards altogether. Instead, a pen is used to interact with graphical data-entry screens. This miniaturization brings the functionality of desktop computing to the point of health care.

Mobilization. Networking technology has evolved to the point that the local area network is an oxymoron, without spatial meaning. Computing communities are defined more by interest and occupation than by location, and it is perfectly possible to join health administrators at opposite ends of the country through virtual private networks. Wireless networks allow all kinds of devices, physically untethered, to remain in contact with health databases. Cellular and satellite networks combined with geographic positioning systems are now preinstalled in many mobile computing devices, allowing precise regional data collection from any location.

Modularization. The most rapidly established computer technology in history, the handheld or palm computer, exemplifies the power of modular computing. The device performs a specific subset of personal computing tasks including contact management, scheduling, task management, and other personal information chores. It does this extraordinarily well, extending the desktop computer with which it synchronizes at the touch of a button.

Point of care computing. A necessary but insufficient condition for the improvement of health care is the ability to detect possible patient care problems, make changes in health care processes, monitor changes in practitioner behaviors, measure health outcomes, and link changes to outcomes with changes in processes. Until recently, process and outcome measurements have been blunt (e.g., duration of hospital stay, drug administration errors), supporting limited deductions about the effectiveness of quality-improvement strategies.

Point of care network devices now permit the capturing of information about health care processes during the course of everyday work. Vital signs become part of the medical record as soon as they are measured; order-entry systems record who requests what services, where and when; and patients can use handheld devices to answer surveys about their health status and health care experience.

The great challenge of the next decade is to harness all of this data, create meaningful linkages between databases, and form deductions that can be used to improve health care efficiency and effectiveness. Point of care computerized data entry devices can analyze data, detect inconsistencies, and prompt the user for additional information. Not only is legible, reliable, and validated information captured, but it also does not have to be reentered into the computer system from paper charts.

Multimedia

The sights and sounds of the health care environment are being digitized. As aging radiology equipment is replaced by digital imaging equipment, x-rays are made and stored as computer graphics files that are easily transferred from place to place. Electrocardiograms, electroencephalograms, ultrasounds, CT scans, MRI scans, pathology slides, photographs, and endoscopic images also are captured and stored in electronic format. Indeed, health care progress notes are digitally recorded at many institutions. Many diagnostic units now use voice-recognition software to package automated reports with digital images. Because these paper-less systems offer significant savings over conventional systems, they will become commonplace.

Modern computer workstations are becoming the eyes and ears of the health care environment. They can manipulate and display millions of colors on large display screens while rendering high-quality video and digital sound. They replace conventional character-based computer monitors and can also replace display devices for most diagnostic and therapeutic interventions. Indeed, the multimedia computer is attracting clinicians to a single, preferred source for data, information, and knowledge. By using these computer workstations, clinicians are able to visit virtual laboratories, imaging units, surgical suites, and libraries—all without leaving the point of care.

CONVERGENCE OF WORK, EDUCATION, AND EN-TERTAINMENT The health information milieu is converging with the education and entertainment milieus. Perhaps the most radical information shift of our time is the move from uni-directional mass media (television, movies, video recordings) to bidirectional mass media (Internet, interactive video, video conferencing) as the preferred method of information exchange. Engaging graphical interfaces present information in ways that resemble televisions more than books. With these changes, expertise from the entertainment and advertising industries is starting to influence the presentation and dissemination of health information. Institutions that tap into the vast powers of multimedia are more likely to reach and influence practitioners and their patients.

NATURAL COMPUTING INTERFACES The traditional health care information culture is oral. Surveys of practitioners show that they prefer having conversations with consultants and peers to finding information in books and computers. Given the hectic work pace of most hospitals, a fundamental barrier to computer use may be the need to sit down, focus, and communicate with a keyboard.

As computers evolve from multimedia output devices to multimedia input devices, they become more compatible with the predominantly oral culture of health care. Voice-recognition software has become usable, inexpensive, and more readily available. In the next few years multimedia computing will merge with tele-health and telemedicine, bringing the information preferences of clinicians into synchrony with the power of modern computer networks.

Information Convenience

Evidence-based informatics is helping to bridge the gap between demand and capacity for information management in two complementary ways: by expanding the range of information sources included in health information systems and by defining the information skills required to use those resources appropriately.

Information Sources

For optimal decision making, health care decision makers must attend to at least four major sources of information:

- Health care research about the effects of health interventions on patients and populations;
- Health services research about the direct and indirect costs of interventions and their effects on the health care system;
- Results of health assessments, laboratory tests, and other clinical measurements; and
- Each patient's unique risks, circumstances, preferences, and ability to comply with interventions.

The first two sources constitute external evidence, derived from the systematic study of defined patient and practitioner populations. Whereas clinical decision makers try to adapt external evidence to the circumstances of individuals at a specific place and time, clinical policy makers consider how the evidence applies to patient and practitioner groups within a particular population or region.

The second two information sources constitute internal evidence, derived from specific observations about the patients and practitioners for whom decisions are being made. Whereas decision makers attend to internal evidence about individuals, policy makers attend to aggregated evidence about the patterns of risk factors and disease in specific populations (see Table 4.2).

Information Systems

Health information systems may be grouped in four categories (see Table 4.3) corresponding to

TABLE 4.2 Health Care Information Sources

Information Source	Content	Comments
External evidence	Health care research	Results of experiments about the effects of health interventions on patients and populations.
	Health services research	Systematic evaluation of the effects of health interventions on health care processes and systems.
Internal evidence	Health practice observations	Individual or group observations from clinical investigations and measurements.
	Health subject observations	Patient-reported observations about health status preferences, and circumstances.

the four information sources described in the previous section:

- Knowledge-based systems that store, summarize, and interpret what is known about the effects of health interventions
- Administrative systems that capture information about health processes and facilitate such tasks as appointment scheduling, billing, and accounting
- Clinical systems that capture, organize, and display clinical observations (history and physical examination) and test results (laboratory reports, procedure notes, etc.)
- Consumer-centered systems that capture, analyze, interpret, and store patient-reported data about health status, preferences, and educational needs

The 1990s saw great advances in the power and sophistication of administrative and clinical health information systems. Consumer-based systems are just beginning to grow. More recently knowledge-based products have proliferated, with many traditional resources such as textbooks, drug information databases, and clinical policies being converted to electronic formats. Although the quantitative tools for amassing health information are impressive, they may cause confusion in practice unless they are linked to qualitative changes in the organization and presentation of information at the point of care.

Information Discrimination

Using each of the four health information sources calls for unique skills in

- *assessing* an initially disorganized information mix in order to recognize and detect important patient or policy problems;
- *asking* specific questions that are directly relevant to the patient or population of interest, suggest an appropriate source of information, and are specific enough to facilitate an efficient search for evidence;
- *acquiring* the most important and convincing evidence from an ever-expanding health literature, diverse clinical measurements, and ever more complex mixes of patient preferences and circumstances;
- *appraising* and synthesizing the best information to expose bias and variability; and
- *applying* useful, valid, and important evidence and monitoring health outcomes to see

TABLE 4.3 Health Information Systems

System Type	Purpose
Knowledge-based	Store, summarize, and interpret research about the effects of health interventions.
Administrative	Capture information about health care processes.
Clinical	Capture, organize, and display clinical observations and interventions.
Consumer-based	Capture, organize, and interpret patient-reported data.

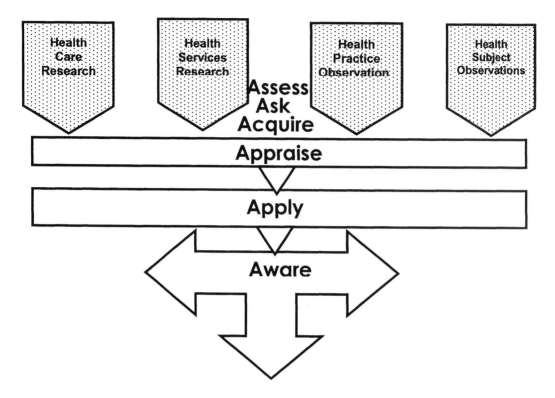

FIGURE 4.1 Clinical Information Tasks

whether the patient or population goals are achieved.

Figure 4.1 shows the five steps of the health information cycle: assess, ask, acquire, appraise, and apply. Evidence-based health information systems favor software and resources that facilitate appropriate use of each of these steps.

Information Integration

Administrative, clinical, consumer, and knowledge-management systems need not be mutually exclusive. Our present and future challenge is to build simple, sustainable, and affordable links between these categories of health information systems.

Integration of information systems can occur at a number of levels (see Figure 4.2):

- *Combined* systems unite one or more components under a common interface. A combined drug prescription system, for example, may include menus that allow the clinician to

search for dosing details or patient-advice handouts before generating prescriptions.
- *Clustered* systems use information about the provider to predetermine which information tools to present to the user. Presentation of a relevant drug database, for example, can be automated upon recognizing that a particular type of physician is logged onto the system.
- *Context*-sensitive systems are "aware" of the clinical context, allowing more efficient use of all context-compatible information systems that may be combined under a common interface. The context includes at least five elements: patient, practitioner, problem, procedure, and policy. A context-sensitive drug prescription support system, for example, would allow the user to view a laboratory result in one software application then immediately switch to a drug database where a search for drug dosing modifications can be made based on prior knowledge of the patient's age and primary medical problems.
- *Coupled* systems automatically link knowledge to observations, given a specific clinical event. A coupled drug prescription system,

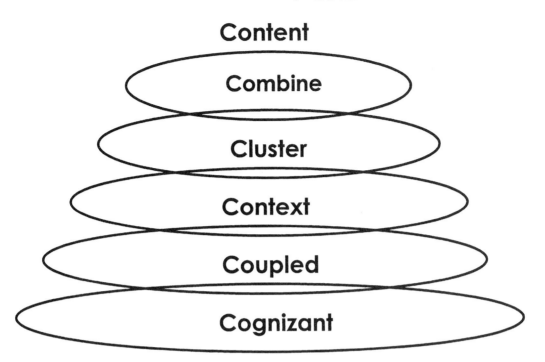

FIGURE 4.2 Health Information Integration (a)

for example, would alert the clinician to alternative, potentially cheaper interventions just before a prescription is generated.

- *Cognizant* systems would use artificial intelligence to respond to clinical events, detect patterns, and determine which knowledge resources are most appropriate for problem solving. No such systems exist today.

The most advanced clinical information environments present users with their own unique mix of software, communications tools, educational resources, and feedback. The user's information persona becomes part of a computing context that all software applications can access. Indeed, a new clinical context object workgroup (CCOW) standard specifies how multitasking computers can set a patient, practitioner, problem, and practice context known to all applications (see Figure 4.3).

Implications

Governments and institutions realize that large investments in infostructure are required. Indeed, investment in information communications technology is a health care expenditure that is expected to steadily increase per capita in the future. As hospitals begin to spend, they meet pent-up demand with relatively large system-wide hardware upgrades. Large investments in software systems follow. The biggest expenditures will be for integrated electronic medical records and the newest expenditures will be for knowledge-based software. Region-wide investment will emphasize interinstitution communication and data exchange at all levels.

In general, available hardware is overpowered for the available software. Current computer hardware poses no functional barriers to health infostructure development. Indeed, from a functional point of view, the rate-limiting factor is availability of useful, integrable computer software.

As software development tools become easier to use and standardized programming languages extend Internet-based information development, a new generation of clinician-informaticians will dilute the power and influence of computer engineers. New software will better reflect the

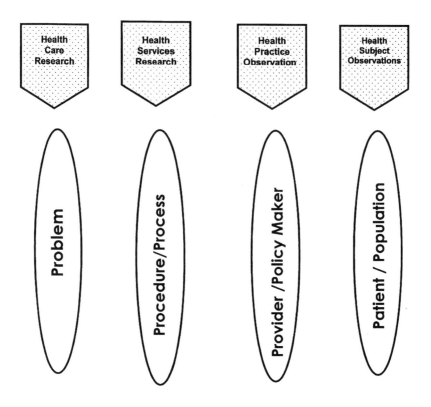

FIGURE 4.3 Health Information Integration (b)

needs of health practitioners while generating byproduct databases that meet the needs of health administrators. Change management and professional development initiatives should alert physicians to emerging specialization and re-treading options in health informatics.

Use of the Internet as a health information source is expanding at an exponential rate. The vision of using the Internet for dissemination, education, and communication is becoming a widespread reality, even among information technology neophytes. Every health care organization is spending money and effort to explore the way it can use the Internet. The unique features of Internet-based projects are their immediacy, ease of access, and interactive nature. Information organizations that want access to the health sector in the immediate future should focus their attention on Internet-based strategies for information and software dissemination. The Internet's power and potential to reach providers and patients, as well as to gather data on populations, will redefine the communication structures of health care and transform expectations

about the quantity and quality of evidence that can be gathered.

Information convenience is the first and most pressing need for busy practitioners. Even the provision of a simple drug information system and a general electronic textbook alongside clinical laboratory results would represent a leap forward in most learners' information access. Stakeholders should not wait for replete, stable information systems to appear or for electronic health records to be developed but should start soon with small, high-impact combinations of existing clinical and knowledge-based systems. These will generate comfort with and demand for more on-line information.

The great promise of health informatics could be marred by a number of nontechnical barriers:

• Overemphasis on technological protections of privacy hamper information access while failing to protect the interests of patients and populations.
• Lack of agreed standards for coding, classification, and communication of health risks,

clinical events, health outcomes, costs, and considerations of validity, importance, and applicability leaves users frustrated.

- Poor connections between regional, provincial, and national databases contribute to inefficient duplication of effort and lost opportunities for distilling intelligence from information.
- The medical profession has enjoyed a monopolistic control over its intellectual territory, demarcated by semantic (medical vocabulary and jargon) and intellectual (restricted distribution of medical knowledge) privileges. The Internet has broken down these barriers, giving full access to medical knowledge to the general public. However, naive database users are equally exposed to casual and reputable sources, without clear distinctions between the two.
- The Internet erodes traditional copyright, publishing, and intellectual property protections. Refined knowledge is in demand, but how can it be sold in ways that preserve both credibility and sustainability?

INFORMATION CULTURE

The organizational charts of most health care institutions feature sections for selecting, installing, maintaining, and enhancing computer systems and software. In the days of mainframe computers, information technology (IT) departments focused on the things of computing—wires and machines—and employed specialized technicians to care for a centralized infrastructure. IT infrastructure was determined by the types and capabilities of computers and the distribution of computing resources in a health care organization.

As personal computers proliferated, new computer users emerged with new demands for training and support. IT departments gave way to information services (IS) departments focused on the people of computing—diverse consumers doing diverse jobs—and employed a new cadre of information specialists to build infostructure throughout the health care institution.

Health care institutions' organizational charts increasingly feature sections for optimizing the flow of information through an organization. Information management (IM) departments treat information as a commodity, intellectual capital that can be acquired, channeled, and warehoused

to improve the efficiency and effectiveness of health care processes. A few leading-edge health institutions are beginning to shift and influence the information culture that determines how organizations build and deploy intellectual capital.

Health Intelligence

An informed information culture emerges from explicit processes that support the following four strata of interpretation (see Figure 4.4):

- *Data* constitutes the raw observations associated with health interventions (e.g., physical examination, laboratory tests, treatment results, etc.).
- *Information* exists when the significance of data is determined for a particular problem, patient, and practitioner (e.g., the physical examination is abnormal, laboratory test elevated, or treatment result successful).
- *Knowledge* is abstracted from information when external evidence is used to anticipate how additional interventions could change the data (e.g., surgery will cure the physical finding, a drug will normalize the laboratory test result and prevent disease).
- *Wisdom* is added to knowledge when internal data and external evidence are integrated with considerations of preference, values, and costs to determine whether and how the primary intervention should have been performed in the first place.

Key trends in information management relate to how internal health data is captured, information is codified, knowledge is coupled, and wisdom is generated.

Data

There is a push to move health data capture to occur as closely as possible to the data source. Instead of having clerical staff in hospital pharmacies enter medication orders to centralized databases, for example, physician and nurse order-entry systems increasingly are used to record information at the source. This reduces duplication. It also allows clinical decision support systems to analyze and influence the medication requests by, for example, automatically identifying drug interactions. By embedding data capture capabilities in tools commonly used during

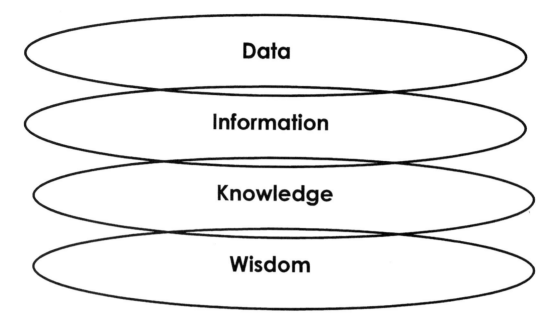

FIGURE 4.4 Information Culture

health care, it becomes possible to observe a much wider range of health care practices.

Data capture will become an integral, implicit part of day-to-day health care. As more and more health care tasks are computerized, information systems will measure and record more information about how health practitioners work. This information can then be analyzed and used to generate feedback that could change health practices.

Information

With the capture of more data about health care processes and outcomes, huge databases accrue. But the data is of little value unless it can be classified and shared between health information systems. Advances in codification of clinical observations, diagnoses, health interventions, and outcomes have, more than any other development, enabled the harvesting of internal evidence from health databases. Standardized vocabularies for describing signs and symptoms (e.g., SNOMED [Systematized Nomenclature of Medicine] index) allow better interpretation of

health observations, converting them to secondary databases of health information. International disease classifications allow the experiences of different health care environments to be compared. Protocols for communicating clinical information (e.g., Health Language 7 [HL-7]) allow different computers running different software to exchange information.

Sophisticated software has been produced to automate much of the yeoman's work of health care document indexing. However, these systems still fail for lack of proven methods for identifying patients, practitioners, and events. The simple act of recognizing a specific patient, provider, time, and place has proved surprisingly difficult; yet this is essential for dredging information from data. The development of regional health information systems has encouraged the creation of central patient registries and general person indexes. These will become increasingly influential for interdatabase communications.

Knowledge

When decision makers seek information about health problems, they need specific details about a health condition or intervention. In addition, they need to hone in on applicable (matching the patient, practitioner, and circumstances of interest), important (reporting something that patients would care about), and valid (satisfying predefined criteria for believing what is reported) information. Most existing knowledge resources are not organized in ways that support clinical decision making.

In general, existing coding and classification schemes emphasize questions of relevance over questions of usability. Some are optimized for describing clinical events, including diseases (e.g., ICD-9 [International Classification of Diseases]) and interventions (e.g., CPT [Current Procedural Terminology]), while others were developed for health knowledge. In order for knowledge-based software to be coupled with other information systems, there needs to be a middle layer of concepts that the clinical software can refer to when linking to the knowledge base.

By mastering the principles and techniques of concept mapping, software vendors will be able to maximize application of knowledge to health information databases.

Wisdom

The most difficult task in information management is to present data, information, and knowledge in ways that facilitate the accrual of wisdom about how to make the entire system perform better. Wisdom is not a derivative attribute; it is not something that can be deduced from observations. Experienced practitioners and policy makers observe growing databases for patterns and connections. This pattern recognition then leads to hypotheses about how data could be interpreted differently or knowledge could be alternately applied. To support the cognitive processes of wisdom generation, management information systems will be developed to help decision makers perceive patterns and trends in large data repositories.

Health Communication

The health care sector prefers oral communication to any other method of information exchange. Physicians, in particular, learn best when in conference with a trusted colleague or "opinion leader." Much of the excitement about the modern health information systems' poten-

tial relates to their emerging ability to combine interprofessional communication with on-line information convenience and filtering. To the extent that electronic mail, discussion forums, electronic knowledge bases, and health data can be seamlessly combined in a common "virtual bedside," there is a greater likelihood that information systems will become an integral part of the health care information culture.

Implications

Improved access to internal evidence will result from investments in more efficient health administration practices:

- Case costing systems will generate information about the frequency and outcomes of health interventions.
- Health claims databases will be linked to hospital, practitioner, and pharmacy databases, yielding new intelligence about health services utilization by health condition, health intervention, and health practitioners and patients.
- Automated patient data-collection devices will improve surveillance of individual health risks, health status, and preferences.

Improved access to external evidence will result from new regulatory requirements that health practitioners and institutions justify choices with best evidence about effectiveness:

- The accreditation of health institutions increasingly will require practitioner and policy maker access to best evidence.
- Access to health practice training programs will become contingent upon rapid access to clinical and research data in clinical teaching environments.

Practitioner interest and adoption of new health information systems will be enhanced by

- simultaneous attention to information communication, convenience, and integration needs in education and practice.
- emphasis on the communicative capabilities of computers and their ability to enhance interprofessional discourse and reflection on health data and knowledge.

Change management initiatives should embrace and extend the emerging information culture in health care by building virtual learning communities that use information technologies to extend learning and communication across time and space.

References

Advisory Council on Health Infostructure. (1999). *Paths to better health.* Ottawa: Health Canada Publications. Retrieved from http://www.hc-sc .gc.ca/ohih-bsi

Alberta wellnet. (2003). *Vendor conformance and usability requirements: Clinical decision support.* Edmonton: Alberta Health and Wellness.

Guyatt, G., & Rennie, D. (2002). *Users' guides to the medical literature: A manual for evidence-based clinical practice.* Chicago: American Medical Association Press.

Harris, J. M., Jr., Salasche, S. J., & Harris, R. B. (2001). The Internet and the globalisation of medical education. *British Medical Journal, 323*(7321), 1106.

Haynes, R. B., Hayward, R. S. A., & Lomas, J. (1995). Bridges between health care research evidence and clinical practice. *Journal of the American Medical Informatics Association, 2*(6), 342–350.

Lau, F., Doze, S., Vincent, D., Wilson, D., Noseworthy, T., Hayward, R. S., et al. (1999). Patterns of improvisation for evidence-based practice in clinical settings. *Information Technology and People, 12*(3), 287–303.

Leape, L. L., Woods, D. D., Hatlie, M. J., Kizer, K. W., Schroeder, S. A., & Lundberg, G. D. (1998). Promoting patient safety by preventing medical error. *Journal of the American Medical Association, 280,* 1444–1447.

National Forum on Health. (1998). *Creating a culture of evidence-based decision making in health.* Ottawa: Health Canada Publications. Retrieved from http://www.hc-sc.gc.ca/english/care/health _forum/forum_e.htm

5   TOWARD COMMON PERFORMANCE INDICATORS AND MEASURES FOR ACCOUNTABILITY IN BEHAVIORAL HEALTH CARE

Gregory B. Teague, Tom Trabin, & Charles Ray

In this chapter we describe an initiative that focuses broadly on organizations and systems of care. Other chapters in this volume focus on implementing specific evidence-based practice models or on developing or using measures to inform clinical practice, together offering practitioners an inviting array of diverse alternatives oriented to the clinical needs of particular groups of clients. Here, in contrast, is a plan to bridge this diversity of measurement by formulating common performance indicators and measures and promoting their widespread use across a wide array of service settings. The Adult Mental Health Workgroup (AMHW) of the Forum on Performance Measures in Behavioral Health and Related Service Systems (Forum) is a nationally representative group that has formulated and now proposes broad adoption of a few organizational performance measures for accountability and quality management in behavioral health care. The measures were carefully selected to reflect key aspects of care—access, quality/appropriateness, and outcomes—in essentially all settings providing mental health services to adults. Although the focus of the AMHW and consequently of this chapter is adult mental health services, the AMHW is working in conjunction with other Forum workgroups with corresponding initiatives in performance measurement for prevention and treatment of mental health and substance use disorders for all age groups.

THE NEED FOR COMMON PERFORMANCE MEASUREMENT

Underlying the movement toward common measurement are two compelling motivations: efficiency and quality. First, the proliferation of reporting requirements compromises efficient delivery of services. Numerous performance measurement systems were developed during the 1990s as services were increasingly provided through large systems or health plans and as computer technology made routine reporting increasingly feasible.[1] In general, these systems were intended to serve as mechanisms for both accountability and quality improvement at organizational and systems levels, as distinct from outcomes management or practice-based research at the client level, but any one system might include data that could serve multiple purposes. However, providers have typically been required to report via several systems as a condition of reimbursement. The duplication imposed by redundant but largely incompatible systems came to impose a significant resource burden on the service delivery system; in response, several initiatives were put forward in hopes of consolidation.[2] These efforts advanced the debate regarding consolidation of redundant reporting requirements and laid some of the groundwork for common measurement but thus far have yielded no tangible impact.

A second and more crucial motivation for common measurement is to help elevate the role of service quality in decisions about resource allocation and to make the overall system more accountable for delivering high-quality services. As in general health care, cost rather than quality often dominates behavioral health care re-source decisions, in part because the field lacks consensus on how to demonstrate the overall quality of care, including the attainment of desirable outcomes (Manderscheid, 1998). To be sure, quality is much more difficult to define and demonstrate than cost; ironically, one impediment to promoting quality is the great diversity in measurement systems intended for quality management. While there are significant areas of agreement and overlap in indicators, the lack of common measures means that behavioral health organizations and systems of care cannot be effectively compared, and the resulting fragmentation limits the capacity of the field as a whole to speak with clarity and authority on the issue of quality. In the absence of generally accepted evidence of quality, it is difficult to counter effectively the proposition that cheaper is better, and the result is a continuing drain of resources from behavioral health care (Lutterman & Hogan, 2000). Consistent use of even a small set of common indicators and measures across large segments of the field would help to establish the credibility of claims about quality of care and in so doing would place behavioral health in a more equitable position in debates about the allocation of health care and other societal resources. Perhaps more important, comparable data derived from common measures would extend the utility of benchmarking for quality improvement and decision support.

KEY CONCEPTS OF A COMMON MEASUREMENT INITIATIVE

Indicators and Measures

In discussing performance measurement it is important to maintain the distinction between indicators and measures. An *indicator* is a quantitative specification, typically expressed as a ratio (e.g., percentage) of a selected aspect of performance. A *measure*—consistent with the use of this term in research—represents the methodology for deriving and calculating quantitative results used in an indicator. For any one indicator, there may be many alternative sets of specifications for source data and calculations, each producing its own set of results. Some earlier plans for shared indicator sets stopped short of recommending common measures, leaving to implementers the detailed decisions about how performance would actually be measured

(American College of Mental Health Administration [ACMHA], 1998). Although this approach would present potential users with minimal requirements for adaptation and thus more easily lead to consensus and wide participation in a common framework, the inevitable variation in instrumentation across settings or populations would make comparisons between groups less precise and therefore largely speculative. Performance measurement systems using unique measures are inevitably local systems, and the AMHW has taken up the necessary if challenging pursuit of commonality of measures.

Inclusion, Not Replacement

The proposed common indicators and measures are intended to complement rather than replace current measurement systems. The plan calls for use of a small number of carefully selected performance indicators and corresponding measures across essentially all settings providing mental health services to adults. For those indicators measured through consumer self-report surveys, the proposal is to include certain specific items within all relevant performance measurement systems rather than to use a single uniform consumer survey instrument. Performance measurement systems reflecting the core needs of specific types of organizations, health care plans, consumer populations, or treatment of specific disorders are vital and should remain in use.

Distinction Between Common and Core

A key distinction for the AMHW's initiative on common performance indicators and measures is the difference between the concepts of *core* and *common*. An organization or group that pays significant attention to performance in service settings could have key or core indicators—that is, indicators representing areas of performance that are central to its mission or fundamental concerns. Because of differences in mission, population, and so on, views of the relative importance of particular areas of substantive performance typically differ across groups. For example, some advocates for adult consumers with serious mental illness focus intensively on reducing use of seclusion and restraint; some advocates for adults with co-occurring disorders focus on integration of care; and some advocates for children focus on increasing family involvement in treatment planning. Each of these

groups sees the core issues for the other groups as being relevant but for various reasons not quite as important as their own, and their respective choices of core performance indicators would differ.

Nonetheless, it is also clear that some interests and concerns are important to virtually everyone and are thus held in common, even if these concerns are only a small subset for any one group. For example, whatever else may be a core issue for any group, it is critical that the population of interest be able to gain access to needed care. Access is thus a domain within which one or more common indicators can be defined. Similarly, there are widely shared concerns within the other domains of quality/appropriateness and outcome. Indicators are defined as common if they are both feasible to measure and shared as indicators across a wide range of stakeholder groups. This focus on a number of common indicators is not intended to suggest that core indicators and measures for specific segments of the field have less value or importance in context. In any given setting, core indicators may have more consequence for improving specific aspects of treatment, but common measures offer the capacity to link findings about practice across settings and impact quality of care more widely.

IDENTIFYING AND OVERCOMING PROBLEMS AND OBSTACLES TO COMMON MEASUREMENT

In the face of an ambitious initiative such as widespread adoption of new measurement practices there are inevitably numerous potential objections and impediments. Although most of them represent real challenges, they are also largely surmountable, depending on environmental incentives and other factors.

Measurement Concerns

The general resistance to quantitative measurement of mental health practices in field settings has—at least overtly—diminished, the publication of this volume being a case in point. However, important methodological and substantive concerns remain and can contribute to resistance if they are not satisfactorily answered.

Concerns about psychometric quality are always in order. The methodological work done in developing the measures proposed here is reassuring in that it grounds the proposed survey items in the most thorough empirical investigation on this topic to date (Eisen et al., 1999; Shaul et al., 2001). However, proponents of item response theory (IRT) would argue that the work done on these measures, like the majority of current mental health measures based on classical test theory (CTT), have inherent limitations that can be ameliorated by exploiting the strengths of more theoretically sophisticated methods (Embretson, 1996). In particular, the interest in embedding a small set of specific items in a wide range of surveys could be significantly supported by having the kind of item-specific and population-independent information that IRT methods generate. Future Forum-sponsored work on surveys may incorporate use of these methods.

Some stakeholders may have concerns about content or perspective. One concern might focus on the scope of measurement. The proposed common measures capture only a few key constructs of care; because they do not constitute a comprehensive measurement model, they would by themselves provide only a partial view of the services and experiences they measure and would therefore ideally be used in conjunction with other measures oriented to quality improvement. At a deeper level there remains considerable variance of opinion among professionals about the value of information obtained from consumers in evaluating practice. Historically, attitudes within the professional community have tended to devalue the views of patients in contrast to professional judgment, and this outlook may weigh against a positive view of the proposed common measures based on consumer surveys. To counter this concern those who encourage use of the proposed common measures in the field will need to convey information about the emerging understanding of the recovery process and the importance of the consumer perspective (Campbell, 1997; Burt, Duke, & Hargreaves, 1998).

Strategic Risk

The proposed indicators and measures are designed to serve both accountability and quality improvement purposes. Few individuals or organizations voluntarily offer themselves up for external accountability, and the mere possession

of standardized data that could be used in this way might seem to present risks to those whose services are measured, even if no current plans or mechanisms exist for such use. Such perceived risks could reinforce resistance to adopting common measures, even for exclusively internal use; the earlier industry-wide resistance to the proposal from the Joint Commission on Accreditation of Healthcare Organizations (JCAHO) for such data requirements illustrates this sensitivity. Widespread adoption of common measures will require assurances in the form of clearly defined protocols to ensure proper confidentiality for organizations, reliable and valid data, and appropriate analysis and reporting of comparisons. These and other assurances will also have to be coupled with the acceptance of the common measures by a few regulatory or accrediting bodies that have the authority to override local risk aversion in the service of a more general interest in concerted quality improvement.

Prior Commitments

The process of undertaking a common project would be much simpler if all participants were starting from scratch. To the contrary, most behavioral health organizations and provider groups have already committed themselves to measurement frameworks, determined their measurement priorities, and invested in measurement systems that are or appear partially inconsistent with participation in a common effort. To that extent, any effort such as the one presented in this chapter faces the same kinds of challenges that have become so vividly apparent in efforts to disseminate evidence-based practices (Drake et al., 2001). The Forum's outreach model, discussed later in this chapter, reflects awareness of both the forces underlying reluctance to change and the dynamics through which change can occur (Rogers, 1995).

Financial commitments are typically identified as primary obstacles. The cost of implementing even minor conversions of information systems that are used on a large scale can be daunting. Depending on the amount of methodological rigor desired, the cost of new data collection—for example, via surveys—could discourage participation. With appropriate incentives, however, the reinvestment could seem worthwhile. As in the case of overcoming risk aversion, widespread adoption of common measurement will likely require endorsement by those organizations whose reporting requirements serve as conditions for access to the material and regulatory benefits their members seek.

An important resource that will significantly defray the cost of revising prior measurement commitments for many organizations is Decision Support 2000+ (DS2K+), a national decision support service for both clinical and management decision making that is being developed through support by the Center for Mental Health Services at the U.S. Substance Abuse and Mental Health Services Administration (SAMHSA). Policy makers, data experts, clinicians, consumers, organizational leaders, and software vendors are collaborating to identify data standards and develop a Web-based plug-in system designed to receive and analyze data against appropriate benchmarks and report back comparative results to the requesting organization. Different types of information for decision support will also be available to individual clinicians and consumers. Measures resulting from the work described in this chapter will be included as available components within DS2K+, making implementation of common measures significantly more useful and affordable for organizations using this system.

Collective Action in a Market Environment

In the context of the U.S. health care market environment, collective action is difficult to orchestrate. At one level, the obstacles to common measurement invoke the classic problem of the common: what seems good for the individual (minimizing risk and expense and maximizing market advantage) may not lead to good for the group (optimizing opportunity for collective quality improvement). Since the proposed common indicators and measures do not typically include the core concerns for specific groups, the gain from using them at the individual level is modest, and thus the intrinsic incentive to adopt them is also modest. As indicated, what will be required is that key opinion leaders and organizations in a position to redefine incentives and reframe perceptions of interest endorse both the underlying assumptions and an initial starting point for common measurement. In this regard, it may be important to bear in mind the general tractability of overt objections. What can be perceived or presented at one point as insurmountable obstacles can be transformed by alternative incentives into readily manageable challenges. The AMHW suggests that the potential benefits of common measurement justify attempting such a transformation.

THE FORUM ON PERFORMANCE MEASURES: HISTORY AND PURPOSE

The AMHW's initiative for common measurement in adult mental health care is presented under the auspices of the Forum on Performance Measures in Behavioral Health and Related Service Systems (Forum). The Forum was established in response to the consensus recommendation of a large group of leaders in the field who attended the Consensus Forum on Mental Health and Substance Use Performance Measures in March 2001 at the Carter Center in Atlanta, Georgia. Sponsored by SAMHSA and growing out of the planning efforts of several groups,[3] the meeting included representatives and stakeholders from the full range of the behavioral health field. The meeting's purpose was to assess the progress made to date on the development and implementation of performance measures in health care and related service systems. It highlighted the considerable efforts made to date by a variety of public and private groups in the development of empirical measures of access, quality/appropriateness, and outcomes of care and also made explicit the tremendous overlap in both content and process that has guided these efforts to date. The meeting concluded with a consensus recommendation that the forum be formally constituted to provide ongoing support, enhancement, and coordination of performance measurement efforts in behavioral health. The three SAMHSA centers agreed to collaborate on furthering this initiative and funding its activities. The resulting Forum articulated a mission with suitable scope and focus:

The mission of the Forum is to improve the delivery of behavioral health treatment and prevention services by supporting the development and adoption of broadly applicable indicators and measures to assess organizational performance and consumer outcomes. These indicators and measures should be designed to serve the needs of both external accountability as well as internal quality improvement. The Forum will provide an ongoing venue for collaboration, coordination, and communication between the various initiatives, both public and private, which are already working separately to measure service access and delivery, quality, and outcomes. The Forum will foster the sharing of information and experiences of provider, government, employer, consumer, and accreditation groups in implementing performance and outcome measurement practices and initiatives. (AMHW, 2003)

Although the Forum's initial vision had allowed for articulation of comprehensively common indicators and measures spanning all age groups and behavioral health treatments, substantive differences in priorities and practices for major subpopulations led to a decision to pursue the Forum's goals initially through five workgroups. They are oriented respectively to adult mental health treatment, adult substance abuse treatment, child and adolescent mental health treatment, child and adolescent substance abuse treatment, and substance abuse prevention. All of the workgroups are articulating indicators and measures within a commonly agreed-upon framework, described later in this chapter. They are finding considerable agreement on the indicators they have formulated, but they differ at the level of measure specifications because of the concerns of the different subpopulations and settings they seek to address.

Each of the five workgroups has adapted its activities to the specific challenges of its focal area. With support from SAMHSA's Center for Mental Health Services, the AMHW has refined a specific set of recommended indicators and measures for adult mental health. On behalf of the Forum this group has also developed a broad outreach strategy for reengaging key groups and individuals in the field to encourage implementation. These products will be described in detail in the remainder of this chapter. The Adult Substance Abuse Workgroup is continuing the agenda laid out by the Washington Circle Group (McCorry, Garnick, Bartlett, Cotter, & Chalk, 2000) and supported by SAMHSA's Center for Substance Abuse Treatment. The long-term goal is refinement and promulgation of a set of indicators and measures for the four domains of alcohol and other drug services representing prevention/education, recognition, treatment, and maintenance; the initial focus is on indicators of identification, treatment initiation, and treatment engagement (Garnick et al., 2002). The Child and Adolescent Mental Health Workgroup

is functioning as a corollary effort of the Outcomes Roundtable for Children and Families (1998), supported by SAMHSA's Center for Mental Health Services. They have facilitated movement to consensus on measurement priorities by the diverse set of stakeholders in this field and are currently testing the applicability of the identification, treatment initiation, and treatment engagement measures to child and adolescent mental health services. Similarly, the Child and Adolescent Substance Abuse Treatment Workgroup is working in concert with the Adult Substance Abuse Workgroup to customize measure specifications for applying these indicators to child and adolescent substance abuse treatment services. The Substance Abuse Prevention Workgroup is adapting indicators excerpted from the Core Measures Initiative sponsored by SAMHSA's Center for Substance Abuse Prevention and is supported by that Center. Supporting and linking these five substantive groups within the Forum are a coordinating committee and an executive committee, as well as several task forces that help to integrate and further refine workgroup products to ensure consistency of proposed terminology and credibility of proposed measurement methods.

In addition to these components, a new, crosscutting Forum workgroup is being formed: the Modular Consumer Survey Workgroup (MCSW). This workgroup will use the products of the AMHW along with input from the Forum workgroups and other experts to articulate preliminary specifications for modular sets of consumer survey items. The concepts underlying this effort are discussed in more detail later in the chapter. Many of the products of the MCSW will be incorporated into the next version of the SAMHSA-sponsored Mental Health Statistics Improvement Program (MHSIP) Consumer Survey, which will be modular in design rather than being a single survey instrument. The close relationship between MHSIP and the Performance Partnership Grants, the primary federal funding mechanism for state behavioral health programs, provides an additional avenue for broad implementation of these proposed common measures. The importance of these linkages is reflected in the fact that both the MCSW and MHSIP are represented on the Forum's executive committee.

SELECTING PERFORMANCE MEASURES

The processes used by the Forum workgroups for identifying common indicators and measures included substantial input from consumers, providers, payers, and purchasers of behavioral health care services. Workgroup members representing these key stakeholder groups carefully reviewed the work of previous groups addressing similar tasks (ACMHA, 1998; 2001 Center for Mental Health Services [CMHS], 1996; Teague et al., 1997; National Association of State Mental Health Program Directors [NASMHPD], 1998). Selection of indicators focused on fundamental concerns within a common framework and was informed by a set of underlying core values and technical criteria.

Fundamental Concerns Within a Common Framework

As components of the Forum, all of the workgroups are working to articulate indicators and measures for their specific combinations of population and service sector within a two-dimensional common framework. One dimension of this framework covers the domains, or content areas, of common performance measurement: access, quality/appropriateness, and outcome. These three domains together reflect a fundamental set of underlying values, critical questions, and expectations about performance:

• Are people in need able to get services?
• Are the services that people receive the ones they need and are these services being provided the way they should be?
• Are services effective in producing the results that people need and in maintaining or improving the mental status of the population?

The second dimension in the common framework is the data source. Data to support identified indicators should come from both administrative databases and primary sources of consumer perceptions and self-report. The potential to use administrative data continues to increase as computing hardware and software expand coverage and enhance technical capability. Large-scale systems relying on such data have been in use for several years, albeit using different reporting systems and under different authorities;[4] the technical challenges here are principally in standardization and integration. There is also increasingly widespread acceptance of the need to consider the consumer perspective as a fundamental component in evaluating the effectiveness of behavioral health care services. Recognition of the central role of consumers' perceptions and choices in treatment is reflected in the surgeon general's report on mental health (U.S. Department of Health and Human Services, 1999), the Institute of Medicine's (IOM) report on the "quality chasm" in health care (IOM, 2001), and in discussions about the interpersonal context of evidence-based practice (Drake et al., in press). Reliable methods to gather primary data from consumers are increasingly available; over the past decade many studies have defined and collected this kind of information, resulting in a number of separate but sound measures of consumer perceptions of important aspects of care across populations, organizational settings, and plans (Teague, 2000).

Technical Criteria

Each indicator proposed by the AMHW met three general criteria, which were derived from or consistent with criteria used in performance measurement efforts by other national organizations and policy groups:

• *Meaningfulness*: Does the proposed indicator address a dimension that relates to a critical aspect of care, has value for consumers and other stakeholders in services, and can differentiate among persons or organizations or over time?
• *Measurability*: Can reliable, accurate, and valid information be obtained to support the proposed indicator?
• *Feasibility*: Can the proposed indicators be used at a reasonable cost using data currently available or readily obtainable?

An additional requirement for any common indicator is that it should have *relevance* across diverse consumer populations as well as across differing types of provider and managed care organizations. Finally, fundamental to any performance indicator is the criterion of *actionability*: Does the indicator measure a construct that is susceptible to identifiable corrective action?

Setting Measurement Priorities

The work of selecting indicators and measures was carried out in several phases. Because common measures will impose at least a modest burden on users, parsimony has been of high value throughout. This is particularly the case for the consumer survey, where a large number of survey items would discourage its adoption. At each point, parsimony was challenged by the value of ensuring adequate coverage of important aspects of care; the AMHW's recommendation of 21 items demonstrates a balance between these two values. Nonetheless, anticipating that the MCSW and other organizations may find 21 items too many to adopt, the AMHW has taken the additional step of identifying the most critical content within each indicator, distinguishing between 12 higher-priority and 9 lower priority items. Further details about the items and their respective priority levels are provided in the measure overview later in the chapter as well as in the appendix.

Collaboration Among Forum Workgroups

Initially much of the Forum's work was carried out separately by the workgroups. Nevertheless, the Forum retained its underlying commitment to identify more broadly based common indicators that might be applicable across the different population settings addressed by each of the workgroups. Consequently, the workgroups sought successfully to identify commonalities between their proposed indicators, even though specifications at the measurement level had to be customized for differing treatment contexts or populations. Instances of this form of commonality were identified for both administrative data–based and consumer survey–based indicators.

The exploratory work on measures for identification, initiation, and engagement in treatment represents a prominent example of the effort to find commonality, in this case using administrative data–based indicators. These measures were initially defined and tested for adult substance abuse treatment. Slight modifications have been made to the original measures to adapt them to the requirements for adult mental health and child/adolescent treatment populations, and they are currently being tested in a variety of administrative datasets.

The pending modular measure development represents another important integrative initiative within the Forum, in this case focusing on consumer survey–based data. Some of the modules will have items measuring content shared across multiple behavioral health care sectors. Even before the MCSW has begun its work, the executive committee has identified at least four of the AMHW consumer survey–based indicators as having this wider commonality—three across all treatment populations and one across both treatment and prevention. These designations are noted in the appendix.

OVERVIEW OF THE AMHW'S PROPOSED INDICATORS AND MEASURES

Common Indicators

A table showing recommended indicators and sample items by domain and data source is located in the appendix to this chapter; the following is a brief overview of content. The first indicators we discuss here are based on measures that have already been tested and validated in the field. In the access domain, an indicator of "timeliness of access to treatment services" is generated by data from consumer survey item responses and indicators of "service use" and "treatment duration" are generated via administrative data. In the quality/appropriateness domain consumer survey data support four indicators: "quality of interaction with counselors and clinicians," "information provided by counselors and clinicians," "perceived overall quality of treatment services," and "perceived cultural sensitivity of treatment services." Another quality/appropriateness indicator is generated from administrative data: "follow-up after hospitalization." In the outcome domain, a single indicator of "perceived improvement" is derived from consumer survey data. In the prioritization of indicators derived from the consumer survey, the outcome indicators were top ranked, followed by the access indicator; the quality/appropriateness indicators were somewhat lower ranked. Each indicator had some high-priority item content, so no indicators were considered to have low priority.

The following indicators are currently under evaluation. Given strong individual and societal interests in employment, there is a consumer survey indicator of "work functioning improvement." There are also three indicators using administrative data corresponding to the common indicators proposed for substance abuse treatment, identification, initial engagement in "treatment," and "continuing engagement in treatment."

Common Measures

The workgroup recognized that only parsimonious scales or other measures tapping general dimensions would be acceptable for widespread implementation, so it relied heavily on material developed and validated in multiple service settings and sectors.

Consumer Survey–Based Measures

A number of proposed survey items are taken from the Experience of Care and Health Outcomes (ECHO) survey (Eisen et al., 1999), which was designed to integrate the best aspects of two national consumer survey measures for evaluating behavioral health care from the perspective of consumers, oriented respectively to private and public sectors. Members of the workgroup participated with developers of the two original surveys in development and extensive testing to optimize the fit between ECHO items and the recommended indicators. Selection of specific items was based on research findings of main item groupings, or factors, from the survey instrument (Shaul et al., 2001) as well as on the preliminary list of target concerns that the precursor to the AMHW had generated prior to the first Carter Center Forum. Next, we briefly describe item content for each survey-generated indicator, with higher and lower priorities indicated.

For the access indicator, the high-priority item asks about timeliness of urgent care; lower-priority items ask about timeliness of regular appointments and availability of help by telephone. For the quality of interaction indicator, higher priority items are used to assess whether practitioners listen carefully and explain things understandably and whether consumers have been sufficiently involved in their treatment; lower priority items ask whether practitioners demonstrate respect for what the consumer says and spend enough time with the consumer and whether consumers feel safe with them. For the information indicator, higher priority questions

ask whether practitioners have provided information about medication side effects, treatment options, and illness self-management; lower-priority items ask whether information has been provided about self-help groups and patient rights. The perceived overall quality of treatment indicator is calculated using a single global rating item. The cultural sensitivity indicator is also calculated from a single item, in this case preceded by a screener question designed to elicit responses only from consumers who deem the issue important. The perceived improvement scale asks for comparison of consumers' current status with their earlier status in four areas: higher priority items tap level of problems and symptoms and ability to deal with daily problems; lower priority items tap respondents' ability to accomplish things they want to do and ability to deal with social situations. The primary question for the work functioning improvement indicator addressing ability to perform paid work is structurally identical to the perceived improvement items and is likely to be included in the latter scale in future analyses.

Administrative Data–Based Measures

The measures based on administrative data are a combination of established and developing measures. The measures of "persons with mental health problems using services" (equivalent to measures of penetration), treatment duration, and time until follow-up after hospitalization are already standard in the field and seeing extensive use. They are consistent with definitions and data in one or more of such influential measurement reporting sets as the National Committee for Quality Assurance's (NCQA) Health Employer Data Information Set (HEDIS) (Druss, Miller, Rosenheck, Shih, & Bost, 2002), those advanced by the National Association of State Mental Health Program Directors (NASMHPD, 1998), and the federal Center for Mental Health Services' (CMHS) Uniform Reporting System (URS).

The three additional measures of identification, initial engagement, and continuing engagement are still in development and testing. These are adaptations of the treatment phase–specific measures put forward by the Washington Circle Group for adult substance abuse treatment in managed care settings (Garnick et al., 2002). They address respectively the rate at which persons having specific conditions of interest are newly identified in claims data; the rate at which these persons receive a subsequent service promptly, indicating that they have been initially engaged in treatment; and the rate at which they receive two additional services in due course, indicating that treatment has continued. Although these concerns have not had the same relative prominence in the mental health field as some of the concerns highlighted in the AMHW indicators of quality/appropriateness and outcome, the importance of access and continuity, particularly for persons with serious mental illness, in combination with historically low performance for this population in both of these areas, warrants widespread application of these measures.

Methods

Use of rigorous, standardized methods for data collection are recommended but not necessarily required of all who might use the measures. The workgroup makes the assumption that there are trade-offs between coverage and rigor: if measures are to be widely used, there will inevitably be great variance in capacity and will to commit resources to data collection. For both consumer survey and administrative data, users may opt to conform to existing standards for collection and analysis, and data voluntarily provided in this way can be used in developing norms. Alternatively, users may opt to use the measures in less standardized but nonetheless internally useful ways.

PLANNED NEXT STEPS

The Forum increasingly has come to realize its role as an ongoing manager and coordinator of key efforts to develop common measures. Its placement and membership enable it, both directly and through its components, for example, the AMHW, to facilitate crucial linkages and to speed up development and implementation of common measures. The project of expanding and evaluating the Washington Circle Group measures of identification, initiation, and engagement in other populations is a case in point. Three important tasks are forthcoming: developing modular measures that build on the AMHW's proposed consumer survey–based measures, thereby extending common measurement across other behavioral health care sectors;

convening representatives of selected national organizations to share information about the Forum's progress and map out specific implementation steps; and conducting additional outreach to the field as an initial step toward implementation. Following are brief descriptions of these three tasks.

Modular Survey

When the Forum was first established, the challenge of articulating common ground across the full range of behavioral health care seemed premature, and the separate workgroups were formed to make initial progress on a more manageable scale. At this point, attention has returned to the task of integrating separate areas through the creation of a new workgroup, the MCSW, charged with the responsibility of developing a modular survey approach. The vision is that it will be possible to achieve a balance between the unifying vision of common measurement and the substantial variation in populations and treatment concerns represented within the Forum. For this purpose the context is the four primary treatment populations defined respectively by the intersections of two age categories, adult and child/adolescent, and two behavioral disorder categories, mental health and substance use. The premise is that critical performance measurement content has some overlap, however small, across adjacent pairs of these groups as well as across all four groups. The goal is to identify measurement modules that will be used in a unique combination for each of the primary populations. Thus, for example, the total common measurement set for adult mental health would include the content of three separate modules: items unique to adult mental health, items shared with adult substance abuse but not used elsewhere, and items used with all populations.

At this stage, the agenda for the MCSW can be outlined only generally. Products and priorities of the current Forum workgroups will serve as critical input. Critical constructs for each treatment population and corresponding items will be identified and if necessary revised over time to optimize the balance among individual modules. As noted, it is already apparent that several AMHW indicators are relevant outside of adult mental health, but it is not yet clear which of the proposed AMHW measures will be applicable to which of the four modules relevant to adult mental health because overlap with other populations at the level of items has not yet been determined. The goal of developing modular measures will entail achieving a significant degree of measurement utility and efficiency, so it is anticipated that use of methods derived from IRT may be helpful in this work.

Outreach

On behalf of the Forum, the AMHW has identified critical elements in a strategy for taking tested and refined common performance indicators and measures back to the field that, through its representatives at the initial consensus meeting, had provided encouragement to undertake the effort. This important step entails disseminating the Forum's work to major constituencies in behavioral health care, inviting feedback, engaging in dialogue, and obtaining endorsement. National organizations to be contacted are of five types: research and policy organizations that influence opinions and that have some interest in using the data derivable from widespread use of the indicators and measures; consumer advocacy groups; professional associations representing individual clinicians; trade associations representing provider and managed care organizations that are likely to be required to collect, analyze, and report on data from these measures; and public and private purchasers of behavioral health care benefits and accrediting organizations that are in positions to require implementation of these measures.

In view of the considerable effort required both to revise the data infrastructure and to reorient behavior, communications in this outreach process will need to do the following:

- Present a compelling argument for the value of this endeavor and the advantages to organizations of implementing the recommended common measures.
- Provide reassurance to people and organizations that the proposed common measurements are intended to supplement, not supplant, their own unique organizational measurement needs and possible proprietary measurement interests.
- Describe the highly inclusive, multiconstituent consensus process by which proposed common indicators and measures were identified, thus helping to establish the credibility and momentum of the enterprise.

- Portray the current common set in the context of a multiphase, incremental, and continuously improving initiative spanning several years, rather than as completed work. Such a perspective invites participation in the larger, ongoing initiative and helps to allay fears of pressure to employ measures beyond their useful life.
- Assess each organization's readiness and willingness to play a role in supporting their own and others' implementation of the measures. Indicators and measures will adapt and become more refined over time, and ongoing feedback will be needed, but there must be general commitment to going forward with an initial set to get the work started.
- Convey a final point about the level of resources behind this initiative that may be critical to persuasion: SAMHSA is committing ongoing support and intends to encourage the field's use of data derived from widespread adoption of common measures for benchmarking and decision support, for example, through such mechanisms as DS2K+.

Consensus Forum

As initial impetus to this distributed outreach dialogue, the second national Consensus Forum on Mental Health and Substance Abuse Performance Measures will be convened. The meeting itself will serve as an important part of the outreach effort, providing representatives of important stakeholders a setting for collective engagement with the now mature Forum to understand the benefits and opportunities of common measurement. While representatives from all of the types of aforementioned stakeholder groups will be invited, there will be a particular emphasis on inviting those organizations that are in positions either to directly require or implement the common measures. Specific products from Forum workgroups will be featured, including work in progress on modular consumer survey measures and the family of identification, initiation, and engagement measures that have been customized for use with specific populations. Conversely, the meeting will also provide Forum representatives the opportunity to refresh their familiarity with the diversity of contexts to which common measures must be adequately adapted and with the related needs of those who will ultimately carry out common measurement.

CONCLUSION

In this chapter we have outlined the rationale, plan, and substance of a proposal to establish a small number of common indicators and measures of key aspects of performance in adult mental health care. This initiative is part of a larger plan for implementation of common performance measurement throughout behavioral health care for the purpose of improving quality and accountability. The plan calls for incorporation of selected indicators and measures within existing systems rather than replacement of current efforts. Indicators and measures have been selected on the basis of broad applicability to services and populations, technical merit, empirical validation, and capacity to reflect the shared values and concerns of a wide range of stakeholders. It is anticipated that widespread implementation of common measures and indicators would yield several benefits, including

- generating compatible performance measurement efforts across all organizations to facilitate appropriate comparisons for accountability to consumers and purchasers;
- providing more informed decision support for consumers and purchasers selecting treatment and/or health plans;

- facilitating collaboration for benchmarking and quality improvement purposes;
- providing guidance on critically important dimensions of performance to those behavioral health care organizations that are in early stages of measuring performance; and
- reducing redundancy in requirements for performance data by accreditation, regulatory, and purchaser organizations, thereby increasing efficiency and reducing costs.

It is premature at this stage to gauge the degree of success of this effort. Additional refinement and actual implementation still lie ahead. Although the proposal is for modest change in any one setting, the industry-wide impact is potentially substantial, and large systems are difficult to move in concert. However, the Forum and its workgroups represent leadership at the intersection of several crucial spheres: public and private, mental health and substance abuse, and treatment and prevention across the life span. There is therefore reason for optimism, at least about significant progress; even if common measures are less widely implemented than envisioned here, the scope of engagement already visible will surely provide a basis for broader consensus at a later stage.

APPENDIX

Common Indicators, Measures, and Data Sources

Domain Data	Indicator	Abbreviated Description or Items
Access		
Consumer survey	Timeliness of access to treatment services[1]	*In the last [ ] months,* when you needed to get counseling or treatment **right away**, how often did you see someone **as soon as you wanted?**[2]
		In the last [ ] months, how often did you get an **appointment** for counseling or treatment **as soon as you wanted?**
		In the last [ ] months, how often did you **get the professional help or advice** you needed **over the phone?**
Admin. database	Identification[1]	Percent of persons in enrolled/eligible population with major depression, schizophrenia, schizoaffective disorder, or bipolar disorder who have had at least one mental health service during the year.

(continued)

Common Indicators, Measures, and Data Sources (*continued*)

Domain Data	Indicator	Abbreviated Description or Items
Admin. database	Persons with mental health problems using services	Percent of persons in enrolled/eligible population with at least one mental health service, broken out by defined categories of age, gender, race/ethnicity, diagnosis, and level of care.

Quality Appropriateness

Consumer survey	Quality of interaction with counselors and clinicians	*In the last [ ] months,* how often did the people you went to for counseling or treatment **listen carefully to you?**[2]
		In the last [ ] months, how often did the people you went to for counseling or treatment **explain things in a way you could understand?**[2]
		In the last [ ] months, how often were you **involved as much as you wanted** in your counseling or treatment?[2]
		In the last [ ] months, how often did the people you went to for counseling or treatment **show respect for what you had to say?**
		In the last [ ] months, how often did the people you went to for counseling or treatment **spend enough time** with you?
		In the last [ ] months, how often did you **feel safe** when you were with the people you went to for counseling or treatment?
Consumer survey	Information provided by counselors and clinicians	*(Screener) In the last [ ] months, did you take any prescription medications as part of your treatment?*
		(If yes . . .) In the last [ ] months, were you told what **side effects of those medications to watch for?**[2]
		In the last [ ] months, were you given information about **different kinds of counseling or treatment** that are available?[2]
		In the last [ ] months, were you given as much information as you wanted about **what you could do to manage your condition?**[2]
		In the last [ ] months, were you told about **self-help or support groups,** such as recipient-run groups or 12-step programs?
		In the last [ ] months, were you given information about **your rights as a patient?**
Consumer survey	Perceived overall quality of treatment services[1]	Using any number from 0 to 10, where 0 is the worst counseling or treatment possible and 10 is the best counseling or treatment possible, what number would you use to rate the counseling or treatment you received in the last 12 months?[2]
Consumer survey	Perceived cultural sensitivity of treatment services[1]	*(Screener) Does your* **language, race, religion, ethnic background, or culture** *make any difference in the kind of counseling or treatment you need?*
		(If yes . . .) In the last [ ] months, was the care you received **responsive to those needs?**[2]

Domain Data	Indicator	Abbreviated Description or Items
Admin. database	Treatment duration	Mean length of service during the reporting period for persons receiving services in each of three levels of care: inpatient/24-hour, day/night structured outpatient programs, and ambulatory.
Admin. database	Follow-up after hospitalization	Percent of persons discharged from 24-hour mental health care who receive follow-up ambulatory or day/night mental health treatment within 7 (30) days.
Admin. database	Initiation of treatment[1] for mental health problems	The percent of persons identified during the year with a new episode of major depression, schizophrenia, schizoaffective disorder, or bipolar disorder who have had *either* an inpatient encounter for treatment of that disorder *or* a subsequent treatment encounter within 14 days after a first outpatient encounter.[3]
Admin. database	Engagement in treatment[1] for mental health problems	The percent of persons identified during the year with a new episode of major depression, schizophrenia, schizoaffective disorder, or bipolar disorder who have had *either* a single inpatient encounter *or* two outpatient treatment encounters within 30 days after the initiation of care.[3]
Outcome		
Consumer survey	Perceived improvement[4]	*Compared to [ ] months ago,* how would you rate your **ability to deal with daily problems** *now*?[2]
		Compared to [ ] months ago, how would you rate your **problems or symptoms** *now*?[2]
		Compared to [ ] months ago, how would you rate your **ability to deal with social situations** *now*?
		Compared to [ ] months ago, how would you rate your **ability to accomplish the things you want to do** *now*?
Consumer survey	Work functioning improvement	*Compared to [ ] months ago,* how would you rate your **ability to perform paid work** *now*?[2, 3]

1. Indicators common to all treatment perspectives
2. Consumer survey–based items designated as having higher priority
3. Measures undergoing development
4. Indicators common to all treatment perspectives as well as prevention
Additional details may be found at the website for the Adult Mental Health Workgroup of the Forum on Performance Measures in Behavioral Health and Related Service Systems, http://mhindicators.org/.

Notes

1. Performance measurement systems: Digital Equipment Corporation's (DEC) Performance Measurement System for HMOs under contract to provide behavioral health care services; National Association of Psychiatric Health Systems (NAPHS)/Association of Behavioral Group Practices (ABGP) performance indicator study; National Committee for Quality Assurance's (NCQA) Health Plan and Employer Data Information Set (HEDIS); Mental Health Statistics Improvement Program's (MHSIP) Consumer-Oriented Report Card; Mental Health Corporation of America (MHCA) consumer survey and performance indicator set; American Managed Behavioral Healthcare Association's (AMBHA) Performance Measurement System (PERMS); Joint Commission on Accreditation of Healthcare Organizations' (JCAHO) Oryx Requirements.

2. Consolidation efforts: Council for Accreditation

of Rehabilitation Facilities' (CARF) Performance Measurement Advisory Council; National Association of State Mental Health Program Directors' (NASMHPD) review of state mental health program performance measures and its subsequent multistate studies using selected performance measures; American College of Mental Health Administration's (ACMHA) multiyear initiative in collaboration with the major accrediting organizations serving the mental health care field to produce a consensus document of recommended common performance indicators (ACMHA, 2001).

3. Planning groups for consensus conference: the Summit Planning Group, which worked closely with and built on related initiatives, particularly the ACMHA-hosted Workgroup of Accrediting Organizations; the Washington Circle Group, which focused on substance abuse treatment measures; the Experience of Care and Health Outcomes (ECHO) consumer survey development team; and the Child and Adolescent Outcomes Roundtable.

4. See note 1.

References

American College of Mental Health Administration (ACMHA). (1998). *Summit 1997: Preserving quality and value in the managed care equation.* Pittsburgh, PA: The American College of Mental Health Administration. Retrieved July 21, 2003, from http://www.acmha.org/summit_1997_1.htm.

American College of Mental Health Administration (ACMHA) (2001). *A proposed consensus set of indicators for behavioral health.* Pittsburgh, PA: The American College of Mental Health Administration. Retrieved July 21, 2003, from http://www.acmha.org/files/acmha_20.pdf.

Adult Mental Health Workgroup (AMHW). (2003). *Mission.* Retrieved July 21, 2003, from http://mhindicators.org/.

Burt, M. R., Duke, A., & Hargreaves, W. A. (1998). The program environment scale: Assessing client perceptions of community-based programs for the severely mentally ill. *American Journal of Community Psychology, 26*(6), 853–879.

Campbell, J. (1997). How consumers/survivors are evaluating the quality of psychiatric care. *Evaluation Review, 21*(3), 357–363.

Center for Mental Health Services (CMHS). (1996, April). *The final report of the Mental Health Statistics Improvement Program Task Force on a Consumer-Oriented Mental Health Report Card.* Washington, DC: Center for Mental Health Services, SAMHSA. Retrieved July 21, 2003, from http://www.mhsip.org/reportcard/reportcard.html.

Drake, R. E., Goldman, H. H., Leff, H. S., Lehman, A. F., Dixon, L., Mueser, K. T., et al. (2001). Implementing evidence-based practices in routine mental health service settings. *Psychiatric Services, 52*(2), 179–182.

Drake, R. E., Rosenberg, S. D., Teague, G. B., Bartels, S. J., & Torrey, W. C. (in press). Fundamental principles of evidence-based medicine applied to mental health care. In Evidence-based practices in mental health. *Psychiatric Clinics of North America.*

Druss, B. G., Miller, C. L., Rosenheck, R. A., Shih, S. C., & Bost, J. E. (2002). Mental health care quality under managed care in the United States: A view from the health employer data and information set (HEDIS). *American Journal of Psychiatry, 159*(5), 860–862.

Eisen, S. V., Shaul, J. A., Clarridge, B., Nelson, D., Spink, J., & Cleary, P. D. (1999). Development of a consumer survey for behavioral health services. *Psychiatric Services, 50*(6), 793–798.

Embretson, S. E. (1996). The new rules of measurement. *Psychological Assessment, 8*(4), 341–349.

Garnick, D. W., Lee, M. T., Chalk, M., Gastfriend, D., Horgan, C. M., McCorry, F., et al. (2002). Establishing the feasibility of performance measures for alcohol and other drugs. *Journal of Substance Abuse Treatment, 23*, 375–385.

Institute of Medicine (IOM) Committee on the Quality of Health Care in America. (2001). *Crossing the quality chasm: A new health system for the 21st century.* Washington, DC: National Academy Press.

Lutterman, T., & Hogan, M. (2000). State mental health agency controlled expenditures and revenues for mental health services, FY 1981 to 1997. In R. W. Manderscheid & M. J. Henderson (Eds.), *Center for Mental Health Services. Mental Health, United States, 2000* (DHHS Publication No. SMA 01-3537). Washington, DC: U.S. Government Printing Office. Retrieved July 21, 2003, from http://www.mentalhealth.org/publications/allpubs/sma01—3537/chapter16.asp.

Manderscheid, R. (1998). From many into one: Addressing the crisis of quality in managed behavioral health care at the millennium. *Journal of Behavioral Health Services and Research, 25*(2), 233–236.

McCorry, F., Garnick, D. W., Bartlett, J., Cotter, F., & Chalk, M. (2000). Developing performance measures for alcohol and other drug services in managed care plans. *Journal on Quality Improvement, 26*(11), 633–643.

National Association of State Mental Health Program Directors (NASMHPD). (2000). *Recommended operational definitions and measures to implement the NASMHPD Framework of mental health performance indicators.* Alexandria, VA: National Association of State Mental Health Program Directors Research Institute. Retrieved July 21, 2003, from http://nri.rdmc.org/PresidentsTaskForce2001.pdf.

Outcomes Roundtable for Children and Families (1998). *Fitting the pieces together: Building outcome accountability in child mental health and child welfare systems.* Washington, DC: Center for Mental Health Services, SAMHSA.

Rogers, E. M. (1995). *Diffusion of innovations* (4th ed.). New York: Free Press.

Shaul, J. A., Eisen, S. V., Clarridge, B. R., Stringfellow, V. L., Fowler, F. J., et al. (2001). *Experience of Care and Health Outcomes (ECHO ™) survey field test report: Survey evaluation.* Retrieved July 21, 2003, from http://www.hcp.med.harvard.edu/echo/home.html.

Teague, G. B. (2000). Patient perceptions of care measures. In A. J. Rush, H. A. Pincus, First, M. B., Zarin, D. A., Blacker, D., Endicott, J., et al. (Eds.), *Handbook of Psychiatric Measures.* Washington, DC: American Psychiatric Association.

Teague, G. B., Ganju, V., Hornik, J. A., Johnson, J. R., & McKinney, J. (1997). The MHSIP mental health report card: A consumer-oriented approach to monitoring the quality of mental health plans. *Evaluation Review, 21*(3), 330–341.

U.S. Department of Health and Human Services. (USDHHS). (1999). *Mental health: A report of the surgeon general.* Rockville, MD: U.S. Department of Health and Human Services, Substance Abuse and Mental Health Services Administration, Center for Mental Health Services, National Institutes of Health, National Institute of Mental Health. Retrieved July 21, 2003, from http://www.surgeongeneral.gov/library/mentalhealth/home.html.

6 AN OVERVIEW OF FOCUS GROUP INTERVIEWING

Mary Anne Casey & Richard Krueger

Robert Merton, the sociologist who pioneered the approach, first wrote about focus groups in *The Focused Interview* (1956). Since the 1950s market researchers have used focus groups to search for ways to improve their products and market them to consumers. In the last 20 years government agencies, NGOs (nongovernmental organizations), universities, and nonprofit organizations have begun using findings from focus group interviews to help make decisions about their products and services.

This chapter provides an overview of focus group interviewing as used in not-for-profit settings. It will outline the characteristics of focus group interviews and the stages/tasks involved in conducting a focus group study. This chapter also provides how-to advice on conducting these studies.

CHARACTERISTICS OF FOCUS GROUP INTERVIEWS

A focus group is not just any group that gets together to talk about a topic. Focus groups have certain characteristics.

Focus groups have carefully recruited participants. To do this

- invite individuals who have the desired characteristics, experiences, or knowledge needed to provide rich information on the topic of discussion.
- limit the size of the group. Invite five to nine people; six to eight participants is the preferred size. Recruit enough people to generate diverse ideas but not so many that participants do not have a chance to share.

- conduct three or four groups with each type of participant about which you want to make statements. Therefore, if you want to compare and contrast how men and women view a particular topic, conduct three to four groups with men and three to four groups with women.
- avoid power differentials among participants. All participants should feel comfortable talking with others in the group.

Focus groups take place in a comfortable environment. To create this

- hold focus groups in settings where the participants will feel comfortable. Focus groups have been held in office buildings, libraries, schools, homes, cafés, and community gathering spots.
- seat people so that they can easily see each other.
- interview people in their first language if possible. Do not use an interpreter in the group. Using an interpreter stilts the discussion, and the process turns into serial interviews rather than a lively discussion among participants. It is better to train someone who knows the language to moderate the groups than to have someone who knows how to moderate work through an interpreter. After the group is over translate the discussion back into the analyst's language if necessary.

Focus groups should have a skillful moderator. To do this

- pick moderators who have a skill for making people feel comfortable and who are good at listening. For groups of people who are used to being in powerful positions, pick a moderator who can keep the group on track and control dominant participants.
- practice the skills mentioned later in this chapter.
- use predetermined questions. The moderator should be prepared to ask a set of questions designed to get the information needed by decision makers.
- establish a permissive environment. It is the moderator's job to create the feeling that it will be OK for participants to freely express themselves in the group.

Focus groups include systematic analysis and reporting. To do this

- record the discussion for analysis. Take field notes and use a tape recorder to make an audio tape recording. Sometimes a laptop computer can be used to make a transcript of the discussion during the focus group. Explain why you are recording and who has access to the data.
- develop a systematic analysis process. Be able to describe the process to others. Several different processes can be used; pick one that is appropriate for your project.
- use a verifiable process. Verifiable means that there is a trail of evidence. Another researcher, given the data and analysis materials, should be able to replicate the analysis and verify the links between the data and the final report.

A focus group is working well when participants begin to talk to other participants and build upon others' comments rather than continually responding directly to the moderator. Participants become engaged, and the discussion becomes their conversation. The moderator begins to play a less central role as participants share experiences, debate ideas, and offer opinions. Some groups arrive at this point quickly. Others never get to this point.

STAGES IN CONDUCTING FOCUS GROUPS

There are different stages or tasks involved in a focus group study. These stages include the following:

- Planning (designing the study and developing questions)
- Recruiting (inviting participants)
- Moderating (leading the groups, capturing the data)
- Analyzing/reporting (reducing the data to a usable form for various audiences)

One person can complete all of these tasks. However, the quality of the results is often improved when a small team of about three to five people works together. For example, one person could plan a study and develop questions, but the plan and the questions are usually stronger when that person involves others in that process who care about the study. The stages are described in the following sections.

Planning

The main challenge during the planning stage is to come up with a study design that will answer the study questions within timeline and budget constraints. You and your team must be clear about the study's purpose. You must decide whether focus groups are the appropriate research method. If focus groups are appropriate, you must decide how many groups to do and what experiences or characteristics participants should have.

First Steps

1. DECIDE WHETHER FOCUS GROUPS ARE APPROPRIATE Focus groups work particularly well for

- understanding how people see needs and assets in their lives and communities.
- understanding how people think or feel about an idea, a behavior, a product, or a service.
- pilot testing ideas, campaigns, surveys, or products. Focus groups can be used to get reactions to plans before money is spent in implementation.
- evaluating how programs/products are working and how they might be improved.
- developing other research instruments such as surveys or case studies.

Focus group interviews are not meant to be used as

- a process for getting people to come to consensus.
- a way to teach knowledge or skills.
- a test of knowledge or skills.

If you answer yes to any of the following questions, you should consider using other methods in conjunction with or instead of focus group interviews.

- Do you need statistical data? Focus groups cannot provide statistical data to project to a population. The number of people interviewed is simply too small.
- Will harm come to people who share their ideas in a group? Although a researcher can promise to keep information shared in the group confidential, it is not possible to guarantee that participants in the group will keep the information that is shared confidential. If harm may come to people who openly share in the group, choose another method such as individual interviews.
- Are people polarized by this topic? People are very passionate about and polarized by some topics. The topics will likely vary by country. In the United States, abortion and the environment are two topics that people have a hard time discussing with others who hold opposing views. Emotions run high, and it is difficult to conduct focus groups when people holding opposing views are in the same group.
- Is there a better, more efficient way to get the information?

2. CLARIFY THE PURPOSE OF THE STUDY Sometimes study team members disagree about what information they want to gather as a result of the study and what they will do with the information once they have it. Having a clear purpose will make planning, conducting the groups, analyzing, and reporting simpler.

3. DECIDE WHAT TYPES OF PEOPLE TO INTERVIEW What types of people have the experiences or characteristics that will serve as a basis for providing input on the study topic? Michael Q. Patton calls these "information rich" cases (*Qualitative Evaluation and Research Methods*, 1990). They may not be the most highly educated or the most influential sources, but they are the people who know something about what you want to know. For example, young people who drop out of school know a lot about what it might take to keep other young people in school. Teachers, counselors, and parents can give different perspectives on the same topic.

Consider the usefulness of listening to

- elected officials.
- influentials—these people are respected by others but may not be elected.
- those most affected by the change being discussed.
- those who must buy into the change being discussed before it can happen.
- employees (both frontline staff and management) of the organizations that may implement programs or services to support the change being discussed.

4. DECIDE HOW MANY GROUPS TO CONDUCT The basic sampling strategy is to conduct three or

four focus groups for each type of person or audience category that is of interest to you. If you want to understand how parents and teenagers feel about a new school policy, you might plan three or four groups with parents and three or four groups with teenagers. Often planners must strike a balance between how many groups they would like to do and how many groups they have the sufficient time and budget to do.

5. LISTEN TO KEY INFORMANTS Find a few people like the people you want to invite to the focus groups. Tell them about the study. Ask for their advice. Ask them questions such as the following: Who can ask these kinds of questions (moderate)? What type of moderator would people feel comfortable with? Where might the groups be held? What days or times might work well for people? How do you find people with these characteristics? What would it take to get people to come?

6. PUT YOUR THOUGHTS IN WRITING Develop a plan that includes purpose, types of people you want to listen to, number of groups, potential questions, a timeline, and a budget. This will help clarify your thinking and provide a basis for further discussions. Share this plan with colleagues. Invite feedback.

Developing a Questioning Route

There are several challenges when developing focus group questions. The aim is to ask questions that address your study's purpose. Although that may sound obvious, many study teams get swept away dreaming about questions that would be fun to ask or nice to know the answer to but do not address the purpose of the study. The questions must be conversational and easy for the participants to understand. You must have the right number of questions—not too many or too few. You must begin with questions that allow the participants to get ready to answer the most important questions.

A questioning route is a set of questions developed for the focus groups. In a two-hour focus group, expect to have about a dozen questions. The following steps are used to develop a questioning route:

1. Hold a brainstorming session. Invite four to six people who are familiar with the study to a one- or two-hour meeting. Ask these people to generate questions that should be answered by the study. Questions may be briefly discussed, but try not to get stuck debating the merits of a single question. Have one person record all of these questions. Adjourn when ideas dry up.

2. Use the questions from the brainstorming session to draft a questioning route. Groups are good at brainstorming but are not efficient at developing the questioning routes. Have one person use the questions generated in the brainstorming session to develop a questioning route. Select the questions that seem most likely to provide useful information. Rephrase these questions so that they are open-ended, conversational, and devoid of jargon. Then sequence the questions in a logical flow from general to specific. Say the questions out loud. Are they easy to ask? Do they seem like questions the participants will be able to answer?

There is no magic to having about 12 questions. However, beginning focus group researchers often develop questioning routes with 20 to 30 questions—far too many. The result of too many questions is shallow data. Participants will not have time to share or discuss in depth. Once you have a draft of the questioning route, estimate how much time the group should spend on each question. Not all questions deserve the same amount of time. Some questions are simple or not as important and can easily be covered in five minutes. Some of the key questions may be complex or include activities. A key question might take 15 to 20 minutes to cover. Once you have estimated times for each of the questions, add up the total amount of time to determine whether to add or delete questions.

3. Send the draft of the questioning route out for feedback. Send the questioning route to the brainstorming team and ask the following questions: Will these questions get us the information we need? What have we missed? What can be deleted? Are these the words participants would use? Does the flow make sense? Revise the questioning route based on the feedback received.

Remember that the same questions should be asked in all of the interviews with the same types of people. However, if separate groups are going to be conducted—for example, with teachers, parents, and students—a slightly different questioning route might be used for each of these audiences (e.g., you might ask students a question that you do not want to ask parents or teachers). Keep a core set of questions the same in each questioning route so that responses can be compared across audiences.

Example of a Questioning Route: Evaluating a Service for Children

1. Introduce yourself and tell us how you learned about these services.
2. Think back to when you first became involved with these services. What were your first impressions of the service?
3. What has been particularly helpful about the services your family has received?
4. What has been frustrating about the services?
5. What has your child liked about the experience?
6. What has your child *not* liked about the experience?
7. Some of you may have had experiences with other services for your child. How does this approach compare with other services you've experienced? Is it any different? How so?
8. What would make the services work better?
9. Is your child any different because he or she has received these services? If so, how?
10. Is your family life any different because you received these services? How?
11. If you had a chance to give advice to the director of this program, what would you say?
12. Based on your experiences, would you recommend these services to other parents?

Recruiting

The next challenge is finding the right people and getting them to attend the focus groups. A basic focus group principle is that the researcher controls attendance. Participants are selected and invited because they have certain experiences or qualities in common. People are not recruited or allowed to come simply because they are interested in attending. You invite people because they meet the *screens*, or qualifications of the study. They all have experiences or characteristics in common. For example, they may have participated in a community program that you are evaluating, or they are residents in the community for which you are doing a needs assessment, or they are farmers who have adopted certain agricultural practices.

One of the challenges of focus group research is how to get people who may be uninterested in your study to participate. These people may be apathetic, indifferent, or may even consider the topic to be irrelevant. If you limit your study only to those who show interest in the topic, you might get biased results. To recruit people who are not committed to your topic, you will need to think about your procedures as well as the incentives for participation.

The Recruiting Procedure

There are two distinct qualities of successful recruiting. First, the process should be personalized. This means that each person feels that he or she has been personally asked to attend and share his or her opinions. Second, the invitation process is repetitive. Invitations are given not just once but two or three times. Here is a typical recruiting process:

1. Set meeting dates, times, and locations for group interviews. Most groups with adults are scheduled for two hours. Focus groups with children are usually shorter. Do not schedule more than two groups in one day unless you have multiple moderators.

2. Recruit potential participants via phone or in person. Before beginning the recruiting, be clear about how you are going to describe the study to people whom you invite. People will want to know the purpose of the discussion, who wants the information, what the sponsor of the study is going to do with the information, and why they are being asked to participate ("Why me?").

We usually do not formally invite people to a "focus group." Such an invitation can be intimidating. Instead, we say we are getting a few people together to talk about the topic. Do not use jargon in the invitation. In most cases you want it to sound like it will be an easy, comfortable, interesting conversation.

Think about who should offer the invitation. People are usually more likely to say yes if someone they know and respect invites them to participate. If that is not possible, it helps to be able to refer to a person they know and respect as supporting the study. For example, it often helps to say something such as, "Maria Smith, the community health nurse [or the name of a person they know and respect], said you might be able to help us. We are getting a few people together to talk about [name of topic]."

3. Soon after the person has agreed to participate, send him or her a personalized follow-up letter. Do not use a generic salutation such as "Dear friend." This letter should thank the person for agreeing to participate and confirm the date, time, and place of the focus group.

4. Phone or contact each person the day before the focus group to remind them of the group. "I'm looking forward to seeing you tomorrow at . . ."

Finding a Pool of Participants

Typically we find a pool of people who meet our selection requirements, and then we randomly select from that pool individuals to invite to participate. For example, we might invite every fifth name on a list or every 10th person who enters a store. Where do you find the pool? Here are several different ways to find a pool:

- Find a list of people who fit your selection criteria. Think about who might have such a list.
- Piggyback on another event that attracts the type of people you want to include. For example, if you want to recruit farmers from a certain area, do all farmers in this area get together for a specific event?
- Recruit on location. For example, invite every fifth person who arrives at the clinic from which you want to recruit your focus group members.
- Work with a school, community center, or faith community to find people who fit the screens. Make a donation to the organization as a thank-you for their help.
- Nominations. Ask key people such as elders, educators, or service providers who they know who would fit the selection criteria.
- Snowball samples. Once you find some people who fit the selection criteria, ask them for names of other people who fit the selection criteria. Put the names in a pool.
- Place ads in newspapers and on bulletin boards.

Getting People to Attend: Incentives

Think about what might make it difficult for people to attend. Try to eliminate these obstacles. If appropriate, provide transportation and child care.

Think about what might entice people to participate. Try to offer some of these things. Ask a few people who are like the people you are trying to attract what it will take to get them to come. Here are some of the things that have been used to encourage people to participate in focus groups:

- money (We will pay you.)
- food (There will be something to eat.)
- gifts (We have a gift for you.)
- compliments (We value your insights.)
- enjoyment (You will have a nice time.)
- community (Your participation will help the community.)

Moderating

The challenge of moderating is to help people feel comfortable enough to share what they think and how they feel while they are in the group. Participants must trust the moderator, the process, and the sponsoring organization and must trust that the results will be used in a positive way. The moderator must know when to wait for more information and when to move on. The moderator must be able to control dominant speakers and encourage hesitant participants. The moderator must respect the participants, listen to what they have to say, and thank them for their views even when he or she may disagree personally.

The moderator does not need to be an expert on the topic but should understand common terms that will be used in the discussion. It sometimes helps to have a moderator who looks like the participants. This can make the participants more comfortable and give the impression that "this person will understand what I have to say." Consider characteristics such as gender, age, race, and ethnicity. For some topics these characteristics may not matter, but for other topics they are very important. For example, women are more willing to talk about breastfeeding with a woman than with a man. Also remember that the moderator should be fluent in the participants' first language.

Other Things the Moderator Should Do

Be mentally prepared:

- Be alert and free from distractions. Arrive early so that you are relaxed and ready to listen.
- Have the discipline to listen. Beginning moderators often are delighted that people are

talking, and they do not notice that the participants are not really answering the question. As you listen, ask yourself, "Are they really answering the question?" If not, refocus their attention on the question.

- Be familiar with the questioning route. Know which questions are the most important. Know which questions can be dropped if you are running out of time.

Work with an assistant moderator:

- An assistant moderator improves the quality of the groups.
- At one level the assistant helps by taking care of details (e.g., taking care of refreshments, monitoring the recording equipment, dealing with latecomers).
- On a more important level the assistant helps ensure the quality of the analysis by taking careful notes, summarizing the discussion at the end, and acting as another set of eyes and ears for analysis.

Greet and talk with participants before the group begins:

- Create a warm and friendly environment.
- Have everything prepared so you can focus your attention on the participants as they arrive, just as you would welcome people to your home.

Record the discussion. The focus group can be recorded in several ways such as with field notes, tape recording, or a laptop computer. The moderator will not be able to take comprehensive notes and guide the discussion at the same time. The assistant moderator is usually responsible for recording the focus group.

Give a short and smooth introduction:

- Welcome everyone.
- Give an overview of the topic.
- Provide any ground rules for the discussion.
- Ask the first question.

Use pauses and probes to draw out additional responses:

- Be comfortable using a five-second pause. Beginning moderators are sometimes uncomfortable with silence. However, pauses encourage people to add to the conversation.
- Use probes to get more detail. Detailed information is often more useful. Consider these: "Can you give an example?"; "I don't understand"; "Tell me more."

Control your reactions to participants:

- Do not lead participants by giving verbal or nonverbal clues as to what you like or do not like. Avoid head nodding and verbal cues such as "that's good," "excellent."
- Do not correct participants during the group. If they share information that is harmful, offer the correct information at the end of the group.
- Do not become defensive if participants tell you they think your program is horrible. Instead, try to get information that will help you understand their perspective.

Use subtle group control:

- Your job is not to make sure that everyone speaks the same amount in a group, but everyone should have the opportunity to share. Some people will have more to say. If they are answering the question and giving new and useful information, let them continue.
- Control dominant talkers by thanking them for their input and asking for others to share. Remind the group that it is important to hear from everyone.
- Call on quiet participants. They are often reflective thinkers and have wonderful things to offer. Invite them to share by saying something such as, "Maria, I don't want to leave you out of the discussion. Is there something you would like to add?"

Use an appropriate conclusion:

- Summarize the key points of the discussion and ask for confirmation. Usually the assistant moderator does this. (Do not summarize the entire focus group. Instead, summarize three to five of the most important points.)
- Review the focus group's purpose and ask if anything has been missed.
- Thank the participants and conclude the session.

Analysis

The analyst must take the focus group data and find what is meaningful to the purpose of the study so that the results can be used. One of the skills that beginning analysts must learn is to match the level of analysis to the problem at hand. Not all studies require the same level of analysis.

It helps to break analysis into manageable chunks so that the analyst is not overwhelmed by the task. The analyst must look for the major themes that cut across groups and those gems that might have been shared by only a few people. The analyst can only do this by being clearly grounded in the purpose of the study. Also, analysis is much easier to do if the analyst has attended the focus groups to see the interactions and hear the discussions.

Systematic Analysis Process

Focus group analysis should be systematic. Being systematic means that the analyst follows a predetermined and verifiable set of steps. There is no single best way but rather many possible ways to have a systematic process. The following is an example of a systematic analysis process. Notice that the process begins while the first group is still being conducted and continues past the final focus group.

1. START WHILE STILL IN THE GROUP

- Listen for vague or inconsistent comments and probe for understanding.
- Consider asking each participant a final preference question.
- Offer an oral summary of key findings and inquire if the summary is correct.

2. CONTINUE IMMEDIATELY AFTER THE FOCUS GROUP

- Draw a diagram of the seating arrangement.
- Spot-check the tape recording to be sure that the recorder picked up the discussion. If the tape does not work, immediately take time to expand your notes. Recreate as much of the discussion as possible.
- Turn the tape recorder back on. Tape the observations of the moderator and assistant moderator.
- Discuss things such as the following: What seemed to be the key themes of this discussion? What was surprising? How did this group compare with prior groups? Do we need to change anything before the next

group? Note hunches, interpretations, and ideas.
- Label and file field notes, tapes, and other materials.

3. SOON AFTER THE FOCUS GROUP—WITHIN DAYS—ANALYZE THE INDIVIDUAL FOCUS GROUP
Option A: Transcript-based analysis

- Make backup copies of the tape(s) and send the tape(s) to a transcriptionist if a transcript is needed.
- The analyst listens to the tape(s), reviews field notes, and reads the transcript, if available.
- Use the transcripts as the basis for the next steps.

Option B: Analysis without transcripts

- Prepare a summary of the individual focus group in a question-by-question format with amplifying quotes.
- For verification share each summary with other researchers who were present at the focus groups.
- Use summaries as the basis for the next steps.

4. LATER—WITHIN DAYS—ANALYZE THE SERIES OF FOCUS GROUPS

- Analyze groups within a category (e.g., first analyze the parent groups, then analyze teacher groups, then analyze student groups).
- Analyze groups across categories (e.g., compare and contrast the parent groups with the teacher and student groups).
- Look for emerging themes by question and then for overall emerging themes.
- Construct typologies or diagram the analysis if appropriate.

5. FINALLY, PREPARE THE REPORT

- Consider narrative style versus bulleted style.
- Use a few quotes to illustrate each important point.
- Sequence could be either question-by-question or by theme.
- Share the report for verification with other researchers.
- Revise and finalize the report.

Things to Consider When Analyzing Focus Group Data

INTERNAL CONSISTENCY Participants in focus groups sometimes change their positions after interaction with others. When there is a shift in opinion, the analyst typically traces the flow of the conversation to find clues that might explain the change. What seems to have prompted the change?

FREQUENCY Frequency tells us how often a comment was made. But frequency alone does not tell us how many different people made this particular comment. Indeed, you might have 10 comments all made by the same person. Do not assume that frequency is an indicator of importance. Some analysts count how many times certain topics were mentioned and believe that those topics discussed most often are more important. This is not necessarily true.

EXTENSIVENESS Extensiveness tells us how many different people made a particular comment. This measure gives you a sense of the degree of agreement on a topic. Unfortunately, it is impossible to determine extensiveness using only the transcript unless names are attached to comments. If you were present in the focus group you will have a sense of the degree of extensiveness, and this can be captured in the field notes. Extensiveness is a more useful concept in focus group analysis than is frequency.

INTENSITY Occasionally participants talk about a topic with a special intensity or depth of feeling. Sometimes the participants will use words that connote intensity or tell you directly about their strength of feeling. Some individuals may speak faster with excitement while others will speak slowly and deliberately. Some may cry. Some may bang their fists on the table. Pay attention to what is said with passion or intensity. Intensity is difficult to gauge with transcripts alone because the tone of voice, speed of speaking, and emphasis on certain words are lost in the transcript.

SPECIFICITY Responses that are specific and based on experiences should be given more weight than responses that are vague and impersonal. To what degree can the respondent provide details when asked a follow-up probe?

Greater attention is often paid to responses that are in the first person as opposed to hypothetical third-person answers. For example, "The new practice is important because I used it and my child is much healthier" has more weight than "These practices are good and people in the area should use them."

CONCLUSIONS

The following suggestions can help you learn more about focus group interviewing:

- Read. There are many good books and articles about using focus groups in social sciences, education, health care, and market research.
- Practice. If you have not conducted focus groups before, consider volunteering to conduct a small study for a group you support (e.g., a community center or place of worship). Start with an easy topic such as reviewing a newsletter or getting input on a youth sports program. Hold about three groups with five or six participants in each. Share your findings with the organization, and then reflect on the process. What went well? What would you do differently?
- Become an apprentice. Watch and work with people who are good at conducting focus group studies.

Further Reading

Debus, M. (1990). *Handbook for excellence in focus group research*. Washington, DC: Academy for Educational Development.

Goldman, A. E., & McDonald, S. S. (1987). *The group depth interview: Principles and practice*. Englewood Cliffs, NJ: Prentice-Hall.

Greenbaum, T. L. (1998). *The handbook for focus group research*. Thousand Oaks, CA: Sage.

Krueger, R. A., and Casey, M. A. (2000). *Focus groups: A practical guide for applied research* (3rd ed.). Thousand Oaks, CA: Sage.

Merton, R. K., Fiske, M., & Kendall, P. L. (1990). *The focused interview* (2nd ed.). New York: Free Press.

Morgan, D. L. (1997). *Focus groups as qualitative research*. Newbury Park, CA: Sage.

Patton, M. Q. (1990). *Qualitative evaluation and research methods* (2nd ed.). Newbury Park, CA: Sage.

7 MENTAL ILLNESS, SUBSTANCE DEPENDENCE, AND SUICIDALITY

Secondary Data Analysis

Kenneth Yeager & Albert R. Roberts

Mental illness, substance dependence, and suicide are three of the most prevalent social and public health concerns throughout North America. Recent estimates indicate that every 20 minutes somewhere in the United States or Canada a suicide occurs. In the United States alone there are 30,000 suicides per year (Bush, Fawcett, & Jacobs, 2003; Institute of Medicine, 2002). This chapter seeks to explain the contributing factors leading to rehospitalization and suicide risk among the psychiatric, substance abuse, and substance dependent populations. Data from a university medical center will be reviewed regarding characteristics of inpatient hospitalization and potential contributing factors increasing the individual's risk of a suicide attempt following inpatient psychiatric/substance dependence hospitalization. In 2001 approximately 15 million adults age 18 or greater were estimated to have suffered from a severe mental illness during the previous year. The population with the highest rate of severe mental illness was the 18-to-25-year-old age group (12%). Persons ages 26–49 demonstrated a rate of approximately 8%, with the 50 or older age group demonstrating a rate of 5%. Females were more likely than males to have a diagnosis consistent with severe mental illness (9% female versus 6% male) (National Institute of Mental Health, 2001; Bush et al., 2003; Institute of Medicine, 2002).

It is important to understand this population and potential diagnostic pattern changes occurring within the population group to provide the most effective psychiatric illness management.

To help facilitate such understanding this chapter outlines an emerging pattern of comorbid diagnosis that emerged in a recent secondary data set review of admissions to a metropolitan psychiatric and substance dependence treatment facility. Within this population the impact of multiple psychiatric diagnoses, dependence on multiple substances among substance dependent individuals, and comorbid psychiatric and substance dependence diagnoses were examined in the context of their contribution to rehospitalization within 31 days of initial hospitalization and the presence and severity of suicidal ideation in those rehospitalized.

Recent research has demonstrated that in many cases severe mental illness can be successfully managed if the affected individual is able to receive treatment; however, in 2001 National Institute of Mental Health data revealed that less than one half (47%) of persons with a severe mental illness received treatment or counseling intervention within the previous year. Within this population adults aged 26 or greater are most likely to receive treatment. Females were more likely to receive treatment (52%) compared with their male counterparts (38%). Whites were more likely to receive mental health treatment or counseling than were Hispanics or blacks (National Institute of Mental Health, 2001).

The National Institute of Mental Health data indicates that adults with a severe mental illness were more likely to have used illicit drugs during the previous year compared with those without a severe mental illness. Incidence of illicit drug use was more than twice as high among adults with an identified severe mental illness (27%) than among the general population without a mental illness diagnosis (11%) (National Institute of Mental Health, 2001; Jacobs, 1999)

DATA COLLECTION

Within the day-to-day function of the psychiatric facility examined in this study data is gathered on an ongoing basis. Data is collected for registration purposes, assessment purposes, and quality and operational improvement purposes. Initially, demographic information is collected during the initial call, emergency department admission, or upon intake. Data collected is utilized to create an electronic file for each patient and stored in the "information warehouse," the medical center's electronic warehousing computer.

The next step in the data collection process is completion of the patient's psychiatric screening. The screening consists of the patient's presenting problem, review of symptoms, suicidal risk assessment, current functionality status, and current life circumstances, including living arrangements, assessment of the individual's ability to care for self and potential risk for self-harm. The initial screen data is reviewed with the attending psychiatrist, and the patient is admitted to the most appropriate level of care. For most patients this process will take approximately 1 hour to 90 minutes. Again, information gathered is stored in the electronic record in the information warehouse.

If the psychiatric prescreeners and the psychiatrist determine that the patient meets criteria for inpatient admission, a complete biopsychosocial assessment is completed by a master of social work (MSW) or psychiatric nurse (RN) as part of the admission process. The patient's diagnosis as previously established during the screening and intake process is confirmed during the more complete biopsychosocial assessment and treatment planning process, which are both electronically recorded. Once the patient's treatment is complete, the length of stay, primary discharge diagnosis, and other rank diagnoses are recorded into the information warehouse. It is important to note that the electronic medical record and categorization is monitored and updated throughout the patient's hospitalization.

This provides for optimal data collection because the data is based on the actual care experience. Utilization of the electronic medical record minimizes commonly occurring errors in electronic data collection such as missing data, data entry errors, and poorly timed data entry secondary to data entry not being given top priority. In addition, data verification included but was not limited to comparing data by patient and encounter, diagnostic coding between billing ICD-9 codes and medical record rank ordering of diagnosis, and frequency analysis to facilitate elimination of multiple entries for the same patient.

Additional uses for the data collected over the length of stay include quality and operational improvement activities. Data collected throughout the patient's stay is analyzed for quality improvement processes. Among the quality indicators measured are patient falls, reported medication errors, observed to expected length of stay, restraint and seclusion episodes, and readmissions within 31 days. Tracking and reporting of this data is a requirement of mental health credentialing entities and accreditation entities such as the Joint Commission on Accreditation of Healthcare Organizations (JCAHO). JCAHO evaluates and accredits nearly 17,000 health care organizations and programs in the United States. An independent, not-for-profit organization, JCAHO is the nation's predominant health care standards-setting and accrediting body. As such, JCAHO seeks to continuously improve the safety and quality of care provided to the public through the provision of health care accreditation and related services that support performance improvement in health care organizations. Examples of quality and safety initiatives include each institution's analysis of trends within high risk areas of behavioral health care such as episodes of restraint and seclusion, patient falls, and medication errors and established action plans to address emergent quality improvement opportunities. For example, readmissions may be representative of issues with length of stay being either too short or longer than necessary given population breakouts. Finally, keeping track of readmissions within a 31-day period is helpful in monitoring psychiatrists' prescribing practices and to increase practice-based evidence designed to facilitate optimal medication management.

SECONDARY DATA ANALYSIS

This secondary data analysis demonstrates how hospital quality assurance programming can be combined with data analysis to determine the presence of an emerging pattern of increasing severity of suicide risk including acts of harm to self and others both prior to and during readmissions to the inpatient psychiatric facility within 31 days of initial hospitalization. Specifically, within the process of quality improvement initiatives three cases of remarkable patient acts of harm to self or others on the inpatient psychiatric facility led to completion of a root cause analysis, which examined potential contributing factors to the emergence of violent actions of harm to self or others in the inpatient psychiatric unit. Figure 7.1 is the simplified fishbone diagram completed as a portion of the root cause analysis documenting common factors among the three cases leading to potential harm to self and others. This analysis led to further investigation into the occurrence of comorbid diagnosis among the presenting population. The findings of this "drill-down" analysis indicated that an identifiable group of nominal variables was present in each case and may be indicative

of a larger force working among the patient population. In the next step of the analysis the patient population of this facility was examined utilizing data collected in the information warehouse to determine the prevalence of high-risk behaviors such as suicidal ideation among those readmitted within 31 days and to determine if there were emerging patterns of increasing comorbid diagnostic categories. Analysis indicated a .79 correlation between the presence of comorbid diagnosis and increasing risk of harm to self and others.

A study was conducted that reviewed secondary data collected over a 6-month period examining a total of 4,467 cases evaluated for inpatient psychiatric and substance dependence disorders. Within the population evaluated 1,942 patients did not present with clearly identifiable diagnostic criteria on Axis 1 within a major diagnostic category or were under 18 years of age, thus excluding these cases from this data set. A total of 2,525 cases met criteria for inclusion in the study, that is, cases presenting with either a substance dependence diagnosis or a major diagnostic category for mental illness as defined by the DSM-IV-TR via mental health assessment by licensed independent social workers and

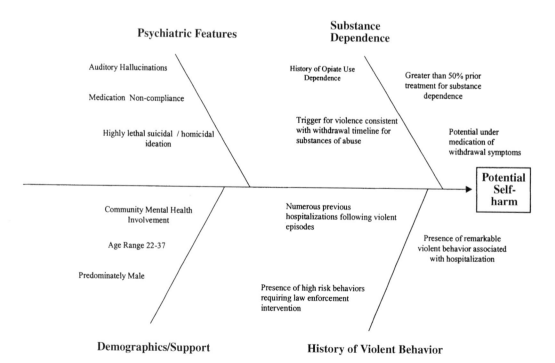

FIGURE 7.1 Analysis of Potential Harm to Self and Others

TABLE 7.1 Inpatient Psychiatric Population
Overview by Primary Diagnosis

Diagnosis	Number of Cases
Alcohol dependence	495
Drug dependence	490
Bipolar disorder	470
Anxiety disorder	436
Major depressive disorder	317
Schizophrenia group	317

Note: Substance abuse was the prevalent secondary diagnosis presenting in 740 cases. Alcohol abuse was identified in 114 cases and was considered to be under-diagnosed. Alcohol abuse was defined as frequent consumption of more than six drinks per occasion with the absence of physical dependence and diagnostic criteria as defined by the DSM-IV-TR.

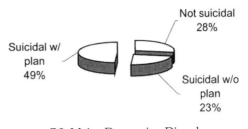

FIGURE 7.2 Major Depressive Disorder Reporting Suicidal Ideation

psychiatric nurses. An overview of the primary diagnostic categories is listed in Table 7.1. In addition, a subpopulation of 740 cases that were in the initial data set and were readmitted within a 31-day period was examined to determine potential trends of suicide risk factors (American Psychiatric Association, 2002).

It is important to note that criteria for inpatient admission to this facility require presence of clear and present risk to self or others or the inability of the individual to care for him- or herself secondary to psychosis or impending substance withdrawal requiring medical intervention. Hence the prevalence of suicidal ideation will be greater than that described above as applying to the general population.

PREVALENCE OF SUICIDAL IDEATION AMONG THE MOOD DISORDER POPULATION

We conducted electronic case reviews of patients presenting for psychiatric and substance dependence treatment. The first group examined was the population presenting with depressive disorder with suicidal ideation. Within this population 72% presented with current suicidal ideation. Of the patients with current suicidal ideation 23% reported ideation without plan or intent, and 49% were able to verbalize plan and intent (see Figure 7.2).

Examination of the prevalence of suicidal ide-

ation among the bipolar I and II population was conducted in much the same manner, demonstrating slightly higher rates of suicidal ideation upon inpatient hospitalization, with 86% of this population presenting with active suicidal ideation at the time of admission. Fifty-seven percent verbalized a plan with intent to carry out, 17% verbalized suicidal ideation, and only 12% were admitted without suicidal ideation (see Figure 7.3). The remaining 14% were omitted secondary to extreme manic and delusional states that made determination of suicide risk impossible.

Among the population presenting with a schizophrenia diagnosis the reporting of suicidal ideation was less than expected, and the reporting of ideation without a plan was higher than expected. In all, 29% of this population verbalized no suicidal ideation but instead were admitted secondary to an inability to care for self. Of those admitted with suicidal ideation 37% reported ideation with no specific plan, and 34% reported specific plan with intent (see Figure 7.4).

EXPRESSED PLANNED METHOD

Within the population that verbalized suicidal ideation we examined the expressed suicide plan.

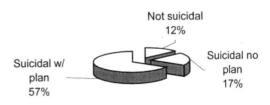

FIGURE 7.3 Bipolar I and II Reporting Suicidal Ideation

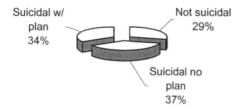

Suicidal w/
plan
34%

Not suicidal
29%

Suicidal no
plan
37%

FIGURE 7.4 Schizophrenia Group Reporting
Suicidal Ideation

Within the population four clear suicide plan categories emerged: poisoning (e.g., taking a known toxic substance or dose of a substance believed to create a toxic and lethal outcome; overdose was included in this area); suffocation, including hanging or suffocation by plastic bag; firearm (the use of a gun as the suicide weapon); and other, which included numerous methods, but cutting and motor vehicle accidents were prominently identified methods (see Figure 7.5).

GENDER AND RACE ISSUES

Among the population examined in this study there were more female admissions than male admissions, but only by 2%: female, 51%; male, 49%. Females had higher rates of verbalizing self-injury than males. Men and women between the ages of 18 and 45 demonstrated the highest rates of verbalizing self-harm. When examined in terms of ethnicity, females of all races and ethnicities verbalized the highest rates of suicidal ideation with plan. Black women had higher rates of verbalized desire for self-harm than white or Hispanic women.

THE IMPACT OF COMORBID DIAGNOSIS ON REHOSPITALIZATION FOR SUICIDE RISK

In this study we examined comorbid diagnosis in a population rehospitalized within 31 days following discharge to determine the impact on suicide risk of comorbid substance abuse and mental health diagnosis. The most significant findings were among the substance dependent population. Within the substance dependence population approximately one-third of initial admissions demonstrated suicidal ideation on admission via verbalization of plan or presence of suicide attempt or gesture.

Opioid-dependent persons verbalized the highest prevalence of suicide risk at 41.5%; alcohol-dependent persons demonstrated the second highest reporting of suicide risk at 39.7%, followed by sedative hypnotic and polysubstance abusers at 34.6% and 16.6% respectively.

Two significant changes occurred within the 31-day rehospitalization population. First, identified suicidal risk via plan or attempted suicide increased by 50 percentage points. The second and possibly more interesting change is that primary diagnosis upon readmission was no longer substance disorders. In fact, 56% of rehospitalizations had a primary psychiatric diagnosis of major depressive disorder (23%), schizophrenia (14%), or bipolar disorder (19%).

IMPLICATIONS FOR PRACTICE

The implications for practice stem from the percentage of those patients presenting with suicidal ideation in relation to the total admissions pop-

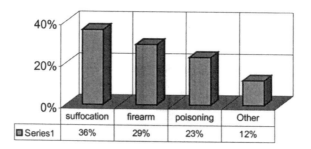

	suffocation	firearm	poisoning	Other
■ Series1	36%	29%	23%	12%

FIGURE 7.5 Verbalized Plan Method

ulation. This study indicated that persons working in psychiatric intake should give strong consideration to the presence of comorbid diagnosis and the potential for suicidal ideation and risk of harm to self and others once patients are hospitalized. Patients presenting to psychiatric intake with severe levels of anxiety and agitation and a history of substance dependence demonstrated the highest risk of harm to self and others, with a 27% greater risk of violent actions in the inpatient unit versus the general admitted populations.

In addition, a cluster of symptoms emerged within the population that indicated that the following components were consistently present in those verbalizing suicidal ideation and demonstrating suicidal risk behaviors:

- Medical illness
- Impulsivity
- Anxiousness
- Irritability
- Access to weapon
- Hopelessness
- Remarkable life stressors
- Family history of suicide
- Substance abuse and psychiatric illness comorbidity

In the population examined by this study it is important to separate two stages within suicidal ideation. The first is best described as thoughts of death: frequently persons reported "fleeting thoughts of death" or thoughts of what the world would be like without them; frequently persons reported justifying the belief that others would be better off without them in the world. The second stage includes the first stage's thought process but adds the intent to die and the planning component. Within this population patients presented with vague to well-thought-out plans of how to commit suicide. It is important to note that there no distinction was made between vague plans and concrete plans because patients were frequently reluctant to reveal their suicide plan, saving it for a later "opportunity" for suicide.

LIMITATIONS AND IMPLICATIONS FOR FURTHER INVESTIGATION

This study is exploratory in nature and provides a baseline examination of psychiatric diagnosis, comorbidity, suicide ideation, and suicide attempts. It was designed to examine emergent trends among persons presenting for initial hospitalization and rehospitalization within 31 days of discharge. Nevertheless, there appears to be an increasing prevalence of comorbid diagnosis emerging among persons at acute risk for suicide. There also appear to be alarming trends demonstrating the impact of comorbid substance and psychiatric diagnosis on risk for suicidal behaviors demonstrated via verbalization of plan and intent and actual suicide attempt.

Further examination is required to document the extent of the impact of comorbid diagnosis on patient suicide risk. Application of standardized measures and statistical analysis to determine correlation and contributing and causal factors should be undertaken in a variety of settings to document national agreement on the presence of identified risk trends. In addition, examination of treatment methodology, medication management, patients' length of stay, follow-up planning, and environmental factors should be considered.

References

American Psychiatric Association. (2002). *Diagnostic and statistical manual of mental disorders* (4th ed.). Washington, DC: Author.

Bush, K. A., Fawcett, J., & Jacobs, D. G. (2003). Clinical correlates of inpatient suicide. *Journal of Clinical Psychiatry, 64*(1), 14–19.

Institute of Medicine. (2002). *Reducing suicide: A national imperative.* Washington, DC: National Academies Press.

Jacobs, D. G. (1999). *The Harvard Medical School guide to suicide assessment and intervention.* San Francisco: Jossey Bass.

National Institute of Mental Health. (2001). *The numbers count: Mental disorders in America* (NIMH Publication No. 01-4584). Retrieved May 17, 2003, from http://www.nimh.nih.gov/publicat/numbers.cfm.

MAKING PARTICIPANT OBSERVATION RESEARCH MATTER

8

A Typology Based on 12,000 Felons

Frederic G. Reamer

During much of my career I have been privileged to wear two hats simultaneously, that of an academician (professor in a graduate school of social work) and that of a practicing professional in various settings. For years I have shuttled—often on the same day—between my academic duties and my positions as a policy analyst on a governor's staff, member of the board of commissioners of a state housing finance agency, and, most recently, as a member of a state parole board. In each instance I have sought to integrate what I have learned about research—formulating research questions, designing quantitative and qualitative empirical inquiries, gathering data, analyzing and interpreting results, and drawing on empirically based literature—with my diverse duties as a practitioner. During the years when I was active in the affordable housing field and on a governor's staff, for example, I spent considerable time using my research knowledge and skills to gain a better understanding of the magnitude and determinants of homelessness and housing shortages, the likely benefits and limitations of various policy responses, and the impact of policy initiatives.

Most recently I have drawn on my research knowledge and skills to enhance my work as a member of a state parole board. What follows is a case study of practice-based research from the vantage point of what anthropologists call a participant observer. That is, I did not embark on my research activities as a dispassionate, "objective" academician motivated primarily by intellectual curiosity and discovery. Rather, initially I sought to collect, analyze, and make use of data for my own very practical purposes—to enhance my understanding of criminal behavior and the quality of my decisions about whether to release incarcerated offenders from prison. Over time I chose to organize this knowledge in a way that might be useful to colleagues in the criminal justice, corrections, and social work fields.

Much has been written about the importance of quantitative and qualitative practice-based research. At this point in history, practitioners should not need to be convinced that they have an ethical duty to draw on the best available knowledge as they seek to understand and respond to diverse social problems such as poverty, mental and physical disability, substance abuse, domestic violence, child abuse and neglect, unemployment, homelessness, and crime and delinquency. By now we have ample evidence of the importance of using research skills to understand more about the extent and nature of the social problems that professionals aim to address and the impact of various interventions, programs, and policies. Both quantitative and qualitative research are vitally important in professionals' efforts to help people by using clinical treatment and to organize communities, administer programs, and design and implement social policy. To enhance the relevance of research and evaluation, we need to supplement traditional academic studies with the application of research methods and skills by practitioners who have compelling problems to solve.

THE CONTEXT

I have spent a considerable portion of my career working in correctional settings—a maximum-security state penitentiary, a state forensic unit (for individuals who have been found not guilty of offenses by reason of insanity or who are not competent to stand trial), and a federal correctional center. In 1992 I was appointed by the Rhode Island governor to the state parole board. As in many states, the Rhode Island Parole Board is made up of members from various disciplines and professions (specified in the state statute) who serve part-time. Each week I coordinate my academic schedule (teaching, research, faculty meetings, etc.) with my parole board schedule. Each month my parole board colleagues and I conduct approximately 150 hearings in Rhode Island's various high-security, maximum-security, medium-security, and minimum-security prisons for men and women who, by law, are eligible for parole.

Prior to each hearing I review the inmate's file (police reports, record of convictions, psychosocial assessments, institutional and disciplinary reports, summaries of inmates' involvement in various rehabilitation and educational programs, and correspondence from inmates, victims, prison officials, police, and other interested parties) and, when feasible, meet personally with victims of the inmates' crimes. The parole hearing itself includes questioning of and testimony by each inmate and, in some instances, the inmate's attorney. Following each hearing the inmate is escorted out of the room and the parole board discusses the merits of the inmate's parole application. The board then votes on whether or not to release the inmate and, if the vote is to release, at what point during the inmate's sentence (release dates range from several weeks from the hearing date to months or years down the road) and with what conditions (such as mandatory residential substance abuse treatment, domestic violence or sex offender counseling, community service, and electronic monitoring) the release should occur.

Historically many parole boards have made their decisions without the formal use of screening or risk-assessment instruments. More recently some parole boards have moved in the direction of drawing more explicitly on research-based knowledge about the correlations between various risk factors (such as age at first conviction, prior incarcerations, employment and education history, criminal history, prison disciplinary record, mental health and substance abuse profile, and marital status) and criminal behavior (Andrews & Bonta, 1998; Burke, 2001; Glancy & Regehr, 2002; Harris & Rice, 1997; Irwin & Austin, 2000; Lidz, Mulvey, & Gardner, 1993; Monahan et al., 2001; Roberts & Rock, 2002). My goal in this project was to move beyond the research literature on individual risk assessment, use aggregate data from my own experience on the parole board to develop a better understanding of the patterns of circumstances that lead to criminal behavior, and use this knowledge to inform parole decisions and design and implement meaningful responses to crime.

THE METHOD

As a member of the Rhode Island Parole Board I have conducted more than 12,000 hearings. Beginning in 2000 I decided to use qualitative research methods to review, organize, and interpret the diverse offenses committed by inmates who had appeared before me, along with the complex circumstances surrounding their crimes. Using grounded theory (Glaser & Straus, 1967; Straus & Corbin, 1990)—which entails discovering theories, concepts, propositions, and new hypotheses from qualitative data collected in the field—I sought to develop a typology of the circumstances that lead offenders to commit crimes and explore the implications of these patterns. The methodology included three principal steps (Creswell, 2002; Holosko, 2001; Reamer, 1998; Sherman & Reid, 1994). First, I developed a comprehensive list of the types of offenses of which inmates had been convicted (e.g., armed robbery, breaking and entering, rape, child molestation, driving under the influence with serious injury or death resulting, murder, arson, automobile theft, embezzlement, sale and distribution of narcotics). Second, using what qualitative researchers call first-level coding (Neuman & Kreuger, 2003), I identified initial conceptual units and placed the diverse circumstances surrounding inmates' offenses into categories. For example, patterns began to emerge with respect to inmates who committed crimes under the influence of alcohol or other drugs, inmates whose offenses appeared to be a function of their mental illness, and inmates whose offenses appeared to be the result of their poor impulse control (domestic violence, for instance) or financial desperation (e.g., chronic shoplifting). Third, I conducted second-level coding (or axial coding), during which I combined a number of smaller conceptual units into broader conceptual categories (this process is the qualitative version of what occurs when quantitative researchers conduct factor analyses where they use statistical software to examine data points in matrix form—using statistical techniques such as principal components analysis, principal factor analysis, orthogonal rotation, and structural equation modeling—to reduce a large number of variables to a smaller set of factors). Finally, I examined the patterns I had identified in an effort to highlight key themes and implications for the prevention of future crimes (Patton, 2001; Tutty, Rothery, & Grinnell, 1996). (See Reamer, 2003, for a detailed discussion of the methodology and results.)

THE RESULTS

First-Level Coding

My first-level coding of parole board cases produced a seven-category typology of the circumstances that appear to lead to criminal conduct. I generated these seven categories based on my assessment of three key dimensions: the causes of the various crimes (e.g., spontaneous conflict between spouses, drug addiction, gambling debt, workplace revenge), the diversity or types of crimes (e.g., crimes of violence, property crimes, drug possession, financial crimes), and the pattern of inmates' criminal careers (e.g., long-standing pattern of violent crimes, onset of criminal activity in middle age, isolated incident). Using these seven broad conceptually oriented categories of crimes I developed what I have named the "Typology of Criminal Circumstances," which is detailed in the following sections.

Crimes of Desperation

People who find themselves in desperate circumstances—for example, as a result of sudden debt or family crises—sometimes engage in desperate acts. Examples of crimes of desperation include burglaries committed by parents living in dire poverty who need money to feed their hungry children, fraud committed by people who are under intense pressure to pay their debt to organized crime figures, and embezzlement by white-collar offenders whose financial world has crumbled around them. Here is a representative example:

Mary L. was 18 and the mother of a severely disabled infant. Mary L. had been involved with Tony, the 31-year-old father of her child, for about 2 years. According to Mary L., Tony physically abused her, mostly when he was drunk. After her baby was born, Mary L. knew she had to leave Tony. After leaving a shelter where she stayed for a short time Mary L. was having a difficult time finding an affordable apartment and paying for food. Mary L. was arrested for shoplifting an expensive video camera from a department store; this violated her probation on earlier shoplifting charges, and the judge sentenced her to eighteen months in prison.

Crimes of Greed, Exploitation, and Opportunism

For a variety of reasons—some psychological, some cultural, and some biochemical—some people prey on others. The people who commit these predatory offenses are willing to take other people's money and property—for instance, by physical theft or identity theft—for selfish purposes. Examples of crimes of greed, exploitation, and opportunism are financial schemes and Internet scams that take advantage of vulnerable people (e.g., the elderly and people who are lonely), corporate fraud, drug deals that generate large profits, racketeering, murder for hire, arson for hire, and warehouse thefts to obtain goods for black-market sales. For example:

Marvin H., 25 years old, dropped out of school when he was in the eleventh grade. He had been suspended from high school two times for fighting and was expelled once for stealing a teacher's pocketbook. Marvin H. spent five months in the state training school for boys after being arrested for automobile theft. Since leaving high school Marvin H. has never held a steady job.

For nearly 2 years Marvin H. sold cocaine to customers around his neighborhood. "I never used the stuff," Marvin H. said. "I was just making a real good living." Marvin H. was arrested after police received a tip from a neighbor. Marvin H. was paroled after serving nine months of a one-year sentence. Two years later he was arrested again on drug-dealing charges.

Crimes of Rage

Some offenses are committed by people who are unable or unwilling to contain their anger. They respond to conflict by lashing out or assaulting others. Examples of crimes of rage include stabbings and murders that result from fierce domestic disputes, assaults resulting from "road rage" conflicts, and spontaneous intergang warfare among adolescents. For example:

Ronald B. married Jenelle B. soon after they learned that she was pregnant with their child. For the first several years of their marriage the couple got along well. More recently, however, the couple had fought constantly. During one of the couple's heated arguments, Ronald B. suddenly flew into a rage, grabbed his wife by the throat, and beat her head against the wall. The police and medical reports show that Jenelle B. had some swelling on the brain as a result. Ronald B. was serving a four-year sentence for aggravated assault.

Crimes of Revenge and Retribution

In contrast to crimes of rage, which are typically spontaneous and impulsive, crimes of revenge and retribution are much more deliberate and more likely to be the result of planning and calculation to "pay back" individuals who have allegedly mistreated the offender. Examples of crimes of revenge and retribution are planned (as opposed to spontaneous or impulsive) murders, assaults, and vengeful thefts. For example:

Belinda W., 18 years old, was dating Hal V., 42. The couple met when they both worked part-time at a county fair. Hal V. was the father of two children and was separated from his wife.

For some time Belinda W. did not tell her parents about Hal V. However, her parents found out about the relationship when they overheard a telephone conversation between the two. Belinda W.'s father became extremely upset and forbade his daughter to see Hal V. Her father said that she should not be involved with a married man 24 years her senior.

For weeks Belinda W. and her father were locked in a bitter dispute about the relationship. She was extremely resentful. One night Belinda W. broke into her father's machine shop, destroyed some of his valuable equipment, and stole cash from his safe.

Crimes of Frolic

Many offenses are committed in the context of people having fun, albeit often excessive, out-of-control fun that leads to serious mischief or mayhem. Examples of crimes of frolic are teenagers' high-speed drag races that lead to critical injury or death, serious vandalism and property destruction that is preceded by heavy drinking or drug use, and death caused by recreational gun play (e.g., Russian roulette). For example:

One night Adam K. and two friends consumed about a six-pack of beer each and drank several shots of whiskey. Toward the end of the evening Adam K. showed his friends his gun collection. He picked up one of his hunting rifles, pointed it playfully at one of his friends, and pulled the trigger, thinking that the rifle was not loaded. The rifle contained one round of ammunition; Adam K. unintentionally shot his friend in the chest, and the friend died instantly.

Crimes of Addiction

A significant percentage of criminal behavior is related to various forms of addiction. Examples of addiction-related crimes include drug possession, prostitution by drug addicts to pay for their habits, pathological gambling, driving under the influence with serious injury or death resulting, and a variety of property crimes committed to obtain goods to sell on the black market to finance addictions (e.g., automobile theft, breaking and entering, burglary, receiving stolen goods). For example:

Lawrence M., 37 years old, lived in a homeless shelter after he was evicted from his apartment for failing to pay the rent. He was a heroin addict; he lived by doing occasional odd jobs and panhandling.

One afternoon Lawrence M. was desperate to buy a bag of heroin but did not have any money. He borrowed a gun from another resident at the homeless shelter and robbed a nearby convenience store.

Crimes of Mental Illness

Many crimes are committed by people with diagnosable mental illness or brain damage. Usually these offenses are committed because of individuals' mental illness and psychiatric problems, which limit the offenders' ability to control their behavior. Examples include sex offenders who have been diagnosed with pedophilia or mental retardation, individuals with bipolar disorder who have been arrested for domestic violence, and people with schizophrenia who have been convicted of murder or assault. For example:

Arlindo P. has a history of mental illness. He was diagnosed with schizophrenia at the age of 16 and hospitalized on several occasions. Arlindo P. functions well when he takes his prescribed neuroleptic (antipsychotic) medication.

Arlindo P. became addicted to cocaine and stopped going to the local community mental health center for his medication. His schizophrenia symptoms, which involved paranoid delusions, returned. One evening Arlindo P. stabbed his roommate and injured him seriously. After his arrest Arlindo P. told police and his lawyer that he believed his roommate was a terrorist agent who was going to poison his food and water.

Second-Level Coding

The results of the first-level coding were quite useful, but my second-level coding made it clear that within each of these seven broad categories are meaningful subtypes or subsidiary patterns within the broader themes. With respect to crimes of addiction, for example, I found it important to distinguish between addictions related to drugs and alcohol and those related to gambling. With respect to crimes of rage it seemed important to distinguish among offenses involving true strangers (road rage, for example) and offenses involving family members and acquaintances (domestic disputes). With respect to crimes of greed, exploitation, and opportunism it seemed important to distinguish among street offenses (such as drug dealing for profit), white-collar financial schemes, and crimes involving serious personal injury (such as murder for hire).

This second stage of coding (axial coding) and data analysis produced various specific subcategories within each of the broad categories of criminal circumstances.

Subcategories Within Crimes of Desperation

FINANCIAL DESPERATION AND POVERTY The close connection between poverty and crime is indisputable. Although most people living in poverty do not commit serious crimes, a significant percentage of offenders are living in poverty when they commit their crimes. Some people respond to poverty by committing crimes to try to extract themselves from their desperate circumstances. For some offenders poverty is a chronic and lifelong condition; for others poverty is more acute, often the result of sudden illness or disability, divorce or separation, or unemployment.

WHITE-COLLAR FINANCIAL DESPERATION Crimes of financial desperation are not limited to people living in poverty. A significant number of financial crimes that occur out of a sense of desperation (e.g., securities or tax fraud, embezzlement) are committed by white-collar workers, people with relatively high levels of education and professional and social status.

CRIMES OF FEAR Not all crimes of desperation are financial in nature. Some offenders commit crimes because of their fear of unwanted and dire circumstances that have nothing to do with money. Examples include individuals who leave the scene of a serious automobile accident because of their fear that they will be charged with vehicular homicide, those who manipulate a company's personnel or financial records under pressure from an intimidating supervisor, and those who engage in prostitution under the coercive direction of a pimp.

DESPERATE PERSONAL CIRCUMSTANCES Many crimes of desperation involve offenders' attempts to resolve personal problems—problems that are not primarily, although they may be indirectly, financial in nature. Typically, these personal problems involve relationships with family, friends, and acquaintances. Examples include individuals who drive an automobile on a suspended license because they feel desperate to get to their jobs (and then get into a serious accident that maims another driver) and inmates who escape from a minimum-security prison to visit their seriously ill relatives.

Subcategories Within Crimes of Greed, Exploitation, and Opportunism

FINANCIAL CRIMES Crimes involving financial exploitation, greed, and opportunism are different from crimes involving financial desperation. Crimes involving financial exploitation, greed, and opportunism—such as scams designed to fleece the elderly, sales of shoddy merchandise, illegal drug sales for profit, racketeering, consumer fraud, securities theft, accounting fraud, commercial bribery, bankruptcy fraud, and computer crimes—are rooted in a sense of entitlement rather than despair. Offenders who commit these crimes tend to be much more calculating, cunning, and manipulative than those who commit crimes as a result of a sense of desperation.

ORGANIZED CRIME Organized crime in the United States dates as far back as the colonial period. Contemporary examples of organized crime that is motivated by greed, exploitation, and opportunism include drug trafficking, firearms smuggling, money laundering, gambling, labor racketeering, loan-sharking, prostitution, pornography, kidnapping, fraud, robbery, stolen property and shipments, and murder.

GANG EXPLOITATION Many communities throughout the United States struggle to cope with problems involving gangs whose activities involve various forms of greed, exploitation, and opportunism. Gangs operate in diverse forms, including street gangs mostly made up of youths and members of racial and ethnic minorities. Some gangs exist for many years and control geographical turf. Other gangs have shorter lives and are less territorial.

SEXUAL EXPLOITATION Some individuals who commit sex-related offenses are better described as exploiters rather than as sexually deviant people or people with sexual disorders (such as pedophilia, exhibitionism, fetishism, and voyeurism), although many sex offenders have some form of major mental illness. Sexual exploiters take advantage of unique circumstances to sexually abuse victims; they are manipulative and disregard the rights and feelings of others in order to pursue their own pleasure (e.g., a mother's boyfriend who fondles the mother's teenage daughter or a college student who date rapes his girlfriend).

Subcategories Within Crimes of Rage

FAMILY AND RELATIONSHIP VIOLENCE A significant portion of violence involves disputes among family members. Such violence tends to take the form of physical attacks, psychological or emotional aggression and abuse, sexual assaults or threatened sexual assaults, and neglectful behavior.

SOCIAL VIOLENCE This form of violence occurs between people who are not members of the same family. Typical situations involving social violence include conflicts among casual acquaintances, "drinking buddies," fellow drug users, and neighbors.

WORKPLACE VIOLENCE Typical incidents of workplace violence involve disputes between coworkers and angry outbursts by employees who

have been disciplined or sanctioned by management.

STRANGER RAGE Many violent incidents occur between strangers who encounter each other. Examples include violence that erupts when strangers exchange words in public places (such as restaurants or stores) or occurs as a result of road rage.

Subcategories Within Crimes of Revenge and Retribution

FAMILY AND RELATIONSHIP REVENGE AND RETRIBUTION Most crimes of revenge and retribution (which may involve physical, emotional, or financial abuse) involve people who have some kind of intimate relationship with each other: spouses, partners, children, parents, siblings, and other relatives. The most common examples involve estranged partners who were involved in an intimate relationship.

ACQUAINTANCE REVENGE AND RETRIBUTION Conflict between friends and acquaintances sometimes leads to intense anger and resentment. When the conflict is protracted and festers over time, one party may feel the need for revenge and retribution that requires far more calculation and planning than a more spontaneous rage-filled response.

COWORKER REVENGE AND RETRIBUTION Although many incidents of workplace violence occur spontaneously, some involve more deliberate, premeditated revenge and retribution. Some vengeful acts involve violence and some involve psychological torment or financial sabotage.

AUTHORITY FIGURE REVENGE AND RETRIBUTION Some crimes of revenge and retribution are directed at people who are or were in influential positions of authority in the offender's life. Examples include students who become infuriated with teachers who assigned a failing grade; criminals who rail against prosecutors, parole board members, or judges who rendered adverse decisions; and prison inmates who want to harm correctional officers who disciplined them.

Subcategories Within Crimes of Frolic

THRILL-SEEKING BEHAVIOR Some crimes of frolic occur when a group of people decides to engage in thrilling, high-risk activity such as drag racing that results in serious injury or malicious vandalism of high-security settings (e.g., a school or construction site).

ENTERTAINMENT Other crimes of frolic take the form of pure entertainment and recreation rather than intense thrill-seeking activity. Thrill-seekers typically aim for some kind of adrenalin rush, whereas those involved in more recreational pursuits often have more capacity for self-control but fail to exercise good judgment.

FROLIC UNDER THE INFLUENCE Alcohol and other drugs are involved in a significant percentage of cases involving frolic. Often these offenders are not bona fide alcoholics or addicts; rather, their excessive use and abuse of substances fueled their criminal conduct.

Subcategories Within Crimes of Addiction

SUBSTANCE ABUSE People with addictions or whose offenses are related to addiction commit a remarkably large percentage of all crimes. Such offenses typically involve possession, distribution, manufacture, or cultivation of drugs; violent acts (such as murder, rape, domestic assault, robbery) that are committed by people who are under the influence of drugs or alcohol; and property crime (such as burglary, larceny, shoplifting, automobile theft) that is committed to obtain goods to sell (fence) for money to buy drugs.

PATHOLOGICAL GAMBLING Access to legalized gambling has grown exponentially in the form of casino betting (blackjack, roulette, poker, baccarat, slot machines, keno, craps, sports betting, etc.), state lotteries, and horse and dog track betting. Many crimes are committed by people who are unable to control their gambling and who, as a result, engage in fraud, drug selling, robberies, shoplifting, and other forms of theft to support their addiction.

Subcategories Within Crimes of Mental Illness

SCHIZOPHRENIA AND PSYCHOTIC DISORDERS A significant percentage of offenders with major mental illness have been diagnosed with schizophrenia (where there is evidence of some combination of delusions, hallucinations, incoherence, and grossly disorganized or catatonic

behavior) or another psychotic disorder (although relatively few people with these disorders commit serious crimes).

MOOD DISORDERS These disorders entail a serious disturbance in the individual's basic mood or affect. Major depression and bipolar disorder are prominent among offenders with major mental illness.

ANXIETY DISORDERS Offenders suffering with anxiety disorders have difficulty managing stress in their lives. Common anxiety disorders among offenders with major mental illness are generalized anxiety disorder and posttraumatic stress disorder (e.g., in offenders whose difficulties are a result of having been sexually abused as a child).

PARAPHILIAS Many sex offenders have been diagnosed with the serious psychiatric disorder of paraphilia. Paraphilias that lead to criminal behavior involve persistent, intense sexually arousing fantasies and urges and behaviors involving children or other nonconsenting individuals.

MENTAL RETARDATION Some individuals commit crimes because of their severely limited intelligence and cognitive ability. These offenders are often very impressionable and vulnerable to pressure from other individuals (and are sometimes referred to as "naive offenders").

DISSOCIATIVE DISORDERS Occasionally offenders manifest symptoms of dissociation, including severe impairment of consciousness, memory, identity, or perception. These symptoms may be solely psychiatric in nature or the function of traumatic brain injury or temporal lobe epilepsy. Examples include people who commit crimes while suffering from amnesia or in the context of a multiple personality disorder (dissociative identity disorder).

PRAXIS: MOVING FROM PRACTICE TO RESEARCH AND BACK

Once I concluded my analysis and data coding and the development of the Typology of Criminal Circumstances, I began thinking about the practical implications of this conceptual framework. As a parole board member I was interested in exploring the relevance of these findings to my decisions about prison inmates. As a social work educator and researcher my principal goal was to generate knowledge that can be applied in various practice settings. More specifically, I was concerned about the ways in which my typology might be helpful to professionals who work with offenders and who are interested in crime prevention: police, judges, social workers, corrections officials, and probation and parole officers. That is, I wanted my research results to be directly relevant to practice.

My primary claim, based on my data analysis, is that meaningful attempts to address the crime problem must take into consideration the diverse circumstances in offenders' lives that contribute to their criminal conduct. My research findings suggest that the vast majority of criminal acts arise from offenders' sense of desperation (financial and interpersonal); greed, exploitation, and opportunism; rage; wish for revenge and retribution; eagerness for frolic and entertainment; addictions to alcohol, other drugs, and/or gambling; and mental illness.

It is not possible in this limited space to provide a comprehensive summary of implications and recommendations. Briefly, my findings seem to suggest that any worthwhile crime prevention strategy must address both clinical and broader policy and environmental issues. For example, many offenders have mental health-, relationship-, and addictions-related problems that require attention if we are to prevent these problems from leading to further crime. In addition, we must also address broader societal and structural issues that involve public policy debates, economic issues, racism, and so on. To prevent crimes of desperation, for example, we must focus on issues of poverty and help vulnerable people enhance their educational and vocational skills. Comprehensive mental health services can help prevent crimes associated with mental illness and with individuals' difficulty controlling their rage and impulses. Programs that challenge so-called criminal thinking and values may help prevent crimes of exploitation, greed, opportunism, and frolic. Also, a very significant percentage of crime will be prevented by the implementation of effective addictions-related services. Some offenders may not be amenable or responsive to treatment and rehabilitation and therefore need to be incarcerated for public-safety purposes.

The main point is that criminal justice professionals should draw on research-based knowledge to enhance their design and delivery of diverse crime prevention and control programs, including evidence-based knowledge concerning the effectiveness of various interventions (probation, intensive supervision, specialized caseloads, curfew restrictions, electronic monitoring, residential programs, incarceration, etc.), public policies (e.g., those related to various policing strategies and the use of drug and gun courts, alternatives to incarceration, and sentencing guidelines), and risk-assessment instruments (Andrews & Bonta, 1998; Monahan et al., 2001; Roberts & Rock, 2002; Siegel, 2000; Tonry, 1998; Wilson & Petersilia, 1995).

LESSONS LEARNED

When I take a step back and reflect on this multiyear research endeavor, several key lessons emerge:

1. It is feasible for human service professionals who are actively involved in practice to use classic participant observer strategies to gather meaningful data.
2. Practitioners can gather data over long periods of time without detracting from their principal professional duties. Data can be collected unobtrusively, without interfering with professional functions and obligations.
3. Data gathered from practice settings can be analyzed and interpreted inductively to generate useful, relevant conceptual frameworks and typologies. These frameworks and typologies can be informally shared with one's immediate colleagues to enhance their practice and decision making. The frameworks can also be introduced more formally into the professional and academic knowledge base through published literature.
4. The process of gathering data as a participant observer can do more than facilitate the generation of knowledge; it can also enhance the quality of the participant observer's own practice. As my data collection unfolded, I found myself conceptualizing about my parole board duties, and the circumstances that led to the inmates' crimes, in novel and fruitful ways. The research process itself helped me to think in new ways about the causes of crime and constructive ways to prevent crime. I believe this process has enhanced my decisions as a parole board member.

5. Conducting practice-based research as a participant observer is an important way for professionals to satisfy their ethical obligation to draw on research-based evidence to enhance the quality of their work. As one prominent code of ethics, the National Association of Social Workers Code of Ethics (1999), states:

> Social workers should base practice on recognized knowledge, including empirically based knowledge, relevant to social work and social work ethics. (standard 4.01[c])

> Social workers should monitor and evaluate policies, the implementation of programs, and practice interventions. (standard 5.02[a])

> Social workers should critically examine and keep current with emerging knowledge relevant to social work and fully use evaluation and research evidence in their professional practice. (standard 5.02[c])

Clearly, earnest attempts to draw on and apply research-based knowledge are consistent with professionals' ethical obligations. Practitioners have a duty to base their practice on relevant research knowledge generated by colleagues and, as in the present study, should actively explore opportunities to generate research-based knowledge from their own work. Anything less undermines professionals' efforts to enhance human well-being and meet the compelling needs of vulnerable people.

References

Andrews, D. A., & Bonta, J. (1998). *The psychology of criminal conduct* (2nd ed.). Cincinnati, OH: Anderson.

Burke, P. (2001). Probation and parole violations: An overview of critical issues. In M. M. Carter (Ed.), *Responding to parole and probation violations* (pp. 5–12). Silver Spring, MD: Center for Effective Public Policy.

Creswell, J. W. (2002). *Research design: Qualitative, quantitative, and mixed methods approaches* (3rd ed.). Thousand Oaks, CA: Sage.

Glancy, G., & Regehr, C. (2002). Step-by-step guidelines for assessing sexual predators. In A. R. Roberts & G. J. Greene (Eds.), *Social workers' desk reference* (pp. 702–708). New York: Oxford University Press.

Glaser, B., & Straus, A. (1967). *The discovery of grounded theory: Strategies for qualitative research*. Chicago: Aldine.

Harris, G. T., & Rice, M. E. (1997). Risk appraisal and management of violent behavior. *Psychiatric Services, 48*, 1168–1176.

Holosko, M. (2001). Overview of qualitative research methods. In B. Thyer (Ed.), *The handbook of social work research methods* (pp. 263–272). Thousand Oaks, CA: Sage.

Irwin, J., & Austin, J. (2000). *It's about time: America's imprisonment binge* (3rd ed.). Belmont, CA: Wadsworth.

Lidz, C. W., Mulvey, E. P., & Gardner, W. (1993). The accuracy of predictions of violence to others. *Journal of the American Medical Association, 269*(8), 1007–1011.

Monahan, J., Steadman, H. J., Silver, E., Appelbaum, P., Mulvey, E., Roth, L., et al. (2001). *Rethinking risk assessment: The MacArthur study of mental disorder and violence*. New York: Oxford University Press.

Neuman, W. L., & Kreuger, L. W. (2003). *Social work research methods: Qualitative and quantitative applications*. Boston: Allyn and Bacon.

Patton, M. (2001). *Qualitative research and evaluation methods* (3rd ed.). Thousand Oaks, CA: Sage.

Reamer, F. G. (1998). *Social work research and evaluation skills: A case-based, user-friendly approach*. New York: Columbia University Press.

Reamer, F. G. (2003). *Criminal lessons: Case studies and commentary on crime and justice*. New York: Columbia University Press.

Roberts, A. R., & Rock, M. (2003). An overview of forensic social work and risk assessments with the dually diagnosed. In A. R. Roberts & G. J. Greene (Eds.), *Social workers' desk reference* (pp. 661–668). New York: Oxford University Press.

Sherman, E., & Reid W. (1994). *Qualitative research in social work*. New York: Columbia University Press.

Siegel, L. (2000). *Criminology: Theories, patterns, and typologies* (7th ed.). Belmont, CA: Wadsworth.

Straus, A., & Corbin, J. (1990). *Basics of qualitative research: Grounded theory procedures and techniques*. Newbury Park, CA: Sage.

Tonry, M. (Ed.). (1998). *The handbook of crime and punishment*. New York: Oxford University Press.

Tutty, L. M., Rothery, M. A., & Grinnell, R. M., Jr. (1996). *Qualitative research for social workers*. Boston: Allyn and Bacon.

Wilson, J. Q., & Petersilia, J. (Eds.). (1995). *Crime: Public policies for crime control*. San Francisco: ICS Press.

9 COMPUTER TECHNOLOGY AND SOCIAL WORK

Carrie J. Petrucci, Stuart A. Kirk, & William J. Reid

Whether technology is utilized is dependent on two things: the characteristics of the technology itself and how receptive the audience is (Schoech, 1999). The use of computer technology in social work is no exception. After much initial reticence social work researchers and practitioners have become increasingly familiar with integration of computer technology in practice, research, and education (see, for example, special journal issues edited by Butterfield, 1983; Raymond, Ginsberg, & Gohagon, 1998; Menon & Coe, 2000; Menon & Brown, 2001). Clearly, the potential uses of computer technology are vast and varied. In recent work in which we took a broad historical view of computer technology and social work, we identified four key "quests" in an attempt to grasp the boundaries of this area (Kirk, Reid, & Petrucci, 2002). These included the quest for efficiency, in which computer technology was seen as a means toward achieving accountability; the quest to integrate research into practice, with single-case research being a prime example; the quest for improved services to clients, which included decision support systems, expert systems, and clinical assessment systems; and the quest for communication, which looked at on-line support groups for clients and professionals as well as information retrieval systems. In our assessment social work practitioners have displayed reluctance to integrate computer technology into their day-to-day practices largely because the technology itself did not directly address their needs, giving credence to Schoech's (1999) notion that the characteristics of the technology and receptivity to the technology are key to utilization. Luckily (or so we would suggest), the characteristics of computer technology continue to improve in their direct application to practice and their ease of use. Applications of interest to practitioners,

such as programs for record keeping, scheduling, monitoring, and clinical assessment and testing are becoming more widely used and more readily accepted (Schoech, 1999).

Increased computer technology use in practice has advantages beyond increasing practitioners' effectiveness and efficiency. Computer technology's inherent record-keeping function also opens the door to a renewed discussion of a practice-based research agenda. Computer technology was initially heralded as the "answer" to agency-based research (Reid, 1978) that would give researchers and administrators the needed documentation and analysis to demonstrate program effectiveness. The technology fell short of this goal as the characteristics of the technology itself made accomplishing this task far more complex than it appeared to be in theory. If we have learned anything, however, it is that computer technology advances more quickly than most of us can keep up with. Almost 30 years after the initial excitement about the potential realization of research-based practice, there is again renewed interest in this topic as the accessibility of computer technology and the receptivity to its use continues to advance.

This chapter will discuss computer technologies specific to social work practice that are applicable in a research-based practice and evaluation context. First, we will look at the social work profession's earliest impressions of computer technology and discuss how two opposing positions, one of a social work educator and another of a practitioner, set up polemical viewpoints of computer technology in the 1960s that remain with us today. We will then discuss how computer technology has assisted the integration of research into practice and how it has changed the way social workers view service provision. Finally, we will look at specific technologies useful in a research-based practice context. These include clinical assessment, on-line therapy groups, single-case research, decision support systems, and expert systems. We will conclude with some predictions of our own that, by the time this chapter reaches publication, may again be outpaced by the ubiquitous changes inherent in computer technology.

EARLY IMPRESSIONS: OPPOSING VIEWS OF COMPUTER TECHNOLOGY

The earliest article we could find about computers in the major social work journals appeared in *Child Welfare* in 1967 and was titled "Social Casework—Science or Art?" (Teicher, 1967). In it, Morton Teicher, a dean of a school of social work, rails against the notion that social casework can be a form of science and that computers have any useful role in practice. He stresses that casework calls for the creative skill of the artist and warns about the dehumanizing effects of computers that will eliminate individual worth, human freedom, and responsibility. He describes game theory as a recent application of computers in the military and business and argues that the use of quantitative data in social work is inappropriate because social workers deal in values that are not reducible to the mathematical language of computers. These machines, he argues, require clear and structured information that is simply not available for most social work situations. Too many idiosyncrasies about the client and the situation are unknown. People are too complex to convert to numbers for processing, and to do so is to ignore individual qualities. Teicher identifies a conflict between intuition and intellect: social work practice is doing and feeling, not scientific investigation. Social work offers skill that is based on knowledge and experience, used with conditional intuition, refined hunches, disciplined instinct, and tempered faith. Computers are to Teicher a threat to the profession.

A year later in *Social Casework*, in the second article about computers to appear in the social work literature, "Developing a Data Storage and Retrieval System" (1968), Ivan Vasey, a physician and director of a mental health agency, waxes enthusiastic about how computerization can benefit social agencies. His article is a case study of how "modern" electronic data-processing techniques can improve the efficiency

and quality of a clinic's social services without increasing the staff workload. Today his description seems elementary: developing common forms, gathering client data, having the data keypunched on cards, involving staff in these developments, and producing simple reports. The clinic he discusses in the article used a time-share computer at another location. His agency entered more than 1,200 cases with up to 400 items per case into a database; it also entered information on 100 control families and then analyzed follow-up data on its clients, thus merging administrative and research functions within a direct practice agency.

Vasey's article traces the process of integrating a computerized data-processing system into social work practice and foreshadows what will become core elements for success: involve all levels of staff from the beginning so that the system is useful and they have a stake in it; and coordinate face-to-face communication between data-processing staff and program staff during development of the system, not only to decrease the possibility of animosity but also to develop a system that is meaningful to program staff and feasible for the computer to run. He also notes the positive "unintended consequence" of the staff's becoming interested in the data produced by the system and pursuing research questions as a result, an embryonic version of the practitioner-as-researcher concept pursued in the following decade. He concludes that a computerized record-keeping system can improve services and save staff time, that clerks are capable of extracting and coding data reliably, and that his staff showed great interest and excitement in being a part of a "forward-looking" agency.

These two early articles offer a glimpse of developments to come. Vasey foreshadows the optimism surrounding computers, and Teicher anticipates the concern for harm to clients and workers and the dehumanization of social services. In fact, much of what was published in the 1960s and 1970s about concerns and implementation issues for computer technology remains pertinent today.

THE EVOLUTION OF COMPUTER TECHNOLOGY IN RESEARCH-BASED PRACTICE SETTINGS

As Vasey's article demonstrates, many commentators saw computers as a means of promoting research within agencies and allowing practitioners to do research. In the early stages, Fuller (1970) was the most optimistic. He believed that the two greatest barriers to research in practice settings were lack of time and lack of statistical competence. He argued that computer technology brought "research within the range of almost every practicing social worker" (p. 608) and saw no reason why every practitioner could not learn the elements of the FORTRAN computer programming language in order to do statistical computations. Others made similar claims, suggesting that with only a few hours' training, agency staff could be taught early versions of SPSS, a statistical package for computerized data analysis (Hoshino & McDonald, 1975).

In the 1970s the very nature of applied research in agencies was thought to be changing. For example, Reid (1974, 1975, 1978) foresaw the agency functioning as a "research machine," which would use computerized information systems to generate a limitless variety of specific studies at a fraction of what they would cost if carried out by traditional methods. Some spectacular examples of this kind of research did appear. For instance, Fanshel (1977) used a multiagency information system in New York City to produce a study of parental visits to children in foster care; the sample consisted of more than 20,000 cases. However, this mode of research did not become the major force that Reid and other computer advocates had predicted. The notion that sophisticated information systems able to generate research studies would rapidly develop turned out to be excessively optimistic for its time. It was believed that computers could support many research functions, but agencies would need specialized personnel to analyze their data quickly in order to provide a feedback loop useful to practitioners (Reid, 1974). Hoshino and McDonald (1975) promoted this research-in-the-practice-setting model, thinking that there would be no additional monetary costs if, in the name of accountability, agencies evaluated their own service delivery on an ongoing basis. Research must be integrated into everyday agency practice, and staff involvement is crucial in identifying important outcome variables and interpreting findings (Hoshino & McDonald, 1975). This advice, first offered by Vasey (1968), would be restated again by many authors in the coming decades.

Relatively early in the evolution of computer technology a few social workers could envision an expansive role for computer technology in practice. For example, Paul Abels offered an upbeat and hopeful view in "Can Computers Do Social Work?" (1972), noting that social workers were well behind psychiatrists and psychologists in using computers for tasks such as interviewing and assessment. He characterized resistance as due to the "antihuman" perception that social workers have of computers. Fred Vondracek and his colleagues (Vondracek, Urban, & Parsonage, 1974) argued that computers can greatly improve service delivery by promoting better coordination and integration across agencies. Computers are tools that liberate direct service practitioners from menial tasks so that they have more time to address humanitarian concerns. Technology can enable and enhance the quality and quantity of services to clients by removing the mounds of paperwork and red tape endemic to bureaucracies (Boyd, Hylton, & Price, 1978; Vondracek et al., 1974). By 1990, with greater practitioner and agency access to computers, there was great optimism that computers would transform practice routines. Although examples of more advanced computer use in practice exist, computers were not yet being used to examine caseloads or to improve practice (Taber & DiBello, 1990). The aforementioned authors represented a small but persistent group of staunch promoters who saw computer technology's potential for assisting with important direct practice tasks such as intake, assessment, record keeping, data analysis, decision making, and coordination of services (Abels, 1972; Fuller, 1970; Hoshino & McDonald, 1975; Schoech & Arangio, 1979; Vondracek et al., 1974). Since their early advocacy, progress has been made in practice-based computer applications.

TECHNOLOGY-BASED SOCIAL WORK PRACTICE METHODS

Twenty years after personal computers entered the mainstream, practitioners now have available to them a steadily growing number of technology options that can be integrated into practice. Although no agreement on how to categorize computer technologies exists, Schoech (1999) broadly categorizes computer applications as generic (database and word processing programs); research (statistical analysis, neural networks, computer-assisted surveys); education (computer-aided instruction and simulations); and assistive technology (technology used to assist mobility, access, communication, sensory aids, etc.). In this discussion, we are most interested in applications that would assist research-based practice.

Schoech (1999) further divides applications related to direct service practitioners into two types: those that help practitioners manage and report their work and those that support the practitioner–client interactions. Two examples of these will be discussed next: clinical assessment and treatment options. A third category, single case studies or single-system designs by definition would be considered both a direct practice application and a research application. Schoech (1999) also identifies five management applications (data processing, management information systems, knowledge-based systems based on artificial intelligence, decision support systems, and performance support systems) of interest to agency administrators and researchers. We will focus on expert systems as an example of knowledge-based systems and decision-based systems because of their potential to contribute to research-based practice. In discussing these, it becomes clear that applications do not always fit easily into one category or another. Applications have attributes that may be of interest to management, researchers, and practitioners. Our review is not exhaustive; we only introduce the capabilities of some of what is currently available.

Clinical Assessment

Computer-Assisted Assessment

The nature of some practice tasks makes it easier to capitalize on computer technology to facilitate them. Initial assessment of clients is one such task, particularly when the primary purpose is informational rather than therapeutic (Schoech, 1999). Computerized assessment has been more easily accepted than the more sophisticated uses of computer technology such as expert systems. Perhaps this is because the role of assessment technology clearly is to assist practitioners rather than to replace them, or because its time-saving capacity is clear. Assessment involves the collection of various small, discrete pieces of information through self-reporting, usually following a structured or semistructured format compatible with computer data entry methods.

Moreover, initially, clients are often more willing to share personal information with a computer than an individual (Schoech, 1999).

The undisputed pioneers in computer-assisted assessment in social work have been Walter Hudson and his associates. Through the development of the Client Assessment System (CAS) they have integrated current computer technology with up-to-date, empirically tested assessment tools. CAS was created with the computer novice in mind and can be used interactively with the client or the social worker. It contains twenty standardized multiple-item assessment scales that have been developed and validated over several decades such as a global screening inventory, partner-abuse checklists, and behavioral checklists for children. Clients can input the intake data, or social workers can do so in an interview format (Nurius & Hudson, 1988a; 1988b). The CAS has a user-friendly interface, so almost anyone who can reach the keyboard and read the screen can perform the assessment. As important, CAS is structured in such a way that agency-specific assessments can be added. Finally, CAS facilitates client monitoring and evaluation and accommodates the many functions necessary throughout the life of a case such as transferring the case, writing progress notes about it, or closing it. Nurius and Hudson (1988a) are quick to point out that a computer cannot replace clinicians. Computers cannot do all that a practitioner can do, such as noting the demeanor of a client or easily recognizing important idiosyncratic contextual factors. In short, CAS was developed by social workers for social workers, and while it has its limitations, its benefits are evident (Franklin, Nowicki, Trapp, Schwab, & Peterson, 1993).

Computer-Assisted Interviews

Social science research shares with social work practice a heavy dependence on respondent/client interviews for relevant information. In survey research the standard method of data collection was face-to-face interviews in which the social worker would use a structured and at times complex written questionnaire to elicit responses from an interviewee. For reasons of cost, many survey and marketing organizations eventually opted for telephone interviews. Then, with the development of computer technology, they began to use computer-assisted telephone interviews (CATI) in which the interviewer follows the prompts on a computer screen in asking questions and recording answers, thereby eliminating the need for a separate data entry step (Baker, 1992). An additional innovation has been computer-assisted personal interviews (CAPI) in which the interviewer uses a small laptop computer in conducting face-to-face interviews. Thus the programmed computer plays a direct role in guiding the interaction between interviewer and respondent, setting the pace of the interview, checking the responses and response patterns immediately, and jumping through the various contingency sections of the questionnaire. And, unlike in computer-assisted telephone interviewing, the computer's presence and role are openly visible to the respondent.

The use of CAPI has some obvious relevance for intake assessments, needs assessment, outcome and follow-up measurement, and studies of client satisfaction with services—traditional clinical tasks that use scientific survey methods. To date, however, CAPI is still primarily a tool of social work researchers rather than a routine practice method. Nonetheless, this computer application could easily be adopted for routine client assessments and evaluation of service outcomes.

Treatment Programs, On-line Support Groups, and Conferencing

On-line Groups and E-therapy

The new modes of communication have been pressed into service relatively quickly to extend the help provided by practitioners. It is only a short leap from e-mail and chat rooms to on-line support groups and therapy sessions (O'Neill, 2001). The fact that many of these applications can document what is taking place in the therapeutic relationship through written e-mail messages creates a potential for tracking the research process for practice-based research purposes. Computers and telephones are being used as the media for self-help and support groups, the latter moderated by a therapist (Meier, 1997; Finn & Lavitt, 1994). An early survey of 213 group workers revealed that only 6 had experience with telephone groups and 7 with computer groups (Schopler, Galinsky, & Abell, 1997). Internet-based therapy may have an uphill climb to be accepted by therapists. In a study that included 378 masters of social work (MSW) students across 4 schools, more than half

of the students said that they did not think that e-therapy could be as effective as in-person counseling (Finn, 2002). Students did see an adjunct and follow-up role for e-therapy. In another study, however, MSW students were exposed to three types of web-based group techniques—discussion group forum, chat room, and a listserve—as part of their computer class for group work (Abell & Galinsky, 2002). Based on a small sample ($n = 38$) pretest/posttest design, students' knowledge and comfort level with computer-based groups increased. Students also reported that they would be more likely to utilize a computer group after exposure to these techniques. It is unclear how common on-line support groups may be today. Finn (2002) groups several Internet-related therapy services under the phrase *e-therapy*. Based on his Internet searches conducted in November 2001, he identified 18 to 36 e-therapists with social work degrees. More than 250 private practice e-therapy Web sites have been counted (Finn, 2002). On-line support groups can occur *simultaneously*, meaning that members can gather via their home computers at the same time to communicate with each other in real time, or *asynchronously*, meaning that members can read and send messages at their convenience (Schopler, Abell, & Galinsky, 1998). The benefits of on-line groups include increased accessibility, convenience, anonymity, and improvements to the group process. The anticipated problems or disadvantages are inability to discern interpersonal cues, technological issues, group process issues, and professional and organizational concerns (Schopler, Galinsky, & Abell, 1997). Of course, on-line support groups are limited to the written word and participants' ability to communicate in writing. Advances in computer technology, such as affordable videoconferencing, may alter how on-line support groups are used in the future.

Virtual Reality

Computers creating virtual environments have been used in treatment. Gary Holden and colleagues (Holden, Bearlson, Rode, Rosenberg, & Fishman, 1999) used STARBRIGHT World, a three-dimensional, multiuser, virtual environment, to link seriously ill, hospitalized children into an interactive, on-line community. The children participated in a cartoon-like world that appeared on their computer screens by selecting a character to represent them and moving that character through the virtual reality to encounter and communicate with other characters (hospitalized children) doing the same thing in real time via voice and videoconferencing technology. The study attempted to determine whether use of such technology in pediatric care would decrease pain intensity, pain aversiveness, and anxiety levels. The results were equivocal, but the intervention represented an application of computer technology to direct practice.

Treatment Programs

Interactive computer programs are also being developed as a "play therapy" approach in counseling (Cowan, 2002). Children's familiarity with and interest in computers can be capitalized on with carefully constructed computer programs that can maintain the child's attention and encourage communication with the therapist. In "Bruce's Multimedia Story" a favorite children's book was converted to a computer program that allowed the child to navigate through a series of choices in the computer program. The story imitates a child welfare placement situation as it follows a dog named Bruce who must find a home with a new family. The author describes another program for slightly older children that emphasizes an action/choice/consequence sequence that deals with behavioral problems and their consequences. Children playing the game can choose from a series of choices that the main character, Billy, is confronted with (for example, he steals money from his foster parents). The children playing also observe the consequences that Billy encounters based on his choices. Both of these programs depend on the interaction of a trained therapist to utilize the computer program as a tool to engage the child in a therapeutic process that deals with the child's own thoughts and feelings (Cowan, 2002).

Single-Case Research

One of the best-known methods for evaluating practice is single case research, also referred to as single-system designs (Bloom, Fischer, & Orme, 1999). Advantages to this approach include the practitioner's ability to specify characteristics of the subject, the setting, and the procedure and relate these to outcomes on a case-by-case basis—something that group research designs often cannot do (Mattaini, 1996).

Clinical researchers interested in promoting the use of single-subject designs to make practice more scientific quickly saw how computers could be employed to inform practice, increase effectiveness, and promote accountability (Benbenishty & Ben-Zaken, 1988; Bronson & Blythe, 1987). Computers would make data analysis faster and easier, thereby circumventing the common barriers of practitioners' lack of statistical know-how, time to input and analyze the data, and agency support (Bronson & Blythe, 1987). Moreover, the data from individual practitioners conducting single-case research potentially can be aggregated at the agency level (Benbenishty, 1996; 1997). It is difficult to say what role single-case design will continue to have in practice, but the potential to bridge the gap between research and practice has been consistently noted (Bloom, Fischer, & Orme, 1999; Kirk & Reid, 2002; Mattaini, 1996). Perhaps as the user-friendliness of computer software continues to advance, practitioners' utilization of this method will also increase.

Over the years, attempts have been made to integrate single-case research strategies, with only modest success (Benbenishty & Ben-Zaken, 1988; Bronson & Blythe, 1987). In a recent study, social work faculty at Yeshiva University in New York dedicated a one-semester course to single-system design for their cohort of MSW students (Conboy, Auerbach, Beckerman, Schnall, & LaPorte, 2000). The authors developed a user-friendly computer program specifically set up to input the data, generate the graphs, and conduct the statistical analyses for students as they conducted single-system designs in their internships. Students overwhelmingly responded positively (95%) when asked whether the computer program added a valuable component to the research. As important, 80% of the students said the program was helpful as a tool to evaluate their practice. Almost all students (89%) found the program easy to use (Conboy et al., 2000).

Decision Support Systems

Decision support systems are a natural outgrowth of data processing and management information systems (MIS), with their main purpose being effectiveness of practice (Schoech, 1995; 1999). A decision support system is a computer-based processing application designed to help professionals make complex decisions

(Schoech & Schkade, 1980) such as those prompted by the question, What if this were the case? The systems answer these questions by using statistical models based on algorithms.

Decision support systems were expected to play a role in organizing and disseminating the profession's knowledge base. Some believed that they could help by translating the knowledge of experienced workers so that it could be utilized by others (Schwab, Bruce, & McRoy, 1986). For example, Schwab and colleagues (1986) explain that expertise in child welfare cannot be easily articulated, captured, stored, and passed on to future generations of child placement practitioners. To remedy this, the authors developed a software program that could make placement recommendations based on a database containing the records of 2,799 children in various types of placements. Boyd and colleagues (Boyd, Pruger, Chase, Clark, & Miller, 1981) developed and studied the integration of a decision support system in a large in-home supportive services agency with the goal of regulating equitable allocation of awards among clients across three county offices. These studies point out various ways that a decision support system can be helpful to caseworkers: in assisting with routine tasks such as filling out and printing forms, helping a worker through decision steps, offering options for unstructured queries, and generating reports that explain decision making. Other studies of decision support systems for child welfare placement decisions (Schwab, Bruce, & McRoy 1985; 1986) and for in-home support services resource allocation (Rimer, 1986) were successful in part because they focused on discrete decisions and allowed staff members to help develop the systems (Schwab et al., 1986).

In a more recent evaluation that tracked decision-support system use for youth probation services over a 3-year period, it was found that probation officers used the decision support system in only about 1 out of 5 cases (Savaya, Monnickendam, & Waysman, 2000). Later analysis of the data revealed that the decision made by the practitioner and the decision made by the decision support system were different in 39% of the cases, but practitioners changed their recommendations in only 7.6% of these cases. Factors found to predict usage of the decision support system included the "probation officer's personal assessment of the relevance of the DSS to his or her work" (p. 10), which explained the greatest amount of variance, followed by the particular office where the probation officers were located, the probation officer's having a rational decision-making style, and the probation officer's overall perception of the system's importance to the agency's national administration. The study's authors highlight three familiar areas in their discussion of barriers to system usage: perceived relevance, staff involvement, and management support. Survey results showed that most probation officers did not understand the purpose or rationale for the decision support system and therefore did not see its relevance. As was suggested by Vasey (1968) and Teicher (1967) many years earlier, probation staff who were involved in the system's development were found to be far more invested in it compared to those who were not. Similarly, when probation staff observed that management did not place a high priority on the usage of the decision support system, many of the workers also placed less importance on it (Savaya et al., 2000).

Expert Systems

Expert systems have been defined as "software applications that mimic processes to perform tasks at skill levels comparable to human experts" (Schoech, 1999, p. 91). Their primary purpose is to organize a knowledge base in a particular area (Schoech, 1999). Expert systems are more advanced than decision support systems because they attempt to model or simulate professional decision-making processes themselves. Few expert systems have gone beyond experimental usage in agencies, although their potential remains strong (Schoech, 1999).

Expert systems grew out of the larger field of artificial intelligence, in which computer-generated behavior imitates how the human mind works (Butterfield, 1987). Other examples in this category of knowledge-based applications include case-based reasoning and neural networks (Schoech, 1999). In case-based reasoning, the details and outcomes in thousands of cases are entered into a computer program. Practitioners can then enter the circumstances of their existing case to see how similar cases were handled. Neural networks are more of a research application and have a more complicated programming structure in which a computer program "learns" how to fit a statistical model based on an existing set of detailed cases. Neural network analysis has been found to discriminate cases better than regression models (Schoech, 1999).

Expert systems were identified as the most promising form of artificial intelligence, and for a brief period there was great enthusiasm among some scholars about their potential role in social work. Promoters of expert systems expected that they could be used to pass on scarce expertise to less experienced workers (Gingerich, 1995; Schuerman, 1987); to train practitioners (Gingerich, 1995; Goodman et al. 1989; Schuerman, 1987); to "guide and monitor" practice through documentation of intervention implementation; to acquire, describe, and refine practice knowledge for later use; and to develop theory by carefully outlining the concepts used to solve problems (Goodman, Gingerich, & deShazer, 1989; Gingerich, 1995). In short, expert systems were viewed as ways to identify the profession's knowledge base, rationalize decision making, and capture for both science and the profession that elusive ghost, practice wisdom.

The necessary steps to develop an expert system are not easy. Schoech (1999) estimates that it can take 3–5 person-years to develop, test, and refine an expert system. For example, in developing a child welfare expert system Schuerman and colleagues (Schuerman, Mullen, Stagner, & Johnson, 1988) identified several intellectual issues that must be considered, including the integration of "common sense" into the knowledge base; consideration of the context of the organization, such as political barriers, caseloads, and resources; dealing with what is actually done in practice versus what may be considered "best practice"; and acknowledging that social work practice is "moderately complicated," which makes integration of an expert system challenging (Schuerman et al., 1988). For instance, care must be taken in gathering the knowledge from the expert staff, and validating the expert system is difficult due in part to conflicting expert opinions about what constitutes a "correct" decision (Schuerman et al., 1988).

Finally, expert systems can only be as good as the knowledge base on which they are built. In social work the knowledge domains are difficult to systematize, practice experts often do not agree, and many times not all facts are known (for discussion, see Mullen & Schuerman, 1990; Stein, 1990; Reamer, 1990; Wakefield, 1990). If expertise has not been developed, then it cannot be translated into an expert system. In addition, expert systems hinge on the necessity of making discrete decisions, for example, whether to remove a child from a home. But often practice is not driven by the need for a specific decision, as when a worker is simply gathering information, making an assessment, and establishing a relationship.

CONCLUSIONS

Social work researchers and administrators have embraced computer technology more willingly than practitioners, perhaps because they see the potential uses of computers to conduct research, make service delivery more rational, and improve practice. And, because the early computers were primarily rapid calculating machines for scientists and engineers, social work researchers believed that the new technology could advance the scientific basis of social work practice by offering a means of forging links between the research and practice worlds. Social work practitioners, in contrast, have been more ambivalent, suspicious, and fearful of creeping impersonalization or of machines replacing people. Admittedly, the technology has taken longer to advance to the point where it offers advantages to practitioners in the same way it has for researchers and administrators. Nevertheless, there is a burgeoning technology literature in social work education and in key social work journals including the *Journal of Social Work Education* and *Social Work*. This takes on a "training the trainers" strategy of sorts in which social work educators expose new social workers to computer technologies available for use in practice during their graduate education. This will likely decrease fear of and resistance to computer technology and increase technology usage in practice. Time will tell to what extent the social work profession embraces computer technology in its practice and research endeavors.

ACKNOWLEDGMENT Portions of this chapter are used with permission from Columbia University Press and were previously published in S. A. Kirk, W. J. Reid, and C. Petrucci's "Computer-Assisted Social Work Practice: The Promise of Technology" (chapter 6) in S. A. Kirk and W. J. Reid's *Science and Social Work: A Critical Appraisal* (2002).

References

Abell, M. L., & Galinsky, M. J. (2002). Introducing students to computer-based group work practice. *Journal of Social Work Education 38*(1), 39–54.

Abels, P. (1972). Can computers do social work? *Social Work* 17(5), 5–11.

Baker, R. P. (1992). New technology in survey research: Computer-assisted personal interviewing (CAPI). *Social Science Computer Review* 10(2), 145–157.

Benbenishty, R. (1996). Integrated research and practice: Time for a new agenda. *Research on Social Work Practice* 6(1), 77–82.

Benbenishty, R. (1997). Outcomes in the context of empirical practice. In E. J. Mullen & J. Magnabosco (Eds.), *Outcome measurement in the human services* (pp. 198–208). Washington, DC: National Association of Social Workers.

Benbenishty, R., & Ben-Zaken, A. (1988). Computer-aided process of monitoring task-centered family interventions. *Social Work Research and Abstracts* 24, 7–9.

Bloom, M., Fischer, J., & Orme, J. G. (1999). *Evaluating practice* (3rd ed.). New York: Free Press.

Boyd, L. H., Jr., Hylton, J. H., & Price, S. V. (1978). Computers in social work practice: A review. *Social Work* 23(5), 368–371.

Boyd, L. H., Jr., Pruger, R., Chase, M. D., Clark, M., & Miller, L. S. (1981). A decision support system to increase equity. *Administration in Social Work* 5(3–4), 83–96.

Bronson, D. E., & Blythe, B. J. (1987). Computer support for single-case evaluation of practice. *Social Work Research and Abstracts* 23(3), 10–13.

Butterfield, W. H. (Ed.). (1983). Computers for social work practitioners [Special issue]. *Practice Digest* 6(3).

Butterfield, W. H. (1987). Artificial intelligence: An introduction. *Computers in Human Services* 3(1/2), 23–35.

Conboy, A., Auerbach, C., Beckerman, A., Schnall, D., & LaPorte, H. H. (2000). MSW student satisfaction with using single-system design computer software to evaluate social work practice. *Research on Social Work Practice* 10(1), 127–138.

Cowan, L. (2002). Interactive media for child care and counseling: New resources, new opportunities. *Journal of Technology in Human Services* 20 (1–2), 31–48.

Fanshel, D. (1977). Parental visiting of children in foster care: A computerized study. *Social Work Research and Abstracts* 13, 2–10.

Finn, J. (2002). MSW student perceptions of the efficacy and ethics of Internet-based therapy. *Journal of Social Work Education* 38(3), 403–419.

Finn, J., & Lavitt, M. (1994). Computer-based self-help groups for sexual abuse survivors. *Social Work with Groups* 17(1/2), 21–46.

Franklin, C., Nowicki, J., Trapp, J., Schwab, A., & Peterson, J. (1993). A computerized assessment system for brief, crisis-oriented youth services. *Families in Society* 74, 602–616.

Fuller, T. K. (1970). Computer utility in social work. *Social Casework* 51(10), 606–611.

Gingerich, W. J. (1995). Expert systems. In R. L. Edwards (Ed.), *Encyclopedia of social work 1995* (19th ed.) (pp. 917–925). Washington, DC: National Association of Social Workers.

Goodman, H., Gingerich, W. J., & deShazer, S. (1989). Briefer: An expert system for clinical practice. *Computers in Human Services* 5(1/2), 53–68.

Holden, G., Bearlson, D., Rode, D., Rosenberg, G., & Fishman, M. (1999). Evaluating the effects of a virtual environment (STARBRIGHT World) with hospitalized children. *Research on Social Work Practice* 9, 365–382.

Hoshino, G., & McDonald, T. P. (1975). Agencies in the computer age. *Social Work* 20(1), 10–14.

Kirk, S. A., & Reid, W. J. (2002). *Science and social work: A critical appraisal.* New York: Columbia University Press.

Kirk, S. A., Reid, W. J., & Petrucci, C. (2002). Computer-assisted social work practice: The promise of technology. In S. A. Kirk & W. J. Reid (Eds.), *Science and social work: A critical appraisal* (pp. 114–150). New York: Columbia University Press.

Mattaini, M. A. (1996). The abuse and neglect of single-case designs. *Research on Social Work Practice* 6(1), 83–90.

Meier, A. (1997). Inventing new models of social support groups: A feasibility study of an on-line stress management support group for social workers. *Social Work with Groups* 20(4), 35–53.

Menon, G. M., and Brown, N. K. (Eds.). (2001). Going the distance: Use of technology in human services education. Proceedings of the 3rd Annual Technology Conference, Charleston SC, September 1999 [Special issue]. *Journal of Technology in Human Services* 18(1/2).

Menon, G. M., & Coe, J. R. (Eds.). (2000). Technology and social work education: Recent empirical studies [Special issue]. *Research on Social Work Practice* 10(4), 397–427.

Mullen, E. J., & Schuerman, J. (1990). Expert systems and the development of knowledge in social welfare. In L. Videka-Sherman and W. J. Reid (Eds.), *Advances in clinical social work research* (pp. 67–83). Washington, DC: National Association of Social Workers.

Nurius, P. S., & Hudson, W. W. (1988a). Workers, clients, and computers. *Computers in Human Services* 4(1/2), 71–83.

Nurius, P. S., & Hudson, W. W. (1988b). Computer-based practice: Future dream or current technology? *Social Work* 33(4), 357–362.

O'Neill, J. V. (2001, January). Online therapy on verge of major launch. *National Association of Social Workers News*, p. 5.

Raymond, F. B., Ginsberg, L., & Gohagan, D. (Eds.). (1998). Information technologies: Teaching to use—using to teach [Special issue]. *Computers in Human Services, 15*(2/3).

Reamer, F. G. (1990). The nature of expertise in social welfare. In L. Videka-Sherman & W. J. Reid (Eds.), *Advances in clinical social work research* (pp. 88–91). Washington, DC: National Association of Social Workers.

Reid, W. J. (1974). Developments in the use of organized data. *Social Work 19*(5), 585–593.

Reid, W. J. (1975). A test of a task-centered approach. *Social Work 20*, 3–9.

Reid, W. J. (1978). The social agency as a research machine. *Journal of Social Service Research 21*, 11–23.

Rimer, E. (1986). Implementing computer technology in human service agencies: The experience of two California counties. *New England Journal of Human Services 6*(3), 25–29.

Savaya, R., Monnickendam, M., & Waysman, M. (2000). An assessment of the utilization of a computerized decision support system for youth probation officers. *Journal of Technology in Human Services 17*(4), 1–14.

Schoech, D. (1995). Information systems. In R. L. Edwards (Ed.), *Encyclopedia of social work 1995* (19th ed.) (pp. 1470–1479). Washington, DC: National Association of Social Workers.

Schoech, D. (1999). *Human services technology: Understanding, designing, and implementing computer and Internet applications in the social services.* New York: Haworth Press.

Schoech, D., & Arangio, T. (1979). Computers in the human services. *Social Work 24*(2), 96–102.

Schoech, D., & Schkade, L. L. (1980). Computers helping caseworkers: Decision support systems. *Child Welfare 59*(9): 566–575.

Schopler, J. H., Abell, M. D., & Galinsky, M. J. (1998). Technology-based groups: A review and conceptual framework for practice. *Social Work 43*(3), 254–267.

Schopler, J. H., Galinsky, M. J., & Abell, M. (1997).

Creating community through telephone and computer groups: Theoretical and practice perspectives. *Social Work with Groups 20*(4), 19–34.

Schuerman, J. R. (1987). Expert consulting systems in social welfare. *Social Work Research and Abstracts 23*(3), 14–18.

Schuerman, J. R., Mullen, E., Stagner, M., & Johnson, P. (1988). First generation expert systems in social welfare. *Computers in Human Services 4*(1/2), 111–122.

Schwab, A. J., Jr., Bruce, M. E., & McRoy, R. G. (1985). A statistical model of child placement decisions. *Social Work Research and Abstracts 21*(2), 28–34.

Schwab, A. J., Jr., Bruce, M. E., & McRoy, R. G. (1986). Using computer technology in child placement decisions. *Social Casework 67*(6), 359–368.

Stein, T. J. (1990). Issues in the development of expert systems to enhance decision making in child welfare. In L. Videka-Sherman & W. J. Reid (Eds.), *Advances in clinical social work research* (pp. 84–87). Washington, DC: National Association of Social Workers.

Taber, M. A., & DiBello, L. V. (1990). The personal computer and the small social service agency. *Computers in Human Services 6*(1/2/3), 181–197.

Teicher, M. (1967). Social casework—science or art? *Child Welfare 46*, 394–395.

Vasey, I. T. (1968). Developing a data storage and retrieval system. *Social Casework, 49*(7), 414–417.

Vondracek, F. W., Urban, H. B., & Parsonage, W. H. (1974). Feasibility of an automated intake procedure for human service workers. *Social Service Review 48*(2), 271–278.

Wakefield, J. C. (1990). Expert systems, Socrates, and the philosophy of mind. In L. Videka-Sherman & W. J. Reid (Eds.), *Advances in clinical social work research* (pp. 92–100). Washington, DC: National Association of Social Workers.

10 PROBLEM FORMULATION, CONCEPTUALIZATION, AND THEORY DEVELOPMENT

Harris Chaiklin

It is common to think of theory, applied research, and practice as separate, distinct entities. While these three entities seem logically dissimilar, in practice the distinctions between them make no difference. It is also common to think of theory as the province of esoteric researchers whose work has little relation to what happens in the "real world." This too is the stuff of myths, but it is an idea with a long history. In 1803 Immanuel Kant railed against anyone denying that theory is related to practice as "exposing himself as an ignoramus in his field" (Kant, 1974, pp. 41–42).

Those who deny the need for theory emphasize the role of ideology in practice. On one side Halmos saw theory and practice as being locked in a necessary and mutually destructive conflict: "While sociology weakens the inspirational elements of professional experience and interpretation, the professional ideology of personal service weakens the positivistic authority of social science" (Halmos, 1971, p. 593). On the other side the Schwendingers see practitioners as corporate liberals who use therapy as a form of social control. According to them, this transforms Freud into an instrument of the corporate state: "With these models, political issues and behavior are regarded as problems of individual adjustment" (Schwendinger & Schwendinger, 1974, p. 347). As long as the relationship between theory and practice is argued on ideological grounds there will be no progress in testing the extent to which theory is necessary and meaningful in advancing practitioners' ability to help people. Bailey puts it clearly and simply: "Theory means and requires practice" (Bailey, 1980, p. 97).

Professionals have an obligation to identify the theory they use. Flyvjberg (2001) laments the loss of influence and enthrallment that once made social science a delight. He sees three things as necessary to change this. First, the social sciences should stop emulating natural science by building a cumulative predictive theory. This is a partial truth. Since a unified theory that explains all behavior may never be attained, all theories and styles of research are potentially useful. His next two points have more merit. One is that important problems must be studied, and the other is that the results of this work must be clearly and effectively communicated.

WHAT IS THEORY AND HOW IS IT BUILT?

At its base theory is a position used to interpret data. Merton uses a bit of verse to show that depending on the theory used, the same behavior can be interpreted differently:

> I am firm,
> Thou art obstinate,
> He is pigheaded (Merton, 1957a, p. 428)

That the theory used to interpret behavior often reflects the viewpoint of the person making the interpretation and the person to whom it is being applied reflects the intricacy and the joy in theory construction. It is intricate because there is no unified theory that can explain all of any behavior and joy when one can be sure that a part of that behavior has been correctly interpreted.

There are a profusion of theories about criminal justice. For example, a National Institute of

Drug Abuse publication classified theories in terms of their relationship to self, others, society, and nature. It then listed 43 theories under these headings and indicated that this was only a selection of existing theories (Lettieri, Sayers, & Wallenstein, 1980).

The large number of available theories gives researchers the freedom to choose an orientation with which they are compatible. To avoid partisan wrangling researchers need to be reminded that any theory used to interpret behavioral findings is only a partial explanation of the total phenomenon.

Theory building can be complex and sophisticated. Those interested in the more advanced aspects of theory building should consult works on the nature of science and theory building that explore the subject more deeply (Blalock, 1984; Cohen & Nagel, 1934; Kaplan, 1964; Nagel, 1961; Popper, 1965; Reynolds, 1971; Willer, 1967; Winton, 1974).

THEORIES OF THE MIDDLE RANGE

The specific concern of this chapter is with contributing to practice theory related to the community reintegration of offenders being released from prison. The contribution that research makes to theory is that it "initiates, reformulates, re-focuses and clarifies" (Merton, 1957b, p. 12). This means that research contributes to the continuous process of reformulating and refining theory.

There are many levels of theory development. The ideal of the tightly controlled experiment with precise measurements of all concepts is rarely possible where practice theory is concerned. There are too many variables that affect any given behavioral act. Correlational studies seldom show that any one factor accounts for a great proportion of a particular behavior (Epstein & Blumenfeld, 2001). Behavioral scientists seldom know enough to make the predictions that characterize hypothesis testing in laboratory research (Schwartz & Jacobs, 1979).

The approach taken to theory development in this project was to use middle range theory. Such theory neither proposes to explain all of society nor build a formal theory of micro behavior. It avoids dealing with either end of the empirical qualitative dichotomy and seeks outcomes that will eventually become one of the discrete theories integrated into larger wholes

(Merton, 1967). Merton says that middle range theories serve to guide empirical research. Once again, this means that they provide a basis for interpreting data. The concepts used are simple and clear and are tested in hypotheses where the aim is to develop empirical generalizations. Merton was not talking about the statistical tests of hypotheses derived from cross-sectional surveys. His approach to data was more in the case study mode, so his concept of hypothesis testing was broad.

THEORIES OF EXPLANATION AND THEORIES OF INTERVENTION

Practice theory is broad. The focus in this chapter is on intervention and not explanation. A theory of intervention justifies procedures used in the attempt to change behavior. A theory of explanation explains behavior but seldom provides a basis for intervention. The explanation for and treatment of lung cancer illustrates the convolutions that practice theory takes. Smoking is one way to get lung cancer. Lung cancer will not be cured with the cessation of smoking. Change requires deciding between surgical, radiological, and chemical treatments. These treatments are complementary, but some physicians favor one treatment theory over the other, and this makes for confusion when people try to decide on treatment. The matter is further complicated because practice has shown that individuals differ in their response to treatment.

While it is fairly easy to show the distinction between explanation and intervention with physical disease, it is more difficult when the same logic is applied to human behavior. One reason for this is that there is a tendency to mix explanation and intervention together. Removing the cause is often assumed to change behavior. One well-known illustration of this has been the ongoing debate in the literature about the relationship between broken homes and delinquency. While there are differences over the size and the meaning of the relationship, there is general agreement that it is a small but significant factor (Rebellon, 2002). Another example concerns the effect on children who experience violence. In reviewing literature for their theory of violence Gelles and Straus (1979) note that one consistent finding is that early experience with violence as a child is associated with being violent as an adult.

What do we know about intervention if we accept that broken homes and experiencing violence are causal factors in deviance? The answer is practically nothing. In both cases low correlation and the possibility that in the time between the presumed cause and the effect so many other causal events can occur means that the initial explanation is practically meaningless. Yet, among the most common actions recommended for dealing with delinquency is to propose preventive programs to make families "healthy." This is one of those goals that is possible but not probable.

Massive prevention programs assume that everyone has the potential to commit a crime. While this may be true in the abstract, the causal social factors of broken homes and early violence do not account for enough of the problem to warrant large-scale expenditure of funds on "prevention." The overwhelming majority of people toward whom these programs are directed would never engage in such behavior.

Theoretically it should be possible to develop good predictors so that early intervention with the correct target population is possible. To date no one has established norms for identifying which family behaviors predict with great certainty what later behavior will be (Freud, 1965). There have been some suggestive lines of inquiry that warrant further attention. Plionis (1977) found that by using family assessment with the families of children who came to the emergency room for accidents she could develop predictors that would differentiate between an accident that was likely to be a single occurrence and one that was likely to be the first in a long series of accidents.

If something is to be done about delinquency and violent behavior, what is necessary is to intervene in the present with factors that can be controlled. Intervention should not be based on historical factors that cannot be changed. Changing behavior means working with current behavior and involving the offenders and their families in work, educational, social, and therapy programs.

While there may be some overlap between theories of explanation and theories of practice, there is not a lot. In sociology, theories of explanation tend to be well developed and numerous. Theories of practice can scarcely be identified because social work does little of its own theorizing and relies on other academic disciplines to supply this content. Social work education has long been identified as having low standards and relying on borrowed knowledge rather than developing its own strong knowledge base (Kadushin, 1976; Stoesz, 2000).

TOWARD A THEORY OF SOCIAL INTERVENTION

When explanations are conceptualized in a diagnostic system they become part of a practice theory where, based on experience, diagnosis indicates something about the intervention that can be undertaken. Regardless of their defects, such systems have been worked out for physical and emotional diagnosis and treatment. They have not been worked out for the social elements in behavior.

The path to developing such a social component starts with Lisansky and Schochet's classic article about interviewing "above the line" and "below the line" (Lisansky & Schochet, 1967). "Above the line" refers to physical symptoms. "Below the line" refers to emotional symptoms. Lisansky later expanded this into a comprehensive piece that showed how sensitive medical interviewing could develop into psychotherapy (Lisansky, 1969). The model for this approach is "Doctor, my ulcer began to bleed . . . after I had a fight with my wife." The implication of this statement is that the patient's physical condition was exacerbated by the nature of his emotional defenses. But the causal chain could be extended further: "Doctor, my ulcer began to bleed . . . after I had a fight with my wife . . . and I had a fight with my wife after I found out that I might lose my job." In each of these "facts"—the bleeding ulcer, the fight, and the threat of job loss—the weight of the physical, emotional, and social components is relative. None of them is pure. For the moment that is not what concerns us. What does is that for the physical and emotional aspects of behavior, medicine has well-developed diagnostic systems that have associated treatment protocols.

The same cannot be said for social diagnosis in social work. In 1955 Greenwood said that "unless and until the social work profession develops typologies of its problems and procedures, its concepts will remain indefinite, its language loose, and its textbooks vague" (p. 28). In the intervening years not much has been done to change this situation. The latest attempt was a large-scale effort by the National Association of Social Workers (Karls & Wandrei, 1994). There is little evidence that the "person-in-environment" (PIE) system suggested as a part of that effort has come into wide use.

TO APPLY THE THEORY IN PRACTICE

The theory under consideration here concerns social intervention. Social behavior reflects commonly accepted definitions and accepted rules for interaction that show that people take account of each other as they relate. To say that one is an accountant by occupation immediately conveys a whole set of definitions and expectations to others. To decide not to use four-letter words in greeting a clergyman reflects the speaker's awareness that the clergyman probably would not find this acceptable.

This approach to the social is rooted in the philosophy of pragmatism. It is America's contribution to philosophy and is typically American in that it proposes no grand overview of the world, is disorganized, and has many different views of what constitutes the philosophy. Its core is reflected in the question, "What difference would it make if this proposition were true?" In terms of a practice question it is, "What leads this person to behave as they do?" It is not, "What is wrong with this person?" To work in this framework means that you do not try to answer ultimate questions such as how to cure delinquency but that you work in the present moment.

What makes pragmatism useful to practitioners is that it is rooted in the tradition and values of democracy. It avoids absolutes. Scheffler calls it a "mediating philosophy" (1974, p. 2). At the same time it is oriented to science so that it is open to new findings. In human affairs this means that value principles are constant but that their enactment and interpretation may vary according to time and place. This leads some to charge it with moral relativism. This is not the case. Take, for example, the history of prison reform where efforts have been made to make incarceration humane. A variety of schemes ranging from transportation to isolation have been tried. They all are behaviorally different, but their values are the same. They are also equally unsuccessful.

There are many varying interpretations of both pragmatism and symbolic interaction. In true pragmatic fashion I shall avoid these niceties of detail and stick with middle range social theoretical assumptions about the nature of the social. This stance on the social and social interaction follows George Herbert Mead's view of pragmatism and symbolic interaction (Rock, 1979; Strauss, 1964). The aim is to clarify and specify practice theory and not to create new theoretical postulates.

Accordingly, the realm of the social has been divided into levels based on the degree of abstraction from the empirical world (Chaiklin, 1978). These include the following:

1. Climate: the worldview of a society, its ethos. It concerns such things as whether people in the society see the future as positive or negative. In working with people it is necessary to take account of the climate, but it is not possible to directly influence it.

2. Institution: the agencies that make up the way a society is organized. It includes such familiar institutions as education, courts, and medicine. Institutional sociology is directly concerned with such institutional categories and is not much in fashion these days. At this level individual actions do little to influence the way institutions function.

3. Social characteristics: social labels usually called statuses. One is born with them—for example, race and religion—or acquires them—for example, a college degree or a job skill. These categories are not pure and exist in many combinations—for example to rise or fall from the social class into which you are born, to obtain a membership in your father's plumbing union, or to become president of the American Legion women's auxiliary that your mother led for many years. The ability to change status is mixed. Some statuses, such as race, cannot be changed; some, such as social class, can be changed slowly; and some, such as religion, can be changed fairly rapidly.

4. Social behavior: expressed through actions widely accepted and understood in a society. There are three subcategories of social behavior:

   • Forms: relates to social behavior that requires no or very little interaction or emotional contact with the other, only knowledge of the rules. For example, people drive cars and for the most part obey stop signs and red lights. In formal affairs such as weddings or religious ceremonies usually one can get by just by following prescribed procedures. This even holds true for the clerk in the supermarket who mechanically wishes that you "have a nice day." Social forms generally change slowly, although there are periodic fads that come and go quickly.

- Interaction: knowledge of the forms is added to a mutual awareness where people who talk to each other take account of their own and others' expectations in the relationship they are having. At this level there is the possibility of rapid behavior change if desired. Changing social behavior at this level does not involve a personality change, only a desire to do something and the ability to learn the new behavior and to find ways to get it accepted by others.
- Transaction: to a knowledge of the norms and mutual awareness is added the idea that in the interaction both of the participants are in some way changed. This goes over the borderline between sociology and psychology because at this level personality change is involved. This occurs very slowly.

Within these levels the focus is on social characteristics and interaction. These are behavioral aspects relatively uninfluenced by either physical or personality considerations. Generally, social characteristics are called "face sheet" information. Almost any kind of case record routinely collects this data and then pays almost no attention to it. In practice research, face sheet data must be action elements. For example, to collect data on family status and composition would mean that with the client's permission family members would be contacted.

To relate to people on an interactional basis means that the manifest is related to before the latent; reality takes precedence over fantasy, and the overt is considered before the covert. The stance that the practitioner takes is that people mean what they say. If they do not, this becomes obvious soon enough. If someone says, "I need help in finding an apartment," that is what the practitioner works on with the client. This does not mean that the client dictates everything that happens in the relationship. The practitioner has a professional obligation to assess whether the request is appropriate and ethical. It does mean that the practitioner does not give a psychotherapeutic response. Psychotherapy is a form of transactional relationship. It takes latent, covert, and fantasy meanings into account. In the practice model that is developed from the social approach, where people's manifest statements are not a true basis for their actions because of either fear or lack of awareness, the practitioner explores the need for a psychotherapy referral. If the client's initial request is a form of testing or gamesmanship the practitioner explores with the client whether they want the service. The aim is to quickly move to working with the client's direct needs.

CONCLUSION

This chapter has presented the way the social element in practice theory can be conceptualized so that it provides a basis for practice. In the human service professions this has been a difficult task (Jacob, 2002). The nature of the social was traced from a foundation in pragmatic philosophy through the symbolic interaction of George Herbert Mead. The way people perceive and respond to each other is a theoretical formulation that is ideally suited for practice. "It is a way of seeking to make the world a better place by incremental changes in small things— not a heroic vision perhaps but maybe all the more effective for that" (Dingwell, 2001, p. 241). It deals with the specifics of human behavior in ways to which practitioners can relate (Fore & del Carmen, 2002).

In developing the specific focus of this exercise in theory building it was stressed that the aim was not to develop a striking new way of looking at data but rather to provide a necessary explication of existing ideas so that they would be more useful for practice. Toward this end the conceptual focus was on middle range theory and within practice theory more on intervention than on explication. "Applied science is oriented to the discovery of new uses for knowledge claims that have been previously evaluated and tentatively accepted" (Cohen, 1989, p. 52). This is as important to developing knowledge as the more prestigious exercises in presenting grand theory.

In practice professions there are many problems connected with both creating and using knowledge. The literature is not organized, practice decisions are often made on the basis of single studies, practitioners draw unsystematized knowledge from a large variety of sources, and there is no structure for making knowledge cumulative (Kirk & Reid, 2002). In sum, well-organized and sound practice theory not only will contribute to knowledge but also will help educate more effective practitioners.

References

Bailey, J. (1980). *Ideas and intervention.* Boston: Routledge and Kegan Paul.

Blalock, H. M. (1984). *Basic dilemmas in the social sciences.* Beverly Hills, CA: Sage.

Chaiklin, H. (1978). Social aspects of behavior. In G. U. Balis, L. Wurmser, E. McDaniel, & R. G. Grenell (Eds.), *The behavioral sciences and the practice of medicine* (Vol. 2, pp. 263–276). Boston: Butterworth.

Cohen, B. P. (1989). *Developing sociological knowledge: Theory and method* (2nd ed.). Chicago: Nelson-Hall.

Cohen, M. R., & Nagel, E. (1934). *An introduction to logic and scientific method.* New York: Harcourt, Brace.

Dingwell, R. (2001). Notes toward an intellectual history of symbolic interactionism. *Symbolic Interaction, 24*(2), 237–242.

Epstein, I., & Blumenfield, S. (Eds.). (2001). *Clinical data-mining in practice-based research: Social work in hospital settings.* New York: The Haworth Social Work Practice Press.

Flyvbjerg, B. (2001). *Making social science matter.* Cambridge: Cambridge University Press.

Fore, H. M., & del Carmen, A. (2002). The "I" and the "me" of criminology and criminal justice students: Symbolic interaction in an educational setting. *Journal of Criminal Justice Education, 13*(2), 351–368.

Freud, A. (1965). Normality and pathology in childhood. In *The writings of Anna Freud* (Vol. 6, pp. 3–9). New York: International Universities Press.

Gelles, R. J., & Straus, M. A. (1979). Determinants of violence in the family: Toward a theoretical integration. In W. R. Burr, R. Hill, F. I. Nye, & I. L. Reiss (Eds.), *Contemporary theories about the family* (Vol. 1, pp. 553–554). New York: Free Press.

Greenwood, E. (1955). Social science and social work: A theory of their relationship. *Social Service Review, 39,* 20–33.

Halmos, P. (1971). Sociology and the personal service professions. *American Behavioral Scientist, 14,* 583–597.

Jacob, A. V. (2002). Translating theory into practice: Self-efficacy and weight management. *Healthy Weight Journal, 16*(6), 86–88.

Kadushin, A. (1976). *Supervision in social work.* New York: Columbia University Press.

Kant, I. (1974). *On the old saw: That may be right in theory but it won't work in practice.* Philadelphia: University of Pennsylvania Press.

Kaplan, A. (1964). *The conduct of inquiry: Methodology for behavioral science.* San Francisco: Chandler.

Karls, J. M., & Wandrei, K. E. (Eds.). (1994). *PIE manual: Person-in-environment system.* Washington, DC: National Association of Social Workers.

Kirk, S. A., & Reid, W. J. (2002). *Science and social work: A critical appraisal.* New York: Columbia University Press.

Lettieri, D. J., Sayers, M., & Wallenstein, P. H. (Eds.). (1980). *Theories on drug abuse: Selected contemporary perspectives.* Washington, DC: Department of Health and Human Services and National Institute on Drug Abuse.

Lisansky, E. T. (1969). History taking and interviewing. In *Tice's practice of medicine* (Vol. 10, pp. 1–32). New York: Harper and Row.

Lisansky, E. T., & Schochet, B. R. (1967). Comprehensive medical diagnosis for the internist: A modification of the associative anamnesis of Deutsch. *Medical Clinics of North America, 51,* 1381–1397.

Merton, R. K. (1957a). The self-fulfilling prophecy. In R. K. Merton (Ed.), *Social theory and social structure* (Rev. ed., pp. 421–436). Glencoe, IL: Free Press.

Merton, R. K. (1957b). *Social theory and social structure.* Glencoe, IL: Free Press.

Merton, R. K. (1967). On sociological theories of the middle range. In R. K. Merton (Ed.), *On theoretical sociology: Five essays old and new* (pp. 39–72). New York: Free Press.

Nagel, E. (1961). *The structure of science.* New York: Harcourt, Brace & World.

Plionis, E. M. (1977). Family functioning and childhood accident occurrence. *American Journal of Orthopsychiatry, 47*(2), 250–263.

Popper, K. R. (1965). *The logic of scientific discovery.* New York: Harper Torchbooks.

Rebellon, C. J. (2002). Reconsidering the broken homes/delinquency relationship and exploring its mediating mechanisms. *Criminology, 40*(1), 103–135.

Reynolds, P. D. (1971). *A primer in theory construction.* Indianapolis, IN: Bobbs-Merrill.

Rock, P. (1979). *The making of symbolic interactionism.* Totowa, NJ: Rowman and Littlefield.

Scheffler, I. (1974). *Four pragmatists: A critical introduction to Peirce, James, Mead, and Dewey.* London: Routledge and Kegan Paul.

Schwartz, H., & Jacobs, J. (1979). *Qualitative sociology: A method to the madness.* New York: Free Press.

Schwendinger, H., & Schwendinger, J. R. (1974). *The sociologists of the chair.* New York: Basic Books.

Stoesz, D. (2000). *A poverty of imagination: Boot-*

strap capitalism, sequel to welfare reform. Madison: University of Wisconsin Press.

Strauss, A. (Ed.). (1964). *George Herbert Mead on social psychology.* Chicago: University of Chicago Press.

Willer, D. (1967). *Scientific sociology theory and method.* Englewood Cliffs, NJ: Prentice-Hall.

Winton, C. A. (1974). *Theory and measurement in sociology.* New York: Wiley.

11 STATISTICS FOR HUMAN SERVICE WORKERS

Gunnar Almgren

The basic purpose of this chapter is to provide a general overview of the fundamentals of statistical reasoning and analysis that are particularly applicable to the evaluation of human services practice. The audience for this chapter is assumed to include social workers and other behavioral practitioners who may have had a course in statistics that is but a distant and regrettable memory and practitioners who have not had a course in basic statistics. While it offers practitioners considerably enhanced opportunities to evaluate practice, the availability of highly sophisticated and user-friendly statistical software over the last decade brings with it the risk of extremely erroneous findings and conclusions that are ultimately far more detrimental to empirically based practice than the profession of honest uncertainty. In this chapter I will review the critical assumptions that are embedded in the application and interpretation of some of the more popular statistical tests employed in the evaluation of human services practice, as well as some of the common errors one can make in test selection and interpretation. Although this chapter will be more conceptual than mathematical, I will walk the reader through some equations essential to statistical reasoning. First, however, I will review some fundamental concepts and terminology.

APPLICATIONS OF STATISTICS: DESCRIPTION, EXPLANATION, AND PREDICTION

Broadly speaking, statistics in the social sciences are used in three ways: description, explanation, and prediction. Used descriptively, statistical indices are typically a convenient way to summarize selected characteristics of a collection of individuals in quantitative terms. In explanation, both statistical indices and procedures are employed as evidence with which to evaluate assumptions, arguments, hypotheses, or conclusions. If used for predictive purposes, statistical indices and procedures are employed as aids in the estimation of the likelihood of a specific outcome or set of outcomes.

It can be shown with a single statistical observation from a hypothetical community agency that all three applications of statistics are critically relevant to the evaluation of practice. The exemplar statistical observation to be used in all three ways is the mean score on a conventional clinical depression scale observed in a cohort of clients entering service during a particular month. Applied purely in the descriptive sense this statistic describes a characteristic of those seeking services from the agency that is highly relevant to accountability and funding concerns. Used in the explanatory sense, the mean score on the depression scale would be an essential baseline for evaluating the relative effectiveness of alternative forms of psychotherapy. It is also conceivable that the mean score on a depression scale for this cohort might be highly useful with respect to the prediction of future utilization of crisis intervention services, depending on the evidence that fluctuations in the level of depression in the client base correspond with fluctuations in the utilization rates of crisis intervention services.

GENERAL TYPES OF STATISTICS

Aside from the different applications, statistical indices and procedures are also categorized as either *descriptive* or *inferential* statistics. Descriptive statistics are based on the assumption that the statistical indices considered (e.g., mean, variance, correlation coefficient) are derived from measurements observed for each member of the reference population. Where this is the case, statistical indices are referred to as *parameters*. Thus the mean IQ (intelligence quotient) of the freshman class of a given college should be treated mathematically as descriptive statistic if and only if it can be assumed that every freshman class member's IQ score was included in the calculation of the mean. Inferential statistics, on the other hand, are based on sampling procedures that permit the investigator to estimate population parameters, within a known probability of error. Using again the example of the freshman class IQ score, a random sample of IQ scores of *N* size would permit the investigator to employ parametric statistical procedures to estimate the mean IQ score of the entire population—again, within a defined probability of error. Although parameter and parameter estimates are both generally referred to as statistics, their properties are quite distinct and critical to the selection of the appropriate statistical procedure.

Statistical procedures that are commonly employed to evaluate practice fall into two broad classes: *parametric statistics* and *nonparametric statistics*. Parametric statistics require quantitative dependent variables and specific assumptions about the distribution of scores on the dependent variable in the population of interest. For example, the widely used independent samples *t* test assumes that the samples are selected randomly and independently; the dependent variable approximates the interval level of measurement and is also normally distributed. Nonparametric statistics are less restrictive with respect to the quantitative properties of the dependent variable and distributional assumptions. Because the parametric tests that are favored for practice evaluation are robust with respect to violations of distributional assumptions (that is, the same conclusion reached is consistent whether or not distributional assumptions are met), this chapter will omit discussion of nonparametric procedures. The exception to this is the chi-square test, which is commonly used both by itself and in conjunction with parametric statistics in practice evaluation.

ANALYSIS OF VARIANCE, COVARIANCE, AND THE DISTINCTION BETWEEN ASSOCIATION AND CAUSAL INFERENCE

Statistics, whether in the context of evaluating social work practice or enabling more efficient industrial production, is largely about analyzing variance. Analysis of variance involves two distinct statistical activities: the estimation of variance in a given variable or set of variables and the estimation of covariance between variables. Used in the general sense the term covariance merely refers to the variation in a given variable being associated with the variation in one or more other variables. An example of this would be the way in which the amount of covariance in the serums level of an antidepressant and the scores on a depression scale might demonstrate the efficacy of the particular medication. Statistically based explanation and prediction both are derived from a plethora of statistical procedures that identify such patterns of covariance.

While variables are referred to as being associated with one another where covariance is present, a critical principle to all statistical analysis is the distinction between association and causality. Where covariance is observed and argued to be causal, this is more properly to be regarded as a claim rather than a complete certainty. It should be kept in mind that while causality can be tested and inferred through observation of covariance, causality is in its essence a theoretical claim that may or may not generally be accepted, dependent in large part on the body of evidence available to link covariance with a credible theoretical basis for causality. Covariance among variables can occur for a number of reasons other than a causal association (i.e., variation in one variable influencing the variation in another), a common one being a spurious relationship where both reference variables covary in response to the influence of a third variable that happens to affect both. A notorious example of this is the relationship between ice cream sales and homicides, which covary with each other as well as with the hours of daylight.

LEVELS OF MEASUREMENT

Thus far we have reviewed the general applications of statistics that are relevant to the generation of human service knowledge, the central interest in analysis of variance and covariance, and the critical distinction between association and causality. A final foundational point before moving on to specific statistical procedures entails a brief discussion of different levels of measurement and their relevance to the correct choice of statistical procedures.

Any property or characteristic of an individual or group that can be expressed in statistical terms first involves the activity of measurement. Measurement refers generally to the quantification of some property or aspect of an object according to whatever explicit rules of measurement are adopted (Borgatta & Kamo, 2000). In this discussion we are referring primarily to the quantification of characteristics of individuals and whatever treatment conditions to which they might have been exposed. The particular measure chosen to represent the property or characteristic in question is typically chosen on the basis of theory, knowledge, and the capacity to observe the property in question. Thus the assignment of "male" or "female" to an individual is typically based on a theoretical conceptualization of sexual types, knowledge of distinct physiologies, and the ability to observe social behavior that is associated with physiological characteristics. Note that although the measure of individuals' sexual identity employed in this case is expressed as a dichotomy, both the distinct physiologies and social behaviors associated with sexual typology are far more accurately expressed as a continuum. This perennial gap between the theoretical conception of an attribute and the measure employed is one fundamental

source of *measurement error;* the other is inaccuracies in the observation of whatever concept measure is employed. Measurement error is mentioned at this juncture because one source of measurement error is highly related to the *level of measurement* assigned to a characteristic being studied and because the degree of measurement error present has a profound effect on all processes related to statistical observation and reasoning.

To a large extent, the choice of the appropriate statistical procedure for a question or problem is predicated on the classification of variables into any one of four levels: nominal, ordinal, interval, and ratio. A variable that is classed at the *nominal level* is treated as though it has no distinct quantitative properties—that is, individuals or treatments are classed differently according to a nominal measure (e.g., male versus female, group versus individual treatment)—but there is no assumption of having more or less of the attribute in question. For example, even though Roman Catholics might in various degrees ascribe to the tenets of their religious affiliation, if religious affiliation is measured at the nominal level (e.g., Roman Catholic, Jewish, Muslim, Protestant, Other), it means that all Roman Catholics are lumped together and treated statistically as having an equal amount of the attribute of being Roman Catholic.

Variables measured at the *ordinal level,* on the other hand, have the quantitative property of being ordered along some abstract continuum (e.g., agnostic, somewhat religious, very religious). While an ordering of the degree to which an attribute is present is the central feature of an ordinal measure, ordinal measures lack the property of being precise in how much difference separates the rankings on an ordinal scale. *Interval level* measures, on the other hand, provide both the capacity to order categories of the variable in question and define precisely and consistently the difference between categories. For example, 5 points on the IQ scale treated as an interval level variable is regarded as representing the same increment in intelligence whether the 5 points separates persons with IQ scores of 100 and 105 or persons with IQ scores of 85 and 90. Variables that are treated as *ratio level* of measures have all of the properties of interval measures plus the property of having an absolute zero (Blalock, 1979). Height, for example, has the property of having an absolute zero. The primary statistical advantage of ratio level measures is the capacity to compare scores through use of ratios, a comparison that is not legitimate where an absolute zero cannot be assumed.

As should be apparent from the preceding discussion of the mathematical distinctions between different levels of measurement, the selection of the appropriate statistical procedure for any given question is in large part determined by the levels of measurement of the variables included in the analysis. One-way analysis of variance, a very common procedure in the evaluation of alternative treatment approaches, is predicated on a nominal level (or in some instances ordinal level) independent variable and on at least one interval level dependent variable. Alternatively, should both variables in question be nominal (e.g., type of treatment and a set of different but unquantifiable responses to treatment), a chi-square test would be feasible whereas a one-way ANOVA would not be. A special note of caution emphasized here: Statistical software programs that are now readily available to human service agencies and practitioners do not by themselves discriminate data in a way that prevents the user from running any number of statistical procedures or tests that are invalid due to the levels of measurement inherent in the data. Therefore, understanding the levels of measurement of the variables employed in the analysis and their relationship to the validity of particular statistical procedures is critical to the exercise of competent statistical analysis.

The remainder of this brief overview of statistics for practitioners will present in more definitive terms some of the more conventional statistical approaches to description, explanation, and prediction that serve as tools for empirically based practice. Again, the presentation will be more conceptual than computational.

PREPARING DATA FOR COMPUTER-ASSISTED STATISTICAL ANALYSIS

There are any number of ways data might be prepared for statistical analysis, and the most popular statistical analysis software programs have a menu of options available to the user to read data and create an analysis file. For most practitioners the most convenient way to enter data for analysis is through the use of a spreadsheet program or a database program that then

can be saved into a file readable by a statistical program. Database files, spreadsheet files, and data analysis files all have the common structure of a two-dimensional matrix, with individual cases on the y axis, variables on the x axis, and the cells available for entry of individual scores on variables. Alternative methods of data entry include ones in which simple text is in a tab-delimited format (where lines represent individual cases and scores on variables are typed in and then separated by a tab-space) or fixed format (where scores on particular variables are entered in exactly designated line spaces). However, the latter is much more prone to error and is not recommended for those who do not do data analysis for a living.

After entering or transforming data into a data analysis file, the next step generally taken is *data cleaning*, where missing data and errors in entry are corrected as much as possible. If the dataset is relatively small (both in cases and variables), this can be accomplished through the "eyeballing" method. However, in many instances it is more convenient and realistic to run a frequencies procedure on all of the variables to identify both the number of missing observations on each variable and to identify scores that seem extreme or improbable as clues to data entry error or errors in observation. The conventional statistical analysis programs all have selection functions that enable the user to generate a list of the case identifiers with missing observations or suspicious scores. Sometimes these problems can be corrected by referring back to the original data collection documents (e.g., case records, questionnaires); at other times the person conducting the analysis either will need to substitute imputed scores or exclude a variable or case from the analysis. Although a complete discussion of the circumstances and trade-offs involved in such decisions are beyond the scope of this chapter, the primary concern should be how exclusion of a particular observation or set of observations might bias the findings of the analysis.

DESCRIBING DISTRIBUTIONS OF VARIABLES

The following discussion is based on the assumption that the researcher is using descriptive statistics rather than their inferential counterparts. Descriptive statistics may be calculated to describe the distribution of a variable in a sample or the distribution in an entire population. The principal statistics for describing distributions of variables fall into two general categories: measures of dispersion and measures of central tendency. The most commonly used measures of dispersion include the range, the variance, and the standard deviation. All of these measures provide information about the magnitude of variability in the distribution of a variable and pertain to variables measured on at least the ordinal level. The range simply refers to the difference between the lowest score in the distribution and the highest, computed by subtracting the lowest from the highest. The variance refers to the sum of squared deviations of individual scores from the mean of all scores being considered (e.g., as in a sample) divided by the number of individual scores, and the standard deviation is simply the square root of the variance. Conceptually as well as mathematically, the standard deviation is the average deviation from the mean of the group of scores being considered. For this reason, the standard deviation is the favored measure of dispersion employed to describe the essential properties of a distribution of scores. Figures 11.1 and 11.2 provide graphic examples of two hypothetical distributions of IQ scores, one representing a sample of fifteen 11th-grade students in a general requirements classroom and the other fifteen students from an 11th-grade calculus class.

Note that the mean IQ in the calculus class is higher than that of the general requirements class while the standard deviation is lower. Both indices confirm that the calculus class is more selective with respect to IQ than the general requirements class, suggesting that the students in the calculus class are measured as having more intellectual ability and that there is less deviation in intellectual ability than is observed in the sample taken from the general requirements class.

The measures of central tendency used to describe a distribution of scores are the mean, median, and mode. In the case of interval level variables all three are useful and appropriate indices of central tendency; where ordinal measures cannot be argued to be a reasonable approximation of an interval scale, only the median and mode are appropriate. In the case of nominal level variables only the mode is available as a measure of central tendency (in essence, one can only observe the category of the variable that appears most often in the distribution). In Figures 11.1 and 11.2 it can be seen that the modal IQ category for the general requirements class is 100 (generally regarded as the average IQ score among high school students) while the modal category for the calculus class is 110.

The mean $\bar{x}$ is the arithmetic average score and is calculated simply as the sum of scores of variable x divided by the N. The mean is also

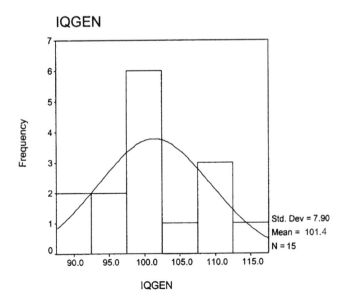

FIGURE 11.1 IQ Distribution in a General Requirements Classroom

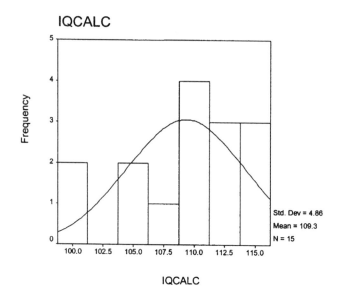

FIGURE 11.2 IQ Distribution in a Calculus Class

the most frequently utilized measure of central tendency. Although the mean is useful as an expression of the average and is a component of a variety of more complex statistics, its limitation for descriptive purposes is its property of being distorted by extreme values. For example, consider a sample of women on public assistance who have an average score on a depression scale that reflects moderate depression. To the extent that the sample is small and has very extreme scores one may get a grossly distorted notion of what the typical level of depression is in the sample. Therefore, one would err badly in claiming that "we found the sample to be moderately depressed." In a macro example consider how the rhetoric of "average income" is sometimes used to mask or ignore extremes of wealth and poverty.

In instances where there are extreme values that distort the shape of a distribution on a variable x from the normal bell shape (that is, where x is not normally distributed), the median is often the preferable alternative to the mean as the measure of central tendency. The median is simply the point in the distribution of scores where 50% of the scores are lower and 50% of the scores are higher. Unlike the mean, the median is not influenced by extreme scores and has a consistent interpretation no matter what the shape of the distribution.

The mode, in addition to having the capacity to reflect the central tendency of the nominal level of data, is also the score that is most likely to be observed in a random draw of all scores in a distribution. The mode answers the question, Which score am I most likely to observe?

It should be noted and emphasized that measures of central tendency and dispersion require each other to convey an understanding of the overall distribution and the proper interpretation of any score. For example, the score of 3.0 on a grade distribution derives some of its meaning from its place relative to both the range and median of all assigned grades. Similarly, an average level of depression has a very different meaning where standard deviation is extreme as opposed to instances where the variance in the distribution is modest.

Positional scores are those that that permit individual raw values on the variable x to be conveniently compared to the distribution of x as a whole. The first two are derived from the frequency distribution and are termed the *percentile rank* and *percentile*. The percentile rank is simply the percentage of scores that are at or below a given raw value of x while the percentile refers to the raw value of x that corresponds to a given percentile rank (Jaccard & Becker, 1997). For example, the fact that a client has a raw score of 25 on a risk scale for child abuse tells you little by itself, but if you know that the range on the scale is 0–40 and that the client's score is actually at the 90th percentile rank of the agency's caseload, you have critical information. Another kind of positional measure, based on a given raw value of x's relationship to the mean and standard deviation of x is the standard score, expressed as

$$\text{standard score} = \frac{X - \mu}{\sigma},$$

where μ stands for the population mean and σ stands for the standard deviation.

When dealing with samples rather than populations, the notation is altered to

$$\text{standard score} = \frac{X - \bar{X}}{S},$$

where s = the sample standard deviation and $\bar{x}$ = the sample mean.

As is shown by these examples, standard scores are nothing more than the ratio of the deviance of a given value of x from its mean and the standard deviation of x. In the next section, devoted to statistical inference and tests of significance, I will show how the most prevalent tests of significance used to compare differences in means are constructed in the same general form.

Nothing has been said thus far about graph-

ical depictions of distributions, which are extremely informative if used properly. Bar charts, as they generally are known, are utilized primarily for data measured at the nominal level such as the distribution of individuals by religion or political affiliation; histograms represent frequencies of quantitative data grouped into categories of magnitude; and line graphs show the general shape of a frequency distribution or might be used to depict the linearity of the relationship between two variables. As an example of a combined scatterplot and line graph, I show the estimated relationship between a maternal depression scale and a child behavior problems scale based a sample of school-aged children born to teenage mothers (see Figure 11.3; Almgren, Yamashiro, & Ferguson, 2002). Note that the data points on the scatterplot show that while child behavior problem scores tend to increase as the level of maternal depression increases, there is a lot of variance in this relationship—indicating that there are many factors aside from maternal depression influencing the child behavior problem score. The line on the graph shows the best-fitting linear estimate of the relationship, based on a bivariate regression estimate.

As a final point of information on graphical data description, the reader should appreciate that it is possible to manipulate the appearance

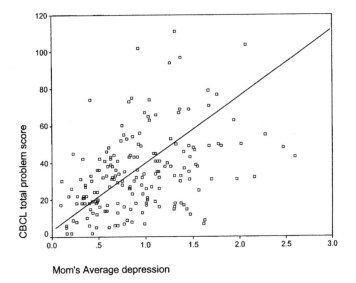

FIGURE 11.3 Linear Estimate of Relationship Between Child Behavior Problem and Mom's Depression

of distributions dramatically by using the formatting options available in graphics software; therefore, the reader is cautioned to examine carefully the categories, gradients, and ranges employed in the graphical representation of distributions.

STATISTICAL INFERENCE, THE MEANING OF STATISTICAL SIGNIFICANCE, AND SELECTION OF TESTS OF SIGNIFICANCE

The fundamental application of tests of significance in social work concerns the analysis of service effectiveness and the fostering of empirically based social work practice. In context tests of significance yield the probability of a single outcome or a limited set of observed outcomes occurring by chance as opposed to as a result of particular interventions. Where we can, by established statistical conventions, reject the argument that the particular outcome or set of outcomes occurred by chance, we can reasonably infer that a relationship exists between the outcomes of interest and the interventions applied— assuming also that we have controlled for other potentially relevant extraneous influences. Such is the process of statistical inference. Tests of significance pit an observed outcome in the form of a test statistic against the probability of the outcome occurring by chance in accordance with a theoretical distribution of probabilities called a *sampling distribution*. The names of particular tests of significance commonly employed in the analysis of social work methods generally refer to the sampling distribution on which they are based, for example, the *t* test, *F* test, chi-square, and *z* test. All of these tests of significance have in common the property of yielding an estimate of the probability of a particular test statistic being observed by chance. Where we are unable to reject the possibility that a test statistic's magnitude occurred by chance (the dominant convention for rejection is a probability of $< .05$), we are unable to reject the *null hypothesis* that the variable that represents our intervention and the variable that measures the outcome are independent from one another. Although the precise wording of the null hypothesis will vary by the type of test employed, this is the basic idea.

Hopefully, at this juncture the reader can appreciate the fact that the notion of "statistical significance" is actually a rather narrow one— that is, that the probability of a given outcome occurring by explicit theoretical rules of chance falls below some specified threshold. Under a wide variety of circumstances, an outcome that appears to be related to a programmatic or clinical intervention can reach statistical significance, even when the actual magnitude of the intervention's effect is rather trivial. This is true because the observation of statistical significance is influenced by the size of the sample, the amount of the variance in the measures analyzed, the actual magnitude of the intervention effect, and the investigator's selected threshold for incorrect rejection of the null hypothesis (Type I error). Thus, the statistical significance of an observed outcome should never be the primary or sole basis for either endorsing or rejecting an intervention's utility (Weinbach, 1989).

Choosing the appropriate test of significance depends on a variety of factors, chiefly the levels of measurement of the variables employed in the analysis, the nature of the study design, the type of hypothesis being tested, the number of cases being used in the analysis, and the distributional properties of the variables employed. Although it is obviously beyond the scope of this short chapter to explicate these issues, even modestly, some general guidance concerning appropriate test selection under a variety of circumstances common to the evaluation of social work services and clinical practice can be offered. In order to make this presentation simple, I will focus on what are often the most critical discriminators in the choice of the appropriate statistical test and limit the discussion to the context of a specific intervention and an observed outcome. The critical discriminators discussed are the level of measurement in the dependent variable, the sample size, the number of levels of the intervention, and whether the study design is a within-subjects or between-subjects design. Also, as mentioned at the beginning of the chapter, the only nonparametric test considered will be the chi-square test of homogeneity.

Chi-Square Test

The chi-square test of homogeneity considers whether or not two nominal level variables are statistically independent, where one has a fixed distribution of cases and the other is allowed to vary. This is typically the kind of analysis in which clients are assigned to contrasting interventions in order to compare their relative effi-

TABLE 11.1 Distribution of 45 Clients by Intervention and Goals Achieved

	All Goals Achieved	Some Goals Achieved	No Goals Achieved	Total
Intervention A	9	1	5	15
Intervention B	3	7	5	15
Intervention C	3	5	7	15
	15	13	17	45

$\chi^2 = 9.58$, df $= 4$
$p < 05$

cacy. This is accomplished through analysis of the distribution of cases on a contingency table, with the columns on the table representing categories of one variable and rows representing categories of the other. If the column variable (which in my example I will label the outcome) is independent of the row variable (labeled the intervention), one would expect the cases employed in the analysis to be distributed across the column variable in a way that is roughly proportionate to their frequency in the row variable. If the departure from the expected frequency is extremely different from what one might expect from chance alone (e.g., less than a probability of .05), then the researcher would reject the hypothesis that the intervention is independent of the outcome. This test's utility for programmatic evaluation and the analysis of clinical interventions should be fairly obvious. Often it is the case, both for interventions and outcomes, that the categories are not quantifiably distinct so much as representative of differences. Another advantage of the chi-square test is that it can accommodate several different categories of both the intervention and the outcome variable while yielding an estimate of the probability that the intervention and the outcome variables are independent. However, the chi-square test cannot by itself offer any information as to which particular categories of either the intervention variable or outcome variable are contributing to the relationship between the variables.

The hypothetical example shown in Table 11.1 illustrates some of these key points. In this example there are three social work interventions labeled A, B, and C. Each intervention is applied to 15 clients, and outcomes are categorized in rough fashion as: (a) all goals achieved,

(b) some goals achieved, and (c) no goals achieved. The question, assuming that there is no relationship between the client's characteristics and the intervention applied, is whether the type of outcome achieved is independent of the intervention. Were this the case, the frequency in each cell on the table would be close to 5. In examining Table 11.1 it appears that there is a relationship, in that Intervention A appears to yield a higher number of favorable results than the other two categories. However, with such a small number of clients in each intervention category some consideration should be given to the possibility that these results might reflect random chance rather than the contrasting effects of the three interventions.

As it happens, the chi-square statistic (χ^2) of 9.58 with 4 degrees of freedom (calculated as rows $-$ 1 x columns $-$ 1) crosses the region of the χ^2 distribution where the probability of the results shown on the table by chance alone are less than .05. Based on this statistical inference we can therefore reasonably reject the argument that the intervention and the outcome variables are independent. Although the χ^2 statistic will not by itself explain which of the particular interventions is responsible for this result, the distribution of cases on the table shows that Intervention A is the one with the highest variance from the results one would expect from chance alone.

The *t* Test

The *t* test has some important variations that will be discussed later in this section, but in general it is applied when the investigator has two categories of the intervention variable, and the outcome variable is assumed to at least approximate the interval level of measurement. In its clinical applications the t test is principally employed to test the difference between the means scores on some outcome variable across two treatment conditions that are hypothesized to have different effects. Where there is a statistically significant difference between the means of the outcome variable across the two treatment conditions that comprise the independent variable, it is inferred that there is a treatment effect—the magnitude of which can be estimated from the ratio that employs the t test statistic and the number of subjects used in the analysis. A distinct advantage of the t test is that it has the property of being robust with respect to violation of its distributional assumptions, even with a small number of subjects. The t test is divided into two general types (although there are multiple additional variations): the independent samples t test and the correlated groups t test. In the former, it is assumed that subjects are randomly assigned to the treatment conditions being contrasted while in the latter the subjects are either the same individuals exposed to all of the treatment conditions being contrasted or are matched by characteristics that are assumed to have an important effect on the dependent variable across the treatment conditions being contrasted. The correlated groups t test is a more efficient test because fewer subjects are required to identify a statistically significant treatment effect on the dependent variable.

In a hypothetical example of a correlated group t test, suppose a group of 10 cancer patients who have similar types of cancer are given a baseline interview and scored on a set of questions pertaining to the amount of knowledge they have concerning their particular diagnosis and their treatment alternatives. After participating in a cancer support group facilitated by a social worker and oncology nurse the patients are again interviewed, and a score is again assigned based on a version of the baseline questions. Table 11.2 shows both the data and the results from a correlated group t test. It is noted that the mean change in scores from the baseline interview to the post–support group interview is 2.40 with a standard deviation of 1.78, indicating a high degree of variation among the group in how much participation in the support group appears to have impacted knowledge of the disease and treatment relative to the average change. Still, is the change in knowledge larger than what might be expected from chance alone?

The short answer to the question is yes. That is, the probability of observing a t statistic of at least 4.27 by random chance with the number of subjects involved in the analysis is less than .05. Note that the numerator in the correlated groups t test is expressed as $\bar{D}$, or the mean change in the dependent variable (knowledge score), while the denominator, $\hat{S}_{\bar{D}}$ is the standard error of the mean of the difference. Conceptually, this is a ratio comprised of the observed change in the level of cancer knowledge over the average amount of variance in an infinite number of estimates of the observed change predicted from the sampling distribution of t.

In order to estimate the magnitude of the effect of the support group intervention, the t score derived from the data can be transformed to a statistic called eta^2, which represents the proportion of the variability in the dependent variable that is explained by treatment effect. A convenient method for the computation of eta^2 is

$$\text{eta}^2 = \frac{t^2}{t^2 + df}$$

and in example given in Table 11.2 is

TABLE 11.2 Post Support Group Change in Cancer Knowledge

Mean Baseline Cancer Knowledge Score	Mean Post–support Group Knowledge Score	Mean Change in Score	Standard Deviation of Change in Score
2.20	4.60	2.40	1.78

$t = \dfrac{\bar{D}}{\hat{S}_{\bar{D}}} = \dfrac{2.40}{.562} = 4.27$, *degrees of freedom* $= N - 1 = 9$

$p < .05$

$$\frac{4.27^2}{4.27^2 + 9} = .67.$$

In other words, in the hypothetical example in Table 11.2, 67% of the variation in the average change in the cancer knowledge base between the pretest and posttest interview score is attributed to the influence of the support group experience.

One-Way ANOVA

The limited purpose and length of this chapter precludes more than a cursory discussion of one-way analysis of variance (ANOVA), which, like the *t* test, is a widely employed method of assessing both statistical significance and magnitude of effect in experimental and quasi-experimental evaluations of clinical and programmatic interventions. One-way ANOVA is a bivariate analysis tool commonly used in situations where the investigator has a set of three or more distinct interventions/treatment conditions and an outcome variable that at least approximates the interval level of measurement. The interventions can be measured at either the nominal or ordinal level, which is one more reason the ANOVA is so widely used. Also like the *t* test, ANOVA yields both test of significance for a difference in means and an estimate of eta², or the proportion of variance in the outcome variable that can be attributed to the interventions.

ANALYSIS OF EFFECTS AND STATISTICAL CONTROL

The earlier discussion of chi-square, *t* tests, and ANOVA all concerned the ideal circumstance in which the investigator is able to assume that there are no extraneous sources that are confounding the relationship between the intervention/treatment variable and the outcome variable. In the hypothetical example of the cancer support group analysis, sources of confound were controlled by having the same subjects exposed to the two different treatment conditions (pregroup and postgroup). However, the conditions for a within-subjects experimental design often are not possible, and the investigator must draw on other methods of controlling for extraneous sources of influence over the interven-

tion–outcome relationship. Multivariate analysis techniques, when properly applied and interpreted, have the advantage of introducing statistical controls in a manner that yields estimates of the variance in the outcome variable while controlling for variables that represent extraneous sources of influence. The most widely used methods of statistical control that are employed in clinical and programmatic analyses are derived from the additive linear model in which the variance in the outcome variable is modeled as the sum of a series of effects of a set of specified independent variables, including both the control variables and the intervention/treatment variable.

A simple exemplar of statistical control techniques involves partial correlation, where the correlation between two interval level variables is observed while controlling for a third. The correlation coefficient in its most common form varies between −1 and +1, with 0 representing no relationship and the extreme values representing either a perfectly linear negative relationship or a perfectly linear positive relationship. As a hypothetical example, I constructed a dataset with three sets of scores of 27 adolescent girls with low self-esteem. The first score varies from 1 to 4 and represents the intensity of individual counseling efforts aimed at self-esteem enhancement while the second variable represents the change in the self-esteem scale that occurred for each child over the course of the counseling intervention. It is noted in my hypothetical example that the bivariate correlation coefficient between these variables is .70 at the $p < .01$ level of statistical significance, indicating a very strong beneficial effect of the counseling. I then introduced a third variable, a 5-point social class scale that introduces the possibility that the self-esteem enhancement benefits attributable to counseling are actually very sensitive to social class differences among the children. When I control for influence of social class via the statistical technique of partial correlation, the estimate of the correlation between the counseling intensity variable and the change in self-esteem variable is reduced to a .30 and also falls well below conventions of statistical significance. The inference is that social class in this context exerts a powerful confounding effect on the beneficial influences of counseling.

While techniques of statistical control that are derived from linear regression models are widely used for statistical control and the analysis of intervention/treatment effects, they are also widely misused. Fundamental errors of misuse and misinterpretation abound both in everyday applications and in published literature. Chief among these errors are errors of specification, for example, a failure to include relevant variables in the model, inclusion of irrelevant variables, or application of a linear model where the relationship between the intervention/treatment variable and the outcome variable is nonlinear (Pedhazur, 1982). Errors of interpretation also abound, in particular due to an inadequate understanding of the factors affecting the partitioning of variance in regression models.

MULTIVARIATE APPLICATIONS TO PROBLEMS OF PREDICTION: A BRIEF NOTE ON STEPWISE REGRESSION AND DISCRIMINANT ANALYSIS

It should be apparent from the preceding discussion that multivariate analysis techniques that are applied to the problem of statistical control can be extended to problems of prediction. Both involve the estimation of the relative degree of influence on a given dependent variable from multiple sources of variance. In prediction, however, the researcher's aim is not to explain cause and effect, but rather to identify the most efficient limited set of predictors from a large set of potential predictors. One might ask, for example, what best predicts the likelihood of a mental health clinic client's risk of hospitalization over a specified observation period from a plethora of factors—for instance, the frequency of outpatient visits, the baseline level of social functioning on a standard scale, the DSM-IVR code assigned to the client, the principal therapist, the type of insurance coverage provided, and so on. Knowing which particular factors are most predictive of hospitalization would enable the agency to target services to those clients who were most likely to be hospitalized. Another clinical application concerns suicide risk and the development of assessment tools that include items that are most highly predictive of suicide. In a recent study researchers applied stepwise regression analysis to data from a sample of clients diagnosed with schizophrenia to identify

the factors that were most predictive of suicide risk. Their findings suggest that younger age and recent traumatic stress each significantly predicted higher suicide risk, independent of the depressive symptoms that might ordinarily be the only dimension closely assessed by many clinicians (Schwartz & Cohen, 2001). In stepwise regression, a criterion variable that represents the event or phenomena of interest is identified as the dependent variable and a set of independent variables specified as predictors are systematically tested against one another in a series of regression equations. In this fashion the variables that are the most predictive of the criterion event are identified. Discriminant analysis is employed where the general aim is to study group differences on several variables simultaneously (Pedhazur, 1982). In clinical application this often translates to a discovery of which variables are relevant to problems of prediction, for example, as in identifying critical differences between violent and nonviolent juvenile offenders. Although explication of these procedures is beyond the scope of this chapter, a general acquaintance with them is highly relevant to the practitioner interested in problems of prediction.

References

Almgren, G., Yamashiro, G., & Ferguson, M. (2002). Beyond welfare or work: Teen mothers, household subsistence strategies, and child development outcomes. *Journal of Sociology and Social Welfare, 29*(3), 125–149.

Blalock, H. M. (1979). *Social statistics: Revised second edition.* New York: McGraw-Hill.

Borgatta, E., & Kamo, Y. (2000). Measurement. In E. Borgatta and R. Montgomery, *Encyclopedia of sociology.* New York: Macmillan.

Jaccard, J., & Becker, M. (1997). *Statistics for the behavioral sciences.* Pacific Grove, CA: Brookes/Cole.

Pedhazur, E. J. (1982). *Multiple regression in behavioral research.* Chicago: Holt, Rinehart, and Winston.

Schwartz, R. C., & Cohen, B. N. (2001). Risk factors for suicidality among clients with schizophrenia. *Journal of Counseling and Development, 79*(3), 314–319.

Weinbach, R. W. (1989). When is a statistical test meaningful? A practical perspective. *Journal of Sociology and Social Welfare, 16*(1), 31–37.

SECTION II
Research Ethics and Step-by-Step Research Grant Guidelines

12 METHODOLOGICAL, PRACTICAL, AND ETHICAL CHALLENGES TO INNER-CITY HEALTH RESEARCH

Stephen W. Hwang, Rochelle E. Martin, & Ahmed M. Bayoumi

Population growth is increasingly concentrated in metropolitan centers, with more than half the world's population expected to be living in cities by the year 2008 (United Nations Human Settlements Programme, n.d.). These large urban centers often consist of geographic communities that span a broad range of social and demographic characteristics, from neighborhoods of affluence and prosperity to those of severe and concentrated poverty. In the latter, sometimes referred to as the *inner city*, residents contend with distinctive environmental, social, and health problems.

Social and economic disadvantage and the associated impact on health are a growing concern in both developed and developing nations (Wilkinson, 1996). As socioeconomic disparities have widened, the health of the poor has worsened (Kawachi, Wilkinson, & Kennedy, 1999). Only some of the factors linking ill health, urbanization, and social disadvantage are understood. The goals of inner-city health research are to gain greater understanding of the social, economic, and health care factors that influence both individual and population health and to evaluate policies and interventions that may lead to improved health and health care delivery among disadvantaged urban populations.

Inner-city health research can present a variety of challenges (Table 12.1). Some issues are methodological, such as how to design research and analyze data. Others are ethical, such as how to obtain informed consent and protect the privacy and confidentiality of participants drawn from vulnerable populations. In this context, we focus on vulnerabilities to poor health, to which inner-city residents may be more prone given the higher than average rates of poverty, social instability, environmental degradation, recent immigration, mental illness, and substance use in these environments (Wasylenki, 2001). Research in the inner city is also associated with special considerations stemming from the unique role of the inner-city health researcher, who may be called upon to balance the roles of investigator, advocate, activist, and caregiver.

PROJECT DESIGN AND DATA ANALYSIS

Definition of the Issues

As with all scientific inquiry, inner-city health research must be demonstrably interesting, relevant, and feasible (Cummings & Hulley, 1988). Research that defines itself in terms of socially disadvantaged regions or populations may raise questions about the motivations propelling the endeavor. Specifically, the inspiration of the study may arise from a desire for social or political change rather than from a scientifically objective pursuit of new knowledge. Whereas some argue that no scientific pursuits are truly value-free, we believe that investigators conducting such "mission-based" research need to

TABLE 12.1 Challenges of Inner-City Health Research

Project design and data analysis	• Definition of the issues • Selection and definition of the research question and study population • Recruitment of study participants • Retention and follow-up of study participants • Data collection and analysis
Ethical considerations	• Informed consent • Participant incentives • Privacy and confidentiality
Role of the researcher	• The researcher as advocate or activist • The researcher's obligation to study participants • Dissemination of findings • Translation of research into action
Policy and practice implications	• Stigma and stereotypes • Observation vs. intervention • Health problems vs. social problems

acknowledge that motivational biases can—and do—exist.

Consider a researcher concerned about the paucity of primary care physicians in low-income neighborhoods. Her primary motivation for research may be a belief in health as a human right, but her research question relates to the association between access to primary care and health status. Accordingly, she designs a study to investigate whether low-income women without primary care are at increased risk of developing undetected cervical cancer. Despite her values and beliefs, the researcher needs to maintain scientific rigor (e.g., by identifying important confounders such as patients' behaviors). In general, researchers should be transparent in the way they conduct scientific inquiry and vigilantly self-critical in reporting both positive and negative results.

Similarly, funding opportunities, rather than values or community needs assessments, often drive research agendas (Freudenberg, 2001). Thus, researchers may feel constrained or compromised when applying for funding. Grant competitions that are thematic in their request for proposals may limit the range of questions that researchers are able to address. Award requirements may also dictate elements of study design, such as researcher-driven versus community agency participation. Furthermore, scientists' perspectives on interesting and important research questions may diverge from those of funding agencies or community members.

Consider a granting agency that has extended a call for proposals to address the risk of prostate cancer among minority men. Consultation with community agencies that work with minority men in the inner city may reveal that these agencies are willing to partner with the researcher, but that prostate cancer is not a leading concern. Instead, economic development and access to primary care may be community priorities, creating tension between expressed needs and what is immediately fundable. Extended dialogue and strategizing may be necessary to reach consensus (Leviton, Snell, & McGinnis, 2000).

Selection and Definition of the Research Question and the Study Population

To appropriately describe and interpret research findings, researchers must clearly define and describe the populations being studied, as well as highlight the assumptions that lie behind the classification of such aggregate groups. For example, how should individuals be aggregated—into neighborhoods, census tracts, or cities? How will these be defined? The definitions used will shape—and, in some cases, will be shaped by—the study design and recruitment strategies. Definitions are also important when considering individual characteristics. For instance, who are the homeless? Does this group include those who are living with friends or family because they cannot afford a place of their own, or only those living on the street and in homeless shelters? Investigators should approach these issues from several perspectives. Pragmatically, restricting the definition to shelter users and street dwellers makes sample selection easier. Scientifically, such restrictions may threaten the generalizability of the findings and introduce misclassification biases. Politically, restricted definitions may be challenged if they are perceived to exclude a significant subgroup of people without stable housing.

Question selection and population definition are not simply matters of semantics. In many cases, the manner in which a question is defined may determine a priori the possible results of the study. Conversely, an incorrectly framed question or poorly selected research methods may produce accurate results but spurious conclusions. This problem has been called getting the "right answer to the wrong question," or Type III error (Schwartz & Carpenter, 1999). Underlying this problem is the fact that predictors of individual differences in health outcome may not be the same as predictors of differences in health between populations (Schwartz & Carpenter, 1999). For example, consider the example of racial differences in infant mortality presented by Schwartz and Carpenter (1999). Studies that focus on interindividual differences, such as risk factors for preterm delivery among African American women, may not answer the question of primary interest, which is the causal factors underlying the infant mortality rate difference between Whites and African Americans. By examining African American women only, characteristics common to African American women (such as discrimination) will not be identified as potential causal factors underlying the between-population differences.

Sometimes the intent of research is to draw conclusions concerning macrolevel processes, such as how neighborhood-level characteristics impact the health of individuals. Again, properly defining the unit of analysis will determine how the research is undertaken and how the results will be interpreted. For instance, administrative data sources, such as hospitals, municipal governments, and community agencies, may vary in their definitions of city boundaries. Some neighborhood-level data are defined by postal or zip code, while others are linked to census tract boundaries. Furthermore, communities may have their own definitions that do not concur with official designations. The degree of overlap between differing definitions will determine the ease and accuracy with which such information can be incorporated into inner-city health research.

Recruitment of Study Participants

Once a research question has been formulated and the population of interest defined, the next step is to begin participant recruitment. In inner-city health research, gaining access to vulnerable and hard-to-reach populations may be challenging due to geographic dispersion or sociocultural constraints. Successful recruitment strategies may include collaborating with community-based organizations, using peer recruiters, or promoting the study in public spaces frequented by the individuals of interest. Each method should be flexible, adaptive, and sensitive to participants' needs (Julion, Gross, & Barclay-McLaughlin, 2000; Lindberg, Solozano, Vilaro, & Westbrook, 2001). Word-of-mouth recruitment strategies may be useful in certain studies for increasing enrollment; however, the potential threat to external validity is great (Julion et al., 2000).

A common reason that inner-city researchers fail to recruit individuals is mistrust on the part of potential participants. Suspicions may originate from individuals' negative experiences with the health care system, a general aversion to authority, experiences with systematic discrimination, or past abuses by health researchers (Jones, 1993). An awareness and appreciation of the potential tensions in the researcher–participant relationship provides a crucial foundation for successful recruitment strategies. Tensions may be eased through partnering with community-based organizations.

Retention and Follow-up of Study Participants

Longitudinal studies are critical in observational research to establish causal links between predictors and health outcomes. They are also important in evaluating the effectiveness of interventions. However, conducting long-term follow-up studies among inner-city populations faces several challenges. For example, inner-city residents are highly mobile, making follow-up and retention difficult. This problem may be exacerbated by the fact that a significant number may lack a home telephone or may change telephone numbers frequently (Senturia et al., 1998; Blumenthal, Sung, Coates, Williams, & Liff, 1995).

Follow-up may also be hampered if participants use pseudonyms or variants of their names. Pseudonyms may be used for a variety of reasons, including cultural preferences, mental illness, or a desire for anonymity (Rendelman, 1998). The names of immigrants may be Anglicized or transliterated into multiple spelling variants. It is important to be cognizant of these issues, particularly when large databases are used to identify individuals for follow-up or to link information between databases. The use of soundex algorithms, which match records based on the way a name sounds rather than the way it is spelled, may aid in minimizing the loss of participant information due to the misspelling of names. In populations in which the use of aliases may be common, such as street culture subgroups, questions regarding known aliases could be included in the data collection process.

Important techniques for successful retention of inner-city residents in research studies include obtaining multiple alternate contacts outside the participant's household, making studies flexible enough to schedule follow-up interviews on evenings and weekends, offering financial incentives for follow-up, and using computerized databases and telephone search methods (Senturia et al., 1998). Longitudinal contact with many population subgroups, such as homeless people, can also be facilitated through community agencies that maintain close ties with these individuals (Pollio, Thompson, & North, 2000).

Data Collection and Analysis

Even when research questions are clearly formulated, the design of data collection may not be straightforward. Surveys administered by an interviewer maintain a degree of consistency between surveys, but individuals may be more forthcoming if self-completed questionnaires are used, particularly when the information sought is of a personal nature. Preselected response categories allow for ease of analysis, as well as facilitating comparability between studies. However, these may miss important subtleties or entire possibilities that an open-ended response may reveal.

Qualitative researchers face their own set of challenges, particularly at the time of data collection. Although qualitative interviewers always need to be aware of how their own biases and beliefs may guide the interview process, such considerations may be particularly important in settings where individuals are in a vulnerable state. One method of demonstrating rigor in qualitative research is to appeal to external standards; an alternative conceptualization of rigor starts from an assessment of inquiry as intrinsically value-laden (Ratcliffe & Gonzalez-del-Valle, 1988). Such a paradigm, which evaluates each choice in the process of inquiry

against the implicit and explicit values behind the decisions, may be beneficial for all health researchers in the inner city.

In recognition of the community's key role in research, conclusions reached through qualitative methods should be brought back to the participating population for validation (Bailey, 1996). After analyzing, evaluating, and summarizing findings, researchers should verify with participants that the synthesized results are accurate reflections of the study participants' responses. Such steps help ensure that conclusions drawn from participants' responses are based not on researchers' biases but on the participants' own experiences and views.

Researchers who perform aggregate-level quantitative analyses need to guard against the ecological fallacy, in which inferences are inappropriately drawn at one analytical level (e.g., individuals) from studies focused on a different unit of analysis (e.g., neighborhoods). For example, if the level of injection drug use is more common in low-income neighborhoods, it does not necessarily follow that individuals with low income are more likely to be injection drug users. Multilevel methods, in which hierarchical systems are used to classify the potential units of analysis, are often an appropriate and appealing method for quantitative statistical analysis of inner-city projects if sufficient data are available (Burton, Gurrin, & Sly, 1998). Researchers planning interventional studies face a related set of concerns, in which the level of intervention may not be the same as the level at which outcomes are measured.

ETHICAL CONSIDERATIONS

Inner-city health research comes with important ethical responsibilities and implications for the researcher. This section examines ethical considerations that are inherent to all investigation but that may be particularly relevant to inner-city health research.

Informed Consent

As part of the recruitment process, all potential study participants must provide informed consent prior to enrollment. Individuals must be provided with sufficient information to allow them to make an informed and uncoerced decision concerning participation. For studies that are complex or associated with substantial risks, this process becomes more involved and potentially more difficult to undertake responsibly.

A central tenet of consent is that it should be voluntary. The U.S. Office for Human Research Protections' definition of voluntary, derived from the Belmont Report, is consent that is "free of coercion, duress, or undue inducement" (National Commission for the Protection of Human Subjects of Biomedical and Behavioral Research, 1978). Issues of coercion and duress (compulsion through the use or threat of force) may be of particular concern for individuals whose autonomy and freedoms are limited due to extreme impoverishment or restrictions imposed by the judicial system. When individuals are recruited from these groups, investigators need to ensure that participants are not consenting for the wrong reasons, for example, because they fear that they will be punished if they do not participate.

Individuals may feel coerced into participation if they perceive that the researcher has significant control over their well-being. Such may be the case when the researcher is also a physician who provides health care to the individual or if there is a partnership between the researcher and a community agency whose services the individual accesses. Effective communication can mitigate the potential power differential between researcher and participant. The researcher's manner of dress, for instance, can either highlight or subdue his or her authority. For example, although hospitalized patients prefer that their doctor wear a white coat because the physician is perceived as being more professional, authoritative, and scientific (Gooden, Smith, Tattersall, & Stockler, 2001), these characteristics could significantly impede uncoerced consent. Similarly, the type of language used when communicating with a potential participant can create ease or tension.

Researchers conducting inner-city health studies may wish to recruit individuals with mental illness or substance abuse problems, or they may conduct studies in populations that have a high prevalence of these conditions, such as homeless people (Fischer & Breakey, 1991). In these circumstances, mental health research has highlighted several important considerations when obtaining consent (Moser et al., 2002). First, the presence of mental illness or addiction per se does not necessarily indicate incapacity to give consent (Poythress, 2002). Furthermore, a diagnosis of severe and persistent mental illness—even one as limiting as schizophrenia—is less important for determining capacity than the presence of specific capacity-limiting symptoms and impairments. Second, capacity to consent can vary in an individual patient at different times. Specific instruments are available to evaluate decisional capacity to consent, but these instruments frequently require modification for specific studies and careful interpretation (Applebaum & Grisso, 2001). Third, such instruments may be most useful in identifying areas of the consent process that require specific remediation. Table 12.2 provides links to information that may be of use to researchers regarding the ethical issue of informed consent.

Other situations that may make obtaining consent difficult include low literacy and lack of fluency in the languages of the research study. Evidence suggests that most consent forms, even those approved by institutional review boards, are written at too high a reading level (i.e., above an eighth-grade reading level; Paasche-Orlow, Taylor, & Brancati, 2003). Researchers in the inner city need to establish explicit procedures to ensure that study participants have the capacity to give consent and that they comprehend the specifics of the consent process (Capron, 1999; McGrady & Bux, 1999). Examples include translating consent forms into languages other than English, rewriting consent forms in low-literacy versions, and using nonwritten methods such as video and multimedia to communicate important messages (Jimison, Sher, Appleyard, & LeVernois, 1998).

Participant Incentives

An issue that often arises in conjunction with informed consent is the use of participant incentives. Payment may be offered to participants for a variety of reasons, including reimbursement for expenses, compensation for time and effort, or as an incentive to participate in a study that may otherwise have difficulty attracting participants (Grady, 2001). Incentives are often monetary payments, but they could also include nonmonetary material rewards, such as vouchers or transportation tokens. Researchers who offer potential recruits payment, whether monetary or in-kind, in exchange for participating in a study need to be particularly careful that consent is not obtained under coercion because some participants may have a difficult time resisting the rewards.

Even when compensation of participants is deemed acceptable, selection of the appropriate

TABLE 12.2 Information Resources on the Ethical Conduct of Research

Resources	Web locator
National Institutes of Health	www.nih.gov
NIH Certificate of Confidentiality	grants.nih.gov/grants/policy/coc/
The Belmont Report: Ethical Principles and Guidelines for the Protection of Human Subjects of Research	206.102.88.10/ohsrsite/guidelines/belmont.html
The President's Council on Bioethics	www.bioethics.gov
Research Involving Persons with Mental Disorders That May Affect Decisionmaking Capacity: Vol. 1. Report and Recommendations of the National Bioethics Advisory Commission	www.georgetown.edu/research/nrcbl/nbac/capacity/TOC.htm
Readability scales (e.g., Fleisch-Kincaid)	Available as part of many word-processing software packages, often as a component of the spell-check or grammar functions

amount may be difficult (Sears, 2001). Suggested methods include setting the monetary amount at a level that is not excessive and that is calculated based on time or contribution (Grady, 2001) or setting the compensation rate at the level of low-wage, unskilled labor (Dickert & Grady, 1999). Yet even low payment rates may sometimes be an undue inducement for inner-city residents because the potential for undue inducement is greatest when "a person is economically destitute and truly has no other options for acquiring comparable amounts of money" (Grady, 2001, p. 42).

Other considerations in setting an appropriate compensation also need to be considered. Whereas a rate that is too high may act as an undue inducement, an overly low rate may introduce a selection bias into a study by dissuading participation among those individuals, such as the working poor, who cannot afford to forgo their regular source of income (Viens, 2001). Practically, researchers, research ethics boards, and community partners will need to determine the "appropriate" compensation rates according to local circumstances, the particulars of a project, and their own sense of fairness (Dickert & Grady, 1999).

Privacy and Confidentiality

It is the responsibility of all research team members, and not only the principal investigator, to ensure the privacy of research participants and to uphold the confidentiality of all garnered information. Privacy and confidentiality are paramount concerns when study participants suffer from potentially stigmatizing conditions, such as human immunodeficiency virus infection, or are engaged in illegal activities, such as the sale of illicit drugs. Researchers collecting sensitive information should consider obtaining a certificate of confidentiality, which is issued by the National Institutes of Health (NIH), to protect research information from forced disclosure in civil, criminal, and other proceedings (see Table 12.2). Although anonymity can be maintained relatively easily in laboratory studies, observational and survey-based research can face more difficult challenges, particularly when answering the research question involves obtaining life history and personal information. If participants are not sufficiently confident that confidentiality will be upheld, the accuracy and completeness of the data will likely be compromised.

Researchers usually inform participants about procedures designed to safeguard confidentiality, but they less frequently discuss the limits of confidentiality (McGrady & Bux, 1999). For example, researchers may be required to break confidentiality if they discover that a research participant is actively homicidal or suicidal or is engaged in child abuse or neglect. Researchers should become informed of current policies and procedures for managing these and other critical events, and protocols should be developed in advance of undertaking any study where these situations could conceivably occur.

Researchers working with secondary data that contain confidential or potentially sensitive information need to balance the issues of privacy and confidentiality against the pursuit of free scientific inquiry. Although advances in data management make collection, storage, and linkage of data much easier than in the past, researchers should practice restraint in the mining of such resources. Real or perceived unfettered access may quickly engender mistrust and disillusionment. Appropriate consultation with community representatives, research ethics boards, and the original data custodians is a prudent and reasonable path for researchers to follow when planning data analyses beyond the scope of the original data collection or research project.

ROLE OF THE RESEARCHER

Inner-city researchers can face personal dilemmas in balancing the potentially conflicting roles of scientist, policy advocate, and political activist. More pointedly, the overarching question is whether investigators who study socially unjust situations are obligated to work for remedial changes.

Researcher as Advocate and Activist

The role of the researcher has been debated in many disciplinary arenas, not solely in that of inner-city health. Some argue that scientific inquiry ought to be conducted with objectivity and that research ought to be free of moral or social ideologies (Savitz, Poole, & Miller, 1999). Others contend that value judgments are inextricable from scientific inquiry and conduct (Krieger, 1999). By its nature, inner-city health research seeks ways to address unsolved problems, whether through policy, practice, or more research. Accordingly, all researchers are proponents of change, but they express this advocacy in different arenas.

The degree of overt activism will vary among researchers. It may range from writing a letter to the editor, to risking arrest in acts of civil disobedience, or even seeking political office or appointment. Although such choices reflect individual values, we believe it is problematic for investigators who conduct research in the inner city to have no sense of political engagement. At a minimum, investigators should acknowledge that the framing of a research question pertaining to the health of the disadvantaged occurs within a specific political and social context.

Researcher's Obligation to Study Participants

Another dilemma that researchers may face relates to their obligations to their research participants. Investigators, particularly those who are also health care providers, may find themselves in situations where they have identified individuals with remediable conditions. Quite often these identified issues will be unrelated to the research topic, but they still pose a real need for the participant. Investigators need to think carefully about what level of involvement they will have in helping their research participants navigate complicated systems—whether in health or social services—to find the care they need, and how this involvement may influence their research project.

From a health services perspective, investigators and funding agencies also need to think carefully about their obligations for facilitating or providing ongoing care that is being delivered within the context of a research project but that ceases when funding expires. For example, consider a study that is examining the effectiveness of a new intervention aimed at improving the access to care and the health status of recent immigrants. Preliminary results show that the program is effective, but when study funding runs out, there are no measures in place to continue providing services to this population. Community agencies may rightly feel a sense of abandonment. Rancor and tension between the investigators and the investigated may ensue. The long-term consequences of carrying out research in the inner city are worth considering at the beginning stages of research design, and potential contingency measures should be drafted *before* study initiation.

Dissemination of Findings

Research conducted in the inner city faces special challenges in the dissemination of findings (Leviton et al., 2000). Community members may express frustration and displeasure at researchers who harvest data but depart without sharing their results. Frontline workers and advocates may favor immediate release of research results through the media, in the hopes of rapidly affecting public policy. However, this strategy may conflict with the relatively slow time line of the academic cycle and may jeopardize publication in a peer-reviewed journal.

Communicating unexpected or unpopular findings can be difficult. Researchers should discuss and negotiate these issues with community representatives at the outset of the research effort. When communicating with the media, both researchers and community members should use concise language that is not prone to misinterpretation, that avoids negative stereotyping, and that states policy implications clearly.

Translation of Research Into Action

In addition to acknowledging the advocacy potential of researchers in the inner city, it is important to note that researchers may not possess the skills necessary to effectively bring about policy changes. Political savvy, communication skills, and knowledge of the social service system are not generally part of a researcher's training, yet these are essential if needed changes are to be effected. Researchers could learn many of these skills from community advocates. Partnerships not only make research more pertinent to the community but also can enhance researchers' ability to advocate effectively on the basis of their findings.

POLICY AND PRACTICE IMPLICATIONS

The importance of inner-city health research does not end with the termination of a study. The generation of knowledge has the potential to effect change in policy and practice, in both the short and the long term. This generally does not happen, however, without insight and planning on the part of the researcher.

Stigma and Stereotypes

Researchers in the inner city are most often motivated by benevolent intentions, such as highlighting issues of inequity and need among individuals and populations. Paradoxically, such initiatives may sometimes stigmatize and stereotype those individuals whom the researcher wishes most to help. The labels used—for example, words such as *poor*, *underprivileged*, or *addiction*—can stigmatize individuals. The extent to which individuals are considered as "participants to study" can be pejorative and potentially dehumanizing. For instance, referring to "the homeless" as a group highlights only one characteristic—an individual's lack of shelter—while neglecting many others that help to define a person. In truth, homeless individuals vary greatly in terms of age, education, family ties, and health status (Hwang, 2001).

The tendency to generalize study results to all members of a population can also result in stereotypes. Not all individuals who lack shelter suffer from mental health conditions, nor do all individuals who live in low-income areas of the city lack higher education. Similarly, stereotypes can obscure the strength and diversity of inner cities. For instance, although urban youth may be more likely to engage in violence than adolescents in rural areas, they also experience less emotional stress, are less likely to attempt suicide, and are less likely to engage in early sexual intercourse than rural youth (Leviton et al., 2000). Despite the positive aspects of urban centers, the "inner city" is often understood to be synonymous with social pathology, addictions, poverty, and homelessness (Andrulis, 1997). Inner cities also differ greatly from one another, and they change over time, as many experience an "urban renaissance" (Andrulis, 2000). More work is needed to understand what works well in inner cities and why, and how these lessons can be applied to alleviating the problems that occur there.

Observation Versus Intervention

Over the past decade, research has provided a great deal of information on the health of inner-city populations. Although much still needs to be examined and better understood, researchers now have a wealth of descriptive and observational data at their disposal. Unfortunately, there has not been a commensurate focus on the development and implementation of interventions that seek to improve the health of inner-city populations (Geronimus, 2000). This is often a more difficult challenge than simply describing the problem. Yet, of what use is knowledge if it is not used to effect positive change?

Advocacy is one means of intervention that has already been addressed. However, researchers should also apply scientific methods to the development and evaluation of interventions to improve the health of inner-city populations. Again, community partnerships, capacity building, and program development are key to developing effective interventions. This may require the participation of researchers and practitioners from disciplines other than health science, such as urban planners, economists, and political scientists, to name a few, who have not traditionally been invited to the table. Doing so can only increase the ability of research to truly effect change.

Health Problems Versus Social Problems

Implicit in inner-city health research is an understanding of the importance of social, economic, and systemic factors in determining the health status of populations. That is, issues apart from traditional biomedical models of disease and the health care system usually undergird health problems in disadvantaged urban populations. However, addressing social and economic issues in terms of their health consequences occasionally has the effect of removing them from the forum of public policy and social responsibility (Meyer & Schwartz, 2000). A further concern arises if social issues are addressed only if they have negative health consequences. As stated succinctly by Meyer and Schwartz, "Would homelessness divorced from its health impact be any less troubling? . . . Is discrimination any less unjust if it does not lead to adverse health outcomes?" (Meyer & Schwartz, 2000, p. 1190). Although socially unjust policies and structures may have deleterious outcomes, poor health is only one such outcome, and it is by no means the only important one.

In short, inner-city health has multiple determinants and dimensions beyond those traditionally studied by health researchers. Because the study and practice of improving health occurs within social and political contexts, and because nonhealth outcomes are important, the solutions to many issues are not likely to be found within the traditional health care sector. Instead, they may be found in "upstream" social and economic policies. Health care delivery is important for addressing an individual's specific health issues, but the provision of adequate

housing, education, and job skills training can improve the well-being of many inner-city residents. Researchers should be aware of both of these dimensions when seeking to make their work relevant to policy.

EXAMPLES OF PRACTICAL DILEMMAS

In practice, issues and challenges are not always easily distinguishable from each other; research design will have ethical implications, and involvement with community agencies will affect the researcher's role. To illustrate the issues that may arise in conducting research among vulnerable populations, the following two examples are presented, based on real-life situations that inner-city health researchers have experienced. Potential approaches to resolving each issue are discussed, bearing in mind that any response must be appropriate to the context in which the research is conducted.

Example 1: Paying Crack Cocaine Users

In conducting a longitudinal study of crack cocaine users, you give participants $20 for each follow-up visit they attend. A caseworker informs you that your participants are high the day after each visit and asks you to stop paying them. He says that you are contributing adversely to the crack epidemic in your city. Do you stop paying participants?

Several issues are highlighted in this example. The use of incentives is presumably intended to improve retention of study participants and to increase the likelihood of successful follow-up. An alternative to using monetary incentives as a retention tool might have arisen from involving community agencies or caseworkers (such as the one voicing concern in this example) in the research development phase. For instance, instead of providing participants with $20 in cash, the research team could have offered food or coffee vouchers of comparable value to participants who return for follow-up interviews.

Hindsight may be twenty-twenty, but the current predicament must be addressed. Several options are available to the researcher. For instance, the investigator may choose to continue with the current protocol. If this study has been approved by a research ethics board, the nature and amount of the incentive were deemed acceptable and appropriate in the context of the study. To discontinue with compensation may also jeopardize the study, eliminating the possibility of potentially important research findings. Alternately, the researcher may choose to discontinue compensation on the basis that the public health and political implications of providing crack users with money to buy drugs override other concerns. A third approach would be to alter the type of incentive offered by the study.

Example 2: Research and Politics

The director of a community agency calls you to express concern regarding a change in welfare policy. The director asks you to collaborate on a study that will demonstrate the negative health effects of the new policy. You are concerned that it will be difficult to demonstrate adverse outcomes because the policy change is recent and the outcomes are difficult to measure, yet you are sympathetic to the director's point of view. What do you say to her?

This example highlights the transscientific motivations that may drive research. Just as research ought to inform policy, policy changes ought to be evaluated for their impact on individuals and communities. Yet how should investigators respond to requests for research that serve a political agenda? One possibility would be to decline participation in the study in order to maintain scientific objectivity. This would not preclude revisiting the issue later, when outcomes resulting from the policy change may be more easily defined and measured. Another possibility is to consider undertaking the study, while insisting on rigorous scientific standards. This option requires a great deal of communication with community agencies that are affected by the policy change. Participants on both sides— research and community partners—must be clear in their intentions and abilities. A third possibility would be for the researcher to offer to speak publicly as an expert in the area, drawing on previous research to address the policy options being proposed.

CONCLUSION

The same issues that make improving the health of inner-city disadvantaged populations compel-

ling also make research in the field challenging. Successfully navigating these challenges requires strict scientific and ethical standards, a clear perception of one's own values and how these could potentially bias research, and sensitivity to political issues at the individual, community, and societal levels. Reaching a consensus on many issues may not be possible. What is imperative, however, is that investigators must explicitly consider issues relevant to their research, engage in dialogue with the inner-city communities in which they work, and develop cogent reasons for the decisions they ultimately make.

References

Andrulis, D. P. (1997). *The urban health penalty: New dimensions and directions in inner-city health care.* (Position paper.) Philadelphia: American College of Physicians.

Andrulis, D. P. (2000). Community, service, and policy strategies to improve health care access in the changing urban environment. *American Journal of Public Health, 90,* 858–862.

Appelbaum, P. S., Grisso, T. (2001). *MacArthur Competence Assessment Tool for Clinical Research.* Sarasota, FL: Professional Resource Press.

Bailey, P. H. (1996). Assuring quality in narrative analysis. *Western Journal of Nursing Research, 18,* 186–194.

Blumenthal, D. S., Sung, J., Coates, R., Williams, J., & Liff, J. (1995). Recruitment and retention of subjects for longitudinal cancer prevention study in an inner-city black community. *Health Services Research, 30*(1, Pt. 2):197–205.

Burton, P., Gurrin, L., & Sly, P. (1998). Extending the simple linear regression model to account for correlated responses: An introduction to generalized estimating equations and multi-level mixed modelling. *Statistics in Medicine, 17,* 1261–1291.

Capron, A. M. (1999). Ethical and human-rights issues in research on mental health disorders that may affect decision-making capacity. *New England Journal of Medicine, 340,* 1430–1434.

Cummings, S. R., & Hulley, S. B. (1988). *Designing clinical research: An epidemiologic approach.* Baltimore: Williams & Wilkins.

Dickert, N., & Grady, C. (1999). What's the price of a research subject? Approaches to payment for research participation. *New England Journal of Medicine, 341,* 198–203.

Fischer, P. J., & Breakey, W. R. (1991). The epidemiology of alcohol, drug, and mental disorders among homeless persons. *American Psychologist, 46,* 1115–1128.

Freudenberg, N. (2001). Case history of the Center for Urban Epidemiologic Studies in New York City. *Journal of Urban Health, 78,* 508–518.

Geronimus, A. T. (2000). To mitigate, resist, or undo: Addressing structural influences on the health of urban populations. *American Journal of Public Health, 90,* 867–872.

Gooden, B. R., Smith, M. J., Tattersall, S. J., & Stockler, M. R. (2001). Hospitalized patients' views on doctors and white coats. *Medical Journal of Australia, 175,* 219–222.

Grady, C. (2001). Money for research participation: Does it jeopardize informed consent? *American Journal of Bioethics, 1,* 40–44.

Hwang, S. W. (2001). Homelessness and health. *Canadian Medical Association Journal, 164,* 229–233.

Jimison, H. B., Sher, P. P., Appleyard, R., & Le-Vernois, Y. (1998). The use of multimedia in the informed consent process. *Journal of the American Medical Informatics Association, 5,* 245–256.

Jones, J. H. (1993). *Bad blood: The Tuskegee syphilis experiment.* Toronto: Free Press.

Julion, W., Gross, D., & Barclay-McLaughlin, G. (2000). Recruiting families of color from the inner city: Insights from the recruiters. *Nursing Outlook, 48,* 230–237.

Kawachi, I., Wilkinson, R. G., & Kennedy, B. P. (1999). Introduction. In I. Kawachi, B. Kennedy, and R. G. Wilkinson (Eds.), *Income inequality and health: The society and population health reader* (Vol. 1, pp. xi–xxxiv). New York: New Press.

Krieger, N. (1999). Questioning epidemiology: Objectivity, advocacy, and socially responsible science. *American Journal of Public Health, 89,* 1151–1153.

Leviton, L. C., Snell, E., & McGinnis, M. (2000). Urban issues in health promotion strategies. *American Journal of Public Health, 90,* 863–866.

Lindberg, C. S., Solozano, R. M., Vilaro, F. M., & Westbrook, L. O. 2001. Challenges and strategies for conducting intervention research with culturally diverse populations. *Journal of Transcultural Nursing, 12,* 132–139.

McCrady, B. S., & Bux, D. A. (1999). Ethical issues in informed consent with substance users. *Journal of Consulting and Clinical Psychology, 67,* 186–193.

Meyer, I. H., & Schwartz, S. (2000). Social issues as public health: Promise and peril. *American Journal of Public Health, 90,* 1189–1191.

Moser, D. J., Schultz, S. K., Arndt, S., Benjamin, M. L., Fleming, F. W., Brems, C. S., Paulsen, J. S., Appelbaum, P. S., & Andreasen, N. C. (2002). Capacity to provide informed consent for participation in schizophrenia and HIV research. *American Journal of Psychiatry, 159,* 1201–1207.

National Commission for the Protection of Human Subjects of Biomedical and Behavioral Research. (1978). *The Belmont Report: Ethical principles and guidelines for the protection of human subjects of research* (DHEW Publication No. OS 78-0012). Washington, DC: U.S. Government Printing Office.

Paasche-Orlow, M. K., Taylor, H. A., & Brancati, F. L. (2003). Readability standards for informed-consent forms as compared with actual readability. *New England Journal of Medicine, 348,* 721–726.

Pollio, D. E., Thompson, S. J., & North, C. S. (2000). Agency-based tracking of difficult-to-follow populations: Runaway and homeless youth programs in St. Louis, Missouri. *Community Mental Health Journal, 36,* 247–258.

Poythress, N. G. (2002). Obtaining informed consent for research: A model for use with participants who are mentally ill. *Journal of Law, Medicine and Ethics, 30,* 367–374.

Ratcliffe, J. W., & Gonzalez-del-Valle, A. (1988). Rigor in health-related research: Toward an expanded conceptualization. *International Journal of Health Services, 18,* 361–392.

Rendelman, N. (1998). False names. *Western Journal of Medicine, 169,* 318–321.

Savitz, D. A., Poole, C., & Miller, W. C. (1999). Reassessing the role of epidemiology in public health. *American Journal of Public Health, 89,* 1158–1161.

Schwartz, S., & Carpenter, K. M. (1999). The right answer for the wrong question: Consequences of Type III error for public health research. *American Journal of Public Health, 89,* 1175–1180.

Sears, J. M. (2001). Payment of research subjects: A broader perspective. *American Journal of Bioethics, 1,* 66–67.

Senturia, Y. D., McNiff Mortimer, K., Baker, D., Gergen, P., Mitchell, H., Joseph, C., & Wedner, H. J. (1998). Successful techniques for retention of study participants in an inner-city population. *Controlled Clinical Trials, 19,* 544–554.

United Nations Human Settlements Programme. (n.d.). Urbanization: Facts and figures [On-line]. Available: http://www.unhabitat.org/mediacentre/documents/backgrounder5.doc.

Viens, A. M. (2001). Socio-economic status and inducement to participants. *American Journal of Bioethics, 1,* 1f–1g.

Wasylenki, D. A. (2001). Inner city health. *Canadian Medical Association Journal, 164,* 214–215.

Wilkinson, R. G. (1996). *Unhealthy societies: The afflictions of inequality.* London: Routledge.

13

QUALITATIVE RESEARCH ETHICS

Thriving Within Tensions

Beverley J. Antle, Cheryl Regehr, & Faye Mishna

Qualitative research methods emerge from a worldview that asserts that subjective experiences and the meanings assigned to those experiences intimately shape notions of reality. Embedded within this broad framework are the expectation that there are multiple perspectives on the same phenomenon, the belief that the values and perceptions of both the researcher and the researched are an integral part of the endeavor, and the application of an inductive approach to investigation that begins with the experiences of participants and moves to ever-increasing layers of analysis and understanding (Cresswell, 1998; Maxwell, 1996; Strauss & Corbin, 1990). Traditional hierarchical barriers between the researcher and "the subject" are altered so that the expertise and subjectivity of both the researcher and the participant are acknowledged and viewed as an essential foundation for fostering a fuller and richer understanding of the phenomenon or issue being explored. These distinctions in worldview and researcher–participant roles have considerable implications for the ethical dimensions of qualitative research, which are more contextually based and render themselves less amenable to a structured set of rules. An emerging body of literature reflects the unique ethical issues that qualitative researchers face (Brownlow & O'Dell, 2002; Burman, 1997; Denzin, 2002; Hadjistavropoulos & Smythe, 2001; Magolda & Weems, 2002; O'Connor, 2001; Punch, 1994; van den Hoonaard, 2001). By examining the reported experiences of qualitative researchers, the research community can become better informed about unintentional harm and unanticipated risks that emerge from this methodology (Boman & Jevne, 2000; O'Connor, 2001; Punch, 1994).

There has been a worldwide effort to improve the ethical underpinnings of research since the Code of Nuremberg in 1947, but these efforts have intensified in the past decade. Researchers in North America who are conducting studies with human subjects are expected to submit their research proposals to independent research ethics boards for approval prior to implementation. To attain approval, they must demonstrate that the benefits associated with any research outweigh the risks; that the research design is scientifically sound and therefore worthy of submitting people to the associated risk and discomfort; that there is an informed consent process for participants; and that each participant's identity will be kept in confidence in all forums such as publication of research results (Council for International Organizations of Medical Sciences, 1993; Tri-Council Working Group, 1996). Indeed, the National Institutes of Health (NIH) in the United States, as a demonstration of their commitment to rigorous ethical review of research they fund, now demand that institutions receiving NIH funding offer a course that certifies the principal investigator's knowledge of the prevailing ethical research responsibilities [National Institutes of Health], 1999).

Although these efforts toward increasing accountability for researchers conducting studies are important and valuable, the prototype on which research ethics frameworks were developed is quantitative, specifically randomized control clinical trials. There are emerging concerns among qualitative researchers that the potentially unique ethical issues they face are not adequately captured either in current debates on research ethics or in institutional ethics review processes. Indeed, van den Hoonaard (2001) suggests that there is pervasive "moral panic" with respect to research ethics that may lead to an overestimation of the level of risks associated with qualitative research, especially if adjudicated by individuals who are unfamiliar with the method.

Further, whereas contemporary biomedical ethics are governed by an emphasis on moral principles (Beauchamp & Childress, 1994; Lantz, 2000), we suggest that qualitative research ethics may be more effectively informed by more contextual forms of ethics, such as reflective equilibrium (Pellegrino, 2000) and feminist ethics (Sherwin, 1992). Reflective equilibrium, derived from Rawls's work on distributive justice, calls upon the person to weigh morally important principles, such as autonomy, beneficence, nonmaleficence and justice, with significant contextual factors and the consequences of acting on these principles in this context. Resolution is achieved by striking a balance between principles, context, and potential outcomes. Indeed, Lantz (2000) suggests that reflective equilibrium is still essentially governed by principles and that what is needed are holistic ethics that are more phenomenologically based: "We must take interest in thick concepts such as health, quality of life, death, life, home, comfort, pain . . . by offering informal definitions in terms of wider contexts, for example by using stories or giving accurate descriptions of whole lives viewed as unitary entities" (p. 25). Feminist ethics places emphasis on appreciating the impact of potential outcomes on others and asserts that a good can be brought about only if the solution considers ways to correct inherent imbalances in the lives of women or other oppressed groups (Sherwin, 1992, 2001). A further hallmark of feminist ethics is the emphasis placed on relationships and the importance of considering the impact of a decision on the nature of key relationships among stakeholders (Mauthner, 2000).

It is of note that social work scholars and professional associations are beginning to specifically address research ethics (Butler, 2002; Reamer, 1998). The Codes of Ethics for Australia (AASW, 1999), Britain (BASW, 2002) and the United States (NASW, 1999) now contain more detailed guidance with respect to research. Indeed, Butler (2002) has proposed a unique code of ethics for social workers, suggesting that social workers should focus on the emancipatory potential of research.

In this chapter, we review the emerging ethical issues for qualitative researchers in the social sciences who engage individuals or human systems in research, viewing them from a more holistic ethics perspective and highlighting the complexity underneath desired ethical standards. We begin with a discussion of the relationship between the researcher and the participant as a foundation for the ethical issues that emerge in qualitative research. From this base, the following issues have been selected for inclusion in this discussion: (a) free and informed consent in the qualitative context; (b) protection of confidentiality with respect to highly personal and descriptive information; (c) balancing the roles of researcher and therapist; and (d) ownership of the story, determination of the outcomes of the research and how it should be disseminated.

POWER IN THE RESEARCH RELATIONSHIP

There are considerable variations among qualitative methods, but a cornerstone of the method is the distinct nature of the relationship between the researcher and participant. Rather than observing from a dispassionate distance, researchers using qualitative methods in the study of people (i.e., human subjects) are expected to immerse themselves in and engage with participants or communities to gain an insider's perspective on the phenomenon of interest. In the social sciences we are often interested in illuminating the experiences of vulnerable groups (children, people living in poverty, those who experience discrimination) and/or sensitive issues (bullying, rape, HIV/AIDS). The aim is to close the gap between the researcher and the participant to illuminate the depth of these experiences, to understand the meanings people and communities form about them, and to assist the voices of those in need to be heard. As is poignantly stated by Catherine MacKinnon (1987), "When you are powerless, you don't speak differently. A lot, you don't speak. Your speech is not just differently articulated, it is silenced. Eliminated, gone" (p. 39). Qualitative researchers often seek to break such silence and provide a forum for unheard voices.

Depending on the type of qualitative design employed, there is a greater or lesser attempt to engage the participant as a partner in various stages of the process. In some models, researchers seek to involve the community in the entire process of research, from formulation of the question, to the interpretation of findings (authenticity), to identification of solutions, and to the mobilization of human resources to effect social change (catalytic validity) (Brydon-Miller, 1997; Comstock & Fox, 1993). However, despite attempts to equalize the power between the researcher and those affected by the issue, there remains an inherent power imbalance in which the researcher, by virtue of role, education, institutional authority, and/or income, has a distinct "advantage" in the relationship. The risks to participants associated with this imbalance include the level of perceived freedom to refuse to engage in the research, the risk of divulging more personal information than they intended, and the control over the outcome of the research and use of their story.

FREE AND INFORMED CONSENT

Concern for the dignity and respect of individual participants is at the heart of research ethics. One important way that this principle is codified is through the doctrine of informed consent. The important elements of informed consent in research are: (a) ensuring that the person has the mental capacity to consent; (b) candidly disclosing sufficient information about the study and its aims to permit a person to weigh the potential risks and benefits of participation and to make a meaningful choice; (c) providing sufficient time and privacy to allow the person to fully consider participation; (d) providing any other safeguard to ensure that consent is given freely and without coercion; (e) ensuring that each person understands what will happen with information collected during the research process, the steps researchers will take to safeguard confidentiality of this material, and the measures to ensure anonymity in any reports of the study; and (f) ensuring that the person is aware that he or she may refuse to participate or may later withdraw consent without any penalty (Antle & Regehr, 2003; CIOMS, 1993; Tri-Council Working Group, 1996).

A challenging aspect of obtaining informed consent in qualitative research is the difficulty in anticipating potential risks. Indeed, Magolda and Weems (2002) mention lack of gatekeeper vigilance in anticipating harms as one of the unforeseen risks in qualitative research. Magolda describes the experience of meeting with a senior administrator of a residential college where he wanted to conduct his research. He was anticipating a discussion of risks and was unprepared for the administrator's ready acceptance of the proposal. Magolda reflected on his professional tensions between wanting to discuss potential risks with the administrator, who as a senior insider might foresee difficulties that could not be anticipated by the researcher, and not wanting to jeopardize the access that he needed to complete his study.

A potential risk for an individual participant is disclosing more information than he or she had anticipated or desired. The question of over-disclosure has been debated in the social science literature particularly with respect to ethnographic studies, where the researcher becomes immersed within the community of interest precisely so that the he or she will come to be seen as an insider and thus gain knowledge that would not otherwise be shared (Baez, 2002; Mauthner, 2000). The opportunity for participants to express their viewpoint about a particular issue or concern may be unprecedented and may result in a watershed of information and emotion. Once information is exposed, the participant may feel highly vulnerable and distressed. An example from one author's experiences in participatory research in the disability community highlights this dilemma. Our research team included consumers and had been approved by a local disability rights group, in addition to undergoing institutional ethics review, and thus had been authorized by important gatekeepers. In the course of sharing the journey to independent living, one participant provided a great deal of information about her/his employer and workplace difficulties. Following the interview, the participant contacted the investigator to express distress about the amount of information revealed. She/he requested the information be deleted from the transcribed version of the tape. Although the team expressed reservations, particularly because the issues were salient to the research, we decided that the most ethical course, given the participatory nature of the project and our guiding theoretical framework that promoted control and choice for persons with disabilities, was to honor this request.

These questions lead to a discussion of the inherent risks in probing deeply sensitive issues. If they have gained the participant's trust, what limits, if any, should qualitative researchers impose with respect to the level of intrusiveness of questions? What signals serve as reliable indicators that the participant is not protecting him- or herself sufficiently? Can these risks be anticipated in advance or during the process to prevent the research from straying into overly sensitive areas of a person's life or a community's experiences? One of the authors, for example, was interested in exploring the experiences of young women who had recovered from an eating disorder, with respect to their perceptions of the recovery process. Consultations with an expert clinician led to a change in the research design to interview young women rather than adolescents, thus increasing the length of time since recovery from the eating disorder. The clinician raised convincing concerns about the potential for relapse as a result of the in-depth retrospective discussions inevitable in a qualitative study.

A further risk to free and informed consent is whether there is a prior or concurrent therapeutic relationship between the researcher and the participant. In an era in which practitioners are encouraged to more rigorously evaluate their work, research and clinical practice are becoming increasingly intertwined. As we have discussed elsewhere (Regehr & Antle, 1997), a prior therapeutic relationship may limit the client's ability to consider carefully risks and benefits. Individuals may feel reluctant to refuse to participate for fear of disapproval or rejection by the researcher–therapist. Further, if the therapeutic relationship has been a helpful one, the client, now the participant, may assume that the research relationship will be similarly helpful, in spite of any warnings to the contrary by the researcher. This may also place participants at additional risk to expose more about themselves and their private perspectives than they might otherwise do if there had not been a preexisting therapeutic relationship.

The final area we wish to explore regarding informed consent is the question of deception in qualitative research. Since Whyte's landmark work *Street Corner Society* (1943), have the expectations changed among the individuals and communities that we hope will benefit from our research? Whyte's classic ethnography carefully documented street corner life and illicit networks that provided unprecedented insights into gang organization. Indeed, Whyte was an early pioneer of participatory action research, as he actively tried to influence community members to

mobilize a protest march addressing their needs and injustices. In a later edition of *Street Corner Society* (1955), Whyte reflected on his methods of gaining entry into and approval of the community, which were greatly assisted by "Doc," a leader of one of the gangs. Doc facilitated Whyte's ability to live with a family and provided explanations to community members who were curious or concerned about Whyte's presence and intentions. Doc, as a local gatekeeper, was an essential component in Whyte's successful integration into this society.

In spite of its tremendous impact, Whyte's study relied on deception, or at least a reduced vigilance by community members, over his 3½-year presence. In reexamining his decisions in this classic study, Whyte stated: "I believed that the themes I was presenting would have greater impact if I could present them about particular individuals, their relations with each other, the relations of group to group and groups to larger organizations. . . . Clearly some people were embarrassed by the book, but I could not find any evidence that I had seriously damaged any of them" (pp. 33–34).

Whyte's study continues to provide a vivid blueprint for the questions raised in contemporary qualitative research. Could Whyte, as an outsider, albeit one who had gained access and trust, adjudicate the extent of the harms to those who would remain in the community? What are the obligations of researchers to anticipate risks such as becoming aware of illegal activity, or indeed becoming an unwitting participants in such activity, when in the role of participant observer? And what role do the many other gatekeepers in both the academic community and the local community have in addressing potential harms to individuals and communities?

PROTECTING CONFIDENTIALITY

Whyte's classic study also leads to the important question of confidentiality in qualitative research. Confidentiality and anonymity are at the heart of an ethical and authentic research process (Council for International Organizations of Medical Sciences, 1993; Tri-Council Working Group, 1996), but they become much more difficult to assure when individuals are describing important and personal details of their experiences. In addition, the reporting of qualitative studies involves the use of quotations directly relating to the individual. Further, tapes of interviews with individuals involved in judicial proceedings, such as families currently involved with the child welfare system, or individuals who are victims of crimes or who are accused in criminal or civil proceeding, may contain damaging information relevant to these proceedings and could clearly reveal the identity of the participants.

Qualitative researchers who seek to gain an in-depth insider's perspective on a phenomenon frequently assert that unless sources perceive they will be protected by anonymity, the researcher will not receive an authentic picture of the insider experience. This was successfully argued by a Canadian criminology student, Russel Ogden, who after great effort successfully defended his perceived obligation to not reveal the identity of his participants in the HIV/AIDS community who discussed their experiences with assisted suicide, in spite of an ongoing coroner investigation (van den Hoonaard, 2001). Van den Hoonaard (2001) points out, however, that Ogden was successful only because he was able to demonstrate that absolute confidentiality and anonymity were essential to the research relationship. Van den Hoonaard asserts that with current standards for confidentiality, which require researchers to disclose the limits to confidentiality at the point of consent (such as a duty to report potential harm to self and others), it is unlikely that researchers can rely on the Ogden case as precedent for withholding participant information in legal proceedings. Ogden's case, though, does open up the specter of qualitative researchers arguing in select situations that institutional research ethics boards approve complete anonymity, thus selectively removing the requirement to present limits to confidentiality upon enrolment. To be effective, this would require the institution granting ethics approval to stand behind the researcher in a court challenge and to support legal costs.

A secondary challenge raised by prevailing ethical guidelines for confidentiality is that participants' stories and direct quotations be edited in such a way as to protect the identity of the participant. Although such changes are viewed as necessary to protect identity, they raise questions about how such modifications affect the overall results of the study, and further whether significant aspects of the phenomenon are lost in the process of alteration or omission (Baez, 2002; Magolda & Weems, 2002; Mauthner, 2000).

Baez (2002), for example, points out the challenges he faced in studying sexism and racism in tenure decisions in one university. The concerns of his colleagues with respect to potential retributions should the depth of their experiences be revealed meant that he could not report extensive examples of the discrimination experiences prevalent among faculty. The conflict for Baez was that he could protect participants' identities, but his research failed to have the transformational impact often sought in qualitative research and thus participants continued to be harmed by the oppressive structures that led them to so vigilantly demand anonymity. Burman (1997) suggests that qualitative researchers might need to be open to the transformational possibilities of other methods, such as questionnaires, that afford more protection for participants by being less intrusive or less revealing of identities in their presentation of results.

Balancing the Roles of Researcher and Therapist

We have already identified a potential conflict that may emerge if the researcher is also a practitioner who has a prior therapeutic relationship with the research participant in terms of undermining the perception of free consent. That is, not only may the participant feel that refusal to consent may jeopardize their relationship with the therapist/researcher, but also due to their trust that the therapist is acting in their best interest, they may not fully consider the risks associated with the research. A further issue that can arise from qualitative interviews conducted by researchers with clinical skills is that through the process of discussing their story, participants may become highly distressed, or reveal information that indicates they are in significant psychological or emotional distress. The challenge of dual relationships becomes imminently clear as the researcher grapples with whether to address the participant's distress in a therapeutic manner or as any research interviewer might, which is to provide referral for support and treatment. If the decision to refer is made, what obligation does the researcher have to ensure that the person has obtained help and is not at personal risk? Further, if the decision to refer is made, does this mean that the researcher can no longer consider the individual as a research participant, because of the researcher's knowledge of the individual's vulnerability?

Although many of the questions and issues discussed in this chapter also apply to conducting research with children and adolescents, some important and difficult ethical issues are unique to children (Graue & Walsh, 1998; Jokinen, Lappalainen, Meriläinen, & Pelkonen, 2002), most of which are beyond the scope of this chapter. Nevertheless, one important ethical consideration consists of the dilemma of children reporting in the course of a research interview that they may be hurt in some way that does not constitute a legal definition of abuse, for example, being bullied by other children or by siblings. The researcher in this case does not have the legal obligation, nor indeed the right, to follow up if a child does not indicate a desire for such intervention. Rather, the researcher is obligated to maintain the child's confidentiality and autonomy as much as possible (Jokinen et al., 2002). However, if they do not act on information that a child is being hurt, adults—in this instance the researchers—are not protecting the children, which raises ethical concerns. Indeed, even in cases where there are clear legal obligations and procedures such as reporting child abuse, and the procedures have been explained to the children and their parents prior to their involvement in the research, there may be ethical questions regarding whether and when to continue the research protocol with this child, after legal procedures are followed. These are pressing issues that require greater attention in the qualitative field, where such disclosures are more likely than in traditional methods.

WHO OWNS THE STORY?

The "place" of the researcher in the whole research endeavor has also opened up questions of ownership and appropriation of story. Whose story is it, and is it fair to expose tragedy and suffering without any direct objective of improving the circumstances of those who have taken the risks to expose their experiences? Can qualitative researchers use direct quotations from study participants without having copyright agreements signed? O'Connor (2001) suggests that qualitative researchers need to acknowledge that the study results are ultimately the researcher's story, one that is cocreated with the participants and ideally representative of their experiences, but that nonetheless is represented through the lens of the researcher and

influenced by his or her own theoretical orientation and worldview. O'Connor captures this process well: "I gradually began to realize that in contrast to where I had begun, I was becoming increasingly present in my work as I attempted to make explicit my interpretations, my positioning. With this realization came the recognition that I could neither write *the* story of another person nor could I write the *whole* story; I could, however, write part of *a* story" (p. 152).

In the wake of a number of communities expressing dissatisfaction with both the nature of the research process and the actual benefit accrued to participants from within these communities, demands have been made to provide participants greater control over the research process. (The disability community has been particularly vocal on this matter; see L'Institut Roeher Institute, 1994; Longmore, 1995; Woodill, 1992.) This demand is further reinforced by questions about the researcher's own stake in the research process. Competition for scarce funding and the value placed by the academic community on external funding for research and on publication of findings in scholarly journals mean that the successful engagement in and completion of studies are an integral part of the researcher's own professional success (von Schroeder, 1997). Further, the desired consumers of research results are often others involved in scholarly endeavors, that is, readers of high-impact, peer-reviewed journals. For instance, in medicine, publication in the *New England Journal of Medicine*, the *Journal of the American Medical Association* (JAMA), or the *Lancet* have become synonymous with success and high impact in the medical community. Yet those involved in the emerging field of knowledge transfer will tell us that publication in peer-reviewed venues alone is not effective in reaching either frontline practitioners or the community of people with whom the study was conducted (Broner, Franczak, Dye, & McAllister, 2001).

Other groups have been highly critical of the ability of researchers, particularly those within the university structure, to accurately reflect their experiences and needs. Heaney (1993) suggests that experts in universities are part of a system that promulgates the established order of society. Participatory research by such experts is, in his opinion, a contradiction in terms. Their mandate to represent the oppressed has been bestowed by legislators, not the subjects of inquiry themselves. Johnson (1996) eloquently raises this question with respect to participatory research with Native populations:

Participatory research under the direction of middle class indigenous leaders has not returned the control of knowledge production to indigenous communities. Rather, control has remained in the hands of the middle class (who represent the status quo). . . . Although the balance of power may be shifted from independent to collaborative research, western thought remains the dominant force in defining why, what and how knowledge is produced. (p. 28)

These groups, then, would not see externally based and funded researchers as capable of representing their needs and instead would see them as appropriating the voices of the oppressed.

ADDRESSING ETHICAL DILEMMAS IN QUALITATIVE RESEARCH

Without minimizing the complexity and seriousness of the questions raised here, we offer potential solutions to the inherent challenges of the research relationship in a qualitative context for practitioners engaged in research. In doing so we attempt to employ a more holistic and contextual approach to ethics such as reflective equilibrium and feminist ethics, which were described earlier. We agree with others in the field who reflect that ethical conduct of qualitative research requires the active engagement of the researcher throughout the research process and does not end with institutional approval and the participant's informed consent (Magolda & Weems, 2002; Punch, 1994; van den Hoonaard, 2001).

We acknowledge that the presence of a power differential between researcher and participant creates an underlying tension that must be attended to by the researcher. We, however, suggest that this differential does not in and of itself present a threat to potential participants or to the authenticity of research results. Indeed, social workers and other social scientists have a longstanding ethos that holds that successful social change often relies on a high-status person or institution using its power for the greater good of those who share neither such a high status nor its benefits (Antle & Regehr, 2003;

Balcazar, Seekins, Fawcett, & Hopkins, 1990; Sheppard, 2002). As eloquently stated by Burman (1997), "The dangers in research of exploitation arise where qualitative research is treated (only) as a method divorced from, wider structures of power" (p. 8).

Ensuring Free and Informed Consent

Applied social researchers, who frequently work with vulnerable populations, must anticipate issues related to accessibility and provide information both verbally and in written form. We recommend that written material be at a standardized grade 6 reading level and be made available in the language of choice of participants.

When studying sensitive issues, researchers are encouraged to reflect carefully and to consult with others regarding potential risks for participants and the broader potential risks to the population being studied (Antle & Regehr, 2003; Regehr, 2000; Burman, 1997). These consultations should include not only experts in qualitative methods and ethics but also experts in the phenomenon under study to diligently anticipate risks. We also encourage researchers to consider including a representative of the community of interest on the research team, even when other aspects of participatory methods are not feasible or desirable. Risks, once determined, should be communicated openly and fairly, both upon consent to participate and throughout the research process (van den Hoonaard, 2001). When there is a dual relationship, researchers should specifically forewarn potential participants of the complications associated with a therapeutic alliance and the potential to "overdisclose" (Antle & Regehr, 2003; Larossa, Bennett, & Gelles, 1981). In addition, participants should be told that not all risks can be anticipated and that should additional concerns arise, these must be addressed openly with participants (Larossa et al., 1981).

We suggest that the need for deception be carefully weighed in relation to the importance of the research question and the limitations in obtaining authentic information without deception, and that key stakeholders in the community of interest be consulted in such deliberations. We take a position that social science researchers should generally avoid the use of deception in research because of its implications for

TABLE 13.1 Ensuring Free and Informed Consent

Risks	Protections
• Individual discloses more information than anticipated • Emotional distress over sharing personal information • Therapeutic relationship overrides skepticism or undermines perceived freedom to refuse • Deception regarding purpose of research or role of researcher in order to obtain "insider" view	• Consultation with experts about possible unanticipated risks • Inclusion of community representative in research design • Ensuring competence to consent • Ensuring individual understands he or she may refuse to participate or withdraw • Full disclosure of risks, including the risk of overdisclosure • No use of deception unless scientifically compelling reason

the public trust in the academic mission. See Table 13.1 for a summary of these points.

Protecting Confidentiality

Preservation of privacy and confidentiality remains a paramount ethical consideration, and participants have a right to know the limitations on confidentiality. When concerns exist about fracturing stories to preserve confidentiality, qualitative researchers are encouraged to actively engage key stakeholders to address their anticipated concerns and to explore possible alternatives, which may need to include consideration of alternative research methods.

Researchers must also have legal counsel available to them address any legal risks to confidentiality of data. For work with groups on highly sensitive issues, we recommend that tapes should be transcribed, transcriptions cleaned of identifiers, and tapes destroyed at the earliest opportunity. See Table 13.2 for a summary of these points.

Balancing the Roles of Therapist and Researcher

When working with vulnerable populations, it is reasonable that the researcher should anticipate that individual research participants might become upset at recalling difficult or traumatic times in their lives. The researcher should therefore be prepared to utilize crisis intervention skills if they discover in the course of a research interview that this is necessary. Arrangement should be made prior to the onset of the research project to ensure that resources will be available for distressed participants. Professional obligations defined by licensing and regulatory bodies demand that professionals ensure that individuals are safe from harm. Researchers should stop immediately if participants become highly distressed or if action, such as a report to

TABLE 13.2 Protecting Confidentiality

Risks	Protections
• Quotes and stories may be identifiable • Tapes reveal identity of person and could be ordered for production in court proceeding • Editing of stories to protect confidentiality undermines authenticity of research data	• Anonymize transcripts • Engage key stakeholders in discussions about balancing authenticity and confidentiality • Consult legal counsel if access to data is required by the courts; take all measures necessary to protect confidentiality

TABLE 13.3 Balancing Roles of Researcher and Therapist

Risks	Protections
• Participant becomes distressed during the course of the research interview • Participant reveals that he or she is experiencing emotional or psychological problems but not not receiving assistance • Children reveal abuse or bullying	• Provide crisis intervention as required • Prearrange counseling support services for vulnerable participant groups • Immediately stop data gathering when participants demonstrate severe distress • Follow up as legally mandated regarding abuse; present to child options for assistance regarding bullying • Provide clear opportunity for children to request support; prearrange counseling should children request support

child welfare, is necessary. See Table 13.3 for a summary of these points.

Preserving and Respecting the Voices of Participants

With respect to the notion of appropriation of stories, we suggest that the question Whose story is it? fails to capture the dynamic and interrelated nature of qualitative work. Depending on the actual method, the researcher's role in the story may be to interpret, coconstruct, or reveal its place in the larger sociopolitical system (O'Connor, 2001). Thus, rather than seeking to represent the truth, we shed light on a dimension of human experience that was otherwise missing, incompletely represented, or inadequately contextualized. In the process, researchers must actively and reflexively consider whether their presence in the story is too influential or does not accurately reflect participants'

reservations about the conclusions we have drawn.

To ensure authenticity, researchers are encouraged to use member checking not only to clarify authenticity of content but also to explore participant reactions to the research process (O'Connor, 2001) and to extend the member-checking process to the final report (Regehr, 2000; van den Hoonaard, 2001). Researchers should also assign research dissemination dollars to provide a meaningful mechanism for sharing research results and recommendations with both participants and the community of interest (Antle et al., 1999), in addition to more formal academic or professional venues such as peer-reviewed conference presentations and journal articles. Increasingly this is becoming a requirement of funding bodies, a change that reflects the general move toward ensuring that research findings are both meaningful and useful. See Table 13.4 for a summary of these points.

TABLE 13.4 Who Owns the Story?

Risks	Protections
• Exposure of hardship and tragedy without change • Researcher's view and interpretation become more valid • Dissemination of findings is not shared or useful for participants	• Active consideration of various interpretations of data • Member checking of research results • Ensuring research results are made available to the affected community and to policy makers who may offer funds or programs to assist the affected community

CONCLUSIONS

Although some authors contend that the concerns presently being raised by research ethics boards and in the professional literature represent a type of overstated "moral panic" with respect to protecting research participants from harm (van den Hoonaard, 2001), qualitative research remains nuanced and fraught with uncertainty. In light of such uncertainty, we ought to proceed with caution and due diligence, drawing on the inherent tensions as a signal of important issues and concerns. In this respect, we believe due diligence requires the researcher to carefully examine, with the benefit of the expertise of others who have knowledge and experiences surrounding the phenomenon under study, the researcher's adjudication with respect to participant harm relative to societal benefits; to address more diligently the issue of informed consent with participants in qualitative studies than might be expected in studies of a more distant, quantitative nature; and to seek advice in balancing confidentiality with authenticity. We believe that a more contextualized holistic form of ethics will better position qualitative researchers to view the ethical issues in the context of their own discipline and other key stakeholders in the research process.

References

AASW (1999). *AASW code of ethics.* Kingston: Australian Association of Social Workers.

Antle, B. J., Frazee, C., Contaxis, G., Forma, L., Nikou, R., Self, H., Tonack, M., & Yoshida, K. (1999). *Creating a life of your own: Experiences with transition to independence among adults with life-long disabilities. Final report of research fellowship in community living.* Toronto: West Park Hospital.

Antle, B. J., & Regehr, C. (2003). Beyond individual rights and freedoms: Metaethics in social work research. *Social Work, 48,* 135–144.

Baez, B. (2002). Confidentiality in qualitative research: Reflections on secrets, power and agency. *Qualitative Research, 2,* 35–58.

Balcazar, F. E., Seekins, T., Fawcett, S. B., & Hopkins, B. L. (1990). Empowering people with physical disabilities through advocacy skills training. *American Journal of Community Psychology, 18,* 281–296.

BASW (2002). *BASW: A code of ethics for social workers.* British Association of Social Workers. [Online]: Available: http://www.basw.co.uk/ [2002, November 9, 2002].

Beauchamp, T. L., & Childress, J. F. (1994). *Principles of biomedical ethics* (4th ed.). New York: Oxford University Press.

Boman, J., & Jevne, R. (2000). Pearls, pith, and provocation: Ethical evaluation in qualitative research. *Qualitative Health Research, 10,* 547–554.

Broner, N., Franczak, M., Dye, C., & McAllister, W. (2001). Knowledge transfer, policymaking and community empowerment: A consensus model approach for providing public mental health and substance abuse services. *Psychiatric Quarterly, 72,* 79–102.

Brownlow, C., & O'Dell, L. (2002). Ethical issues for qualitative research in on-line communities. *Disability & Society, 17,* 685–694.

Brydon-Miller, M. (1997). Participatory action research: Psychology and social change. *Journal of Social Issues, 53,* 657–666.

Burman, E. (1997). Minding the gap: Positivism, psychology, and the politics of qualitative methods. *Journal of Social Issues, 53,* 785–801.

Butler, I. (2002). A code of ethics for social work and social care research. *British Journal of Social Work, 32*(2), 239–248.

Council for International Organizations of Medical Sciences. (1993). *International Ethical Guidelines for Biomedical Research Involving Human Subjects.* Geneva: Author.

Comstock, D., & Fox, R. (1993). Participatory research as critical theory: The North Bonneville, USA, Experience. In M. P. Park, Brydon-Miller, B. Hall, & T. Jackson (Eds.), *Voices of change: Participatory research in the United States and Canada* (pp. 103–124). Toronto: OISE Press.

Cresswell, J. W. (1998). *Qualitative inquiry and research design: Choosing among five traditions.* Thousand Oaks, CA: Sage.

Denzin, N. K. (2002). Social work in the seventh moment. *Qualitative Social Work, 1,* 25–38.

Graue, M. E., & Walsh, D. J. (1998). *Studying children in context: Theories, methods, and ethics.* Thousand Oaks, CA: Sage.

Hadjistavropoulos, T., & Smythe, W. E. (2001). Elements of risk in qualitative research. *Ethics and Behavior, 11,* 163–174.

Heaney, T. (1993). If you can't beat 'em join 'em: The professionalization of participatory research. In M. P. Park, Brydon-Miller, B. Hall, & T. Jackson (Eds.), *Voices of change: Participatory research in the United States and Canada* (pp. 41–46). Toronto: OISE Press.

Johnson, P. (1996). *Mohawk voices.* Waterloo, Canada: Wilfid Laurier University.

Jokinen, P., Lappalainen, M., Meriläinen, P., & Pelkonen, M. (2002). Ethical issues in ethnographic nursing research with children and elderly people. *Scandinavian Journal of Caring Sciences, 16,* 165–170.

Lantz, G. (2000). Applied ethics: What kind of ethics

and what kind of ethicist? *Journal of Applied Philosophy, 17,* 21–28.

Larossa, R., Bennett, L. A., & Gelles, R. J. (1981). Ethical dilemmas in qualitative family research. *Journal of Marriage and the Family, 43,* 303–313.

L'Institut Roeher Institute. (1994). *Disability is not measles: New research paradigms in disability.* Toronto: L'Institut Roeher Institute.

Longmore, P. K. (1995, September/October). The second phase: From disability rights to disability culture. *Disability Rag and Resource,* 4–11.

MacKinnon, C. (1987). *Feminism unmodified.* Cambridge, MA: Harvard University Press.

Magolda, P., & Weems, L. (2002). Doing harm: An unintended consequence of qualitative inquiry? *Journal of College Student Development, 43,* 490–507.

Mauthner, M. (2000). Snippets and silences: Ethics and reflexivity in narratives of sistering. *International Journal of Social Research Methodology, 3,* 287–306.

Maxwell, J. A. (1996). *Qualitative research design: An interactive approach* (Vol. 41). London: Sage.

National Institutes of Health. (1999). *Educating for the responsible conduct of research: NIH guide.* Author. [Online]: Available: http://grants2.nih.gov/grants/guide/notice-files/not99-044.html [2003, February 18, 2003].

NASW (1999). *Code of Ethics.* Washington, DC: National Association of Social Workers.

O'Connor, D. (2001). Journeying the quagmire: Exploring the discourses that shape the qualitative research process. *Affilia, 16,* 138–158.

Pellegrino, E. D. (2000). Bioethics at century's turn: Can normative bioethics be retrieved? *Journal of Medicine and Philosophy, 25,* 655–675.

Punch, M. (1994). Politics and ethics in qualitative research. In N. K. Denzin & Y. S. Lincoln (Eds.), *Handbook of qualitative research* (pp. 83–97). Thousand Oaks, CA: Sage.

Reamer, F. G. (1998). The evolution of social work ethics. *Social Work, 43*(6), 488–500.

Regehr, C. (2000). Action research: Underlining or undermining the cause. *Social Work and Social Sciences Review, 8,* 194–206.

Regehr, C., & Antle, B. J. (1997). Coercive influences: Informed consent and court-mandated social work practice. *Social Work, 42,* 300–306.

Sheppard, M. (2002). Mental health and social justice: Gender, race and psychological consequences of unfairness. *British Journal of Social Work, 32,* 779–797.

Sherwin, S. (1992). *No longer patient: Feminist ethics and healthcare.* Philadelphia: Temple University Press.

Sherwin, S. (2001). Moral perception and global visions. *Bioethics, 15,* 175–188.

Strauss, A., & Corbin, J. (1990). *Basics of qualitative research.* London: Sage.

Tri-Council Working Group. (1996). *Code of conduct for research involving human subjects.* Ottawa, Canada: Medical Research Council of Canada, Natural Sciences and Engineering Research Council of Canada, Social Sciences and Humanities Research Council of Canada.

van den Hoonaard, W. C. (2001). Is research-ethics review a moral panic? *Canadian Review of Sociology and Anthropology, 38,* 19–36.

von Schroeder, H. (1997). The altruistic medical researcher: Gone and forgotten? *Annals of the Royal College of Physicians and Surgeons of Canada, 30,* 353–358.

Whyte, W. F. (1955). *Street corner society* (2nd ed.). Chicago: University of Chicago Press.

Woodill, G. (1992). *Independent living and participatory research: A critical analysis.* Toronto: Centre for Independent Living in Toronto.

14 THE FINE ART OF GRANTSMANSHIP

David L. Streiner

For most people, the three R's means reading, 'riting, and 'rithmetic. For many in academia, though, it could easily stand for 'riting grants, rewriting grants, and rewriting the bloody things yet again. Grant writing is an integral part of a researcher's life, but surprisingly, few graduate schools offer formal courses in it. It is a skill that some people pick up through painful trial and error. Based on my many years as a reviewer, grant panel member, and committee chair, however, I can safely say that some people never pick it up at all (although that does not stop them from applying). Once we leave aside grants that address "who cares" types of questions, part of the problem is that proposals serve two purposes, one overt and one covert. The overt purpose—telling the review panel what you want to do, why it is important, and how you will go about it—is the relatively easy part. The covert message—convincing the panel that you are able to carry out the project—is equally important but often overlooked by applicants, to their detriment. This chapter will discuss how to address both issues in a proposal and, equally important, how to deal with rejection.

THE GRANT REVIEW PROCESS

To learn how to write a grant, it is necessary to know what happens to it and who reads it once it leaves your desk. It often seems that we rush at the last minute to meet the agency's deadline, and then there's an interminable wait before we hear back yea or nay. Despite the belief of some researchers that the delay is due solely to the gross ineptitude and bureaucracy of the agency, in fact much is happening behind the scenes. Although each agency follows a different set of procedures, most elements are shared by all of them; these are shown in Figure 14.1.

The first step is that the grant is quickly looked at by someone within the agency to determine if it falls within the agency's terms of reference (TOR). Some agencies, especially those that are funded by the national government in the United States and Canada, have very broad TORs, covering basic and applied research in a wide variety of areas. Others, especially those supported by organizations or private foundations, have much narrower foci (e.g., Alzheimer's disease, or where the principal investigator is a member of the organization or has certain credentials). If the grant falls within the TOR, it is assigned to a *review committee*, which may also be called a *panel* or *study section*, depending on the agency.

Smaller agencies may have only one grant review panel, whereas larger agencies may have two, three, or a even few dozen. Some of these panels deal with salary support (e.g., pre- and postdoctoral fellowships, awards for scientists at various levels); others focus on specific research topics or methodologies. The applicant can often ask that the grant go to a certain panel, but this request can be overridden by a staff person who may feel that it better fits with a different panel or by the chair of the panel itself.

The proposal is then sent to a number of *external reviewers*. With some agencies, the applicant is asked to suggest reviewers, but the agency is not obligated to use these people or to limit itself to people on the list. (Some agencies also allow you to name people to whom the grant should *not* be sent, because you feel they may be biased, or you do not want to tip off a rival to your new, hot idea.) For reasons that are discussed later under the language used in the grant, it is extremely important to keep in mind who these external reviewers are and why they were selected. Some of them may be content ex-

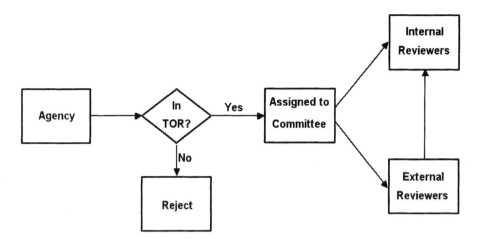

FIGURE 14.1 Flow Diagram of the Agency's Duties

perts, who are asked to comment on your grasp of the field, your knowledge of recent developments, and the significance and importance of your research question. Other external reviewers may be sent the protocol because of their expertise in research methodology, statistics, or the specific technique you will be using. Bear in mind that some people in this latter group will know nothing about your content area, so you cannot assume that they know the jargon or why this topic is so crucial to the health and happiness of the entire world.

Some time later, the committee meets as a whole. The membership of the committee again is variable, but it usually includes between 10 and 15 senior researchers, methodologists, and perhaps community representatives. As with the external reviewers, some members may speak your language, and others may know little or nothing about your research area. One person, who is usually a scientist, will chair the meeting. Another person acts as a secretary, recording the discussion that takes place. In some agencies (e.g., the Canadian Institutes of Health Research [CIHR]), the secretary is another researcher; in others (e.g., the National Institutes of Health [NIH]), he or she is an employee of the agency. In Canadian granting bodies and in some smaller U.S. agencies, the grant will have been assigned to two or more members, who act as *internal reviewers*. Their job is to review the proposal carefully and write an in-depth review of it. At the large federal agencies in the United States, this job is done by external reviewers alone. The reviewers are directed to address a number of points:

- the scientific *significance* of the proposal;
- its *originality*;
- the *methodology* used in the study;
- the *qualifications* of the research team, and especially the principal investigator;
- the adequacy of the *facilities* (e.g., lab space, patient flow, availability of colleagues);
- the *budget*;
- *ethical concerns*; and
- *other issues*

The reviewers then give the protocol a numerical rating. In some agencies, they must agree on the number; in others, the two ratings may differ. At the meeting, the reviews are read, and the discussion is thrown open to include all the members of the committee. After the discussion, which may last from 5 to 30 minutes, each panel member assigns his or her own numerical rating. Again, practices differ among agencies; some allow the members to use the entire range of values, but others constrain the ratings within certain limits. For example, at the CIHR, if the two internal reviewers had agreed on a rating of 3.5 (out of 5), then the individual ratings must be in the range of 3.5 ± 0.5.

A number of aspects of this process are worth noting because they can be potential traps for the unwary. First, some agencies have altered the procedure in order to deal with an increasing workload. In this new arrangement, the internal reviewers are asked, before reading out their critiques, what the bottom line is: reject or accept. If all the reviewers say reject, and no one else on the panel disagrees (and we will soon see why

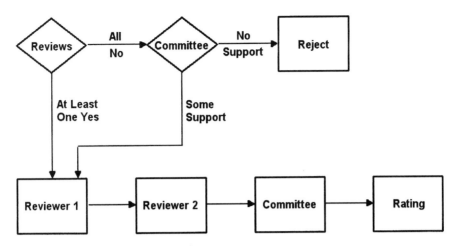

FIGURE 14.2 Flow Diagram of a Typical Review Process Used by the Canadian Instittues of Health Research

there are rarely dissenting voices at this stage), then the lead reviewer gives only a brief outline of the "fatal flaws," and the committee moves on to the next proposal (a process that the CIHR refers to with the euphemism *triaging*). So, the protocol that you labored over for so many months is dealt with in 30 seconds. This means that you cannot rely on the collective wisdom of the other panel members to rescue your grant from oblivion; if you have not made the case strongly enough yourself, it will not be made by anyone else.

The second point to remember is the situation of the reviewers. Agencies are very canny; the request for us to sit on a committee often is made during a slack period, usually 3 to 6 months before the meeting. We are flattered by the recognition and, unable to believe that this period of relative ease will ever end, agree to serve. Then, just when we are at our busiest trying to get our own grants out the door, and starting to teach a new semester, a delivery person arrives at our office, lugging boxes large enough to house two elephants, a washing machine, and a compact car. Inside are the dozen or so grants for which we are the primary reviewer, as well as all the others that the panel must deal with. We are asked to prepare written comments on those assigned to us and to read all the others so that we can knowledgeably participate in the discussions. So, while all applicants hope that their grants are reviewed by a person who has nothing else to do except

carefully read every word in the body of the proposal and the appendixes at least twice, in truth it will looked at as one of a dozen grants, read at night when we would much prefer to be working on our own grant or simply relaxing.

Third, and the reason that objections by the other panel members to the "reject" decision are relatively infrequent, is that the committee members barely have time to complete their reviews (it is amazing how many are written on the plane flight to the meeting), much less read the texts of grants not assigned to them. *If the proposal is opened at all, most likely all that is read is the summary, which means that this may be one of the most crucial parts of the protocol.* I will return to this later in the discussion of the various parts of the grant.

THE PARTS OF THE GRANT

Before discussing the various sections of the proposal, let me elaborate on the earlier point about the overt and covert purposes of the grant. The *overt* task of the application is to tell the reviewers what you want to do, why it is important, and how you will carry it out. The other, *covert*, task, which is rarely acknowledged, is to convince the reviewers that you are able to manage the project through all its phases; this is particularly important for young researchers who do not have established track records they can hold up to demonstrate their competence in this re-

TABLE 14.1 A Checklist for Writing Grants

1. Summary
2. Progress to date/Preliminary data
3. Introduction
    A. Are the objectives clear?
    B. Is the problem significant?
    C. Is the literature review:
        i. Up-to-date?
        ii. Comprehensive?
        iii. Balanced?
    D. Are the hypotheses or questions clearly stated?
4. Methods
    A. Design
        i. Is the design clearly specified?
        ii. Is the design the most rigorous one possible?
        iii. Does it adequately test the hypotheses?
        iv. Are appropriate control groups included?
        v. Are potential confounding variables recognized and accounted for?
    B. Participants
        i. Are inclusion and exclusion criteria stated?
        ii. Are these criteria necessary and sufficient?
        iii. Are sampling procedures adequately described?
        iv. Will the sampling strategy ensure representativeness?
        v. Is the sample size justified?
        vi. Are sufficient participants available?
    C. Procedures
        i. Are the procedures described in detail?
        ii. Are the dependent variables fully described?
        iii. Do the measures relate to the hypotheses?
        iv. Is the time line realistic?
5. Data analysis
    A. Are the exact statistical methods described?
    B. Does each analysis relate to one of the hypotheses or questions?
    C. Are the assumptions of the tests met by the data?
    D. Are you aware of potential pitfalls?
6. Relevance
    A. Have you explained the relevance of the proposal in lay terms?
    B. Is it relevant for this agency?
7. Budget
    A. Are there funds for
        i. Research staff plus benefits?
        ii. Trainees?
        iii. Supplies?
        iv. Printing and mailing forms?
        v. Travel for participants?
        vi. Travel to conferences?
        vii. Computers?
        viii. Other equipment?
    B. Have all expenses been justified?
    C. Are all categories allowed by the agency?
8. Appendixes
    A. Are copies of all scales and questionnaires appended?
    B. Is there institutional approval for
        i. Human ethics?
        ii. Animal care?
        iii. Radiation protection?
        iv. Biohazards?
        v. Investigational drugs?
    C. Have you attached letters of support from collaborating units or labs?
    D. Have you attached letters of participation from consultants?

gard. However, it is also true for experienced researchers. The committee may be willing to cut them some slack if the proposal is vague on some points, because there is evidence from previous research that they know what they're doing. On the other hand, the panel may feel that the researcher is getting lazy or arrogant (or both) and may send him or her a message by turning down the proposal.

When running a study, the issue is not *whether* things will go wrong but *how many* and *which ones* will go wrong. Subjects will be lost to follow-up, forms will be misplaced, equipment will break down, and everything will take twice as long to implement as was planned. You have to demonstrate to the internal and external reviewers that these inevitable mishaps will not derail the entire project; that you and your collaborators are aware they will happen; and that you have the necessary expertise to account for them in the analyses.

In a similar vein, all research, especially when it uses human participants, and most particularly when it uses patients, involves compromises. The ideal design may be infeasible because of logistics, the most precise assay or interview schedule may be too costly, or the best control group may be too difficult to recruit. When you are forced to make major concessions, do not try to disguise it; on the contrary, *let the reviewers know*. If you do not spell out your reasoning for making specific decisions, the reviewers will likely conclude that you are not aware of the problems or are trying to hide them; and thus lose confidence in your ability. On the other hand, if you make your reasons clear, they may disagree with your choice, but they will be more inclined to offer suggestions on how to modify the proposal, rather than reject it outright.

Now let us turn to the individual sections. Table 14.1 provides a checklist of the key elements, which are described in more detail in the text. In referring to this table, keep in mind two things. First, the elements apply primarily to quantitative research proposals; qualitative studies have different criteria, especially regarding sample size, sample recruitment, and analysis. Second, not all the elements are germane for every study; if you are doing a survey to estimate the prevalence of a disorder, to evaluate attitudes toward some event, or to explore the relationship among different variables, you may pose questions rather than hypotheses, for example, or may not need control groups.

Summary

The summary is often written at the last minute and as an afterthought, seen as another bureaucratic necessity, akin to signatures from the administrators or quotations from equipment manufacturers. Leaving this section for the last minute and filling it in without adequate thought is a mistake of the first order. As mentioned earlier, this may be the only part of the proposal looked at by administrators determining if the

protocol fits within the agency's TOR and by other members of the review panel. If they are going to join in the discussion and either leap to your defense or roundly criticize your ideas, it will be on the basis of reading just the summary. So put as much time and thought into this section as into the other parts of the grant.

Progress to Date

Some agencies, such as CIHR, ask you to begin with a one- or two-page section in which you report on your progress to date. Do not misinterpret this to mean you should report only progress for a renewal application. You can, and should, use this part to show how your previous studies lead naturally to the one you are proposing. You should tell a story—the story of your research to date—and like all good stories, it should be interesting and make the reader want to read more. For most U.S. organizations, this section is called *preliminary studies* and serves a somewhat different purpose. It is where you *must* report the results of pilot studies that have demonstrated the feasibility of the design; this is discussed in more detail later in the section on the role of pilot studies.

If the submission is a renewal, you should list all the goals you hoped to achieve and what their status is: met and a paper prepared; not reached because of the following difficulties; or not pursued for the following reasons. Do not forget that reviewers *expect* that your research will evolve as you get into it; some leads will turn out to be blind alleys, and serendipitous results, which warrant further investigation, may pop up. You are not obligated to follow your original proposal in every regard, but you have to justify why the project changed.

Introduction

The introduction sets the stage for everything else that follows. Much has to be conveyed at both an overt and a covert level in relatively few pages. The primary task is to indicate your objectives—what you are interested in and why. You also have to indicate why the problem is an important one; a study can be well designed, but if it elicits nothing but yawns in the reviewers, your chances of having it funded are far from good. The introduction is not a novel; do not make the reviewers wait until the very end to discover what the story is about. Begin by stating what you are researching in a short, to-the-point paragraph.

The statement of objectives has to be buttressed by a literature review that achieves a balance between being comprehensive yet brief enough to allow sufficient room for the other sections of the proposal. The review itself must satisfy a number of criteria. First, it must be up-to-date; if the most recent publication cited is 5 years old, it is a sign to the reviewers that you have not been keeping up with the literature. If you are submitting a previously rejected proposal, be sure to update your review with any significant publications that may have appeared since the previous application. Second, the review must mention the important articles in the field; the covert message that you are trying to get across is that you know the area and the key issues. It is an excellent idea to mention your own publications in order to demonstrate your own expertise, but not to the exclusion of other players; be humble (and realistic)—you probably are not the only person who has had these brilliant insights. Third, the review must be balanced. If there are authors whose theories or findings contradict your own, do not pretend they do not exist. Assume that at least one of the reviewers knows the field better than you do; he or she will notice the omission and attribute it to either stupidity or cupidity, and you do not want either label attached to you.

The introduction should end with a clear and simply worded statement of your hypotheses or the questions you are posing. Statisticians like to phrase issues in terms of the null hypothesis (i.e., there is no difference between the interventions or groups). Do not do this in the application; state what you hope to find, not what your worst fears are.

Methods

The methods portion of the grant has a number of subsections. A good place to start is with the design, where you spell out the overall structure of the study: whether it is a cross-sectional survey, a longitudinal study, or an experimental factorial design; the number of groups there will be; and how often the participants will be seen. This section need be no longer than one or two sentences, to orient the reader to the strategy you will be taking. Some designs are more prone to biases than others (Streiner & Norman,

1996), so you should indicate that you are aware of the potential for bias, how you will try to control for it, and why the design you have chosen is the best for your purposes. Each design is a trade-off among competing pressures. For example, a randomized controlled trial controls for bias better than a cohort study but is far more expensive; cohort studies allow better control of bias than case-control studies but may be infeasible for studying disorders with a very low prevalence; and cross-sectional surveys are less expensive than longitudinal ones but do not provide data from which you can conclude causality. Let the reviewers know, first, that you are aware of the limitations and, second, that you had sound reasons for choosing the design you did.

In the subsection on participants, you should spell out who the participants will be. Among psychologists, the favored choice is undergraduate students who must participate in studies as a course requirement. Indeed, over 50 years ago, McNemar (1946) called psychology "the science of the behavior of sophomores." It is clear why this is the case: They are available, numerous, and, according to some, give important information about the behavior of the pigeon and white rat. However, they may not be appropriate participants if the aim is to validate scales that are to be used in clinical populations or to assess the attitudes of the "average" person. In fact, one secondary-source journal refuses to abstract articles that use students in "analog" studies of therapy or scale development (Reynolds & Streiner, 1998). If the participants are patients with a given diagnosis, how and by whom will the diagnosis be made? The inclusion and exclusion also have to achieve a balance between competing aims. You do not want to include people who cannot complete scales, because of either low intellectual ability or poor command of the language; those who will not be compliant with treatment recommendations; or those whose outcomes may be affected by coexisting disorders. By the same token, though, the selection criteria should not be so stringent that you cannot generalize your results beyond this narrowly defined group (Streiner, 2002b). Similarly, the control or comparison group must be chosen carefully, with reasons given about entry criteria. This is usually not an issue when participants are randomly assigned to groups, since both groups then come from the same population, but can be quite problematic in cohort or

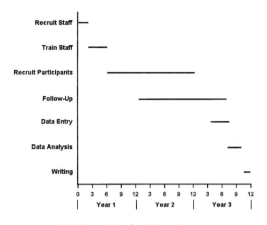

FIGURE 14.3 Sample of a Time-line

case-control studies. For example, if the question is about early loss in depression, with whom will the depressed patients be compared: randomly selected nondepressed people, normals with the same number of losses, patients with disorders other than depression, or some other group? A case can be made for each, and the important point is to state your reasons. Again, the reviewers may disagree with you, but they will be more inclined to give you the benefit of the doubt if you have shown that you have thought through the implications of selecting certain groups and not others.

A rationale must also be given for the sample size. There must be enough participants to show a meaningful difference, a few more to compensate for those who will inevitably be lost or drop out, and no more. A number of books and articles are available to help you determine sample size (e.g., Cohen, 1990; Kraemer, 1987; Streiner, 1990), as well as commercial and free software packages through the Web. If you are looking at a relatively rare condition and are unable to recruit more than a fixed number of patients in a reasonable length of time, do not try to fool the reviewers by "fudging" the sample size calculation with a lower value for the power (the probability of finding statistical significance when in fact the groups differ) or a very large effect size. Be honest, and work backward: Say that with the number of patients who are likely to be available, the study would have a given amount of power to detect a difference this large between the groups. Again, you are letting the reviewers know that you are cognizant of the potential dif-

ficulty, and then the decision is whether it is worth the risk of funding an interesting proposal with a known probability of finding nothing rather than funding an incompetent researcher with whom the chances of a poor outcome are even higher. You must also show that, given the flow of patients through the unit or the number of people in the community who fit your criteria, it is feasible to find a sufficient number of participants within the allotted time.

In the subsection on procedures, you spell out what you want to do in detail. The basic rule is that anyone else reading the proposal should be able to replicate the study: what is done to the participants, who is doing it, how they will be trained (if necessary), what will be measured, and how. If the outcome measures are other than well-established scales or assays, you must provide information about their reliability and validity and include copies of the scales in an appendix. Avoid the temptation to administer every scale ever developed. This not only increases the burden on the participants (the tests truly become a *battery*) but also leads to problems when it comes to analyzing the results: What do you do if Scale A shows a change but Scale B does not, and how will you handle the problem of highly correlated dependent variables (an issue called *multicollinearity*; Streiner, 1994)? It is better to use judgment than a shotgun. Also, the main dependent variable should not be a scale you are currently developing because there is too much risk that you will come up with negative findings, simply because the scale does not have sufficient reliability or validity (Streiner & Norman, 2004). You should also clearly indicate how each measure is tied to one of the hypotheses, and that each of the hypotheses is linked to one or more of the dependent measures.

If the study has a number of phases or extends for a substantial time, it is worthwhile to include a figure showing its time line, such as that shown in Figure 14.3. The x axis marks off the months of the study, and there are a number of horizontal lines, one for each phase. So, for example, recruiting and training the research assistant may extend from the first through the third month; the next line down may show the recruitment of participants from months 3 through 15; another line will show the data analysis; and one will indicate when you plan to write up the results (do not forget to include these last two steps; the funding should extend beyond the last testing date, or else your ability to get the results into press will be jeopardized). This will show both you and the reviewers that you are being realistic in your scheduling.

Data Analysis

One way to ensure that your grant will be rejected is to simply write that "the data will be analyzed with appropriate parametric and non-parametric tests using SPSS/PC for Windows, Version 11.1" (or SAS, Stata, or whatever) and leave it at that. If you want to be more sophisticated, but still have your proposal turned down, say only that "multivariate procedures will be used." Few phrases are as telling as these in letting the reviewers know that you do not have the foggiest idea what you are doing. They do not care which package, and especially which version, you will be using to analyze the data (unless you plan to use a highly sophisticated analysis that requires specialized software), much less into what spreadsheet the data will be entered. What they do want to know is which *specific* tests you will be running and why. It is a good idea to describe how you will screen the data for missing values, outliers, and deviations from the assumptions of the tests, such as normality or equality of variances. Unless you are using lab animals for subjects (e.g., rats, hamsters, undergraduates), where you can easily replace missing data, you should say how missing values will be dealt with, such as replacement with the mean, multiple imputation, and so forth (Streiner, 2002a). Then you should indicate which statistical tests you will run for the first hypothesis, and so on for each of the hypotheses. If you are out of your depth, do not try to fake it; find a statistician who will act as a consultant or coinvestigator, and have him or her write this section.

Relevance

The relevance section, like the summary, is often left to the last minute and seen as unnecessary and irrelevant. This, too, is a mistake. With calls by politicians for greater accountability for research dollars, agencies must demonstrate the relevance of what they are funding (we may deplore the move toward "targeted" research and agency-initiated calls for proposals, but they are becoming a fact of life). Use this section to jus-

tify why your project is important and meaningful rather than simply well designed (leading to the dreaded "ho-hum" review). Finally, do not try to demonstrate the significance of the study by stating that this topic has not been previously investigated; there may be a good reason for this, such as no one really cares.

Budget

The details that should be included in the budget are listed in Table 14.1 and in the manuals published by the different agencies. Again, a balance is called for. You do not want to overlook or underestimate an expense that can jeopardize the execution of the project, such as long-distance telephone calls to contact participants, printing of forms, postage, computer resources, and the like. On the other hand, remember that a grant is awarded in order to conduct a study, not as a way of underwriting the cost of running a clinical service. If psychological assessments are routinely done on all children, for example, then the cost of the supplies and the staff should not be charged to the grant. They are allowable expenses only if they are done solely for the purposes of the study.

It is also important to justify your expenses. If you are asking for a research assistant (RA), spell out how his or her time will be spent: how long it will take to find the participants, enlist them in the study, assess them, and enter the data into the computer. Rest assured that the reviewers will be questioning this. If you are anticipating seeing 50 patients in a year, most reviewers are capable of deducing that this works out on average to one person per week, so it would be hard to justify hiring a full-time RA, a secretary, and a graduate student. If in doubt, err on the side of including too much detail rather than too little.

It is rare for a grant to be turned down solely on the basis of the budget, unless the reviewers feel that you are trying to pull the wool over their eyes, and an obviously padded budget could tip the balance against you. Also remember that the reviewers have had more experience than you in trying to pad a budget, so they are wise to most tricks.

Appendixes

Some appendixes are mandatory. If the study involves human participants or animals as subjects; if you will be using radioactive isotopes for scanning or any other hazardous material; or if the study uses new investigational drugs, you must append forms from the appropriate committees at your institution or the regulatory body (some agencies allow ethics approval to be sent after the proposal is funded, so that the ethics board doesn't waste its time reviewing rejected projects; read the manual). Because everything is always done at the last moment, it sometimes happens that you do not have the necessary forms when it is time to send off the grant. Write a covering letter indicating that they are coming, but be sure they arrive at the agency before the grant is reviewed.

If you are relying on community agencies, hospital units, or other organizations to gain access to patients, attach letters from them stating that they will cooperate. Similarly, any consultants to the study should send letters of support. These must be specific; they should not simply say, "Your idea is interesting," but "I look forward to working with you, and this is what I am prepared to do." As mentioned earlier, you should also include copies of any scales or questionnaires that are not widely known, especially if you developed them yourself. If you can include any data about reliability and validity, so much the better.

As for what else you should or could include, break with tradition and read the manual. Some agencies allow or even encourage you to include copies of previous publications to show what you have done; others expressly forbid it. If you have done a comprehensive literature review, but it is too long to use for the introduction, you may be able to include it as an appendix. At the very least, some reviewers may be grateful to you for having saved them a lot of time when they prepare their own grant. Some agencies want your full curriculum vitae; others restrict you to a form or a fixed number of pages. The moral is: Read the instructions (or, as computer consultants like to say, "RTFM—read the flippin' manual").

GETTING IT TOGETHER

There is more to a grant that simply the component parts of the proposal. How you put the package and the research team together also plays a role, and, as with the individual sections, there are overt and covert messages.

Who Should Be on the Team

Many areas have moved past the stage where one person has all the requisite skills to carry out any except the simplest research project. A study often requires knowledge of the content area itself, quantitative or qualitative methodology skills, and statistics. Sometimes specialized techniques are required, such as brain imaging, health economics, neuropsychological assessment, different forms of therapy, and so forth. It is highly unlikely that one person would have the necessary expertise in all these fields. One question all agencies ask reviewers to address is whether the researchers have the necessary skills to carry out the project. If your curriculum vitae can leave any doubt in the reviewers' minds, and especially if your track record is limited, think seriously of having coinvestigators or consultants whose areas of expertise complement your own. Being the sole investigator is usually reserved for four types of people: brilliant polymaths; people who think they are brilliant polymaths; those with more chutzpah than brains; and people with schizoidal personality disorders. Since few of us fall in the first category, it is best to find collaborators.

The Role of Pilot Studies

For grants sent to the NIH, it is almost mandatory that you conduct some pilot work and include the results in the application; this is less true at CIHR, but it is still an excellent idea to do so. Pilot data show the reviewers that you have thought about the area for more than the past week, that the methodology is feasible, and that the preliminary results (hopefully) look promising and worthy of support. However, you want to avoid giving the impression that you have done so much work without support that you should be able to complete the study on your own. It takes some skill to achieve this balance, but it is an important skill to master.

The Language to Write In

In the United States, grants must be written in English; in Canada, either English or French may be used. Notice which languages are not listed here—psychologese, medicalese, statistics, nursing theory, and other obscure dialects. The following are actual quotations from research proposals (citations have been omitted to protect the guilty):

Manifestations of speeding up of human field rhythms are coordinate with higher frequency environmental field patterns. Radiation increments of widely diverse frequencies are common household accompaniments of everyday life. Atmospheric and cosmological complexity grows.

For example STEAM will be used to shim a Voxel several times larger than where the pathology is believed to be located followed by an SI experiment.

Does anyone have the foggiest idea what these mean? Needless to say, we are talking about achieving a compromise. Specialized terms exist because they make communication easier, but only among specialists who know the jargon. Remember that not all the reviewers who will evaluate your proposal have content expertise in your area; some are methodologists or statisticians; if the agency is relatively small, some may be content experts in other fields. A good model to follow is *Scientific American*, which contains articles that are aimed at intelligent but ignorant readers; that is, readers who are bright enough to understand what the authors are saying, as long as the terms and concepts have been defined. It is a good idea to ask a colleague from a completely different field to read your grant proposal. If he or she does not understand what you are talking about, at least one of the reviewers probably will not either. Do not forget that the primary reviewers must act as your ambassadors and salespeople for your proposal; if they do not understand what you will be doing, they are doomed to fail (along with the grant).

Color Within the Lines

Strictly speaking, your proposal should be evaluated on the basis of its scientific merit and significance, not spelling and neatness. Nevertheless, do not forget that you are trying to create an impression of being competent to carry out the research. If you cannot spell (especially with the availability of spell checkers in word processors) and are sloppy about packaging the proposal, you are jeopardizing your chances. One grant I reviewed asked for less than $3,000; that amount would cover miscellaneous expenses for some proposals, and the general feeling was that the risk of funding the project would be very

small. However, there were three places where the investigators had to specify the total amount requested, and all three were different. The grant was ultimately turned down because the committee felt that if the researchers were so careless in this regard, they could not be trusted to look after the details of running a study and ensuring the fidelity of the data. By the same token, avoid "lavish covers and elaborate ornamentation [that] make readers suspect you are trying to hide something" (Sultz & Sherwin, 1981, p. 20). Bull excrement may baffle brains in the corporate world, but it rarely works with grants.

When All Else Fails, Read the Instructions

The importance of reading the manual cannot be emphasized too strongly. Every agency has its own rules (or quirks, depending on your perspective), and these should be followed assiduously. If you are allowed 20 pages, do not try to get away with 21; if the instructions say to use double spacing and 12-point type, do not attempt to squeeze in more by using 1½ spacing and an 11-point font; and so on. Keep in mind the perspective of the reviewers; they are wading through a dozen or more grants and resent anything that makes their work more onerous. If they become annoyed with you for making them read more than what is allowed, the chances of getting a positive review are lessened, so keep them happy. Even worse, some organizations, such as NIH, won't even send the proposal out.

Allow Yourself Enough Time

In many ways, writing the body of the grant is the easiest and least time-consuming part. Before submitting your proposal, though, it should be read by at least three people: one who is a content expert, one who knows nothing about the area, and one who has experience sitting on review panels. The first person should comment on your hypotheses, methods, and knowledge of the area; the second on the understandability of the language; and the third on the more covert aspects of grantsmanship. Then you must get ethics approval (which may take 4 to 8 weeks, at best); the signature of your department chair (who probably will be out of town); letters from collaborators (who are all at conferences); up-to-date curricula vitae for yourself and your coin-vestigators (at least one of whom will just have had a computer crash and be unable to retrieve it quickly); quotations for equipment (their fax machine just broke); and salary figures for the staff (from a person who is on sick leave). Finally, you must make 12 or so copies (and the copying machine is being serviced). It is often these "extras" that take two or three times as long as the actual writing, so always allow yourself at least twice as much time to put the grant together as you originally anticipated (unless you are new to the game, in which case you should allow yourself three times as much time).

DEALING WITH REJECTION

Even if you follow all these steps religiously, the prospects of funding are not great. In both the United States and Canada, only 25% or so of new proposals are accepted. Some agencies use somewhat more lenient criteria for new re-searchers, so the chances of being funded by those agencies are higher. Even so, if you are going to submit grants, be prepared to handle rejection.

A word, first, on what you will hear from the organization. Most agencies will send you a summary of the reviews and discussion, pre-pared by the panel's secretary or scientific offi-cer. You may also get the anonymous internal and external reviews themselves, depending on the policy of the agency. Very often there is a disparity between seemingly positive reviews and a negative final decision. The reason is that the reviews are written prior to the meeting. During the discussion, flaws may emerge that may have been missed by the reviewers. The dynamics of a committee are such, especially given the limited amount of funding, that it is easier to criticize a project than to rescue it. Also, an internal study done for the CIHR (Thorngate, Faregh, & Young, 2002) showed that if one re-viewer gives a proposal a high rating and the other a low one, the final committee consensus is most often closer to the lower value.

When you get the notice of rejection, you should immediately write an angry letter to the agency, highlighting what the reviewers, in their haste or ignorance, failed to notice and demand-ing an appeal. Print out the letter, sign it, and throw it away; then put their letter on the shelf for at least a week until you calm down. At that time, you may be in a better frame of mind to acknowledge that you may have missed some-thing, or that what you thought was perfectly clear could in fact be misinterpreted or over-looked.

The resubmission should address each point raised by the reviewers, both internal and exter-nal. By all means, emphasize any positive com-ments, such as the originality of the ideas or that the grant addresses an important area. Then give a synopsis of the criticism and how the proposal has been modified in light of it. If you disagree with any of the criticisms, acknowledge the wis-dom of the reviewers (nastiness and sarcasm may feel good, but they do little to improve your chances) and give a rationale for the choice you made. Most reviewers are flexible and are willing to change their minds when given a proper explanation.

SUMMARY

Grants, for most people, are an inescapable part of academic life. What differentiates a so-so pro-posal from an excellent one is a combination of an interesting research idea and a presentation that communicates your ability to carry it out successfully. Nothing can rescue a grant that is pedestrian or commits a Type III error (answer-ing a question that nobody is asking), but there are many ways to undermine an otherwise good proposal. Being aware of these covert messages may improve your chances. It is always a good idea to keep in mind Hodgson and Rollnick's (1996) eight "rules" of research:

- Getting started will take at least as long as the data collection.
- The number of available subjects will be one tenth of your first estimate.
- Completion of a research project will take twice as long as your last estimate and three times as long as your first estimate.
- A research project will change twice in the middle.
- The help provided by other people has a half-life of 2 weeks.
- The tedium of research is directly propor-tional to its objectivity.
- The effort of writing up is an exponential function of the time since the data were col-lected.
- Evidence is never enough.

ACKNOWLEDGMENT Portions of this paper were modified from Streiner (1996), with permission from the *Canadian Journal of Psychiatry*.

References

Cohen, J. (1990). *Statistical power analysis for the behavioral sciences* (2nd ed.). Mahwah, NJ: Erlbaum.

Hodgson, R., & Rollnick, S. (1996). More fun, less stress: How to survive in research. In G. Parry & F. N. Watts (Eds.), *Behavioural and mental health research: A handbook of skills and methods* (2nd ed., pp. 3–14). East Sussex, UK: Erlbaum.

Kraemer, H. C. (1987). *How many subjects?* Thousand Oaks, CA: Sage.

McNemar, Q. (1946). Opinion-attitude methodology. *Psychological Bulletin, 43,* 289–374.

Orlich, D. C. (1996). *Designing successful grant proposals.* Alexandria, VA: Association for Supervision & Curriculum Development.

Reif-Lehrer, L. (1982). *Writing a successful grant application.* Boston: Science Books International.

Reynolds, S., & Streiner, D. L. (1998). Why we do not abstract analogue studies of treatment outcomes and scale development. *Evidence-Based Mental Health, 1,* 101–102.

Streiner, D. L. (1990). Sample size and power in psychiatric research. *Canadian Journal of Psychiatry, 35,* 616–620.

Streiner, D. L. (1994). Regression in the service of the superego: The do's and don'ts of stepwise regression. *Canadian Journal of Psychiatry, 39,* 191–196.

Streiner, D. L. (1996). "While you're up, get me a grant": A guide to grant writing. *Canadian Journal of Psychiatry, 41,* 137–143.

Streiner, D. L. (2002a). The case of the missing data: Methods of dealing with drop-outs and other vagaries of research. *Canadian Journal of Psychiatry, 47,* 68–75.

Streiner, D. L. (2002b). The two Es of research: Efficacy and effectiveness trials. *Canadian Journal of Psychiatry, 47,* 347–351.

Streiner, D. L., & Norman, G. R. (1996). *PDQ epidemiology* (2nd ed.) Toronto, Canada: B. C. Decker.

Streiner, D. L., & Norman, G. R. (2004). *Health measurement scales: A practical guide to their development and use* (3rd ed.). Oxford: Oxford University Press.

Sultz, H. A., & Sherwin, F. S. (1981). *Grant writing for health professionals.* Boston: Little, Brown.

Thorngate, W., Faregh, N., & Young, M. (2002). Mining the archives: Analyses of CIHR research grant adjudications [On-line]. Available: http://www.cihr-irsc.gc.ca/services/funding/peer_review/thorngate_shtml.

Further Readings

Allen, E. M. (1960). Why are research grant applications disapproved? *Science, 132,* 1532–1534.

Barrett, E. (1995). Hints for writing successful NIH grants [On-line]. Available: http://chroma.med.miami.edu/research/Ellens_how_to.html.

Bauer, D. G. (1999). *The "how to" grants manual: Successful grantseeking techniques for obtaining public and private grants* (4th ed.). Phoenix, AZ: Oryx Press.

Brown, L. G., Brown, M. J., & Nichols, J. E. (2001). *Demystifying grant seeking: What you REALLY need to do to get grants.* Hoboken, NJ: Wiley.

Browning, B. A. (2001). *Grant writing for dummies.* Hoboken, NJ: Wiley.

Carlson, M. (1995). *Winning grants step by step: Support Centers of America's complete workbook for planning, developing, and writing successful proposals.* Hoboken, NJ: Jossey-Bass.

Hall, M. S., & Hall, M. K. (1988). *Getting funded: A complete guide to proposal writing* (3rd ed.). Portland, OR: Continuing Education Press.

Lefferts, R. (1978). *Getting a grant: How to write successful grant proposals.* Englewood Cliffs, NJ: Prentice-Hall.

15

APPLYING FOR RESEARCH GRANTS

Step-by-Step Guidelines

Carol T. Mowbray

Perhaps nothing strikes more terror in the hearts of new assistant professors, professionals in their first jobs, or even graduate students as being told that they *must* write a research grant application. Unfortunately, for individuals in these situations, who have limited or no research or evaluation experience, such demands are increasingly likely to occur. The reasons for this are multiple: In academia, faculty are now expected to get and maintain research funding from grants and contracts, starting at an early point in their careers (Ries & Leukefeld, 1998). In addition, budget cuts at universities and human service agencies have fueled constant searches for outside funding, especially for new initiatives. Finally, the push toward evidence-based practice has improved the climate for research on practice; in fact, a professor, clinician, or administrator who has developed an innovative service knows that getting recognition from his or her colleagues and from funding sources virtually *requires* several studies of the program's efficacy and effectiveness.

So what is the assistant professor, practitioner, or student faced with the demand to get a grant to do? One solution might be to produce excuses for why this is an impossible task. Neither the academic department chair, agency director, or supervisor is likely to buy such excuses for very long, however—he or she is under the gun as well, from the dean, the board, the funding source, and so forth, to get research and evaluation going, get more money, show more products. We (the editors and I) hope this chapter may be at least a partial solution to the dilemma. The purpose of the chapter is to take the reader through a step-by-step process in preparation, planning, and developing a success-

ful grant application and thereby to demystify the process, break it down into its component parts, and allow future principal investigators (PIs) to take steps forward in the grant-writing process, feeling knowledgeable about and competent in what they are doing. This chapter will also provide some "readiness" guides. It may indeed be that some of you *do* have excellent excuses for why pursuit of a research grant *is* inappropriate; the chapter will provide you with specific reasons and a reference to back up your argument for why this is the case.

As a caveat, based on my own situation and experiences advising practitioners, new faculty, agency administrators, and students, I do feel that one objective of graduate training and professional socialization should be to give students practice, role models, and experience in developing and writing grant applications. I believe that everyone who considers him- or herself a professional should want to do practice-based research, in order to systematically evaluate the effectiveness of his or her services. Since funding for human services never seems to be adequate, we need to get special funding for practice-based research. We also need to do research and development, as in business and industry, to innovate and to rigorously assess the impact of new service models. In the future, if graduate education does become more centered on the necessity of employing evidence-based practice, perhaps guides like the present chapter will not be so necessary, as emerging professionals will have grant-writing experience before they enter the field.

Much of the focus of this chapter will be on the steps leading up to the development of a grant application. Perhaps even more so in fund-seeking than in other endeavors, almost nothing replaces good solid planning and investigation. Thus, the first section of this chapter concerns preparation—to be or not to be a PI. The next section addresses planning a grant submission, including specifying the research questions, selecting the funding source, obtaining necessary information, establishing time lines, identifying necessary tasks, and dividing up the labor for putting together a proposal. The third section discusses developing the grant application—general guidelines as well as suggestions for the major sections expected to be included in most requests for research funding. Finally, I discuss what to do when a resubmission is necessary.

Before proceeding, a few caveats are necessary. I have attempted to write this chapter to encompass as broad an array as possible of practice-based research topics and potential funding sources. However, breadth usually sacrifices depth, so important details about some aspects of the grant application process are not covered. In these instances, for example, obtaining a major grant from the National Institutes of Health or from a large foundation, I refer the reader to other sources, as available. However, for readers who are experienced grant writers and want a high degree of specific, technical advice, this is probably the wrong chapter. The focus here is on relatively new investigators, seeking research funding for the first or second time, with a moderate amount of money being requested.

PREPARATION: TO BE OR NOT TO BE A PI

Ries and Leukefeld (1995) provide a "research strengths inventory" (pp. 13–15) for new PIs to assess their readiness to apply for funding. They stress the importance of research experience as a PI or co-PI, formal coursework in research, evaluation design, and statistical methods, having research or evaluation publications and professional presentations, and so forth. This advice is important. However, having none of the above does not preclude an individual from applying for some *modest* amount of funds from *some* external source. At this point in time, there is a wide array of funding sources at many different levels to enable an individual who is motivated and competent in his or her field to get started. The major sources of start-up funding are usually state or local government authorities or foundations. The federal level is usually considered to be the most challenging source of funds, as might be expected because selection means national recognition; funding amounts are usually larger and also provided over a longer period; and federal sources usually pay the highest indirect cost rates (the percentage an institution is allowed to add on to a funding request in acknowledgment of institutional expenses involved in administering the grant—for example, costs of maintaining a laboratory, administrative costs associated with personnel/payroll, accounting systems, security, or insurance, and other infrastructure expenses).

An important assessment in the preparation stage is whether you, personally, would be seen as competitive to the funder. To make this determination, talk to colleagues who have received external research funding, people from potential funding sources, or your agency or institutional development office. Sometimes more extensive consultation is necessary from a wider array of sources. For example, an investigator may be relatively inexperienced, but given his or her area of practice, there are only limited potential funders, reducing the latitude of decision making. In such cases, an investigator is usually advised to collaborate with a more senior investigator in his or her own or a similar field (Ries & Leukefeld, 1995).

An equally important consideration is the amount of resources available to investigators from their own agency or institution. Potential PIs should find out if there is a development office and what services it provides. These services might encompass budget preparation, final formatting, completing required checklists and assurances, getting needed signatures, and so forth. The potential PI should also talk to his or her agency director or academic chair or dean to investigate the situation at that level. What about in-kind matches? Could agency resources be used to supply space, provide a dollar match, donate time from support personnel? Investigators should also know about the availability of technical skills and expertise needed for some grant submissions: Is there an experienced support person who has prepared grant applications? Are there statistical consultants who can advise on sample size (power), sampling, and statistical methods?

Third, and perhaps most important, because we are focused on practice research, the investigator should thoroughly investigate the willingness and capability of administrative and clinical personnel from the program you plan to research, or those who would need to be involved in developing a new program, to participate in research. Given all the requirements associated with research and the stresses and strains that research may impose on ongoing treatment, a lukewarm reception may red-flag a program that should be avoided. The last thing a new investigator needs is to spend 6 months developing a research application only to confront a resistant agency that refuses to provide a needed support letter.

In summary, in the preparation stage, potential PIs should carefully examine their own capabilities and credentials, as well as the resources of their institution and the willingness of the program to be studied. If review of all three areas produces very low ratings, the advice would be to go very slowly or, better yet, find a different subject or program to study. Alternatively, you might consider being a co-PI to another investigator or doing some small-scale research with internal funding to increase your experience. If ratings are low to midrange, foundation or state or local government funding sources may be most appropriate. PIs situated in institutions with a lot of capabilities may wish to pursue federal funding options, making their selection based on their own credibility and experience. Having made a decision to proceed, you should follow three pieces of advice as you move forward (McCabe & McCabe, 2000): (a) Have confidence, focus, and persistence; (b) expect that submitting a grant will take a lot of time and effort, and that you will have to reapply; and (c) even though you may not get funded on the first or second try, you will never get a grant if you do not apply!

PLANNING: WHAT, WHEN, WHO, AND HOW?

The Research Question

Obviously, a major issue in obtaining practice-based research funding is what to study. Some investigators may have more or less latitude than others in coming up with an answer to this question; for example, an individual working for a traditional agency with only one new innovation worth studying or willing to be studied

may not have any choice. Investigators in academic settings may have more possibilities. In fact, new assistant professors are often faced with a dilemma about what their research question should be. This should be less of a problem than it is; that is, new Ph.D.s should have a line of research continuing from their dissertation study. However, possibilities may be reduced because of a geographic shift (it is difficult to study Alaskan native culture in Kentucky), problems getting access to data from a dissertation supervisor, or any of a number of other issues. For ideas about getting ideas, consult McGuire (1998), who provides a range of methods for selecting topics—from those that are rational and need-based to ones that are highly creative.

Choosing a Funder

The next "what" question is about the funding source. At this stage, you have narrowed your focus and chosen state or local government, foundations, or federal sources. Now you need to identify a specific funder and sometimes the specific request for proposals (RFP) to which you plan to respond. The development office at your institution should be of great assistance at this point, by doing searches for you through relevant databases on funding opportunities. Usually this involves meeting with the development office staff, telling them what you want to study, as well as where the boundaries are (what you do not intend to study, and other exclusion criteria). For example, you need to exclude funders that give most of their grants outside your geographic area; funders that give to only certain types of institutions, such as religious organizations or businesses; funders that focus on populations other than those you are interested in (e.g., many foundations fund only applications on children and youth, or elderly, or disability groups); or funders that specifically exclude research. Other search criteria might be the amount of funding you need (many funders specify funding ranges or maximum funding levels) or the funding purpose (some funders will not support services, some may have funds only for videos, conferences, training, etc.). For foundations, there are numerous directories (in your public or university library) and the Foundation Center in New York. There are also funding newsletters that cover corporate and charitable foundations as well as federal sources (contact Aspen Publishers in Alexandria, Virginia, or CD Publications in Silver Spring, Maryland). The Internet is a valuable aid to locating funding sources. You can search for charitable and corporate foundations, as well as government grants and contracts; a federal Web locator service and a United States government manual are available on-line. State and local government sources are probably most easily identified through your institution's development office or through the sources' Web sites. State and local government funders will usually have mailing lists of potential vendors; if you are interested in this source, you should submit the necessary documentation to get on their lists.

Your purpose in the funding search should be to narrow down the possibilities to a few best candidates. Once you have done this, you need to do more homework. Consult your institutional development office and see if any grants have been received from that source; follow up with the PI. Request information from the funder that describes the focus of its funded research grants, grantees, and typical funding amounts, as well as the percentage of applications funded and in what areas. Is the funder switching priorities or about to distribute a new announcement? What are the submission dates and the time lines for review? How are funding decisions made? Annual reports from agencies may be good sources of information. If a funder provides the name of a contact person, do not hesitate to contact him or her. But be well prepared—remember that initial impressions are often permanent, and this may be a person who can be a critical resource in your grant seeking.

Being prepared means carefully reading written materials in advance (do not ask a question that has already been answered) and having specific and appropriate questions written down. You will want to ask whether the stated priorities are still in place and if the funder actually has funds to expend within the near future. You want to get feedback concerning the probability that a quality proposal in your area of interest could get funded. Also, if not readily available to you from other sources, ask about the possibility of receiving copies of highly rated and funded applications in your area. Finally, ask about what types of assistance the funder can provide to you in developing your proposal; some funders are glad to read and review concept papers or application drafts; some are not.

If they are willing, you need to find out how much lead time they require before submission.

The next step should be to pick the most appropriate funding source. Ideally, you will have some resources to assist you with this decision: colleagues, more experienced investigators, the agency director or academic department chair, your supervisor, the development office, and so forth. There are usually no clear-cut right or wrong answers—it is more a matter of the match between your research topic, your credentials and those of your institution or agency, and what the funder expects and prioritizes. Do not disregard personal connections (especially to foundations); an extremely interested foundation or program officer might provide sufficient help to get something funded, even though it was not previously funded or not currently a high priority.

The final steps in planning get down to the nitty-gritty. Having selected a funding source, obtain the materials required for a grant application. Read them carefully; reread them carefully; have your collaborators, mentors, and research development office read them carefully. There is no excuse for putting a lot of time and effort into a grant application, only to find that it does not get through the funder's front door because of length, format, focus, submitting agency, or important requirements that are missing.

With all this knowledge about your funding source, you now need to specify and develop your project idea. This really needs to be done in a group. If no operating research work groups are available where you are located, you need to construct one.

Who to Involve in the Research Group

Start with someone knowledgeable at your agency or institution to get suggestions about who to involve, as well as interested colleagues. Research work groups should have a seasoned investigator and an experienced grants writer from a research area as close to your own as possible; this might be one person or two. You should also decide whether you want or need coinvestigators. One book on writing grants (McCabe & McCabe, 2000) advises that "modern science requires collaborators" (p. 45). The authors go on to write that, no matter how qualified, the PI cannot be an expert with demonstrated skill in every method. Collaborators are needed to provide these skills to the research endeavor, to provide services, or to assure availability of key components (such as clients, records, program data) necessary to accomplish the proposed research. Hohman (n.d.) suggests considering people with different professional training and scientific perspectives because they can help you see new and creative ways to look at a problem or issue. McCabe and McCabe (2000) also advise choosing collaborators carefully—not just on expertise or status but also on management style, values, motivation, and even personality.

Besides coinvestigators, the research team should include students and key representatives from the program or service you will be researching. As you assemble this group, be clear in your own mind why you are involving each person: What do you expect them to do? Students may work on literature searches, copying, or other support tasks; they may need to be paid. For coinvestigators, it should be clear why they are involved in this project. Are they interested in doing data collection or analysis? Dissemination? What can they do in writing the proposal? Also be clear what you expect from the service providers involved in the group: Providing a support letter? Helping overcome agency hurdles to research participation? Accessing client records and/or administrative data? Providing detailed information about agency operations to work out logistics and timing? As you develop a specific proposal, other individuals may need to be added—for example, an advocacy group representing consumers, another state or local agency whose records you need, and so forth.

The first step for your group is to produce a concept paper. (For some foundation funders, this is much like the initial letter of inquiry.) The purpose of the concept paper is to clarify and focus the project by having you describe it in a few pages, and to provide you with valuable feedback before you put time and energy into writing a full proposal. Although many funders and grant-writing authorities advise new investigators to produce a concept paper (e.g., Pincus, 1995), with one exception, reference books and articles are generally silent about its details. The first directive is that it should be readable; that means short, a maximum of five pages. The concept paper should be seen as a promotional document. It should get the readers (who include potential funders) excited about the project and eager to see a full proposal. But it should not be a schmooze job, either. You want to get good feedback from your reviewers if your ideas are not fundable or are off-base, as well as suggestions for what you need to fill in for a full proposal.

Start with a brief description of your institution and of the organization providing the service (if different); include its history, purpose, and activities, emphasizing its capacity to carry out the proposal. It should give the message that you, as the PI, are competent and have expertise in what you propose to study. Your concept paper should include the specific aims and hypotheses of the research project, the background and significance of the project, and an outline of the methodology and planned analyses (Hohmann & Larson, n.d.). You should describe the practice to be studied in enough detail to enable the reader to decide on its appropriateness, value, potential impact, and feasibility. The overview of the research design should describe the constructs you will examine as outcomes (not the specific measures) and provide some information on the source of data: secondary analysis of agency databases, client or staff self-report, observations, and so on. Finally, you should give some idea of the time line for this practice research proposal and an estimate of the total funding required. Be sure to end with a statement summarizing the significance of the research and its utilization—to improve practice, to disseminate or replicate this innovative practice, and so forth.

Once you have a concept paper that satisfies the research group, send it to inside and outside experts to get feedback. This group could include the contact person from the funding agency and experienced colleagues at your institution or elsewhere. Sometimes individuals who have previously served on the funder's review board, or who have received funding themselves from this source, are good choices. Note, though, if you contact someone with a high level of expertise (except for the funding agency contact) and you have no personal relationship with that individual, you should expect to pay a small honorarium for having him or her critique the concept paper and give you feedback. Sometimes experts will agree to do a review, which then gets put at the bottom of a big pile of prior commitments; reimbursements can improve priorities!

When and How? An Operations Time Line

While the concept paper is being reviewed by outside experts, take advantage of this time to set up your operations timeline. First look at what could be a reasonable upcoming date for submissions, according to the funder's guidelines. At least five months is recommended, but an initial application almost always takes longer to prepare than expected (McCabe & McCabe, 2000). Another source suggests planning 6 to 12 months to develop a submission (Pincus, 1995); obviously this depends on how much money you are requesting, for what duration, and how complicated the project is. An exception to such an extended time line can be made for so-called opportunity announcements, which are one-time RFPs that come up, usually without any prior announcement, and often with a very short time line for submissions. If your research objective matches the RFP, this may indeed be a golden opportunity and worth the chaos and extra work involved in pulling a proposal together on short notice. McCabe and McCabe (2000) note, "The first time an announcement is made, there may be less competition due to the inability of some groups to mobilize and submit a proposal in time" (p. 32). But beware, there is also the chance that an unexpected announcement is really tailored for one specific applicant agency—so be sure that you have a good contact person at the funding source who can advise you whether the announcement is relevant to your area.

Once you have a potential future submission date for your proposal, work backward to the present. Consider the time required for processing, review, and obtaining signatures by your agency or institution. Next consider the time needed to get outside experts to review and comment on a final draft and how long it may take you to make suggested revisions. Now look at how much time there is between the present date and the date when you need to send the final draft to reviewers. List all the tasks that need to be done between now and then. A comprehensive checklist is provided by McCabe and McCabe (2000). Necessary tasks include doing the literature review, writing sections of the proposal, collecting support letters from sites and consultants, collecting biographical sketches for key personnel, developing the budget, completing forms and required checklists, submitting applications for human subjects review, writing

a letter of transmittal, and assembling material for the appendix. Go over this list with your collaborators and try to assign dates. If the time line is too tight to allow input from important sources, or if you or your collaborators have too many other current commitments to write a quality proposal, you may need to pick another submission date. Also, if you get feedback from multiple sources, at any point (concept paper, proposal draft, etc.), that what is being proposed is inappropriate, seriously flawed, or logistically impossible, you will probably need to meet in depth with your collaborators and consultants to make revisions and to consider necessary alterations in the time line. It is better to submit an initial high-quality proposal, even if it takes another 3 to 6 months, than to hurriedly submit a proposal that is suboptimal. It is hard enough getting proposals funded, and much harder if the applicant has a strike against him or her because of an unacceptable first submission.

Once you have your time line, you need to assign specific responsibilities. Maybe several people are working on a task, but one needs to have primary responsibility for getting it done. Giving students primary responsibility is usually not a good idea; they often have too many other pressures and demands and not enough experience. Besides writing sections of the proposal, other tasks are just as important—for example, contacting agencies or consultants for letters of support, finding relevant literature, compiling a bibliography, preparing the budget and budget justification, and so forth. You will probably need to negotiate so that all your collaborators feel their contributions are fairly assigned; if they do not the assignments may not be done on time or be of high quality. The proposal submission also requires that you specify who will do what if and when the project is funded; these roles should be negotiated early on.

Especially in the United States, a final item of negotiation, especially where the applicant agency is a university, can be overhead or indirect cost (IDC) rates. (Outside the United States, federal funding sources may not allow overhead or may pay overhead only on contracts.) When IDC is paid out, returns usually go back to the unit submitting the proposal, but if you are in social work and your colleague is in nursing, giving all the IDC to social work is probably not fair. Thus, investigators (or sometimes research administrators on their behalf) have to decide how to split the IDC. Usually a fair way to do this is on the basis of the proportion of work that each unit does. If nursing is responsible for doing all the interviewing for the study, it should have a subaccount that includes all the funding necessary to get this done. The proportion of the funding included in this subaccount would then be its proportion of the IDC.

Another important activity that can be accomplished while waiting for feedback on the concept paper is contacting, meeting, and negotiating with field sites for the research study. Besides your collaborators, there are probably other relevant individuals who will need to provide information or approval for the research to be conducted, or even for the grant application to be submitted. Agencies may have their own research committees (sometimes required by accreditation bodies). An umbrella agency or corporate structure that funds the program you are researching may need to approve access to the management information system. In your research design, you may be including a comparison program or population. Agreements with this place or group would have to be negotiated and finalized before proposal submission.

Finally, you should be in contact with the funder to share information about your progress and to keep on top of funding priorities. You will want to know the composition of the group that will be reviewing proposals. For government funders, this is public information that is often listed on the agency's Web site. Ries and Leukefeld (1995) note, "An important step toward producing a quality application is determinng the expectations guiding those who will review and judge your application" (p. 27). More concretely, if some of the reviewers have established expertise in your research area, be sure to include and cite their publications in your literature review. However, under no circumstances should you ever contact potential reviewers directly, for any reason, either before or after the review. This is an unethical practice that puts you and the reviewers in jeopardy.

THE RESEARCH PROPOSAL: GENERAL GUIDELINES

First, make sure you are thoroughly familiar with and follow the funding agency's requirements. Some funders have strict rules for font size, characters per inch, lines per inch, margins, and so forth—not just page length. They may have requirements for biolerplate language required in the proposal or the budget. Several people, not just the PI, should review and re-review the funder's guidelines.

The proposal should be visually attractive, neat, clean, and easy to read. Use indentations, bullets, and subheadings to break up pages; avoid pages that are "walls of text" (McCabe & McCabe, 2000, p. 53). Use different typefaces and double spacing, if possible. Make your proposal as brief and concise as possible, but make sure you cover all the required points, and in the order indicated. The time of the reviewers is valuable and should be respected. Use short paragraphs (4 to 6 lines), clear and easy-to-read sentences, and the active rather than the passive voice. Try to make the proposal interesting. Write for an educated nontechnician, someone who is not an expert in your field (Hohman, n.d.). In addition, make sure that the proposal flows logically from section to section: The problem solution should emerge from the problem statement, the methods should flow from the solution, and the budget should be clearly tied to the methods. Be positive and check for completeness. These are the don'ts:

- Don't assume that the reader knows what you know! You have to be convincing.
- Don't overpromise, but don't raise too many doubts, either.
- Don't apologize, but don't brag.
- Don't call attention to your mistakes unnecessarily.
- Use alternative methods to present statistics, such as tables within the narrative.
- Don't irritate the reviewers!

The last point may be the most important: Some of the things that really annoy reviewers are tables that are erroneously labeled, not being able to find items in the appendix, or cross-references to pages in the narrative that are wrong. Your rating will not benefit if the reviewer gets a headache from reading your proposal; nor will the reviewer think highly of your organization or attention to detail.

THE RESEARCH PROPOSAL: SPECIFIC COMPONENTS

Requirements for research submissions may vary greatly—among federal funding agencies;

between federal agencies, state and local government, and foundations; and among foundations. You need to carefully review the application instructions. And after you receive feedback on your concept paper but before you start writing your proposal is a good time to do this. However, in most proposals, the following topics need to be addressed. (How these sections are labeled and their order may differ, as well as the required length; other specific sections may be required, such as dissemination and replication, hypotheses and objectives). The topics are title; abstract; introduction (specific aims, purpose, objectives); statement of the problem (background/literature review); solution to the problem (how the practice you are researching addresses the problem); prior relevant work; research or evaluation methods (sample, measures, research design, data collection methods, statistical analysis plan); significance and benefits; time line; and budget. For NIH applications, Ries and Leukefeld (1998, pp. 26–31) provide an excellent discussion of what to include in each section.

The Title

Carefully select the title to reflect the main focus of the proposal and the kind of study you are conducting. Titles should be short (10 to 13 words) and descriptive. Catchy titles may mislead readers and may not be considered scholarly or serious. Ries and Leukefeld (1995) also advise the following about titles: The first word should categorize, and the title should be interesting and informative. It should not be necessary to read through an abstract or the beginning of a proposal to find out what it is about.

The Abstract

The abstract is probably the most neglected part of the proposal, but also the most read, according to Rhein (1996), who advises that it should be written last, when the writer knows exactly what is in the rest of the proposal. The abstract is of critical importance because it sets the tone for the entire proposal. If the application does not specify length, the abstract should be no more than one page. Make sure that the abstract includes, succinctly, all the important points in the full proposal. Especially important are the rationale, the overview of what you want to do, and the significance of the proposed activities. Ries and Leukefeld (1995) indicate that the ab-

stract is additionally important because it may affect decisions about the disposition of your proposal at some funding agencies; and that the abstract should include a statement of the relationship between the proposed project and the mission of the funding source. *Mental Health News Alert* (1998) writes that foundation staffers may use the abstract verbatim in describing the proposed project to their boards.

Specific Aims

Where funders require this section, it usually will encompass some of the material in the abstract, as well as objectives and hypotheses. The purpose of this section is to indicate how the proposed project addresses a problem or need. Hohmann (n.d.) advises this format: Briefly describe the problem, describe what we do and do not know; and describe the niche your research will fill in the theoretical or empirical literature. Use bullets to highlight the specific aims (what you propose to do—statements of expected research accomplishments). There should be no more than three to five specific aims, followed by your research hypotheses. The rest of the proposal should be based on and organized around the specific aims.

Statement of the Problem

This section reviews the relevant published literature (make sure you cite major authorities from the relevant fields, especially those on the review committee; also make sure that you read entire articles that you cite, not just the abstracts; and that the citations are up-to-date). According to one expert, nothing is so damning as a misinterpretation of the literature (Rhein, 1996). The purpose of the literature review is to make a case for the practical or theoretical importance of what you are proposing, to lay the foundation for how your research will contribute to existing knowledge, and to convince readers that you have a solid grasp of the field (Ries & Leukefeld, 1995) and that you understand the research questions in the larger scientific context (Hohmann, n.d.).

The literature review should set up a theoretical and conceptual framework for your research (especially in applications to the federal level). The literature review does not have to be exhaustive. If you bring up gaps in the prior literature, you will have to state in your proposal how you will address those gaps (e.g., non-diverse populations, small clinical samples, unreliable measures, lack of follow-up). This section provides the logical foundation for what you are proposing as a solution. Do not get so carried away with having a comprehensive literature review that you include needs or problems that your proposal cannot or will not address. Do not engage in circular reasoning either: "The problem in this community is that we have no stress reduction programs. So what we are proposing is a new stress reduction program." Rather, "The problem in this community is that stress levels are high and increasing due to high unemployment, increasing work demands, bigger families, and a dwindling supply of experienced workers. Further, neither employers nor health care providers have mounted any efforts to decress stress levels."

The Proposed Solution

Describe the activities or services that you plan to undertake and why they are likely to address the problem described. Include objectives, which need to be specific, time-limited, and measurable. Objectives should tell who (to or for whom) is doing what, when, how much, and how it will be measured. Make sure that all the objectives flow out of the problem statement and are problem-related. Objectives should focus on outcomes (benefits for consumers) as much as possible, not just process (what is going on). The objectives should be as quantifiable as possible, which makes writing the evaluation section more clear-cut. Finally, do not overpromise; maintaining credibility is more important.

Besides stating objectives, this section needs to clearly justify the program or the practice that is the subject of the research and explain its underlying rationale. Some funders (NIH) expect the PI to include the theory behind the intervention—that is, what are the underlying causal mechanisms for the intervention selected?—and this information definitely enhances most proposals. This could be empirically based (e.g., pilot data indicate that people in this consumer-run program feel that they are getting more social support, which increases their confidence and their willingness to go out and find a job) or, preferably, theory-based (e.g., on the transtheoretical theory of change, or Anderson's model of health care service utilization). Part of describing how the program is theory driven

should involve presenting the rationale for why this intervention model will work, why this theory is relevant, and what the theory predicts. Are there other sites that have a similar program which has proven success? How about sites that have attempted some other models and failed? This section should provide enough descriptive information so that a nonexpert reader will understand what the program does and how it should be able to achieve the proposed ends. Also, make sure that the scope of the program presented is reasonable and can be accomplished within the time frame and the budget constraints. Finally, it is very helpful if, at the end of this section, the proposal identifies some possible barriers that might emerge and how these will be overcome. It is particularly useful if you can cite prior agency success in overcoming obstacles.

Prior Relevant Work

The purpose of this section is to provide evidence of your ability to do the kind of research you are proposing. To do so, it must show how your previous work is relevant to this proposal and/or how your current skills and experience have prepared you to carry out the proposed project. This section also provides investigators with an opportunity to demonstrate the feasibility of what they are proposing. In large federal studies, proposals are almost always expected to have some pilot test data—to show the feasibility of the intervention, enrollment in the intervention, data collection, follow-up of participants, and so forth. The pilot data need to be strategically tied to anticipated questions that reviewers may have.

Research and Evaluation Methods

Of course, in a research proposal, this should be the main section; it describes how you intend to do the work. It is usually divided into descriptions of participants, research design, method, measures, and statistical analysis plans. The research activities should be tied to and flow from the objectives for the program, specified earlier. In general, the research should encompass process as well as outcome evaluation. Process refers to the measure of whether the expected type and number of participants were served, in the manner specified, within the time frame delineated; and were community involvement, staffing, and other aspects of the program congruent with what was proposed? Outcome evaluation is also necessary, answering questions such as whether the participants receive the expected benefits from the program. Is it clear that outcomes are the result of the program, not historical events, other simultaneous interventions, or selection factors? In large grants, especially those funded by the NIH, the evaluation design is expected to utilize randomized control trials (RCTs)—that is, random assignment to a control and to a treatment condition. RCTs are considered the only definitive way to rule out other explanations for program effects. For a discussion of RCTs and alternative research designs, see Shadish, Cook, and Campbell (2002).

Subjects/Participants

Describe the participants, the expected number, how their recruitment will take place, whether they will be compensated, and the time frame for recruitment. If recruitment involves some screening or applying selection criteria, you need to describe this in detail and provide the measures you propose to use. Many practice research studies involve a follow-up period; you need to provide a rationale for why a specific time (e.g. 6 or 12 months) is necessary for the follow-up and some justification for expecting to see benefits from the intervention at that point. Further, you need to outline the methods that you will use to locate or track participants to minimize attrition (see Ribisl et al., 1996). Be sure to include some reasonable expectations regarding attrition; provide evidence to the extent possible. Finally, investigators need to justify their sample size. In applications for large-scale funding, especially for experimental designs, proposals must include a power analysis—a justification for the fact that the sample size is sufficient to detect a given effect size. In providing the rationale for your proposed sample size, make sure you take attrition into account.

Methods

All your data collection methods must be justified, especially in terms of their feasibility and reliability. In using existing management information system data, you need to prove that you will have access to data on the appropriate participants, over the relevant time periods, and you need to demonstrate that the data are complete, reliable, and valid. If you are doing primary data

collection, describe criteria for selecting interviewers, how they will be trained and supervised, the trainers' credentials, quality control procedures, and so forth. Ries and Leukefeld (1995) advise that if there are alternative research procedures in the literature, you should justify why the procedure you selected is most appropriate for your purposes. Also, you should anticipate problems in data collection that might be experienced and how these will be handled; for example, what if your recruitment sources do not produce enough participants? What if the attrition or refusal rates are higher than you anticipated?

Measures

It is helpful to list measures according to the domains or constructs they represent. *All* the constructs you are measuring must flow from the literature review; if they show up here for the first time, it is a problem. The constructs may reflect the independent variables (characteristics of the intervention, "dosage" level, duration, etc.) or the dependent variables (expected outcomes, as specified in the program objectives) or, probably, both. The measures selected for most research studies are less likely to raise questions if they have been previously published and have established reliability and validity, particularly in populations similar to the ones you will be studying (Have they been used with racial or ethnic minorities? Low-literacy populations? Persons with mental illness?). Generally, investigators should avoid constructing their own measures unless this is absolutely necessary. If this is the case, funders (especially at the federal level) will probably want to see pilot data on the measures' psychometrics. Avoid measures that are extremely dated, make sure that the number of measures you are proposing to use can credibly be administered in the time frame you propose, and address sensitivity to participant reporting bias, if relevant.

Data Management

The proposal's section on research should also indicate how data will move from primary instruments (interviews, questionnaires) into an electronic format ready for analysis. This includes how data will be entered and coded (with tests for interrater reliability), quality controls for accuracy, how confidentiality will be assured, and what will be done about missing data.

Statistical Analysis Plan

Ries and Leukefeld (1995) advise investigators to describe their statistical plan in as much detail as possible. It should include information on how you will check for representativeness of the sample and for possible attrition bias. It should also address expected data transformations, including scale construction, handling missing data, and so forth. For each aspect of the analysis, describe the specific test statistic to be used; anticipate any problems that might alter this (distributional problems, smaller-than-expected samples), and indicate what will be done. It is also a good idea to tie specific statistical analysis plans with each of the proposal's hypotheses, along with a rationale for selection of that approach. The selection of the statistical methods should be based on their appropriateness in providing answers to the research questions, not because they are in vogue or because the PI or collaborators are knowledgeable about them.

Significance and Benefits

It is usually a good idea to have a strong concluding section to a proposal. You might summarize the positive impacts of the program or practice for your community or for participants. Planned dissemination of research results to other programs and professionals might also be addressed here. The importance of dissemination varies with the funding source, for example, whether it has a national or local focus.

Bibliography

Putting together an accurate listing of all the sources cited in a grant application, in a consistent reference style, is probably one of the most tedious aspects of any grant application. However, it is still important. A bibliography that is incorrect or incomplete, which has entries that are not cited or citations that are not included, can be seen as a sign of carelessness and an indication that the PI is not competent to do the proposed research. The reference format of the American Psychological Association is often recommended (see Ries & Leukefeld, 1995).

Timetable

You need to include a timetable for carrying out your research project, particularly to demonstrate to funders its feasibility. The timetable should focus on major benchmarks; it should also include developmental activities (e.g., hiring, contracts and agreements, recruiting participants) to show that you have thought about these things. An agreed-upon timetable is useful in guiding relationships after an application is funded; it should be sufficiently detailed so that it can be used to direct the project (Ries & Leukefeld, 1995). Although it may be tempting to do so because of page limitations, be advised that it is often problematic to put the time line in an appendix. Some federal applications specifically indicate that this is not to be done (this is considered to be inappropriately using the appendix to extend the length of the application). Further, in many reviews, copies of appended material are not distributed to all the reviewers, in which case most of the reviewers will not even know that you have constructed a timetable.

Letters of Support

Letters of support are absolutely necessary for most proposals. You have to have such letters from your consultants and people you may have for an advisory group. This shows that the individuals are in fact willing to do this. If your research is being conducted at an agency other than the applicant, support letters are also critical. Form letters are little better than no letters at all. The "best" support letters, in terms of enhancing funding possibilities, are those that are individualized and specific: where the writer clearly understands what the research is all about, describing in detail the role he or she will play in the research and indicating why and how this research is important and needed.

Budget

Experts advise that investigators do not pay enough attention to the budget. Make sure you determine far in advance whether the funder requires match amounts, whether certain items cannot be funded (e.g., equipment, international travel, time of existing agency staff, construction or renovation) and any other restrictions. You will need to find the funding sources to pay for these items—and this may take quite a while. In terms of the total funding request, asking for less than you need is not likely to improve your funding prospects; in fact, reviewers may think that you do not know what it takes to do research (Rhein, 1996). The budget should be basically realistic; some generous budgeting may be acceptable as long as rationales are provided. Further, researchers should be aware that many federal and other funding sources typically make postaward, proportional reductions in project budgets (sometimes 10 to 20%). Thus, PIs are advised to be sure that all personnel and materials required to complete the project are included in the budget, including inflationary and other to-be-expected cost increases (e.g., announced increases in tuition, staff benefits). The budget categories that are typical for research projects are listed below. However, if the funder provides specific categories for use in its applications, definitely use them instead.

Typical research budget categories include salaries and wages, travel, contractual (including consultants), consumable supplies, copying, telecommunications (mail, phone), phones and other utilities, equipment (usually over $5,000), research participant fees, training and professional development (for staff), and indirect costs (if allowable, these are set by the funder).

In many settings, as allowable by funding sources, it is appropriate to include requests to fund the time of the PIs on the grant. (In some contexts, the submitting institution is expected to cover the time investment of the PI.) Hohmann (n.d.) says that small allocations of time among a large number of investigators are to be avoided; adequate time commitment of the PI is seen as assuring the necessary accountability. According to Ries and Leukefeld (1995), PIs are expected to devote at least 20 to 25% effort (compensated) to any given project. They further advise that every research project should have a professional statistician in the budget or engage a statistical consultant, as needed. In terms of other budget categories, they indicate that travel to professional meetings by the PI and co-PI to present findings is an acceptable expenditure, limited to one trip per year. Supply items need to be itemized only when the cost for any single category (such as stationery, computer supplies, audiotapes) exceeds $1,000.

The budget should be accompanied by a narrative that ties the funding type and amount requested to the activities in the proposal: position descriptions for staff indicating who will be responsible for specific research activities. At least the major budget items (or categories of items) must be justified as to their need and tied into the specific aims, objectives, and proposed activities. For major project personnel, make sure that you delineate each person's unique responsibilities and how these complement those of other members. Equipment purchases are often sensitive items and need to be well justified. In fact, some funders feel that equipment purchases should be the responsibility of the applicant agency because they are usually not returned to the funder and contribute to the general infrastructure.

Cover Letter

While not necessarily mentioned in the application instructions, some experts (Rhein, 1996) advise that applications, even to the NIH, should include a cover letter. Use this to suggest particular review groups or the type of expertise required for review. The cover letter could also identify any reviewers who would be unsuitable because of conflict of interest, documented disputes, or other issues.

Human Subjects Protection

All research involving human subjects is covered by international directives, such as the World Medical Association's Declaration of Helsinki, the United Nations General Assembly statement "The International Covenant on Civil and Political Rights," and the Council for International Organizations of Medical Sciences' "International Ethical Guidelines for Biomedical Research Involving Hhuman Subjects." In the United States, human subjects protection has been articulated within the Belmont Report and in Canada by the "Tri-Council Policy Statement on Ethical Conduct for Research Involving Humans." The policies and procedures for review are quite similar in all these guidelines. Generally, in addressing issues of human subjects protection, you will need to describe how you will obtain informed consent, assuring that participation is informed, voluntary, and not coerced. You also need to explain how you will assure the confidentiality and anonymity of the data; how the data will be stored; and how participants' safety, including adverse reactions, will be monitored. Many of these issues can affect the research design; thus it is appropriate that human subjects protection be addressed up front, before funding is received.

In the United States, all federal grant applications and guidelines for many other funding sources require investigators to address human subjects protections, following specified criteria and procedures. Usually this involves a two- to three-page writeup for a grant application, as well as seeking approval from an institutional review board (IRB), operated by a college or university or by the program sponsor or fiduciary. Guidelines should be available from funders and from IRBs. Most have specific formats. You may also need approvals from other agencies, depending on the practice you are researching. Research participants in U.S. correctional facilities have special protections; individuals in other institutional settings (such as psychiatric hospitals) may also. Other special populations include pregnant women and minors.

PROPOSAL REVIEWS

Ries and Leukefeld (1995) recommend not having colleagues review a proposal until the PI has a good handle on his or her methods and procedures. A colleague might suggest including additional variables or altering methods, which may not be appropriate given a thorough understanding of the subject population or the data collection circumstances. They write, "Listen to these suggestions and use what you can, but do not feel compelled to significantly modify your plan unless a colleague points out a fatal flaw" (p. 155)—then it's back to the drawing board. They also advise, at the point of finishing a proposal draft, rereading the application instructions and making sure that all have been followed.

The investigator should then distribute the proposal to a limited number of outside reviewers, probably including proposed consultants and the funder's contact person. If the proposal is distributed too widely, you may get more comments than you can handle, just producing confusion. Consider identifying a neutral reader, perhaps someone who has served on a committee similar to the one reviewing your proposal, and ask for his or her verbal or written review. Expert readers should be compensated for their time, at a fair rate. All expert readers should have been lined up in advance and should be included as part of the operational time line—not just when the proposal happens to get completed. Finally, after all the substantive changes have been made, have someone who has not been closely involved with the proposal and who is also a good editor read the proposal carefully for errors in spelling, grammar, formatting, cross-referencing, and so forth.

AFTER PROPOSAL SUBMISSION: NEXT STEPS

Proposal reviews can take anywhere from a few weeks (in many foundations) to nearly a year (federal funders). In the meantime, you might capitalize on the experience of putting together the grant application by continuing relationships established with service providers or conducting a small pilot study. You might also use the time to further develop or refine your literature review, especially keeping it current.

Do not be surprised if your proposal is rejected—most are the first or second time they are submitted. At the NIH, 88% of R-01 type applications are not funded; in fact, two thirds of all continuations are not funded. But the success rates vary even within the NIH—from 7 to 29% across different institutes (Ries & Leukefeld, 1998). The major reasons for grants not getting funded are that the research is risky, which includes ideas that are unconventional, as well as an investigator with a short or disputed track record; the statement of the problem is inadequate—not well documented or does not seem significant; the project objectives are too ambitious or do not match the funder's objectives; the proposal is poorly written or unclear; consumers were not involved in the project development, or the project has not been coordinated with other programs in the field; and guidelines of the funder are not followed, including the budget being too large.

An appeal process is available if you feel the review was seriously flawed. But whatever you do, do not give up; make a plan for resubmission (if it is allowed) or for submission to a new funding source. Both approaches will probably require extensive revisions. Try to get all the information you can about why you did not get funded and the weaknesses in the proposal. Federal funding authorities usually do this as a stock practice; some foundations may give no feedback at all, but you could try calling and asking to talk to someone about your review. Remember, now you have momentum and people geared up to do this activity—do not let it go to waste. *Aid for Education Report* (1996) notes that any idea with merit eventually will be funded.

References

Aid for Education Report. (1996, September 27). Grant tips: Secret of gaining funding: Keep trying, Don't give up on request rejection. Silver Spring, MD: CD Publications.

Hohmann, A. A. (n.d.). Tips on developing an NIMH grant application. Rockville, MD: National Institute of Mental Health, Division of Epidemiology and Services Research.

Hohmann, A. A., & Larson, D.B. (n.d.). Grant funding in mental health services research: Methods and mechanisms. Rockville, MD: National Institute of Mental Health, Division of Epidemiology and Services Research.

McCabe, L. L., & McCabe, E.R.B. (2000). *How to succeed in academics.* San Diego, CA: Academic Press.

McGuire, W. J. (1998). Creative hypothesis generating in psychology: Some useful heuristics. *Annual Review of Psychology, 48,* 1–30.

Mental Health News Alert. (1998, August 17). Grant and funding tips. Silver Spring, MD: CD Publications.

Pincus, H. A. (1995). *Research funding and resource manual: Mental health and addictive disorders.* Washington, DC: American Psychological Association.

Rhein, R. (1996). Dollars and grants: Information about funding for biomedical researchers. *Journal of NIH Research, 8,* 29–30.

Ribisl, K. M., Walton, M. A., Mowbray, C. T., Luke, D. A., Davidson, W. S., & BootsMiller, B. J. (1996). Minimizing participant attrition in panel studies through the use of effective retention and tracking strategies: Review and recommendations. *Evaluation and Program Planning, 19*(1), 1–25.

Ries, J. B., & Leukefeld, C. G. (1995). *Applying for research funding: Getting started and getting funded.* Thousand Oaks, CA: Sage.

Ries, J. B., & Leukefeld, C. G. (1998). *The research guide funding guidebook: Getting it, managing it, and renewing it.* Thousand Oaks, CA: Sage.

Shadish, W. R., Cook, T. D., & Campbell, D. T. (2002). *Experimental and quasi-experimental designs for generalized causal inference.* Boston: Houghton Mifflin.

16   SETTING THE STAGE FOR ACCOUNTABILITY AND PROGRAM EVALUATION IN COMMUNITY-BASED GRANT-MAKING

Cindy A. Crusto & Abraham Wandersman

Community-based organizations are increasingly being looked to and funded to address local social welfare, health care, and mental health needs. They are relied upon to develop and implement innovative programs to be delivered to individuals and communities they serve. However, the lack of staff and other resources available to these agencies often challenges their ability to develop high-quality grant proposals and programs to achieve desired outcomes. Moreover, few agencies have the capacity for evaluating the short- and long-term effects and impacts of their efforts (Morley, Hatry, & Cowan, 2002); therefore, in many instances the potential programmatic benefits remain unknown. In a study to explore foundation performance and effectiveness, foundation CEOs indicated that although the provision of nonmonetary assistance (e.g., management advice, advice about the field) to grantees during the course of the grant could contribute to grantee satisfaction and program impacts, this was rarely provided (Center for Effective Philanthropy, 2002b). Some foundations have attempted to build the capacity for achieving realistic grantee outcomes through creating a more trusting relationship between grant makers and grant seekers that allows for mutual learning (Center for Effective Philanthropy, 2002a). Building the capacity of potential grantees to develop high-quality grant applications and programs and to evaluate their programs is crucial to successful funding initiatives. This capacity helps ensure the promise of grantees to accomplish their own and the funder's desired outcomes and to positively influence communities. The purpose of this chapter is to describe a grant-making and grant-implementation system that is designed to assist community-based organizations build their capacity to develop grant proposals and implement programs from a results-based accountability perspective. The chapter presents an example of how such a system was used in a state-initiated, community-based grant program to address juvenile delinquency, providing evaluation results from the first attempt to evaluate the benefits of the grant-proposal phase of the system. The chapter concludes with suggestions for professionals working with community-based organizations to develop the capacity for effective grant-making and grant implementation.

RESULTS-ORIENTED GRANT-MAKING AND GRANT-IMPLEMENTATION (ROGG) SYSTEM

The Results-Oriented Grant-making and Grant-implementation (ROGG) System incorporates results-based accountability concepts and practices into program development, implementation, and evaluation of the granting process. The system is rooted in several years of our university-based evaluation team's work with

state and federally funded community partnerships designed to address local problems such as alcohol, tobacco, and other drug use and community violence (Goodman & Wandersman, 1994; Goodman, Wandersman, Chinman, Imm, & Morrissey, 1996; Wandersman et al., 1998; Yost & Wandersman in W. K. Kellogg Foundation, 1999). In this work the team partnered with local project staff, community members, and other participants to develop formative, outcome, and impact evaluations. In our experience with these community initiatives and agencies, we found that they were often ill equipped to carry out the large mandates for impacting communities and the expectations for evaluating their efforts. This served as an important precursor to the development of the ROGG System. Equally important was work we undertook with funders who stressed a desire to develop and support programs from an accountability perspective and with the best chances of positively influencing communities (Yost & Wandersman in W. K. Kellogg Foundation, 1999).

The system provides community-based program developers with an empowerment evaluation approach to improve planning, implement with quality, evaluate outcomes, and develop a continuous quality improvement system—thereby increasing the probability of achieving positive program results (Yost & Wandersman in W. K. Kellogg Foundation, 1999). As described in Figure 16.1, ROGG is divided into two phases: the grant proposal process and the grant-implementation process. The first column of the figure lists the five tools ROGG provides to influence the capacity of community-based organizations and their members to develop successful grant proposals and programs, including continuous quality programming (CQP) and empowerment evaluation (EE) concepts, accountability questions, technical assistance, workshops, and guidebooks. The ROGG System uses the CQP approach to accountability (Wandersman et al., 1998). This approach emphasizes an empowerment evaluation orientation (Fetterman, Kaftarian, & Wandersman, 1996) and provides a framework by asking nine accountability questions (see Table 16.1) to build the capacity of program developers to achieve positive results (Yost & Wandersman in W. K. Kellogg Foundation, 1999; Wandersman et al., 1998;[1] Wandersman, Imm, Chinman, & Kaftarian, 2000).[2]

The ROGG accountability system depends on a partnership among the funder, evaluator, and

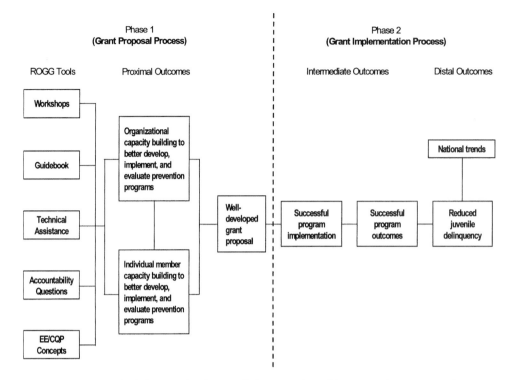

FIGURE 16.1 Model of the Results-Oriented Grant-Making/Grant-Implementation System Intervention

funded program staff (see Figure 16.2; Yost & Wandersman, 1998). This partnership provides the system's foundation, and each partner has roles and responsibilities for carrying out the work of the granting and accountability process. To be successful, the funder provides the resources for the granting process, the programs, and the work of the evaluator *and* sets the tone and expectations for the results-based accountability process and empowerment evaluation value system. The funder's commitment and buy-in to the results-based accountability process help ensure that the applicant and ultimately the funded programs understand its importance and establish their commitment to the accountability process. Through participation in the granting program, applicants agree to participate in the system during proposal development (Phase 1) and implementation once funding has been awarded (Phase 2). Through this system the funder provides ongoing technical assistance (TA) to develop the capacity of community groups or agencies to plan, implement, and evaluate their programs.

An important area of concern that often emerges in grant-making is the political nature of some processes (e.g., funding decisions that are based on factors other than proposal merits or predetermined priority areas of need). ROGG implicitly addresses political concerns by describing expectations for successful program completion and award criteria well in advance of the grant program's implementation. Second, all parties (i.e., funders, proposal reviewers, TA providers) involved in the grant-making phase are trained in the initiative goals and the objective scoring criteria. Third, independent, voluntary grant proposal reviewers are enlisted to numerically score grant proposals based on objective scoring criteria, provide qualitative comments on the proposal strengths and weaknesses, and make recommendations for funding based on the relative merits of the proposals. It is believed that individuals who are not intimately involved in the granting program will provide unbiased ratings. Finally, given the funders' level of buy-in, involvement, and support for the accountability system, it is expected that

TABLE 16.1 Accountability Questions

Question	Description
1. How do you know you need this program?	Programs are more effective when they address identified needs.
2. What is your local council trying to accomplish?	It is important to specify the mission, goals, and outcomes for programs to provide a clear direction and rationale for the program.
3. How does this program incorporate the "science/best practice" information regarding interventions for youth?	Knowledge generated by the "science/best practice" information in prevention science regarding effective interventions for youth should be used to select a program.
4. How will this program link and fit with other programs already offered in the community?	A determination of how programs duplicate, complement, or interfere with existing programs is related to success.
5. How will this program be carried out?	Sound program planning that specifies what, where, when, and how program activities will be delivered is important.
6. How will the quality of implementation (process evaluation) be carried out?	Assessing the quality of implementation allows for the identification of program difficulties and for midcourse corrections.
7. How well did the program work (outcome evaluation)?	Assessing the outcomes is an important aspect in determining the program's utility in addressing a particular problem and in making midcourse corrections.
8. What can be done to improve the program (continuous quality improvement)?	Given what was learned about the program, how can it be improved?
9. If this program (or its components) is successful, what can be done to continue or expand the program in the future?	What can be done to help sustain the program beyond initial funding?

they will adhere as closely as possible to reviewer recommendations in making funding decisions.

The evaluators in this system may (a) provide assistance to applicants about the ROGG process (e.g., conduct workshops to teach the results-based principles and concepts, develop a guidebook for presenting results-based information and assistance for completing the grant proposal) and (b) establish an empowerment evaluation system and tools that would be used to assess results.

Capacity-building efforts via the ROGG tools focus on increasing awareness of accountability issues and developing competencies to apply accountability practices to grant development and implementation. Through this capacity building, the organization and/or individuals become better prepared to write a grant proposal and develop a program (see Figure 16.1, proximal outcomes). We believe that a well-developed grant proposal and program, coupled with continuing TA, develop the foundation for a successful Phase 2 of the system—a program that is well implemented and that will achieve the desired outcomes (see Figure 16.1, intermediate outcomes), ultimately achieving desired results (see Figure 16.1, distal outcomes). At the center of Figure 16.2 are results. All parties overlap and help each other to obtain meaningful results.

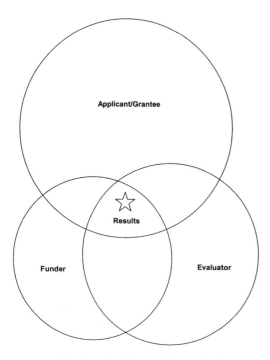

FIGURE 16.2 Results-Oriented Grant-Making/
Grant-Implementation Partnership Model

CASE STUDY

We present an example depicting a statewide
grant-funded initiative to illustrate how the
ROGG System can be utilized. In the 1990s, the
governor of a southeastern state created a Juvenile Justice Task Force to address the root
causes of juvenile crime and to take a compassionate but critical look at the problem of juvenile justice in the state. The task force recommended the creation of Governor's Community
Youth Councils in each of the state's 16 judicial
circuits with the goal of addressing juvenile justice system reform at the local level. The primary goal of the Youth Councils was to develop
partnerships and volunteerism through community collaboration to reduce the rate of incarceration among youth in the state. To this
end, Youth Councils were to (a) identify effective programs for the diversion, intervention,
and probation of juveniles in the justice system;
(b) replicate effective programs throughout the
judicial circuit; (c) make policy recommendations
to the governor and the task force regarding juvenile justice issues; and (d) heighten public
awareness on issues of prevention and intervention in youth crime. Youth Councils were to

consist of individuals who could garner resources
to address juvenile justice issues, such as family
court judges, solicitors, public defenders, human
service agencies, educators, and elected officials.
The governor's office and the state's Department
of Juvenile Justice provided $500,000 for local
juvenile delinquency intervention and prevention programs, and each Youth Council had the
opportunity to apply for program planning or
implementation funding via a granting process
administered by the Center for Family Policy.

Our university-based evaluation team partnered with the governor's office, the Center for
Family Policy, and the Department of Juvenile
Justice to develop a grant-making process
(ROGG System) so that money would be distributed using an accountability approach. This
partnership was rooted in previous evaluation
and consultation work the university-based team
provided to two of the agencies. The partnership
among the funders, grantees, and evaluators allowed for mutually beneficial relationships and
the shared goal of reducing the number of youth
in the state juvenile justice system. The Center
for Family Policy and the Department of Juvenile Justice Prevention and Intervention staff
provided TA to the Youth Councils. The Youth
Council members were invited to attend a workshop that provided an orientation to the granting
process and an overview of the accountability
and the results-oriented concepts and framework
they were to use in developing programs and
writing proposals. During the workshop, Youth
Council staff received a guidebook, which outlined all the grant requirements, provided examples of highly rated and less highly rated
grant proposals that were developed by the evaluators, and answered questions about the grant
process. In addition, participants received the
grant application, which was customized for the
granting process using the ROGG System. Finally, the funders recruited volunteer grant proposal reviewers, such as university professors
and state agency staff, and the evaluators oriented them to the accountability principles and
the granting process and trained them to work
as grant proposal reviewers. In addition, the evaluators provided the volunteer reviewers with
the examples of the highly rated and less highly
rated grant proposals, from which they reviewed
specific ROGG scoring criteria.

As mentioned earlier, the ROGG System implicitly addresses some political aspects of traditional granting programs. In this particular

case, although the director of one of the partner agencies had not been formally trained in the accountability system, the individual was well informed of the ROGG approach and how it had been applied to the granting process. By all accounts, a high level of buy-in and support for the granting program had been achieved at all levels of management and leadership. With respect to the applicants, the staff provided a clear message that applicants could seek as much TA as needed to submit the best proposal possible. To this end, potential grantees were encouraged to seek assistance or advice on any aspect of the proposal development phase of the granting program. In addition, the granting program provided them with samples of highly rated grant proposals to demonstrate the kinds of proposals sought. Finally, the competitive nature of the granting program was de-emphasized but not totally eliminated. There was a mandate that all 16 judicial circuits would receive some level of funding, but the level varied according to the merits of the proposal.

CASE STUDY EVALUATION

The case study describes how the ROGG System worked in practice. Since the ROGG System had been under initial development and refinement before its implementation with the youth councils, the developers had not yet systematically evaluated it. In addition, several methodological challenges made evaluation of the granting system difficult, including lack of random assignment of ROGG recipients and a lack of developed methods. Consistent with Chelimsky's (1997) description of the three purposes of evaluation, the ROGG evaluation was conducted to (a) improve the ROGG System, (b) evaluate accountability in the grant proposal phase (Phase 1) of ROGG, and (c) generate research knowledge for understanding granting processes. This study is significant because it provides a description of a comprehensive results-oriented approach to grant-making and is the first attempt to systematically assess aspects of the system, including the tools and the proximal outcome of the development of sound grant proposals. We used a case study method to evaluate the grant proposal development phase of the ROGG System in which multiple sources of evidence were triangulated to establish facts about the phenomenon under study (Merriam, 1988; Yin,

1994, 1998). We provide "mundane" results about the many facets of the system because we think it is valuable to describe what different key participants thought and did in working with a grant system. This chapter presents results on the evaluation that assessed Phase 1, including strengths and areas needing improvement, by converging qualitative (interview) and quantitative (survey) data from multiple sources and informants. This case study shows that the ROGG System possesses several strengths and has promise for leading to better grant proposal scores. Table 16.2 presents aspects of the ROGG System that were evaluated (Column A), the ROGG participants providing data (Column B), the methods for gathering evaluative data (Column C), and a summary of study findings (Column D).

PARTICIPANTS

Survey Respondents

Prior to completing the ROGG grant proposal, 22 prospective applicants completed a survey to assess their individual accountability skills (e.g., how often they conducted needs assessments, process evaluations, outcome evaluations). Following submission of the grant proposal, the researchers surveyed those completing pretests and additional individuals who were involved in the grant development process but who had not completed the initial assessment. A total of 49 posttest surveys were mailed out, and 21 were returned, for a 43% response rate. Of the 21 surveys returned, 10 individuals had completed the pretest; and the remaining 11 assessed their pre-ROGG and post-ROGG accountability skills at posttest only (following grant proposal submission).

Pre-grant Workshop Participants

Nineteen Youth Council members (e.g., council chairs, members) evaluated a pre-grant workshop. They were employed by state and community-based organizations.

Interviewees

Twenty individuals representing various roles within the ROGG System participated in group or individual interviews. Fifteen were Youth

Council members and represented seven Youth Councils. The Youth Council members were employed by state agencies and community-based organizations. Four of those interviewed had also participated in and evaluated a pre-grant workshop. Other individuals interviewed were members of the proposal reviewer group and the ROGG development group.

Grant Proposal Reviewers

Seven individuals participated in the system as volunteer grant proposal reviewers. They were employed by state agencies, including a state university. Their employment positions included grants manager, program directors, professor, prevention coordinators, and an administrative assistant.

PROCEDURE

Interviews

The first author and two doctoral candidates in psychology conducted the 10 in-person interviews (five group interviews and five individual interviews). Interviewers were trained in qualitative research and general interviewing techniques. Interviews ranged from 45 to 90 minutes and were audiotaped and transcribed. In addition to audiotaping, interviewers took notes from which they verified main points with participants at the conclusion of each interview. Interviewers produced written notes and audiotaped impressions, which were also transcribed. The researchers checked each transcript against tape-recorded interviews. To further assess the strengths and weaknesses of the system, the ROGG team and the Center for Family Policy met twice following submission of the grant proposals to discuss the strengths and weaknesses of the ROGG System.

Surveys

Accountability skills were assessed prior to and following submission of the grant proposals. Participants completed evaluation surveys prior to and following each workshop or training.

INSTRUMENTS AND MEASURES

The university-based evaluation team developed all ROGG assessment surveys and interview guides with feedback from the grant program partners. Interview guides were developed to help ensure more systematic and consistent gathering of information about key ROGG components.

Accountability Survey

A survey was developed to assess individual member capacity to better develop, implement, and evaluate programs. This assessment included the degree to which the Youth Council members used results-oriented principles and practices in the development of previous programs and during the planning and writing of the ROGG grant proposal. Respondents answered items using a Likert scale, ranging from 1 (not at all) to 5 (frequently). The survey included items such as "How often have you consulted the scientific literature or experts to determine which programs have worked or been successful in the past before designing a program for your population?" and "How often have you consulted the scientific literature on the best way to evaluate or assess your program?"

Pre-grant Workshop Evaluation Form

Following each pre-grant workshop, participants evaluated workshops using a 12-item survey. The survey included rating scale and open-ended items. Rating scale items assessed the overall quality of the presentations ("Overall, how would you rate the organization of the workshop?") and participant knowledge acquisition ("Overall, how would you rate the workshop on increasing your personal knowledge of results-based accountability"), ranging from 1 (low) to 5 (high). Items assessing the difficulty of sharing and implementing the information ranged from 1 (high) to 5 (low). Open-ended items solicited feedback about the grant proposal examples ("What did you think of the mentoring example as a successful grant? How could it be improved?"); grant application ("What do you think of the Governor's Community Youth Council 1998 Incentive Grant Program Application? How could it be improved?"); guidebook ("What do you think of the guidebook to the Governor's Community Youth Council 1998 Incentive Grant Program? How could it be improved?"); and the kind of assistance they believed they would need to complete the grant application.

Grant Proposal Reviewer Surveys

In addition to asking information about previous grant proposal writing and reviewing experience, the reviewer survey evaluated several aspects of the each of the two reviewer trainings. Open-ended and structured items asked how well the training had prepared the reviewers to rate grant proposals, if they needed more training on the application of the scoring criteria, and if they would have preferred to rate a sample grant proposal during the training.. Finally, the survey assessed perceptions and experiences of the award determination process.

DATA ANALYSIS

Consistent with a constant comparative method of data analysis (Strauss & Corbin, 1990; Glasser & Strauss, 1967), the researchers reviewed transcripts of the 10 interviews, using notes, phrases, and key words to identify emergent themes. The data were coded according to the memos and emerging themes. Non-numerical Unstructured Data Indexing Searching and Theorizing (Q-NUDIST) was used to further code and categorize the data.

Information from the open-ended survey responses was analyzed by placing responses on note cards. The first card was drawn from the pile, and its content became the first category theme. Subsequent cards were drawn, and if their themes did not match any previously identified theme, then new thematic categories were developed.

RESULTS

The evaluation results are summarized in Table 16.2, Column D.

ACCOUNTABILITY SKILLS

From pre- to post-ROGG assessment, pre-grant workshop participants indicated that eight of their accountability-related skills increased, and two decreased. An increase was reported in (a) consultation of the scientific literature or experts to determine which programs have worked or been successful in the past before designing a program for your population; (b) identification of other programs in the community to assess

whether your program would be a duplication of others' efforts; (c) collaboration with other agencies or organizations in planning programs; (d) documentation of the program goal; (e) documentation of your desired results or outcomes for the program; (f) monitoring of the number of sessions or services provided by your program; (g) monitoring changes in your target populations; and (h) development of a budget. The largest reported increase from pre- to post-assessment was the frequency with which they monitored the changes in their target population, identified other programs in the community to assess duplication of efforts, and monitored program sessions or services. A decrease in skill was found for (a) monitored the number of people who attended your program and (b) conducted a structured planning process before implementing the program, and three behaviors remained the same. For the 11 individuals who did not attend a pre-grant workshop, there was a reported increase for one accountability behavior (identification of other programs in the community to assess whether your program would be a duplication of others' efforts) and a decrease on nine behaviors; one behavior remained the same. Due to the small sample size, statistical differences between pre and post-ROGG accountability skills were not determined.

ROGG SYSTEM STRENGTHS AND WEAKNESSES

Six general ROGG system strengths and weaknesses themes emerged from the data: ease and simplicity; workshops and training; technical assistance; logistics; program evaluation; and review and award process.

Ease and Simplicity

A majority (70%) of the transcribed interview documents referenced the ease and simplicity of the granting process. One interviewee said that the ROGG System made the grant process "digestible." In addition, a participant with no formal grant-writing training brought a professional grant writer to a pre-grant workshop to help him understand the process. After participating in the workshop, the participant with little prior training said:

When you talk about your proposal, everything was simplified. A lot of these things you go to you kind

TABLE 16.2 ROGG System Evaluation Design and Results

Column A ROGG Component	Column B Data Source	Column C Evaluation Technique	Column D Results: Strengths and Improvements
ROGG System (overall evaluation)	• Applicants • ROGG developer • Proposal reviewers • Technical assistance providers • Grant program administrators	• Surveys • Interviews	Strengths • Ease/simplicity of system • Workshops/trainings • Technical assistance Improvements • Logistics (short proposal review time) • Need for more program evaluation assistance • Political proposal review and award process
Accountability skills	• Applicants	• Accountability survey	• 8 skills increased • 2 skills decreased • 3 skills remained unchanged
Pre-grant workshops	• Applicants	• Pre-grant workshop evaluation form • Interviews	Strengths • Pre-grant workshops highly rated Improvements • Need for planning grant information • No new information for experienced grant writers • Need for ongoing workshops to shape and reinforce accountability concepts and skills • Poor attendance (workshop was optional but recommended)

Proposal reviewer trainings	• Proposal reviewers	• Grant proposal reviewer surveys
		• Interviews
			Strengths
			• Few granting systems provide reviewer training
			• Good framework for outlining how the granting process would proceed
			Improvements
			• Rated moderately well
			• Needed additional information/practice regarding
			  • scoring planning grants
			  • scoring budgets
			  • accountability conceptual training
			  • rating actual grant proposals
			  • scoring ambiguities

Technical assistance	• Applicants	• Interviews	Strengths • Tangible assistance • Information • Emotional support

Column A ROGG Component	Column B Data Source	Column C Evaluation Technique	Column D Results: Strengths and Improvements
			Improvements • More decentralized • Needed more frequently, on an ongoing basis
Grant application	• Applicants	• Surveys • Interviews	Strengths • Simple, direct, straightforward • Well organized and explained Improvements • Need to include planning grants • Need more clarity in using and applying accountability questions in grant proposal
Guidebook	• Applicants	• Surveys • Interviews	Strengths • Easy to follow • Helpful • Good resource • Informative, purposeful Improvements
Sample grant	• Applicants	• Surveys • Interviews	Strengths • Good, excellent • Adequate Improvements • None provided
Quality of ROGG grant proposals	• Independent grant proposal reviewers	• Grant comparison survey	• No significant difference between ROGG and non-ROGG grant proposals

of have to stand back if you are not familiar with what's going on, sometimes you never grasp the idea. It was very plain. A kid could know what's going on . . . after I got there, I found the process was so simple, I understood it. If I thought it was that simple, I wouldn't need her [professional grant writer].

The data revealed several factors that contributed to the ease and simplicity of the process, including (a) the provision of a clear structure, an outline, and a "mental" and "written" framework from which applicants could shape their ideas; (b) training and TA at all levels for how the proposal was to be completed; (c) the provision of sample grant proposals; (d) the ease of the word processing program used for grant submission; (e) sufficient time to complete the grant proposal; (f) fewer requirements than other

granting systems for obtaining and gathering background information; and (9) the perception that it was a less daunting and complicated process and structure than other granting processes.

Workshops and Trainings

Pre-grant workshop and reviewer training data revealed both strengths and weaknesses of ROGG. Survey data indicated that the pre-grant workshops were well received, with all ratings falling in the two highest possible scores (the 4- to 5-point range). The most highly rated aspects of the pre-grant workshops were clarity of the information about the granting or funding time line ($M = 4.68$, $SD = 0.47$); the feeling that the participants would share the information with other members of their Youth Council ($M =$

4.63, $SD = 0.59$); and the belief that they would use the material from the workshop ($M = 4.63$, $SD = 0.59$).

Nine out of 10 responses to an open-ended item regarding the sample grant proposal indicated that it was good to excellent, and the remaining response indicated that it was adequate. With respect to the grant application, 11 of 14 (79%) responses focused on positive aspects of the application, including comments that it was simple and direct, very straightforward, very easy to understand, and well organized. Two (14%) responses suggested improving particular aspects of the application process (e.g., examples of planning grants, clarifying utilization of some application questions). All 11 responses about the guidebook were favorable. It was seen as excellent, very easy to follow, helpful, a good resource, informative, and purposeful, and no suggestions for improvements were offered.

Results of interviews indicated that of the four individuals who attended the pre-grant workshop and wrote a grant proposal, two indicated that the workshop helped them feel as if they could complete the proposal themselves. In addition, the Department of Juvenile Justice staff indicated that the workshops were extremely well done, particularly because the completed and submitted proposals followed the outlined structure well.

Suggestions for workshop improvements emerged in about one third of the interviews. These suggestions centered on the need to include planning grant information; a feeling that for experienced grant writers the training was less useful because it failed to provide new information; the assessment that the provision of one workshop was inadequate and ongoing workshops and/or TA was needed to obtain the desired benefits of results-based accountability; and the observation that Youth Council member attendance at the workshops was poor.

Results of survey data indicate that the grant proposal reviewer training was rated moderately well. The most favorable aspects were the time for discussion ($M = 5.00$, $SD = 0.00$); the knowledge of the trainers ($M = 4.5$, $SD = 0.54$); and time for questions and answers ($M = 4.83$, $SD = 0.40$). Although still in the satisfactory range, the least favorably rated aspects of the training were clarity of the overheads ($M = 2.50$, $SD = 0.31$); a feeling that reviewers were satisfactorily prepared to rate the grants given the material provided ($M = 3.0$, $SD = 0.89$); and

the presentation style of the trainers ($M = 3.50$, $SD = 0.54$).

Reviewers were asked additional qualitative survey items to help evaluate the utility of the prerating training workshop, and five of the seven (71%) provided comments. Two indicated that the grant rater workshop failed to prepare them for rating planning grants, two indicated that it failed to adequately prepare them for rating budgets, and one indicated that the training would have been improved if the raters had been given conceptual training followed by the opportunity to rate actual grant proposals and time to discuss the ambiguities of scoring.

Once the grant proposals were individually rated, reviewers were asked how well the first training had prepared them. Ratings fell in the middle range, indicating that the training and preparation were moderately helpful in rating the grant proposals.

The grant proposal reviewer who was interviewed commented that it was beneficial to provide training to the reviewers because most processes do not do so. She also indicated that the training presented a good framework for how the grant proposal review process was going to proceed.

Technical Assistance

Sixty percent of the documents referenced the strength of the TA provided by the Center for Family Policy. Further content analysis yielded three major themes that characterized the positive aspects of the TA: tangible assistance, informational assistance, and emotional support. Tangible assistance refers to the provision of specialized aid, services, and resources that helped participants to complete the final product (grant proposal), complete other programmatic requirements, and secure additional funding. The tangible assistance helped Youth Council members with the more technical aspects of the proposal.

Informational assistance included the feeling that the Center for Family Policy TA providers were a resource to provide information and answer questions about the application, help Youth Council members understand the application, and provide information about other grant opportunities. One participant commented:

With other grants, if you call and keep calling the person who is handling the grant, they can't be real specific. But Jennifer and Tina[3] were real specific. You can do this and this or you can't do this and how about if you try this or write about this. Whereas other grants people seem to be real cautious and guarded about not telling you.

Emotional support related to the personal characteristics of Center for Family Policy TA staff and their style of interacting with participants. Members of the TA staff were described as helpful, very patient, encouraging, available, supportive, able to provide guidance, easy to contact and talk to, willing to attend meetings and conduct site visits, able to develop personal relationships, and responsive in a timely manner.

Logistics

Logistical issues were raised in 30 percent of the interviews. The grant proposal reviewer indicated that there was not a lot of time to review grants. Although she did not mind, she read most of the proposals during her personal time due to the short turnaround time. One proposal writer indicated that the application format on the floppy disk did not match the hard copy application, and that the disk version became available in the middle of the process, which was late in the grant-writing process. The Center for Family Policy office had difficulty with receiving too many faxes at one time as the deadline approached, resulting in some incomplete proposals.

Program Evaluation

The data in 30 percent documents indicated that Youth Council members would have benefited from additional evaluation assistance, particularly in developing and conducting outcome evaluations. The university-based ROGG staff person indicated:

We were asking them about how they're going to evaluate their program. I think we need to provide them more information or assistance, rather than just asking how they're going to evaluate the program. I'd like to do some of that through an example, you know, with all of it, use an example.

The Center for Family Policy staff indicated that the evaluation criteria were developed for implementation grants, and they recognized the need to develop evaluation criteria specifically for planning grants.

Review and Award Processes

Discontent with the proposal review process surfaced in 30 percent of the interviews. Political influences were thought to negatively impact the grant proposal review or award determination process. Once grant proposals were submitted and scored using the accountability approach, the director of one of the partnership agencies reviewed the funding decisions and asked for modifications to some proposed programs. A Youth Council member was concerned about the modifications because the Youth Council had not developed the modified proposal and program, and it was anxious about a potential audit. The Youth Council had developed the original program and understood how to manage it, but with a new project, it felt disconnected and unsure about managing the program. A member of the university-based grant-writing team felt that the changes in programs negated the spirit of the ROGG process and demonstrated that the leadership of the partner agency was not committed to using data to drive decisions or to an agency accountability process.

EXPLORATORY SUPPLEMENTAL STUDY COMPARING PROPOSALS FROM ROGG SYSTEM VERSUS NON-ROGG SYSTEM

To assess the final proximal outcome of Phase 1 (quality of grant proposals), a study was conducted to determine how grant proposals produced by the ROGG System compared with those produced by a different granting system.

Participants

Independent Grant Proposal Reviewers

Following the award determinations, four independent, non-ROGG System reviewers were recruited to rate four ROGG and four non-ROGG grant proposals matched on key criteria (e.g., type and scope of program, budget, target group). All raters had previously participated in the same grant-writing and certification course from which they were recruited. All four reviewers were female and were employed by a private consulting firm and a community foundation. Three of the raters returned completed surveys.

Procedure

Independent Reviews of Proposals

Independent grant reviewers were selected, contacted by phone, and given a brief explanation of the study. Once they agreed to participate, each was sent two ROGG and two non-ROGG proposals. Included in the package of information sent were a consent form and a definition page explaining key accountability terms (e.g., needs assessment, outcome evaluation, continuous quality improvement) to help ensure uniformity.

Instruments

Grant Comparison Survey

A survey was developed to compare ROGG and non-ROGG proposals in which the raters used a 6-point Likert scale (0 = element not included in the grant proposal, 1 = poor, 2 = fair, 3 = good, 4 = very good, 5 = excellent) to rate aspects of the proposal (e.g., quality of the problem statement, quality of the proposed program evaluation). Several items also assessed how well the proposal addressed accountability-related issues such as the use of science-based programming, the quality of the proposed evaluation, and the underlying theory of how the program would affect the target population.

Independent Reviews

Due to the subjectivity involved with rating grant proposals, an estimation of interrater reliability measurement error was conducted before an analysis of differences between the two types of proposals was conducted. In this study, interrater reliability was determined using an intraclass correlation coefficient using two thirds of raters who rated a subset of overlapping grant proposals (four of the six proposals). A two-way mixed effect model was used to estimate interrater reliability. Results indicated that although there was a wide range ($\alpha = 0$–.88), the majority of variables reached an acceptable level of consistency.

The next step in examining the potential dif-

ferences between the two sets of grants was to determine scores for each of the 34 items of comparison. To obtain composite scores, for grants with more than one rater, the mean score was calculated for each item. For those with one rater, those scores were entered into the analysis. The results of the independent t tests indicated that there were no significant differences between the two types of grant proposals on the total scores or for any of the survey items.

In relation to the ROGG and non-ROGG granting program comparison, the comparison group used was the best comparison group available at the time of this study; however, there are several significant methodological limitations. A small number of grant proposals were rated, which may have influenced the ability to detect real differences. Although the ROGG intervention was available to all 16 Youth Councils, they differed in the degree to which they participated in the system, and this was not assessed. Thus, included in the analysis were proposals from Youth Councils that likely did not participate to a large extent in the ROGG accountability process. Furthermore, a consultant could have written proposals, and this was not assessed. Also unknown were the nature, type, and frequency of the assistance provided to the non-ROGG program participants. Finally, some of the proposals submitted to the non-ROGG system may have been continuation and/or modified grant proposals; thus the comparison of these proposals with first-time proposals may not be appropriate.

DISCUSSION

Although this study set out to explore one component (granting program) of a larger statewide initiative (Youth Councils), the evaluation of ROGG System highlighted several factors that can be important for working with community-based agencies and for developing and implementing community-based granting and funding initiatives.

1. *Minimize the complexity of the grant-making process.* A major goal of the ROGG System was to develop a grant-making system that included results-oriented principles but that was not overly complicated and complex such that community groups and individuals, regardless of their previous knowledge and experience, could complete the process. The feedback from indi-

viduals at all levels of the system (Youth Council members, TA providers, grant proposal reviewers) indicated that this goal was achieved—the most consistent strength being the ease and simplicity of the system. Factors contributing to the uncomplicated and straightforward process included simplified grant application questions, provision of grant-making tools and assistance (sample grant proposals, TA), and provision of a framework (results orientation) from which ideas could be shaped.

2. *Provide grant-making assistance.* The pre-grant workshops and technical assistance were seen as strengths of the system. The utility of the pre-grant workshops was apparent from the qualitative and quantitative data. Information provided in the workshops regarding the proposal-writing process (e.g., whom to call for questions, the need to answer application questions thoroughly) appeared most salient. This finding points to the need to balance information provided about the specific granting process or program with communicating the more general accountability principles and concepts during the workshops. Feedback indicated that workshops could be strengthened in several ways to ensure maximum access and utilization, such as offering them at remote sites and at various times to bolster attendance and access.

A second important system tool was the TA that addressed multiple needs of grant writers and applicants, including tangible resources, information, and emotional support. Particularly for individuals with less grant experience or Youth Council support, the provision of emotional support to complete the grant-writing process seemed to be as important as providing tangible resources. The suggested TA improvements provided in the evaluation of this program are useful to informing other granting systems and programs. Participants saw the potential benefits of making the TA more widely and frequently available and providing it on-site during the grant-making phase to reduce barriers to participation.

The finding that ongoing TA and information were very important aspects of this grant-making system is consistent with Shaw, Furnari, and Odendahl's (2000) study of the policies and procedures that foster greater accountability in foundations. The researchers indicated that foundation staff should be accessible by telephone and/or e-mail, and employees at all levels should be educated to handle inquiries about the application and grant-making process. In addition, communication with applicants and grantees should be respectful, interactive, and responsive.

3. *Ensure adequate training for grant proposal reviewers.* Training for the proposal reviewers is essential to attain standardization and reinforce the principles of accountability. In this particular program, the grant proposal reviewer workshops were rated moderately well and could have been improved to better prepare reviewers for rating proposals. Raters wanted more information about planning grants, including a sample planning grant proposal, a discussion of how to score budgets, and the opportunity to score and discuss sample proposals. In addition to developing raters' skill, the inclusion of practice scoring during the training can also help to increase consistency and interrater reliability.

4. *Obtain system-level buy-in.* Commitment to an accountability process at all levels of the granting initiative is essential for success. A lack of buy-in from a partner agency for the accountability process was apparent in the award determination process (i.e., after the grant proposal was submitted). Although the grant scoring process was based on objectively stated and enforced requirements and guidelines at the applicant and reviewer levels, the director of one funding and partner agency modified some funding decisions based on the perceived agency need. In some instances, it was strongly suggested that applicants change the nature, focus, scope, or budget of their programs in ways that were inconsistent with the accountability questions. By most accounts, this undermined the granting process, particularly because accountability principles were at the foundation. This raises serious questions about such an accountability process in which several agencies are involved but with seemingly different levels of commitment and understanding. It also highlights the potential political aspects of grant-making. Initially, some participants felt that the granting system was depoliticized due to the support of the TA, the consistent messages communicated to potential grantees that funding was available, the availability of clear guidelines for obtaining funding, and the goal of giving everyone an equal chance at succeeding. However, some who were asked to make seemingly arbitrary modifications felt confused by the process and struggled with the decision to accept the award. A major issue that granting systems should address is how to func-

tion in what is often a political system, particularly in this case where the overall project may be mandated by political leaders who have specific ideas for successful programming. A second issue this raises is the inclusion of upper-level agency management in the development and implementation of a process in which accountability principles may be a new and/or different way of managing grants programs. This inclusion and adoption of accountability in organizations and systems will require ongoing training and involvement at all levels of decision making.

5. *Provide program evaluation assistance.* Evaluation issues emerged as an area of the system that needed improvement. A major criticism by one grant writer was that the evaluation expectations were unrealistic and elaborate, particularly if the funding was to be used for discrete, add-on services. In addition, the results indicated that more consideration should have been given to the development of evaluation strategies for planning grants. There should be assistance with planning and carrying out evaluation-related work, which is a highly technical and skilled area of grant-making and implementation. For many grant-making entities that already face inadequate numbers of staff, it is common not to have evaluation staff and/or to have staff who lack formal evaluation training (Alie & Seita, 1997; Carter, 1992); thus evaluation is likely to be left undone. Granting entities should ensure that there are enough staff members to assist with program evaluation in the planning stages of grant development and programming at both the agency and grantees levels (Chelimsky, 2001).

6. *Develop clear criteria for grant quality.* The exploratory comparison of grants produced by the ROGG and non-ROGG systems was not significant, in part due to the small sample size (four reviewers). Nevertheless, the approach and measures can be useful for future studies of grant quality.

STUDY LIMITATIONS

Although the study highlights some important factors to consider in developing and implementing a community-based grants program, there are some limitations.

1. Monitoring and tracking participants over time was difficult. For instance, those who participated in the pre-grant workshops

were not necessarily those who participated in writing the grant proposal. Measuring the attitudes of different individuals receiving different components of the intervention at different times compromised the continuity of the evaluation.

2. The researchers developed all instruments (because there were no studies like this in the literature). Although the study provided necessary evaluation information, the validity and reliability of the measures are not established. However, the measures are straightforward and rely on face validity.

3. Given the amount of time to develop and implement systemic outcomes-based changes (Julian, 2001), the benefits (changes in accountability behaviors) and strengths of the system may not have been apparent during the limited period of the study.

ACKNOWLEDGMENT We thank Pam Imm, Michelle Andra, Patrick McCarty, the South Carolina Center for Family Policy, the South Carolina Governor's Office, the South Carolina Department of Juvenile Justice, and members of the Governor's Youth Councils who kindly volunteered to participate in this study. We would also like to thank Barbara Nangle and the Investigators Group in the Division of Prevention and Community Research, Yale University School of Medicine, for helpful comments on the manuscript.

This work is based on the first author's dissertation, completed in the Department of Psychology at the University of South Carolina, Columbia, South Carolina.

Correspondence concerning this article should be addressed to Cindy A. Crusto, the Consultation Center and Division of Prevention and Community Research, Department of Psychiatry, Yale University School of Medicine, 389 Whitney Avenue, New Haven, CT 06511. Electronic mail may be sent to cindy.crusto@yale.edu.

Notes

1. Original article includes eight accountability questions. With input from ROGG partners, a ninth accountability question—"What is your local council trying to accomplish?"—was added to meet the needs of the community-based granting initiative.

2. The Comprehensive Quality Programming approach was incorporated into the broader Getting To Outcomes Approach in this article.

3. Names have been changed to protect anonymity of staff.

References

Alie, R. E., Seita, J. R. (1997, October). Who's using evaluation and how? *Nonprofit World, 15*(5), 40–49.

Carter, J. (1992). Evaluation in foundations. *Evaluation Practice, 13*(1), 33–38.

Center for Effective Philanthropy. (2002b). *Indicators of effectiveness: Understanding and improving foundation performance.* Boston: Author.

Center for Effective Philanthropy. (2002a). *Assessing foundation performance: Current practices, future possibilities.* Boston: Author.

Chelimsky, E. (1997). The coming transformation in evaluation. In E. Chelimsky & W. Shadish (Eds.), *Evaluation for the 21st century: A handbook* (pp. 1–26). Thousand Oaks, CA: Sage.

Chelimsky, E. (2001). What evaluation could do to support foundations: A framework with nine component parts. *American Journal of Evaluation, 22,* 13–28.

Fetterman, D. M., Kaftarian, S. J., & Wandersman, A. (Eds.). (1996). *Empowerment evaluation: Knowledge and tools for self-assessment & accountability* (pp. 3–46). Thousand Oaks, CA: Sage.

Glasser, B. G., & Strauss, A. L. (1967). *The discovery of grounded theory.* Chicago: Aldine.

Goodman, R. M., & Wandersman, A. (1994). FORECAST: A formative approach to evaluating community coalitions and community-based initiatives. In S. Kaftarian & W. Hansen (Eds.), *Improving methodologies for evaluating community-based coalitions for preventing alcohol, tobacco, and other drug use. Journal of Community Psychology* (CSAP special issue), 6–25.

Goodman, R. M., Wandersman, A., Chinman, M., Imm, P., & Morrissey, E. (1996). An ecological assessment of community-based interventions for prevention and health promotion: Approaches to measuring community coalitions. *American Journal of Community Psychology, 24*(1), 33–61.

Julian, D. A. (2001). A case study of the implementation of outcomes-based funding within a local United Way system: Some implications for practicing community psychology. *American Journal of Community Psychology, 29,* 851–874.

Merriam, S. B. (1988). *Case study research in education: A qualitative approach.* San Francisco: Jossey-Bass.

Morley, E., Hatry, H., & Cowan, J. (2002). *Making use of outcome information for improving services: Recommendations for nonprofit organizations.* Washington, DC: Urban Institute.

Shaw, A., Furnari, E., & Odendahl, T. (2000). *Preserving the public trust: A study of exemplary practices in grant-making.* Washington, DC: Aspen Institute.

Stamler, B. (2000, November 20). Charities award grants, then pay to evaluate how the money is spent. *New York Times.*

Strauss, A., & Corbin, J. (1990). *Basics of qualitative research: Grounded theory procedures and techniques.* Newbury Park, CA: Sage.

Wandersman, A., Imm, P., Chinman, M., & Kaftarian, S. (2000). Getting to outcomes: A results-based approach to accountability. *Evaluation and Program Planning, 23,* 389–395.

Wandersman, A., Morrissey, E., Davino, K., Seybolt, D., Crusto, C., Nation, M., Goodman, R., & Imm, P. (1998). Comprehensive quality programming and accountability: Eight essential strategies for implementing successful prevention programs. *Journal of Primary Prevention, 19,* 3–30.

W. K. Kellogg Foundation. (1999). *Empowerment evaluation and foundations: A matter of perspectives.* Battle Creek, MI: Author.

Yin, R. K. (1994). *Case study research: Design and methods.* (2nd ed.). Thousand Oaks, CA: Sage.

Yin, R. K. (1998). The abridged version of case study research: Design and method. In L. Bickman & D. Rog (Eds.), *Handbook of applied social research* (pp. 229–259). Thousand Oaks, CA: Sage.

Yost, J., & Wandersman, A. (1998, November). Results-oriented grant-making/grant-implementation: Mary Black foundation's experience. Paper presented at the annual meeting of the American Evaluation Association. Chicago, IL.

17 CONDUCTING COST-BENEFIT ANALYSIS IN HUMAN SERVICES SETTINGS

Carol Harvey, Michael J. Camasso, & Radha Jagannathan

The pressure on social work practitioners to engage in accountable service provision has increased dramatically over the past two decades. At all levels of practice, from clinical care and case management to program administration and executive decision making, interventions once viewed as demonstrations of human compassion and social justice are increasingly subject to the hard questions about treatment effectiveness, service costs, and accrued benefits that arise in an environment of managed care, public–private partnerships, and contracted-out services. Cost-benefit analysis provides a useful framework within which human services administrators and supervisors can measure the relationship between effort expended and results achieved.

The social work response to the call for economic evaluation has been halting and, at times, antagonistic. A number of recently published social work evaluation texts, however, acknowledge the importance of cost-benefit analyses (Grinnell, 1997; Posavac & Carey, 1997; Royse & Thayer, 1996; Yegidis & Weinbach, 2002; Unrau, Gabor, & Grinnell, 2001). Extensive treatments of the monetary valuation of human services are found in the work of non–social workers as well (Gold, Siegel, Russell, & Weinstein, 1996; Rossi, Freeman, & Lipsey, 1999; Yates, 1996).

The principal focus of a cost analysis of any intervention is to assess the opportunity cost of the intervention from a societal perspective. *Opportunity costs* are defined as the benefits that the resources expended for that intervention would yield in their next best alternative use. Cost-effectiveness analysis compares the incremental monetary cost of an intervention to the incremental nonmonetary outcome (i.e., number of clients employed, number of inpatient hospital days avoided, postsentencing recidivism rate, and the like). Results are typically expressed as a ratio of costs to outcome, for example, in terms of costs per client employed. Cost-benefit analysis compares the opportunity cost of an intervention with all benefits achieved by its implementation; both costs and benefits, in this instance, are expressed in monetary terms. The results of a cost-benefit analysis are typically presented either as the ratio of benefits to costs (i.e., as a benefit-cost ratio) or as the difference between benefits and costs, or "net benefits" (see French, 2000; Thompson, 1980). Cost-benefit analyses are preferred to cost-effectiveness analyses when diverse interventions with multiple treatment goals or outcomes are under consideration.

In the real world of social work, the application of cost analysis, either cost-effectiveness or cost-benefit analysis, is no simple task. It is certainly difficult to place a dollar value on intervention outcomes such as relief from addiction, poverty, illness, infirmity, and victimization, yet if these consequences are not addressed, the benefits of social interventions may be seriously underestimated. Moreover, the very notion that one should attempt such a task runs counter to the basic working philosophy of many social work practitioners. Also at issue is our ability to measure the exact treatment (dosages prescribed, administered to, and consumed by recipients) delivered by the intervention. Finally, as Yates (1996) points out, the outcomes attributed to the intervention may actually be the result of other processes specific to the client, practitioner, agency, or community. Of course, this last issue can be avoided if the cost analysis is performed within the framework of an experimental design, where outside processes are controlled through random assignment. While we recognize that classic experimental design is a luxury not often afforded to the evaluation of social work practice, this evaluation methodology provides one of the most unclouded vantage points from which to frame a cost analysis. The cost analysis we present in this chapter is based on data generated from a welfare reform experiment undertaken in New Jersey from 1992 through 1996 called the Family Development Program (Camasso, Harvey, & Jagannathan, 1998). In previous work, we have shown that random assignment in this experiment was successfully implemented (Camasso, Jagannathan, Harvey, & Killingsworth, 2003; Jagannathan and Camasso, 2002).

The underlying premise of welfare reform demonstrations that began in the 1980s and continued into the mid-1990s was that a significant number of recipients of public assistance could be made more self-sufficient if they could acquire more or better job skills and/or if job search costs and other barriers to employment could be minimized. Many of these welfare demonstration projects had other objectives as well, including the formation and maintenance of two-parent households, better family functioning, and better health outcomes for children on welfare.

Reductions in long-term reliance on public assistance, increases in employment and earnings, and improved family structure and other outcomes among welfare recipients and their households were some of the anticipated benefits of these experiments. However, costs were also incurred as financial incentives to work and to marry were implemented and as additional services and benefits were provided to welfare recipients.

The positive impacts of these initiatives must be balanced against the higher costs associated with their operation. A cost-benefit analysis provides a systematic calculation and comparison of the costs and benefits attributable to the implementation of a specific welfare intervention. This type of analysis identifies and quantifies (to the extent possible) specific costs and benefits associated with program implementation and operation, providing a practical framework for assessing the economic impacts of the program or policy.

Cost-benefit analysis has long been used to assess the overall economic effect of social policy in the context of manpower programs and policies. Early applications of this analytical tool include an assessment of the Upward Bound program (Garms, 1971), analyses of the economic efficiency of various manpower programs to train dislocated workers (Cain & Stromsdorfer, 1968; Hardin & Borus, 1966), and assessments of the effectiveness of education (Carnoy & Marenbach, 1975). More recently, cost-benefit analysis has been used to demonstrate the positive payback on various types of welfare-to-work initiatives. The demonstration projects evaluated by Manpower Demonstration Research Corporation (MDRC) throughout the 1980s indicate small but significant net positive impacts associated with specific programs designed to enhance employment options and incentives for recipients of Aid to Families with Dependent Children (AFDC) (Gueron & Pauly, 1991). Welfare reform evaluations conducted since 1987 generally included a cost-benefit analysis and typically employed an experimental design methodology (see, e.g., Camasso, et al., 1998; Gordon & Martin, 1999; Kemple, Friedlander, & Fellerath, 1995; Riccio, Friedlander, & Freedman, 1994).

COST-BENEFIT ANALYSIS: SOME BASIC CONCEPTS AND METHODOLOGY

Cost-benefit analysis is, first and foremost, an economic tool. From an economic perspective, the question that arises in the evaluation of any public policy initiative or intervention is that of economic or allocative efficiency. Social work interventions are expected to improve some aspect of individual or social well-being. However, these interventions typically require additional resources (i.e., personnel, equipment, or materials) for their implementation and operation, and the allocation of these resources toward one use precludes their productive use elsewhere. Do the improvements in well-being produced by a specific welfare reform intervention justify the expenditure of resources in that direction? Could these resources have been employed more productively in another intervention, providing a greater increase in well-being?

An efficient use of resources (i.e., labor, equipment, and other productive resources) is that use which provides, at least potentially, the greatest amount of well-being or benefit. If the current allocation or use of resources cannot be changed to improve the lot of one or more parties without simultaneously reducing another party's well-being, then the current use of resources is *efficient*.[1] Cost-benefit analysis is the traditional analytical framework for evaluating the allocative efficiency of public programs, regulations, or interventions.

Cost-benefit analysis is an especially useful tool at the programmatic level, where there is typically more than one approach to achieving a given objective. A cost-benefit analysis of competing approaches designed to reduce welfare dependency, for example, can identify the approach that makes the most productive use of the additional resources required for this activity. The following list describes the various tasks or steps involved in conducting a cost-benefit analysis.

- Step 1: Define/describe the program(s) or intervention(s) to be evaluated

- Step 2: Identify all possible costs and benefits for each alternative

- Step 3: Measure costs and benefits

- Step 4: Compare costs and benefits. When appropriate, adjust for time distribution of costs/benefits

Step 1: Defining and Describing Alternative Programs or Interventions

The initial step in cost-benefit analysis requires that the analyst develop a clear understanding of how alternative programs or interventions work, and what impacts are to be expected from each program's implementation. This focus on impact takes the analyst beyond a mere description of alternative program measures and objectives to a detailed comparison of what happens when the program in question is implemented versus what would happen without the program (or with an alternative intervention).

A thorough description of program alternatives requires the consideration of four types of factors or variables: program structure, process, outcomes, and the characteristics of the recipient population. Program structure factors are the personnel, facilities, technologies, treatments, and related instrumentalities that constitute the actual intervention. Program process factors are

changes in the social, educational, or psychological states of program recipients that occur as a result of an intervention. Examples would include increased feelings of self-esteem or empowerment, learning a new skill, or controlling anger. Program process factors may be outcomes of an intervention. More often, they are measures of the treatment taking effect.

Program outcomes represent desired life-changing behaviors engaged in by program recipients. These include such behaviors as completion of an education or training program, successful employment, remaining drug-free, and/or avoiding unwanted pregnancies. Identifying the characteristics of the program's target population, such as level of education, racial or ethnic composition, level of income, family structure, work history, and other features, is the fourth factor critical to program description. This information allows the analyst to assess both how the program and its outcomes compare with similar interventions elsewhere and, more to the point, how readily the evaluation finding can be generalized to other circumstances.

Step 2: Identifying Costs and Benefits

Costs and benefits represent, conceptually, losses and gains in well-being. Benefits are any and all positive effects of a program or policy on society's well-being. The benefits or gains associated with any policy or program are usually identified with reference to that program's objectives. For example, benefits associated with training programs for welfare recipients or other dislocated or disadvantaged workers include enhanced employment and earnings opportunities for the program participants.

Costs represent losses in well-being attributable to a given program or policy. The concept of cost is defined in terms of forgone consumption opportunities. More specifically, the economic cost of producing any desired outcome, such as improving employment and earnings opportunities among welfare recipients, is the value of all other goods or services that must be forgone by allocating resources, such as materials or personnel, away from other uses and into training programs.

Costs or benefits may be either internal or external. Internal effects, whether costs or benefits, are anticipated by the intervention and are typically deliberate or planned outcomes or losses. External effects are more complex; they are side effects produced by the program or activity. These external effects are more difficult to identify and measure than the direct effects of a given program or policy. They also tend to affect third parties, that is, groups or individuals who are not direct participants or agents in the program. To the extent possible, all costs and benefits (both internal and external) associated with a given program or policy should be considered within a cost-benefit analysis.

The process of identifying specific cost and benefit items is a tricky business when, as is the case in welfare reform programs, one party's cost is another party's benefit. Reductions in cash assistance received by welfare recipients as their earnings from employment increase will be viewed as a benefit from the perspective of state and federal budgets; these are budgetary resources that can be utilized elsewhere. From the welfare recipient's perspective, however, reduced cash assistance is a cost, reflecting a reduction in consumption opportunities. From a global or societal perspective, changes in cash assistance received or paid out as a result of welfare reform program cancel each other out and have no net impact on real consumption opportunities.[2] Cost-benefit analyses should be conducted from the societal or global perspective if the intent of the evaluation is to gauge the allocative efficiency of proposed or implemented programs. However, when actually classifying a particular item as either a cost or a benefit, particularly when dealing with pure transfers that involve no change in production or consumption of real resources, the cost-benefit analyst may need to arbitrarily choose a particular perspective.

Step 3: Measuring Costs and Benefits

If benefits represent gains and costs losses in well-being, how do we measure the value that individuals or society attaches to these losses or gains? Conceptually, willingness to pay forms the basis for evaluation of both benefits and costs. In its simplest terms, willingness to pay can be measured by the amount of income that an individual would be willing to give up (accept) to gain (relinquish) some desirable outcome.[3] In a very simple example of a private market transaction, the price that we pay for a gallon of gasoline reflects our willingness to pay for it, and this provides a first approximation of the value that we as consumers place on that item. Willingness to pay is most easily explained

using examples of simple market transactions, in a well-organized and competitive market setting, where the individual who bears the cost of a particular action or transaction also enjoys the full benefits of this activity. Willingness to pay is usually not so easily observed and measured, and typical operational measures, based on observed market prices, only approximate the true conceptual measure of benefits from the willingness-to-pay perspective.

The notion of opportunity cost also provides an operational basis for valuation. Losses in well-being associated with the provision of job training services for welfare recipients are measured as the value of the output that is lost as resources are allocated to these training programs and away from their most productive alternative use. Market prices (i.e., wages paid to case managers and instructors, and other input costs) are typically taken as a measure of productivity in alternate uses.[4]

Certain costs and benefits cannot be easily observed, let alone quantified. For example, training programs may also have some (unintended) external costs if the workers who graduate from these programs take jobs away from existing workers. These labor market effects are difficult to measure in practice and are highly dependent on local labor market conditions. Increased job skills and employment opportunities arising from job-training programs may also provide intensely personal benefits of increased self-esteem and self-satisfaction. Perhaps better employment prospects ultimately improve marital and household stability. There are all sorts of possible psychosocial effects (such as higher self-esteem or increased motivation) that may be perceived as beneficial outcomes (intended or not) of manpower training programs but cannot easily be valued in monetary terms. However, even if some benefits (or costs) cannot easily be valued, they should be identified and, if possible, measured in nonmonetary terms.

Data that measure costs and benefits can come from a variety of sources, including administrative records on programmatic participation and fiscal records, as well as surveys of program workers and program clients.

Step 4: Comparing Costs and Benefits

Strictly speaking, we should be comparing marginal, rather than average, effects. What does this mean? In making any choice (i.e., how much of a particular item to purchase, how many hours of labor to provide, how many years of education to attain, how much resource to devote to a specific intervention), we weigh the additional (or marginal) gains from an incremental increase or decrease in the contemplated activity against the additional (or marginal) costs involved. As long as the marginal gains outweigh the marginal losses, we increase our well-being by continuing to purchase more of the item in question, or by working more, or by continuing our education. All this is, of course, subject to any constraints imposed by budgets, time, or other factors. At some point, however, the additional cost to an individual of, for example, working an extra hour will exceed the additional gain from doing so. At this point, working more hours will actually produce a decline in overall well-being. Well-being is maximized when the marginal cost of pursuing a given objective equals the marginal gain from doing so.

Cost-benefit analysts, in practice, frequently measure and compare average costs and benefits. This practice is sometimes dictated by program complexities; it is difficult to conceptualize marginal costs and benefits if intervention outcomes or treatments are not easily divisible into small units, or in the presence of multiple program objectives. It may also be driven by data deficiencies; analysis of marginal changes requires much more detailed data than analysis at the average level. Too often, however, the measurement and comparison of average cost and benefits is done with little understanding of the underlying implications.

Comparisons of average costs and benefits do provide some information of economic value. If average benefits exceed average costs, then overall gains exceed total losses. In economic terms, this tells us that the program or policy in question is feasible, in other words, that it pays for itself. However, a whole range of scenarios may be feasible; only one is most desirable from an economic perspective. Comparisons of average costs and average benefits do not tell us whether overall well-being has reached a maximum. Comparisons of marginal costs and benefits (or the calculation of marginal net benefits) associated with incremental movements in program or policy initiatives allow the policy analyst to judge whether or not to continue, expand, or contract the program. Among a range of options, that which maximizes net benefits is preferred.

Those who reap benefits from a specific intervention do not necessarily bear the costs. Furthermore, many social policy initiatives are directed specifically at assisting certain groups within the general population. Cost-benefit analysis will assign equal weight to gains and losses, no matter who is affected. However, a policy or program that exhibits tremendous efficiencies from an allocative perspective but that appears to confer large benefits on the wealthy may be seen as appropriate to some policy interests but may also draw considerable criticism from other quarters. If acceptable methods of weighing gains and losses within the cost-benefit framework cannot be derived analytically, policy makers should be informed of the distributional consequences of their actions.[5]

The distribution of costs and benefits over time presents a somewhat more tractable problem, from an analytical perspective, but one that is not completely free of subjective elements. Taking our manpower training example, programmatic costs associated with training are incurred immediately, whereas the benefits of this training occur later and can conceivably last a lifetime. Individuals generally prefer present gains over future gains and thus place a higher value on a dollar of benefits received (or costs incurred) today vis-à-vis a dollar received (or costs incurred) several years into the future (even after adjusting for inflation). Operationally, we allow for this pattern of time preferences by using an appropriate factor to discount future gains and losses to their current value. Higher discount rates reflect a higher preference for (and place a higher weight on) changes in current consumption possibilities relative to the future (see Poister, McDavid, & Magoun, 1979, for the discounting formula and an example of its application).

In the case of private investment projects, where gains and losses accrue solely to private individuals, market-determined real interest rates in private capital markets provide a good indicator of the rate of time preference of private investors.[6] However, for programs and policies that have broader social implications, the appropriate discount rate is one that reflects society's evaluation of the trade-off between present and future consumption. This social discount rate is probably not accurately captured by the operation of private capital markets.

Difficulties in both conceptualizing and measuring the society's rate of time preference have led to a wide range of rates used in cost-benefit analyses. The federal Office of Management and Budget (OMB) currently suggests a 7% discount rate, under the assumption that this rate approximates the marginal pretax rate of return on a typical investment in the private sector.[7] However, OMB also urges analysts to test the sensitivity of their results to a range of discount rates around this 7%.

Finally, all costs and benefits, no matter when incurred, should be measured using prices, wages, and other costs from a given year. The rationale behind this is quite simple: Cost-benefit analysis seeks to measure real, as opposed to purely inflationary, changes in consumption or production. Measurement of real program effects in monetary terms requires that we use a fixed price measure.

COST-BENEFIT ANALYSIS OF NEW JERSEY'S FAMILY DEVELOPMENT PROGRAM

We now apply the procedures for conducting a cost-benefit analysis to the New Jersey Family Development Program.

Defining and Describing the Family Development Program and Its Alternative

The Family Development Program (FDP) was signed into law in New Jersey in January 1992. A major objective of the FDP was to reduce welfare dependency and to move clients from the welfare rolls into employment. The program was also intended to improve household stability and family functioning and to encourage a stronger sense of responsibility among recipients of AFDC for their childbearing decisions.

The FDP included several provisions waivered under Section 1115 of the Social Security Act. The most well-known and the most controversial element of the program was its "family cap" provision, which precluded an AFDC recipient from receiving additional cash benefits for a child conceived while the mother was on welfare. Other important program elements included an enhanced earned income disregard for households with "capped" grants, a reduction in the

financial penalties for (re)marriage, 2 years of transitional Medicaid benefits for AFDC recipients who left the welfare rolls for employment, a requirement that women with children aged 2 or older participate in education or training programs designed to improve their labor market opportunities (under the Job Opportunities and Basic Skills, or JOBS program), and more immediate sanctions for failure to participate in the JOBS program.

The mandated evaluation strategy for this waivered program consisted of an experimental design in which two samples of recipients were selected from New Jersey's AFDC caseload. One sample, designated as a control group, included 1,440 cases selected at random from the AFDC caseload as of October 1, 1992 (ongoing cases), and another 1,056 cases selected at random from new AFDC applications from October 1, 1992, through December 31, 1994 (new applicants). AFDC cases in this control group were *not* subject to any of the program components that characterized the FDP.

A second sample was selected and designated as an experimental group. This sample included 2,882 cases selected at random as of October 1, 1992 (ongoing cases), and another 1,876 cases selected from new AFDC applications received on or after October 1, 1992, through December 31, 1994 (new applicants). These cases were subject to all provisions and waivers under the FDP. Analyses were conducted separately for new and ongoing cases because in the former instance experimental cases were less likely to have experienced prior welfare spells under a different set of welfare rules.

This research design, with its reliance on comparisons between an experimental and a control group, does provide some distinct advantages. In principle, it should allow us to observe the direct costs and benefits associated with the FDP. If all evaluation cases are truly selected at random, and if control group cases are treated correctly (i.e., treated strictly under the provisions of New Jersey's prior welfare program, Reaching Economic Achievement, or REACH),[8] then any differences in costs or benefits between the experimental and control groups can be attributed to the implementation of the FDP, and not to differences in the characteristics of the evaluation subjects. There are practical difficulties in maintaining the integrity of the control group; however, these issues appear to have been dealt with successfully in this experiment (Camasso et al., 2003).

Identifying Program Costs and Benefits

Anticipated program costs associated with the implementation and operation of the FDP in New Jersey included the following:

- Possible additional case management costs for AFDC clients who were referred to the FDP.
- Possible additional costs of assessments and educational and employment-directed activities (such as remedial education, job training, job search, and the like) under the JOBS program to FDP clients.
- Additional reimbursement for training-related expenses, including transportation, child care, and work-related expenses for FDP participants.
- Additional costs of providing child care information and referral services to FDP clients.
- The costs of providing an additional year of Medicaid coverage for former FDP participants who left AFDC for employment. This additional coverage could be regarded as a benefit to former recipients, but it was certainly an additional program cost as far as the state and federal governments are concerned. We take the government perspective in this evaluation for purposes of classifying transfers as costs or benefits, and thus identify programmatic impacts on Medicaid as a cost of the FDP intervention.
- Costs incurred for processing eligibility (re)determination and benefits for AFDC and food stamp recipients. To the extent that FDP decreased (increased) recipience among AFDC clients, these costs declined (increased).
- Any additional general administrative costs associated with the FDP.

One goal of most welfare reform programs, either stated or implicit, was to reduce welfare dependency and, ultimately, to reduce welfare caseloads. If the FDP was successful in moving AFDC recipients into the labor market and making them less dependent on public assistance, expenditures on various types of public assistance, including AFDC cash benefits and food stamps, should have declined. The family cap provision also could have affected AFDC cash payments, if not food stamps or Medicaid. Measurable anticipated benefits attributable to FDP include the following:

- Reductions in AFDC cash payments and food stamp benefits. Although this was a potential program cost from the perspective of the individual AFDC client, it was a potential benefit as far as the federal and state government was concerned. Taking the government perspective, we classify reductions in reliance on cash assistance or food stamps as a potential benefit of the FDP.
- Increased earnings received by AFDC recipients as they moved off the welfare rolls and into productive employment.
- Increased tax revenues paid to federal and state government from additional earnings received by (former) AFDC recipients

If it is successful in meeting its objective of improving family functioning in AFDC households, the FDP could be expected to generate a host of benefits to these families, which cannot be assigned a monetary value. Such intangibles as improved quality of life, improved sense of familial responsibility, or a decline in single-parent households may be observed and measured, either from administrative data or from data collected directly from our evaluation subjects. However, while we can assign a dollar value to reduced benefit streams or to increased earnings attributable to FDP, we cannot easily value changes in attitudes, family functioning, or household formation.

Measuring Costs and Benefits

For each case in our experimental and control groups, we measured (in dollars) each of the costs and benefits over a 4-year period, from 1993 through 1996. Administrative welfare or Medicaid data provided ready measures of the following data elements:

- Cash assistance payments received
- Food stamp assistance received
- Payments on Medicaid claims reported
- Support payments received by each case for child care, transportation, and work-related expenses

Information on earnings for occupations or employers required to report employee earnings to the state (under federal legislation governing coverage for unemployment compensation) was obtained for AFDC recipients in our sample from the New Jersey Wage Reporting System.[9] Some agricultural and domestic employees, persons who are self-employed, who work for their families, and some other types of workers are not included in this data because they are not eligible for unemployment compensation. Clearly, this data also excludes evaluation subjects who were working and earning "off the books."[10]

Average costs of providing case management services and child care information and referral services to evaluation subjects were determined using reported quarterly costs (from administrative fiscal records) divided by the AFDC caseload, as were average program and general administrative costs per case. Average costs of education and job training services received by evaluation subjects were based on fiscal and level-of-service reports filed by individual contractors providing these services, fiscal records maintained by the Job Training Partnership Act program, and college tuition costs (for those subjects who utilized Pell grants and other forms of financial assistance to attend college).

Comparing Costs and Benefits

The evaluation's experimental design had distinct implications for the calculation and comparison of program costs and benefits. Unequal sample sizes required that we compare *unit* or *per case* costs (benefits) per experimental case with *unit* or *per case* costs (benefits) per control group case, and *not* the difference in total costs (benefits) incurred by each group. For each cost and benefit category, we calculated average costs (benefits), averaged over *all* cases in each evaluation sample, whether or not each case actually incurred specific types of costs or benefits. Thus, for each evaluation group (i.e., experimental and control samples for both new applicants and ongoing cases), we calculated the average costs and benefits per case on an annual basis over a 4-year time horizon (1993 through 1996).

We then calculated annual net benefits (costs) under the FDP as the difference between benefits (costs) per case for experimental group cases and control group cases. These net benefits (costs) measure the incremental impact of FDP on each cost or benefit item (and in total) compared with

the prior program, REACH/JOBS. Net benefits and costs, summed over 1993 through 1996, are presented in Table 17.1. In addition to societal net impacts, Table 17.1 includes separate estimates of the net cost or benefit per case to the FDP client and to various governmental units at the federal, state, and county levels.

There was a tendency for experimental group cases to remain on the AFDC and/or food stamp rolls longer; this tendency was more pronounced among our sample of new applicants. We observed lower AFDC household unit sizes (defined as the number of household members included in the calculation of the cash grant) among recipient cases in our experimental sample, probably as a result of the family cap. These smaller household units translated into smaller amounts of cash assistance paid per case, which only partially offset the effect of higher AFDC recipience among experimental cases. In the case of food stamps, higher recipience rates among experimental group cases and lower cash assistance amounts paid to experimental cases that received cash benefits both contributed to higher food stamp payments to experimental group cases compared with controls.

We found no evidence that the FDP Program had any systematic positive impact on employment, employment stability, or earnings among AFDC recipients.

Among longer term (ongoing) AFDC recipients, program costs exceeded program benefits from all perspectives. On average, over the period between 1993 and 1996, society lost $1,042 per case under FDP compared with the control group. Most of the loss was caused by lower employment and earnings of FDP participants compared with their control group counterparts. Lower earnings among FDP participants were slightly offset by gains in food stamps; the net loss to FDP participants amounted to $665 per case. Higher benefits paid to FDP participants and the costs of program services and supports under FDP amounted to $377 per case out of federal, state, and county budgets.

Among new AFDC applicants, increased cash assistance, food stamp, and Medicaid benefits received by our experimental sample resulted in a net 4-year benefit to this group of $468 per case compared with their control group counterparts. However, the overall impact on society was a net loss of $1,600 per case, reflecting both the lower earnings reported for experimental group sub-

TABLE 17.1 Four-Year Net Benefits (+) and Net Costs (−) of the Family Development Program, 1993–1996[a]

Ongoing Cases (Dollars Per Case)			
Benefit-Cost Component	Society	AFDC Recipient	Government
Employment benefits			
Gross earnings	−954	−954	0
Employment costs			
Taxes	0	+250	−250
Recipience			
Cash assistance	0	−2	+2
Food stamps	0	+124	−124
Medicaid	0	−83	+83
Support and service costs			
FDP administrative costs	+1	0	+1
IM/FS administrative costs	−52	0	−52
Case management	+11	0	+11
Child care			
Referral services	+2	0	+2
Payments	−100	0	−100
Transportation/work-related	−1	0	−1
Education/training	+51	0	+51
NET GAIN (or LOSS) Per Case	−1,042	−665	−377

New Applicants (Dollars Per Case)			
Benefit-Cost Component	Society	AFDC Recipient	Government
Employment benefits			
Gross earnings	−1,318	−1,318	0
Employment costs			
Taxes	0	+399	−399
Recipience			
Cash assistance	0	+468	−468
Food stamps	0	+391	−391
Medicaid	0	+528	−528
Support and service costs			
FDP administrative costs	−4	0	−4
IM/FS administrative costs	−164	0	−164
Case management	−15	0	−15
Child care			
Referral services	−3	0	−3
Payments	+4	0	+4
Transportation/work-related	−24	0	−24
Education/Training	−76	0	−76
NET GAIN (or LOSS) Per Case	−1,600	+468	−2,068

[a] No significance tests are available.

TABLE 17.2 FDP Net Impact, Present Discounted Value (1993 Dollars)

	Discount Rate		
	4%	6%	10%
All counties	−$941	−$914	−$867
New applicants	−$1,367	−$1,306	−$1,198

jects and the higher costs of providing support and services to this group.

The cost-benefit results presented here were aggregated over the 4-year evaluation period by simply summing our annual results. No adjustments were made for the impact of inflation or for the unequal distribution of costs and benefits over time.

FDP net impacts are deflated using regional consumer price indices for urban consumers produced by the U.S. Department of Labor.[11] Furthermore, we account for the time rate of preference by summing discounted estimates for 1993, 1994, 1995, and 1996. Given the uncertainty regarding the appropriate choice of discount rate, we provide discounted estimates of FDP impacts using three possible rates: 4%, 6%, and 10%.

Table 17.2 summarizes our findings regarding the net monetary impact of the FDP for longer term welfare recipients and new AFDC applicants, respectively.

DISCUSSION

The FDP did not result in any net gains overall compared with the alternative welfare program as experienced by the control group. In fact, our results indicate that the additional costs associated with the FDP exceeded the additional (measurable) benefits of this program. However, our 4-year observation period may be too short to assess possible favorable longer term FDP impacts on employment, earnings, and recipience especially for those in the experimental group who participated primarily in educational or human capital investment activities. It is also possible that the results were affected by some contamination of the control group subjects, although our analyses of the contamination

through both actual delivery of treatment and misperception by recipients of treatment group status indicates this is unlikely (Camasso et al., 2003).

Cost-benefit analysis, in its practical form, falls short of theoretical perfection in a number of areas. First of all, it has little to say about the formulation of policy ends; it is best applied after ends have been completely thought through (Richardson, 2002). Even as a tool to compare various means to an end, cost-benefit analysis may prove wanting. In practice, analysts may not be able to identify all the gains and losses associated with a given program or policy initiative. They may be unable to attach a monetary value to all identified costs and benefits. Limitations in available data, as well as deviations between conceptual measures and their operational counterparts, contribute to errors in measuring both costs and benefits. So why bother with cost-benefit analysis?

The advantage offered by cost-benefit analysis is a structured, systematic framework to cataloging, valuing, and comparing all the economic effects, both positive and negative, associated with the implementation of a specific program or policy. To the extent possible, cost-benefit analysis should lay out and quantify all relevant cost and benefits, as well as offer some assessment of those costs and benefits that cannot be assigned a monetary value. The distributional consequences of the program under analysis should be explicitly recognized and documented.

CONCLUSION

Economic efficiency may not be the only criterion to use in determining whether a particular program or policy should be implemented or continued. A particular policy or program may not produce positive net gains overall but may have a strong and socially desirable impact on specific groups within the general population. The outcome of a cost-benefit analysis, with its focus on economic efficiency, is but one piece of information to be used in policy evaluation. Nonetheless, cost-benefit analysis is an increasingly important element in today's social work practice and policy environment and should be an integral component in every human services and health care organization that must account for both resource inputs and client outcomes.

Notes

1. In more technical terms, cost-benefit analysis utilizes the criteria of potential Pareto superiority as a decision rule. A reallocation of resources is Pareto superior if it expands consumption possibilities (and thus improves well-being) for an individual or group. A program or policy is potentially Pareto superior if both consumption gains and losses are realized, but if those who gain from the activity could potentially provide adequate compensation to the losers for their loss and still retain an overall net gain in well-being.

2. This assumes that the value of the loss experienced by one party is equivalent to the value of the gain experienced by another party. We will have more to say about measuring these distributional impacts later.

3. There are other measures of willingness to pay, as well. This concept of willingness to pay also carries over into the realm of costs. The value of some loss in well-being associated with a given outcome is the payment that must be made to return the affected individual(s) to their original level of well-being. A complete discussion of the theoretical foundations that underlie welfare measurement on both the cost and benefit sides is provided by Milberg (1988).

4. Although wages and other market-determined input prices are usually taken as indicative of their social value, imperfections in labor and resource markets may cause market-determined input prices to diverge from their social value. This may occur, for example, in resource markets where buyers or sellers exercise undue influence on market prices. When no organized market exists for a particular resource, economic theory calls for the use of shadow prices, which measure the value of the change in some specified performance index induced by the use (or loss) of an incremental unit of that input. In practice, however, these shadow prices are usually difficult to calculate.

5. The debate over whether or not the distributional effects of a given program or policy lie outside the realm of cost-benefit analysis altogether has a long history. Mishan (1971) flatly rejects the notion that cost-benefit analysts should inject social norms into their analysis. Another objection is raised by Harberger (1971), who maintains that cost-benefits analysts do not have the expertise to make these types of judgments. Others disagree, and there have been attempts to develop methods of weighting gains and losses to take explicit account of the value of distributional effects. Hettich (1976) maintains that cost-benefit analysis must take explicit account of distributional impacts. Failure to do so is tantamount to assuming that the increase in well-being that an additional dollar of income brings to one party is equivalent to the loss in well-being brought about the loss of a dollar by another party. Hettich acknowledges that there is no simple way to value the distributional consequences

of policy gains and losses, but he does review attempts by others to do so.

6. Note that a real interest rate excludes the effect of expected future price inflation.

7. This directive regarding the mandated discount rate for federal projects dates back to 1992 (Office of Management and Budget, 1992).

8. REACH/JOBS did not have a family cap provision. Other REACH/JOBS program elements that were modified under FDP included a 1-year transitional medical benefit (FDP extended this benefit for 2 years), higher financial penalties for marriage (FDP reduced these financial disincentives), and a requirement that women with children aged 3 or under participate in the JOBS program (FDP required participation for women with children aged 2 or under). FDP made sanctions for noncompliance with the JOBS program less stringent but more easily implemented, compared with REACH/JOBS.

9. The New Jersey Wage Reporting System is an administrative database maintained by the New Jersey Department of Labor. This database includes wages and other information collected from employers for those employees who are covered by the Federal Unemployment Tax Act and subsequent legislation, and who may be eligible to receive unemployment benefits.

10. We also could not identify those evaluation subjects who were working in another state.

11. See U.S. Department of Labor, Bureau of Labor Statistics, *CPI Detailed Report* (various issues).

References

Cain, G. G., & Stromsdorfer, E. W. (1968). An economic evaluation of government retraining programs in West Virginia." In Gerald G. Somers (Ed.), *Retraining the unemployed* (pp. 299–332). Madison, WI: University of Wisconsin Press.

Camasso, M. J., Harvey, C., & Jagannathan, R. (1998). *Cost-benefit analysis of New Jersey's Family Development Program.* Trenton, NJ: New Jersey Department of Human Services.

Camasso, M. J., Jagannathan, R., Harvey, C., & Killingsworth, M. (2003). The use of client surveys to gauge the threat of contamination in welfare reform experiments. *Journal of Policy Analysis and Management, 22,* 207–223.

Carnoy, M., & Marenbach, D. (1975). The return to schooling in the United States, 1939–69. *Journal of Human Resources, 10,* 312–331.

French, M. T. (2000). Economic evaluation of alcohol treatment services. *Evaluation and Program Planning, 23,* 27–39.

Garms, W. I. (1971). A benefit-cost analysis of the Upward Bound program. *Journal of Human Resources, 6,* 206–220.

Gold, M. R., Siegel, J. E., Russell, L. B., & Weinstein,

M. C. (1996). *Cost effectiveness in health and medicine*. New York: Oxford University Press.

Gordon, A. R., & Martin, T. J. (1999). *Cost-benefit analysis of Iowa's Family Investment Program: Two-year results*. Princeton, NJ: Mathematica Policy Research.

Grinnell, R. M. (1997). *Social work research and evaluation* (5th ed.). Itasca, IL: F. E. Peacock.

Gueron, J., & Pauly, E. (1991). *From welfare to work*. New York: Russell Sage Foundation.

Harberger, A. C. (1971). Three basic postulates for applied welfare economics: An interpretive essay. *Journal of Economic Literature, 9*, 785–797.

Hardin, E., & Borus, M. E. (1966). An economic evaluation of the Retraining Program in Michigan: Methodological problems of research. *Proceedings of the 1966 Social Statistics Section Meetings* (pp. 133–137). Washington, DC: American Statistical Association.

Hettich, W. (1976). Distribution in benefit-cost analysis: A review of theoretical issues. *Public Finance Quarterly, 4*, 123–150.

Jagannathan, R., & Camasso, M. J. (2002). Family cap and nonmarital fertility: The racial conditioning of policy effects. *Journal of Marriage and Family, 5*, 52–71.

Kemple, J. J., Friedlander, D., & Fellerath, V. (1995). *Florida's Project Independence: Benefits, costs, and two-year impacts of Florida's JOBS program*. New York: Manpower Demonstration Research Corporation.

Milberg, W. (1988). Welfare measurement for cost-benefit analysis. In M. Berkowitz (Ed.), *Measuring the efficiency of public programs: Costs and benefits in vocational rehabilitation* (pp. 28–45). Philadelphia: Temple University Press.

Mishan, E. J. (1971). *Cost-benefit analysis*. London: Allen and Unwin.

Office of Management and Budget (1992). *Discount rates to be used in evaluating time-distributed costs and benefits* (Circular A-94, revised). Washington, DC: U.S. Government Printing Office.

Poister, T. H., McDavid, J. C., & Magoun, A. H. (1979). *Applied program evaluation in local government*. Lexington, MA: Lexington Books.

Posavac, E. J., & Carey, R. (1997). *Program evaluation: Methods and case studies* (5th ed.). New York: Prentice Hall.

Riccio, J., Friedlander, D., & Freedman, S. (1994). *GAIN: Benefits, costs and three-year impacts of a welfare-to-work program*. New York: Manpower Demonstration Research Corporation.

Richardson, H. S. (2002). *Democratic autonomy: Public reasoning about the ends of policy*. New York: Oxford University Press.

Rossi, P. H., Freeman, H. E., & Lipsey, M. W. (1999). *Evaluation: A systematic approach* (6th ed.). Thousand Oaks, CA: Sage.

Royse, D., & Thayer, B. A. (1996). *Program evaluation* (2nd ed.). Chicago: Nelson-Hall.

Thompson, M. S. (1980). *Benefit-cost analysis for program evaluation*. Thousand Oaks, CA: Sage.

Unrau, Y. A., Gabor, P. A., & Grinnell, R. M. (2001). *Evaluation in the human services*. Itasca, IL: F. E. Peacock.

U.S. Department of Labor, Bureau of Labor Statistics (various years). *CPI Detailed Report*. Washington, DC: U.S. Government Printing Office.

Yates, B. T. (1996). *Analyzing costs, procedures, processes and outcomes in human services*. Thousand Oaks, CA: Sage.

Yegidis, B. L., & Weinbach, R. W. (2002). *Research methods for social workers* (4th ed.). Boston: Allyn and Bacon.

SECTION III

Evidence-Based Practice: Diagnosis, Interventions, and Outcome Research

18

CONCISE STANDARDS FOR DEVELOPING EVIDENCE-BASED PRACTICE GUIDELINES

Enola K. Proctor & Aaron Rosen

The central challenge now confronting the profession of social work is ensuring and demonstrating that its services are effective. In our view, agencies and individual practitioners can best enhance their effectiveness by using treatment approaches that are evidence-based. Practicing on the basis of scientifically tested evidence is responsible, consistent with social work's values and commitment to client welfare and improvement, and responsive to societal expectations and National Association of Social Workers (NASW) aspirations for effective and accountable practice. Yet we recognize the many challenges inherent in the application of evidence-based approaches in day-to-day practice. Our chapter addresses some of those challenges and lays out steps through which practitioners' ability to apply evidence-based practice can be enhanced.

MEANING OF EVIDENCE-BASED PRACTICE

Evidence-based practice (EBP) has been described in terms of a number of attributes. Most simply, it is the use of treatments for which there is sufficiently persuasive evidence to support their effectiveness in attaining the desired outcomes (Rosen & Proctor, 2002). Consistent with but not exhaustive of definitions by others (Gam-

brill, 1999; Gonzales, Ringeisen, & Chambers, 2002), we emphasize here three attributes of evidence-based practice: (a) Empirical, research-based support for the effectiveness of interventions is the most persuasive evidence for practice decisions (Rosen, 2002); (b) empirically supported interventions must be critically assessed for their fit to and appropriateness for the practice situation at hand and must be supplemented or modified according to the practitioner's experience and knowledge; and (c) practice should be regularly monitored, and revisions to the course of treatment should be based on a recursive process of outcome evaluation (Proctor & Rosen, in press; Rosen, 2002).

BACKGROUND AND CONTEXT

Evidence-based practice originated as evidence-based medicine (EBM) and subsequently influenced clinical psychology and social work as EBP. Within social work, EBP was first and more widely embraced in Great Britain. Although practitioners have long been urged to apply research in their day-to-day practice and to use approaches with demonstrated effectiveness, the work of Eileen Gambrill (e.g., 1999) could be credited with advancing the concept of EBP in social work in the United States. Evidence-based practice is lodged within broader, long-standing premises about social work practice. First, EBP is consistent with the expectations that practitioners need to identify, explicate, and provide a persuasive rationale for their practice decisions. In evidence-based practice, those decisions must be based, to the fullest extent possible, on the best available and most appropriate research evidence. While managed care accelerated practitioners' need to describe and justify their treatment plans, practitioners have long been encouraged to systematize their treatment plans and provide a rationale for their decisions (Rosen, Proctor, & Livne, 1985; Rosen, Proctor, Morrow-Howell, & Staudt, 1995).

Evidence-based practice is also consistent with a long-standing emphasis within social work on testing and demonstrating practice effectiveness. Research on effective social work practices has grown markedly (Reid & Fortune, in press), increasing the supply of evidence-based practices for practitioners' selection and use (cf. Thyer & Wodarski, 1998). Another recent trend supporting the application of EBP is the increased use of treatment manuals (Fraser, in press). Treatment manuals detail the interventions that have been found to be effective in research studies. Their clear and detailed descriptions of the relevant worker actions and behavior facilitate the application of EBP.

Evidence-based practice is further lodged within an assumption that social work practice should be focused on outcomes and its success evaluated in terms of actually attaining the desired outcomes (Rosen & Proctor, 1978, 1981). As such, it is important that the research upon which practice is based clearly demonstrates the linkages between interventions and the outcomes toward which they are directed (Rosen & Proctor, 2002). Finally, EBP is consistent with the movement to develop and make available guidelines for practice or constellations of practice approaches that, based on current evidence, are deemed to be most effective in addressing certain problems or attaining certain targeted outcomes.

Although practitioners have long been exhorted to use the findings of research, proponents of evidence-based social work practice have grown in number and strength. A fundamental challenge for EBP is practitioners' acceptance of pretested, standardized, empirically supported treatments (ESTs) as a legitimate foundation for practice. This chapter identifies and addresses the steps necessary to identify, select, and apply in day-to-day practice those interventions that have a base of empirical support.

STRATEGIES FOR IMPLEMENTING EVIDENCE-BASED PRACTICE

Although our chapter focuses on the selection, modification, and application of interventions, the treatment process begins with assessment. Vandiver (2002) describes a process for applying practice guidelines, commencing with assessment, making a diagnosis, identifying problems, and deciding the goals or targets of change, which we refer to as treatment outcomes (Proctor & Rosen, in press; Rosen & Proctor, 2002). The reader is encouraged to refer to Vandiver's (2002) discussion, for our strategies commence at the point in the treatment process where assessment, diagnosis, and problem formulation have resulted in designating the desired ultimate and intermediate outcomes to be pursued through intervention. It is important to underscore the point that practice should focus on outcome. The purpose of intervention is to achieve desired outcomes, and interventions should be selected for their potential to attain the outcomes.

Once problem assessment and formulation of desired outcomes are accomplished, the use of empirically tested knowledge necessitates four types of actions: (a) identify potential empirically supported treatments (ESTs) that are relevant to the outcomes to be pursued; (b) select the best-fitting intervention (EST) in view of the client problems, situation, and outcome; (c) supplement and modify the EST as needed, drawing on practitioner experience and knowledge; and (d) monitor and evaluate intervention effectiveness.

Step 1:   Locate evidence-based interventions relevant to the outcomes for pursuit.

The first challenge in implementing EBP is identifying and obtaining information about interventions that have been empirically tested and supported. In the search for EBPs, practitioners should use as their point of departure the outcomes they are striving to achieve with and for a given client. For example, when working to achieve an outcome "to increase client's skills of conflict resolution," the practitioner should search for interventions for which there is research evidence as to their effectiveness in attaining this outcome. The practitioner should seek to identify not just one intervention but rather a repertoire or set of alternative interventions that have solid empirical support for attaining the outcome.

Identifying relevant evidence-based interventions is made challenging by the fact that much of the practice literature is written and organized around problems addressed, not necessarily outcomes sought. That is, while research may report on interventions for the client's relevant population, presenting problem(s), or both, the practitioner must look closely to ascertain that effectiveness was assessed in terms of the outcomes that are actually being pursued.

Where can such evidence be found? First, and in our view ideally, practice guidelines can be a valuable source of empirically supported interventions (Proctor & Rosen, in press). Various practice, professional, and public health organizations have approved and published guidelines and treatment recommendations for a variety of problems and outcomes. Guidelines have a number of advantages: They are well focused around particular practice issues, are oriented to practitioners, may refer to specific client populations or practice conditions, and are worded specifically enough to offer practitioners clear guidance and direction as to the steps to be taken in treatment. To the extent that guidelines are based on empirical research, they offer the considerable advantage of having already been subjected to extensive guideline-development processes that weighed and compared evidence and selected the most effective approaches. Guidelines thereby ease this burden for practitioners. However, at present, three factors may serve to limit the usefulness of some guidelines for social workers. First, some extant guidelines may not be based on empirical support but instead on a consensual process that integrates and summarizes accumulated practice wisdom and expertise in a particular area. To the extent that they are not based on research, their use may not advance evidence-based practice. Second, as noted previously with regard to research studies, some guidelines are not outcome focused but rather address diagnostic categories, probably leaving unclear the specific outcome for which the intervention can be appropriately used. Third, some medicine- and psychiatry-oriented guidelines may emphasize pharmacological treatment.

However, guidelines increasingly contain interventions relevant to social work, including psychosocial, behavioral, and family system interventions. Proctor and Rosen (in press) present a model of practice guidelines for social work and the organizational, professional, and research efforts needed to foster their development. Examples of research-based guidelines with high relevance to social work practice can be found at a number of Internet Web sites. The National Guideline Clearinghouse at http://www.guidelines.gov lists practice guidelines, organized by problem/disorder or treatment/intervention. This site lists 46 psychotherapy guidelines, such as for the treatment of school-age children with attention-deficit/hyperactivity disorder, depression treatment, and treatment of sexual dysfunction. The American Psychological Association Web site also provides recommendations and information about empirically supported treatments (ESTs) (http://www.apa.org/divisions/div12/rev_est/), including for anxiety disorder, posttraumatic stress disorder, obsessive-compulsive disorder, and stressful events. Finally, the National Institute of Drug Abuse's (NIDA) Web site provides EBP recommendations for treating a variety of addictions (http://www.drugabuse.gov/TXManuals/).

Systematic critical reviews of intervention studies in a given area are a second valuable source of empirically supported interventions. For the practitioner, critical reviews have several advantages: The relevant research literature has been carefully canvassed, the goodness of the evidence has already been assessed systematically and carefully, and the findings are succinctly summarized. However, as with practice guidelines, practitioners must carefully ascertain the fit between the outcomes they target for pursuit and the outcomes evaluated in the research studies. Systematic reviews of research supporting interventions are widely published in psychology, and their number is growing in social work. The Campbell Collaboration provides an umbrella for the conduct of systematic reviews of research in the areas of criminal justice, education, and social welfare, and it summarizes the information in a relatively consumable form (http://www.campbellcollaboration.org/Fralibrary.html). Critical reviews are currently being prepared on such topics as the impact of welfare reform on family structure, cognitive and behavioral interventions for sexually abused children, psychosocial interventions for adolescents with anorexia nervosa, and group-based parent training programs.

Journal articles reporting the results of studies testing the effectiveness of interventions are a third source of evidence-based practices. For practitioners needing guidance about how to treat a particular case, the tasks of locating relevant studies and evaluating their scientific merit and validity may be very challenging. However, agencies and individual practitioners engaged in highly specialized areas of practice, with routine access to research-based journals and time to read them, might avail themselves of knowledge about interventions with a high degree of research support, even before that knowledge is included in systematic reviews and practice guidelines. The Program on Assertive Community Treatment (PACT model) is an example of an intervention program whose effectiveness has been supported in a number of research studies. Indeed, PACT's solid base of evidence has earned it the endorsement of the National Association for the Mentally Ill (NAMI) as the treatment of choice.

Textbooks and edited volumes containing chapters about practice are a fourth source of evidence-based practices. Many such books are based on and also provide detail about the extent of empirical support. For example, Thyer and Wodarski (1998) have published a two-volume book organizing evidence-based interventions around various social problems and psychiatric diagnoses. Reid and Fortune (in press) overview the extent of support for 130 social work intervention programs that were studied in the decade of the 1990s. And in the area of marriage and family therapy, a recent book compiles empirically supported interventions for the problems frequently addressed by family therapists (Sprenkle, 2002).

Practitioners can increasingly find treatment manuals that detail and behaviorally specify interventions and their components, formulated on the basis of a systematic program of research and testing. Treatment manuals facilitate implementation and consistent application across clients and practitioners. The National Association of Social Workers (NASW) Press has begun publishing manuals and handbooks that provide specific guidance on practice strategies. The first such manual addresses social problem-solving skills for use with children (Fraser, Nash, Galinsky, & Darwin, 2000). To the extent that these manuals are evidence-based, they provide an excellent tool by which practitioners can select and use empirically tested interventions. The National Institute of Drug Abuse Web site (http://www.drugabuse.gov/TXManuals/) provides manuals for a variety of evidence-based interventions in the area of addictions.

Individual practitioners and social work agencies can facilitate the evidence-based practices with some preparation and resource gathering. It is advantageous to develop an in-house collection or compilation of empirically supported interventions for the outcomes most frequently pursued in their settings. Handbooks, research journals, and computers with "bookmarks" to Internet sites containing relevant guidelines or manuals can enhance practitioners' access to ESTs relevant to their practice.

Step 2: Select the best fitting intervention in view of the particular client problems, situation, and outcomes.

Even when well specified in treatment manuals, interventions studied and found effective through research remain generalized formulations that have been tested with samples of clients. The practitioner's own client is not likely to share with the clients in the research samples all the characteristics that are relevant to the effective intervention. Hence, having a solid foundation of empirical support does not guarantee that a given intervention will meet the needs of a particular client. Thus, after identifying an array of alternative interventions with empirical support, the practitioner must select from that array the intervention most appropriate to the client and practice task at hand. The second step in evidence-based practice, then, is to select the best fitting intervention from a repertoire of interventions with a solid evidence base. This task requires the practitioner to critically assess the fit between each of the alternative (evidence-based) interventions, on the one hand, and the client's needs and goals on the other hand.

Using assessment skills and critical thinking, the practitioner must bring to the task of selecting the most appropriate intervention from within an array familiarity with the client and circumstances; appreciation of the problem's duration, severity, and co-occurring conditions; knowledge of resources available for implementing the intervention; appreciation of client strengths and preferences; and knowledge of the circumstances that will bear on the implementation of the intervention. Client personal qualities and context, culture, preferences for process, and the service environment and its culture must all be assessed and understood. All that knowledge and understanding is then juxtaposed against the characteristics of the samples and circumstances of the research through which the interventions were supported, and then the practitioner must gauge their similarity to the client and practice context at hand. This assessment and comparison process should enable the practitioner to select from among the alternative interventions the evidence-based intervention that is most appropriate for the task at hand.

Step 3: Supplement and modify the most appropriate and best supported treatments, drawing on practitioner experience and knowledge.

Even with a careful assessment of intervention appropriateness, it is unrealistic to expect a perfect fit between an empirically supported, standardized intervention and the needs of a particular client. If the practitioner doubts the goodness of fit of an evidence-based treatment to the needs of the client and situation at hand, a third critical step in EBP is supplementing or modifying the chosen intervention. That is, the best research-based knowledge must be applied in relation to the particular client and be attuned to "local knowledge" (Stricker & Trierweiler, 1995), knowledge of the agency and community setting, prior experience, and theory. Although sometimes given short shrift, local knowledge is an important complement to research-based knowledge.

When the selected empirically based interventions require adaptation, the practitioner's task will involve modifying the intervention by supplementing or revising it in accordance with local knowledge to create a new "blended" or "composite" intervention. This task is likely to be facilitated by the degree of specification typical of empirically supported interventions; specification may be related to their components, recommended order, dosage, and intensity. This level of detail of ESTs would enable the practitioner to discern what elements need to be modified in relation to a particular practice situation. This process of adapting empirically supported treatments to the needs of particular clients and practice situations relies on practitioners' best judgment, as informed by their knowledge and practice experience.

The practitioner should carefully assess the similarity between the conditions under which the EST was tested and shown to be effective and the conditions characterizing the particular practice situation in which the EST is to be applied. Differences between these two sets of conditions do not necessarily preclude application of the EST, nor do they signal the necessity of modifying the EST in order to apply it. Among the differences between the conditions that might signal a need for modifying the standardized, evidence-based interventions are that (a) the client's problem configuration, personal characteristics, or situation differs from the samples that were studied in testing the ESTs; (b) the specific outcomes pursued with the client, while within the same general category, differ somewhat from the outcomes that were tested (for example, the empirically supported treatment was tested in relation to enhancing assertiveness with colleagues at work, whereas the practitioner is working toward enhancing the client's assertiveness with a spouse); and (c) the EST was tested in a different practice setting or with different types of practitioners than those characterizing the practice situation at hand.

When the practice situation differs from the context in which the supporting research was conducted, the following elements in the EST may require modification: (a) intermediate outcomes may need to be added or omitted; (b) the frequency, intensity, or duration of the treatment inputs may need to be altered; (c) changes to the tasks given to clients, such as homework assignments, may be called for; and (d) because many manualized ESTs do not specify procedures for establishing and maintaining a facilitative helping relationship, the practitioner may need to supplement an EST with his or her own knowledge and skills in developing a good relationship with the client. The particular modification to be made depends, of course, on the practitioner's knowledge and the reasons for undertaking the modification.

Modification of established evidence-based treatments carries two risks. First, as practitioners are aware, there is the risk of overcommitting to standardized interventions, applying them "as is" without considering the issue of fit to the client. Doing so may be "taking the easy way out." Second, there is risk associated with changing empirically standardized treatments. Our encouragement to modify and revise ESTs should not be taken as a call to freely change the intervention. Rather, modifications must be careful and well reasoned, or the practitioner could not assume that the modified intervention would retain the effectiveness of the EST. Therefore, both adherence to and modification of evidence-based treatments should always be accompanied by ongoing evaluation, as we discuss later. However, it is critical to recognize that any modification of the original empirically supported intervention introduces substantial change that therefore may affect its effectiveness. Hence ongoing evaluation, as addressed in Step 4, is very important.

Step 4:   Monitor and evaluate the effectiveness of
          the intervention.

Fundamentally, evidence-based practice means that practice decisions should be made on the basis of the best evidence available. In this discussion, we have implicated two types of evidence. First is the evidence on the basis of which practitioners evaluate and select the appropriate intervention to use, as discussed previously. The second type of evidence is that for deciding whether the intervention implemented is having its predicted results, whether it should be further modified or abandoned, or whether treatment has reached its desired outcome. This type of evidence is contained in the feedback that has to be obtained from evaluation of treatment.

Evaluation is especially critical when empirically supported treatments have been modified. When some of the ingredients of the original intervention have been changed, the practitioner cannot assume that the modified intervention retains the effectiveness of the original EST. Accordingly, feedback from evaluation must be used to inform further modification and all other treatment decisions. Recognizing the importance of practicing on the basis of feedback from systematic evaluation, the Council on Social Work Education requires that professional social work education must include training in practice evaluation.

A number of sources provide good information pertaining to practice evaluation. Among them are Roberts and Green's *Social Workers' Desk Reference* (2002), particularly Part 13, and what is by now the classic textbook by Bloom, Fischer, and Orme (1999). Recognizing the limited scope of our discussion here, we underscore three points that are critical in evaluation. First, all the outcomes being pursued need to be defined operationally and assessed as specifically as possible by clinically meaningful indicators. Second, when available, clinically relevant standardized measures with acceptable reliability and validity should be used (cf. Fischer & Corcoran, 1994). Third, although some outcomes are categorical in nature (e.g., obtaining housing, avoiding pregnancy, finding employment), the attainment of many commonly pursued outcomes can be appropriately measured by continuous scales. Such measurement affords a more discriminating evaluation of change and enables assessment of outcome attainment over time—including comparisons of treatment with pretreatment status, assessment of progress during and maintenance of change after treatment, and other comparisons of interest. Constant monitoring and recursive evaluation and revision of treatment should lessen practitioner concern that EBPs may be insensitive to clients and their needs.

CONCLUSION

Increased research activity in social work is yielding a growing number of treatments that meet criteria of effectiveness and appropriateness, address a broader range of issues confronting practitioners, and have been tested in settings that serve more diverse and varied client groups. Concomitantly, considerable progress is evident in distilling research knowledge and packaging and communicating this information for better retrieval and application by practitioners. In this chapter, however, we focused mostly on practitioners and the challenges they face in attempting to apply evidence-based treatments to their individual clients. Undoubtedly, the successful application of EBPs will be greatly affected by the knowledge, skills, and critical judgment of the practitioner. A major factor that we have not addressed that should nonetheless be mentioned here is the auspices under which practice is conducted. As Mullen and Bacon (in press) have suggested, agency administrators and supervisors have a distinct and necessary role in creating an agency culture that encourages, supports, and lends legitimacy to practitioners' efforts to use EBP.

References

Bloom, M., Fischer, J., & Orme, J. G. (1999). *Evaluating practice: Guidelines for the accountable professional* (3rd ed.). Englewood Cliffs, NJ: Prentice Hall.
Fischer, J., & Corcoran, K. (1994). *Measures for clinical practice* (2nd ed.). New York: Free Press.

Fraser, M. W. (in press). Intervention research in social work: A basis for evidence-based practice and practice guidelines. In A. Rosen & E. K. Proctor (Eds.), *Developing practice guidelines for social work intervention: Issues, methods, and research agenda.* New York: Columbia University Press.

Fraser, M. W., Nash, J. K., Galinsky, M. J., & Darwin, K. M. (2000). *Making choices: Social problem-solving skills for children.* Washington, DC: National Association of Social Workers.

Gambrill, E. (1999). Evidence-based practice: An alternative to authority-based practice. *Families in Society, 80,* 234–259.

Gonzales, J. J., Ringeisen, H. L., & Chambers, D. A. (2002). The tangled and thorny path of science to practice: Tensions in interpreting and applying "evidence." *Clinical Psychology: Science & Practice, 9*(2), 204–209.

Mullen, E. J., & Bacon, W. F. (in press). Practitioner adoption and implementation of practice guidelines and issues of quality control. In A. Rosen & E. K. Proctor (Eds.), *Developing practice guidelines for social work intervention: Issues, methods, and research agenda.* New York: Columbia University Press.

Proctor, E. K., & Rosen, A. (in press). The structure and function of social work practice guidelines. In A. Rosen & E. K. Proctor (Eds.), *Developing practice guidelines for social work interventions: Issues, methods, and research agenda.* New York: Columbia University Press.

Reid, W. J., & Fortune, A. E. (in press). Empirical foundations for practice guidelines in current social work knowledge. In A. Rosen & E. K. Proctor (Eds.), *Developing practice guidelines for social work intervention: Issues, methods, and research agenda.* New York: Columbia University Press.

Roberts, A. R., & Green, G. J. (2002). *Social workers' desk reference.* New York: Oxford University Press.

Rosen, A. (2002). *Evidence-based social work practice: Challenges and promise.* Invited address at the Society for Social Work and Research, San Diego, CA.

Rosen, A., & Proctor, E. K. (1978). Specifying the treatment process: The basis for effectiveness research. *Journal of Social Service Research, 2*(1), 25–43.

Rosen, A., & Proctor, E. K. (1981). Distinctions between treatment outcomes and their implications for treatment evaluation. *Journal of Consulting and Clinical Psychology, 49,* 418–425.

Rosen, A., & Proctor, E. K. (2002). Standards for evidence-based social work practice: The role of replicable and appropriate interventions, outcomes, and practice guidelines. In A. R. Roberts & G. J. Greene (Eds.), *Social workers' desk reference* (pp. 743–747). New York: Oxford University Press.

Rosen, A., Proctor, E. K., & Livne, S. (1985). Planning and direct practice. *Social Service Review, 59,* 161–167.

Rosen, A., Proctor, E. K., Morrow-Howell, N., & Staudt, M. (1995). Rationale for practice decisions: Variations in knowledge use by decision task and social work service. *Research on Social Work Practice, 5,* 501–523.

Sprenkle, D. H. (2002). A therapeutic Hail Mary. In D. A. Baptiste (Ed.), *Clinical epiphanies in marital and family therapy: A practitioner's casebook of therapeutic insights, perceptions, and breakthroughs* (pp. 20–28). New York: Hawarth Press.

Stricker, G., & Trierweiler, S. J. (1995). The local clinical scientist: A bridge between science and practice. *American Psychologist, 50*(12), 995–1002.

Thyer, B. A., & Wodarski, J. S. (1998). First principles of empirical social work practice. In B. A. Thyer & J. S. Wodarski (Eds.), *Handbook of empirical social work practice* (pp. 1–21). New York: John Wiley & Sons.

Vandiver, V. L. (2002). Step-by-step practice guidelines for using evidence-based practice and expert consensus in mental health settings. In A. R. Robert & G. J. Greene (Eds.), *Social workers' desk reference* (p. 131). New York: Oxford University Press.

19

HEALTH CARE EVIDENCE-BASED PRACTICE

A Product of Political and Cultural Times

Sophia F. Dziegielewski & Albert R. Roberts

We firmly believe that practice accountability through quality assurance measures and operational improvement, utilization of outcome measures, systematic research, and evidence-based practice will become the dominant challenge for all health care and human service professionals in the current decade. "Increasingly federal, state, and foundation funding sources will demand proof of the effectiveness of specific service interventions" (Austin & Roberts, 2002, p. 826) in health care and human service agencies. We predict that there will be intense pressures on professionals in mental health and substance abuse treatment managed care programs to document and measure quality of service, program, and client outcomes. Effectiveness and outcome data will come from rapid assessment measures, case observations, case records, and multiple methodologically rigorous, randomized clinical research trials in different settings (see Chapters 1, 2, 3, 18, 20, 21, 23, 24, and the chapters by Corcoran and Streiner).

In the area of health care practice, managed behavioral health care, first introduced in the early 1990s, presents a type of health care delivery never before experienced. As the chapters in this book reinforce, health care professionals are expected to show that the services provided are both short term and evidence-based. If this stance is not adopted, health care professionals will be replaced with other professionals who do adopt this stance. In current health care practice, it is crucial to realize that effectiveness must go beyond just helping the client (Dziegielewski & Holliman, 2001). For evidence-based practice to occur, it must also involve validation that the

greatest concrete and identifiable therapeutic gain was achieved, in the quickest amount of time, and with the least amount of financial and professional support. This means that not only must the interventions that professional practitioners provide be socially acknowledged as necessary but also they must be therapeutically effective (Franklin, 2002), specific, and individualized to guide all further intervention efforts (Maruish, 2002). In addition, these services must be professionally competitive with other disciplines that claim similar treatment strategies and techniques. This has led to the rebirth of all efforts for client betterment to be evidence-based in order to be acknowledged as effective (Donald, 2002).

EVOLUTION OF EVIDENCE-BASED PRACTICE

Health care practice has changed dramatically over the years. In addition, the clarity of a definition of what the health care professionals do has been further complicated by basic changes in the health care environment that include scope of practice, the roles served, and the expectations within the client–practitioner relationship. Furthermore, this definition, along with the focus of care, is shifting (Dziegielewski, 2002). Health care practice is changing from a focus on "inpatient acute, tertiary, and specialty/subspecialty care, to ambulatory and community-based care, and to physician's offices, group practices and health maintenance organizations" (Rock, 2002, p. 13). This focus-shifting environment requires that health care practitioners constantly battle "quality-of-care" issues versus "cost-containment" measures, while securing a firm place as a professional provider in the health care environment. Barry Rock (2002) aptly recommends an evidence-based agenda for social workers under the primary care and managed health care environment:

1. Develop job descriptions and skill/knowledge/task inventory for primary care–based social work practice.
2. Develop refined, concise high-risk screening instruments for biopsychosocial assessment, treatment, and outcome measurement.
3. Create treatment protocols—much in demand by managed health and managed behavioral health organizations—linking psychosocial and medical comorbidities, such as diabetes with depression and hypertension with anxiety, in systematic treatment guidelines.
4. Establish psychosocial and medical outcome linkages.
5. Further refine screening tools, assessment instruments, and high-risk indicators appropriate for value-added psychosocial intervention. (Rock, 2002, p. 13)

Today, the health care worker has become essential as the professional "bridge" that links the client, the multidisciplinary or interdisciplinary team, and the environment. For future marketability and competition, it is believed that all health care professionals will need to move beyond the traditional definition and subsequent roles occupied in the past (Dziegielewski, 2002). In the area of clinical practice and as emphasized in each section of this book, new or refined methods of service delivery need to be established and used. By joining the researcher and the practitioner together, the models of evidence-based practice described in this book become manageable.

BECOMING MARKETABLE IN UNCERTAIN TIMES

Many events over the last 15 years have truly transformed health care delivery and the professional expectations of health care workers. For survival in this environment, Dziegielewski (2002) suggests several steps: (a) All health care professionals need to continue to market the services they provide and link them to cost–benefit measurement; (b) all practitioners need to present themselves as essential team members on the health care interdisciplinary and multidisciplinary teams; (c) all health care workers should never forget the importance of anticipating the environment and the role that political and social influences can have on service delivery; and (d) all health care professionals need to adopt a researcher–practitioner stance that looks beyond traditional expectations and assumptions historically noted as clinical professional practice.

This requires all methods of service delivery to incorporate new and innovative ideas and methods that allow for rethinking foundation issues in terms of human growth and development (Farley, Smith, Boyle, & Ronnau, 2002), while applying these concepts in an evidence-based framework (Wodarski & Dziegielewski, 2001). In evidence-based practice, new and revitalized models to guide practice are needed to remain competitive in today's health care environment. Therefore, health care remains a changing environment that requires resilient professionals willing to ebb and flow with the changes.

ROLES AND STANDARDS FOR ALL HEALTH CARE PRACTITIONERS

All health care workers, whether in the role of clinical practitioner, supervisor, administrator, or advocate, have been challenged to anticipate our current health care system. Incremental changes involve compromising and implementing service agreements that are based on the needs and wishes of various political forces. For all health care workers, evidence-based practice must entail some degree of controlling the rising health care costs, whether they have the ultimate power to control this trend or not.

Responsibility for high-quality service delivery in this cost-containment climate has placed greater emphasis on macropractice. This means that health care workers must take an active role in ethical practice while advocating for social action and social change (Strom-Gottfried & Dunlap, 1999). For evidence-based practice to be effective, there must also be advocacy that seeks to help society understand, while controlling and regulating the health care industry. Therefore, regardless of the health care setting, all health care workers must help to develop and present a format for approaching problems in the current system and establishing means for addressing them.

CONCEPTS ESSENTIAL TO CLINICAL PRACTICE

In health care, the behaviorally based biopsychosocial approach continues to be the model of choice to integrate the biomedical and the psychosocial approaches to practice. In this approach, health care professionals such as social workers are considered leaders regarding understanding and interpreting the "behavioral," "psycho," and "social" factors in a client's condition. Teamwork and collaborative efforts are now required in health care service delivery (Abramson, 2002). Practicing professionals on interdisciplinary teams not uncommonly encounter blurred definitions and diffused boundary distinctions (Dziegielewski, 1996). This does not have to be viewed as problematic. Abramson (2002) identifies and discusses the typology of physician–social worker teams that she developed with Terry Mizrahi in 1994. Typologies provide useful frameworks for comparing professional roles of different professions, allocation of control over decision making, opening up of active communication patterns, facilitating a clinical focus and shared responsibility for patient care, and utilizing information from the team meetings (Abramson, 2002). To creative practitioners, it can be viewed as a way to expand roles and services as part of the team. To exemplify this concept, health care practitioners are encouraged to become leading professionals in the quality review process. It is also recommended that efforts toward solid evidence-based practice must highlight the issues related to informed consent that stipulate that health care providers reveal to clients the nature of the medical treatments as well as potential risks and benefits. Practice-based research with solid research designs should be strongly encouraged in order to study the impact of health care teams on patient outcomes (Abramson, 2002). Evidence-based practice can guide this process, while ensuring that high-quality care services are provided.

PRINCIPLES FOR EVIDENCE-BASED PRACTICE

Prior to the publication of this book, there were no specific guidelines that were entirely comprehensive and inclusive of the different health care disciplines. For the first time, this inclusive desk reference addresses the formulation and execution of evidence-based practice, the different levels of evidence-based practice, quantitative and qualitative practice research exemplars, and empirically based guidelines that have recently been developed. For an understanding of the components, definitions, and step-by-step methods of evidence-based practice, see Chapters 1, 2, and 3 in this book. To learn more about informatics and Internet technology in the dissemination of evidence-based practice guidelines, see Chapter 4. To see specific guidelines and applications of these principles, the reader is referred to the chapters in Part 3, especially Chapters 18, 20, 22, 24, 25, 27, 28, 31, 33, 34, and 35.

It is crucial to remember that when creating these guidelines all the resulting practice principles must include three primary sources: (a) information from the client, (b) information from informed sources of practice, and (c) information based on the latest available research. This will require constant evaluation and reevaluation for practical and scientific rigor, as well as sensitivity to the needs of the individual client being served.

For the researcher–practitioner developing these principles and guidelines, the Centre for Health Evidence (2003) suggests considering the following questions:

Were all important options and outcomes clearly identified?
Was an explicit and sensible process used to identify, select, and combine evidence?
Was an explicit and sensible process used to consider the different outcomes?
Is the guideline likely to account for recent developments?
Has the guideline been subjected to peer review and testing?

Furthermore, according to the Centre for Health Evidence (2003), in examining the results the following questions should always be considered:

Can practical, clinically important recommendations be made on the information that was gathered?

How strong are the recommendations that are being made?

What is the impact or the uncertainty associated with the evidence gathered from the use of these guidelines?

In addition, these authors suggest that the following questions be added to ensure that a comprehensive and client-centered approach is conducted.

Does the particular problem being addressed by the client seem to be best addressed by the standardized protocol developed?

If not, what needs to be added to assist the client in terms of self-empowerment, thereby maximizing self-determination?

CHANGING THE HEALTH CARE ENVIRONMENT: DOCUMENTATION, QUALITY ASSURANCE, AND EVIDENCE-BASED PRACTICE

For the worker in health care practice, the process of recording needs to go beyond the traditional bounds of documentation. Documentation to support and justify evidence-based practice is pivotal. Systematically coordinating research and practice yields the type of record keeping employed in the medical setting to facilitate quality assurance (see Chapters 96, 98, 99, and 103 in Section X of this volume). This mix should consider the need to achieve both high-quality service and cost-effectiveness. Although this union may, at times, be an awkward one, the combination is essential to ensure delivery of efficient and effective services.

The health care environment is changing rapidly, and with the tremendous increase in allied health professionals (Flood, Shortell, & Scott, 1994), it is thought that only the strongest will survive. Not only is this survival important for the professions of health care social work, nursing, and medicine but also it is essential for the clients who are served. Each day and with every task the health care specialist completes, the client's lifestyle and expectations are influenced. Health care professionals help to make their cli-

ents better able to relate to their environments. To continue to adequately address the client–environment match in the health care setting, there is no choice—practice and research must be one. When practice and research combine, evidence-based practice results (Dziegielewski, 2002; Wodarski & Dziegielewski, 2001). It is this type of evidence-based practice that will be best suited to withstand the rigor and instability of the managed care practice environment in which the health care professional must survive.

Today, the concept of behaviorally based managed care services is creating a whole new practice revolution, in which the provision of research-based practice leading to evidence-based interventions is germane (Bolter, Levenson, & Alverez, 1990; Dziegielewski, 1997). For a strategic practice approach, attention might best be placed on intermittent or crisis-oriented treatment as a form of brief intervention in which each session stands alone and is conducted as if it is the only client contact that will occur (Dziegielewski, 2002; Roberts, 2000). Crisis intervention, health maintenance organizations, and employee assistance programs generally favor highly structured brief forms of intervention, and as they continue to proliferate, so will use of the time-limited models they support (Roberts, 2000; Wells, 1994). To take this a step further, it is suggested that health care practitioners will need to continue to learn and use psychosocial education in achieving behavioral outcomes.

Furthermore, the goal for insight-oriented intervention and cure-focused therapy seems to have given way to the acquisition of outcomes-based behavioral change that is considered more realistic and practical (Dziegielewski, 2002). This becomes evident since most health care providers (similar to physicians) generally do not cure the problems clients suffer from. What is expected, however, is to help clients realize and use their own strengths to diminish or alleviate symptoms or states of being that cause discomfort or dysfunctional patterns. Emphasis on evidence-based practice and outcomes-based behavioral changes should be not only expected but also mandated for state-of-the-art practice.

The need for time-limited practice strategies has been clearly established, and the models and methods of service delivery, such as those presented throughout this book, only begin to open the door on evidence-based practice and what is yet to come. Practice environments crisp with managed health care policies, capitation, and so on will continue. Evidence-based practice must demonstrate effectiveness and cost containment (Gibelman, 2002). It is important for all health care practitioners to realize, whether they like it or not, that professional survival dictates change. In general, no matter what the setting, the health care worker needs to embrace a more eclectic approach to practice—in which allegiance to one particular model or method is discouraged (Colby & Dziegielewski, 2001). In closing, (a) evidence-based practice approaches need to include a time-limited intervention approach; (b) such approaches must always stress mutually negotiated goals and objectives; (c) all practice should include efforts to make it evidence-based, and objectives should be behaviorally linked, outcomes-based, and measurable; (d) there should always be an emphasis on client strengths and self-development; (e) the focus of intervention should always be concrete, realistic, and obtainable; and (f) it should be changeable, based on the needs and desires of the client being served—not the preference of the practitioner (Dziegielewski, 2002).

CONCLUSION

Rapid change in health care delivery is well under way. Now physicians, nurses, and social workers must decide whether we want to take an active part in the controversial and adversarial evidence-based practice debate or whether we just want to sit at the "gate" and make sure the other business managers or hospital administrators get through and become the ultimate patient care decision makers. If we decide that the role of the health care specialist is essential to the delivery of competent, effective, and efficient health care services, we will have to strongly advocate for it. By building coalitions and strong advocacy efforts, we believe that we will benefit our clients and ourselves as a profession. If we decide not to advocate for ourselves and assume a position of hesitance and apathy for too long, the importance and strength of the evidence-based physician or social worker as a crucial member of the health care delivery team will go untold, and more assertive professions will be free to claim what once was our turf.

References

Abramson, J. S. (2002). Interdisciplinary team practice. In A. R. Roberts & G. J. Greene (Eds.), *Social workers' desk reference* (pp. 44–50). New York: Oxford University Press.

Austin, D. M., & Roberts, A. R. (2002). Clinical social work research in the 21st century: Future, present, and past. In A. R. Roberts & G. J. Greene (Eds.), *Social workers' desk reference* (pp. 822–828). New York: Oxford University Press.

Bolter, K., Levenson, H., & Alverez, W. (1990). Differences in values between short-term and long-term therapists. *Professional Psychology, 21,* 285–290.

Centre for Health Evidence. (2003). *Users' guides to evidence-based practice.* Retrieved June 15, 2003, from http://www.cche.net/usersguides/main.asp

Colby, I., & Dziegielewski, S. F. (2001). *Social work: The people's profession.* Chicago: Lyceum.

Donald, A. (2002). Evidence-based medicine: Key concepts. *Medscape Psychiatry & Mental Health eJournal, 7*(2), 1–5. Retrieved June 15, 2003, from http://www.medscape.com/viewarticle/430709

Dziegielewski, S. F. (1996). Managed care principles: The need for social work in the health care environment. *Crisis Intervention and Time-Limited Treatment, 3,* 97–110.

Dziegielewski, S. F. (1997). Should clinical social workers seek psychotropic medication prescription privileges? Yes. In B. A. Thyer (Ed.), *Controversial issues in social work practice* (pp. 152–165). Boston: Allyn & Bacon.

Dziegielewski, S. F. (2002). *DSM-IV-TR® in action.* New York: Wiley.

Dziegielewski, S. F., & Holliman, D. (2001). Managed care and social work: Practice implications in an era of change. *Journal of Sociology and Social Welfare, 28*(2), 125–138.

Farley, O. W., Smith, L. L., Boyle, S. W., & Ronnau, J. (2002). A review of foundation MSW human behavior courses. *Journal of Human Behavior and the Social Environment, 6*(2), 1–12.

Flood, A. B., Shortell, S. M., & Scott, W. R. (1994). Organizational performance: Managing for efficiency and effectiveness. In S. M. Shortell & A. D. Kaluzny (Eds.), *Health care management: Organizational behavior and design* (3rd ed., pp. 316–351). Albany, NY: Delmar.

Franklin, C. (2002). Developing effective practice competencies in managed behavioral health care. In A. R. Roberts & G. J. Greene (Eds.), *Social workers' desk reference* (pp. 1–9). New York: Oxford University Press.

Gibelman, M. (2002). Social work in an era of managed care. In A. R. Roberts & G. J. Greene (Eds.), *Social workers' desk reference* (pp. 16–22). New York: Oxford University Press.

Maruish, M. E. (2002). *Essentials of treatment planning*. New York: Wiley.

Roberts, A. R. (Ed.). (2000). *Crisis intervention handbook: Assessment, treatment and research* (2nd ed.). New York: Oxford University Press.

Rock, B. (2002). Social work in health care in the 21st century. In A. R. Roberts & G. J. Greene (Eds.), *Social workers' desk reference* (pp. 10–16). New York: Oxford University Press.

Strom-Gottfried, K., & Dunlap, K. M. (1999). Unraveling ethical dilemmas. *The New Social Worker, 6*(2), 8–12.

Wells, R. A. (1994). *Planned short-term treatment* (2nd ed.). New York: Free Press.

Wodarski, J., & Dziegielewski, S. F. (2001). *Human behavior and the social environment: Integrating theory and evidence-based practice*. New York: Springer.

20   FACILITATING PRACTITIONER USE OF EVIDENCE-BASED PRACTICE

Edward J. Mullen

This chapter discusses ways to support social work practitioners in their attempts to use evidence-based practice to assess, intervene with, and better understand clients. Although social work practitioners report little use of evidence-based practices, many express a desire to use methods that are considered to be valid (Drake et al., 2001; Mullen & Bacon, 2000, 2003; U.S. Department of Health and Human Services, 1999). There is an emerging literature addressing implementation of evidence-based practices in organizations, but little attention has been given to how individual practitioners can be helped to use evidence-based practice (Addis & Krasnow, 2000; Torrey et al., 2001). While implementation strategies that seek system change by focusing on specific service delivery systems or organizations are important, there are limitations to such efforts. The sheer number of organizations defies any attempt to change them one by one. Also, many practitioners provide services outside such organizational settings, such as in private practice. Accordingly, in ad-

dition to implementation strategies directed at service systems and organizations, attention needs to be paid to how practitioners themselves can be helped to implement evidence-based practices. This is the focus of this chapter. This chapter describes evidence-based practice, approaches to dissemination and implementation of best practices that can be of benefit to practitioners, organizational and environmental supports needed for practitioners to function as evidence-based practitioners, and suggestions for training social work practitioners in evidence-based practice.

EVIDENCE-BASED PRACTICE

An *evidence-based practice* is considered to be any practice that has been established as effective through scientific research according to a set of explicit criteria (Drake et al., 2001). For example, in 1998 a Robert Wood Johnson Foundation consensus panel concluded that research findings identify six evidence-based treatment practices for the treatment of persons with severe mental illness: assertive community treatment (ACT), supported employment, family psychoeducation, skills training, illness self-management, and integrated dual-disorder treatment. To be considered an evidence-based practice, four selection criteria were used: the treatment practices had been standardized through manuals or guidelines; the practices had been evaluated with controlled research designs; through the use of objective measures, important outcomes were demonstrated; and the research was conducted by different research teams (Torrey et al., 2001). Accordingly, we can say that evidence-based practices or best practices were identified for the treatment of persons with severe mental illness through efficacy trials meeting these four criteria.

The term *evidence-based practice* is used also to describe a way of practicing, or an approach to practice. For example, evidence-based medicine has been described as "the conscientious, explicit and judicious use of current best evidence in making decisions about the care of individual patients" (Sackett et al., 1996, p. 71). Evidence-based medicine is further described as the "integration of best research evidence with clinical expertise and patient values" (Sackett, Straus, Richardson, Rosenberg, & Haynes, 2000, p. 1). Sheldon described evidence-based social care as "the conscientious, explicit and judicious use of current best evidence in making decisions regarding the welfare of service-users and carers" (Sheldon, 2002). Accordingly, evidence-based practice is a decision-making process in which judgments are made on a case-by-case basis by using best evidence. In addition, evidence-based social work practice would incorporate the following characteristics:

- Rather than a relationship based on asymmetrical information and authority, in evidence-based practice the relationship is characterized by a sharing of information and of decision making. The practitioner does not decide what is best for the client, but rather the practitioner provides the client with up-to-date information about what the best evidence is regarding the client's situation, what options are available, and likely outcomes. With this information communicated in culturally and linguistically appropriate ways, clients are supported to make decisions for themselves whenever and to the extent possible.

- There is a focus on fidelity in implementation of client-chosen interventions rather than an assumption that selected interventions will be provided as intended. Fidelity of implementation requires that the specific evidence-based practice be provided as it was tested when research supported its effectiveness. Too often serious distortion occurs during implementation.

- There is a critical, inquisitive attitude regarding the achievement of valued outcomes and unintended negative effects rather than an unquestioning belief that only intended outcomes will be achieved (and therefore a failure to secure information about actual outcomes, or permitting prior expectations to color achievements).

- Rather than relying on static prior beliefs, practitioners aggressively pursue new information about outcomes. This new information is derived from researching what occurs when interventions are implemented and new research findings promulgated by others.

- Ongoing knowledge revision is based on this new information, which in turn is communicated to clients.

- A relative weighing of information occurs, placing information derived from scientific inquiry as more important than information based on intuition, authority, or custom.

Social work practitioners need to know what has been identified as best practices, and they need to be prepared to be evidence-based practitioners. Social workers can benefit greatly from clear identification of interventions that work, through such efforts as seen in the systematic reviews conducted and disseminated through the Cochrane and Campbell Collaborations, as well as the work of the many evidence-based practice centers around the world. These collaborations and centers are using systematic reviews to identify effective interventions. What is learned through such reviews needs to be effectively disseminated and made available to practitioners (Eisenstadt, 2000; Nutley & Davies, 2000b; Nutley, Davies, & Tilley, 2000; Torrey et al., 2001). Dissemination and implementation of evidence-based practices present special challenges when the intended users are social work practitioners and their clients.

TWO APPROACHES TO DISSEMINATION AND IMPLEMENTATION OF EVIDENCE-BASED PRACTICE

As noted by Nutley and Davies, two major approaches to dissemination and implementation of best practices have been used, namely, *macro* and *micro*, or what I call *top-down* and *bottom-up* strategies (Nutley & Davies, 2000a).[1] In top-down strategies, findings are disseminated for use by frontline practitioners through agency directives, guidelines, manualized interventions, accreditation requirements, algorithms, tool kits, and so forth. Top-down or macro strategies can serve to get the word out about what works or what those in authority favor, but such methods do not guarantee adoption of best practices on the front lines. To increase the likelihood of adoption, a bottom-up approach is needed. In contrast to the top-down approach, social work practitioners need to be prepared to engage in a process of critical decision making with clients about what this information means when joined with other evidence, professional values and ethics, and individualized intervention goals. A bottom-up approach recognizes the importance of engaging the practitioner and the client in a critical, decision-making process.

ORGANIZATIONAL AND ENVIRONMENTAL SUPPORTS NEEDED FOR PRACTITIONERS TO FUNCTION AS EVIDENCE-BASED PRACTITIONERS

Implementation of evidence-based practice in social work organizations depends on many parts fitting together into a coherent whole (National Health Service Centre for Reviews and Dissemination, 1999). The team for the Implementing Evidence-Based Practices for Severe Mental Illness Project developed a model for achieving organizational change by using implementation tool kits (Torrey et al., 2001). This model provides steps to address a range of stakeholders, including funders, administrators, clinicians, and consumers and their families. Nevertheless, as Sackett and others have noted, there may be insurmountable barriers to implementing evidence-based practice guidelines in individual circumstances (Sackett et al., 2000, pp. 180–181).

For successful implementation, a number of components need to be in place, including:

- Organizational culture, policies, procedures, and processes must provide opportunities and incentives supporting evidence-based practice (e.g., financial incentives, funding, openness to change, workload adjustments, information technology supports, and legal protection).
- The organization's external environment must provide similar opportunities and incentives supporting evidence-based practice (e.g., national, regional, and local authorities; funders and accrediting groups).
- Applied practice research and evaluation must provide scientific evidence about assessment, intervention, and outcomes pertinent to the organization's practice domain.
- Systematic reviews that synthesize research findings must be conducted to assess the weight of the evidence generated by current research and evaluation studies.
- Prescriptive statements based on these syntheses must be developed and communicated in user-friendly forms (e.g., practice guidelines, manuals, and tool kits).
- Organizational procedures need to be put in place to assure fidelity of implementation of these prescriptions.
- Systematic, structured evaluation processes capable of providing timely feedback to various stakeholders as to the fidelity of implementation and outcomes must be designed and implemented as an ongoing process.
- The organization must have social workers available who are trained as evidence-based practitioners capable of functioning in evidence-based practice organizations.

TRAINING FOR EVIDENCE-BASED PRACTICE

Unless social work practitioners are trained for evidence-based practice, it is unlikely that organizations will be capable of providing such services to clients (Goisman, Warshaw, & Keller, 1999; Mullen & Bacon, 2000, 2003; Weissman & Sanderson, 2001). Furthermore, as accountable professionals, social workers must be prepared to engage in evidence-based practice even when working in organizations and environments without such supports, as well as when working in nonorganizational environments, such as in private practice.

Unfortunately, for the most part, social work practitioners are currently not engaged in evidence-based practice (Mullen & Bacon, 2000, 2003; Sanderson, 2002; Weissman & Sanderson, 2001), nor are social work educational programs currently training students for evidence-based practice (Weissman & Sanderson, 2001). In health care there has been much discussion of evidence-based education and how it differs from traditional education (Gray, 2001; Sackett et al., 2000; Willinsky, 2001). We are only beginning to have this discussion in social work (Gambrill, 2003; Howard, McMillen, & Pollio, 2003).

The future of evidence-based practice in social work rests on the profession's capacity and willingness to provide current practitioners and future generations of practitioners with training in evidence-based practice. In the immediate future, evidence-based practice training will need to be provided both for new social work students and for professional social workers already in practice. For the latter group, social workers who are engaged in practice, employing organizations need to make training opportunities available if the organizations are to adopt evidence-based practice. They will need to make a large investment in continuing education and other in-service training programs. Furthermore, especially for private practitioners and others not working in organizational settings conducive to evidence-based practice training, continuing education in such practice methods will need to be put in place. But, for practitioners in training, educational programs will need to provide a foundation in evidence-based practice content and methods. Regrettably, such training is generally absent from current educational programs. As noted by Weissman and Sanderson in discussing training for psychotherapy:

One major obstacle to the use of evidenced-based treatments is their near absence in many training programs for psychologists and social workers and in residency training programs for psychiatrists. This lag may be due in part to the recency of the evidence, although some is due to ideologic differences. Training efforts are more vigorous in Canada, Great Britain, Holland, Iceland, Germany and Spain where calls for workshops, individual training and supervision in EBT by psychiatrists, general practitioners (in Canada) and psychologists have been overwhelming. (Weissman & Sanderson, 2001, p. 18)

They also note:

Clinicians trained ten years ago are unlikely to be up-to-date with the newer, evidence-based psychotherapies, since the data supporting EBTs have appeared in the past 10 to 15 years. Continuing Education (CE) Programs have the potential to fill this void. (Weissman & Sanderson, 2001, p. 23)

Because few social work educational programs in the United States now provide training in evidence-based practice, a major curricular challenge lies ahead (Weissman & Sanderson, 2001). Nevertheless, there are indications that this situation may be changing. For example, the George Warren Brown School of Social Work at Washington University in St. Louis has recently adopted evidence-based practice as one of two approaches to graduate education (Howard et al., 2003). Leonard Gibbs has published the first evidence-based social work practice text, which builds on his many years of experience in teaching evidence-based practice (Gibbs, 2003). Gambrill's writings provide useful suggestions for teaching evidence-based practice, with special emphasis on critical thinking skills (Gambrill, 1999, 2003). In the years ahead, the profession needs to experiment with innovative evidence-based practice curricula. Practitioners need to be prepared to engage in a process of information gathering, analysis, and decision making with clients about what would be a best practice for a given client situation. This idea is in agreement with Lawrence Green's notion that it is *best processes* rather than *best practices* that should be advocated in public health promotion (Green, 2001).

Students preparing for evidence-based practice will need training in critical thinking skills (Gambrill, 1999); evidence-based practice as a framework for and requirement of contemporary social work practice; practice guidelines, manuals, tool kits, and other forms currently used to translate evidence into practice prescriptions; information retrieval and critical assessment skills; systematic review methods, data syntheses, and meta-analytic procedures; methods of social intervention research as a process for developing, testing, refining, and disseminating scientifically validated social work practices; foundations of scientific thinking; research and evaluation methods, as well as quantitative and qualitative modes of inquiry and analysis; and skills for adapting general research findings and guidelines to individualized client circumstances, preferences, and values (Mullen, 1978; Mullen & Bacon, 2003).

CONCLUSION

This chapter has discussed ways to support social work practitioners in their attempts to use evidence-based knowledge to assess, intervene with, and better understand clients. While there is an emerging literature addressing implementation of evidence-based practices in organizations, little attention has been given to how individual practitioners can be helped to use evidence-based knowledge in everyday practice. Accordingly, in addition to dissemination and implementation strategies directed at service systems and organizations, attention needs to be paid to how practitioners themselves can be helped to implement evidence-based practice. This chapter has provided suggestions toward that end.

ACKNOWLEDGMENT This chapter is adapted from: Mullen, E. J. (2002). Evidence-based knowledge: Designs for enhancing practitioner use of research findings. Paper presented at the fourth International Conference on Evaluation for Practice, University of Tampere, Tampere, Finland.

Note

1. The Cochrane Effective Practice and Organization of Care Group (EPOC) focuses on what has been learned through research about effective dissemination and implementation interventions (Cochrane Effective Practice and Organization of Care Group. 2000). Retrieved July 26, 2003, from http://www.epoc.uottawa.ca.

References

Addis, M. E., & Krasnow, A. D. (2000). A national survey of predicting psychologists' attitudes toward psychotherapy treatment manuals. *Journal of Consulting and Clinical Psychology, 68*(2), 331–339.

Drake, R. E., Goldman, H., Leff, H. S., Lehman, A. F., Dixon, L., Mueser, K. T., et al. (2001). Implementing evidence-based practices in routine mental health service settings. *Psychiatric Services, 52*(2), 179–182.

Eisenstadt, N. (2000). Sure start: Research into practice; practice into research. *Public Money & Management, 20*(4), 6–8.

Gambrill, E. (1999). Evidence-based practice: An alternative to authority-based practice. *Families in Society: The Journal of Contemporary Human Services, 80*(4), 341–350.

Gambrill, E. D. (2003). Evidence-based practice: Sea change or the emperor's new clothes? *Journal of Social Work Education, 39*(1), 3–23.

Gibbs, L. E. (2003). *Evidence-based practice for the helping professions: A practical guide with integrated multimedia.* Pacific Grove, CA: Brooks/Cole–Thompson Learning.

Goisman, R. M., Warshaw, M. G., & Keller, M. B. (1999). Psychosocial treatment prescriptions for generalized anxiety disorder, panic disorder, and social phobia, 1991–1996. *American Journal of Psychiatry, 156,* 1819–1821.

Gray, J. A. M. (2001). *Evidence-based healthcare* (2nd ed.). New York: Churchill Livingstone.

Green, L. W. (2001). From research to "best practices" in other settings and populations. *American Journal of Health Behavior, 25*(3), 165–178.

Howard, M. O., McMillen, C. J., & Pollio, D. E. (2003). Teaching evidence-based practice: Toward a new paradigm for social work education. *Research on Social Work Practice, 13*(2), 234–259.

Mullen, E. J. (1978). Construction of personal models for effective practice: A method for utilizing research findings to guide social interventions. *Journal of Social Service Research, 2*(1), 45–63.

Mullen, E. J., & Bacon, W. F. (2000, May 3–5). *Practitioner adoption and implementation of evidence-based effective treatments and issues of quality control.* Paper presented at the Evidence-Based Practice Conference: Developing Practice Guidelines for Social Work Interventions—Issues, Methods, & Research Agenda, George Warren Brown School of Social Work, Washington University, St. Louis, MO.

Mullen, E. J., & Bacon, W. F. (2003). Practitioner adoption and implementation of evidence-based effective treatments and issues of quality control. In A. Rosen & E. K. Proctor (Eds.), *Developing practice guidelines for social work interventions: Issues, methods, and a research agenda.* New York: Columbia University Press.

National Health Services Centre for Reviews and Dissemination, University of York. (1999). Getting evidence into practice. *Effective Health Care Bulletin 5*(1). Retrieved July 26, 2003, from www.york.ac.uk/inst/crd/ehcb.htm.

Nutley, S. M., & Davies, H. T. O. (2000a). Making a reality of evidence-based practice. In H. T. O. Davies, S. M. Nutley, & P. C. Smith (Eds.), *What works? Evidence-based policy and practice in public services.* Bristol: Policy Press.

Nutley, S., & Davies, H. T. O. (2000b). Making a reality of evidence-based practice: Some lessons from the diffusion of innovations. *Public Money & Management, 20*(4), 35–42.

Nutley, S., Davies, H. T. O., & Tilley, N. (2000). Editorial: Getting research into practice. *Public Money & Management, 20*(4), 3–6.

Sackett, D. L., Straus, S. E., Richardson, W. S., Rosenberg, W., & Haynes, R. B. (2000). *Evidence-based medicine: How to practice and teach EBM* (2nd ed.). New York: Churchill Livingstone.

Sackett, D. L., Rosenberg, W. M. C., Gray, J. A. M., Haynes, R. B., & Richardson, W. S. (1996). Evidence based medicine: What it is and what it isn't—It's about integrating individual clinical expertise and the best external evidence. *British Medical Journal, 312*(7023), 71–72.

Sanderson, W. C. (2002). Are evidence-based psychological interventions practiced by clinicians in the field? *Medscape Psychiatry and Mental Health eJournal, 7*(1). Retrieved from http://www.medscape.com/viewarticle/414948©

Sheldon, B. (2002). *Brief summary of the ideas behind the Centre for Evidence-Based Social Services.* Retrieved July 26, 2003, from http://www.ex.qc.uk/cebss@introduction.html.

Torrey, W. C., Drake, R. E., Dixon, L., Burns, B. J., Flynn, L., Rush, A. J., et al. (2001). Implementing evidence-based practices for persons with severe mental illnesses. *Psychiatric Services, 52*(1), 45–50.

U.S. Department of Health and Human Services. (1999). *Mental health: A report of the Surgeon General.* Rockville, MD: U.S. Department of Health and Human Services, Substance Abuse and Mental Health Services Administration, Center for Mental Health Services, National Institutes of Health, National Institute of Mental Health.

Weissman, M. M., & Sanderson, W. C. (2001, October). *Promises and problems in modern psychotherapy: The need for increased training in evidence based treatments.* Paper presented at the Josiah Macy Jr. Foundation conference: Modern Psychiatry: Challenges in Educating Health Professionals to Meet New Needs, Toronto, Canada.

Willinsky, J. (2001). Extending the prospects of evidence-based education. *InSight, 1*(1), 23–41.

IMPLEMENTATION OF PRACTICE GUIDELINES AND EVIDENCE-BASED TREATMENT

21

A Survey of Psychiatrists, Psychologists, and Social Workers

Edward J. Mullen & William Bacon

Evidence-based practice and the associated use of practice guidelines have become important emphases in recent years within social work, psychology, and psychiatry (e.g., Gibbs, 2003; Weissman & Sanderson, 2001). These emphases stress practitioner use of methods that have been empirically demonstrated to be effective. This movement within the human service professions is a reaction to the widespread use of methods that have not been empirically tested, as well as the variability in practice of methods used.

Clinical practice guidelines have been described by the Institute of Medicine as "systematically developed statements to assist practitioner and patient decisions about appropriate health care for specific clinical circumstances" (Field & Lohr, 1990). Professional organizations and governmental agencies have formulated practice guidelines for various clinical conditions (e.g., American Academy of Child and Adolescent Psychiatry, 1994; American Psychiatric Association, 1993, 1994, 1997). These guidelines prescribe how clinicians should assess and treat clients. Sometimes the guidelines are based on research findings. Sometimes research is not available, and, therefore, the guidelines are based on professional consensus. Although practice guidelines have been promoted for several decades in medicine, this topic has received attention in social work only recently (e.g., Mullen, 2002a, 2002b; Mullen & Bacon, 2002; Rosen & Proctor, 2002; Sackett, Straus, Richardson, Rosenberg, & Haynes, 2000). Not examined is the question of how agencies and practitioners view this development. Prior research has indicated that practitioners are not likely to use research in practice (Kirk, Osmalov, & Fischer, 1976; Kirk & Reid, 2002, Chapter 8). Little is known about the use of guidelines in social work practice and how social work practitioners view the use of guidelines (Sanderson, 2002). Accordingly, this chapter presents findings of one of the few studies examining practitioner attitudes toward and use of practice guidelines and other aspects of evidence-based practice (Addis & Krasnow, 2000).

We conducted a survey examining practitioner awareness of practice guidelines, specification of guidelines known about and used by individual practitioners, practitioner attitudes toward the use of guidelines, and their preferences for guidelines based on expert consensus or based on empirical research findings. In addition, the survey examined a variety of aspects of research use for practice. The survey was conducted in a large, urban, nonprofit social agency.

METHOD

The agency surveyed is among the largest of its type in the United States. It is noted for the high quality of its services and training programs. Master's-level social workers are the primary providers of service, although the staff is multidisciplinary, including psychologists, psychiatrists, and other mental health professionals. At the time of the survey, the agency employed a professional staff of 697. Of this number, 500 were engaged in provision of clinical services, including 42 psychiatrists, 53 psychologists, 386 social workers, and 19 other mental health professionals. This was the population surveyed. The organization provided a list of all professional staff employed by the agency at the time of the survey, August 1999. A questionnaire was sent by the organization to each staff member addressed to his or her home. A cover letter from the agency executive director stressed the importance of the survey and asked for cooperation. The cover letter explained that the study was seeking information regarding clinical practice and that it was being conducted by a university-based social work research center. Respondents were asked not to write their names on the questionnaire. They were assured that their questionnaires and responses would be anonymous. The questionnaires were to be returned to the research center. Questions were to be directed to the center rather than to the employing organization. Because of the assurance of anonymity and the methods employed, we assume that practitioners provided honest answers.

SAMPLE CHARACTERISTICS

Of the 500 questionnaires mailed to the practitioners' homes, 124 usable ones were returned (24.8%). Of these 124 respondents, 65.3% (81) were social workers, 12.9% (16) were psychologists, 13.7% (17) were psychiatrists, and 8.1% (10) were other mental health professionals (e.g., art therapists). Relative to the population distribution, social workers were somewhat less likely to have responded to the survey (21%, 81 of 386) than the other professions (38%, 43 of 114). With an overall return rate of approximately 25%, one cannot be confident that the respondents are representative of the total population of clinicians at the agency. It is reasonable to suppose that on average respondents were more favorably disposed to research than their nonresponding colleagues. One might also assume that respondents were less likely to be those who felt overburdened by paperwork and administrative demands. The number of respondents who were psychologists or psychiatrists was especially small, and conclusions pertaining to those professions must be made with caution. Because the 10 respondents classified as "other mental health professionals" are from a range of professions, it is not possible to treat them as a homogeneous professional group. Accordingly, they are excluded in the following analyses; subsequently, we report on a total set of 114 respondents. While no claim of representativeness can be made, the findings do provide initial information regarding an important and unresearched area of pertinence to practice. Nevertheless, the low response rate must be recognized as a serious limitation, and generalizations from this sample to professional groups can be made only with extreme caution.

Nearly three fourths (71.9%, $N = 82$) of the respondents reported their highest academic degree to be a master's degree, 14.9% ($N = 17$) reported an MD, and 13.2% ($N = 15$) reported a PhD or its equivalent (13.2%, $N = 15$). All social workers and one psychologist held the master's degree as the highest degree. Of the 112 respondents providing information, the large majority of respondents were employed in an outpatient clinic (61.6%, $N = 69$) or a residential facility (23.2%, $N = 26$). Other reported locations were scattered-site facility (3.6%, $N = 4$), day treatment program (5.4%, $N = 6$), school-based program (1.8%, $N = 2$), and other type of facility (4.5%, $N = 5$). Nearly all the respondents (95.6%, $N = 109$) were engaged in direct practice, and some were also engaged in clinical supervision, clinical training, and administration of clinical services. Most of the respondents reported full-time employment (63.2%, $N = 72$). The length of time employed by this agency ranged from 2 months to 40 years. The median was 3 years, whereas the mode was 1 year. Approximately 28% (28.6%, $N = 15$) of the respondents had worked for the organization 1 year or less, whereas 25% ($N = 36$) had worked at the organization for 6 or more years. The number of years since licensure or certification ranged from 1 to 49. The median was 7 years, whereas the mode was 1 to 2 years. About a quarter (24.6%) of the respondents had received licensure or certification within the past 2 years, whereas 26.4% had received licensure or certification 16 or more years earlier.

ABOUT PRACTICE GUIDELINES

We asked about the practitioners' knowledge of and attitudes toward practice guidelines. As an introduction to these questions, we provided a brief description of what we meant by practice guidelines. Because we found that there were systematic differences among the professions, the findings are presented by profession.

Heard About Practice Guidelines

We asked the respondents if they had ever heard of practice guidelines before this survey. Nearly all of the psychiatrists (94.1%) had heard about practice guidelines, and the overwhelming majority of psychologists (81.3%) had also heard about guidelines, but fewer than half of the social workers had heard of them (42.3%).

Know of a Particular Guideline

When asked if they were aware of a particular guideline, most psychiatrists said they were aware of at least one (87.5%), but relatively few psychologists (12.5%) or social workers (18.4%) reported awareness of even one guideline. For those who said that they were aware of a guideline, we asked them to specify the organization that had developed the guideline and/or what disorder or situation it addressed. Fourteen of the 17 psychiatrists said they knew of a particular guideline, and 12 of these listed the American Psychiatric Association and the American Academy of Child and Adolescent Psychiatry. Just 2 of the 16 psychologists reported knowing a guideline, and no psychologist actually listed an organization. Only 14 of the 81 social workers reported knowing a particular guideline, and just 3 of these listed organizations.

Twelve of the 17 psychiatrists responded that they were aware of guidelines pertaining to a range of mental disorders, including schizophrenia, substance abuse, eating disorders, bipolar disorder, major depression, dementia, anxiety disorders, panic disorder, and borderline personality disorders. Eight of 81 social workers listed disorder-specific or situation-specific guidelines. These were guidelines pertaining to child abuse and neglect reporting, suicide intervention, depression therapy, trauma assessment, posttraumatic stress disorder, how to treat and transfer juvenile sex offenders, teenagers in residential care with conduct disorders, borderline personality disorder, and treatment of depression in residential treatment centers. One of the 16 psychologists indicated awareness of a guideline pertaining to depression evaluation for medication.

Used Guideline

Respondents were asked if they had ever used any practice guideline to help them plan treatment. The majority of psychiatrists (64.3%) said they had, only one psychologist (6.3%) had, and about one in five social workers (18.7%) had used a guideline. For those who said they had used a guideline, we asked what the guideline was and what their experience had been with the guideline's use. For those who said they had not used a guideline, we asked why they had not used one. Most of the social workers who had used a guideline reported vague comments about why a guideline had been used. Only three of the comments could be classified as indicating that the guideline was considered to have been useful to improve treatment. Two indicated that the reason for use was that the guideline was required. One psychologist who had used a guideline commented, "I followed a guideline and have found it helpful." Three guideline-using psychiatrists provided vague or neutral comments, and one commented that it improved treatment ("I have used the dementia guidelines to look for treatment options for family members with a particular client").

Among social workers who had *not* used a practice guideline, the majority of the comments related to being unaware of the existence of guidelines. Some social workers provided vague or neutral comments. Two expressed a lack of need for guidelines ("I have followed the guidance of supervisors & colleagues who have extensive knowledge working with clients experiencing depression"; "agency administrative guidelines from beginning contact with a client to discharge have been clear—changed and/or modified in time and work well"). One said guidelines were not relevant ("sometimes it seems like guidelines don't incorporate culturally relevant issues + what to do"). No social worker volunteered a strongly negative opinion of guidelines' potential usefulness, a sentiment expressed frequently by psychologists ("I don't like following a formula if it doesn't feel right

for the patient"; "I am mistrustful of guidelines that seem to encourage cost-saving procedures, or exclude patient/clinician from decision"; "I'm very much a believer in the complexity of development, individual difference, and the fact that the same symptom/syndrome meant very different things in different people—and thus required different intervention"). Among other psychologists' responses, some pertained to guideline irrelevance ("didn't feel that such guidelines were relevant to the cases I was treating"; "didn't apply to the population working with"). Only one psychologist mentioned not being aware of guidelines, and three provided vague or neutral comments as to lack of use. Four psychiatrists commented on reasons for not using guidelines ("I have read the guidelines but don't necessarily look them up for each and every case"; "haven't had enough time or opportunities to use yet"; "Already had information"; "not needed").

Inclination to Use Guidelines

We asked whether respondents were inclined to use guidelines, regardless of whether they had used them in the past. Most psychiatrists (86.7%) and social workers (81.4%) were inclined to use guidelines, whereas about half of the psychologists were so inclined (54.5%). When asked to say why they were or were not inclined to use guidelines, several reasons were common. For social workers who were inclined to use guidelines, the most common type of response (10 of 24 responses) related to guidance. These respondents indicated that they thought guidelines would help them in conceptualizing or planning treatment. Two others specifically mentioned that guidelines would increase their knowledge or skills. Four said that guidelines would improve treatment. Four social workers mentioned or implied that they were attracted to practice guidelines because of their research basis. The remaining comments made reference to willingness to use guidelines if they were not burdensome and if they were easily accessible.

Four psychologists commented on why they would be inclined to use guidelines. They referred to guidance ("if clear and helpful"), their research base ("I'm interested in effective techniques based on empirical data"), and other qualifications ("contingent on the care and guideline restrictions"; "I nevertheless reserve the right to use my clinical judgment in specific cases"). Six psychiatrists commented on why they would use guidelines, mostly making reference to their value in providing guidance ("for reference and guidance"; "They are helpful in approach to patient case"; "standardized consensus"; "as a guide to my own thinking"; "useful in client planned treatment"; "Only because they comply with my practice").

Among social workers who were *not* inclined to use practice guidelines, explanatory comments were usually vague rather than expressing concern about the validity of practice guidelines. On the other hand, psychiatrists and psychologists were more likely to describe a specific objection to practice guidelines.

Guideline Preference

Respondents were asked which type of guideline they would be more inclined to use: those based on research findings or those based on professional consensus (whether or not research supported the consensus). A number of the respondents selected both answer choices (43.8% of psychiatrists, 13.4% of social workers, and 7.1% of psychologists). Of those who selected only one choice, psychiatrists most often said they would be most inclined to use those supported by research (50% for research-only; 6.3% for consensus-only), whereas both social workers and psychologists said they would be most inclined to use those based on professional consensus (social workers: 50.7% for consensus-only vs. 35.8% for research-only; and for psychologists 50.0% for consensus-only vs. 42.9% for research-only).

Practice Conforms to Guidelines

We asked respondents if they thought their current practice conformed to what existing guidelines prescribe. All of the psychologists and most psychiatrists (85.7%) responded affirmatively, whereas about three fourths of social workers (74.1%) thought this. When asked why they thought that their practice did or did not conform, they gave a range of answers. Those who thought their practice did not conform mentioned that the guidelines probably were not promulgated by other social workers, that guidelines probably emphasized short-term treatments, or that practice guidelines are not generally consulted for treatment planning. For those who believed that their practice probably did conform to practice guidelines, most made general statements about their professional competence or the apparent effectiveness of their work.

OTHER INDICATORS OF EVIDENCE-BASED PRACTICE

We asked about other indicators of an evidence-based approach to practice, including frequency of reading professional publications, especially research publications; use of single-subject designs; use of assessment instruments in practice; and seeking consultation from the literature, supervisors, and colleagues regarding research evidence for practice decisions.

Reading or Referring to Journal Articles

We asked how often respondents read or referred to journal articles in their field. The modal responses were strikingly different across professions: one or two times a month for social workers, about once a week for psychologists, and a few times a week for psychiatrists. The response distribution is shown in Table 21.1 under the columns labeled *Articles*.

Reading Other Professional Literature

We also asked how often they read professional literature other than journal articles (e.g., books, newsletters). These responses are shown in Table 21.1 under the columns labeled *Other*.[1] Nearly one quarter of social workers replied that they did this less than once or twice a month (24.6%), with 9.8% reporting doing this once or twice a year or less. About half (51.8%) reported reading or referring to other professional literature at least weekly. No psychiatrist reported such low frequency, with nearly half saying they did this daily or a few times a week (47.0%). Nearly three quarters (70.5%) reported reading or referring to other professional literature at least weekly. Psychologists reported a pattern somewhere in between, with somewhat more than half (56.3%) responding about once a week or once or twice a month and more than one third (37.5%) responding at least weekly.

TABLE 21.1 Reading or Referring to Publications

| Frequency | Social Workers | | | | Psychologists | | | | Psychiatrists | | | |
| | Articles | | Other | | Articles | | Other | | Articles | | Other | |
	N	%	N	%	N	%	N	%	N	%	N	%
Daily or nearly so	5	6.3	7	8.6	0	0.0	0	0	3	17.6	3	17.6
A few times a week	11	13.8	17	21.0	3	18.8	4	25.0	7	41.2	5	29.4
About once a week	14	17.5	18	22.2	6	37.5	2	12.5	3	17.6	4	23.5
Once or twice a month	26	32.5	19	23.5	5	31.3	7	43.8	4	23.5	4	23.5
Several times a year	13	16.3	12	14.8	1	6.3	3	18.8	0	0.0	1	5.9
Once or twice a year	7	8.8	4	4.9	1	6.3	0	0.0	0	0.0	0	0.0
Less than once a year	4	5.0	4	4.9	0	0.0	0	0.0	0	0.0	0	0.0

Reading or Referring to Research Journal Articles

We asked what types of articles respondents read. Listed were case studies, clinical theory, research articles on populations or clinical problems, research articles on clinical assessment or interventions, and research articles on outcomes or effectiveness of particular therapeutic techniques. We report here on their responses about research articles only, combining the three types of research articles into a single measure. Accordingly, a respondent who reported reading all three types of research articles would receive a score of 3, if two types a score of 2, if one type a score of 1, and if none a score of 0. As shown in Table 21.2, the modal responses were 3 for psychiatrists, 1 for psychologists, and bimodal for social workers, with approximately 29% reporting 0 and 29% reporting 3. There was considerable variation among social workers, whereas the other professionals tended to be less varied in their responses.

TABLE 21.2 Reading or Referring to Research Journal Articles

| Number of Types Read | Social Workers | | Psychol- ogists | | Psychia- trists | |
	N	%	N	%	N	%
0 (none)	23	29.1	3	18.8	3	17.6
1 (reads 1 type)	17	21.5	1	6.3	7	41.2
2 (reads 2 types)	16	20.3	4	25.0	3	17.6
3 (reads 3 types)	23	29.1	8	50.0	4	23.5

Using Research Literature for Practice Decisions

We asked if the practitioners ever consulted the research literature when they needed to make a decision about how to proceed in treating a particular case. Most of the psychiatrists (94.1%) and psychologists (87.5%) said they did, but only 64.6% of the social workers said this. For those who said they did consult the research literature, we asked how often they did so. The modal response for all professionals was "several times a year" (32% of social workers, 50% of psychiatrists, and 42.9% of psychologists). Of those social workers who responded that they did consult the research literature, 24.5% said they did this at least weekly, whereas only 14.3% of the psychiatrists consulted this frequently and none of the psychologists reported this frequency.

Using Research Methods in Practice

We asked about the practitioners' use of single-subject designs and assessment instruments in their own practice during the preceding 2 years. No psychologist reported conducting a single-subject design study, and only about 1 in 10 of the social workers (11.3%) and psychiatrists (11.8%) reported doing so. Of those saying they had conducted such studies, the number of studies conducted during the 2-year period was almost always one.

Practitioners were asked if they had used the results from any standardized assessment instrument to help them assess a client's symptoms or response to treatment. Psychologists almost always responded that they had (87.5%), nearly three fourths of the psychiatrists said they had (70.6%), but somewhat less than a third of the social workers said they had (30.4%). Of those who said they had, we asked if they themselves had administered any of these instruments. Nearly all of the psychologists (90.9%) and psychiatrists (100%) said they had, whereas only a little over half of the social workers said they did (58.3%). Of those who said they had used standardized assessment instrument results, we asked them to name those instruments they had used most often. Social workers and psychiatrists most frequently cited simple symptom checklists such as the Beck Depression Inventory. Multisymptom instruments such as the Achenbach were also relatively common. Psychologists were much more likely to employ personality tests such as the Rorschach, along with cognitive and achievement tests.

Reasons for Changing Practice

We asked practitioners if research findings of favorable or unfavorable outcomes with a certain technique ever caused them to change their practice, such as starting or stopping a particular treatment technique with some or all of their clients. We also asked if such changes had ever been brought about by their own experience of what works and what doesn't work or by demands of administration or the mental health care marketplace. If they said any of these three had caused a change, we asked them to specify what the change was and when the most recent change had occurred.

Almost all psychiatrists said that research findings had changed their practice (93.8% or 15 of 16), whereas 42.9% of psychologists (6 of 14) and 40.6% of social workers (26 of 64) said this. In contrast, demands of administration or of the mental health care marketplace were said to have changed practice for approximately three quarters of social workers (76.8%) and psychologists (73.3%) but for only about half of the psychiatrists (56.3%). Nearly all reported that their own experiences had changed their practice (87.1% of social workers, 93.8% of psychologists, and 94.1% of psychiatrists).

Regarding what aspect of their practices had been changed by research findings, all the psychiatrists who answered the question ($N = 6$) mentioned medications. Social workers and psychologists gave a much wider variety of answers,

most mentioning particular techniques or treatment modalities that they had begun to use, such as behavioral techniques for learning disabilities or eating disorders, cognitive techniques for anger management, or eye movement desensitization and reprocessing for trauma.

Using Supervisors and Colleagues for Practice Decisions

As noted previously, we had asked if the practitioners ever consulted the research literature when they needed to make a decision about how to proceed in treating a particular case. We also asked if, when needing to make a decision about how to proceed in treating a particular case, they ever consulted with a supervisor or colleague. Respondents were then asked to estimate the degree to which their consultations were directed at the consultant's knowledge of research findings, knowledge of clinical theory, clinical wisdom or experience, or knowledge of administrative requirements. With the exception of a few psychiatrists, all respondents reported using consultation. Most social workers (80.6%) said they sought consultation a few times a week (32.5%), weekly (24.7%), or one or two times a month (23.4%). By contrast, the majority of psychiatrists said they did so only several times a year (57.1%), and none reported more often than once a week. Psychologists' modal response was one or two times a month. Consultation was sought at least weekly by 70.1% of social workers, 50% of psychologists, and 21.4% of psychiatrists.

One third of the respondents (41 of 124) said they sought the consultant's knowledge of research findings. The distribution differed little among the professions. Sixty-nine percent of the respondents said they sought the consultant's knowledge of clinical theory (85 of 124). This was true for approximately three quarters of social workers and psychologists but only 41% of the psychiatrists. Seeking consultation regarding administrative requirements was common for all professionals (67.9% of social workers, 50.0% of psychologists, 41.2% of psychiatrists). With few exceptions, respondents also sought the consultant's clinical wisdom and experience.

IMPLICATIONS

These findings have implications for developing and using practice guidelines and evidence-based practice in social work. Viewed from the perspective of how practitioners working in organizations such as the one surveyed in this study think of practice guidelines and other aspects of evidence-based practice, we draw a number of conclusions. The three mental health professions represented in this survey were strikingly different in their knowledge of practice guidelines. Psychiatrists appeared to be relatively well informed about relevant practice guidelines, whereas social workers were poorly informed, typically not even aware of the meaning of practice guidelines. Psychologists were somewhere in between. Once told what practice guidelines were, social workers were inclined to be open to their use.

Social workers generally were not using research findings or research methods in their practice. Psychiatrists and, to a lesser extent, psychologists were using findings and methods of assessment. Many social workers did not often read the research literature or even other professional literature. Psychiatrists read this literature frequently. Social workers were heavy users of consultation, much more so than the other professionals, who functioned more autonomously. Social workers frequently sought guidance and direction from supervisors and other consultants, who were viewed as repositories of knowledge based on experience and as spokespersons for organizational policy.

Given the low use of research methods and infrequent reading of professional literature, it is not likely that social work practitioners will be influenced significantly through these routes. Rather, supervisors and consultants seem to be the most promising conduit for knowledge regarding practice guidelines and other forms of evidence-based practice for social workers. Social workers appeared to be open to guidelines, so long as they are perceived as helping them improve practice, but their preference was for guidelines that represent professional consensus rather than research evidence. A few social work practitioners deviated from this norm, appearing to function more autonomously through behaviors more like those of the psychiatrists in the sample. These social workers expressed preference for evidence-based guidelines, and they have higher frequencies of reading research articles and professional publications. It is likely that they use supervisors and consultants differently as well. These types of social workers may be important resources for dissemination of evidence-based practice knowledge within social work organizations. It is likely that their training has provided them with research skills of relevance to practice.

The reported findings have implications for technologies needed to assist practitioners in identification and use of evidence-based practice guidelines, for quality control and accountability, and for education. Future work is needed to develop and test technologies that can facilitate the use of evidence-based practice. Because of the crucial role played by social work supervisors regarding information, dissemination research is needed to further understand how this resource can be better used to advance evidence-based practice in social work. Also, research is needed to better understand the characteristics of those social workers who are high users of research, as well as how these types of social workers might be used as agents of research dissemination in social work organizations. Finally, because the study reported here is limited to one agency, studies are needed examining additional practitioners in a wide range of settings to determine how representative our findings are of the larger group of human service practitioners and to identify characteristics of situations wherein evidence-based practice and empirically based practice guidelines have been adopted.

Note

1. Missing information is excluded from the tabulated results in Tables 21.1 and 21.2, accounting for variation in the sample sizes shown.

References

Addis, M. E., & Krasnow, A. D. (2000). A national survey of practicing psychologists' attitudes toward psychotherapy treatment manuals. *Journal of Consulting and Clinical Psychology, 68*(2), 331–339.

American Academy of Child and Adolescent Psychiatry. (1994). Practice parameters for the assessment and treatment of children and adolescents with schizophrenia. *Journal of the American Academy of Child and Adolescent Psychiatry, 33,* 616–635.

American Psychiatric Association. (1993). Practice guideline for major depressive disorder in adults.

American Journal of Psychiatry, 150(Suppl. 4), 1–29.

American Psychiatric Association. (1994). Practice guideline for treatment of patients with bipolar disorder. *American Journal of Psychiatry, 151* (12), 1–36.

American Psychiatric Association. (1997). Practice guideline for the treatment of patients with schizophrenia. *American Journal of Psychiatry, 154*(12), 1–63.

Field, M. J., & Lohr, K. N. (Eds.). (1990). *Clinical practice guidelines: Directions of a new program.* Washington, DC: National Academy Press.

Gibbs, L. E. (2003). *Evidence-based practice for the helping professions: A practical guide with integrated multimedia.* Pacific Grove, CA: Brooks/Cole–Thompson Learning.

Kirk, S. A., Osmalov, M., & Fischer, J. (1976). Social workers' involvement in research. *Social Work, 21,* 121–124.

Kirk, S. A., & Reid, W. J. (2002). *Science and social work: A critical appraisal.* New York: Columbia University Press.

Mullen, E. J. (2002a). *Evidence-based knowledge: Designs for enhancing practitioner use of research findings.* Paper presented at the fourth International Conference on Evaluation for Practice, University of Tampere, Tampere, Finland.

Mullen, E. J. (2002b). *Evidence-based social work— theory & practice: Historical and reflective perspective.* Paper presented at the fourth International Conference on Evaluation for Practice, University of Tampere, Tampere, Finland.

Mullen, E. J., & Bacon, W. F. (2003). Practitioner adoption and implementation of evidence-based effective treatments and issues of quality control. In A. Rosen & E. K. Proctor (Eds.), *Developing practice guidelines for social work interventions: Issues, methods, and a research agenda.* New York: Columbia University Press.

Research on Social Work Practice. (1999). *9*(3).

Rosen, A., & Proctor, E. (Eds.). (2003). *Developing practice guidelines for social work interventions: Issues, methods, and a research agenda.* New York: Columbia University Press.

Sackett, D. L., Straus, S. E., Richardson, W. S., Rosenberg, W., & Haynes, R. B. (2000). *Evidence-based medicine: How to practice and teach EBM* (2nd ed.). New York: Churchill Livingstone.

Sanderson, W. C. (2002). Are evidence-based psychological interventions practiced by clinicians in the field? *Medscape Psychiatry and Mental Health: A Medscape eMed Journal, 7*(1). Retrieved from http://www.medscape.com/viewarticle/414948

Steketee, G. (1999). Yes, but cautiously. *Research on Social Work Practice, 9,* 343–346.

Weissman, M. M., & Sanderson, W. C. (2001). *Promises and problems in modern psychotherapy: The need for increased training in evidence based treatments.* Unpublished manuscript.

22

MEASURING SKILLS AND REASONING SCIENTIFICALLY AND CRITICALLY ABOUT PRACTICE

Len Gibbs & Eileen Gambrill

IMPORTANCE OF CRITICAL THINKING

Critical thinking skills should contribute to making well-reasoned decisions in practice regarding, for example, accurate assessments of client circumstances and presenting problems, assessing risk (e.g., new sex offense, violence), making generalizations about clients, and selecting effective methods. Research on cognitive biases in decision making (e.g., Baron, 2000; Hastie & Dawes, 2001; Nisbett & Ross, 1980) suggests that certain biases may result in faulty decisions across a broad array of contexts. Such errors and biases in thinking can be costly. Measures that test skills in spotting fallacies in newspaper reports, editorials, and debates may not be valid when applied to clinical situations. Tousignant and DesMarchais (2002) reported that self-assessments by medical students did not correlate well with performance on an oral examination. Their study involved 91 medical students enrolled in a problem-based learning program. Beck, Bennett, McLeod, and Molyneaux (1992) reviewed 13 studies that examined the relationship between clinical reasoning ability in nursing and scores primarily on the Watson-Glaser Critical Thinking Appraisal. They found mixed to negative results, suggesting that the Watson-Glaser test does not validly reflect clinical reasoning in nursing. Such findings support the need for measures of critical thinking about practice that are specific to practice. Here we briefly review some measures that have been used to assess critical thinking and describe some recently designed measures used to assess decision making in professional contexts.

CONCEPTUAL DEFINITIONS OF CRITICAL THINKING

As many writers in this area note, there is no one definition of critical thinking that everyone agrees on. Nickerson (1986) defines *critical thinking* as arriving at well-reasoned actions and beliefs. Facione (1990a), as quoted in Bondy et al. (2001) defines *critical thinking* as "the purposeful, self-regulatory judgment which results in interpretation, analysis, evaluation, and inference, as well as explanation of the evidential, conceptual, methodological, criteriological, or contextual considerations upon which that judgment is based" (Facione, 1990a, p. 310). Some use Ennis's definition: "*critical thinking* is reasonable and reflective thinking that is focused on deciding what to believe or do" (Norris & Ennis, 1989, p. 3). Ennis's conception of critical thinking has been the basis for the creation of the Cornell Critical Thinking Test (Ennis & Millman, 1985) and the Ennis-Weir Critical Thinking Essay Test (Ennis & Weir, 1985).

SOME COMMON MEASURES OF CRITICAL THINKING

A search of the Health and Psychological Instruments (HAPI) database for "critical thinking" on

November 25, 2002, found 34 documents. Among these 34, 16 concern the Watson-Glaser Critical Thinking Appraisal. Among the 34, only the Pediatric Clerkship Clinical Performance Measure (used by clerkship instructors to rate student doctors' performance on a 6-point scale) directly measured thinking about practice (Deterding et al., 1999). The rest were generic measures of critical thinking not specific to practice reasoning (e.g., Cornell Critical Thinking Test, $N = 4$; California Critical Thinking Skills Test, $N = 3$; Ennis-Weir Critical Thinking Test, $N = 2$).

The Watson-Glaser Critical Thinking Appraisal Test (forms A and B) are two parallel forms of a multiple-choice test to assess the following critical thinking dimensions: (a) Inference (discriminating among degrees of truth or untruth of inferences), (b) Recognition of Assumptions, Deduction, Interpretation (weighing evidence and deciding whether generalizations based on the given data are warranted), and (c) Evaluating Arguments. Eighty items are included, and a total score is derived from five subscales. The Watson-Glaser (1980) can be machine scored and has norms for ninth grade through college. Its Spearman-Brown split-half reliability ranges from .69 to .85, and alternate forms reliability is .75 (Watson & Glaser, 1980, p. 10). See the earlier discussion by Beck et al. (1992) regarding validity.

The Cornell Critical Thinking Test Level Z is a multiple-choice test of general thinking skills that asks respondents to choose among three possible answers for each item (Ennis & Millman, 1985). Its 50 items concern interpretation, analysis, evaluation, and inference. Frisby (1992) reports a split-half internal consistency of .74 to .80 and differences found across ability levels.

Facione and Facione developed the California Critical Thinking Skills Test (CCTST) and the California Critical Thinking Disposition Inventory (CCTDI) (Facione & Facione, 1993; Facione, Facione, & Sanchez, 1994). The definition of *critical thinking* used was based on a 46-member Delphi panel consensus (Facione, 1990a). The test includes 34 multiple-choice items distributed across five areas: interpretation, analysis, evaluation, inference, and explanation. Bondy, Koenigseder, Ishee, and Williams (2001) report poor stability for this measure. Facione (1990c) reported a positive correlation between scores on this test and student-related indicators of academic ability and success, such as grade point average and SAT scores.

The Ennis-Weir Critical Thinking Essay Test (Ennis & Weir, 1985) consists of a brief nine-paragraph essay that asks respondents to react, paragraph by paragraph, within a time limit of 40 minutes and includes a key for scoring each paragraph. The nine paragraphs concern the following: getting the point, seeing the reasons for assumptions, seeing other possibilities, responding appropriately to and/or avoiding equivocation, irrelevance, circularity, reversal of if-then, the straw man fallacy, overgeneralizing, excessive skepticism, credibility problems, and the use of emotive language. Ennis and Weir (1985, p. 2) report interrater reliability of .86 and .82 on two trials. In conducting a randomized controlled trial of a critical thinking program for faculty at a university, Gibbs, Browne, and Keeley (1989) corroborated Ennis-Weir's reliabilities (Pearson $r = .86$).

SOME EVALUATIONS OF CRITICAL THINKING IN SOCIAL WORK

At present, other than those in Table 22.1, we know of no measures of critical thinking specific to social work practice, but evaluations of critical thinking have been done in social work. Plath, English, Connors, and Beveridge (1999) did a pretest–posttest of a 32-hour, 4-week block of instruction in an MSW program ($N = 19$ students). Measures included the Cornell Critical Thinking Test, Ennis-Weir Essay Test, and a "self-appraisal measure" (open-ended questions about their definition of critical thinking and its application to their practice). Plath and her colleagues suggest that "while these measures cannot test outcomes in terms of actions and social work practice, what they do test is a number of components of decision-making" (p. 208). Huff's (2000) pretest–posttest of 62 MSW students who participated in a policy course showed improvement on the California Critical Thinking Skills Test at posttest. Whyte (1998) did a Solomon Four Group randomized design to evaluate effects of a critical thinking game on PRIDE1 and PTF scores (see Table 22.1). His subjects were 136 MSW students in research classes. He found positive effects.

SOME MEASURES SPECIFIC TO CLINICAL REASONING

Space limits what we can say here, but measures of clinical reasoning have been developed to fill a need for measures specific to it. Elstein et al. (1978) were among the first to recognize this need. They found that the subject's knowledge concerning a particular medical problem, not general problem-solving skills, related to effective performance. Luck and Peabody (2002) investigated the use of standardized patients to assess physicians' practice. This was a validation study using audio recordings involving 144 randomly selected consenting physicians in four primary care clinics in California. Videotaped recordings were made of 40 visits, one per standardized patient. Agreement between standardized patients' checklists and independent assessments of audio recordings was 91%. The authors concluded: "Properly trained standardized patients compare well with independent assessment of recordings of the consultations and they justified their use as a 'gold standard' in comparing the quality of care across sites or evaluating data obtained from other sources such as medical records and clinical vignettes" (p. 679). Glassman, Luck, O'Gara, and Peabody (2000) reviewed the literature describing use of standardized patients in measuring quality of care. They identified five important issues: (a) developing scenarios, (b) selecting exclusion criteria, (c) standardizing patient (actor) training, (d) creating subterfuges, and (e) assuring reliability and validity of measures. They found that standardized patients could accurately assess physician practice by using evidence-based criteria. Twenty physicians and 27 actor patients were involved in assessing care, using eight clinical cases divided into five clinical domains. To our knowledge, except for Cobb (1987), social work has not taken advantage of the use of standardized clients to assess practice skills. Neville, Cunnington, and Norman (1997) developed a clinical reasoning exercise for use in the problem-based curriculum consisting of short cases that can be used both in oral and written examination format. Fritsche, Greenhalgh, Falck-Ytter, Neumayer, and Kunz (2002) have developed a multiple-choice questionnaire designed to evaluate skills and knowledge in evidence-based practice. Theirs is the first study to offer reliability and validity data concerning related skills and knowledge. Other tests of skills in evidence-based medicine have attempted to assess students' abilities in formulating questions, searching, and quantitative understanding (see Smith et al., 2000). White et al. (1997) found that self-assessment is not a good guide to clinical competence. In a study involving 165 medical students, who completed a clinical assessment examination after an internship and then were asked to rate their performance on a scale ranging from 1 (extremely poor) to 5 (extremely well), they reported correlations that varied from −.49 to .94, with an overall correlation of .34 for the class between actual performance and self-assessments of performance.

FIVE MEASURES DESCRIBED IN GIBBS (2003) AND GIBBS AND GAMBRILL (1999)

Ideally, a measure of reasoning critically about practice should accurately reflect the realities of practice and should be accessible, cheap, and reliably scored. The following five measures are designed to assess critical thinking in social work practice and related helping professions. We describe these measures in Table 22.1 relative to these criteria. None of these measures have been compared to quality of decisions made in real-life practice situations. This remains to be explored.

SUMMARY

Because practitioners' reasoning affects what they say and do to help their clients, studying practitioners' reasoning assumes great importance. Assessing the relationship between critical thinking and the quality of professional decision making has generated much interest; however, many measures, although applied to practice reasoning, have not been developed specifically to measure practice reasoning. The health area has led the way in using measures that simulate and use real-life situations. This format has promise as a way to explore decision making in social work. Our brief look at measures to evaluate practice reasoning suggests that measures should be specific to practice situations and real-to-life to contribute to their validity.

TABLE 22.1 Five Measures of Ability to Reason Critically and Scientifically About Practice (Gibbs, 2003; Gibbs & Gambrill, 1999)

Hospital Interactive Team Thinking Test (HITTT)

Description	Recorded on an active neurosciences ward at Luther Hospital in Eau Claire, WI, this interactive CD pauses 10 times to prompt the user to enter a name and definition for any fallacies in reasoning in the dramatization. The CD also defines and illustrates steps in evidence-based practice. Actors portray physicians, social worker, nurse, occupational therapist, patient, and family member. Useful for training these professions.
Availability and cost	Free (if examined for possible use as text) enclosed in the back cover of Gibbs, L. (2003). *Evidence-Based Practice for the Helping Professions: A Practical Guide with Integrated Multimedia*. Pacific Grove, CA: Brooks/Cole–Thomson Learning. Call 1-800-354-9706 or http://www.brookscole.com/
Time required to administer	Twenty-one minutes, plus 10 or 20 minutes for responses, depending on whether respondents get 1 or 2 minutes for each response. The pauses on the CD are automatic. A videotape may become available that follows script in the instructors' manual; this videotape could be paused.
Materials required	For groups, use a computer with CD-ROM player and sound plus a data projector with sound and screen; for individuals, just use computer with CD player and sound (the program creates a file of answers for scoring). For groups via videotape (if it becomes available), you will need the instructors' manual with HITTT script and pauses, a remote control for VCR, the book's answer sheets, and scoring key.
Validity	Fallacy items are documented with clinical reasoning and informal logic literature in Chapter 2 of *Evidence-Based Practice for the Helping Professions* and elsewhere (Gambrill, 1990; Gibbs, 1991; Gibbs & Gambrill, 1999). We have no norms for this measure. We have no data correlating performance on this measure with quality of decision making in practice. This remains to be explored.
Reliability	All interrater reliability checks in Methods of Social Work Research course labs at University of Wisconsin–Eau Claire with less than 10 minutes of training for raters: December 2000, $N = 15$, $r = .53$ (with outlier score of nauseated student), .80 (without outlier score); October 2001, $N = 21$, $r = .83$; February 12, 2002, $N = ?$, $r = .32, .71, .96$; October 19, 2002, Lab 1, $N = 12$, $r = .95$, $p < .000$; Lab 2, $N = 9$, $r = .73$, $p < .029$; Lab 3, $N = 12$, $r = .77$, $p < 004$.

Courtroom Interactive Testimony Thinking Test

Description	Recorded in Judge Wahl's courtroom at the Eau Claire County Courthouse, this interactive CD pauses 7 times to prompt the user to name and to define fallacies or no fallacy in reasoning. The CD also demonstrates principles of effective testimony by contrasting ineffective testimony versus effective testimony. Actors portray a judge, defense attorney, district attorney, expert witnesses (social worker, psychologist, probation and parole agent), and defendant.
Availability and cost	Same as HITTT above.
Time required to administer	Fifteen minutes, plus 7 or 14 minutes for responses, depending on whether respondents get 1 or 2 minutes for each response. The pauses on the CD are automatic, and a file is made for scoring the respondent's answers. A videotape may become available that follows the script in the instructors' manual; this videotape could be paused according to the script as a measure.

Materials required	See HITTT above.
Validity	See HITTT above.
Reliability	All interrater reliability checks in Methods of Social Work Research course labs at University of Wisconsin–Eau Claire with less than 10 minutes of training for raters: April 15, 1999, $N = 2$ (rating 17 responses), $r = .89$; April 15, 1999, $N = 6$ raters, $r = .52$; April 15, 1999, $N = 7$ raters (24 responses), $r = .77$; November 19, 2002, $N = 21$ raters paired, $r = .83$.

Multidisciplinary Interactive Team Thinking Test (MITTT)

Description	Recorded in a classroom at Lowes Creek School in Eau Claire, this interactive CD pauses nine times to prompt the user to name and to define fallacies or no fallacy in reasoning. The CD also demonstrates group dynamics in a school's individual education plan team meeting. Actors portray an IEP team leader (social worker), school psychologist, school nurse, occupational therapist, physical therapist, and speech therapist.
Availability and cost	Same as HITTT.
Time required to administer	Ten minutes, plus 9 or 18 minutes for responses, depending on whether respondents get 1 or 2 minutes for each response. The pauses on the CD are automatic and record the user's responses on a file. A videotape may become available that follows the script in the instructors' manual; this videotape could be paused according to the script as a measure.
Materials required	See HITTT.
Validity	See HITTT.
Reliability	All interrater reliability checks in Methods of Social Work Research course labs at University of Wisconsin–Eau Claire with less than 15 minutes of training for raters: Fall 1998, lab member paired to right, my rating, paired to left, $r = .81$, .84, and .85, respectively; November 7, 1999, $N = 29$, $r = .72$; spring 1999 in three labs, $N = 11$, 11, and ? respectively, $r = .67$, .80, and .64; April 13, 2000, three labs, $r = .73$, .16, and .93.

Principles of Inference, Decision Making, Evaluation 1 (PRIDE1)

Description	PRIDE1 tests a practitioner's ability to avoid being taken in by human service propaganda. This measure relies on a vivid filmed description of a delinquency prevention program at Rahway Prison in New Jersey that was run by inmates there. The measure tests whether a practitioner would recommend adopting the program based purely on the propagandistic argument and whether the respondent can identify elements of propaganda.
Availability and cost	There are three components of the measure: (a) items found in Gibbs, L., & Gambrill, E. (1999); (b) instructions for administration and scoring in the instructors' manual for this book; (c) videotape available at http://www.amazon.com under *Scared Straight*, Peter Falk, VHS, $89.
Time required to administer	The VHS videotape takes 52 minutes. Respondents can be given 10 to 15 minutes to record their answers to three questions.
Materials required	The VHS videotape, two sheets of 8.5 × 11 lined paper (one for answers and one for notes), questions from the exercise in Gibbs and Gambrill (pp. 65–70), and scoring instructions (in the instructors' manual) are all the materials required.

(continued)

TABLE 22.1 (*Continued*)

Validity	Criteria for scoring answers to question 3 reflect critical thinking and informal logic literature. On the face of it, the *Scared Straight* video stands at the polar opposite of scientific reasoning as an argument regarding treatment effectiveness. PRIDE1 score was not statistically significantly correlated with knowledge of research concepts, suggesting that research knowledge does not protect students from propagandistic appeals (Gibbs et al., 1995). Whyte (1998) has tested the effects of critical thinking training on PRIDE1 and PTF scores with positive results.
Reliability	Two undergraduate research assistants independently scored students in graduate and undergraduate research classes in social work and psychology with these results: $r = .96$, $N = 19$; $r = .89$, $N = 17$; $r = .83$, $N = 18$; $r = .87$, $N = 35$; $r = .90$, $N = 26$ (Gibbs et al., 1995).

Professional Thinking Form (PTF)

Description	The PTF is a paper-and-pencil measure. PTF presents 25 brief vignettes from practice in many helping professions. Each vignette may or may not contain a fallacy in reasoning. The respondent is instructed to react to each item from the standpoint of critical thinking and to state what is wrong with fallacious items, label the item OK, or label it questionable if uncertain.
Availability and cost	PTF's items are in Gibbs, L., & Gambrill, E. (1999). Scoring instructions are in the instructors' manual for this workbook. The text may be available on an examination copy basis from the publisher. The instructors' manual is free for those adopting the text or from the authors.
Time required to administer	Respondents take approximately 30 minutes to write their responses to all 25 items. Scoring takes about 5–7 minutes for each respondent's answers, depending on familiarity with the key.
Materials required	This paper-and-pencil measure requires only a copy of the instructions to respondents, 25 vignettes (thirteen 8.5 × 11 pages), and the scoring key.
Validity	The scoring key makes reference to critical thinking, informal logic, and clinical reasoning literature. Most vignettes come from professional practice or from practice literature. We have no norms for this measure.
Reliability	Trials were done to test interrater reliability on responses from nursing students: Gibbs, L. E., & Werner, J. S. (unpublished, 1988). *Integrating Research Into Practice: Measuring Ability to Detect Common Clinicians' Fallacies.* University of Wisconsin–Eau Claire; Pearson $r = .89$, $p < .0001$, $N = 21$ for total test score. Spearman's Rho for earlier 20-item version ranged from .46 to .99 for items, mean Rho $= .78$, SD $= .13$; second trial $r = .89$, $p < .0001$, $N = 31$, items Rho ranged from .65 to .95, with mean Rho $= .80$, SD $= .08$.

References

Baron, J. (2000). *Thinking and deciding* (3rd ed.). New York: Cambridge University Press.

Beck, S. E., Bennett, A., McLeod, R., & Molyneaux, D. (1992). Review of research on critical thinking in nursing education. In L. R. Allen (Ed.), *Review of research in nursing education* (pp. 1–30). New York: National League of Nursing.

Bondy, K. N., Koenigseder, L. A., Ishee, J. H., & Wil-

liams, B. G. (2001). Psychometric properties of the California Critical Thinking Tests. *Journal of Nursing Measurement, 9,* 309–328.

Cobb, N. H. (1987) Analysis of judgments in psychosocial and behavioral casework (Doctoral dissertation, University of California, Berkeley, 1987). *Dissertation Abstracts International, 48*(5-A), 1317.

Deterding, R., Kamin, C., Barley, G., Adams, L., Dwinnell, B., & Merenstein, G. (1999). Effects of a longitudinal course on student performance in clerkships. *Archives of Pediatric and Adolescent Medicine, 153,* 755–760.

Elstein, A., Shulman, L. S., Sprafka, S. A., Allal, L., Gordon, M., Jason, H., et al. (1978). *Medical problem solving: An analysis of clinical reasoning.* Cambridge, MA: Harvard University Press.

Ennis, R. H., & Millman, J. (1985). *Cornell Critical Thinking Test Level Z.* Pacific Grove, CA: Midwest.

Ennis, R. H., & Weir, E. (1985). *The Ennis-Weir critical thinking tests.* Pacific Grove, CA: Midwest Publications.

Facione, N. C., Facione, P. A., & Sanchez, M. A. (1994). Critical thinking disposition as a measure of competent clinical judgment: The development of the California Critical Thinking Disposition Inventory. *Journal of Nursing Education, 33*(8), 345–350.

Facione, P. A. (1990a). *Technical report #1: CCTST experimental validation and content validity.* East Lansing, MI: National Center for Research on Teacher Learning. (ERIC Document Reproduction Service No. ED 327 549.)

Facione, P. A. (1990b). *Executive summary of critical thinking: A statement of expert consensus for purposes of educational assessment and instruction, the "Delphi Report."* Millbrae, CA: California Academic Press.

Facione, P. A. (1990c). *Technical report #2: Factors predictive of CT skills.* East Lansing, MI: National Center for Research on Teacher Learning. (ERIC Document Reproduction Service No. ED 327 550).

Facione, P. A., & Facione, N. C. (1993). *Test manual: The California critical thinking skills test, form A and form B* (2nd ed.). Millbrae, CA: California Academic Press.

Frisby, C. L. (1992). Construct validity and psychometric properties of the Cornell Critical Thinking Test (Level Z): A contrasted group analysis. *Psychological Reports, 71,* 291–303.

Fritsche, L., Greenhalgh, T., Falck-Ytter, Y., Neumayer, H.-H., & Kunz, R. (2002). Do short courses in evidence based medicine improve knowledge and skills? Validation of Berlin questionnaire and before and after study of courses in evidence based medicine. *British Medical Journal, 325,* 1338–1341.

Gambrill, E. (1990). *Critical thinking in clinical practice.* (2nd ed.). San Francisco: Jossey-Bass.

Gibbs, L., (1991). *Scientific reasoning for social workers.* New York: Macmillan.

Gibbs, L. (2003). *Evidence-based practice for the helping professions.* Pacific Grove, CA: Brooks/Cole–Thomson Learning.

Gibbs, L., & Gambrill, E. (1999). *Critical thinking for social workers: Exercises for the helping professions.* Thousand Oaks, CA: Pine Forge.

Gibbs, L., Gambrill, E., Blakemore, J., Begun, A., Kensington, A., Peden, B., et al. (1995). A measure of critical thinking about practice. *Research on Social Work Practice, 5*(2), 193–204.

Gibbs, L. E., Browne, M. N., & Keeley, S. M. (1989). Critical thinking: A study's outcome. *Journal of Professional Studies, 13*(1), 44–59.

Glassman, P. A., Luck, J., O'Gara, E. M., & Peabody, J. W. (2000). Using standardized patients to measure quality: Evidence from the literature and a prospective study. *Joint Commission Journal of Quality Improvement, 26,* 644–653.

Hastie, R., & Dawes, R. M. (2001). *Rational choice in an uncertain world: The psychology of judgment and decision making.* Thousand Oaks, CA: Sage.

Huff, M. T. (2000). A comparison study of live instruction versus interactive television for teaching MSW students critical thinking skills. *Research on Social Work Practice, 10*(4), 400–416.

Luck, J., & Peabody, J. W. (2002). Using standardized patients to measure physicians' practice: Validation study using audio recordings. *British Medical Journal, 325,* 679–683.

Neville, A. J., Cunnington, J. P. W., & Norman, G. R. (1997). Development of clinical reasoning exercises in a problem-based curriculum. In A. J. Scherpbier, C. P. van der Vleuten, J. J. Rethans, & A. F. van der Steeg (Eds.), *Advances in medical education* (pp. 377–379). Dordrecht: Kluwer Academic Publishers.

Nickerson, R. S. (1986). *Reflections on reasoning.* Hillsdale, NJ: Erlbaum.

Nisbett, R., & Ross, L. (1980). *Human inference: Strategies and shortcomings of social judgment.* Englewood Cliffs, NJ: Prentice-Hall.

Norris, S. P., & Ennis, R. H. (1989). *Evaluating critical thinking.* Pacific Grove, CA: Critical Thinking Press Software.

Plath, D., English, B., Connors, L., & Beveridge, A. (1999). Evaluating the outcomes of intensive critical thinking for social work students. *Social Work Education, 18*(2), 207–217.

Smith, C. A., Ganschow, P. S., Reilly, B. M., Evans, A. T., McNutt, R. A., Osei, A., et al. (2000). Teaching residents evidence-based medicine skills: A controlled trial of effectiveness and assessment of durability. *Journal of Internal Medicine, 15*(10), 710–715.

Tousignant, M., & DesMarchais, J. E. (2002). Accuracy of student self-assessment ability compared to their own performance in a problem-based learning medical program: A correlation study. *Advances in Health Sciences Education, 7,* 19–27.

Watson, G., & Glaser, E. M. (1980). *Watson-Glaser critical thinking appraisal manual.* San Antonio, TX: Psychological Corporation.

White, C., Fitzgerald, J. T., Davis, W. K., Gruppen, L. D., Regehr, G., McQuillan, et al. (1997). Medical students' ability to self assess knowledge and skill levels: Findings from one class of seniors. In A. J. Scherpbier, C. P. van der Vleuten, J. J. Rethans, & A. F. van der Steeg (Eds.), *Advances in medical education* (pp. 395–396). Dordrecht: Kluwer Academic Publishers.

Whyte, D. T. (1998). The effect of an educational unit on the critical thinking skills of social work students. Unpublished doctoral dissertation, College of Social Work, University of South Carolina.

TASK-CENTERED PRACTICE

23   *An Exemplar of Evidence-Based Practice*

William J. Reid & Anne E. Fortune

The task-centered model (TC) is a short-term, problem-solving approach to social work practice (Doel & Marsh, 1992; Reid, 1992, 2000; Reid & Epstein, 1972; Reid & Fortune, 2002). Originally designed for practice with individuals and families, the model has been adapted for work with groups (Fortune, 1985; Garvin, 1974) and larger systems (Tolson, Reid, & Garvin, 2003).

THE DEVELOPMENT OF TC AS A RESEARCH-BASED FORM OF PRACTICE

The task-centered approach was developed as a form of research-based practice. It originated from a randomized experiment conducted in the mid-1960s that suggested that brief intervention might provide a more efficient means of helping individuals and families with many problems than conventional, long-term forms of practice (Reid & Shyne, 1969). Using that brief service approach as a starting point, Reid and Epstein (1972) collaborated on developing a more comprehensive, systematic, and effective model of short-term intervention. The research orienta-

tion of the model was expressed in several ways. Preference was to be given to methods and theories tested and supported by empirical research. Hypotheses and concepts about the client system were to be grounded in case data obtained through such means as client self-report, observation, and rapid assessment instruments. Speculative theorizing about the client's problems and behavior was to be avoided. Assessment, process, and outcome data were to be systematically collected and recorded for each case. This conception fits well with current definitions of evidence-based practice (Thyer, 2001).

The intent was to create an approach to practice that would evolve in response to continuing research and to developments in research-based knowledge and technology consonant with its basic principles. The model was designed to be an open, pluralistic practice system that would integrate theoretical and technical contributions from diverse sources. In keeping with this design, the model did not adopt a particular theory of human functioning or any fixed set of intervention methods. Rather, it provided a core of values, theory, and methods that could be augmented by compatible approaches.

We launched a program of research that has continued to the present, research to which numerous investigators worldwide have contributed. Early studies suggested that more flexible time limits, 8 to 12 interviews within a 4-month period, may work better than a fixed number of sessions (Reid & Epstein, 1972). A subsequent controlled experiment established the effectiveness of a set of methods in the session for preparing the client to undertake actions or tasks outside the session (Reid, 1975).

Additional controlled experiments have demonstrated the efficacy of the model for treating problems of psychiatric outpatients and children at risk of school failure (Gibbons, Butler, & Bow, 1979; Reid, 1976; Reid & Bailey-Dempsey, 1995; Reid, Epstein, Brown, Tolson, & Rooney, 1980). A number of other studies have shown the model to be promising for work with a variety of other populations, including parents in child welfare settings (Rooney, 1981; Rzepnicki, 1985), delinquents (Larsen & Mitchell), and people who are frail and elderly (Dierking, Brown, & Fortune, 1980; Naleppa & Reid, 1998).

As it has matured, the model has integrated methods from other approaches, notably behavioral, cognitive-behavioral, cognitive, and family structural therapies. The pluralistic, integrative nature of TC enables it to incorporate almost any empirically supported approach that focuses on client action as a means of change. In sum, TC is an evidence-based model in three senses: (a) It is in itself a well-tested model of practice, (b) it provides a framework for incorporating other empirically supported methods, and (c) it makes use of case data as a means of providing feedback to practitioners and clients about progress toward problem resolution.

In the sections to follow, we will summarize the steps of TC as it is used with individuals and families, giving particular attention to the use of evidence-based principles and procedures. Fuller explication of TC for individuals and families, as well as variations for work with groups and other systems, can be found in Tolson, Reid, and Garvin (2003). For a tutorial and a comprehensive bibliography, visit the TC Web site at http://www.task-centered.com.

INITIAL PHASE: PROBLEM EXPLORATION, ASSESSMENT, AND THE SERVICE CONTRACT

Client-acknowledged target problems, usually up to a limit of three, are explored and assessed. If the client is nonvoluntary, the practitioner discloses the reason for the referral and then determines if there are issues the client wants to work on. The social worker's role is to enable the client to express the problem in terms that he or she can comprehend and agree with. Assessment data are obtained on the frequency and severity of the problem for a retrospective baseline period, and current manifestations of the problem are spelled out in specific, measurable terms. Factors that may be contributing to the difficulty are examined collaboratively with the client. The social worker and client also consider resources and strengths that may aid in its resolution. In case management variations (Naleppa & Reid, 2003; Reid & Bailey-Dempsey, 1995), problems may be further explored and assessed by a team consisting of the client(s), the social worker, and others.

The practitioner makes use of research or research-based theory to enhance understanding of the client and his or her problems, as well as to ascertain the most effective means of establishing a therapeutic alliance. For example, in work with a suicidal adolescent, the social worker would make use of empirical knowledge of indicators of suicidal intent (Ivanoff & Reidel, 1995). If the client is a substance abuser "in denial," the social worker, guided by research on reactance (Brehm & Smith, 1986; Rooney, 1992) and engagement of substance abusers (Miller, Andrews, Wilbourne, & Bennett, 1998), would avoid a confrontational approach and make clear that the client had a choice about whether to accept treatment.

The client and practitioner form a revisable service contract that covers the problems to be addressed, the kind of intervention to be used, the number of sessions, and the duration of service. Research on the relative efficacy of planned short-term treatment for a wide range of problems has been an important source of evidence in the use of TC (Bloom, 2000). An effort is made to discriminate between those problems for which there is empirical support for use of brief service (e.g., Reid & Shyne, 1969) and those for which there is not, for example, the adjustment problems of persons with schizophrenia (Hogarty et al., 1997).

From its beginnings, TC has encouraged sharing of information with clients, a characteristic of the model that fits well with the emphasis in evidence-based practice on involving clients as informed decision makers (Gambrill, in press). In using TC the social worker shares with the client evidence that might be important to consider in collaborative decisions concerning the service contract. For example, if the client presented with a problem of chronic grief, the social worker might suggest, as one option, the use of "guided mourning" (Artelt & Thyer, 1998). The social worker would then inform the client about the nature of the intervention, especially its use of sustained exposure to grief-invoking stimuli, which might cause the client some discomfort, and discuss evidence about its effectiveness (which is largely positive). Other options, and evidence for them, would also be considered. The final decision about what option to use would be the client's.

The baseline characteristics of each of the client's problems are recorded on a target problem schedule. Progress on each problem is recorded weekly. Additional assessment data may be obtained through rapid assessment instruments, structured observation, and client self-monitoring devices.

MIDDLE PHASE: TASK PLANNING AND IMPLEMENTATION

The core of TC is helping clients select and carry out tasks that address their problems. A key intervention is the task planning and implementation sequence (TPIS), a set of systematic procedures designed to facilitate the client's task work. The client is helped to select a task, plan it in appropriate detail, anticipate any obstacles to its implementation, and rehearse or practice it, if indicated. Tasks that are successful in alleviating the client's problem are repeated; those that are less successful may be revised or replaced. Frequently, however, it is more strategic to resolve obstacles preventing task accomplishment than to change the task. Thus another major emphasis in the model involves the resolution of obstacles. In this process a variety of methods may be used, including practitioner intervention in the environment (if the obstacle is

external) or cognitive-restructuring or insight-oriented techniques (if the obstacle is internal).

The use of an evidence-based approach is incorporated into task selection. Tasks are developed collaboratively with the client (rather than "assigned"). Both clients and practitioners suggest ideas for tasks. In making their suggestions, practitioners give first priority to possible client actions that have research support. This process is facilitated by using task planners, which provide menus of client tasks for a wide variety of clinical problems. One such resource is Reid (2000), which contains task planners for more than 100 frequently encountered problems. Task planners have been developed for specific populations, such as frail elderly people (Naleppa & Reid, 2003) and families receiving temporary financial assistance (TANF) (Reid & Kenaley, 2001). Task planners incorporate empirically supported tasks when such tasks can be located. For example, in a task planner on problems of anger control in children, tasks such as use of self-verbalizations to control angry reactions were drawn from empirically supported cognitive-behavioral programs, with a brief summary of the research support for these programs.

The extraction of tasks from such programs rather than the use of the entire program raises some issues because the evidence of effectiveness applies to the program and not to specific components. However, the extracted tasks are part of an effective program, which gives them priority over tasks lacking any research evidence. Moreover, in practice, social workers usually do not have access to full intervention protocols and, even when they do, are selective in what they draw from them (Richey & Roffman, 1999). Task planners are only one source of evidence-based tasks. Practitioners may have other research-based knowledge or can search for it by using information retrieval procedures, such as those outlined by Gibbs (2002). Most empirically supported interventions are compatible with a task-centered framework.

Once the client has agreed to a task, the details of its implementation are planned. Collaboration between practitioner and client continues in the planning process. The result should be a task plan that is customized to fit the client's abilities, one that should result in progress toward problem alleviation but is not so difficult as to make success unlikely. Possible obstacles to the plan are then considered through "what if" questions. For example, Jon agrees to ask his partner to help him remain sober. The practitioner might ask, "What if she starts to lecture you about your drinking?" Such questions enable the client to anticipate complications that might occur in carrying out the task and to develop ways of handling them.

When appropriate, tasks are rehearsed and practiced in the session through role plays or in vivo exercises. The latter are used extensively in work with couples and families and may take the form of in-session problem solving, communication training, or conflict resolution. Essentially, clients interact, with the practitioner serving as a facilitator. Such tasks draw on evidence-based methods tested in a range of couples and family programs (Robin, Bedway, & Gilroy, 1994; Stern, 1999).

In-session work on tasks (including those involving couple or family interaction) is then followed by clients' implementation in their life situations. Each task is reviewed in the session following its attempt. Progress is recorded on a 4-point task review scale, which specifies if the task has been completely, substantially, partially, or not achieved. The scale may be completed by the practitioner, the client, or both together. This scale, and the one measuring problem change, provides both practitioner and client with a record of progress on each task and its related problem. The information can be used as a guide to case evaluation and planning. When aggregated across cases, the data can provide insight into the relative success of the model with different types of problems and shed light on which types of tasks work best for particular kinds of problems (Reid, 1994). The model's emphasis on tracking problems and tasks also lends itself to the use of case data in agency information systems (Benbenishty & Ben-Zaken, 1988).

Task reviews may identify obstacles preventing task accomplishment. The obstacles may then become the focus of intervention. In helping clients analyze and resolve obstacles, social workers may, as noted, make use of a wide variety of methods. Again, preference is given to those with empirical support. A well-tested method for internalized obstacles is cognitive restructuring (Kuehlwein, 1998). The obstacle is first identified as occurring within the client's cognitive functioning. Through the practi-

tioner's questioning and comments, cognitive distortions are clarified, and the client is helped to develop more functional cognitions. Thus Tom was unable to complete his task of using his wheelchair in a public place because he didn't want others pitying him. Cognitive restructuring helped him to see that people might not necessarily view him that way, given the positive images in the media of people in wheelchairs (e.g., athletes completing in special Olympics) and that he might apply those images to himself. External obstacles may involve individuals in the client's social network, organizations, or lack of resources, among other possibilities. Use is made of the modest research literature on interventions addressed to the client's environment, including research on task-centered methods of linkage (Weissman, 1977), advocacy (Fellin & Brown, 1989), and case management (Madden, Hicks-Coolick, & Kirk, 2002; Naleppa & Reid, 1998).

In TC, methods used to help clients overcome obstacles, whether internal or external, are centered on helping them move ahead with tasks. In this way TC can draw on a wide range of interventions while still maintaining focus on the client's actions as a means of problem resolution.

Practitioners as well as clients can take on tasks to effect changes in the client's environment. Calling such activities *tasks* provides a concrete expression of the collaborative nature of the relationship—both client and practitioner have tasks and are accountable to each other for carrying them out. When a case management team is used, all members, including service providers and peers, may take on tasks.

TERMINATION

The termination phase takes place in the last session or last two sessions. The client and practitioner review changes in target problems and the client's overall problem situation, identify successful problem-solving strategies, discuss ways of maintaining and generalizing client gains, and consider strategies for resolving remaining problems. In some cases, there may be need for further service. If the client requests further help and there is reason to suppose that additional progress can be made, extensions are normally made, usually for time-limited periods, to accomplish specific goals. The client's feelings about the loss of a relationship are dealt with, but these are less likely to occur in short-term than in long-term treatment (Fortune, 2002). The evidentiary base of work in the termination phase includes studies of client reactions to termination (Fortune, 1987; Fortune, Pearlingi, & Rochelle, 1992), of the role of treatment duration on outcome (Howard, Kopta, Krause, & Orlinsky, 1986), and of methods of promoting maintenance and generalization (Karoly & Steffen, 1980; Luiselli, 1998).

CASE ILLUSTRATION

Josie, age 12, was referred by her English teacher to an agency-based case management TC program serving a middle school. Josie was failing English and math and was frequently truant. Initial interviews with the child and her parents were held to explore the problem and develop a tentative service contract. The service typically consisted of meetings with a case management team and concurrent family sessions. The child and parents decided who was to be on the team. In Josie's case, the team was Josie, the social worker, Sarah (Josie's mother, a single parent), Josie's math teacher, and a peer who was not in difficulty in school. Josie and Sarah agreed to work on the problems of Josie's poor academic performance and attendance. In addition, another problem was identified: conflict between Josie and Sarah about Josie's friends (most of whom Sarah considered to be a bad influence).

The TC case management program was developed through a systematic program of studies that began with preliminary tests of the model and culminated in a randomized trial (Bailey-Dempsey & Reid, 1996). In that trial, families assigned to the case management program ($N = 33$) surpassed families assigned to a no treatment control ($N = 38$) and to an alternative monetary incentives condition ($N = 41$) (Reid & Bailey-Dempsey, 1995).

After preparatory interviews with the referring teacher and the math teacher selected for Josie's team, the initial case management team meeting was held. In conducting the session, the social worker used guidelines developed through a process study of case management meetings (Reid & Bailey-Dempsey, 1994). In this and subsequent (twice-monthly) meetings, the team worked together to understand the basis for Jo-

sie's problems and to develop possible solutions. Team members undertook tasks to implement the solutions. For example, because Josie had difficulty communicating with her English teacher, the math teacher on the team agreed to talk to the English teacher about a plan for Josie to make up work in that class. Josie and Sarah agreed to set up a structured homework program for both the English and math classes. The peer on the team (who lived close to Josie) agreed to the task of going to Josie's home in the morning and riding with her on the bus, as a way of helping her avoid the temptation to cut classes. Elements of the TPIS were used to help participants formulate and plan the tasks.

Between the case management meetings, the social worker met with Josie and Sarah. The structured homework task had gone well for a few days but broke down after Josie and Sarah began to quarrel over Josie's taking calls from friends and "spending her homework time gabbing." Such interruptions of Josie's homework were taken up as an obstacle to the task. After some discussion, Josie agreed to let her mother answer the phone during her homework period and advise callers that Josie would call them back. A task relating to the truancy problem (suggested by *The Task Planner* [Reid, 2000]) was developed and planned with Josie and her mother. Josie contracted with Sarah that she would miss no more than one class during the week. If Josie was able to do this, Sarah would allow her to choose the programs they would watch on TV during the weekend. Finally, the conflict concerning Josie's friends was worked on through in-session problem solving by Josie and Sarah. With the social worker's help, they worked out an agreement. Josie would stop seeing the individual that Sarah objected to the most, but in exchange Sarah would stop nagging Josie about her other friends and would allow her to invite them over. The agreement was used as a basis for tasks that they both carried out during the following week.

The practitioner worked with Josie and Sarah over a 14-week period (until the end of the school year). The final assessment of the three problems they had worked on was based on client self-report and school records and summarized on 10-point scales. Josie was able to raise her grades in math and English at least to a passing level, and her attendance improved moderately. The conflict between Josie and Sarah over Josie's friends had been largely resolved, and their relationship was on the whole better. Assessment of their overall situation revealed no new problems in other areas.

The case can be considered successful in that all three target problems showed improvement, accompanied by positive contextual change (e.g., the improved mother–daughter relationship). Findings from controlled studies can be used to help evaluate progress in such cases. Thus the limited improvement in grades and attendance becomes more significant, given evidence that untreated children at risk of failure are likely to show declines on such measures (Reid & Bailey-Dempsey, 1995).

References

Artelt, T. A., & Thyer, B. A. (1998). Treating chronic grief. In B. A. Thyer & J. S. Wodarski (Eds.), *Handbook of empirical social work practice: Vol. 1* (pp. 341–356). New York: Wiley.

Bailey-Dempsey, C., & Reid, W. J. (1996). Intervention design and development: A case study. *Research on Social Work Practice, 6*(2), 208–228.

Benbenishty, R., & Ben-Zaken, A. (1988). Computer-aided process of monitoring task-centered family interventions. *Social Work Research and Abstracts, 24,* 7–9.

Bloom, B. L. (2002). Planned short-term psychotherapies. In C. R. Snyder & R. E. Ingram (Eds.), *Handbook of psychological change* (pp. 429–454). New York: Wiley.

Brehm, S., & Smith, T. (1986). Social psychological approaches to psychotherapy and behavior change. In S. L. Garfield & A. E. Bergin (Eds.), *Handbook of psychotherapy and behavior change* (pp. 69–116). New York: Wiley.

Dierking, B., Brown, M., & Fortune, A. E. (1980). Task-centered treatment in a residential facility for the elderly: A clinical trial. *Journal of Gerontological Social Work, 2,* 225–240.

Fellin, P., & Brown, K. S. (1989). Application of homelessness to teaching social work foundation content. *Journal of Teaching in Social Work, 3*(1), 17–33.

Fortune, A. E. (1987). Grief only? Client and social worker reactions to termination. *Clinical Social Work Journal, 15*(2), 159–171.

Fortune, A. E. (2002). Terminating with clients. In A. R. Roberts & G. J. Greene (Eds.), *Social workers' desk reference* (pp. 458–463) New York: Oxford University Press.

Fortune, A. E., Pearlingi, B., & Rochelle, C. (1992). Reactions to termination of individual treatment. *Social Work, 37*(2), 171–178.

Gambrill, E. (2000). Evidence-based practice: Implications for knowledge development and use in social work. In A. Rosen & E. Proctor (Eds.), *Developing practice guidelines for social work intervention: Issues, methods, and research agenda.* New York: Columbia University Press.

Gibbons, J., Butler, J., & Bow, I. (1979). Task-centered casework with marital problems. *British Journal of Social Work, 8,* 393–409.

Gibbs, L. E. (2003). *Practice for the helping professions.* Pacific Grove, CA: Brooks/Cole.

Hogarty, G., Greenwald, D., Ulrich, R., Kornblith, S., DiBarry, A., Cooley, S., et al. (1997). Three-year trials of personal therapy among schizophrenic patients living with or independent of family. *American Journal of Psychiatry, 154,* 1514–1524.

Howard, K. I., Kopta, S. M., Krause, M. S., & Orlinsky, D. E. (1986). The dose-effect relationship in psychotherapy. *American Psychologist 41,* 159–164.

Ivanoff, A., & Riedel, M. (1995). Suicide. In R. Edwards et al. (Eds.), *Encyclopedia of social work* (19th ed., pp. 2358–2372). Washington, DC: NASW Press.

Karoly, P., & Steffen, J. J. (Eds.). (1980). *Improving the long-term effects of psychotherapy: Models of durable outcome.* New York: Gardner.

Kuehlwein, K. T. (1998). The cognitive therapy model. In R. Dorfman (Ed.), *Paradigms of clinical social work: Vol. 2* (pp. 125–148). New York: Brunner/Mazel.

Luiselli, J. K. (1998). Maintenance of behavioral interventions. *Mental Health Aspects of Developmental Disabilities, 1*(3), 69–76.

Madden, L. L., Hicks-Coolick, A., & Kirk, A. B. (2002). An empowerment model for social welfare consumers. *Lippincott's Case Management, 7,* 129–136.

Miller, W. R., Andrews, N. R., Wilbourne, P., & Bennett, M. E. (1998). A wealth of alternatives. In W. R. Miller & N. Heather (Eds.), *Treating addictive behaviors* (pp. 203–216). New York: Plenum Press.

Naleppa, M. J., & Reid, W. J. (1998). Task-centered case management for the elderly: Developing a practice model. *Research on Social Work Practice, 8,* 63–85.

Naleppa, M., & Reid, W. J. (2003). *Gerontological social work: A task-centered approach.* New York: Columbia University Press.

Reid, W. J. (1975). A test of a task-centered approach. *Social Work, 20,* 3–9.

Reid, W. J. (1994). Field testing and data gathering on innovative practice interventions in early development. In J. Rothman & E. J. Thomas (Eds.), *Intervention research* (pp. 245–264). New York: Haworth.

Reid, W. J. (2000) *The task planner.* New York: Columbia University Press.

Reid, W. J., & Bailey-Dempsey, C. (1994). Content analysis in design and development. *Research on Social Work Practice, 4,* 101–114.

Reid, W. J., & Bailey-Dempsey, C. (1995). The effects of monetary incentives on school performance. *Families in Society, 76,* 331–340.

Reid, W. J., & Epstein, L. (Eds.). (1972). *Task-centered casework.* New York: Columbia University Press.

Reid, W. J., Epstein, L., Brown, L. B., Tolson, E. R., & Rooney, R. H. (1980). Task-centered school social work. *Social Work in Education, 2,* 7–24.

Reid, W. J., & Kenaley (2001). *Task planners for TANF families.* Prepared under contract for the Professional Development Program, University at Albany, State University of New York.

Reid, W. J., & Shyne, A. (1969). *Brief and extended casework.* New York: Columbia University Press.

Richey C. A., & Roffman, R. A. (1999). On the sidelines of guidelines: Further thoughts on the fit between clinical guidelines and social work practice. *Research on Social Work Practice, 9,* 311–321.

Robin, A. L., Bedway, M., & Gilroy, M. (1994). Problem-solving communication training. In C. W. LeCroy (Ed.), *Handbook of child and adolescent treatment manuals* (pp. 92–125). New York: Lexington Books.

Rooney, R. H. (1981). A task-centered reunification model for foster care. In A. N. Malluccio & P. A. Sinanoglu (Eds.), *The challenge of partnership: Working with parents of children in foster care* (pp. 101–116) New York: Child Welfare League of America.

Rooney, R. H. (1992). *Strategies for work with involuntary clients.* New York: Columbia University Press.

Rzepnicki, T. L. (1985). Task-centered intervention in foster care services: Working with families who have children in placement. In A. E. Fortune (Ed.), *Task-centered practice with families and groups* (pp. 172–184). New York: Springer.

Stern, S. B. (1999). Anger management in parent-adolescent conflict. *The American Journal of Family Therapy, 27,* 181–193.

Thyer, B. (2002). Principles of evidence-based practice and treatment development. In A. R. Roberts & G. J. Greene (Eds.), *Social workers' desk reference* (pp. 739–747). New York: Oxford University Press.

Tolson, E. R., Reid, W. J., & Garvin, C. D. (2003). *Generalist practice: A task-centered approach.* New York: Columbia University Press.

Weissman, A. (1977). In the steel industry. In W. J. Reid & L. Epstein (Eds.), *Task-centered practice* (pp. 235–241). New York: Columbia University Press.

TREATMENT EVIDENCE IN A NON-EXPERIMENTING PRACTICE ENVIRONMENT

24

Some Recommendations for Increasing Supply and Demand

Michael J. Camasso

Evidence-based practice has become a fashionable theme in contemporary discussions of social work interventions. Gambrill's (1999, 2001) important essays calling for a social work practice built upon a bedrock of empirical research are among the spate of recent publications that feature "evidence-based" or "empirical-based practice" (Corcoran, 2000; Cournoyer & Powers, 2002; Lloyd, 1998; Thyer & Wodarski, 1998; Vandiver, 2002). This is not to say that empirical research has become the sole or even main source that guides client intervention; the broad consensus in social work would appear to indicate otherwise. Evidence-based practice, defined as practice based on empirical studies preappraised for scientific validity and prescreened for clinical relevance (Gambrill, 2001), remains far less common than practice that stems from authority, face validity, practice wisdom, common practice, and the principle of the respectable minority (Beutler, 2000; Gambrill, 1999; Reid, 1997; Rosen, Proctor, Morrow-Howell, & Staudt, 1995).

This paper sets out to answer two questions that need to be addressed if empirically derived, evidence-based social work practice is to flourish:

1. Why has scientific evidence been so slow to penetrate into the profession?
2. How can the generation of scientific evidence and its utilization by practitioners be increased?

To answer the first question, the current supply and demand for empirically based evidence is briefly examined. Increasing the supply and demand for empirically derived evidence is then discussed as a three-pronged initiative: the need for an emphasis on intervention impacts, the widespread use of research designs that can actually detect impacts, and the creation of professional and institutional incentives that can help to ensure the utilization of findings from impact research.

SCIENTIFIC EVIDENCE: SHORT SUPPLY AND LOW DEMAND

Empirical studies in social work that provide clear and convincing proof of an intervention's positive or negative effect on client functioning are indeed rare. Studies that purport to demonstrate scientific validity are required to establish clear, verifiable, and replicable impact estimates (Mohr, 1995; Orr, 1999; Shadish, Cook, & Campbell, 2002). Impact studies establish the marginal change in client functioning caused by program or therapeutic intervention. The crux of impact analysis is a comparison of what happened to the client because of the intervention with what would have happened to the client had the intervention been withheld. How well this latter condition, termed the *counterfactual condition*, is established in an impact study determines to a great extent the amount of scientific validity the impact estimates carry. Impact studies can take one of two forms: effectiveness estimates, where the focus is an overall program impact, and efficacy assessments, where specific intervention activities, implementation strategies, or dosages are assessed (Nathan & Gorman, 2002; Rosenbaum, 2002; Sommer & Zeger, 1991). As Rosenbaum (2002) notes, efficacy is the impact an intervention would have if used the way it was intended to be used, whereas effectiveness is the impact an intervention would have when used in actual practice.

An examination of research texts written by social workers for social work use reveals that the terms *impact, effectiveness and efficacy assessment*, and *counterfactual condition* receive almost no attention (Bloom, Fischer, & Orme, 1999; Grinnell, 1997; Rubin & Babbie, 2001; Unrau, Gabor, & Grinnell, 2001; York, 1998). When the subject of impact is discussed in social work research texts, it is often referred to as *outcome analysis* (Ginsberg, 2001; Unrau, Gabor, & Grinnell, 2001; Yegidis & Weinbach, 2002).

Scientifically validated research on practice efficacy and effectiveness has never been an especially popular topic in social work's professional journals either (Fraser, Taylor, Jackson, & O'Jack, 1991; Tyson, 1995; Yegidis & Weinbach, 2002). Yegidis and Weinbach (2002) and Tyson (1995) cite literature reviews showing that the greatest percentage of published reports on research are reviews and commentaries, reports on surveys, or program implementation studies. The publication of a new professional journal in 1991, *Research on Social Work Practice*, was designed to stimulate the production of scientifically validated practice evidence. In a review I conducted, only about 30% of the nearly 350 articles published from 1991 through the end of 2002 could be classified as studies that produce estimates of intervention impact where *impact* is defined as the marginal or net change in client functioning due to intervention exposure. About 8% of the studies were experiments, and 20% were simple pre–post comparison group studies or other weak quasi-experimental designs.

When the focus of research is on the marginal or net effect of an intervention on a change in client outcome, there is a clear hierarchy among methods, and this has been unambiguously acknowledged in medicine (Agency for Health Care Research, 2002; Sackett, Robin-son, Rosenberg, & Haynes, 1997), psychology (Chambless et al., 1998; Nathan & Gorman, 2002), and occasionally in social work (Thyer, 2002). Based on this work and assessments of broader statistical and social science literature (Rosenbaum, 2002; Rossi, Freeman, & Lipsey, 1999; Shadish, Cook, & Campbell, 2002), the scientific validity of treatment effectiveness and efficacy evidence can be ranked as follows:

Level 1 Proof

This is evidence that results from randomized, prospective experiments or randomized clinical trials (RCTs). This source of evidence uses assignment rules to treatment and counterfactual conditions to ensure that assignment per se is not directly correlated with treatment outcome(s).

Level 2 Proof

Here the evidence is gleaned from observational studies, "natural experiments," or quasi experiments, where assignment rules are unclear, where assignment may be directly correlated with treatment outcome in the absence of any real treatment, but where the selection process itself can be examined and counterfactual inference(s) can be made. Designs that can provide level 2 proof are regression discontinuity, interrupted time series, or panel studies of substantial length, nonequivalent comparison group studies that incorporate internal controls (i.e., cohorts) and statistical adjustments for possible selection.

Level 3 Proof

Observational studies, "natural experiments," case control studies, and weak quasi experiments where assignment may be directly correlated with treatment outcome in the absence of treatment and where the selection process cannot be adequately examined provide level 3 proof. Designs that use external comparison groups, posttest-only comparisons, case control studies, and group or single-subject pre–post studies can provide a great deal of information but are prone to the problems of retrospective recall (case control studies), uncontrolled selection (comparison group designs), and unstable baselines (short pre–post series) that greatly limit inference about the counterfactual condition.

Level 4 Proof

Really no proof of impact at all is provided by level 4 proof. Ex post facto studies, case studies, reviews and commentaries, histories, and opinion papers where inferences about a counterfactual condition are impossible to make except through speculation comprise this level.

Few researchers or practitioners in the profession would disagree that the amount of evidence produced in level 1 or 2 research endeavors is in short supply.

Reviews of studies with meta-analyses or other systematic review systems can also be ranked in an analogous fashion. The level of evidence produced by such reviews is a function of the design qualities of the studies included in the review. Meta-analysis relying solely or primarily on RCTs provide more compelling evidence of intervention impact than meta-analyses comprised solely or primarily of observational studies, strong quasi experiments, or natural experiments for the reasons outlined previously.

Perhaps more troubling than the low supply of scientifically validated evidence is the low demand for such evidence. Here the market appears to be driven by the twin perceptions of impracticality and irrelevancy. Practitioners place little value on the stock of current research and seem quite willing to substitute other (lower level) sources of evidence into their practices (Gambrill, 1999; McCartt-Hess & Mullen, 1995; Reid, 1997; Tyson, 1995; York, 1998). Strong research designs, especially experiments, are typically perceived as unworkable in most social work settings because of ethical issues around randomization in a scarce resource environment, the withholding of potentially effective intervention, the imposition of undesirable interventions, and the possibility of legal action resulting from these ethical issues (Orr, 1999; Shadish, Cook, & Campbell, 2002; Unrau, Gabor, & Grinnell, 2001). On the other hand, social workers are required by ethics to employ practice interventions that are scientifically valid and that demonstrate clinical effectiveness (Gambrill, 2001; York, 1998).

The current state of scientifically validated practice in social work relies sparingly on research programs that produce proof at levels 1 or 2. Instead, an emphasis has been placed on the ethical, organizational, or researcher costs of impact assessment designs that are mainstays for generating evidence of effectiveness in medicine. The substitution of weaker designs, moreover, has done little to counter the widespread perception among practitioners, students, and many social work academics that most social work research has little value for them (Furman, 2001; Reid, 1997; Tyson, 1995; Yegidis & Weinbach, 2002). Methodological relativism, if it has accomplished anything, has increased skepticism in the capacity of social work research to scientifically inform practice. The discussion now turns to the second question and some steps that the profession needs to take if the current situation is to change.

A PASSION FOR UNDERSTANDING INTERVENTION IMPACT

The first essential step for increasing scientifically validated practice is placing impact assessment at the center of the profession's attention. Needs assessment, process on evaluability evaluations, commentaries, and opinion pieces concerning the ontology and epistemology foundations of research hold an important place for social work knowledge building; however, none of these endeavors can address the question "Are we making a difference?" with the clarity and simple elegance of a well-designed impact study. Unfortunately, this quality of simple explanation, the hallmark of levels 1 and 2 evidence, has been often derided in social work as merely simplistic (Hartman, 1990; Heineman, 1981; Tyson, 1995). It may well be that practice effectiveness and efficacy are the consequences of complex and interacting determinants, as these critics claim. Such arguments, however, do not undermine the practice credibility or scientific validity of strong evidence that demonstrates the marginal effect of a single or small set of treatments (Cook & Campbell, 1979; Shadish, Cook, & Campbell, 2002). Marginal effect analyses emanating from levels 1 and 2 research designs continue to produce practice-relevant results in the fields of medicine, psychology, education, job training, housing, income maintenance, and criminal justice. Some examples are informative:

- Smaller class sizes ($N \leq 20$) have been found to increase the reading, language arts, and mathematics scores of elementary school children; the employment of teacher aides, on the other hand, has not (Krueger, 1998).

- A strategy stressing labor force attachment and rapid entry into the job market has been found to increase the earnings of low-income and no-income individuals; educational and vocational training is less effective (Riccio & Orenstein, 1996).
- A Section 8 housing program that encourages a family's relocation outside poor neighborhoods increases the academic achievement of children (Goering, Kraft, Feins, McInnis, & Holin, 1999).
- A case management program designed to increase employment among persons with disabilities reduced client reliance on Supplemental Security Income (SSI) and Disability Insurance (DI) benefits for a 30- to 42-month follow-up period (Kornfeld & Rupp, 2000).
- Selective serotonin reuptake inhibitors (SSRIs) have consistently been shown to reduce symptoms of unipolar depression without the safety issues associated with equally effective tricyclic antidepressants (TCAs) (Nemeroff & Schatzberg, 2002).
- Behavior therapy (BT) and cognitive behavior therapy (CBT) have been shown to significantly decrease depression severity of clients diagnosed with major depression disorder (MDD) (Craighead, Hart, Craighead, & Ilardi, 2002).
- A comprehensive supplemental food and nutrition program (Women, Infants, and Children [WIC]) directed at pregnant, breastfeeding, and postpartum women increased birth weights of newborns and lowered the incidence of newborns with low birth weight (Devaney, 1998).
- The imposition of a family cap in a Temporary Assistance for Needy Families/Aid to Families with Dependent Children (TANF/AFDC) program—that is, the exclusion of children conceived while the mother is on welfare from the TANF/AFDC grant—reduced births while increasing the number of abortions (Camasso, Jagannathan, Killingsworth, & Harvey, 2003).

These oversimplifications and many others from the medical, behavioral, and social sciences may not provide a comprehensive explanation for student achievement, employment and dependency, depression, or fertility behavior, but it would be difficult to argue that such evidence is not relevant to practice and intervention policies. Nor does impact analysis need to stop at the simple cause–effect relationship between intervention and client outcome. Subgroup, mediator, and other forms of contingency analysis can both qualify the conditions of impact and embed evidence in more causally complex and theoretically satisfying systems of explanation. The family cap research (Camasso et al., 2003) proceeded in this fashion. Building on level 1 evidence of an overall treatment effect, these researchers proceeded to specify the conditions and mechanisms that led to the observed outcomes. Subsequent analyses revealed that the birth reduction impacts of a family cap occurred primarily among African American women, especially African American women living in predominantly non–African American neighborhoods (Jagannathan & Camasso, 2003). African American women, moreover, made more use of abortion than of contraception when responding to the family cap (Jagannathan, 2003). Such elaboration of causal explanation need not be rare in the levels 1 and 2 treatment effectiveness and efficacy literature; in fact, it has become an increasingly essential feature of investigation.

Of course, the evidence from levels 1 and 2 designs is not above reproach; scientific validity can be weakened by threats of client noncompliance, selective compliance, attrition, and a host of other problems that are discussed in social work research texts and journal commentaries. What is not always pointed out is that all research designs or evidence-gathering plans are subject to many of the same threats, with the added disadvantage that these weaker designs usually produce little or no information on the counterfactual condition of clients.

PRACTICAL DESIGNS FOR DETECTING INTERVENTION IMPACT

The generally acknowledged preeminence of random clinical trials (RCTs) in providing unbiased estimates of intervention impacts can be directly traced to this design's capacity to create an "internal" control group—that is, nontreated comparisons from a random subset of would-be participants (Bell, Orr, Blomquist, & Cain, 1995; Shadish, Cook, & Campbell, 2002). External controls, which are often used in observational studies, draw nontreated comparisons from a pool of individuals that can be very different from the pool used to draw treatment cases. Impact estimates from quasi-experimental designs that use external controls do not compare well with estimates from randomized experiments in studies where both randomized and external controls are used (Fraker & Maynard, 1987; Friedlander & Robins, 1995). Fortunately, social work is blessed with a variety of internal comparison options, including waiting lists, multiple program entry cohorts, intakes, program-eligible nonapplicants, no-shows, and screened-out applicants. Placed in a strong observational or quasi-experimental design, these internal comparison groups provide the profession with opportunities to conduct credible impact assessments when RCTs are impractical. Four research designs are proposed for this purpose.

Regression Discontinuity

The regression discontinuity design (Mohr, 1995; Shadish, Cook, & Campbell, 2002; Trochim, 1984) creates an internal control group not through random assignment but through the use of an assignment variable. This variable can be any preintervention measure where a cutoff value is used to determine which clients receive treatment and which clients do not. Hence, in a study of the effectiveness of a new treatment on depression, clients scoring 50 or higher on the Hamilton Depression Scale would be assigned to the treatment while clients with lower scores would be placed on a no-treatment waiting list. Or in a study of the efficacy of an intensive job search program, clients with a yearly income of less than or equal to $15,000 would receive the program while those above $15,000 would be placed on a waiting list (control group). The assignment variable does not have to be a pretest measure and can be unrelated to the outcome(s), a condition that can increase this design's statistical power (Shadish, Cook, & Campbell, 2002). Clients, for example, can be assigned on the basis of their date of application or intake, with the first 100 registrants placed in treatment. Assignment could also be made on the basis of the last 2, 3, or 4 digits of a client's social security number. If two digits are used, any values greater than or equal to 50 could assign clients to treatment, and any below 50 to a control group. Random assignment guards against selection because each client has a .5 probability of receiving treatment, and chance assignment can't be systematic. Regression discontinuity addresses selection

by modeling an explicit, prospective, well-understood selection mechanism. Such modeling is possible because the probability of receiving treatment, while not .5, is still known. In a typical two-group design, for example, the probability for assignment into treatment is always 1.0 if the client scores above (or below) the designated cutoff and 0 if the client scores below (or above).

To gain a better understanding of how the regression discontinuity design can be used to obtain unbiased estimates of intervention impact, it is useful to contrast the design with a random experiment. In a simple linear regression model, an experiment has this form:

$$(1) \quad Y_i = a + B_T T_i + B_X X_i + e_i$$

where Y is an outcome of interest; T is a dummy variable with two values, 1 denoting treatment and 0 denoting control; and X is a pretest measure. Then a, B, and e represent the intercept, slopes, and residuals produced by the regression, with B_T providing the treatment impact estimate. The inclusion of a pretest measure (or, for that matter, any covariate) is largely superfluous because randomization rules out the likelihood that X is confounded with T. The linear model depicting a regression discontinuity design for this study would have this form:

$$(2) \quad Y_i = a + B_T T_i + B_X (X_i - X_c) + e_i$$

where the assignment variable X is an assignment measure in this case, a pretest. Here B_X estimates the effect of the assignment variable on the outcome and adjusts the regression equation to estimate the treatment effect (B_T) from the cutoff point (X_C). If the cutoff point is 0—in effect, no cutoff—Equation 2 reduces to a simple pre–post model with uncontrolled selection.

In cases where regression discontinuity designs use assignment variables that are clearly unrelated to the outcome variable, such as dates of intake or client social security number, the results produced should be virtually identical. This correspondence is illustrated in Figure 24.1 for a hypothetical case of an effective treatment for depression producing a positive impact. The assignment variable here is the last two digits of the client's social security number. In panel A, the digits are placed in a lottery, with any two-digit number having a .5 chance of assignment into a treatment group, and one would expect all

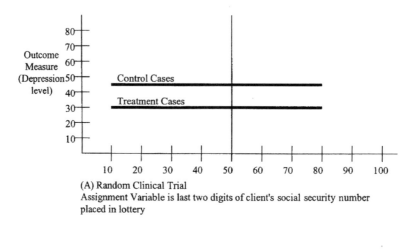

(A) Random Clinical Trial
Assignment Variable is last two digits of client's social security number placed in lottery

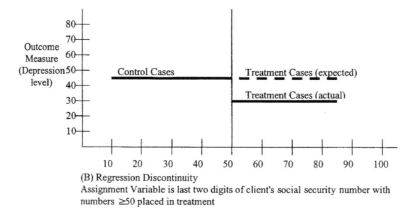

(B) Regression Discontinuity
Assignment Variable is last two digits of client's social security number with numbers ≥50 placed in treatment

FIGURE 24.1 Random Clinical Trials and Regression Discontinuity Designs Illustrating Positive Treatment Effects

two-digit sets to be equally represented in both treatment and control groups. The distance between the two regression lines in panel A represents a 17-unit average treatment impact—that is, the B_T effect in Equation 1.

In panel B, the same two-digit numbers are assigned on the basis of a cutoff point at 50. Clients with social security numbers ending in 50 or higher are assigned to treatment; clients with lower numbers become controls. The dashed line indicates the expected regression line for clients with two-digit sets 50 or greater, while the solid line after the cutoff illustrates a discontinuity, or a B_T effect in Equation 2 of 17 units.

The regression discontinuity design possesses two qualities that should make it more desirable than RCTs in the development of levels 1 and 2

evidence. Since treatment can be assigned on the basis of need, regression discontinuity is not subject to the ethical arguments that have made random assignment so unpopular in social work evaluations. Thoughtful cutoff points or intervals can ensure that clients with the most problems and/or fewest resources are given priority for service intervention. Administratively, regression discontinuity designs provide a much closer fit with managerial practices for prioritizing, rationing, delivering, and discontinuing agency services. All that is required is that the assignment measures used to identify ineligibles, the wait-listed, the screened-out, no-shows, and other potential nontreated comparison groups be ordinal, well measured, and used consistently by agency staff.

Multiple Cohorts

Another observational design that can furnish an internal group counterfactual is the multiple cohort comparison. A cohort is a group of clients who share a common program experience for a specified time period. This experience could begin as a common eligibility, recipiency, intake, or birth date and end when the group has reached a common graduation, program completion, or financial end date. The group is then succeeded by a second and subsequent cohorts. Training and school programs come immediately to mind when considering a multiple cohorts design; however, any program with a cyclical or successive feature is a candidate.

Multiple cohorts can be used in effectiveness or efficacy studies if the treatment has not been given to all the cohorts. Shadish, Campbell, and Cook (2002) note that cohorts serve as especially good control groups if three conditions are met:

- Cohorts differ in only minor ways from their contiguous cohorts.
- Organizations insist that a treatment be given to everybody in a cohort, thus precluding simultaneous controls and making possible only historical controls.
- An organization's archival records can be used for constructing and then comparing cohorts. (p. 149)

The advantage of this design over a pre–post approach is that the threat of aging, maturation, or natural life course effects that occur in a group of clients over time is greatly reduced (Moffitt & Ver Ploeg, 1999). And unless a program dramatically changes its mission, program objectives, target population, or service complement, successive cohorts should be subject to the same agency and client selection process.

In Table 24.1, the structure of a multiple cohort design used to evaluate evidence of effectiveness for a hypothetical school-based counseling program is given. This demonstration program was made available to two of the eight cohorts depicted (i.e., the classes of 2002 and 2003). Program outcomes included school dropouts, absence and tardiness days, standardized test scores, and grade point average. The linear regression model that can be estimated for the quantitative outcomes of interest has the form:

$$(3) \quad Y_i = a + B_t T_i + B_z Z_i + B_X X_i + e_i$$

where Y is an outcome of interest; T is a dummy variable with two values, 1 denoting membership in the treated classes of 2002 and 2003 and 0 denoting membership in the untreated classes of 2000, 2001, and 2004; Z is a measure of time trend; and X is a k-1 dummy measuring class or age effects. Once again, a, B, and e represent the intercept, slopes, and residuals from the statistical model estimation. If the assumption of small difference in selection between cohorts is justified, B_T is an unbiased estimator of the school-based counseling program's impact.

As alluded to earlier, the multiple cohort design can be applied both prospectively and retrospectively. In the latter instance, of course, the quality of the organization's historical data is the

TABLE 24.1 Overall Multiple Cohort Design for Assessing the Effectiveness of a School-Based Program: Program Available to Classes of 2002 and 2003

Class	School Year							
	1996–1997	1997–1998	1998–1999	1999–2000	2000–2001	2001–2002	2002–2003	2003–2004
Freshman	Class of 2000	Class of 2001	**Class of 2002**	**Class of 2003**	Class of 2004	Class of 2005	Class of 2006	Class of 2007
Sophomore	Class of 1999	Class of 2000	Class of 2001	**Class of 2002**	**Class of 2003**	Class of 2004	Class of 2005	Class of 2006
Junior	Class of 1998	Class of 1999	Class of 2000	Class of 2001	**Class of 2002**	**Class of 2003**	Class of 2004	Class of 2005
Senior	Class of 1997	Class of 1998	Class of 1999	Class of 2000	Class of 2001	**Class of 2002**	**Class of 2003**	Class of 2004

determining factor. As in the case of the regression discontinuity design, multiple cohorts have an ethical and administrative appeal lacking in RCTs. A cohort provides the natural program participation dynamic for many human services organizations and does not separate clients into "treated" and "untreated" segments. Organizations, moreover, have both ethical and fiduciary responsibilities to maintain the client participation and outcome data required for this type of impact assessment. In sum, the multiple cohort design has the potential to increase management efficiency, as well as produce credible scientific evidence.

NONEQUIVALENT CONTROLS WITH STATISTICAL ADJUSTMENTS

Nonequivalent control group designs have great difficulty in generating levels 1 or 2 evidence of treatment effectiveness, primarily because the rules for assignment to treatment and comparison groups are unclear. Hence, the probability of any individual client receiving or not receiving treatment is never known perfectly and must somehow be estimated and, if possible, be balanced. This, of course, is not the case with RCTs, regression discontinuity, and multiple cohorts, which meet the assumptions outlined earlier.

Of the many approaches that have been used to deal with selection bias in nonequivalent control groups, two could help boost credible impact assessments in social work. The first of these is selection adjustment through the estimation of propensity scores—that is, the estimation of the conditional probabilities of exposure to treatment for a group of clients, given a set of observed covariates (Joffe & Rosenbaum, 1999; Rosenbaum, 2002; Rosenbaum & Rubin, 1983). The second is the two-step selection modeling advanced by Heckman and his colleagues (Heckman & Hotz, 1989; Heckman & Todd, 1996).

The logic underpinning propensity scores builds on the work of Cochran (1968), who proposed removing selection bias from observation studies through the technique of retrospective subclassification adjustment. The first step is the estimation of a logistic regression of this form:

(4) $Ln(P/1 - P) = a + B_x X_i$

where P is the probability of a client receiving treatment and X_i represents a relatively large set

of variables measured prior to treatment (covariates) and a and B represent regression intercept and slope coefficients. The model is estimated for all treated clients and all untreated individuals who comprise the nonequivalent comparison group pool. The logistic regression provides a predicted probability (a predicted propensity score) for each of the treated and untreated. Once the propensity scores are calculated, the next step is to match treated and untreated cases. Matching can be one to one where each treated (untreated) case with a propensity score (PS_i) is paired to one or more untreated (treated) cases with identical or similar scores. Matching can also be done by grouping scores into strata (5 to 10) and matching treated and untreated scores within each stratum (Rosenbaum, 2002; Shadish, Cook, & Campbell, 2002). Once the matching is complete, tests of equivalence can be performed for each covariate used in Equation 4. When equivalence or balance is achieved, a regression model (Equation 1) can be estimated for the outcome of interest, or an impact model of the following form can be estimated:

(5) $Y_i = a + B_T T_i + B_x X_i + B_S S_i + e_i$

where S indicates a client's membership in one of the 5 (quintile) or 10 (decile) strata.

The method of propensity scores is limited by a reliance on achieving group equivalence through observed covariates. It is possible, even with a large set of covariates, that treated and untreated cases could differ on unmeasured characteristics. Heckman (Heckman & Hotz, 1989; Heckman & Todd, 1996) proposes a two-stage approach to adjust for the possibility of hidden or unmeasured selection bias between groups of treated and untreated clients.

The first step here is to estimate a probit regression for the probability of an individual receiving treatment from a set of covariates by using the entire pool of treated and untreated cases:

(6) $P = a + B_x X_i$

The results from this probit model are used to calculate a statistic for each individual, called variously the inverse Mills ratio or the hazard rate (λ). The bigger the value λ has, the greater the likelihood that a case will be excluded from treatment.

The second step in the Heckman approach is

the estimation of an impact equation that incorporates the selection correction factor (λ). This model has the form:

$$(7) \quad Y_i = a + B_T T_i + B_\lambda \lambda_i + B_x X_i + e_i$$

where B_λ estimates the expected values of sample selection effect. If B_λ is significant, it indicates that individuals are selected into the treatment in a manner that makes a difference with respect to the outcome. Incorporation of λ into Equation 7 can produce unbiased estimates of B_T (the treatment) by controlling for this source of hidden bias.

Propensity scores and selection modeling provide statistical "fixes" for balancing nonequivalent control groups. These methods, however, do not guarantee equivalence because bias may stem from a covariate(s) not included in the statistical estimation process.

Interrupted Time Series

The interrupted time series (ITS) design does not establish a counterfactual with an internal control group, as do the RCT and the other observational approaches discussed in this chapter. It is, however, a very powerful approach for examining interventions' impacts and can produce level 2 proof of effectiveness (Cook & Campbell, 1979; Glass, Willson, & Gottman, 1975; Shadish, Cook, & Campbell, 2002). The interrupted time series design is especially well suited to assess the "time path" or "effect pattern" of an intervention across time; however, it is also possible to examine treatment decay or intensification by extending internal control group designs as well (Orr, 1999). ITS can be employed with a large number of observations on the same set of cases or on sets of similar but different cases. The crucial factor is that the number of observations must be large, typically 50 or more time periods (Bowerman & O'Connell, 1987; Pindyck & Rubinfeld, 1981). Of course, this type of impact assessment can be undertaken only in organizations where historical data on program operations and outcomes are recorded consistently and where aggregate program statistics can be trusted to reflect case level transactions.

A simple form of the linear regression model for estimating an impact from ITS data is:

$$(8) \quad Y_t = a + B_1 T_t + B_2 TIME_t$$
$$+ B_3 SEASON + B_4 AR + e_t$$

where t indicates aggregate observations measured on a monthly, quarterly, or yearly basis and B_1 is the treatment effect (T), B_2 the effect of time trend ($TIME$), B_3 is the effect of seasonality ($SEASON$), and B_4 estimates the first-order autoregression correction for correlated serial errors.

In Figure 24.2, impact estimates from an ITS assessment of a hypothetical welfare-to-work program is presented. The graphic shows that data were available for 50 quarters on the total number of clients working full time. A new jobs program intervention was put into place in quarter 25. In panel A, a positive treatment effect (B_1) of about 200 additional employed workers per quarter is shown. The impact here is the result of an intercept change from projected values of past time trend (the dotted line), which serves as the counterfactual. In panel B, a positive average treatment effect (T x $TIME$) of about 200 employed per quarter is also shown, but in this instance the effect reflects an abrupt slope change after quarter 25.

Inasmuch as the counterfactual condition in the ITS design is established by modeling time trend (and seasonal variation), it is critical that a long observational period precede any introduction of new intervention(s). Short baselines make it very difficult, if not impossible, to rule out time as a reason for client change. Short time series baselines can also lead to unstable estimates of B_4, increasing the risk of a biased estimate of the treatment effect.

CREATING AN EVIDENCE-BASED CULTURE

It is not enough for the profession—its practitioners, academics, and students—to gain an appreciation for impact assessment and the types of research that will increase empirically derived evidence. The institutions of social work—National Association of Social Workers (NASW), Council of Social Work Education (CSWE), state licensing boards, schools of social work, funded research centers—need to go through a cultural transformation on a rather dramatic scale if evidence-based practice is to become a defining feature of what it means to be a social worker. Cultural transformation in this case is defined as change "in the way we do things around here" (Deal & Kennedy, 1982) and requires professional structures and strategies constructed and

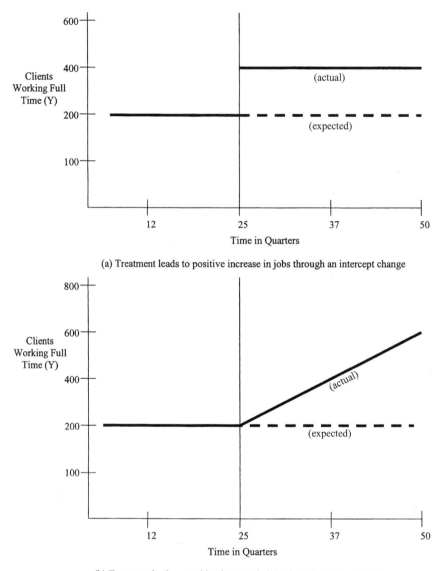

(a) Treatment leads to positive increase in jobs through an intercept change

(b) Treatment leads to positive increase in jobs through a slope change

FIGURE 24.2 Effective Treatment in a Workfare Program Identified With Interrupted Time-Design Series

maintained by true believers. And if the evolution of evidence-based practice in medicine is any indication, the change cannot be expected to come solely from within the profession.

There are several developments in the field of social work that have increased awareness of the need for evidence-based practice. One of these is the proposed integration of evaluation and practice through single-system designs (Bloom, Fischer, & Orme, 1999; Tripodi, 1994). The hope here is that practitioners themselves will take the lead in supplying scientifically validated evidence for practice effectiveness, one client at a time. The logic of single-subject design closely follows that outlined in the discussion of interrupted time series, except that instead of an aggregate data source, one individual's outcomes are repeatedly observed. This individual focus, in fact, is viewed as one of the design's great strengths. Bloom, Fischer, and Orme (1999), for example, make this observation about single-subject research:

> The closeness of the measures to the client's problems produces a type of validity that cannot be matched in group designs. (p. 30)

Perhaps this is true; however, single-subject designs as they are typically used in social work practice have serious shortcomings that limit their evidence-producing capacity. These designs are described with the language of ITS, but their implementation more closely parallels extended pre–post group designs without any adjustment for selection bias. The repeated observation sequence is almost always too short to adjust for serial dependence (Bloom, Fischer, & Orme, 1999), and a nonequivalent outcome variable (i.e., a variable not expected to change with an intervention) is seldom monitored as a counterfactual check.

Placing such technical issues aside, a legitimate question arises as to the feasibility of placing the practitioners in the role of examining their practice without broader institutional oversight. Some critics find the juxtaposition of the scientist–practitioner to be untenable, with both roles suffering (Wakefield & Kirk, 1996). This approach certainly treats practice context as ignorable (Camasso, 2002) and fails to address the well-established fact in medicine that the poorest quality of care and documentation occurs in solo and small practices (Hornbrook & Berki, 1985; Hulka, Kupper, Cassel, & Babineau, 1975).

Another initiative in social work aimed ostensibly at increasing scientific evidence and closing the gap between research and practice is the university-based research center (Austin & Roberts, 2002; McCartt-Hess & Mullen, 1995). In the 1990s several well-established centers were complemented by eight National Institute of Mental Health Social Work Research Development Centers. At the heart of this research center creation is the voluntary partnership among university researchers, agencies, and practitioners.

It is unlikely that universities working with willing agency or practitioner collaborators will profoundly increase either the supply or the demand for scientifically based evidence. Research agendas stem from a variety of sources: theory, social policy, personal interests, with the evaluation of specific agency or practitioner outcomes low on the scholarship totem pole. Without some compelling impetus from within or outside the profession, university researchers will continue to engage in the types of research that have been successful in garnering academic rewards.

If not the practitioners or the academe, where can we expect to see the significant sparks of culture transformation? If Gambrill (2001) is correct, the place is not the CSWE, at least CSWE as currently structured. Gambrill argues persuasively that CSWE, the National Association of (Social Work) Deans and Directors, and (I would include) NASW continue to rely on surrogate indicators for evidence of scientifically validated practice. In short, measures of structure (degrees, licenses held) or process (type of therapy used, caseload size, participation rates) substitute for true impact in definitions of quality in social work like the Educational Policy and Accreditations Standards (EPAS). Gambrill's call for evidence-based standards has raised awareness of the profession's problem, as well as a good deal of resistance to any change (Hoffman & Albers, 2002; Mohan, 2001). The following from Hoffman and Albers is especially revealing:

> She [Gambrill] seems to favor miring social work education in at least 33 measures of quality professional education and thus create a new role for CSWE as an FDA look alike. (p. 184)

While the FDA analogy is overdrawn and CSWE may never rise to a leadership role as an advocate for evidence-based practice, some sort of organizational structure is needed to change the current culture. It is suggested here that a model similar to the Agency of Healthcare Research and Quality (AHRQ) in the U.S. Department of Health and Human Services be seriously explored. Through its evidence-based practice centers (EPCs), AHRQ sponsors the development of evidence reports and technology assessments to assist public and private practitioners in improving the quality of health care across the country (Agency for Healthcare Policy and Research, 2002). In social work, EPCs could be existing university research centers, private for-profit or nonprofits comprised of social work researchers, practitioners, *and* statisticians, economists, experimental psychologists, and medical professionals who understand levels of evidence and the types of research designs required to reach these levels in social work. The EPC evidence reports could provide practitioners, researchers, third-party payers, licensure boards, accrediting bodies, and teaching institutions and their clients with treatment effectiveness evidence that the field itself neither supplies nor demands. It is a model that, if fully implemented, can change "the way we do things around here."

References

Agency for Healthcare Research and Quality. (2002). *Systems to rate the strength of scientific evidence* (Evidence Report/Technology Assessment No. 47, 02.E016). Washington, DC: U.S. Department of Health and Human Services.

Austin, D. M., & Roberts, A. R. (2002). Clinical social work in the 21st century. In A. R. Roberts & G. J. Greene (Eds.), *Social workers' desk reference* (pp. 822–828). New York: Oxford University Press.

Bell, S. H., Orr, L. L., Blomquist, J. D., & Cain, G. G. (1995). *Program applicants as a comparison group in evaluating training programs*. Kalamazoo, MI: W. E. Upjohn Institute.

Beutler, L. E. (2000) Empirically-based decision making in clinical practice. *Prevention and Treatment 3*, 1–15.

Bloom, M., Fischer, J., & Orme, J. G. (1999). *Evaluating practice: Guidelines for the accountable professional* (3rd ed.). Boston: Allyn & Bacon.

Bowerman, B. L., & O'Connell, R. T. (1987). *Time serves forecasting*. Boston: Duxbury.

Camasso, M. J. (2002). Practice ecology of clinical decision making. In A. R. Roberts & G. J. Greene (Eds.), *Social workers' desk reference* (pp. 807–813). New York: Oxford University Press.

Camasso, M. J., Jagannathan, R., Killingsworth, M., & Harvey, C. (2003). New Jersey's family cap and family size decisions: Findings from a five-year evaluation. *Research in Labor Economics, 22,* 71–112.

Chambless, D. L., Baker, M. J., Baucom, D. H., Beutler, L. E., Calhoun, K. S., & Crits-Christoph, R. (1998). Update on empirically validated therapies, II. *The Clinical Psychologist, 51,* 3–16.

Cochran, W. G. (1968). The effectiveness of adjustment by subclassification in removing bias in observational studies. *Biometrics, 24,* 295–313.

Cook, T. D., & Campbell, D. T. (1979). *Quasi-experimentation design and analysis: Issues for field settings*. Chicago: Rand McNally.

Corcoran, J. (2000). *Evidence-based social work practice with families*. New York: Springer.

Cournoyer, B. R., & Powers, G. T. (2002) Evidence-based social work: The quiet revolution continues. In A. R. Roberts & G. J. Greene (Eds.), *Social workers' desk reference* (pp. 798–807). New York: Oxford University Press.

Craighead, W. E., Hart, A. B., Craighead, L. W., & Ilardi, S. S. (2002). Psychological treatments for major depression disorder. In P. E. Nathan & J. M. Gorman (Eds.), *A guide to treatments that work* (pp. 245–261). New York: Oxford University Press.

Deal, T. E., & Kennedy, A. A. (1982). *Corporate cultures: The rites and rituals of corporate life.* Reading, MA: Addison-Wesley.

Devaney, B. (1998). The special supplemental nutrition program for women, infants and children. In J. Crane (Ed.), *Social programs that work* (pp. 184–200). New York: Russell Sage.

Fraker, T., & Maynard, R. (1987). Evaluating comparison group designs with employment-related programs. *Journal of Human Resources, 22,* 194–227.

Fraser, M., Taylor, M. J., Jackson, R., & O'Jack, J. (1991). Social work and science: Many ways of knowing. *Social Work Research and Abstracts, 27,* 5–15.

Friedlander, D., & Robins, P. K. (1995). Evaluating program evaluations: New evidence on commonly used nonexperimental methods. *American Economic Review, 85,* 923–937.

Furman, R. (2001). Letter to editor: Relevance of social work scholarship to practitioners. *Journal of Social Work Education,, 37,* 411–412.

Gambrill, E. (1999). Evidence-based clinical practice: An alternative to authority-based practice. *Families in Society, 80,* 341–350.

Gambrill, E. D. (2001). Editorial: Educational policy and accreditation standards: Do they work for clients? *Journal of Social Work Education 37,* 226–239.

Ginsberg, L. H. (2001). *Social work evaluation: Principles and methods.* Boston: Allyn & Bacon.

Glass, G. V., Willson, V. L., & Gottman, J. M. (1975). *Design and analysis of time-series experiments.* Boulder: Colorado University Press.

Goering, J., Kraft, J., Feins, J., McInnis, D., & Holin, M. J. (1999). *Moving to opportunity for fair housing demonstration program.* Washington, DC: U.S. Department of Housing and Urban Development, Office of Policy Development and Research.

Hartman, A. (1990). Editorial: Many ways of knowing. *Social Work, 35,* 3–4.

Heckman, J. J., & Hotz, V. J. (1989). Choosing among alternative nonexperimental methods for estimating the impact of social programs: The case of manpower training. *Journal of the American Statistical Association, 84,* 862–874.

Heckman, J. J., & Todd, P. E. (1996). *Assessing the performance of alternative estimations of program impacts: A study of adult men and women in JTPA.* Chicago: University of Chicago, Department of Economics.

Heineman, M. (1981). The obsolete scientific imperative in social work research. *Social Service Review, 55*, 371–397.

Hoffman, K., & Albers, D. A. (2002). Letter to editor: Do educational policy and accreditation standards work for clients? *Journal of Social Work Education 38*, 181–185.

Hornbrook, M. C., & Berki, S. E. (1985). Practice mode and payment method: Effects of use, costs, quality and access. *Medical Care 23*, 484–511.

Hulka, B. S., Kupper, L. L., Cassel, J. C., & Babineau, R. A. (1975). Practice characteristics and quality of primary medical care. *Medical Care, 13*, 808–820.

Jagannathan, R. (2003). New Jersey's family cap and welfare births: An examination of racial differences in fertility within the framework of proximate determinates. *Journal of Urban Affairs, 25*, 357–375.

Jagannathan, R., & Camasso, M. J. (2003) Family cap and nonmarital fertility: The racial conditioning of policy effects. *Journal of Marriage and Family, 66*, 220–240.

Joffe, M., & Rosenbaum, P. R. (1999). Invited commentary: Propensity scores. *American Journal of Epidemiology, 150*, 327–333.

Kornfeld, R., & Rupp, K. (2000). The net effects of the project NETWORK return-to-work case management experiment on participant earnings, benefit receipt and other outcomes. *Social Security Bulletin, 63*, 12–33.

Krueger, A. B. (1998). *Experimental estimates of education production functions* (working paper #379). Princeton, NJ: Princeton University, Industrial Relations Section.

Lloyd, E. (1998). Introducing evidence-based social welfare practice in a national child care agency. In A. Buchanan & B. Hudson (Eds.), *Parenting, schooling and children's behavior* (pp. 161–177). Aldershot, United Kingdom: Ashgate.

McCartt-Hess, P., & Mullen, E. J. (Eds.). (1995). *Practitioner–researcher partnerships*. Washington, DC: NASW Press.

Moffitt, R. A., & Ver Ploeg. M. (1999). *Evaluating welfare reform: A framework and review of current work*. Washington, DC: National Academy Press.

Mohan, B. (2001). Letter to editor: Educational policy and accreditation standards. *Journal of Social Work Education, 37*, 591–592.

Mohr, L. B. (1995). *Impact analysis for program evaluation*. Thousand Oaks, CA: Sage.

Nathan, P. E., & Gorman, J. M. (Eds.). (2002). *A guide to treatments that work* (2nd ed.). New York: Oxford University Press.

Nemeroff, C. B., & Schatzberg, A. F. (2002). Pharmacological treatments for unipolar depression. In P. E. Nathan & J. M. Gorman (Eds.), *A guide to treatments that work* (pp. 229–243). New York: Oxford University Press.

Orr, L. L. (1999). *Social experiments: Evaluating public programs with experimental methods*. Thousand Oaks, CA: Sage.

Pindyck, R. S., & Rubinfeld, D. L. (1981). *Ecometric models and economic forecasts* (2nd ed.). New York: McGraw-Hill.

Reid, W. J. (1997). Long-term trends in clinical social work. *Social Service Review, 71*, 200–213.

Riccio, J. A., & Orenstein, A. (1996). Understanding best practice for operating welfare-to-work programs. *Evaluation Review, 20*, 3–28.

Rosen, A., Proctor, E., Morrow-Howell, N., & Staudt, M. (1995). Rationales for practice decisions: Variations in knowledge use by decision task and social work service. *Research in Social Work Practice, 5*, 501–523.

Rosenbaum, P. R. (2002). *Observational studies* (2nd ed.). New York: Springer-Verlag.

Rosenbaum, P. R., & Rubin, D. B. (1983). The central role of the propensity score in observational studies for causal effects. *Biometrika, 70*, 41–55.

Rossi, P. H., Freeman, H. E., & Lipsey, M. W. (1999). *Evaluation: A systematic approach* (6th ed.). Thousand Oaks, CA: Sage.

Rubin, A., & Babbie, E. (2001). *Research methods for social work* (4th ed.). Belmont, CA: Wadsworth/Thomson.

Sackett, D. L., Robinson, W. S., Rosenberg W., & Haynes, R. B. (1997). *Evidence-based medicine: How to practice and teach EBM*. New York: Churchill Livingston.

Shadish, W. R., Cook, T. D., & Campbell, D. T. (2002). *Experimental and quasi-experimental designs for generalized causal inference*. Boston: Houghton Mifflin.

Sommer, A., & Zeger, S. L. (1991). On estimating efficiency from clinical trials. *Statistics in Medicine, 10*, 45–52.

Thyer, B. A. (2002). Principles of evidence-based practice and treatment development. In A. R. Roberts & G. J. Greene (Eds.), *Social workers' desk reference* (pp. 739–742). New York: Oxford University Press.

Thyer, B. A., & Wodarski, J. S. (Eds.). (1998). *Handbook of empirical social work practice: Vol. 1. Mental disorder*. New York: Wiley.

Tripodi, T. (1994). *A primer in single-subject design for clinical social workers*. Washington, DC: NASW Press.

Trochim, W.M.K. (1984). *Research design for program evaluation: The regression discontinuity approach*. Newbury Park, CA: Sage.

Tyson, K. (1995). *New foundation for scientific social and behavioral research: The heuristic paradigm*. Boston: Allyn & Bacon.

Unrau, Y. A., Gabor, P. A., & Grinnell, R. M. (2001). *Evaluation in the human services.* Itasca, IL: F. E. Peacock.

Vandiver, V. L. (2002). Step-by-step practice guidelines for using evidence-based practice and expert consensus in mental health settings. In A. R. Roberts & G. J. Greene (Eds.), *Social workers' desk reference* (pp. 731–738). New York: Oxford University Press.

Wakefield, J., & Kirk, S. (1996). Unscientific thinking about scientific practice: Evaluating the scientist-practitioner model. *Social Work Research, 20*(2), 83–95.

Yegidis, B. L., & Weinbach, R. W. (2002). *Research methods of social workers* (4th ed.). Boston: Allyn & Bacon.

York, R. O. (1998). Conducting social work research: *An experiential approach.* Boston: Allyn & Bacon.

25

EVIDENCE-BASED PRACTICE AND MANUALIZED TREATMENT WITH CHILDREN

Scott K. Okamoto & Craig Winston LeCroy

In social work and allied disciplines, there has been a growing interest in identifying psychosocial treatments for children and adolescents that have demonstrated clinical efficacy and effectiveness. This chapter focuses on illustrating various treatments that have been shown through rigorous, controlled research to be efficacious for child and adolescent mental health problems. Additionally, this chapter focuses on recent literature that addresses the movement of these clinical research studies into the "real world," or what has been described as *transportability* (Schoenwald & Hoagwood, 2001), *diffusion of innovation* (Henggler & Lee, 2002), or *effectiveness* (APA Task Force on Psychological Intervention Guidelines, 1995). While there has been much progress in identifying "what works" with children and adolescents, the issue of implementing these studies into practice remains a challenge for the field of child and adolescent therapy.

HISTORY

Evidence-based treatments for children and adolescents began to garner attention in the mid to late 1990s. For example, during this time period, comprehensive reviews of effective school-based programs (Derzon, Wilson, & Cunningham, 1999) and violence prevention programs (Tolan & Guerra, 1994) were published in efforts to identify the best practices for children and adolescents. Concurrently, organizations such as the Center for the Study and Prevention of Violence (CSPV, 2002) and the Center for Substance Abuse Prevention (CSAP, n.d.) began to examine the research literature to identify model programs for children and adolescents.

One of the arguably most careful examinations of evidence-based practices, however, was conducted in 1995 by the Division 12 Task Force on Promotion and Dissemination of Psychological Procedures. Using the rubric of "empirically validated" treatments, this task force published a report that outlined (a) the minimum criteria for a psychosocial treatment to be considered "well established" or "probably efficacious" and (b) a comprehensive list of treatments (including child and adolescent treatments) that met their strict criteria within these categories. "Well-established" treatments are primarily manualized treatments that have been shown to be superior to a psychological placebo or to another treatment in at least two studies conducted by different investigative teams. "Probably efficacious" treatments are primarily those that have been shown to be more effective than a control group in at least two studies, but they do not necessarily have to be manualized or to have been evaluated by two different investigative teams (see Task Force on the Promotion and Dissemination of Psychological Procedures, 1995, for review). Since the publication of the 1995 report, several updates have been published (Chambless et al., 1996, 1998), and articles have identified and discussed specific programs that meet the task force's criteria for child and adolescent externalizing disorders, such as conduct problems (Brestan & Eyberg, 1998), and internalizing disorders, such as anxiety disorders (Ollendick & King, 1998) and depression (Kaslow & Thompson, 1998). Most recently, several books (e.g., Christophersen & Mortweet, 2001; Corcoran, in press; Rapee, Wignall, Hudson, & Schniering, 2001) and Web sites (e.g., Campbell Collaboration, 2002; Cochrane Library, 2002) have sought to direct practitioners in their use of empirically supported treatments.

EFFICACY

The focus of this section is on several clinical practices with children and adolescents that have met the strict criteria of Division 12 for "well-established" or "probably efficacious" treatments (Task Force, 1995). Several of these programs have been included in other published lists of model programs (e.g., Chorpita et al., 2002; CSAP, n.d.; CSPV, 2002). This section examines evidence-based practices for both internalizing disorders (e.g., anxiety disorders and depression) and externalizing disorders (e.g., conduct disorder, attention-deficit/hyperactivity disorder).

Internalizing Disorders

Anxiety

Evidence-based practices for the treatment of child and adolescent anxiety disorders (e.g., separation anxiety disorder, social phobias) include cognitive behavioral therapy and exposure therapy. For example, Barrett (1998) and Silverman et al. (1999) both compared cognitive behavioral therapy (CBT) conducted in a group format with accompanying parent training sessions against waitlist control groups. In both studies, significantly fewer youth in the therapy group than in the control group were diagnosed with an anxiety disorder at posttest and at 12-month follow-up. Silverman's treatment protocol is 12 sessions in which participants develop fear hierarchies and reward contingencies for achieving goals (sessions 2 and 3); conduct group in-session exposure, using the group to provide feedback, modeling, and reinforcement (sessions 4–11); and identify faulty cognitions (session 7). Parent–child contingency management and contracting are used in the early stages of treatment to facilitate the child's exposure to increasingly anxiety-provoking situations (Silverman & Kurtines, 1996; Silverman et al., 1999). The findings from these studies suggest that group CBT for anxiety disorders may be a cost-effective and time-efficient alternative to individual CBT for youth.

Depression

Evidence-based practices for the treatment of adolescent depression or dysthymia include cognitive behavioral or relationship enhancement approaches. Cognitive behavioral therapy for depression typically focuses on changing adolescents' pessimistic or negative thoughts, depressotypic beliefs and biases, and negative causal attributions (e.g., blaming oneself for failures but not taking credit for successes). Reinforcement schedules are used to eliminate behaviors that support these thoughts (Lewinsohn, Clarke, Rohde, Hops, & Seeley, 1996). The adolescent coping with depression (CWD-A) program is one example of an empirically supported treatment for depression (Chorpita et al., 2002). Components of this program incorporate social skills training, relaxation training, and cognitive therapy that focuses on identifying, challenging, and changing negative thoughts and irrational beliefs (Clarke, Lewinsohn, & Hops, 1990; Lewinsohn et al., 1996). Efficacy research on CWD-A indicates that it yields higher depression recovery rates and a greater reduction in self-reported depression than waitlist control groups (Clarke, Rohde, Lewinsohn, Hops, & Seeley, 1999; Lewinsohn, Clarke, Hops, & Andrews, 1990).

Relationship enhancement therapies, such as interpersonal psychotherapy (IPT-A; Mufson, Moreau, & Weissman, 1996; Mufson, Moreau, Weissman, & Kerman, 1993), emphasize the interpersonal nature of depression and actively attempt to change adolescents' communication, affect, and social skills. IPT-A incorporates three phases of treatment. In the initial phase, problem areas and depressive symptoms are addressed, and a treatment contract is developed. The middle phase of treatment focuses on effective strategies to attack the problem by using techniques such as role play to address issues related to communication, affect, and social skills. The termination phase of treatment focuses on establishing a sense of competence to deal with future problems (Mufson et al., 1996). Compared with a waitlist control group, one study found that youth who received IPT-A reported a significantly greater decrease in depressive symptoms and improvement in social functioning (Mufson, Weissman, Moreau, & Garfinkel, 1999).

Externalizing Disorders

Conduct Problems

Evidence-based practices for conduct problems include behavioral parent training and multisystemic therapy. Behavioral parent training assumes that antisocial behavior is learned and sustained by positive and negative reinforcement, and it seeks to shift social contingencies such that children's prosocial behaviors receive positive parental reinforcement, while negative behaviors are consistently punished or ignored (Serketich & Dumas, 1996). Webster-Stratton's videotape-based parent training program is one example of behavioral parent training (Webster-

Stratton & Hancock, 1998). Using videotaped vignettes of parents and children interacting in natural situations (e.g., during mealtime), group therapists discuss topics such as limit setting, using praise and incentives, and ignoring negative child behaviors. Videotaped scenes depict both negative and positive examples of parenting behaviors. One study of videotape-based parent training indicated that parents participating in the program reported significantly fewer oppositional or noncompliant behaviors and exhibited significantly fewer critical statements and more praise toward their children than a waitlist control group (Webster-Stratton, 1984).

Multisystemic therapy (MST) is an individualized family- and home-based treatment grounded in an ecosystemic framework (Henggler & Borduin, 1990; Henggler, Melton, & Smith, 1992). MST therapists implement a range of therapeutic interventions (e.g., structural family therapy, cognitive behavioral therapy) that reflect the treatment goals identified by the family. Its present-focused and action-oriented interventions target specific and well-defined problems (Henggler, Melton, Brondino, Scherer, & Hanley, 1997). Efficacy research on MST indicates that the program results in improved family functioning and significantly fewer arrests and self-reported offenses than alternative treatments (e.g., probation, individual therapy; Borduin et al., 1995; Henggler et al., 1992).

Attention-Deficit/Hyperactivity Disorder

Evidence-based practices for attention-deficit/hyperactivity disorder (ADHD) include behavior management and pharmacotherapy. Behavior management typically involves the use of positive reinforcement, where children and adolescents earn tokens or points for positive behaviors, and response cost, where negative behaviors cost tokens or points, in order to shape behavior (Pelham & Hoza, 1996). Behaviors that are commonly addressed for youth with ADHD include following rules, paying attention, and remaining on task. Pharmacotherapy involves the use of medications (e.g., methylphenidate) to control ADHD symptomatology.

An example of the combined use of behavior management and pharmacotherapy for ADHD is the summer treatment program (Carlson, Pelham, Milich, & Dixon, 1992; Pelham & Hoza, 1996; Pelham et al., 1993). The program is an intensive summer day treatment program for youth with ADHD that combines behavior management in the classroom (e.g., point system or token economy, time-out procedures), social skills training, daily report cards, and pharmacotherapy (Pelham & Hoza, 1996). Research on the separate and combined effects of behavior management and methylphenidate for youth in the program indicate that both treatments are more effective than no treatment (Carlson et al., 1992; Pelham et al., 1993). Further, one study found that the use of behavior management with lower doses of methylphenidate was as effective as the use of higher doses of methylphenidate alone (Carlson et al., 1992).

EFFECTIVENESS

Recently, critiques of the efficacy literature on evidence-based child and adolescent programs have focused on their effectiveness (i.e., clinical utility) as real-world practices. Much of this literature has focused on dissemination and implementation of these programs (Goldman et al., 2001; Schoenwald & Hoagwood, 2001), or what some have called "diffusion of innovation" (Henggler & Lee, 2002). Three factors described in the literature have been thought to influence the diffusion of evidence-based practices: (a) philosophical differences as to the importance of evidence-based practices versus effective "practice principles," (b) structural characteristics of the intervention, and (c) systemic or political issues.

Philosophical Differences

One of the issues impeding the dissemination and implementation of evidence-based practices relates to the therapeutic value of these practices compared with effective "practice principles." Rather than focusing solely on specialized protocols for specific disorders, advocates of this model suggest that it may be more important to examine the common factors that cut across these treatment protocols and contribute to their effectiveness. For example, Bickman (2002) and Drisko (2002) suggest that therapeutic alliance (i.e., agreement on clinical tasks and goals, an affective bond with the therapist) is a common factor that cuts across all therapeutic techniques for different child and adolescent disorders and has been shown to have a relationship to clinical outcomes. In fact, Drisko indicates that treat-

ment protocol (e.g., CBT) accounts for only about 15% of the therapeutic outcome variance, while common factors, including therapeutic alliance and factors related to the characteristics of the agency and client, account for about 70% of the outcome variance. Clearly, conceptualization of evidence-based practice within this paradigm would influence the direction of clinical research and subsequent implementation in the field. As an example of research within this paradigm, Sapyta, Karver, and Bickman (2000) describe preliminary test development procedures on a therapeutic alliance measure focused on practitioners working with children, which would have relevance for measuring this construct in the practice setting. While research in the area of common factors is promising, Bickman notes that there has been very little research in this area, and therefore very little is known about its relationship to effective and efficacious practice.

Structural Characteristics

Henggler and Lee (2002) identify several characteristics of evidence-based practices that influence their probability for implementation into real-world settings. They suggest that evidence-based practices that have a perceived advantage over current practices, do not deviate far from current practices, are simple to administer, and can be implemented in stages have a higher probability for adoption. Others have suggested that the structural characteristics of evidence-based practices and their relative "fit" into the existing child and adolescent service system need much more research. In fact, well-conducted, randomized, controlled trials that are strong in internal validity are often weak in external validity. Often, serious questions emerge regarding the transportability of these studies into real-world settings. Bickman (2002) suggests that research should focus on the needs and perceptions of service providers and families in order to identify the feasibility of implementation of evidence-based practices. He suggests that there is a need to know which treatments are acceptable to clinicians, based on the ways in which they practice. Further, there is also a need to know how evidence-based practices vary according to within-subject characteristics, such as gender, ethnicity or culture, severity of disorder, and contextual factors. Thus far, research examining such differences has been minimal.

Further, evidence-based practices have been

criticized for having limited applicability to youth with comorbid disorders (Bickman, 2002; Hawley & Weisz, 2002). While youth in the research samples used to establish evidence-based practices have been carefully screened for comorbid disorders, youth receiving services in the real world typically have more than one disorder. How does one implement these practices to meet the needs of the multiproblem youth who are seen in community-based agencies and institutions? Further, how do these practices hold up to other real-world practice constraints (e.g., managed care, lack of intense supervision to ensure treatment fidelity)? Clearly, much more research needs to be conducted to adapt the structural characteristics of these interventions to meet the complex needs of existing child and adolescent service systems.

Systemic and Political Issues

Henggler and Lee (2002) identify characteristics of the service system that influence the probability for the implementation and dissemination of evidence-based practices. They state that, while authoritarian decisions to adopt an evidence-based practice (e.g., directive from a CEO) result in the fastest implementation of the practice, collective decisions to adopt the practice are more likely to be sustained. Further, they suggest that the culture of an organization influences decisions to adopt evidence-based practices. These factors point to the importance of involving key stakeholders in the process of implementing evidence-based practices in order to ensure the success of the process. Further, these factors suggest that successful implementation of these practices may be a lengthy process, as it typically requires a shift in the organizational culture for the practices to be accepted. Perspectives of consumers, clinicians, and administrators will most likely influence this culture and its readiness to accept the interventions.

CONCLUSIONS

This chapter reviewed several evidence-based practices for internalizing and externalizing child and adolescent disorders and reviewed some of the issues related to dissemination and implementation of these interventions. While research has identified treatment techniques that have demonstrated clinical efficacy (e.g., CBT), there is still ambiguity as to how to best incorporate these techniques into the field. Recently, there have been documented efforts toward integrating evidence-based practices into the real world. Chorpita et al. (2002), for example, describe one state's efforts toward this goal by establishing the Empirical Basis to Services Task Force (EBS). EBS is a consortium of researchers from different disciplines (e.g., social work, psychiatry, psychology), clinicians in the field, and parents of youth receiving services, whose goal is to identify efficacious programs that have a high probability of utilization in the field. The next logical step might be for consortiums such as EBS to develop and evaluate programs for youth that have a focus on both efficacy and effectiveness. For now, however, more research is needed to examine aspects of the service system, perceptions of consumers and clinicians, and the unique clinical attributes related to diverse populations in order to successfully "fit" evidence-based practices into the field.

References

APA Task Force on Psychological Intervention Guidelines. (1995). *Template for developing guidelines: Interventions for mental disorders and psychosocial aspects of physical disorders.* Washington, DC: American Psychological Association.

Barrett, P. M. (1998). Evaluation of cognitive-behavioral group treatments for childhood anxiety disorders. *Journal of Clinical Child Psychology, 27,* 459–468.

Bickman, L. (2002). The death of treatment as usual: An excellent first step on a long road. *Clinical Psychology, 9,* 195–199.

Borduin, C. M., Mann, B. J., Cone, L. T., Henggler, S. W., Fucci, B. R., Blaske, D. M., et al. (1995). Multisystemic treatment of serious juvenile offenders: Long-term prevention of criminality and violence. *Journal of Consulting and Clinical Psychology, 63,* 569–578.

Brestan, E. V., & Eyberg, S. M. (1998). Effective psychosocial treatments of conduct-disordered children and adolescents: 29 years, 82 studies, and 5,272 kids. *Journal of Clinical Child Psychology, 27,* 180–189.

Campbell Collaboration. (2002). Retrieved November 16, 2002, from http://campbellcollaboration.org

Carlson, C. L., Pelham, W. E., Milich, R., & Dixon, J. (1992). Single and combined effects of methylphenidate and behavior therapy on the classroom performance of children with attention-deficit hyperactivity disorder. *Journal of Abnormal Child Psychology, 20,* 213–232.

Center for Substance Abuse Prevention. (n.d.). Retrieved October 20, 2002, from http://www.samhsa.gov/centers/csap/csap.html

Center for the Study and Prevention of Violence. (2002). Retrieved October 20, 2002, from http://www.colorado.edu/cspv/

Chambless, D. L., Baker, M. J., Baucom, D. H., Beutler, L. E., Calhoun, D. S., Crits-Christoph, P., et al. (1998). Update on empirically validated therapies II. *The Clinical Psychologist, 51,* 3–16.

Chambless, D. L., Sanderson, W. C., Shoham, V., Johnson, S. B., Pope, K. S., Crits-Christoph, P., et al. (1996). An update on empirically validated therapies. *The Clinical Psychologist, 49,* 5–18.

Chorpita, B. F., Yim, L. M., Donkervoet, J. C., Arensdorf, A., Amundsen, M. J., McGee, C., et al. (2002). Toward large-scale implementation of empirically supported treatments for children: A review and observations by the Hawaii Empirical Basis to Services Task Force. *Clinical Psychology, 9,* 165–190

Christophersen, E. R., & Mortweet, S. L. (2001). *Treatments that work with children: Empirically supported strategies for managing childhood problems.* Washington, DC: American Psychological Association.

Clarke, G., Lewinsohn, P., & Hops, H. (1990). *Adolescent coping with depression.* Eugene, OR: Castalia.

Clarke, G. N., Rohde, P., Lewinsohn, P. M., Hops, H., & Seeley, J. R. (1999). Cognitive-behavioral treatment of adolescent depression: Efficacy of acute group treatment and booster sessions. *Journal of the American Academy of Child and Adolescent Psychiatry, 38,* 272–279.

Cochrane Library. (2002). Retrieved November 16, 2002, from http://www.cochrane.org

Corcoran, J. (in press). *Clinical applications of evidence-based family interventions.* New York: Oxford University Press.

Derzon, J. H., Wilson, S. J., & Cunningham, C. A. (1999). *The effectiveness of school-based interventions for preventing and reducing violence.* Nashville, TN: Vanderbilt Institute for Public Policy Studies, Center for Evaluation Research and Methodology.

Drisko, J. W. (2002, January). *Common factors in psychotherapy effectiveness: A neglected dimension in social work research.* Paper presented at the sixth annual conference of the Society for Social Work and Research, San Diego, CA.

Goldman, H. H., Ganju, V., Drake, R. E., Gorman, P., Hogan, M., Hyde, P. S., et al. (2001). Policy implications for implementing evidence-based practices. *Psychiatric Services, 52,* 1591–1597.

Hawley, K. M., & Weisz, J. R. (2002). Increasing the relevance of evidence-based treatment review to practitioners and consumers. *Clinical Psychology, 9,* 225–230.

Henggler, S. W., & Borduin, C. (1990). *Family therapy and beyond: A multisystemic approach to treating behavior problems of children and adolescents.* Pacific Grove, CA: Brooks/Cole.

Henggler, S. W., & Lee, T. (2002). What happens after the innovation is identified? *Clinical Psychology: Science and Practice, 9,* 191–194.

Henggler, S. W., Melton, G. B., Brondino, M. J., Scherer, D. G., & Hanley, J. H. (1997). Multisystemic therapy with violent and chronic juvenile offenders and their families: The role of treatment fidelity in successful dissemination. *Journal of Consulting and Clinical Psychology, 65,* 821–833.

Henggler, S. W., Melton, G. B., & Smith, L. A. (1992). Family preservation using multisystemic therapy: An effective alternative to incarcerating serious juvenile offenders. *Journal of Consulting and Clinical Psychology, 60,* 953–961.

Kaslow, N. J., & Thompson, M. P. (1998). Applying the criteria for empirically supported treatments to studies of psychosocial interventions for child and adolescent depression. *Journal of Clinical Child Psychology, 27,* 146–155.

Lewinsohn, P. M., Clarke, G. N., Hops, H., & Andrews, J. (1990). Cognitive-behavioral group treatment of depression in adolescents. *Behavior Therapy, 21,* 385–401.

Lewinsohn, P. M., Clarke, G. N., Rohde, P., Hops, H., & Seeley, J. R. (1996). A course in coping: A cognitive-behavioral approach to the treatment of adolescent depression. In E. D. Hibbs & P. S. Jensen (Eds.), *Psychosocial treatments for child and adolescent disorders* (pp. 109–135). Washington, DC: American Psychological Association.

Mufson, L., Moreau, D., & Weissman, M. M. (1996). Focus on relationships: Interpersonal psychotherapy for adolescent depression. In E. D. Hibbs & P. S. Jensen (Eds.), *Psychosocial treatments for child and adolescent disorders* (pp. 137–155). Washington, DC: American Psychological Association.

Mufson, L., Moreau, D., Weissman, M. M., & Kerman, G. (1993). *Interpersonal psychotherapy for depressed adolescents.* New York: Guilford.

Mufson, L., Weissman, M. M., Moreau, D., & Garfinkel, R. (1999). Efficacy of interpersonal psychotherapy for depressed adolescents. *Archives of General Psychiatry, 56,* 573–579.

Ollendick, T. H., & King, N. J. (1998). Empirically supported treatments for children with phobic and anxiety disorders: Current status. *Journal of Clinical Child Psychology, 27,* 156–167.

Pelham, W. E., Carlson, C., Sams, S. E., Vallano, G., Dixon, M. J., & Hoza, B. (1993). Separate and combined effects of methylphenidate and behavior modification on boys with attention deficit-hyperactivity disorder in the classroom. *Journal of Consulting and Clinical Psychology, 61,* 506–515.

Pelham, W. E., & Hoza, B. (1996). Intensive treatment: Summer treatment program for children with ADHD. In E. D. Hibbs & P. S. Jensen (Eds.), *Psychosocial treatments for child and adolescent disorders* (pp. 311–340). Washington, DC: American Psychological Association.

Rapee, R. M., Wignall, A., Hudson, J. L., & Schniering, C. A. (2001). *Treating anxious children and adolescents: An evidence-based approach.* New York: New Harbinger.

Sapyta, J. J., Karver, M. S., & Bickman, L. (2000). Therapeutic alliance: Significance in non-psychotherapy settings. In C. Liberton, C. Newman, K. Kutash, & R. Friedman (Eds.), *The 12th annual research conference proceedings, a system of care for children's mental health: Expanding the research base* (pp. 183–186). Tampa, FL: University of South Florida, The Louis de la Parte Florida Mental Health Institute, Research and Training Center for Children's Mental Health.

Schoenwald, S. K., & Hoagwood, K. (2001). Effectiveness, transportability, and dissemination of interventions: What matters when? *Psychiatric Services, 52,* 1190–1197.

Serketich, W. J., & Dumas, J. E. (1996). The effectiveness of behavioral parent training to modify antisocial behavior in children: A meta-analysis. *Behavior Therapy, 27,* 171–186.

Silverman, W. K., & Kurtines, W. M. (1996). *Anxiety and phobic disorders: A pragmatic approach.* New York: Plenum.

Silverman, W. K., Kurtines, W. M., Ginsburg, G. S., Weems, C. F., Lumpkin, P. W., & Carmichael, D. H. (1999). Treating anxiety disorders in children with group cognitive-behavioral therapy: A randomized clinical trial. *Journal of Consulting and Clinical Psychology, 67,* 995–1003.

Task Force on the Promotion and Dissemination of Psychological Procedures. (1995). Training in and dissemination of empirically-validated psychosocial treatments: Report and recommendations. *The Clinical Psychologist, 48,* 3–23.

Tolan, P., & Guerra, N. (1994). *What works in reducing adolescent violence: An empirical review of the field.* Boulder, CO: University of Colorado, Institute for Behavioral Sciences.

Webster-Stratton, C. (1984). Randomized trial of two parent-training programs for families with conduct-disordered children. *Journal of Consulting and Clinical Psychology, 52,* 666–678.

Webster-Stratton, C., & Hancock, L. (1998). Training for parents of young children with conduct problems: Content, methods, and therapeutic processes. In J. M. Briesmeister & C. E. Schaefer (Eds.), *Handbook of parent training* (pp. 98–152). New York: Wiley.

26 EVIDENCE-BASED TREATMENT FOR TRAUMATIZED AND ABUSED CHILDREN

Carlton E. Munson

The basic premise of this chapter is that intervention with traumatized children must have a developmental focus, using a scientific perspective that relies on evidence that is grounded in a therapeutic relationship. There have been few efforts to link the concepts of a developmental perspective, evidence, and the science of relationship in work with traumatized children. The research literature regarding child trauma is generally not presented or described in a way that is usable for the average practitioner. This chapter provides information that can assist in specifying and measuring relationship in ways that have not been systematically applied in the past and explains uses of evidence in work with traumatized children. This chapter uses a practical but comprehensive approach to child trauma treatment that can be easily understood and applied by practitioners.

Even though awareness of childhood trauma in its modern form has been described since the late 1800s, the treatment of childhood trauma is not well validated, empirically derived, or clearly codified (Kazdin, 1998). There is no generally accepted definition of childhood trauma that can be applied to clinical situations. The American Psychiatric Association's *DSM-IV-TR* (American Psychiatric Association, 2000a) contains a general and nonspecific definition of trauma within the diagnostic criteria for posttraumatic stress disorder that is generally applied to children, but it is not sensitive to the effects of trauma on the developmental process. In order to use an evidence-based approach to child trauma practice, the intervention must be derived from a clear definition of the phenomenon that is to be treated. For this chapter, a child-focused definition of trauma is used. Reactions to traumatic events can be variable, and the criteria for deciding whether a child has met the threshold of being traumatized are based on the following definition: Child trauma can result from any event or series of events that overwhelms, overstimulates, or creates subtle or extreme fear in a child that causes temporary or permanent interruption of normal developmental processes or tasks that occur with or without physical or psychological symptoms and behavioral change (Munson, 2001). Child intervention that focuses exclusively on trauma events or reactions to trauma is limited because the treatment must address the developmental issues (Amster, 1999; Law, 2000) and the caregiver role (see, for example, Carr, 2000; Denton, Walsh, & Daniel, 2002; Reddy & Pfeiffer, 1997; Ryburn, 1999). From an evidence perspective, the effect of trauma can be established by direct measures of traumatic reactions and by developmental measures that identify levels of functioning before and after trauma.

THE SCIENTIFIC METHOD

Collins (1994) has provided a succinct definition of the *scientific method* that is an effective guide for evidence-based child trauma practice:

Science means knowledge about the objective world that is true because that is the way things are, not just because we have imagined it. (p. 3)

The key to the scientific method is to compare, to look for the conditions under which something happens by contrasting them with the conditions under which it does not happen. The scientific method is the search for a set of mutually consistent causal generalizations that are based on the systematic comparison of conditions associated with a varying range of outcomes. (p. 183)

Evidence is the product of science. Evidence is "something that tends to prove" and provide "grounds for belief" (McKechnie, 1983, p. 633). Evidence can be produced in nonscientific ways. For example, in the law there are specific rules for producing evidence, but these rules do not necessarily result in the evidence being true or reliable. When evidence is produced from standard scientific procedures that strive for objectivity, reliability, and validity, evidence is more acceptable and closer to reality. There is a growing trend of merging conceptions of evidence collected through scientific methods and clinical practice activity and outcomes (Monette, Sullivan, & DeJong, 2002).

RELATIONSHIP AND THE LIMITS OF EVIDENCE

Evidence to inform intervention cannot be the exclusive focus of treatment (Benbenishty, Segev, Surkis, & Elias, 2002; Shaw, 2003). The practitioner's relationship with and advocacy for the child client is a critical aspect of effective and accurate assessment and positive outcome of intervention (Proctor, 2002; Sheldon, 2001; Soldz & McCullough, 2000; Webb, 2001, 2002). In this chapter, *clinical professional relationship* is defined as a dynamic collaborative process of interaction between a clinician and a client based on openness and honesty, which is designed to explore, assess, and promote change through recognized theoretical orientations and generally accepted practical interventions derived from scientific research.

Historically, studies have shown that relationship is the key to intervention outcome (Shirk & Russell, 1996), and assessment skills have been added because they are inherently essential to successful intervention. At the same time, relationship cannot be the only measure of outcome. Clinical anecdotal case reports that cannot be replicated and have no generalizability (Wicks-Nelson & Israel, 2002) can hamper effective therapy outcomes if applied by others (for example, see Spiegelman, 2002). Relationship has been described as dealing with the "nonspecifics" of intervention that are difficult to observe, describe, and teach (Kamphaus & Frick, 2001). Research methodology is increasingly being applied to the concept of therapeutic relationship, and the research has quantified relationship-based concepts such as personal attributes, in-session activities, technical activity, alliance activities, instillation of confidence and trust, positive connectedness, therapist training, consistency, nonverbal gestures, verbal expressions, empathy, congruence, positive regard, understanding, and outcome. For a review of the empirical referent studies for these relationship concepts, see Ackerman and Hilsenroth (2003). These relationship indicators can be applied to a number of roles common to child trauma work, such as networker, broker, support provider, educator, clinician, mediator, expert witness, and advocate (Anderson, Weston, Doueck, & Krause, 2002). Through using empirical referents and role concepts, relationship concepts can be transferred from the research world to the practice arena through a practical process of systematically and scientifically assessing skills grounded in an evidence orientation that includes:

• Identifying and reviewing practitioner natural interpersonal relationship skills
• Assessing educationally acquired professional relationship skills
• Surveying for inherent lack of professional relationship skills
• Providing learning that promotes development of relationship skills when they are deficient
• Documenting strategies that connect specific intervention techniques, relationship skills, and evidence-based outcomes
• Identifying intervention strategies that promote fostering trust between client and practitioner

The assessment of relationship skills should be continuously monitored through evaluation of three critical intervention requirements essential to fostering ongoing positive, effective relationship and evidence-focused intervention. To be successful, the practitioner must demonstrate capabilities in each of these areas:

• Articulated, compassionate, and nonjudgmental attitude that is operationalized and communicated to the child and caregivers
• Acquired skill at doing evidence-based objective assessment (nonsuggestive information gathering) and subjective scientific intervention (techniques that suggest, recommend, and motivate the child and caregivers to change or achieve mastery)
• Keen ability to accurately interpret the behavior and communication of the child, caregivers, and self (countertransference) through use of evidence

These intervention requirements set the stage for change. Relationship itself does not produce change, and evidence does not produce change. The use of relationship and evidence through interaction with the child and caregivers produces change, and scientific methods are used to measure the quality of the change (outcomes).

ETHICS, RELATIONSHIP, AND EVIDENCE

Practice based on evidence-related tasks and outcomes has ethical implications. There must be a rational connection between relationship and evidence use in child treatment. The vast expansion of child trauma research and child development research requires evidence-based interventions (Jellinek, 1999). To ignore empirical evidence can be harmful to clients. At the same time, concern must be shown for how practitioners conduct tasks and how outcomes are achieved. There must be monitoring for the subtle belief that only evidence-based tasks or outcomes have value. In child therapy, ethics are central to the process, because children lack the capacity or facility to confront unwanted interventions. Children have expectations of how one should behave toward the other, regardless of expected outcomes, but do not always have the ability to express their desires in power-based relationships such as treatment. The lack of expressive capacity in children that can result from traumatic experience is a strong argument for evidence-based interventions because evidence can aid in avoiding misinterpretation of children's intentions. At the same time, lost expressive capacity in a child requires scientifically derived relationship skills in the practitioner, who must patiently provide direct and indirect forms of alternative expression.

Professional ethics mandates evidence-based, relationship-focused intervention that should be monitored. The increased emphasis on techniques and tasks requires supervisors to monitor the use of techniques to ensure that (a) techniques used are related to problem assessment and resolution, (b) the practitioner is thoroughly trained in the techniques that are being applied, and (c) the techniques are generally accepted and appropriate. Techniques that have not been subjected to empirical analysis or are not subject to regular and consistent monitoring should not be used under current child intervention practice standards. For example, statements made by children during symbolic play should not be interpreted by a therapist without corroboration through independent evidence. Nondirective child therapy and symbolic play used in child abuse cases can lead to expressions of fantasy that are often misinterpreted (Dickinson & McCabe, 1991; Guerney, 1983; Reif & Stollak, 1972), especially in the case of very young children (Hewitt, 1999). In child trauma intervention, clinical symbolic or anecdotal information should not be interpreted without supportive evidentiary information.

INTERVENTION GUIDELINES

Collins's (1994) description of the scientific method reflects the activities and analysis that promote applying the scientific model to practice activity. Therapy has not traditionally been a scientific endeavor, but increasingly interaction and content are focused on promoting the scientific method in the practice situation. General intervention guidelines for promoting evidence-based relationship-focused practice are as follows.

- An intervention can be identified by the practitioner and can be understood by the client.

- An established connection between the intervention and the problem can be articulated by the practitioner (in some cases the child can also make the connection based on developmental level).
- The practitioner and client can implement the intervention with reasonable effort.
- The client has an identifiable reason/motivation to comply with the intervention.
- Along with the proposed intervention an alternate intervention can be identified by the practitioner.
- Possible outcomes (intended and unintended, positive and negative) of intervention can be identified in advance of applying the intervention.
- The intervention can be observed and measured. (Munson, 2003, p. 5)

All the principles do not have to be met in every situation, but the higher the number met, the more likely it is that the intervention will be successful. Applying these simple guidelines clinically can be much more effective than citing a series of research studies regarding the outcome of competing theoretical orientations that can be confusing to the average practitioner.

TYPES OF EVIDENCE

In the scientific method, there are four research goals: description, prediction, explanation, and evaluation (Monette et al., 2002). These four goals also apply directly to the evidence-based clinical situation, and intervention can be conceptualized in this framework. *Description* applies to the database information gathered during the assessment phase that precedes treatment. Historically, it was held that treatment begins at the moment of first contact with the client and that problems and solutions are inseparable (Selekman, 1997). In the actual process of assessment, diagnosis, and treatment, there is a merging and interaction of these functions. The increased emphasis on evidence-based practice has produced the standard that treatment does not deliberately begin until a thorough assessment has been completed, and treatment is connected to and derived from diagnostic and assessment data with respect to exploring the connection between each of these functions (Blythe & Reithoffer, 2000; Jongsma & Peterson, 2000). This does not mean that treatment impact does not occur at the initial contact, but a logical, scientific approach to intervention consists of *conscious* acts that occur after the situation is understood and assessed, based on known events, symptoms, behaviors, and risk factors.

The extensive literature regarding children who have had trauma experience (see, for example, Wolchik & Sandler, 1997) necessitates that clinicians be familiar with and utilize risk factors in assessment and treatment protocols. The concepts of risk factors and protective factors (Rutter, 1987,1998; Vance, Bowen, Fernandez, & Thompson, 2002) are established in child trauma and relate to the second scientific concept of *prediction*. In evidence-based child treatment, there are two forms of prediction. Type 1 prediction is associated with risk factors and protective factors related to the child that occur outside the intervention process and can be compared with scientific literature to establish future risk of symptoms or behavioral outcomes for a specific child (Milner, Murphy, Valle, & Tolliver, 1998). Risk factors serve as guides for the clinician to target areas for immediate intervention and other areas with a prevention focus (Sox, 1993). Type 2 prediction occurs within the treatment and relates to the prediction of the expected outcome of a specific intervention or an intervention strategy. For example, research has shown that Type 1 prediction is associated with early- or late-onset conduct disorder. Family dysfunction, family size, and severe aggression are more prevalent in the early-onset conduct disorder subtype. Type 2 prediction is associated with the fact that research has shown a more positive treatment outcome for the late-onset conduct disorder subtype when problem-solving skills training, parental management training, and multisystemic therapy are used (Kazdin, 1998). Other general examples of Type 1 prediction are low family income, parental chronic mental illness, parental availability, parental criminality, and poor parental supervision. Other examples of Type 2 prediction are that use of anatomically correct dolls in a sex abuse treatment protocol can have interpretive value when based on existing research (Ceci & Bruck, 1995). There is research evidence that child trauma treatment takes approximately 16 to 20 sessions to produce symptom resolution (Finkelhor & Berliner, 1995) and that the use of cognitive behavioral approaches are more effective in reducing symptoms of trauma (Cohen & Mannarino, 1998). Listings of risk factors and theoretical orientation outcomes are not alone sufficient for evidence use. The relevance of theoretical orientations and a set of risk factors and their interactions must be considered in the context of the individual case (Kazdin, 1998).

The concept of *explanation* is related to the interpretations of the child's situation, symptoms, or behavior. Explanation is different from prediction in that predictions can be made without an explanation (Monette et al., 2002). Explanations should be based on empirical support. For example, in a case where a child has symptoms of posttraumatic stress disorder (PTSD) but does not meet the *DSM-IV-TR* criteria, the therapist should make reference to the literature showing that only a small portion (approximately 13%) of children who experience trauma meet PTSD criteria (Merry & Andrews, 1994; Scheeringa, Pebbles, Cook, & Zeanah, 2001; Scheeringa & Zeanah, 2001; Scheeringa, Zeanah, Drell, & Larrieu, 1995; Scheeringa, Zeanah, Myers, & Putnam, 2003; Stoppelbein & Greening, 2000). Lack of understanding of the role of evidence in disorders like PTSD can result in failure to differentially diagnose other debilitating disorders, such as major depression (Weissman, 2001). Diagnostic and treatment explanations that cannot be derived from or supported by empirical literature or standardized measures (Cohen & Mannarino, 2002) should be based on hypothesis testing. This occurs most often in child abuse investigations. Hypothesis testing is applied to the speculative information of the situation to confirm or refute the speculation.

Hypothesis testing has evolved as a standard methodology in child sex abuse allegations (Bowlby, 1988; Ceci & Bruck, 1994, 1995; Faller, 2002; Jones, 1997; Nurcombe & Partlett, 1994). Hypothesis testing has become more essential in child trauma practice since the incidence of abuse allegations has increased in the last three decades (Hobbs, Hanks, & Wynne, 1999), especially in intrafamily sex abuse. The increase of divorce and the decline of adultery as a basis for obtaining a divorce have been paralleled by increasing use of abuse allegations as grounds for divorce (Ehrenberg & Elterman, 1995; Eminson & Postlethwaite, 2000).

Hypothesis testing is used to rule out other plausible explanations once a child has made a disclosure of abuse or in the absence of a disclosure (Ceci & Bruck, 1995; Faller, 1999; House, 2002; Lamb & Johnson, 2002; Ney, 1995; Pezdek, 1994). Faller (2002) states, "The evaluator begins the assessment process with a series of competing hypotheses. . . . The process of decision-making is best described as a process of ruling out hypotheses. The goal is to arrive at one or more most likely explanations for the concerns about abuse" (p. 15). This process is the clinical equivalent of Collins's (1994) scientific principle of establishing when an event has or has not occurred. Ceci and Bruck (1995), in their detailed analysis of the literature on suggestion of abuse, view hypothesis testing as essential to accurately assess abuse allegations, and hypothesis-related questions used in establishing the credibility of abuse allegations have been identified (Adams, 2000).

The concept of *evaluation* applies to the measurement of the outcomes of the interventions (see, for example, Cohen & Mannarino, 1997, 1998). Evaluation occurs when the intervention is being contemplated, as well as postintervention. Evaluation can relate to a single technique, a single session, or a course of therapy. A model for technique intervention guidelines was described in the previous section titled "Intervention Guidelines."

SOURCES OF EVIDENCE

The sources of evidence are observed evidence, reported evidence, and research evidence. *Observed evidence* is most important during the assessment phase and includes nonintrusive informal observations to evaluate children while engaged in routine interactions, as well as formal assessment through the use of standardized instruments (Horton & Bowman, 2002; Ohan, Myers, & Collett, 2002). Observations should be compared with reported evidence. *Reported evidence* is provided by caregivers or other collateral sources, such as teachers, social service workers, or probation officers (Apel, 2001; Lynagh, Perkins, & Schofield, 2002). For example, corroborative evidence can be in the form of structured clinical interviews, standardized scales or checklists (Schaefer, Gitlin, & Sandgrund, 1991) completed by a teacher, or a nonnormed or normed checklist completed by a foster parent. Reported evidence should be compared with observed evidence. *Research evidence* is data

that can be used to assess the child in comparison to scientifically accepted research reports. Included in this type of evidence are practice parameters and research reviews, such as those published by the American Academy of Child and Adolescent Psychiatry that are summary guidelines for understanding and treating various disorders or conditions (Dunne, 1997). For example, 46 review articles and 70 parameters papers have been published. Some of these have direct relevance to child trauma, such as items for child sexual abuse (Bernet, 1997; Shaw, 1999), posttraumatic stress disorder (Cohen, 1998; Pfefferbaum, 1997), oppositional defiant disorder and conduct disorder (Burke, Loeber, & Birmaher, 2002; Loeber, Burke, Lahey, Winters, & Zera, 2000), childhood depression (Boris & Brent, 1998), and language disorders (Beitchman, 1998).

Over the past five decades, there have been various efforts from an organizational and administrative perspective to develop forms of evidence-based outcomes (Manela & Moxley, 2002). These efforts have been variously called management by objectives, program planning and budgeting systems, agency accountability systems, integrated client information systems (Dobmeyer, Woodward, & Olson, 2002), and managed care (Alperin & Phillips, 1997; Austad, 1996; Stout, 2001). The tendency to equate clinical evidence-based intervention with these administrative methods has resulted in confusion about the basis of clinical evidence-based practice. The question is whether clinical evidence-based practice is an individual or organizational endeavor. The answer is that it is both (Hernandez & Hodges, 2001), but there must be a clear distinction about the individual and organizational components of evidence-based practice. Organizational guidelines for evidence-based practice are formalized, structured, procedural guidelines such as practice protocols, whereas individual clinical practice aids are compilations of information to inform clinical decision making, including practice guidelines, standards of practice, and standards of care. Concepts like best practices tend to merge individual and organizational orientations. These models are not necessarily based on evidence but are more effective and useful when grounded in evidence. These models are convenient vehicles for organizing and presenting evidence for use in clinical practice.

FORMATS FOR ORGANIZING EVIDENCE

Evidence-based measures should be applied within the context of a practice protocol. The earliest efforts to devise practice protocols for children were Gardner's (1992, 1995, 2002) in the 1980s regarding sex abuse investigations. A practice protocol is a set of standard procedural guidelines that are applied to all cases in a given area of practice (Munson, 2003). In the current environment of individual and agency accountability for all aspects of practice activity, professionals are being called upon to use standardized protocols to justify interventions (Munson, 2002). Accrediting organizations, private payers, and courts are requiring practice protocols for specific areas of practice. Each practice setting should have intervention practice protocols established by supervisors, practitioners, and agency administrators.

Practice protocols are different from practice guidelines (also referred to as *practice parameters* and *best practices*), standards of care, and standards of practice. These terms are often confused and used interchangeably in ways that can be confusing and inappropriate. Practice guidelines are a set of client care strategies and methods to aid practitioners in making clinical decisions (for more details about and examples of practice guidelines, see American Psychiatric Association, 2000b). Standards of care are precise performance expectations for the level and type of intervention that are provided to a specific child population (for example, sexually abused children) or a specific condition (for example, an anxiety disorder). Standards of care are used to manage risk for the client and liability for the practitioner (Bongar, Berman, et al., 1998). Standards of care are usually based on available clinical data and are subject to change as research and knowledge advance (American Psychiatric Association, 2000a). Standards of care are measured as the degree of care a reasonable professional should use in the same or similar circumstances, and deviations from a standard of care are usually considered negligence or gross negligence (Bongar, Maris, Berman, & Litman, 1998). Child trauma intervention based on this standard has lagged behind other practice areas, but a consensus is gradually emerging. Standards of practice are general guidelines set by professional organizations to guide practitioners in day-to-day professional activities in relation to clients. The current standards of practice use the principle of "professional expectations," which judge professional actions on the basis of the question, "Did the act of a given professional, in a given situation, conform to expectations of practice as defined by the general consensus of professionals working in that area of practice in the same locale?" This principle is also used by courts in deciding professional liability (Flach, 1998; Nurcombe & Partlett, 1994).

The concept of best practices is increasingly being used to assure others that agencies are of high quality and worthy of being considered on the forefront of practice knowledge. What constitutes best practice in organizations is not clear. Currently there are no standards for determining best practices, and they can be based on research evidence, expert testimonials, lobbying, marketing, or other efforts to promote their acceptance (Manela & Moxley, 2002). There is no standard format for establishing and describing best practices. Before the concept of best practices can be considered evidence-based, there must be clarification of the criteria and procedures for determining what constitutes a best practice in clinical settings.

EVIDENCE LIMITATIONS

The use of evidence-based practice is limited by the lack of widely accepted criteria for assessing the reliability and validity of research studies (Salzer, 1996) and the lack of standardized measures for observed and reported evidence use. No organized systems of meta-analysis of outcome research exist (Chang, Sanacora, & Sanchez, 1996). There are no methodologies in place to reconcile conflicting research findings focused on the same problem (see Bolen, 2000; Buttell & Pike, 2002). For example, two widely cited studies found significant differences in the amount of psychotherapy needed to produce effective outcomes for children with psychiatric illness (Petti, 2000). Evidence use is limited by the variation in availability of evidence. In some areas such as conduct disorder, there is limited evidence available (Kazdin, 1998), while there is an array of measures in other areas such as sexual abuse and childhood depression.

After 15 years of delivery systems basing outcomes on managed care cost criteria, professions are faced with how to orient practitioners to pursuing outcomes based on science (Coble,

2002; Jellinek, 1999; Showalter, 1995). For evidence-based practice to become the basis for child trauma intervention, there must be a more concerted effort to teach this approach in graduate training programs (Hodes, 1998), and there must be better systems for making research findings and standardized measures readily available and accessible to practitioners (Card, 2001; Kronenberger & Meyer, 2001; Randall, Cowley, & Tomlinson, 2000). Developing effective standardized intervention protocols is dependent on the dissemination of research findings. Technology has assisted somewhat in the dissemination of knowledge, but many practitioners do not have access to the evidence-based material described in this chapter that promotes empirically grounded child trauma intervention. The increase in research and knowledge about child trauma has led to some codification of evidence, but much more work needs to be done to ensure effective practice based on good evidence (Weber & Sergeant, 2003).

CONCLUSION

The main view of this paper is that evidence-based practice must be balanced with a relationship model. Practice cannot be grounded only in evidence, just as it cannot be formulated solely on relationship. Evidence-based practice is more than compiling supportive research evidence, more than setting up research centers (Iwaniec & McCrystal, 1999), and more than cataloging outcomes. Evidence-based tasks without relationship-based structure in child intervention can lead to outcome errors. For evidence-based practice to be successful, there cannot be an approach of imposing the evidence on the child, but useful evidence can be applied and generated through a facilitated and collaborative relationship with the child. In 1934, Vygotsky (1986) observed that child psychology was a method of exploring human consciousness rather than elementary behavioral acts. We now know that intervention includes both, and only when evidence and relationship are used in combination is effective, scientifically informed practice achieved.

References

Ackerman, S. J., & Hilsenroth, M. J. (2003). A review of therapist characteristics and techniques positively impacting the therapeutic alliance. *Clinical Psychology Review, 23,* 1–33.

Adams, J. A. (2000). How do I evaluate suspected sexual abuse in the adolescent female? In H. Dubowitz & D. DePanfilis (Eds.), *Handbook for child protection practice* (p. 206). Thousand Oaks, CA: Sage.

Alperin, R. M., & Phillips, D. G. (1997). *The impact of managed care on the practice of psychotherapy: Innovation, implementation, and controversy.* New York: Brunner/Mazel.

American Psychiatric Association. (2000a). *Diagnostic and statistical manual of mental disorders* (4th ed., text revision). Washington, DC: Author.

American Psychiatric Association. (2000b). *Practice guidelines for the treatment of psychiatric disorders: Compendium 2000.* Washington, DC: Author.

Amster, B. J. (1999). Speech and language development of young children in the child welfare system. In J. A. Silver, B. J. Amster, & T. Haecher (Eds.), *Young children and foster care* (pp. 117–157). Baltimore: Brookes.

Anderson, L. E., Weston, E. A., Doueck, H. J., & Krause, D. J. (2002). The child-centered social worker and the sexually abused child: Pathway to healing. *Social Work, 47* (4), 368–378.

Apel, K. (2001). Developing evidence-based practices and research collaborations in school settings. *Language, Speech, and Hearing Services in Schools, 32,* 196–198.

Austad, C. S. (1996). *Is long-term psychotherapy unethical? Toward a social ethic in an era of managed care.* San Francisco: Jossey-Bass.

Beitchman, J. H. (1998). Summary of the practice parameters for the assessment and treatment of children and adolescents with language and learning disorders. *Journal of the American Academy of Child and Adolescent Psychiatry, 37,* 1117–1119.

Benbenishty, R., Segev, D., Surkis, T., & Elias, T. (2002). Information-search and decision-making by professionals and nonprofessionals in cases of alleged child-abuse and maltreatment. *Journal of Social Service Research, 28,* 1–18.

Bernet, W. (1997). Practice parameters for the evaluation of children and adolescents who may have been physically or sexually abused. *Journal of the American Academy of Child and Adolescent Psychiatry, 36,* 37s–56s.

Blythe, B., & Reithoffer, A. (2000). Assessment and measurement issues in direct practice in social work. In P. Allen-Meares, & C. Garvin (Eds.). *The handbook of direct social work practice* (pp. 551–564). Thousand Oaks, CA: Sage.

Bolen, R. M. (2000). Validity of attachment theory. *Trauma, Violence and Abuse, 1,* 128–153.

Bongar, B., Berman, A. L., Maris, R. W., Silverman, M. M., Harris, E. A., & Packman, W. L. (Eds.).

(1998). *Risk management with suicidal patients.* New York: Guilford.

Bongar, B., Maris, R. W., Berman, A. L., & Litman, R. E. (1998). Outpatient standards of care and the suicidal patient. In B. Bongar, A. L. Berman, R. W. Maris, M. M. Silverman, E. A. Harris, & W. L. Packman (Eds.), *Risk management with suicidal patients* (pp. 4–33). New York: Guilford.

Boris, M. D., & Brent, D. (1998). Practice parameters for assessment and treatment of children and adolescents with depressive disorders. *Journal of the American Academy of Child and Adolescent Psychiatry, 37,* 46s–62s.

Bowlby, J. (1988). *A secure base: Parent–child attachment and healthy human development.* New York: Basic Books.

Burke, J. D., Loeber, R., & Birmaher, B. (2002). Oppositional defiant disorder and conduct disorder: A review of the past 10 years, part II. *Journal of the American Academy of Child and Adolescent Psychiatry, 41* (11), 1275–1293.

Buttell, F. P., & Pike, C. K. (2002). Investigating predictors of treatment attribution among court-ordered batterers. *Journal of Social Service Research, 28,* 53–68.

Card, J. J. (2001). The sociometrics program archives: Promoting the dissemination of evidence-based practices through replication kits. *Research on Social Work Practice, 11,* 521–527.

Carr, A. (2000). Evidence-based practice in family therapy and systemic consultation in child focused problems. *Journal of Family Therapy, 22,* 29–61.

Ceci, S. J., & Bruck, M. (1994). How reliable are children's statements? . . . it depends. *Family Relations, 43,* 255–257.

Ceci, S. J., & Bruck, M. (1995). *Jeopardy in the courtroom: A scientific analysis of children's testimony.* Washington, DC: American Psychological Association.

Chang, R., Sanacora, G., & Sanchez, R. (1996). The need for outcome studies. *Journal of the American Academy of Child and Adolescent Psychiatry, 35,* 557.

Coble, Y. (2002, December 27). Medicine is more than science. *USA Today,* p. A11.

Cohen, J. A. (1998). Summary of the practice parameters for the assessment and treatment of children and adolescents with posttraumatic stress disorder. *Journal of the American Academy Child and Adolescent Psychiatry, 37,* 997–1001.

Cohen, J. A., & Mannarino, A. P. (1997). A treatment study for sexually abused preschool children: Outcome during a one-year follow-up. *Journal of the American Academy of Child and Adolescent Psychiatry, 36,* 1228–1235.

Cohen, J. A., & Mannarino, A. P. (1998). Factors that mediate treatment outcome of sexually abused preschool children: Six- and 12-month follow-up.

Journal of the American Academy of Child and Adolescent Psychiatry, 37, 44–51.

Cohen, J. A., & Mannarino, A. P. (2002). Addressing attributions in treating abused children. *Child Maltreatment, 7,* 82–86.

Collins, R. (1994). *Four sociological traditions.* New York: Oxford University Press.

Denton, W. H., Walsh, S. R., & Daniel, S. S. (2002). Evidence-based practice in family therapy: Adolescent depression as an example. *Journal of Marital and Family Therapy, 28,* 39–46.

Dickinson, D., & McCabe, A. (1991). The acquisition and development of language: A social interactionist account of language and literacy development. In J. F. Kavanagh (Ed.), *The language continuum: From infancy to literacy* (pp. 1–40). Parkton, MD: York Press.

Dobmeyer, T. W., Woodward, B., & Olson, L. (2002). Factors supporting the development and utilization of an outcome-based performance measurement system in a chemical health case management program. *Administration in Social Work, 26*(4), 25–44.

Dunne, J. E. (1997). History and development of the practice parameters. *Journal of the American Academy of Child and Adolescent Psychiatry, 36,* 1s–3s.

Ehrenberg, M. F., & Elterman, M. F. (1995). Evaluating allegations of sexual abuse in the context of divorce, child custody, and access disputes. In T. Ney (Ed.), *True and false allegations of child sexual abuse: Assessment and case management* (pp. 209–230). New York: Brunner/Mazel.

Eminson, M., & Postlethwaite, R. J. (Eds.). (2000). *Munchausen syndrome by proxy abuse: A practical approach.* Oxford: Butterworth Heinemann.

Faller, K. C. (1999). Questioning children who may have been sexually abused: An integration of research into practice. In K. C. Faller (Ed.), *Maltreatment in early childhood: Tools for research-based intervention* (pp. 37–58). New York: Haworth.

Faller, K. C. (2002, April). *Update on allegations of sexual abuse in divorce.* Paper presented at National Child Advocacy Center conference, Huntsville, AL.

Finkelhor, D., & Berliner, L. (1995). Research on treatment of sexually abused children. *Journal of the American Academy of Child and Adolescent Psychiatry, 34,* 1408–1423.

Flach, F. (Ed.). (1998). *A comprehensive guide to malpractice risk management in psychiatry.* New York: Hatherleigh.

Gardner, R. A. (1992). *The psychotherapeutic techniques of Richard A. Gardner.* Cresskill, NJ: Creative Therapeutics.

Gardner, R. A. (1995). *Protocols for the sex-abuse evaluation.* Cresskill, NJ: Creative Therapeutics.

Gardner, R. A. (2002). *Sex-abuse trauma? Or trauma*

from other sources. Cresskill, NJ: Creative Therapeutics.

Guerney, L. F. (1983). Client-centered (nondirective) play therapy. In C. E. Schaefer & K. J. O'Connor (Eds.), *Handbook of play therapy* (pp. 21–64). New York: Wiley.

Hernandez, M., & Hodges, S. (Eds.). (2001). *Developing outcome strategies in children's mental health.* Baltimore: Paul H. Brookes.

Hewitt, S. K. (1999). *Assessing allegations of sexual abuse in preschool children: Understanding small voices.* Thousand Oaks, CA: Sage.

Hobbs, C. J., Hanks, H. G. I., & Wynne, J. M. (1999). *Child abuse and neglect: A clinician's handbook* (2nd ed.). London: Churchill Livingstone.

Hodes, M. (1998). A core curriculum for child and adolescent psychiatry. *European Child and Adolescent Psychiatry, 7,* 250–255.

Horton, C., & Bowman, B. T. (2002). *Child assessment at the preprimary level: Occasional paper number 3.* Chicago: Erickson Institute.

House, A. E. (2002). *The first session with children and adolescents: Conducting a comprehensive mental health evaluation.* New York: Guilford.

Iwaniec, D., & McCrystal, P. (1999). The Centre for Child Care Research at the Queen's University of Belfast. *Research on Social Work Practice, 9,* 248–260.

Jellinek, M. S. (1999). Changes in the practice of child and adolescent psychiatry: Are our patients better served? *Journal of the American Academy of Child and Adolescent Psychiatry, 38,* 115–117.

Jones, D. P. H. (1997) Assessment of suspected child sexual abuse. In M. E. Helfner, R. S. Kempe, & R. D. Krugman (Eds.), *The battered child* (5th ed., pp. 297–312). Chicago: University of Chicago Press.

Jongsma, A. E., & Peterson, L. M. (2000). *The child psychotherapy treatment planner.* New York: Wiley.

Kamphaus, R. W., & Frick, P. J. (2001). *Clinical assessment of child and adolescent personality and behavior.* Boston: Allyn & Bacon.

Kazdin, A. E. (1998). Psychosocial treatments for conduct disorder in children. In P. E. Nathan & J. M. Gorman (Eds.), *A guide to treatments that work* (pp. 65–89). New York: Oxford University Press.

Kronenberger, W. G., & Meyer, R. G. (2001). *The child clinician's handbook.* Boston: Allyn & Bacon.

Lamb, N. B., & Johnson, M. (2002, April). Combating defense strategies in child sexual abuse cases. Paper presented at the National Child Advocacy Center conference, Huntsville, AL.

Law, M. (2000). Strategies for implementing evidence-based practice in early intervention. *Infants and Young Children: An Interdisciplinary Journal of Special Care Practices, 13,* 32–41.

Loeber, R., Burke, J. D., Lahey, B. B., Winters, A., &

Zera, M. (2000). Oppositional defiant disorder and conduct disorder: A review of the past 10 years, part I. *Journal of the American Academy of Child and Adolescent Psychiatry, 39,* 1468–1484.

Lynagh, M., Perkins, J., & Schofield, M. (2002). An evidence-based approach to health promoting schools. *Journal of School Health, 72,* 300–303.

Manela, R. W., & Moxley, D. P. (2002). Best practices as agency-based knowledge in social welfare. *Administration in Social Work, 26*(4), 1–24.

McKechnie, J. (Ed.). (1983). *Websters' new twentieth century dictionary* (2nd ed.). New York: Simon & Schuster.

Merry, S. N., & Andrews, L. K. (1994). Psychiatric status of sexually abused children 12 months after disclosure of abuse. *Journal of the American Academy of Child and Adolescent Psychiatry, 33,* 939–944.

Milner, J. S., Murphy, W. D., Valle, L. A., & Tolliver, R. M. (1998). Assessment issues in child abuse evaluations. In J. R. Lutzker (Ed.), *Handbook of child abuse research and treatment* (pp. 75–115). New York: Plenum.

Monette, D. R., Sullivan, T. J., & DeJong, C. R. (2002). *Applied social research: Tool for the human services* (5th ed.). New York: Harcourt Brace.

Munson, C. (2002). *Handbook of clinical social work supervision.* New York: Haworth.

Munson, C. E. (2001). *The mental health diagnostic desk reference: Visuals, guides and more for learning to use the Diagnostic and Statistical Manual, DSM-IV-TR* (2nd ed.). New York: Haworth.

Munson, C. E. (2003). Evolution and trends in supervision. In M. J. Austin & K. M. Hopkins (Eds.), *Human service supervision in the learning organization.* Thousand Oaks, CA: Sage.

Ney, T. (Ed.). (1995). *True and false allegations of child sexual abuse: Assessment and case management.* New York: Brunner/Mazel.

Nurcombe, B., & Partlett, D. F. (1994). *Child mental health and the law.* New York: Free Press.

Ohan, J. L., Myers, K., & Collett, B. R. (2002). Ten-year review of rating scales IV: Scales assessing trauma and its effects. *Journal of the American Academy of Child and Adolescent Psychiatry, 41,* 1401–1422.

Petti, T. A. (2000). Commentary: More outcome studies are needed. *Journal of the American Academy of Child and Adolescent Psychiatry, 39,* 169–171.

Pezdek, K. (1994). Avoiding false claims of child sexual abuse: Empty promises. *Family Relations, 43,* 258–260.

Pfefferbaum, B. (1997). Posttraumatic stress disorder in children: A review of the past 10 years. *Journal of the American Academy of Child and Adolescent Psychiatry, 36*(11), 1503–1511.

Proctor, E. K. (2002). Social work, school violence, mental health, and drug abuse: A call for evidence-based practices. *Social Work Research, 26*, 67–69.

Randall, J., Cowley, P., & Tomlinson, P. (2000). Overcoming barriers to effective practice in child care. *Child and Family Social Work, 5*, 343–353.

Reddy, L. A., & Pfeiffer, S. I. (1997). Effectiveness of treatment foster care with children and adolescents: A review of outcome studies. *Journal of the American Academy of Child and Adolescent Psychiatry, 36*(11), 581–588.

Reif, T., & Stollak, G. (1972). *Sensitivity to children: Training and its effects.* East Lansing, MI: Michigan State University Press.

Roberts, A. R. (Ed.). (2002). *Handbook of domestic violence intervention strategies: Policies, programs, and legal remedies.* New York: Oxford University Press.

Rutter, M. (1987). Psychosocial resilience and protective mechanisms. *American Journal of Orthopsychiatry, 57*, 316–331.

Rutter, M. (1998). Routes from research to clinical practice in child psychiatry: Retrospect and prospect. *Journal of Child Psychology and Psychiatry, 39*, 805–816.

Ryburn, M. (1999). Contact between children placed away from home and their birth parents: A reanalysis of the evidence in relation to permanent placements. *Clinical Child Psychology and Psychiatry, 4*, 505–519.

Salzer, M. S. (1996). Interpreting outcome studies. *Journal of the American Academy of Child and Adolescent Psychiatry, 35*, 1419.

Schaefer, C. E., Gitlin, K., & Sandgrund, A. (Eds.). (1991). *Play diagnosis and assessment.* New York: Wiley.

Scheeringa, M. S., Pebbles, C. D., Cook, C. A., & Zeanah, C. H. (2001). Toward establishing procedural, criterion, and discriminant validity for PTSD in early childhood. *Journal of the American Academy of Child and Adolescent Psychiatry, 40*, 52–60.

Scheeringa, M. S., & Zeanah, C. H. (2001). A relational perspective on PTSD in early childhood, *Journal of Traumatic Stress, 14*, 799–815.

Scheeringa, M. S., Zeanah, C. H., Drell, M. J., & Larrieu, J. A. (1995). Two approaches to the diagnosis of posttraumatic stress disorder in infancy and early childhood. *Journal of the American Academy of Child and Adolescent Psychiatry, 34*, 191–200.

Scheeringa, M. S., Zeanah, C. H., Myers, L., & Putnam, F. W. (2003). New findings on alternative criteria of PTSD in preschool children. *Journal of the American Academy of Child and Adolescent Psychiatry, 42*, 561–570.

Selekman, M. D. (1997). *Solution-focused therapy with children: Harnessing family strengths for systemic change.* New York: Guilford.

Shaw, I. F. (2003). Cutting edge issues in social work research. *British Journal of Social Work, 33*(1), 107–111.

Shaw, J. A. (1999). Practice parameters for the assessment and treatment of children and adolescents who are sexually abusive of others. *Journal of the American Academy of Child and Adolescent Psychiatry, 42*, 119–120.

Sheldon, B. (2001). The validity of evidence-based practice in social work: A reply to Stephen Webb. *British Journal of Social Work, 31*, 801–809.

Shirk, S. R., & Russell, R. L. (1996). *Change processes in child psychotherapy: Revitalizing treatment and research.* New York: Guilford.

Showalter, J. E. (1995). Managed care: Income to outcome. *Journal of the American Academy of Child and Adolescent Psychiatry, 34*, 1123.

Soldz, R., & McCullough, L. (Eds.). (2000). *Reconciling empirical knowledge and clinical experience: The art and science of psychotherapy.* Washington, DC: American Psychological Association.

Sox, H. C. (1993). Evidence-based practice guidelines from the U.S. Preventive Services Task Force. *Journal of the American Medical Association, 269*, 2678.

Spiegelman, C. (2002, Summer). The power of magic in working with traumatized children. *Access: Clinical Social Work Federation*, 12–13.

Stoppelbein, L., & Greening, L. (2000). Posttraumatic stress symptoms in parentally bereaved children and adolescents. *Journal of the American Academy of Child and Adolescent Psychiatry, 39*, 1112–1119.

Stout, C. E. (2001). A broadened vision of accountability for our children. *Behavioral Health Accreditation and Accountability Alert, 6*, 8.

Toppelberg, C. O., Medrano, L., Pena Morgens, L., & Nieto-Castanon, A. (2002). Bilingual children referred for psychiatric services: Associations of language disorders, language skills and psychopathology. *Journal of the American Academy of Child and Adolescent Psychiatry, 41*(6), 712–722.

Vance, J. E., Bowen, N. K., Fernandez, G., & Thompson, S. (2002). Risk and protective factors as predictors of outcome in adolescents with psychiatric disorder and aggression. *Journal of the American Academy of Child and Adolescent Psychiatry, 41*, 36–43.

Vygotsky, L. (1986). *Thought and language.* Cambridge, MA: MIT Press.

Webb, S. A. (2001). Some considerations on the validity of evidence-based practice in social work. *British Journal of Social Work, 31*, 795–800.

Webb, S. A. (2002). Evidence-based practice and decision analysis in social work: An implementa-tion model. *Journal of Social Work, 2,* 45–63.

Weber, J. B., & Sergeant, A. J. (2003). Review of find-ing the evidence: A gateway to the literature in child and adolescent mental health. *Journal of the American Academy of Child and Adolescent Psychiatry, 38*(11), 55s–76s.

Weissman, M. M. (2001). *Treatment of depression:*

Bridging the 21st century. Washington, DC: American Psychiatric Press.

Wicks-Nelson, R., & Israel, A. C. (2002). *Behavioral disorders in children* (5th ed.). Upper Saddle River, NJ: Prentice Hall.

Wolchik, S. A., & Sandler, I. N. (Eds.). (1997). *Hand-book of children's coping: Linking theory and in-tervention.* New York: Plenum Press.

27 TREATING JUVENILE DELINQUENTS WITH CONDUCT DISORDER, ATTENTION-DEFICIT/ HYPERACTIVITY DISORDER, AND OPPOSITIONAL DEFIANT DISORDER

David W. Springer

Juvenile delinquents with externalizing disorders are a challenging, yet rewarding, population to treat. The externalizing disorders—namely, at-tention-deficit/hyperactivity disorder (ADHD), conduct disorder (CD), and oppositional defiant disorder (ODD)—are some of the most common encountered by practitioners working with ju-venile delinquents (Kazdin, 2002; Kronenberger & Meyer, 2001). In studies of community and clinic samples, a large percentage of youths with CD or ADHD (e.g., 45% to 70%) also met cri-teria for the other disorder (Fergusson, Hor-wood, & Lloyd, 1991), and comorbidity between CD and ODD, anxiety disorders, and depression

is common as well (Kazdin, 2002). In a recent epidemiological study that examined psychiatric disorders in juvenile delinquents (Teplin, Abram, McClelland, Dulcan, & Mericle, 2002), the most common disorders were substance use disorders and disruptive behavior disorders (ODD and CD), with more than 40% of males and females meeting criteria for a disruptive be-havior disorder. Accordingly, this chapter pre-sents a case exemplar of treating a juvenile de-linquent dually diagnosed with conduct disorder and alcohol abuse.

First, it is important to highlight the differ-ence between juvenile delinquency and CD.

Many readers may be aware of the behaviors associated with a diagnosis of CD, such as aggressive behavior toward others, using a weapon, fire setting, cruelty to animals or persons, vandalism, lying, truancy, running away, and theft (American Psychiatric Association [APA], 2000). The *DSM-IV-TR* allows for coding a client with one of two subtypes of CD: childhood-onset type (at least one criterion characteristic occurs prior to age 10) and adolescent-onset type (absence of any criteria prior to age 10). While an adolescent may be considered a "juvenile delinquent" after only one delinquent act, to warrant a diagnosis of CD, that same adolescent must be engaged over an extended period (at least 6 months) in a pattern of behavior that consistently violates the rights of others and societal norms. It is critical, therefore, that practitioners take painstaking care in their diagnostic assessments of conduct disorder, as both false positives and false negatives carry potentially serious consequences for both the offender and society (Springer, McNeece, & Arnold, 2003).

Part of what makes treating juveniles with conduct disorder so challenging is the multifaceted nature of their problems. Fortunately, in recent years, significant advances in psychosocial treatments have been made in treating children and adolescents with disruptive behavior disorders. Some of these evidence-based practices are applied to the case example of Matt that follows. For purposes here, Rosen and Proctor's (2002) definition of *evidence-based practice* (EBP) has been adopted, whereby "practitioners will select interventions on the basis of their empirically demonstrated links to the desired outcomes" (p. 743).

CASE EXAMPLE: MATT

Matt is a 16-year-old Anglo male who was recently picked up by a police officer and taken to the local juvenile assessment center for truancy, vandalism (graffiti), and underage drinking. Earlier that morning, Matt had beaten up a classmate at school. This physical altercation was unprovoked. His case was formally adjudicated through the county juvenile drug court. Rather than being expelled, he is now attending the alternative learning center (ALC). Following the recommendation from the multidisciplinary treatment team, the judge has ordered Matt to receive substance abuse and mental health treatment while on probation. Matt lives with his mother and stepfather. Matt's father committed suicide when Matt was 8 years old, and his mother married Matt's stepfather when Matt was 10. His mother and stepfather have been having difficulty in parenting Matt since he was 13. He does not respect the rules at home, such as abiding by curfews and completing chores. Matt often loses his temper and takes little responsibility for his behavior, and he has a pattern of stealing and lying. His IQ falls within the normal range, and his medical history is uncomplicated.

Matt's social worker was interested in helping Matt and his family by using interventions that gave them the best shot at a successful outcome. While there were many interventions from which to choose, the social worker wanted to use only those that had a solid evidence base. Vandiver (2002) outlines seven steps in applying evidence-based practices with clients: (a) Conduct a biopsychosocial assessment, (b) arrive at a diagnosis and select diagnostic specific guidelines, (c) identify problems, (d) develop goals or planned targets of change, (e) develop an intervention plan, (f) establish outcome measures, and (g) evaluate. As best as she was able, the social worker used these seven steps as a framework to guide her work with Matt and his family.

Biopsychosocial Assessment

As the first active phase of treatment, a thorough assessment is the cornerstone of a solid treatment plan (Springer, 2002a). During their initial session together, the social worker conducted a complete biopsychosocial assessment with Matt and his parents. (For a more detailed overview of the biopsychosocial interview, see, for example, Austrian, 2002; Springer, 2002a.)

As part of this initial assessment, the Child and Adolescent Functional Assessment Scale (CAFAS) (Hodges, 2000) was also administered. The CAFAS is a standardized multidimensional assessment tool that is used to measure the extent to which the mental health and substance use disorders of youth age 7 to 17 impair functioning. It is completed by the clinician and requires specialized training. A major benefit of the CAFAS in helping practitioners determine a youth's overall level of functioning is that it covers eight areas: school/work, home, community, behavior toward others, moods/emotions, self-harmful behavior, substance use, and thinking. The adolescent's level of functioning in each of these eight domains is scored as severe (score of 30), moderate (20), mild (10), or minimal (0). Additionally, an overall score can be computed. These scores can be graphically depicted on a one-page scoring sheet that provides a profile of the youth's functioning. An appealing feature of recent versions is that the CAFAS now includes strength-based items. While these items are not used in the scoring, they are useful in treatment planning (Springer, McNeece, & Arnold, 2003). The psychometric properties of the CAFAS have been demonstrated in numerous studies (cf. Hodges & Cheong-Seok, 2000; Hodges & Wong, 1996). One study on the predictive validity of the CAFAS supported the notion that this scale is able to predict recidivism in juvenile delinquents (Hodges & Cheong-Seok, 2000). Higher scores on the CAFAS have been associated with previous psychiatric hospitalizations, serious psychiatric diagnoses, restrictive living arrangements, below-average school performance and attendance, and contact with law enforcement (Hodges, Doucette-Gates, & Oinghong, 1999).

The CAFAS was selected for a few reasons. It is clinician rated (as opposed to a self-report pencil-and-paper scale), which is especially important, given that adolescents with CD often suffer from low insight and underreport problematic behavior (Kronenberger & Meyer, 2001; Teplin et al., 2002). The CAFAS is also standardized, covers several areas of functioning, provides clinical cutting scores, and includes strength-based items. For these reasons, it is used widely in communities across the United States. Of course, other scales would have also been excellent choices, such as the widely used Eyberg Child Behavior Inventory (ECBI), a 36-item parent-rating scale that measures conduct-problem behaviors in children and adolescents (Burns & Patterson, 1990; Robinson, Eyberg, & Ross, 1980).

In addition to the CAFAS, the timeline follow-back procedure (Sobell & Sobell, 1992) was used specifically to assess Matt's substance abuse history (his primary substance of choice was alcohol). This procedure is a structured interview technique that samples a specific period of time. A monthly calendar and memory anchor points were used to help Matt reconstruct daily use during the past month. Whereas adult studies have found that direct self-report mea-

sures have high levels of sensitivity in detecting substance use problems and compare favorably with biomedical measures (blood and urine tests) (National Institute on Alcohol Abuse and Alcoholism, 1990), the timeline follow-back may offer the most sensitive assessment for adolescent substance abusers (Leccese & Waldron, 1994). (As part of his probation, Matt also had to submit to random urine screens.)

Diagnose and Review Corresponding Evidence Base

After ruling out medical causes, and based upon the collective results of the biopsychosocial assessment, the CAFAS, and the timeline follow-back, the social worker diagnosed Matt as follows:

Axis I.	312.82	Conduct Disorder, Adolescent-Onset Type, Moderate
	305.00	Alcohol Abuse
Axis II.	V71.09	No diagnosis
Axis III.	None	
Axis IV.	V61.20	Parent–Child Relational Problem; V62.3 Academic Problems; Involvement with juvenile justice system

Once the initial assessment had been conducted, the social worker began working collaboratively with Matt and his parents to decide the best course of action. Through a search of the literature and key databases (cf. Fonagy, Target, Cottrell, Phillips, & Kurtz, 2002; Kazdin, 2002; http://www.effectivechildtherapy.com; http://www.samhsa.gov), the social worker was able to learn the following.

Several recent meta-analyses suggest that the most effective approaches for treating juvenile offenders are those with a cognitive-behavioral component combined with close supervision and advocacy. There is evidence that more positive treatment effects are realized in community settings than in institutional settings (Deschenes & Greenwood, 1994). More recently, Lipsey and Wilson (1998) conducted a meta-analysis of experimental or quasi-experimental studies of interventions for serious and violent juvenile delinquents. They reviewed 200 programs, which were further divided into programs for institutionalized juveniles ($N = 83$) and noninstitutionalized juveniles ($N = 117$). McBride, VanderWaal, Terry, and VanBuren (1999, p. 58) nicely synthesized the findings of Lipsey and Wilson's meta-analysis.

Noninstitutionalized programs that demonstrate good evidence of effectiveness include behavioral therapies (family and contingency contracting), intensive case management (including system collaboration and continuing care), multisystemic therapy (MST), restitution programs (parole- and probation-based), and skills training. Institutionalized programs that demonstrate good effectiveness include behavioral programs (cognitive mediation and stress inoculation training), longer term community residential programs (therapeutic communities with cognitive-behavioral approaches), multiple services within residential communities (case management approach), and skills training (aggression replacement training and cognitive restructuring).

More specifically, the social worker found that expert consensus exists that treatments with the strongest evidence base (as demonstrated in randomized controlled clinical trials) for treating children and adolescents with conduct disorder include parent management training, multisystemic therapy, cognitive problem-solving skills training, brief strategic family therapy, and functional family therapy (Fonagy & Kurtz, 2002; Kazdin, 2002).

Parent Management Training

Parent management training (PMT) is a summary term that describes a therapeutic strategy in which parents are trained to use skills for managing their child's problem behavior (Kazdin, 1997), such as effective command-giving, setting up reinforcement systems, and using punishment, including taking away privileges and assigning extra chores. While PMT programs may differ in focus and therapeutic strategies used, they all share the common goal of enhancing parental control over children's behavior (Barkley, 1987; Cavell, 2000; Eyberg, 1988; Forehand & McMahon, 1981; Patterson, Reid, Jones, & Conger, 1975; Webster-Stratton & Herbert, 1994). To date, parent management training is the best treatment for youth with oppositional defiant disorder (Brestan & Eyberg, 1998; Hanish, Tolan, & Guerra, 1996), and the effectiveness of parent training is well documented and, in many respects, impressive (Serketich & Dumas. 1996).

Yet, studies examining the effectiveness of PMT with adolescents are equivocal, with some studies suggesting that adolescents respond less well to PMT than do their younger counterparts (Dishion & Patterson, 1992; Kazdin, 2002). In Brestan and Eyberg's (1998) review of studies that examined the effectiveness of psychosocial interventions for child and adolescent conduct problems, two interventions were considered to be "well-established treatments," according to the stringent criteria set forth by the Division 12 (Clinical Psychology) Task Force on Promotion and Dissemination of Psychological Procedures: the videotape modeling parent-training program (Spaccarelli, Cotler, & Penman, 1992; Webster-Stratton, 1984, 1994) and parent-training programs based on Patterson and Gullion's (1968) manual, *Living with Children* (Alexander & Parsons, 1973; Bernal, Klinnert, & Schultz, 1980; Wiltz & Patterson, 1974). These two approaches target parents with children ages 3 to 8 and 3 to 12, respectively.

Multisystemic Therapy

Multisystemic therapy (MST) (Henggeler & Borduin, 1990; Henggeler, Schoenwald, Borduin, Rowland, & Cunningham, 1998) is a family- and community-based treatment approach that is theoretically grounded in a social-ecological framework (Bronfenbrenner, 1979) and family systems (Haley, 1976; Minuchin, 1974). A basic foundation of MST is the belief that a juvenile's acting out or antisocial behavior is best addressed by interfacing with multiple systems, including the adolescent's family, peers, school, teachers, neighbors, and others (Brown, Borduin, & Henggeler, 2001). Thus, the MST practitioner interfaces not just with the adolescent but with various individuals and settings that influence the adolescent's life. Services are delivered in the client's natural environment, such as the client's home or a neighborhood center. There have been numerous studies demonstrating the effectiveness of MST with high-risk youth (cf. Borduin et al., 1995; Brunk, Henggeler, & Whelan, 1987; Henggeler et al., 1986). According to Brown, Borduin, and Henggeler (2001), "To date, MST is the only treatment for serious delinquent behavior that has demonstrated both short-term and long-term treatment effects in randomized, controlled clinical trials with violent and chronic juvenile offenders and their families from various cultural and ethnic backgrounds" (p. 458).

Problem-Solving Skills Training

Problem-solving skills training (PSST) (Spivak & Shure, 1974) is a cognitively based intervention that has been used to treat aggressive and antisocial youth (Kazdin, 1994). The problem-solving process involves helping clients learn how to produce a variety of potentially effective responses when faced with problem situations. Regardless of the specific problem-solving model used, the primary focus is on addressing the thought process to help adolescents address deficiencies and distortions in their approach to interpersonal situations (Kazdin, 1994). A variety of techniques are used, including didactic teaching, practice, modeling, role playing, feedback, social reinforcement, and therapeutic games (Kronenberger & Meyer, 2001). The problem-solving approach typically includes six steps for the practitioner and client to address: (a) defining the problem, (b) identifying the goal, (c) brainstorming, (d) evaluating the alternatives, (e) choosing and implementing an alternative, and (f) evaluating the implemented option (Kazdin, Esreldt-Dawson, French, & Unis, 1987). Several randomized clinical trials (Type 1 and 2 studies) have demonstrated the effectiveness of PSST with impulsive, aggressive, and conduct-disordered children and adolescents (cf. Baer & Nietzel, 1991; Durlak, Furhman, & Lampman, 1991; Kazdin, 2000; cited in Kazdin, 2002).

Brief Strategic Family Therapy

Brief strategic family therapy (BSFT) has developed out of a programmatic series of studies with Hispanic youths (Coatsworth, Szapocznik, Kurtines, & Santisteban 1997; Szapocznik & Kurtines, 1989). With its strong grounding in a cultural frame of reference, this approach considers factors such as family cohesion, parental control, and communication. Treatment strategies focus on changing concrete interaction patterns in the family, with the therapist challenging interaction patterns to help the family consider alternative ways of dealing with one another. A unique aspect of this approach is that Szapocznik and his colleagues assert that family therapy is a way of conceptualizing problems and interventions but that seeing the entire family may not be necessary (Kazdin, 2002). Several studies (Type 1 and 2) have demonstrated improvements in child and family functioning compared with other treatment and control conditions (cf. Coatsworth et al., 1997; Szapocznik & Kurtines, 1989).

Functional Family Therapy

Functional family therapy (FFT) (Alexander & Parsons, 1973, 1982), like MST, is an integrative approach that relies on systems, behavioral, and cognitive views of functioning. Clinical problems are conceptualized in terms of the function they serve for the family system and for the individual client. Research underlying FFT has found that families with delinquents have higher rates of defensiveness and blaming and lower rates of mutual support (Alexander & Parsons, 1982). The goal of treatment "is the achievement of a change in patterns of interaction and communication, in a manner that engenders adaptive family functioning" (Fonagy & Kurtz, 2002, p. 158). Treatment is grounded in learning theory. FFT has clinically significant and lasting effects on recidivism. In nine studies conducted on FFT between 1973 and 1997, a 25% to 80% improvement was found in recidivism, out-of-home placement, or future offending by siblings of the treated youth (Fonagy & Kurtz, 2002).

Select Intervention Plan

According to Gambrill (1999), in EBP

> social workers seek out practice-related research findings regarding important practice decisions and share the results of their search with clients. If they find that there is no evidence that a method they recommend will help a client, they so inform the client and describe their theoretical rationale for their recommendation. Clients are involved as informed participants. (p. 346)

Accordingly, the social worker shared as much as she knew about all of these approaches back with Matt and his parents, with the decision making taking place as follows. Given that Matt was 16 years old, that the outcome findings on PMT with adolescents were equivocal, and that his pattern of behavior was rather entrenched, the social worker and his parents decided against PMT as a primary treatment option. While MST is probably the most effective treatment available for treating high-risk juvenile offenders like Matt, MST was not being used in the social worker's setting, or even in the local community. Thus, this treatment was not considered an option for Matt's family. Both PSST and FFT were implemented with Matt and his family. Both of these approaches have been demonstrated to be effective with clients like Matt, and the social worker had been trained in both approaches. While BSFT was also considered, the social worker was not trained in this sophisticated family therapy approach.

Establish Treatment Goals and Targets for Change

Now that the primary interventions, PSST and FFT, had been selected, treatment goals had to be established. The following guidelines are helpful in establishing treatment goals: The goals should be clearly defined and measurable, feasible and realistic, set collaboratively by the practitioner and the client, stem directly from the assessment process, and stated in positive terms, focusing on client growth.

The practitioner worked collaboratively with Matt and his parents to come up with the following treatment goals: (a) Matt's parents will set firm and consistent limits, using natural rewards and consequences; (b) Matt and his parents will improve communication and establish a behavioral contract; (c) Matt will follow the rules at home, as spelled out in the behavioral contract, at least 90% of the time; (d) Matt will follow the rules at school, as evidenced by earning 3 points a day in every class for doing so; (e) Matt will meet all the terms of his probation; (f) Matt will learn alternative ways of dealing with his anger; and (g) Matt will abstain from using alcohol or other drugs. Matt and his family agreed to these terms for a 2-week period, at which time they would be reexamined and modified if needed. The 2-week time limit on these goals was set because doing something for 2 weeks seems more feasible to many adolescents than agreeing to such conditions indefinitely. For an example of a more detailed and comprehensive treatment plan, see Springer (2002b).

Implement Intervention Plan

With treatment goals in place, the social worker began working with Matt and his family in family therapy. In the early phase of treatment, the social worker engaged all of the family members in the therapeutic process, in part by using a "nonblaming message." The social worker stressed the need for active participation on the part of everyone in the family and addressed the effect that Matt's behavior had on the entire family system.

The patterns of blaming in the family were first addressed. Matt often got blamed for all of the family's problems. In other words, Matt has assumed (or been assigned) the family role of scapegoat. Matt's behavior was reframed; he was praised by the social worker for doing too good of a job in acting out the family's problems, and he was relieved of this responsibility for the time being. The social worker introduced cognitive aspects commonly associated with the FFT approach, including behavioral components, communication skills training, behavioral contracting, and contingency management. Positive reinforcement among family members was also encouraged.

It was also important for the social worker to provide Matt with as much one-on-one time as possible early on in treatment to help establish therapeutic rapport (cf. Todd & Selekman, 1994). By joining with Matt, the social worker did not lose him when it came time to empower his parents to set limits. To this end, she also used empathy and humor with Matt.

As Matt's family progressed through treatment, they sometimes had difficulty in translating their treatment goals into actions. For example, when Matt's behavior began to improve, issues that the family had been pushing aside began to surface. The social worker helped the family gradually shift toward more interpersonal issues. Recall that a key assumption of the FFT approach is that clinical problems are couched in terms of the function they serve for the family and for the individual. During one session, Matt shared that he sometimes wondered if his dad had the right idea (by killing himself). The family had never discussed the suicide of Matt's father. This was explored at length in the next couple of family therapy sessions, which served several purposes. It allowed all of them to express their thoughts surrounding this tragic event, and it also gave the family an opportunity to practice some of the new communication skills that they had learned by discussing a sensitive and emotionally charged topic.

As the family examined Matt's alcohol abuse, the social worker avoided the use of labels such as addict or alcoholic. Labels like this often do more harm than good when working with adolescent offenders (Todd & Selekman, 1994). Instead, during individual sessions (with Matt) and family sessions, techniques commonly used in PSST (e.g., role playing, feedback, and in vivo practice) were used to help Matt generate alternative solutions to interpersonal problems (e.g., becoming angry with others) that triggered his drinking.

To help specifically with anger management, which many of her other clients at the ALC also struggled with, the social worker started an anger management therapy group. The Substance Abuse and Mental Health Services Administration, Center for Substance Abuse Treatment (Reilly & Shopshire, 2002), has issued a 12-week cognitive-behavioral anger management group treatment manual, titled *Anger Management for Substance Abuse and Mental Health Clients: A Cognitive Behavioral Therapy*, that is available at no cost from the National Clearinghouse on Alcohol and Drug Information (NCADI) (http://www.samhsa.gov/). This treatment group is a cognitive-behavioral therapy (CBT) approach that employs relaxation, cognitive, and communication skills. The approach presents clients with options that draw on these different interventions and then encourages them to develop individualized anger control plans by using as many of the techniques as possible. The social worker used this treatment manual to successfully facilitate the anger management group with her clients at the ALC. It is important to note that only a few of the adolescents in this group had a diagnosis of conduct disorder. Having too many conduct-disordered youths in the same treatment group can actually be counter-therapeutic (Feldman, Caplinger, & Wodarski, 1983).

Matt's anger management plan reflects many of the interventions used in the 12-week group therapy manual, including five primary treatment goals along with corresponding interventions. See Table 27.1 for a listing of the treatment goals and a sampling of some of the corresponding interventions related to Matt's anger management plan. Of course, this list of interventions is not exhaustive, and there is some overlap across treatment goals and interventions. For a more detailed example of an anger management plan that includes long-term goals and corresponding short-term objectives and interventions, the reader is referred to Dulmus and Wodarski (2002).

Monitor Treatment Progress

As the termination of treatment approached, the social worker introduced longer intervals be-

TABLE 27.1 Treatment Goals and Corresponding Interventions for Matt's Anger Management Plan

Treatment Goals	Interventions
1. Become aware of intense anger outbursts	1. Monitor anger using the "Anger Meter" 2. List positive payoffs that Matt gets from angry outbursts and aggressive actions
2. Stop violence or the threat of violence (physical and verbal)	1. Explore events that trigger anger and cues to anger 2. Explore, role-play, and practice alternative coping strategies (e.g., take a time-out, exercise, deep breathing, conflict resolution model, progressive muscle relaxation)
3. Develop self-control over thoughts and actions	1. Review the aggression cycle 2. Use Ellis's A-B-C-D model of cognitive restructuring 3. Model and practice thought stopping
4. Accept responsibility for own actions	1. Confront Matt in group when he does not accept responsibility for his actions, and reward him when he does 2. Record at least two irrational beliefs during the week and how to dispute these beliefs, using Ellis's A-B-C-D model
5. Receive support and feedback from others	1. Use the here-and-now of the group experience to provide feedback to Matt 2. Discuss Matt's progress in family therapy sessions

tween sessions, treating the final sessions as once-a-month maintenance sessions when the family reported on how things were going. Matt and his family made considerable progress on the desired treatment outcomes, which are "the targets toward which interventions are directed" (Rosen & Proctor, 2002, p. 744). Over the course of 4 months, this was evidenced across several areas of functioning. Matt performed well enough at the ALC that he was allowed to transition back into his mainstream school. For the most part, he continued to meet the terms of probation. This included producing clean urine drug tests. However, on two separate occasions, Matt did report drinking a six-pack of beer at a party. On both occasions, Matt was angry at his parents. Using a harm-reduction approach to substance abuse treatment (cf. McNeece, Bullington, Arnold, & Springer, 2002), the social worker encouraged the family to view this as a normal part of the treatment process. She worked with Matt on identifying the anger that triggered his drinking and, using PSST, problem-solved with him on what he could do differently the next time he was feeling angry. Matt had no incidents of physical violence at school or in the neighborhood, although he did sometimes still "lose his temper" at home when his parents enforced rules.

Matt's therapeutic gains were also monitored by using the CAFAS, which was administered at intake and at termination (see Table 27.2). Based on the scores for each domain, Matt's impairment in functioning could be interpreted as follows: severe (score of 30), moderate (score of 20), mild (score of 10), or minimal (score of 0). The overall scores can also be computed as se-

vere (140–120), marked (100–130), moderate (50–90), mild (20–40), or minimal to no (0–10) impairment in functioning. In sum, then, it seems that Matt made significant progress over the course of treatment, moving from "severe impairment in functioning" at intake to the low range of "moderate impairment in functioning" 4 months later.

CONCLUSION

In the treatment of adolescents, cognitive-based interventions are generally most effective when combined with behavioral contingencies in the child's natural environment (Ervin, Bankert, & DuPaul, 1996). It makes little sense to treat an adolescent in isolation from his or her natural environment. Pearson, Lipton, Cleland, and Yee (2002) encourage policy makers to consider adopting cognitive skills training programs such as those reviewed in this chapter.

The first three treatments reviewed (PMT, MST, and PSST) have more extensive (Type 1 and 2 studies) and follow-up data supporting their effectiveness. FFT has controlled clinical trials supporting its efficacy, but the scope of this evidence is not as solid as it is for the other approaches. Nevertheless, these approaches are all quite promising, and their empirical base places them ahead of other approaches available for treating children and adolescents with conduct problems (Kazdin, 2002). It is worth noting that all but PSST place a primary emphasis on the family.

Despite the promising treatment effects produced by the interventions reviewed here, existing treatments need to be refined and new ones developed. We cannot yet determine the short- and long-term impact of evidence-based treatments on conduct-disordered youths, and it is sometimes unclear what part of the therapeutic process produces change. In the meantime, practitioners can use the existing knowledge base to guide their work with this complex and challenging population.

TABLE 27.2 Matt's CAFAS Results: Intake and Termination

CAFAS Domain	Intake	Termination
School/work	30	10
Home	30	10
Community	30	0
Behavior toward others	30	10
Moods/emotions	20	10
Self-harmful behavior	0	0
Substance use	30	10
Thinking	10	0
Overall functioning	180	50

References

Alexander, J. F., & Parsons, B. V. (1973). Short-term behavioral intervention with delinquents: Impact on family process and recidivism. *Journal of Abnormal Psychology, 81,* 219–225.

Alexander, J. F., & Parsons, B. V. (1982). *Functional family therapy.* Monterey, CA: Brooks/Cole.

American Psychiatric Association. (2000). *Diagnostic and statistical manual of mental disorders* (4th ed., text revision). Washington, DC: Author.

Austrian, S. G. (2002). Guidelines for conducting a biopsychosocial assessment. In A. R. Roberts & G. J. Greene (Eds.), *Social workers' desk reference* (pp. 204–208). New York: Oxford University Press.

Baer, R. A., & Nietzel, M. T. (1991). Cognitive and behavioral treatment of impulsivity in children: A meta-analytic review of the outcome literature. *Journal of Clinical Child Psychology, 20*, 400–412.

Barkley, R. A. (1987). *Defiant children: A clinician's manual for parent training.* New York: Guilford.

Bernal, M. E., Klinnert, M. D., & Schultz, L. A. (1980). Outcome evaluation of behavioral parent training and client-centered parent counseling for children with conduct problems. *Journal of Applied Behavior Analysis, 13*, 677–691.

Borduin, C. M., Mann, B. J., Cone, L. T., Henggeler, S. W., Fucci, B. R., Blaske, D. M., et al. (1995). Multisystemic treatment of serious juvenile offenders: Long-term prevention of criminality and violence. *Journal of Consulting and Clinical Psychology, 63*, 569–578.

Brestan, E. V., & Eyberg, S. M. (1998). Effective psychosocial treatments of conduct-disordered children and adolescents: 29 years, 82 studies, and 5,272 kids. *Journal of Clinical Child Psychology, 27*, 180–189.

Bronfenbrenner, U. (1979). *The ecology of human development: Experiences by nature and design.* Cambridge, MA: Harvard University Press.

Brown, T. L., Borduin, C. M., & Henggeler, S. W. (2001). Treating juvenile offenders in community settings. In J. B. Ashford, B. D. Sales, & W. H. Reid (Eds.), *Treating adult and juvenile offenders with special needs* (pp. 445–464). Washington, DC: American Psychological Association.

Brunk, M., Henggeler, S. W., & Whelan, J. P. (1987). A comparison of multisystemic therapy and parent training in the brief treatment of child abuse and neglect. *Journal of Consulting and Clinical Psychology, 55*, 311–318.

Burns, G. L., & Patterson, D. R. (1990). Conduct problem behaviors in a stratified random sample of children and adolescents: New standardization data on the Eyberg Child Behavior Inventory. *Psychological Assessment, 2*, 391–397.

Cavell, T. A. (2000). *Working with parents of aggressive children: A practitioner's guide.* Washington, DC: American Psychological Association.

Coatsworth, J. D., Szapocznik, J., Kurtines, W., & Santisteban, D. A. (1997). Culturally competent psychosocial interventions with antisocial problem behavior in Hispanic youths. In D. M. Stoff, J. Breiling, & J. D. Maser (Eds.), *Handbook of antisocial behavior* (pp. 395–404). New York: Wiley.

Deschenes, E. P., & Greenwood, P. W. (1994). Treating the juvenile drug offender. In D. L. MacKenzie & C. D. Uchida (Eds.), *Drugs and crime: Evaluating public policy initiatives* (pp. 253–280). Thousand Oaks, CA: Sage.

Dishion, T. J., & Patterson, G. R. (1992). Age effects in parent training outcomes. *Behavior Therapy, 23*, 719–729.

Dulmas, C. N., & Wodarski, J. S. (2002). Parameters of social work treatment plans: Case application of explosive anger. In A. R. Roberts & G. J. Greene (Eds.), *Social workers' desk reference* (pp. 314–319). New York: Oxford University Press.

Durlak, J. A., Furhman, T., & Lampman, C. (1991). Effectiveness of cognitive-behavioral therapy for maladapting children: A meta-analysis. *Psychological Bulletin, 110*, 204–214.

Ervin, R. A., Bankert, C. L., & DuPaul, G. J. (1996). Treatment of attention-deficit/hyperactivity disorder. In M. A. Reinecke, F. M. Dattilio, & A. Freeman (Eds.), *Cognitive therapy with children and adolescents* (pp. 38–61). New York: Guilford.

Eyberg, S. (1988). Parent–child interaction therapy: Integration of traditional and behavioral concerns. *Child and Family Behavior Therapy, 10*, 33–45.

Feldman, R. A., Caplinger, T. E., & Wodarski, J. S. (1983). *The St. Louis conundrum: The effective treatment of antisocial youths.* Englewood Cliffs, NJ: Prentice Hall.

Fergusson, D. M., Horwood, L. J., & Lloyd, M. (1991). Confirmatory factor models of attention deficit and conduct disorder. *Journal of Child Psychology and Psychiatry, 32*, 257–274.

Fonagy, P., & Kurtz, A. (2002). Disturbance of conduct. In P. Fonagy, M. Target, D. Cottrell, J. Phillips, & Z. Kurtz (Eds.), *What works for whom? A critical review of treatments for children and adolescents* (pp. 106–192). New York: Guilford.

Fonagy, P., Target, M., Cottrell, D., Phillips, J., & Kurtz, Z. (2002). *What works for whom? A critical review of treatments for children and adolescents.* New York: Guilford.

Forehand, R. L., & McMahon, R. J. (1981). *Helping the noncompliant child: A clinician's guide to present training.* New York: Guilford.

Gambrill, E. (1999). Evidence-based practice: An alternative to authority-based practice. *Families in Society: The Journal of Contemporary Human Services, 80*, 341–350.

Haley, J. (1976). *Problem solving therapy.* San Francisco: Jossey-Bass.

Hanish, L. D., Tolan, P. H., & Guerra, N. G. (1996). Treatment of oppositional defiant disorder. In M. A. Reinecke, F. M. Dattilio, & A. Freeman

(Eds.), *Cognitive therapy with children and adolescents* (pp. 62–78). New York: Guilford.

Henggeler, S. W., & Borduin, C. M. (1990). *Family therapy and beyond: A multisystemic approach to treating the behavior problems of children and adolescents.* Pacific Grove, CA: Brooks/Cole.

Henggeler, S. W., Rodick, J. D., Borduin, C. M., Hanson, C. L., Watson, S. M., & Urey, J. R. (1986). Multisystemic treatment of juvenile offenders: Effects on adolescent behavior and family interactions. *Developmental Psychology, 22,* 132–141.

Henggeler, S. W., Schoenwald, S. K., Borduin, C. M., Rowland, M. D., & Cunningham, P. B. (1998). *Multisystemic treatment of antisocial behavior in children and adolescents.* New York: Guilford.

Hodges, K. (2000). *The Child and Adolescent Functional Assessment Scale self training manual.* Ypsilanti: Eastern Michigan University, Department of Psychology.

Hodges, K., & Cheong-Seok, K. (2000). Psychometric study of the Child and Adolescent Functional Assessment Scale: Prediction of contact with the law and poor school attendance. *Journal of Abnormal Child Psychology, 28,* 287–297.

Hodges, K., Doucette-Gates, A., & Oinghong, L. (1999). The relationship between the Child and Adolescent Functional Assessment Scale (CAFAS) and indicators of functioning. *Journal of Child and Family Studies, 8,* 109–122.

Hodges, K., & Wong, M. M. (1996). Psychometric characteristics of a multi-dimensional measure to assess impairment: The Child and Adolescent Functional Assessment Scale. *Journal of Child and Family Studies, 5,* 445–467.

Kazdin, A. E. (1994). Psychotherapy for children and adolescents. In A. E. Bergin & S. L. Garfield (Eds.), *Handbook of psychotherapy and behavior change* (4th ed., pp. 543–594). New York: Wiley.

Kazdin, A. E. (2000). *Psychotherapy for children and adolescents: Directions for research and practice.* New York: Oxford University Press.

Kazdin, A. E. (2002). Psychosocial treatments for conduct disorder in children and adolescents. In P. E. Nathan & J. M. Gorman (Eds.), *A guide to treatments that work* (2nd ed., pp. 57–85). New York: Oxford University Press.

Kazdin, A. E., Esveldt-Dawson, K., French, N. H., & Unis, A. S. (1987). Effects of parent management training and problem-solving skills training combined in the treatment of antisocial child behavior. *Journal of the American Academy of Child and Adolescent Psychiatry, 26,* 416–424.

Kronenberger, W. G., & Meyer, R. G. (2001). *The child clinician's handbook* (2nd ed.). Boston: Allyn & Bacon.

Leccese, M., & Waldron, H. B. (1994). Assessing adolescent substance abuse: A critique of current measurement instruments. *Journal of Substance Abuse Treatment, 11,* 553–563.

Lipsey, M. W., & Wilson, D. B. (1998). Effective intervention for serious juvenile offenders: A synthesis of research. In R. Loever & D. Farrington (Eds.), *Serious and violent juvenile offenders: Risk factors and successful interventions* (pp. 313–344). London: Sage.

McBride, D. C., VanderWaal, C. J., Terry, Y. M., & VanBuren, H. (1999). *Breaking the cycle of drug use among juvenile offenders.* Retrieved October 24, 2002, from http://www.ncjrs.org/pdffiles1/nij/179273.pdf

McNeece, C. A., Bullington, B., Arnold, E. M., & Springer, D. W. (2002). The war on drugs: Treatment, research, and substance abuse intervention in the twenty-first century. In R. Muraskin & A. R. Roberts (Eds.), *Visions for change: Crime and justice in the twenty-first century* (3rd ed., pp. 11–36). Upper Saddle River, NJ: Prentice Hall.

Minuchin, S. (1974). *Families and family therapy.* Cambridge, MA: Harvard University Press.

National Institute on Alcohol Abuse and Alcoholism. (1990). *Seventh special report to the U.S. Congress on alcohol and health.* Rockville, MD: U.S. Department of Health and Human Services.

Patterson, G. R., & Gullion, M. E. (1968). *Living with children: New methods for parents and teachers.* Champaign, IL: Research Press.

Patterson, G. R., Reid, J. B., Jones, R. R., & Conger, R. E. (1975). *A social learning approach to family intervention: Vol. 1, Families with aggressive children.* Eugene, OR: Castalia.

Pearson, F. S., Lipton, D. S., Cleland, C. M., & Yee, D. S. (2002). The effects of behavioral/cognitive-behavioral programs on recidivism. *Crime and Delinquency, 48*(3), 476–496.

Reilly, P. M., & Shopshire, M. S. (2002). *Anger management for substance abuse and mental health clients: A cognitive behavioral therapy.* Washington, DC: U.S. Department of Health and Human Services, Substance Abuse and Mental Health Services Administration.

Robinson, E. A., Eyberg, S. M., & Ross, A. W. (1980). The standardization of an inventory of child conduct problem behaviors. *Journal of Clinical Child Psychology, 9,* 22–29.

Rosen, A., & Proctor, E. K. (2002). Standards for evidence-based social work practice: The role of replicable and appropriate interventions, outcomes, and practice guidelines. In A. R. Roberts & G. J. Greene (Eds.), *Social workers' desk reference* (pp. 743–747). New York: Oxford University Press.

Serketich, W. J., & Dumas, J. E. (1996). The effectiveness of behavioral parent training to modify antisocial behavior in children: A meta analysis. *Behavior Therapy, 27,* 171–186.

Sobell, L. C., & Sobell, M. B. (1992). Timeline followback: A technique for assessing self-reported alcohol consumption. In R. Z. Litten & J. P. Allen (Eds.), *Measuring alcohol consumption: Psychosocial and biochemical methods* (pp. 41–72). Totowa, NJ: Humana Press.

Spaccarelli, S., Cotler, S., & Penman, D. (1992). Problem-solving skills training as a supplement to behavioral parent training. *Cognitive Therapy and Research, 16,* 1–18.

Spivak, G., & Shure, M. B. (1974). *Social adjustment of young children.* San Francisco: Jossey-Bass.

Springer, D. W. (2002a). Assessment protocols and rapid assessment instruments with troubled adolescents. In A. R. Roberts & G. J. Greene (Eds.), *Social workers' desk reference* (pp. 217–221). New York: Oxford University Press.

Springer, D. W. (2002b). Treatment planning with adolescents: ADHD case application. In A. R. Roberts & G. J. Greene (Eds.), *Social workers' desk reference* (pp. 731–738). New York: Oxford University Press.

Springer, D. W., McNeece, C. A., & Arnold, E. M. (2003). *Substance abuse treatment for criminal offenders: An evidence-based guide for practitioners.* Washington, DC: American Psychological Association.

Szapocznik, J., & Kurtines, W. M. (1989). *Breakthroughs in family therapy with drug-abusing problem youth.* New York: Springer.

Teplin, L. A., Abram, K. M., McClelland, G. M., Dulcan, M. K., & Mericle, A. A. (2002). Psychiatric disorders in youth in juvenile detention. *Archives of General Psychiatry, 59,* 1133–1143.

Todd, T. C., & Selekman, M. (1994). A structural-strategic model for treating the adolescent who is abusing alcohol and other drugs. In W. Snyder & T. Ooms (Eds.), *Empowering families, helping adolescents: Family-centered treatment of adolescents with alcohol, drug abuse, and mental health problems* (pp. 79–89). Rockville, MD: U.S. Department of Health and Human Services, Center for Substance Abuse Treatment.

Vandiver, V. L. (2002). Step-by-step practice guidelines for using evidence-based practice and expert consensus in mental health settings. In A. R. Roberts & G. J. Greene (Eds.), *Social workers' desk reference* (pp. 731–738). New York: Oxford University Press.

Webster-Stratton, C. (1984). Randomized trial of two parent-training programs for families with conduct-disordered children. *Journal of Consulting and Clinical Psychology, 52,* 666–678.

Webster-Stratton, C. (1994). Advancing videotape parent training: A comparison study. *Journal of Consulting and Clinical Psychology, 62,* 583–593.

Webster-Stratton, C., & Herbert, M. (1994). *Troubled families: Problem children.* New York: Wiley.

Wiltz, N. A., & Patterson, G. R. (1974). An evaluation of parent training procedures designed to alter inappropriate aggressive behavior of boys. *Behavior Therapy, 5,* 215–221.

28

EVIDENCE-BASED TREATMENTS FOR OBSESSIVE-COMPULSIVE DISORDER

Deciding What Treatment Method Works for Whom

Jonathan S. Abramowitz & Stefanie A. Schwartz

Effective treatments for obsessive-compulsive disorder (OCD) can be divided into two broad categories: biological and cognitive-behavioral. Biological treatments include pharmacotherapy with serotonin reuptake inhibitors (SRIs) and neurosurgery. Cognitive-behavioral treatment (CBT) includes exposure, response prevention, and cognitive therapy. These procedures can be delivered on an individual, group, or inpatient basis. Moreover, the frequency of therapy sessions may vary from weekly to daily. We begin this chapter with a brief description of the strengths and limitations of the principal treatment approaches. Next, we review the factors to be considered in deciding which treatment may be most beneficial for a given patient (Table 28.1). A brief discussion of decision factors that are less specific to OCD patients is followed by a more extensive examination of factors specifically related to OCD.

SEROTONIN REUPTAKE INHIBITORS

Although they are the most widely used treatment for OCD, SRIs produce a modest 20% to 40% reduction in symptoms (Rauch & Jenike, 1998). The major strength of a pharmacological approach for OCD is its convenience. Limitations include the relatively modest improvement, the likelihood of residual symptoms, a

high rate of nonresponse (40% to 60% of patients show little response), and the prospect of unpleasant side effects. Moreover, once SRIs are terminated, OCD symptoms typically return rapidly (Pato, Hill, & Murphy, 1990).

INDIVIDUAL OUTPATIENT CBT

Traditional behavioral treatment for OCD involves exposure and response prevention (ERP). Exposure entails repeated and prolonged confrontation with obsessional stimuli; response prevention means refraining from compulsive rituals. Cognitive therapy, a newer approach to OCD, emphasizes cognitive change through education and rational discourse, although "behavioral experiments" involving exposure procedures are almost always performed to reinforce accurate beliefs and assumptions about probability and risk. Because of the procedural and conceptual overlaps (i.e., ERP and cognitive methods both aim to modify dysfunctional cognitions), we collectively refer to these procedures as CBT here and differentiate between ERP and cognitive techniques only when discussing their implementation in specific circumstances.

Research demonstrates that ERP is a highly effective therapy for OCD: Typical improvement rates are in the 60% to 70% range (e.g., Franklin, Abramowitz, Kozak, Levitt, & Foa, 2000).

TABLE 28.1 Considerations for Choosing a Treatment Modality for Patients with Obsessive-Compulsive Disorder

SRI Medication Alone	Individual Outpatient Cognitive-Behavioral	Inpatient Cognitive-Behavioral	Group Cognitive-Behavioral	Supportive Therapy	No OCD Treatment
• If CBT unavailable • If patient prefers medication to psychotherapy • If patient has poor insight • If noncompliance with CBT	• If residual symptoms after SRI trial • If primary OCD • If good support from family/friends • Consider intensive therapy if rituals are severe • Consider loop-tape exposure for severe obsessions • Consider cognitive therapy if hoarding • Consider personality disorders • Consider severity of comorbid anxiety or mood disorder	• If outpatient therapy unsuccessful • If patient has poor insight • If social environment is obstructive of outpatient therapy • If additional severe psychopathology (e.g., suicidal depression) • If comorbid medical condition is present • Consider costs	• Consider patient's comfort and willingness to share symptoms with others	• If symptoms persist despite adequate trials of SRIs and CBT • For long-term symptom management	• If OCD is clearly secondary to another disorder (e.g., generalized anxiety, substance abuse, bipolar disorder, psychosis), address the primary problem before beginning OCD treatment

Initial studies show that cognitive therapy is also beneficial, yet whether it is as effective as ERP is still unknown. Strengths of CBT in general include its brevity (most programs involve 16 sessions), short-term effectiveness, and long-term maintenance of treatment gains. A drawback of this approach is that patients must confront their fear-evoking stimuli and resist urges to ritualize to obtain symptom reduction. Because CBT requires compliance with such procedures, a number of patients refuse this therapy or terminate prematurely. Moreover, CBT is highly focused and does not typically directly address comorbid problems such as personality disorders that often accompany OCD. Finally, only a small percentage of mental health treatment providers are trained in the provision of CBT for OCD.

A few OCD–anxiety disorders specialty clinics offer *intensive* outpatient CBT, meaning 15 daily outpatient treatment sessions over 3 weeks. Abramowitz, Foa, and Franklin (2003) found that this intensive schedule was more effective than 15 sessions of twice-weekly ERP (delivered over 8 weeks) immediately after treatment. However, at 3-month follow-up, these differences were no longer apparent. A practical advantage of the intensive approach over less intensive schedules is that massed sessions allow for regular therapist supervision and therefore rapid correction of subtle avoidance, rituals, or suboptimal exposure practice that might otherwise compromise outcome. The primary disadvantage is the inherent scheduling demands for both the clinician and the patient.

GROUP CBT

Group CBT programs have been found effective in reducing OCD symptoms (McLean et al., 2001). Strengths include the support and cohesion that are nonspecific effects of group therapy. Potential weaknesses to a group approach include the relative lack of attention to each individual's symptoms, particularly given the heterogeneity of OCD symptoms.

INPATIENT CBT

Although most inpatient psychiatric hospitals are equipped to provide standard care for patients with OCD, programming is often limited by the short duration of stay. Therefore, the initial focus is often on stabilizing patients via medication and nonspecific psychotherapy (e.g., supportive counseling). Only a few specialized inpatient treatment programs for severe OCD exist. These residential OCD programs typically include individual and group CBT, medication management, and supportive therapy for comorbid psychiatric conditions. Length of stay may vary from a few weeks to a month or more.

One strength of specialized inpatient OCD programs is that they provide constant supervision for patients requiring help with implementing treatment (i.e., conducting self-directed ERP). This may be helpful to the patient who lacks family or friends to assist with treatment. A shortcoming of inpatient treatment for OCD is that it is often costly. Because patients with obsessions and compulsions regarding specific places or stimuli (e.g., bathrooms at home) may have difficulty reproducing these feared situations within the hospital setting for the purposes of exposure, generalization of treatment effects must be considered. The only study to directly compare inpatient to outpatient CBT for OCD found no differences in outcome between 20 sessions of outpatient and 5.4 months of inpatient treatment (van den Hout, Emmelkamp, Kraaykamp, & Grietz, 1988).

NEUROSURGICAL TREATMENT

Currently there are four different types of neurosurgical interventions for OCD: subcaudate tractotomy, limbic leucotomy, cingulotomy, and capsulotomy. These procedures involve severing interconnections between areas of the brain's frontal lobes and the limbic system. Recommended only in cases where severe OCD and depressive symptoms persist despite all other available treatments having been tried, neurosurgery has risks that include alterations in cognitive functioning and personality. Although clinical improvement has been observed in some cases, it remains unknown why these procedures are successful for only a subset of OCD patients (Jenike, 2000). There is also an increased risk of suicide following failure with this approach.

NONSPECIFIC FACTORS TO CONSIDER WHEN DECIDING ON TREATMENT

Age, Gender, and Race

Age

For different reasons, children, adolescents, and the elderly may have more difficulties with adherence to medication regimens than do young and middle-aged adults. Missed doses or overdoses may result in reduced benefit or unpleasant side effects. Older adults may be subject to more adverse side effects from SRIs because of reduced metabolic rates and interactions with medicine prescribed for other conditions. Thus, CBT is the best initial treatment option for younger children and older adults. Evidence that CBT is highly effective for children with OCD is accumulating (Abramowitz, Whiteside, & Deacon, 2002), and initial studies with elderly populations are encouraging as well (Calamari & Cassiday, 1999). Nevertheless, family conflict occasionally interferes with the effects of CBT in children with OCD. Also, older individuals may feel more comfortable with medication than with attending outpatient psychotherapy. This issue should be discussed openly with such patients.

Gender

Research has not identified gender as a variable to consider when making treatment decisions for OCD. Nevertheless, some patients may feel more comfortable with therapists of their same sex, especially if they have obsessions or compulsions regarding uncomfortable sexual or contamination concerns (e.g., public restrooms). For example, a same-sex therapist would be necessary to accompany the patient during exposure to public restrooms.

Race

Some members of minority groups perceive an increased stigma in presenting for mental health treatment and thus may be more likely to opt for pharmacotherapy over psychotherapy, as there is typically less stigma associated with medication treatment (Williams, Chambless, & Steketee, 1998). This sense of shame can also interfere with CBT by hindering patients' self-report of symptoms and their performance of ERP exercises in public settings. Despite these issues, Williams et al. (1998) reported clinically significant improvement for African-American patients with OCD who completed CBT.

Educational Level

Successful CBT requires that the patient comprehend a theoretical conceptual model of OCD and a rationale for treatment. Moreover, patients must be able to consolidate information learned during exposure practice and implement treatment procedures on their own. This may be difficult for individuals who are very concrete in their thinking. Because group CBT may proceed at a pace that is too rapid for individuals with cognitive impairment, individual therapy is recommended. For those OCD patients too cognitively impaired to comprehend or profit from CBT, it may be more fruitful to explore pharmacotherapy options.

Availability of Treatment

Geographic location limits the availability of CBT but not medication for OCD. Although the number of professionals trained in CBT is increasing, access to qualified therapists is limited, especially in rural areas. Thus, many patients must travel for adequate treatment. Insurance coverage may also dictate the availability of both CBT and pharmacotherapy because some providers do not adequately cover mental health treatment.

Two CBT self-help programs have been developed and tested for OCD. Fritzler, Hecker, and Losee's (1997) 12-week bibliotherapy program uses Steketee and White's (1990) self-help book, *When Once Is Not Enough,* and five sessions with a therapist to review information presented in the book. Improvement among the nine patients in this study was modest, yet three obtained clinically significant benefit. Greist et al. (2002) described an interactive (over the telephone) computerized self-help behavior therapy program for OCD (*BT Steps*). The intervention included education about OCD, treatment planning, ERP instructions, and relapse prevention. Greist et al. (2002) found that patients receiving this program improved about 25% in their OCD symptoms. These findings suggest that some degree of benefit may be obtained from self-help programs, absent a therapist. However, the lack of therapist assistance is likely to jeopardize the integrity of exposure and may compromise long-term outcome.

Patient Preference

It is important to weigh the patient's treatment preferences when considering therapeutic recommendations. We typically review the pros and cons of both CBT and pharmacotherapy and address any concerns when helping a patient decide which treatment(s) they will receive. Greater adherence can be expected if the patient is agreeable with the particular treatment plan. For example, some patients may not be willing to confront anxiety-evoking situations as in ERP.

Availability of Support System

Relatives and friends of OCD sufferers may play a role in maintaining the patient's symptoms by engaging in rituals or avoidance. In some cases family members are aware of this fact, yet in others relatives believe they are helping the patient or that they must avoid conflict over symptoms at all costs. Although it is useful for CBT to involve a support person to help with therapy exercises outside the session, it is a certain kind of support that is helpful in CBT. Several studies suggest that nonanxious, empathetic, firm family members are more successful than anxious, critical, argumentative, and inconsistent ones in providing support during CBT (Mehta, 1990; Steketee, 1993). Chambless and Steketee (1999) found that relatives' emotional overinvolvement, criticism, and hostility predicted higher rates of dropout from CBT. Thus, how individual family members interact with the patient should be assessed before requesting their assistance with CBT. If family members are not supportive and empathetic, involving them in CBT may be counterproductive and is discouraged. For patients who need additional support, group or inpatient CBT may be better options.

OCD-RELATED VARIABLES TO CONSIDER WHEN DECIDING ON TREATMENT

Symptom Presentation

Primacy and Severity of OCD Symptoms

A characteristic of CBT is that treatment methods target specific symptoms. Thus, we recom-

mend CBT for OCD only when obsessions and compulsions are among the patient's primary complaints. Because ERP requires a fairly generous commitment, we typically do not initiate this treatment if patients are concurrently undergoing simultaneous therapies likely to compete for their time and energy. Instead, we advise patients seeking treatment who have additional therapeutic undertakings to delay therapy for OCD, or begin with SRIs, until their schedule can accommodate CBT.

For the most part, clinical severity itself should not be a factor in the decision of whether to pursue medication or CBT. We tend to recommend CBT as the first-line treatment before SRIs. However, more severe symptoms may require a more intense regimen of whichever treatment is offered: a higher dose of medicine or more frequent CBT sessions. In cases where patients are extremely impaired or present a danger to themselves or to others, inpatient treatment is recommended. Where possible, however, we recommend CBT be conducted on an outpatient basis to maximize generalizability of treatment gains to the patient's own personal surroundings.

Symptom Theme

Because of the heterogeneity of OCD, there has been interest in whether patients with different symptom presentations (e.g., checking, hoarding) respond preferentially to certain treatments. Research suggests that both ERP and SRIs are of reduced benefit for hoarding symptoms (Abramowitz, Franklin, Schwartz, & Furr, in press; Mataix-Cols, Rauch, Manzo, Jenike, & Baer, 1999; Saxena et al., 2002). Novel CBT interventions for hoarding symptoms have been developed and tested in preliminary studies (e.g., Hartl & Frost, 1999). Thus, although still experimental, we recommend consideration of these newer procedures when patients present with primarily hoarding symptoms.

Some have suggested that OCD patients with severe obsessions and mental rituals ("pure obsessionals") fare less well in treatment than those displaying overt compulsive rituals (Baer, 1994). However, recent developments in the conceptualization of obsessions have led to a highly effective form of CBT for such patients involving exposure to the obsessional thought itself (i.e., via loop tape) and abstinence from neutralizing or mental rituals. Freeston et al.

(1997) found that more than 70% of patients evidenced clinically significant improvement in obsessions with this regimen.

Insight

There exists a range of insight into the senselessness of OCD symptoms (Foa et al., 1995). It appears that patients with poor insight about their symptoms improve less with ERP than those who have more insight (Foa, Abramowitz, Franklin, & Kozak, 1999). Perhaps patients with poor insight have difficulty deriving changes from exposure exercises. Alternatively, those with poor insight may be more reluctant to confront obsessional situations during therapy because of their fears. While we recommend a trial of ERP even for patients with poor insight, those who struggle with ERP may benefit from the addition of cognitive techniques (Salkovskis & Warwick, 1985). A second augmentative approach in such cases is pharmacotherapy with SRIs, and some psychiatrists even prescribe antipsychotic medication for such patients.

Comorbidity

Certain comorbid Axis I conditions may impede the effects of CBT for OCD. Major depressive disorder (Abramowitz & Foa, 2000; Abramowitz, Franklin, Kozak, Street, & Foa, 2000; Steketee, Chambless, & Tran, 2001) and generalized anxiety disorder (Steketee et al., 2001) are particularly associated with poorer response to ERP. Perhaps seriously depressed patients become demoralized and experience difficulties in complying with CBT instructions. Strong negative affect may also exacerbate OCD symptoms and limit treatment gains. For generalized anxiety patients, pervasive worry concerning other life issues probably detracts from the time and emotional resources available for learning skills from ERP treatment (Steketee et al., 2001).

Other Axis I conditions likely to interfere with ERP are those with psychotic and manic symptoms, which involve alterations in perception, cognition, and judgment. Active substance abuse or dependence is also an exclusion from CBT. These problems presumably impede patients' ability to follow treatment instructions on their own or attend to the cognitive changes that CBT aims to facilitate. Our recommendation is that patients receive treatment to bring these other conditions under control before attempting CBT for OCD.

Research also suggests that both CBT and medication are negatively affected by severe Axis II psychopathology (e.g., schizotypal personality disorder; De Haan et al., 1997; Steketee et al., 2001). Different personality disorder (PD) clusters may differentially influence the process and outcome of CBT. For example, anxious (e.g., obsessive-compulsive PD) and dramatic (e.g., histrionic PD) traits seem to interfere with developing rapport; however, if a therapeutic relationship can be developed, success is possible. If patients gain reinforcement for their OCD symptoms, CBT is unlikely to succeed because patients do not perceive themselves as achieving rewards for their efforts in therapy. In contrast, patients with personality traits in the odd cluster (e.g., schizotypal PD) present a challenge to CBT because of their reduced ability to consolidate corrective information during exposure or cognitive interventions.

Treatment History

For the most part, patients who have received an adequate length and dosage of one SRI (see March, Frances, Carpenter, & Kahn, 1997, for recommended doses) are unlikely to respond to others or to combinations of SRIs. Thus, for medicated patients who have not tried psychotherapy, CBT is the optimal next choice. If, however, patients report that they have undergone CBT, the adequacy of this therapy course should be assessed before making additional recommendations. If previous ERP was inadequate (i.e., infrequent sessions, lack of adequate exposure or response prevention), another course of CBT involving ERP should be considered. Noncompliance with prior ERP due to extreme fear may necessitate the use of cognitive techniques before initiating exposure. However, a history of noncompliance due to motivational factors may suggest the need for inpatient treatment or a supportive approach. Similarly, for patients who have failed adequate trials of both pharmacotherapy and intensive CBT, we recommend supportive therapy, OCD support groups, or, if symptoms are unremitting and insufferable, psychosurgery.

References

Abramowitz, J. S., & Foa, E. (2000). Does comorbid major depressive disorder influence outcome of exposure and response prevention for OCD? *Behavior Therapy, 31,* 795–800.

Abramowitz, J. S., Foa, E. B., & Franklin, M. E. (2003). Exposure and ritual prevention for obsessive-compulsive disorder: Effectiveness of intensive versus twice-weekly treatment sessions. *Journal of Consulting and Clinical Psychology, 71,* 394–398.

Abramowitz, J. S., Franklin, M. E., Kozak, M. J., Street, G. P., & Foa, E. B. (2000). The effects of pretreatment depression on cognitive-behavioral treatment outcome in OCD clinic patients. *Behavior Therapy, 31,* 517–528.

Abramowitz, J. S., Franklin, M. E., Schwartz, S. A., & Furr, J. M. (in press). Symptom presentation and outcome of cognitive-behavior therapy for obsessive-compulsive disorder. *Journal of Consulting and Clinical Psychology.*

Abramowitz, J. S., Whiteside, S. P., & Deacon, B. J. (2002). *Treatment of pediatric obsessive-compulsive disorder: A comprehensive meta-analysis of the outcome research.* Manuscript submitted for publication.

Baer, L. (1994). Factor analysis of symptom subtypes of obsessive-compulsive disorder and their relation to personality and tic disorders. *Journal of Clinical Psychology, 55,* 18–23.

Calamari, J. E., & Cassiday, K. L. (1999). Treating obsessive-compulsive disorder in older adults: A review of strategies. In M. Duffy (Ed.), *Handbook of counseling and psychotherapy with older adults: A review of strategies* (pp. 526–538). New York: Wiley.

Chambless, D. L., & Steketee, G. (1999). Expressed emotion and behavior therapy outcome: A prospective study with obsessive-compulsive and agoraphobic outpatients. *Journal of Consulting and Clinical Psychology, 67*(5), 658–665.

De Haan, E., van Oppen, P., van Balkom, A., Spinhoven, P., Hoogduin, K., & van Dyck, R. (1997). Prediction of outcome and early vs. late improvement in OCD patients treated with cognitive behavior therapy and pharmacotherapy. *Acta Psychiatrica Scandanavica, 96,* 354–361.

Foa, E. B., Abramowitz, J. S., Franklin, M. E., & Kozak, M. J. (1999). Feared consequences, fixity of belief, and treatment outcome in patients with obsessive-compulsive disorder. *Behavior Therapy, 30,* 717–724.

Foa, E., Kozak, M., Goodman, W., Hollander, E., Jenike, M., & Rasumssen, S. (1995). DSM-IV field trial: Obsessive-compulsive disorder. *American Journal of Psychiatry, 152,* 90–96.

Franklin, M. E., Abramowitz, J. S., Kozak, M. J., Levitt, J., & Foa, E. B. (2000). Effectiveness of exposure and ritual prevention for obsessive compulsive disorder: Randomized compared with non-randomized samples. *Journal of Consulting and Clinical Psychology, 68,* 594–602.

Freeston, M. H., Ladouceur, R., Gagnon, F., Thibodeau, N., Rheaume, J., Letarte, H., et al. (1997). Cognitive-behavioral treatment of obsessive thoughts: A controlled study. *Journal of Consulting and Clinical Psychology, 65,* 405–413.

Fritzler, B. K., Hecker, J. E., & Losee, M. C. (1997). Self-directed treatment with minimal therapist contact: Preliminary findings for obsessive-compulsive disorder. *Behaviour Research and Therapy, 35,* 627–631.

Greist, J. H., Marks, I. M., Baer, L., Kobak, K., Wenzel, K., Hirsch, J., et al. (2002). Behavior therapy for obsessive-compulsive disorder guided by a computer or by a clinician compared with relaxation control. *Journal of Clinical Psychiatry, 63,* 138–145.

Hartl, T., & Frost, R. (1999). Cognitive-behavioral treatment of compulsive hoarding: A multiple baseline experimental case study. *Behaviour Research and Therapy, 37,* 451–461.

Jenike, M. (2000). Neurosurgical treatment of obsessive-compulsive disorder. In W. Goodman, M. Rudorfer, & J. Maser (Eds.), *Obsessive-compulsive disorder* (pp. 457–482). Mahwah, NJ: Lawrence Erlbaum.

March, J., Frances, A., Carpenter, D., & Kahn, D. (1997). The expert consensus guidelines for the treatment of obsessive-compulsive disorder. *Journal of Clinical Psychiatry, 58* (suppl 4), 11–72.

Mataix-Cols, D., Rauch, S., Manzo, P., Jenike, M., & Baer, L. (1999). Use of factor-analyzed symptom subtypes to predict outcome with serotonin reuptake inhibitors and placebo in obsessive-compulsive disorder. *American Journal of Psychiatry, 156,* 1409–1416.

McLean, P. D., Whittal, M. L., Thordarson, D., Taylor, S., Sochting, I., Koch, W. J., et al. (2001). Cognitive versus behavior therapy in the group treatment of obsessive-compulsive disorder. *Journal of Consulting and Clinical Psychology, 69,* 205–214.

Mehta, M. (1990). A comparative study of family-based and patient-based behavioural management in obsessive-compulsive disorder. *British Journal of Psychiatry, 157,* 133–135.

Pato, M. T., Hill, J. L., & Murphy, D. L. (1990). A clomipramine dosage reduction study in the course of long-term treatment for obsessive-compulsive disorder. *Psychopharmacology Bulletin, 26,* 211–214.

Rauch, S., & Jenike, M. (1998). Pharmacological treatment of obsessive-compulsive disorder. In P. Nathan & J. Gorman (Eds.), *Treatments that work* (pp. 358–376). New York: Oxford University Press.

Salkovskis, P., & Warwick, H. (1985) Cognitive therapy of obsessive-compulsive disorder: Treating treatment failures. *Behavioural Psychotherapy,* *13*, 243–255.

Saxena, S., Maidment, K. M., Vapnik, T., Golden, G., Rishwain, T., Rosen, R. M., et al. (2002). Obsessive-compulsive hoarding: Symptom severity and response to multimodal treatment. *Journal of Clinical Psychiatry, 63*, 21–27.

Steketee, G. (1993). Social support and treatment outcome of obsessive compulsive disorder at 9-month follow-up. *Behavioural Psychotherapy, 21*(2), 81–95.

Steketee, G., Chambless, D., & Tran, G. (2001). Effects of axis I and II comorbidity on behavior therapy outcome for obsessive-compulsive disorder and agoraphobia. *Comprehensive Psychiatry, 42,* 76–86.

Steketee, G., & White, K. (1990). *When once is not enough.* Oakland, CA: New Harbinger.

Van den Hout, M., Emmelkamp, P., Kraaykamp, H., & Grietz, E. (1988). Behavioral treatment of obsessive-compulsives: Inpatient vs outpatient. *Behaviour Research and Therapy, 26,* 331–332.

Williams, K. E., Chambless, D. L., & Steketee, G. (1998). Behavioral treatment of obsessive-compulsive disorder in African Americans: Clinical issues. *Journal of Behavior Therapy and Experimental Psychiatry, 29,* 163–170.

29 THE IMPLICATIONS OF CONTROLLED OUTCOME STUDIES ON PLANNED SHORT-TERM PSYCHOTHERAPY WITH DEPRESSIVE DISORDERS

Bernard L. Bloom, Kenneth R. Yeager, & Albert R. Roberts

Depressive disorders are the major component of what are referred to in the *DSM-IV-TR* (American Psychiatric Association, 2000; see also Mays & Croake, 1997a, Chapter 4; Morrison, 1995) as mood disorders—periods of time when patients feel abnormally and pathologically happy or sad. The term *depressive disorder* is reserved to describe a person who has had multiple depressive episodes, periods of time of 2 weeks or longer when they feel depressed, cannot enjoy life, and have problems with eating and sleeping, guilt feelings, loss of energy, trouble concentrating, and thoughts about death. Most depressive disorders are recurrent and lifelong.

Depressive disorders are divided into three major subcategories: major depressive disorders, which tend to be relatively severe but relatively short in episode duration (although there is some growing belief that these disorders may also be chronic in nature); dysthymic disorders, which are less severe but chronic; and depressive disorders not otherwise specified, in which symptoms of depression are present but do not meet the criteria for depressive diagnoses or for any other diagnosis in which depression is a major feature.

Symptoms of depression are often found as a direct biological consequence of substance abuse or of a variety of medical conditions or medications, and they can accompany other psychiatric disorders such as schizophrenia, eating disorders, anxiety disorders, panic disorders, or gender identity disorders. In these cases, the depression is thought of as secondary in importance.

The term *adjustment disorder* is usually applied when some stressor (such as illness, normal aging, chronic marital tension, or occupational difficulties) can be identified that appears to serve as a psychological rather than biological precipitant of depressive symptoms. This type of depression was formerly called *reactive depression* (Goodwin & Guze, 1996, pp. 8–10; see also Hudson-Allez, 1997, p. 53; Kasl-Godley, Gatz, & Fiske, 1998).

It has been estimated that as many as 8 million individuals in the United States are afflicted with a major depressive illness in a given year and that the lifetime probability of developing a major depressive disorder may be as high as 25% for women and about half that for men (Biggs & Rush, 1999). The economic burden of depression in the United States alone exceeds $40 billion per year (Biggs & Rush, 1999). Depressive conditions are "common, costly, disabling, typically recurrent, and not infrequently chronic" (Biggs & Rush, 1999, p. 125).

A large literature—larger than for any other single diagnostic category—examines the effectiveness of brief episodes of psychotherapy in their treatment (see, for example, Bemporad & Vasile, 1999; Freeman & Oster, 1999; Mays & Croake, 1997a, 1997b; Swartz, 1999). This chapter reviews controlled outcome studies of brief psychotherapy in the treatment of depression that have been published since 1990. Readers might find it useful to read the papers that have described the results of the National Institute of Mental Health Treatment of Depression Collaborative Research Program (Elkin, Parloff, Hadley, & Autry, 1985; Elkin et al., 1989) and the National Institute of Health Consensus Development Conference on the Diagnosis and Treatment of Depression in Late Life (Schneider, Reynolds, Lebowitz, & Friedhoff, 1994).

In addition, the practice guidelines for the treatment of depressive disorders promulgated by the American Psychiatric Association (American Psychiatric Association, 1993) and the Depression Guideline Panel of the Agency for Health Care Policy and Research (Depression Guideline Panel, 1993), along with their associated commentaries (Blatt, 1995; Blatt, Quinlan, Pilkonis, & Shea, 1995; Lazar, 1997; Persons, Thase, & Crits-Christoph, 1996; Schneider & Olin, 1995; Schulberg et al., 1996; Scogin & McElreath, 1994; Scott, Tacchi, Jones, & Scott, 1997; Zeiss & Breckenridge, 1997), should be examined. Underlying these commentaries is a persistent controversy regarding the relative merits of psychological as opposed to biological approaches to the treatment of depressive disorders (Biggs & Rush, 1999; Feinberg, 1999; Markowitz, 1999).

EVIDENCE-BASED PRACTICE FOR DEPRESSION

Increasingly, practitioners are challenged to justify and improve treatment processes for those presenting with resistant and chronic mental illness. At the same time, practitioners are inundated with a flurry of information surrounding treatment approaches and new medication developments. Application of evidence-based practice can provide decision support based in current practice and outcome research. Eight questions that have been asked and answers from the current literature follow.

1. Is brief psychological treatment, regardless of type (social support, cognitive or behavioral treatment, or psychodynamic treatment), consistently superior to no-treatment or usual-care control conditions in its clinical effectiveness?
2. What happens to the client rate of improvement when treatment is time-limited?
3. Is cognitive and behavioral psychotherapy helpful in the brief treatment of depression?
4. Of all the orientations to psychodynamic psychotherapy, which is the most helpful?
5. Is the outcome of drug treatment for depression enhanced by the addition of brief psychotherapy to the treatment program?
6. Is long-term treatment superior to brief treatment in the case of some particularly severe depressions when outcome is assessed at the termination of treatment?
7. Is there is evidence that patients who do not

improve significantly in brief psychotherapy respond better to longer-term treatment?

8. What is the best and most consistent predictor of outcome of psychotherapy for depression?

CONTROLLED PSYCHOTHERAPY OUTCOME STUDIES

Controlled outcome studies involve the collection of outcome data in at least two groups who differ with respect to some salient characteristics upon entry into the study. The groups may differ by demographic characteristics, diagnosis, severity of disorder, type of treatment, or duration of treatment. The important aspect of controlled outcome studies is that groups of clients who differ in some important way can be contrasted. Controlled outcome studies permit the investigator to examine whether outcome is meaningfully related to specific characteristics of the therapist, the therapy, or the client, and they are thus more informative than uncontrolled outcome studies that simply report on degree of change in a single group of treated clients.

DEPRESSIVE DISORDERS

Shapiro et al. (1994) examined the extent to which initial severity of depression, treatment approach (cognitive-behavioral or psychodynamic-interpersonal psychotherapy), and duration of treatment (8 or 16 sessions) affected treatment outcome in a study of 117 depressed clients whose degree of change was assessed at intake, at the end of treatment, and at 3-month and 12-month follow-ups. Virtually all clients made substantial overall gains that were maintained at follow-up assessments. The cognitive-behavioral and psychodynamic-interpersonal therapies yielded generally equivalent results. Clients with relatively severe depressions who participated in the longer treatment seemed to do better at the end of treatment and at the 3-month follow-up than those in the shorter treatment group, and clients assigned to psychodynamic-interpersonal treatment seemed to be doing better at the 12-month follow-up than clients assigned to cognitive-behavioral treatment.

In a subsequent replication of this study with 36 clients in more varied settings, Barkham, Rees, Shapiro, et al. (1996) found that results were in general about the same as in the first study, but the overall findings were somewhat attenuated. While initial gains were impressive, clients generally failed to maintain their gains. Cognitive-behavioral treatment and psychodynamic-interpersonal treatment yielded equivalent results. Longer therapy duration resulted in generally greater improvement at the end of therapy, but the differences at the follow-up assessments were considerably diminished in comparison with the original study. There were no significant treatment type by treatment duration by initial severity interaction effects.

In a further study of dose–effect relations in time-limited psychotherapy for depression, Barkham, Rees, Stiles, et al. (1996) contrasted outcome in 212 depressed clients randomly assigned to either 8 or 16 sessions of time-limited treatment in order to determine whether (a) there is a negatively accelerated dose–effect curve and (b) there is a differential response rate for acute, chronic, and characterological or interpersonal components of depression. Improvement was found to be negatively accelerated, with change occurring more rapidly earlier in treatment and when tighter time limits were imposed, and certain symptoms were relieved more quickly than others. Changes in remoralization (subjectively experienced well-being) occurred first, followed by remediation (reductions in symptomatology), and finally rehabilitation (enhanced life functioning)—a finding also reported by Howard, Lueger, Maling, and Martinovich (1993).

More recently, Barkham, Shapiro, Hardy, and Rees (1999) evaluated their three-session model of brief psychotherapy for depression (two sessions 1 week apart, followed by a third session 3 months later) in a sample of 116 mildly depressed adults stratified by severity of depression, type of treatment (cognitive-behavioral or psychodynamic-interpersonal), and presence or absence of a 1-month delay before inaugurating treatment. Outcome assessments took place shortly after the conclusion of the final treatment session and again about 8 months later.

Virtually all patients made significant gains between the beginning and end of treatment and final follow-up. Effects of treatment delay were short-lived, with the delay group catching up quickly. Differences in treatment modality were small and insignificant whenever assessed. There was some evidence that time alone was most helpful to the least depressed and that the third session was most helpful to the most depressed in this group.

Because panic disorders have a high relapse rate if treated by drugs alone, Wiborg and Dahl (1996) sought to determine whether adding brief dynamic psychotherapy to the drug treatment would reduce the relapse rate in panic disorder patients as compared with those treated by drugs alone. Two treatment groups of 20 patients each were formed, with one randomly selected group assigned to 9 months of drug treatment and the other assigned to the same drug treatment regimen plus 15 weekly sessions of brief dynamic psychotherapy. Anxiety and depression were assessed at intake and at 6, 12, and 18 months after beginning treatment. All patients in both groups became free of panic attacks within 26 weeks of the start of treatment. Addition of brief dynamic psychotherapy to treatment with clomipramine significantly reduced the relapse rate of panic disorders compared with the group receiving clomipramine treatment alone. Between the end of medication treatment and the 18-month follow-up, the relapse rate was 20% in the drug and psychotherapy group and 75% in the drug treatment alone group.

PROBLEM-SOLVING TREATMENT

Mynors-Wallis (1996) described and evaluated problem-solving treatment, a brief cognitive-behavioral psychotherapy for patients with mild to moderate mental disorders, particularly involving depression, in primary care. Problem-solving treatment involved three steps: (a) Symptoms were linked with their problems, (b) problems were defined and clarified, and (c) attempts were made to solve the problems in a structured way. The treatment program was conceptualized as passing through seven stages: (a) explanation of the treatment and its rationale, (b) clarification and definition of the problems, (c) choice of achievable goals, (d) generation of alternative solutions, (e) selection of a preferred solution, (f) clarification of the necessary steps to implement the solution, and (g) evaluation of progress.

After 4 weeks of treatment with explanation, reassurance, and advice, a total of 47 patients who had high scores (12 or more) on the Present State Examination were randomly assigned to three sessions of problem-solving treatment or usual care. After 7 weeks, both groups had improved significantly, but the reduction in scores was significantly greater for the problem-solving group than for the control group. At 28 weeks, the problem-solving treatment group showed nonsignificant further improvement.

In a second study, problem-solving treatment was used to treat major depression and contrasted with patients receiving antidepressant medication and standard clinical management and a third group receiving drug placebo with standard clinical management. Each treatment was given in six sessions over 12 weeks, with the first session lasting 60 minutes and all others lasting 30 minutes. With about 30 patients in each group, problem-solving treatment was found to be significantly more effective than placebo but not significantly different from amitriptyline both at 6 weeks and at 12 weeks. Average total duration of treatment was about 3 hours. Problem-solving treatment was judged to be as effective as amitriptyline and more effective than placebo, feasible in practice, and acceptable to patients.

A final study examined effectiveness of problem-solving treatment administered by community nurses. Six nurses were recruited and trained. Problem-solving treatment was found to reduce sickness-related days off work, but otherwise the outcomes were the same as those obtained by usual primary care treatment. When indirect costs were included, problem-solving treatment was found to produce significant savings. More recent studies reported by this research group—contrasting problem-solving treatment in primary care with and without accompanying use of antidepressants—demonstrate substantial improvement in all groups, with no advantage attributable to the addition of antidepressant medication to the treatment program (Hegel, Barrett, & Oxman, 2000; Mynors-Wallis, Gath, Day, & Baker, 2000).

Rudd et al. (1996) evaluated an intensive, structured, time-limited outpatient group format for the treatment of suicidal patients based on a problem-solving and social competence paradigm targeting fundamental skill development and improved social and adaptive randomized functioning and coping. These authors contrasted 143 patients randomly assigned to the treatment group and 121 patients randomly assigned to a treatment-as-usual control group. All patients were in the military, and most patients were white men. Follow-up assessments were done at 1, 6, 12, 18, and 24 months posttreatment with a variety of measures: suicidal ideation, life stress, negative expectations, depression, problem-solving behavior and attitudes, personality, symptomatology, diagnoses, intellectual functioning, and psychosocial history. Treatment took place in a day hospital format for 9 hours per day for 2 weeks, and it included three components: a traditional experiential-affective group, psychoeducational classes, and an extended problem-solving group. Treatment and control participants exhibited significant improvement across all outcome measures throughout the follow-up period.

Improvement was generally rapid at first, after which it tapered off. The experimental treatment was more effective than treatment as usual at retaining the highest risk participants. Nonsignificant superiority in clinical improvement was found for the experimental group: 64% versus 48%.

In a study conducted in the United Kingdom, Friedli, King, Lloyd, and Horder (1997) contrasted self-reported outcome and level of satisfaction in a sample of 136 depressed patients randomly assigned to either routine general practice care or to routine care plus between 1 and 12 sessions of nondirective Rogerian psychotherapy provided over a 12-week time period. The mean number of sessions per patient was 7.7.

Follow-up data were collected 3 and 9 months after inauguration of treatment. While patients assigned to the psychotherapy group were more satisfied with the help they received than those assigned to the general practitioner, there were no significant differences in judged outcome, with all patients improving significantly over time.

Weisz, Thurber, Sweeney, Proffitt, and LaGagnoux (1997) reported on the development of an eight-session, small-group, cognitive-behavioral therapeutic intervention program designed to enhance primary control (changing objective conditions to fit one's wishes) and secondary control (changing oneself to buffer the impact of objective conditions) among mildly to moderately depressed elementary school children and contrasted the results of their program with those found in an untreated control group. Scores on measures of childhood depression decreased significantly in both the treated and untreated groups, with score reductions among the treated children significantly greater (averaging

two to three times greater) than among the untreated children, both immediately posttreatment and at a 9-month follow-up.

Blatt, Zuroff, Bondi, and Sanislow (2000) have examined previously unanalyzed data from the Treatment for Depression Collaborative Research Program (see Elkin et al., 1985) to determine whether any additional differences in outcome could be found other than symptom reduction. This study contrasted depressed patients who had been assigned to four treatment groups: antidepressant medication (imipramine), cognitive-behavioral therapy, interpersonal therapy, and placebo. While previous studies showed superior symptom reduction at the 8-week midtreatment assessment for the group receiving imipramine, no significant differences in symptom reduction were found at termination or at the 18-month follow-up. Blatt et al. (2000) found, however, that significant treatment differences emerged at the time of the 18-month follow-up in patients' ratings of the effects of treatment on their life adjustment. Patients in the interpersonal therapy group reported significantly greater satisfaction with treatment at the 18-month follow-up than any of the other groups, and patients in both the interpersonal therapy and cognitive-behavioral therapy groups reported significantly greater effects of the treatment on their capacity to establish and maintain interpersonal relationships and to recognize and understand sources of their depression than did patients in either the placebo or imipramine groups.

These recent controlled outcome studies, all fairly well designed, suggest that depressive symptoms are responsive to most brief psychotherapy treatment approaches. Both cognitive-behavioral and interpersonal-psychodynamic approaches to brief psychotherapy appear to be as effective as pharmacological treatment, particularly in the case of mild to moderate depression. In addition, brief psychotherapy often has a significant additive effect when used in conjunction with psychotropic drugs.

DEPRESSIVE ADJUSTMENT DISORDERS

A number of controlled outcome studies have been reported in which depressions associated with a variety of identifiable stress-inducing precipitating events were treated. These events range from life-threatening illnesses to family caregiving, earthquakes, HIV infection, miscarriage, and infertility. A particularly interesting background paper in this area is that of Cohen, Stokhof, van der Ploeg, and Visser (1996) that describes a brief scale useful in identifying patients recovering from acute myocardial infarctions who require and would accept psychological care.

Fawzy et al. (1990; see also Spiegel, 1999) developed and evaluated a structured 6-week psychiatric intervention for cancer patients that included health education, enhancement of problem-solving skills, stress management, and psychological support. A group of postsurgical patients with malignant melanomas were randomly divided into an experimental sample of 38 patients and 28 controls. By the end of the intervention, patients in the experimental group exhibited higher vigor and greater use of active-behavioral coping. Differences were more pronounced at the 6-month follow-up, at which time the intervention group showed significantly lower depression, fatigue, confusion, and total mood disturbance, as well as higher vigor and more active-behavioral and active-cognitive coping, than did the controls. In general, the intervention program reduced psychological distress and enhanced longer-term effective coping.

Stewart et al. (1992) provided eight 2-hour weekly support group sessions to 64 infertility patients (usually couples) and evaluated their effectiveness by contrasting results with 35 similar patients not offered the support group. Patients in the support group had significantly greater entry than exit scores on several measures of psychological distress and depression. Patients in the comparison group had similar scores at the start of the program but showed no change over 8 weeks. Support groups were found to be highly acceptable and effective.

Greer et al. (1992) examined the effectiveness of adjuvant psychological therapy for patients with cancer. An 8-week course of weekly cognitive-behavioral psychotherapy that was problem focused and designed for individual cancer patients produced significant improvement in various measures of psychological distress at the conclusion of therapy and at 4 months when contrasted with a randomly selected no-psychotherapy control group. Patients receiving adjuvant psychological therapy showed significantly greater improvement than control patients—less anxiety, helplessness, fatalism,

and anxious preoccupation with cancer; less depression; and a more positive adjustment toward their disease and its treatment. At 4 months, significant improvement persisted, and treated patients experienced significantly less anxiety and psychological distress than did the untreated controls.

Kelly et al. (1993) evaluated the effects of brief cognitive-behavioral or social support group therapy with depressed HIV-infected patients. A total of 68 patients were randomly divided into three groups: eight-session cognitive-behavioral groups, eight-session support groups, or a usual-care comparison condition. Group sessions lasted 90 minutes per meeting and included two coleaders. Considerable data were collected before the start of the programs, and patients were studied at the conclusion of the experimental program and at a 3-month follow-up. Both interventions produced reductions in depression, hostility, and somatization when compared with the usual-care group. Social support intervention produced reductions in overall psychiatric symptoms and tended to reduce maladaptive interpersonal sensitivity and anxiety, as well as frequency of unprotected receptive anal intercourse. While the cognitive-behavioral intervention resulted in less frequent illicit drug use during the follow-up period, the social support intervention produced greater evidence of clinically significant change. Thus, the two forms of therapy resulted in both shared and unique improvements in functioning (see also McDermut, Miller, & Brown, 2001).

Gallagher-Thompson and Steffen (1994) randomly assigned 66 clinically depressed family caregivers of frail elderly relatives to 16 to 20 sessions of either cognitive-behavioral or brief psychodynamic individual psychotherapy. Treatment was conducted twice per week for the first 4 weeks and then once per week thereafter. In cognitive-behavioral therapy, caregivers were taught to challenge their dysfunctional thoughts and to develop more adaptive ways to view problematic situations. They were also taught behavioral strategies to enhance mood. Brief psychodynamic therapy was based on the theory that caregivers' past conflicts over dependence and independence were reactivated by the caregiving situation. Therapy focused on understanding past losses and conflicts in separation and individuation.

Assessments were conducted at entry into treatment, 10 weeks later, at the end of treatment, and at 3 months and 12 months after completing treatment. At posttreatment, 71% of the caregivers were no longer clinically depressed, with no differences found between the two treatments. Clients who had been caregivers for shorter periods of time showed greater improvement in the brief psychodynamic condition, while those who had been caregivers for at least 44 months improved most with cognitive-behavioral therapies (see also Niederehe, 1994, pp. 305ff.; Steffen, Futterman, & Gallagher-Thompson, 1998).

Evans and Connis (1995) studied a group of 72 depressed patients undergoing radiation treatment for cancer who were divided into three groups: cognitive-behavioral group treatment, social support, or no-treatment control. Treatments averaged about eight sessions in duration. The cognitive-behavioral groups focused on the use of cognitive and behavioral strategies to reduce maladaptive anxiety and depression. The social support groups encouraged members to describe their feelings about having cancer, to identify and discuss shared problems, and to adopt supportive roles toward others in the group. Patients were assessed with a variety of measures of symptom distress at the beginning and end of treatment and at a 6-month follow-up. Relative to the comparison group, both the cognitive-behavioral and the social support therapies resulted in less depression, hostility, and somatization. The social support intervention resulted in fewer psychiatric symptoms and less maladaptive interpersonal sensitivity and anxiety, and it had longer effectiveness than did the cognitive-behavioral treatment group.

Lee, Slade, and Lygo (1996) tested the effectiveness of a 1-hour psychologically oriented debriefing provided in the home by a female psychologist 2 weeks after a miscarriage by contrasting two groups of women: those who received the debriefing and those who did not (total N = 39). Levels of anxiety and depression were assessed 1 week and 4 months after miscarriage. While women exhibited considerable anxiety and depression following the miscarriage and exhibited reduction in anxiety and depression as time went on, the debriefing program did not significantly influence emotional adaptation.

Noting that palliative care (treatment designed to reduce pain and discomfort without curing the underlying condition) involves relief of emotional symptoms as well as control of physical symptoms, Wood and Mynors-Wallis (1997; see also Mynors-Wallis, 1996) contrasted outcomes in two groups of dying patients undergoing hospice home care: patients receiving traditional hospice care and those who also were provided with three to five sessions of problem-solving treatment. This latter form of treatment was designed to help patients formulate ways of dealing with emotional and psychosocial symptoms induced by their illnesses by helping patients clarify and define the problem, set achievable goals, consider alternative solutions, select a preferred solution, implement the solution, and evaluate progress.

In a small, randomized, controlled clinical trial, the authors reported that the few patients in the problem-solving treatment group found the treatment to be acceptable and helpful. These authors hope to undertake a larger study to determine more definitively the efficacy of problem-solving treatment.

Goenjian et al. (1997) contrasted brief psychotherapy focused on trauma and grief among early adolescents exposed to the 1988 earthquake in Armenia with untreated groups on posttraumatic stress and depressive reactions. The intervention program included classroom group psychotherapy and an average of two 1-hour individual sessions (maximum of four sessions), which were conducted over a 3-week period. All treatment began 18 months after the earthquake and was completed within a 6-week period. Data collected pretreatment, posttreatment, and 3 years after the earthquake revealed that severity of symptoms decreased in the treated group and increased in the untreated group. Symptoms of posttraumatic stress disorder decreased following treatment, while depressive symptoms increased in the untreated group and remained stable in the treated group.

With the single exception of the 1-hour debriefing session provided to women who had suffered a miscarriage 2 weeks earlier, these recent studies, also quite well designed, provide consistent support for the effectiveness of brief psychotherapeutic approaches in the treatment of stress-induced depression.

DEPRESSION AMONG THE ELDERLY

The category of geriatric depression occupies some middle ground between depressive disorders of unknown origin and depressive adjustment disorders that are reactions to some identifiable psychological precipitating event. The extent to which depression can be precipitated as a psychological reaction to normal aging versus its development as a component of the physiology of the aging process is a complex question, but what is clear from the literature is that brief psychotherapeutic approaches have commonly been used in the treatment of such depressions (Coon, Rider, Gallagher-Thompson, & Thompson, 1999; Gatz et al., 1998; Nordhus, Nielsen, & Kvale, 1998).

Useful background papers have been prepared by Sadavoy and Thompson. Sadavoy (1994) contrasted three approaches to treating depression in the elderly—brief psychodynamic, interpersonal, and cognitive-behavioral therapies—and discussed the strengths of each approach. Suggesting that age, per se, is not an impediment to change and may in fact be an important asset in motivating the patient to overcome resistance and work more quickly, Sadavoy outlined an integrated treatment strategy that can help in the tasks of assessment, diagnosis, and selection of treatment modality.

Thompson (1996) provided a clinical description of cognitive and behavioral techniques used in treating elderly depressed patients. These techniques provide the older patient with a broad range of skills to use in coping with stressful life events once the therapy is completed. Thompson described and contrasted cognitive and behavioral theory and described techniques that have been used for the past decade. The paper also described the typical cognitive and behavioral therapy session, as well as the phases of cognitive and behavioral therapy, and discussed special considerations to keep in mind when working with elderly clients.

Niederehe (1994) has provided a very useful review of controlled outcome studies published between 1974 and 1990 in which depressed elderly patients were treated, objective outcome assessments were undertaken, and some comparison or control group was used for comparative analysis. Psychodynamic therapies (examined in six studies) were found to be clinically efficacious in reducing symptoms in elderly depressed patients. Effectiveness of psychodynamic therapy was found to be equivalent to cognitive-behavioral therapies, both in acute phases and in terms of its longer-term impact, with follow-up data available for as long as 2 years.

In a related review, Scogin and McElreath (1994) examined the efficacy of psychosocial treatments of geriatric depression in 17 studies published between 1975 and 1990. In each of these studies, the psychosocial treatments were contrasted with either a no-treatment comparison group or some other psychosocial treatment. Treatments were reliably more effective than no treatment, and effect sizes were significant for both major and less severe levels of depression. The psychosocial treatments averaged 12 sessions in duration. While the type of treatment could not be evaluated because there were too few studies of any specific treatment approach, psychosocial interventions for older adults experiencing depressive symptoms were found to be quite effective and about as successful as pharmacotherapy.

Another useful review of the literature on acute treatment efficacy for geriatric depression was prepared by Schneider and Olin (1995). Their review was based on 30 placebo-controlled clinical trials published between 1982 and 1994 with randomized depressed patients who were not suicidal, not severely ill, and without significant medical illness. Psychotherapy was found to be more effective than waitlist controls, no treatment, or pill-placebo and equivalent to antidepressant medications in geriatric outpatient populations with both major and minor depression. About half of the studies involved group interventions. Therapy orientations were cognitive, interpersonal, reminiscent, psychodynamic, and eclectic.

As for recent controlled outcome studies, Gallagher-Thompson, Hanley-Peterson, and Thompson (1990) contrasted three approaches to psychotherapy with a sample of 91 older adults with a mean age of 67 years initially diagnosed as cases of major depressive disorder. Patients were randomly assigned to 16 to 20 sessions over a 4-month period of either cognitive, behavioral, or psychodynamic psychotherapy and were followed for 2 years. Improvement increased with time, and treatment gains were maintained by the majority of patients. There were no significant differences in response by therapy modality.

Mossey, Knott, Higgins, and Talerico (1996) contrasted the effectiveness of 6 to 8 sessions of interpersonal counseling (IPC) versus usual care (UC) for a sample of 76 randomized subdysthymic patients age at least 60 who did not meet *DSM-III-R* criteria for major depression or dysthymia. Data from the initial assessment as well as from the 3-month and 6-month follow-ups are presented. Geriatric Depression Scale (GDS) scores, health ratings, and measures of physical and social functioning were collected at each data collection point. At 3 months, IPC group members showed nonsignificantly greater improvement than UC group members on all outcome variables. At 6 months, significant differences in the rate of improvement in GDS scores and on self-rated health measures were observed for IPC compared with UC members. The self-rated health of the IPC group members improved, while it deteriorated in the UC group.

Empirical studies evaluating treatment outcome with elderly depressed patients consistently demonstrate the effectiveness of brief psychotherapy. All psychotherapeutic treatment approaches examined in these studies appear to have equal effectiveness and to be as effective as pharmacological approaches and significantly more effective than usual-care control-group treatment.

CONCLUDING COMMENTS

This review of controlled outcome studies of planned short-term psychotherapy in the treatment of depression published since 1990 suggests that:

1. Brief psychological treatment, regardless of type (social support, cognitive or behavioral treatment, or psychodynamic treatment), is consistently superior to no-treatment or usual-care control conditions in its clinical effectiveness.
2. Rate of improvement is negatively accelerated; that is, improvement is more rapid early in treatment than later in treatment and appears to be greater when time is more stringently limited.
3. Cognitive and behavioral psychotherapy has been found to be consistently helpful in the brief treatment of depression. Of all the orientations to psychodynamic psychotherapy, the most helpful has been interpersonal psychotherapy (Bloom, 1997, pp. 100ff.; Hinrichsen, 1997, 1999; Klerman, Weissman, Rounsaville, & Chevron, 1984). These conclusions are similar to those found in the review of controlled outcome studies con-

ducted during and before the 1980s. Marks (1999) has called attention to the fact that these two helpful approaches have both been shown to be valuable in the treatment of depressive disorders, but it is not clear whether similarities in these two approaches account for the similarities in results or whether different but equally effective treatment pathways account for the similarities of results.

4. Outcome of drug treatment for depression is generally enhanced by the addition of brief psychotherapy to the treatment program.
5. Long-term treatment has occasionally been found to be superior to brief treatment in the case of some particularly severe depressions when outcome is assessed at the termination of treatment, but that superiority is often no longer in evidence at the time of follow-up assessments.
6. Relapse rate is high among depressed patients treated by brief psychotherapy. There is evidence that some patients who do not improve significantly in brief psychotherapy do improve with longer-term treatment and that relapse rate can be reduced by providing maintenance treatment.
7. The best and most consistent predictor of outcome of psychotherapy for depression is the level of severity of depression at the start of treatment. The most severely disturbed patients at the start of treatment tend to be the most severely disturbed at the end of treatment (Luborsky et al., 1996; Shea, Elkin, & Sotsky, 1999).

Given that degree of improvement is negatively accelerated in psychotherapy and that maintenance treatment seems to be helpful in reducing relapse rate, there is continuing reason to believe that patients should be encouraged to enter or reenter psychotherapy when needed while episodes of psychotherapy are kept as short as possible. More generally, as Jarrett and Rush have suggested, "the challenge is to determine how to best use the psychotherapies that appear to reduce depressive symptoms, when to use pharmacotherapy alone or in combination with psychotherapy, and how to innovate or adapt psychosocial interventions to reduce the human suffering, as well as the economic cost, of depressive disorders" (1994, p. 128).

References

American Psychiatric Association. (1993). Practice guideline for major depressive disorder in adults. *American Journal of Psychiatry, 150*(Suppl. 4), 1–26

American Psychiatric Association. (1994). *Diagnostic and statistical manual of mental disorders* (4th ed.). Washington, DC: Author.

American Psychiatric Association. (2000). *Diagnostic and statistical manual of mental disorders* (4th ed., text revision). Washington, DC: Author.

Barkham, M., Rees, A., Shapiro, D. A., Stiles, W. B., Agnew, R. M., Halstead, J., et al. (1996). Outcomes of time-limited psychotherapy in applied settings: Replicating the second Sheffield Psychotherapy Project. *Journal of Consulting and Clinical Psychology, 64,* 1079–1085.

Barkham, M., Rees, A., Stiles, W. B., Shapiro, D. A., Hardy, G. E., & Reynolds, S. (1996). Dose-effect relations in time-limited psychotherapy for depression. *Journal of Consulting and Clinical Psychology, 64,* 927–935.

Barkham, M., Shapiro, D. A., Hardy, G. E., & Rees, A. (1999). Psychotherapy in two-plus-one sessions: Outcomes of a randomized controlled trial of cognitive-behavioral and psychodynamic-interpersonal therapy for subsyndromal depression. *Journal of Consulting and Clinical Psychology, 67,* 201–211.

Bemporad, J. R., & Vasile, R. G. (1999). Dynamic psychotherapy. In M. Hersen & A. S. Bellack (Eds.), *Handbook of comparative interventions for adult disorders* (2nd ed., pp. 91–107). New York: Wiley.

Biggs, M. M., & Rush, A. J. (1999). Cognitive and behavioral therapies alone or combined with antidepressant medication in the treatment of depression. In D. S. Janowsky (Ed.), *Psychotherapy indications and outcomes* (pp. 121–171). Washington, DC: American Psychiatric Press.

Blatt, S. J. (1995). The destructiveness of perfectionism: Implications for the treatment of depression. *American Psychologist, 50,* 1003–1020.

Blatt, S. J., Quinlan, D. M., Pilkonis, P. A., & Shea, M. T. (1995). Impact of perfectionism and need for approval on the brief treatment of depression: The National Institute of Mental Health Treatment of Depression Collaborative Research Program revisited. *Journal of Consulting and Clinical Psychology, 63,* 125–132.

Blatt, S., Zuroff, D. C., Bondi, C. M., & Sanislow, C. A. (2000). Short- and long-term effects of medication and psychotherapy in the brief treatment of depression: Further analyses of data from the NIMH TDCRP. *Psychotherapy Research, 10,* 215–234.

Bloom, B. L. (1997). *Planned short-term psychotherapy: A clinical handbook* (2nd ed.). Boston: Allyn & Bacon.

Cohen, L., Stokhof, L. H., van der Ploeg, H. M., & Visser, F. C. (1996). Identifying patients recovering from a recent myocardial infarction who require and accept psychological care. *Psychological Reports, 79,* 1371–1377.

Coon, D. W., Rider, K., Gallagher-Thompson, D., & Thompson, L. (1999). Cognitive-behavioral therapy for the treatment of late-life distress. In M. Duffy (Ed.), *Handbook of counseling and psychotherapy with older adults* (pp. 487–510). New York: Wiley.

Depression Guideline Panel. (1993). *Clinical practice guideline No. 5: Depression in primary care, 2: Treatment of major depression* (USDHHS Publication No. AHCPR 93-0551). Rockville, MD: Agency for Health Care Policy and Research.

Elkin, I., Parloff, M., Hadley, S., & Autry, J. (1985). NIMH Treatment of Depression Collaborative Research Program: Background and Research Plan. *Archives of General Psychiatry, 42,* 305–316.

Evans, R. L., & Connis, R. T. (1995). Comparison of brief group therapies for depressed cancer patients receiving radiation treatment. *Public Health Reports, 110,* 306–311.

Fawzy, F. I., Cousins, N., Fawzy, N. W., Kemeny, M. E., Elashoff, R., & Morton, D. (1990). A structured psychiatric intervention for cancer patients: I. Changes over time in methods of coping and affective disturbance. *Archives of General Psychiatry, 47,* 720–725.

Feinberg, M. (1999). Pharmacotherapy. In M. Hersen & A. S. Bellack (Eds.), *Handbook of comparative interventions for adult disorders* (2nd ed., pp. 156–177). New York: Wiley.

Freeman, A., & Oster, C. (1999). Cognitive behavior therapy. In M. Hersen & A. S. Bellack (Eds.), *Handbook of comparative interventions for adult disorders* (2nd ed., pp. 108–138). New York: Wiley.

Friedli, K., King, M. B., Lloyd, M., & Horder, J. (1997). Randomised controlled assessment of non-directive psychotherapy versus routine general practitioner care. *Lancet, 350* (9092), 1662–1665.

Gallagher-Thompson, D., Hanley-Peterson, P., & Thompson, L. W. (1990). Maintenance of gains versus relapse following brief psychotherapy for depression. *Journal of Consulting and Clinical Psychology, 58,* 371–374.

Gallagher-Thompson, D., & Steffen, A. M. (1994). Comparative effects of cognitive-behavioral and brief psychodynamic psychotherapies for depressed family caregivers. *Journal of Consulting and Clinical Psychology, 62,* 543–549.

Gatz, M., Fiske, A., Fox, L. S., Kaskie, B., Kasl-Godley, J. E., & McCallum, T. J. (1998). Empirically validated psychological treatments for older adults. *Journal of Mental Health & Aging, 4,* 9–46.

Goenjian, A. K., Karayan, I., Pynoos, R. S., Minassian, D., Najarian, L. M., Steinberg, A. M., et al. (1997). Outcome of psychotherapy among early adolescents after trauma. *American Journal of Psychiatry, 154,* 536–542.

Goodwin, D. W., & Guze, S. B. (1996). *Psychiatric diagnosis* (5th ed.) New York: Oxford University Press.

Greer, S., Moorey, S., Baruch, J. D. R., Watson, M., Robertson, B. M., Mason, A., et al. (1992). Adjuvant psychological therapy for patients with cancer: A prospective randomised trial. *British Medical Journal, 304,* 675–680.

Hegel, M. T., Barrett, J. E., & Oxman, T. E. (2000). Training therapists in problem-solving treatment of depressive disorders in primary care: Lessons learned from the "Treatment Effectiveness Project." *Families, Systems, & Health, 18,* 423–435.

Hinrichsen, G. A. (1997). Interpersonal psychotherapy for depressed older adults. *Journal of Geriatric Psychiatry, 30,* 239–257.

Hinrichsen, G. A. (1999). Treating older adults with interpersonal psychotherapy for depression. *Journal of Clinical Psychology, 55,* 949–960.

Howard, K. I., Lueger, R. J., Maling, M. S., & Martinovich, Z. (1993). A phase model of psychotherapy outcome: Causal mediation of change. *Journal of Consulting and Clinical Psychology, 61,* 678–685.

Hudson-Allez, G. (1997). *Time-limited therapy in a general practice setting: How to help within six sessions.* London, Sage.

Jarrett, R. B., & Rush, A. J. (1994). Short-term psychotherapy of depressive disorders: Current status and future directions. *Psychiatry, 57,* 115–132.

Kasl-Godley, J. E., Gatz, M., & Fiske, A. (1998). Depression and depressive symptoms in old age. In I. H. Nordhus, G. R. VandenBos, S. Berg, & P. Fromholt (Eds.), *Clinical geropsychology* (pp. 211–217). Washington, DC: American Psychological Association.

Kelly, J. A., Murphy, D. A., Bahr, R., Kalichman, S. C., Morgan, M. G., Stevenson, L. Y., et al. (1993). Outcome of cognitive-behavioral and support group brief therapies for depressed, HIV-infected persons. *American Journal of Psychiatry, 150,* 1679–1686.

Klerman, G. L., Weissman, M. M., Rounsaville, B. J., & Chevron, E. S. (1984). *Interpersonal psychotherapy of depression.* New York: Basic Books.

Lazar, S. G. (1997). The effectiveness of dynamic psychotherapy for depression. *Psychoanalytic Inquiry* (Suppl), 51–57.

Lee, C., Slade, P., & Lygo, V. (1996). The influence of psychological debriefing on emotional adaptation in women following early miscarriage: A preliminary study. *British Journal of Medical Psychology, 69,* 47–58.

Luborsky, L., Diguer, L., Cacciola, J., Barber, J. P., Moras, K., Schmidt, K., & DeRubeis, R. J. (1996). Factors in outcomes of short-term dynamic psychotherapy for chronic vs. nonchronic major depression. *Journal of Psychotherapy Practice and Research, 5,* 152–159.

Markowitz, J. C. (1999). Interpersonal psychotherapy: Alone and combined with medication. In D. S. Janowsky (Ed.), *Psychotherapy indications and outcomes* (pp. 233–247). Washington, DC: American Psychiatric Press.

Marks, I. (1999). Is a paradigm shift occurring in brief psychological treatments? *Psychotherapy and Psychosomatics, 68*(4), 169–170.

Mays, M., & Croake, J. W. (1997a). *Treatment of depression in managed care.* New York: Brunner/Mazel.

Mays, M., & Croake, J. (1997b). Managed care and treatment of depression. In S. R. Sauber (Ed.), *Managed mental health care: Major diagnostic and treatment approaches* (pp. 244–278). Bristol, PA: Brunner/Mazel.

McDermut, W., Miller, I. W., & Brown, R. A. (2001). The efficacy of group psychotherapy for depression: A meta-analysis and review of the empirical research. *Clinical Psychology: Science and Practice, 8,* 98–116.

Miller, I. J. (1996). Time-limited brief therapy has gone too far: The result is invisible rationing. *Professional Psychology: Research and Practice, 27,* 567–576.

Morrison, J. (1995). *DSM-IV made easy: The clinician's guide to diagnosis.* New York: Guilford.

Mossey, J. M., Knott, K. A., Higgins, M., & Talerico, K. (1996). Effectiveness of a psychosocial intervention, interpersonal counseling, for subdysthymic depression in medically ill elderly. *Journal of Gerontology: Medical Sciences, 51A,* M172–M178.

Mynors-Wallis, L. (1996). Problem-solving treatment: Evidence for effectiveness and feasibility in primary care. *International Journal of Psychiatry in Medicine, 26,* 249–262.

Mynors-Wallis, L. M., Gath, D. H., Day, A., & Baker, F. (2000). Randomised controlled trial of problem solving treatment, antidepressant medication, and combined treatment for major depression in primary care. *British Medical Journal, 320*(1), 26–30.

Niederehe, G. T. (1994). Psychosocial therapies with depressed older adults. In L. S. Schneider, C. F. Reynolds, B. D. Lebowitz, & A. J. Friedhoff (Eds.), *Diagnosis and treatment of depression in late life: Results of the NIH consensus development conference* (pp. 293–315). Washington, DC: American Psychiatric Press.

Nordhus, I. H., Nielsen, G. H., & Kvale, G. (1998).

Psychotherapy with older adults. In I. H. Nordhus, G. R. VandenBos, S. Berg, & P. Fromholt (Eds.), *Clinical geropsychology* (pp. 289–311). Washington, DC: American Psychological Association.

Persons, J. B., Thase, M. E., & Crits-Christoph, P. (1996). The role of psychotherapy in the treatment of depression: Review of two practice guidelines. *Archives of General Psychiatry, 53,* 283–290.

Rudd, M. D., Rajib, M. H., Orman, D. T., Stulman, D. A., Joiner, T., & Dixon, W. (1996). Effectiveness of an outpatient intervention targeting suicidal young adults: Preliminary results. *Journal of Consulting and Clinical Psychology, 64,* 179–190.

Sadavoy, J. (1994). Integrated psychotherapy for the elderly. *Canadian Journal of Psychiatry, 39*(Suppl. 1), S19–S26.

Schneider, L. S., & Olin, J. T. (1995). Efficacy of acute treatment for geriatric depression. *International Psychogeriatrics, 7,* 7–25.

Schneider, L. S., Reynolds, C. F., Lebowitz, B. D., & Friedhoff, A. J. (1994). *Diagnosis and treatment of depression in late life: Results of the NIH consensus development conference.* Washington, DC: American Psychiatric Press.

Schulberg, H. C., Block, M. R., Madonia, M. J., Scott, C. P., Rodriguez, E., Imber, S. D., et al. (1996). Treating major depression in primary care practice. *Archives of General Psychiatry, 53,* 913–919.

Scogin, F., & McElreath, L. (1994). Efficacy of psychosocial treatments for geriatric depression: A quantitative review. *Journal of Consulting and Clinical Psychology, 62,* 69–74.

Scott, C., Tacchi, M. J., Jones, R., & Scott, J. (1997). Acute and one-year outcome of a randomised controlled trial of brief cognitive therapy for major depressive disorder in primary care. *British Journal of Psychiatry, 171,* 131–134.

Shapiro, D. A., Barkham, M., Rees, A., Hardy, G. E., Reynolds, S., & Startup, M. (1994). Effects of treatment duration and severity of depression on the effectiveness of cognitive-behavioral and psychodynamic-interpersonal psychotherapy. *Journal of Consulting and Clinical Psychology, 62,* 522–534.

Shea, M. T., Elkin, I., & Sotsky, S. M. (1999). Patient characteristics associated with successful treatment. In D. S. Janowsky (Ed.), *Psychotherapy indications and outcomes* (pp. 71–90). Washington, DC: American Psychiatric Press.

Spiegel, D. (1999). Psychotherapeutic intervention with the medically ill. In D. S. Janowsky (Ed.), *Psychotherapy indications and outcomes* (pp. 277–300). Washington, DC: American Psychiatric Press.

Steffen, A. M., Futterman, A., & Gallagher-Thompson, D. (1998). Depressed caregivers: Comparative outcomes of two interventions. *Clinical Gerontologist, 19*(4), 3–15.

Stewart, D. E., Boydell, K. M., McCarthy, K., Swerdlyk, S., Redmond, C., & Cohrs, W. (1992). A prospective study of the effectiveness of brief professionally-led support groups for infertility patients. *International Journal of Psychiatry in Medicine, 22,* 173–182.

Swartz, H. A. (1999). Interpersonal psychotherapy. In M. Hersen & A. S. Bellack (Eds.), *Handbook of comparative interventions for adult disorders* (2nd ed., pp. 139–155). New York: Wiley.

Thompson, L. W. (1996). Cognitive-behavioral therapy and treatment for late-life depression. *Journal of Clinical Psychiatry, 57*(Suppl. 5), 29–37.

Weisz, J. R., Thurber, C. A., Sweeney, L., Proffitt, V. D., & LaGagnoux, G. L. (1997). Brief treatment of mild-to-moderate child depression using primary and secondary control enhancement training. *Journal of Consulting and Clinical Psychology, 65,* 703–707.

Wiborg, I. M., & Dahl, A. A. (1996). Does brief dynamic psychotherapy reduce the relapse rate of panic disorder? *Archives of General Psychiatry, 53,* 689–694.

Wood, B. C., & Mynors-Wallis, L. M. (1997). Problem-solving therapy in palliative care. *Palliative Medicine, 11,* 49–54.

Zeiss, A. M., & Breckenridge, J. S. (1997). Treatment of late life depression: A response to the NIH consensus conference. *Behavior Therapy, 28,* 3–21.

30

EVIDENCE-BASED PRACTICE WITH ANXIETY DISORDERS

Guidelines Based on 59 Outcome Studies

Bernard L. Bloom, Kenneth R. Yeager, & Albert R. Roberts

While the number of well-designed, controlled, clinical outcome studies is not large, brief psychotherapeutic interventions appear to play a useful role in the treatment of anxiety spectrum disorders. Such interventions not only appear to be effective in their own right but also add a significant component to the benefits of medication. This chapter summarizes and describes the time-limited interventions and outcomes from 59 studies. This database includes 11 recent outcome studies that measured the effectiveness of crisis intervention and brief therapy approaches with posttraumatic stress disorder (PTSD) precipitated by gunshot injuries, sexual assaults, terrorist attacks, vehicular accidents, and violent crimes.

REVIEW OF EVIDENCE

Several recent outcome studies reviewed in this chapter suggest that psychological approaches to the treatment of anxiety disorders are remarkably effective in their own right and usually add a significant component to the effectiveness of more traditional psychopharmacological treatments. The evidence suggests that brief psychotherapy not only helps reduce symptoms but also serves to reduce relapse rate. Controlled outcome studies are not common, however. The evidence appears to indicate the following:

- *Brief psychotherapeutic treatments of anxiety disorders*: Brief psychotherapeutic treatments of anxiety disorders usually appear to

be no less effective than longer-term treatments.
- *Brief cognitive-behavioral therapy*: Generally seems to be more efficacious than brief psychodynamic therapy, supportive psychotherapy, or nondirective therapy.
- *Brief psychotherapy*: Is not invariably helpful, however. Longer-term psychotherapy may be recommended when brief symptom-focused treatment is not sufficient, although it is not yet clear whether longer treatment yields a consistently superior result (Shear, 1995).

There is need, however, for additional and better-designed controlled outcome studies to solidify our understanding of the overall effectiveness of approaches to the treatment of anxiety.

As to accounting for the effectiveness of cognitive-behavioral therapy in the treatment of anxiety disorders, Harvey and Rapee (1995) have suggested that cognitive-behavioral therapy involves treating the anxiety by "teaching patients to identify, evaluate, and modify the chronically worrisome danger-related thoughts and associated behaviors" (pp. 862–863; see also Wright & Borden, 1991).

Brief cognitive-behavioral psychotherapeutic treatment has been provided in both individual and group formats, as well as by self-help, bibliographic, and other limited therapist-contact procedures. Outcome studies indicate that:

- Therapist-directed programs are usually superior to other formats but that virtually all cognitive-behavioral approaches are superior to waitlist controls.

- There is some evidence that there is a generalized component to psychotherapeutic effectiveness in that treatment conducted with dual-diagnosis patients that include anxiety disorders appear to be just as helpful as treatments designed for single-diagnosis patients.
- Finally, there is consistent evidence that the success of physician treatment for anxiety disorders related to generalized medical conditions can be significantly enhanced by the addition of a psychotherapeutic component to the treatment program.

Significant elements in cognitive and behavioral treatment appear to include:

- Informational and educational components (understanding the disorder and the treatment rationale)
- Somatic management skills (relaxation and breathing training)
- Cognitive restructuring (understanding the role of catastrophic thoughts in anxiety development; psychological debriefing)
- Controlled graded exposure to settings that tend to precipitate symptoms.
- Cognitively based homework assignments

If these positive findings regarding the effectiveness of brief psychological treatments for the anxiety disorder spectrum are corroborated by additional controlled outcome studies, the inclusion of a psychotherapeutic component in the treatment of these conditions should become the recognized treatment standard.

ANXIETY AND EVIDENCE-BASED TREATMENT

Anxiety disorders, affecting some 16% of the population at any given moment, are divided into two subordinate diagnostic categories. The first group includes generalized anxiety disorder, anxiety disorder due to a general medical condition, panic disorder, agoraphobia, specific phobia, social phobia, and acute stress disorder. The second group includes obsessive-compulsive disorder, substance-induced anxiety disorder, and

posttraumatic stress disorder (American Psychiatric Association, 1994). Patients in the first group are commonly treated by primary care physicians (see, for example, Catalan et al., 1991). In contrast, patients in the second group are usually thought of as more disabled and are more often treated by mental health professionals (Choy & de Bosset, 1992; Walley, Beebe, & Clark, 1994).

Principal symptoms of anxiety disorders include excessive anxiety and worry, self-limiting panic attacks, irrational avoidance of situations that present the possibility of embarrassment or humiliation, obsessive thoughts and compulsive behavior, cardiopulmonary symptoms (chest pain, hyperventilation, tachycardia and palpitations, tremulousness, dizziness, light-headedness, faintness, headache, and paresthesias), gastrointestinal symptoms (nausea, vomiting, diarrhea, abdominal pain, and anorexia), depressive symptoms, and sexual dysfunction.

The growing importance of treatment outcome evaluation has been recognized by most writers in the field (see, for example, Lane, 2000), and a number of overviews of empirically validated brief treatments for the anxiety disorders are now available in the literature (see Ballenger, 1999; Barlow, Esler, & Vitali, 1998; Gatz et al., 1998; Hersen & Biaggio, 2000; McCullough, 2000; Newman, 2000; Stanley & Averill, 1999).

This chapter examines recent outcome studies of brief psychotherapy treatments designed to be of help with many of these anxiety disorders. Very few empirical outcome studies have been reported in the case of the more severe anxiety disorders, with the exception of posttraumatic stress disorder, although a number of interesting reviews and clinical case reports are in the literature (e.g., Franklin, Foa, & Kozak, 1999; Marks, 1990; Marmar, 1991; Sifneos, 1985; Starcevic & Durdic, 1993; Weiss & Marmar, 1993; see also Schmidt & Harrington, 1995).

While a variety of pharmacotherapeutic agents, including benzodiazepines, azapirones, tricyclics, monoamine oxidase inhibitors, beta-blockers, and serotonin reuptake inhibitors, are employed in the treatment of anxiety disorders (see, for example, Gross & Rosen, 1997; Sutherland, Tupler, Colket, & Davidson, 1996; Warneke, 1985), psychotherapeutic interventions are being increasingly recognized as having a significant therapeutic role as well.

There are three reasons for the growing interest in alternatives to exclusively pharmacological treatment of anxiety disorders:

- First, many medications have undesirable side effects.
- Second, medications appear to have decreasing effectiveness with time.
- Third, discontinuance of medication results in relapse rates that are far higher than in the case of psychotherapeutic approaches (Harvey & Rapee, 1995; Juster & Heimberg, 1995; Otto & Whittal, 1995).

PANIC DISORDER

The synergistic effectiveness of psychological and biological approaches to the treatment of anxiety disorders is evident in the case of panic disorders. Pollack and Smoller (1995) noted that many patients treated with pharmacotherapy, while improved, remain symptomatic despite treatment. Adding cognitive-behavioral psychotherapy to the pharmacotherapy appears to improve both acute and long-term outcome.

Wiborg and Dahl (1996) studied 40 patients with panic disorders and found that 15 weekly sessions of combined dynamic psychotherapy and treatment with clomipramine significantly reduced the relapse rate, when compared with the clomipramine-only group at the 9-month blind follow-up.

Otto and Whittal (1995) suggest psychological treatments, especially cognitive-behavioral therapy. Findings suggest such treatments offer patients with panic disorders "the potential for . . . efficacy equal to pharmacologic treatment, without the risk of exposure to drug-related side effects or discontinuation effects, or the need for ongoing medication treatment" (Otto & Whittal, 1995, p. 816; see also Craske, Maidenberg, & Bystritsky, 1995).

Beck, Sokol, Clark, Berchick, and Wright (1992) contrasted focused cognitive therapy with brief supportive psychotherapy in a sample of patients with panic disorders. They found that the cognitive therapy yielded significantly superior results in terms of reductions of panic symptoms and general anxiety in comparison with those obtained by brief supportive psychotherapy, both at the conclusion of the therapeutic episode and at the time of a 1-year follow-up.

Additionally, Westling and Öst (1999) developed a four-session, 1 hour per week format that also included keeping a panic diary, reading about the treatment rationale, and thinking about how the patient's own panic problems could be explained by the cognitive treatment model presented to them. Data that were collected pretreatment, posttreatment, and at a 6-month follow-up included independent assessor ratings, self-observation, and self-report scales. A total of 10 patients were involved in this pilot study from whom complete data were obtained.

Compared with pretreatment assessments, posttreatment and follow-up assessments showed significant drops in full panic attacks and in limited symptom attacks, highly significant decreases in virtually all self-report measures, and significant decreases in levels of pathology as judged by independent assessors. All improvements noted at the time of the posttreatment assessment were maintained at the time of the follow-up.

In a similar study, Clark et al. (1999) developed a very brief (up to five sessions during a 3-month period) cognitive therapy approach for the treatment of panic disorder that included between-session self-study modules. They examined its effectiveness by contrasting results with a more traditional cognitive "full" therapy approach (up to 12 1-hour treatment sessions during a 3-month period) and a 3-month waitlist control. Patients in the 3-month waitlist control were randomly assigned to one of the two cognitive treatment programs at the conclusion of the waitlist period.

A total of 42 patients were randomly assigned to the treatment or waitlist groups and completed the treatment sequence. Total therapy and booster-session time was 11.9 hours for patients receiving traditional cognitive therapy and 6.5 hours for patients receiving brief cognitive therapy. Mean age of the patients was 34 years. Mean duration of the current panic episode was 3.7 years. About 60% of the patients were female. About three fourths of the patients were on stable doses of a psychotropic medication (either low-potency benzodiazepines or beta-blockers).

While there were no differences in assessment scores at the start of the treatment program between any of the three groups, at the end of treatment scores on all of the various assessments were significantly less pathological in both of the treatment groups than in the waitlist control, and there were no significant differences between the two treatment groups' scores. The gains made by the members of the two treatment groups were maintained at the time of the 12-month posttreatment follow-up assessment, with no difference in gain maintenance between the two treatment groups.

In these studies, brief interventions have clearly been found to be useful in the treatment of panic disorders in their own right, as well as providing significant supplementary help to patients being treated with psychotropic medication.

GENERALIZED ANXIETY DISORDERS

Crits-Christoph, Connolly, Azarian, Crits-Christoph, and Shappell (1996) have noted that generalized anxiety disorders are characterized by a high level of chronicity and a significant degree of impairment in functioning. Average duration of this disorder, which often begins in the teens or early twenties, is between 6 and 10 years. While pharmacological treatment appears to be efficacious, there are a number of adverse side effects, including attentional, psychomotor, cognitive, and memory-impairing symptoms, reduced coping and stress response capabilities, and physical dependence and withdrawal reactions.

In the case of patients with generalized anxiety disorders, brief cognitive-behavioral therapy has been found to be superior to results with waitlist controls. Treatments accentuating cognitive components have been found to be equal in effect to treatments accentuating behavioral components. Regardless of emphasis, cognitive-behavioral treatments have been generally found to be superior to nondirective treatment methods and to the use of benzodiazepines, particularly when long-term follow-up assessments have been undertaken (Harvey & Rapee, 1995), although the degree of superiority is quite modest.

Crits-Christoph et al. (1996) have explored the potential therapeutic role of interpersonally oriented psychodynamic therapy for generalized anxiety disorders. Their studies examined the ef-

fectiveness of a 16-session treatment program conducted on a weekly basis, followed by three monthly booster sessions. The treatment program was oriented toward understanding the anxiety symptoms in the context of interpersonal and intrapsychic conflicts. Initial research design involved five therapists and a total of 26 patients. Contrasted pre–post measures on a variety of self-report instruments indicated statistically significant changes on all outcome measures. Large decreases were found in interpersonal problems and in anxiety, with smaller decreases found in measures of depression. Controlled outcome studies and long-term follow-up evaluations are envisioned for the future.

In a particularly informative study, Durham et al. (1994) contrasted three brief treatments in a sample of 110 outpatients with generalized anxiety disorders who were randomly assigned to either cognitive therapy, psychoanalytic psychotherapy, or anxiety management training. The cognitive therapy and psychoanalytic psychotherapy groups were further randomly assigned to brief (8 to 10 sessions within 6 months) or longer term (16 to 20 sessions within 6 months) treatment episodes. Assessments by senior staff blind to patients' therapists and treatment conditions used a variety of assessment instruments before treatment, after treatment, and 6 months following the conclusion of treatment.

Cognitive therapy was found to be significantly more effective than psychoanalytic psychotherapy, with about 50% of patients considerably better at follow-up. There were no significant outcome differences associated with length of treatment. Patients receiving anxiety management training improved as much as patients in cognitive therapy when assessed immediately at the conclusion of the treatment episode, but their levels of improvement deteriorated somewhat by the time of the follow-up assessment. The authors suggest:

Cognitive therapy is likely to be more effective than psychodynamic psychotherapy with chronically anxious patients. . . . The superiority of cognitive therapy at follow-up suggests that the greater investment of resources required for this approach is likely to pay off in terms of more sustained improvement. There is no evidence that 16–20 sessions of treatment is more effective, on average, than 8–10 sessions. (Durham et al., 1994, p. 315)

Noting that there is considerable overlap in the diagnoses of anxiety disorder and depression, Kush and Fleming (2000) developed a brief cognitive group therapy approach to the simultaneous treatment of depression and anxiety. Their 12-session group program met weekly for 90 minutes and was based on a curriculum that synthesized cognitive psychoeducational approaches to the treatment of depression and anxiety, cognitive modification, and problem-solving training.

Patients in this pilot program included 29 adult outpatients, of whom 26 completed the curriculum. Diagnoses included depressive mood disorder ($N = 18$) and anxiety disorder ($N = 8$), including generalized anxiety disorder. Assessments were obtained at the beginning and end of the treatment program and included the Beck Depression Inventory, the Beck Anxiety Inventory, and the Dysfunctional Attitudes Scale. Significant reductions in all three scores were found, with scores on the Beck Depression Inventory showing the most significant drop.

PHOBIAS

Two reports have documented the effectiveness of brief interventions for phobias. Hellstrom and Öst (1995; see also Öst, 1989) contrasted five cognitive approaches in a sample of 52 patients with spider phobias. One approach involved a single 3-hour session of therapist-directed graded exposure. The other approaches involved either specific or general manual-based treatments conducted in either the home or the clinic. The therapist-directed exposure was found to be significantly more effective than three of the four manual-based treatments, both immediately after treatment and at a follow-up assessment that included behavioral, physiological, and self-report measures. The specific manual-based treatment conducted in the clinic was significantly superior to the other three manual-based treatments but only at follow-up. Clinically significant improvement levels were 80% at follow-up for the therapist-directed treatment program, 63% for the manual-based treatment program conducted at the clinic, and 10% or less for the other programs.

Three cases of cognitive-behavioral treatment for choking and swallowing phobias were described by Ball and Otto (1994). This treatment was conducted for 11 to 13 sessions and involved psychoeducational, cognitive restructuring, interoceptive, and in vivo exposure techniques. All three patients responded well, as measured by their food hierarchy progressions and by weight gain.

In their recent review of cognitive-behavioral treatment programs, Juster and Heimberg (1995) reported that in the case of patients with social phobias, exposure-oriented treatments seem superior to drug treatments in terms of both degree and duration of improvement. Multicomponent treatment programs (e.g., cognitive restructuring and exposure) do not tend to be superior to single-component programs.

ANXIETY DISORDERS DUE TO A GENERALIZED MEDICAL CONDITION

A number of outcome studies conducted in medical settings have examined the effectiveness of adding brief psychological treatment to traditional medical treatment for anxiety reactions related to medical disorders. Greer et al. (1992) found that an 8-week brief problem-focused cognitive-behavioral treatment program, added to traditional medical treatment in a sample of 174 randomized cancer patients, resulted in significantly decreased helplessness, preoccupation, fatalism, and anxiety symptoms, as well as significantly increased fighting spirit, when the experimental and control groups were contrasted. At the time of a 4-month follow-up, patients receiving the brief psychological treatment program had significantly lower scores than controls on anxiety, psychological symptoms, and psychological distress.

Baldoni, Baldaro, and Trombini (1995) found that adding short-term dynamic psychotherapy to traditional medical treatment in a sample of 13 female patients suffering from urethral syndrome resulted in dramatic superiority in treatment effectiveness when they were contrasted with a sample of 23 patients who received only traditional medical treatment.

In a sample of 68 depressed men with HIV infection randomly assigned to eight-session cognitive-behavioral treatment, eight-session social support groups, or a control group, Kelly et al. (1993) found that both the cognitive-behavioral and social support group therapies produced reductions in overall psychiatric symptoms and tended to reduce maladaptive interpersonal sensitivity, anxiety, and frequency of unprotected intercourse when contrasted with the control group. The two forms of therapy resulted in both shared and unique improvements in functioning.

Harrison, Watson, and Feinmann (1997) provided an 8-week group therapy experience to a total of 19 patients with chronic idiopathic facial pain that had ranged from 1 to 5 years in duration and that had been unresponsive to a variety of prior medical treatments. Four groups of four or five patients met in weekly 3-hour sessions. The therapeutic orientation was cognitive-behavioral and included relaxation exercises during and between group sessions. Significant reductions in reported pain, anxiety, and depression were obtained, along with improved abilities in coping.

In a particularly striking study of the use of cognitive-behavioral interventions, de Jongh et al. (1995) examined the effectiveness of this treatment in a sample of 52 patients suffering from dental phobias. These patients were randomly assigned to a cognitive restructuring group, an educational group, and a waitlist control condition. Neither of the interventions lasted longer than 1 hour. Cognitive restructuring was designed to modify negative cognitions associated with dental treatment, while the educational intervention provided information about oral health and dental treatment. Compared with the waitlist control and the educational intervention, the patients in the cognitive restructuring condition showed a significant decrease in frequency and believability of negative cognitions and in dental anxiety following the intervention. One year later, patients in the two intervention conditions were reexamined. Further reductions in dental anxiety were found in both intervention groups, and the reductions were so great in the case of the educational intervention condition that differences in treatment effectiveness between the two intervention groups no longer were found.

Two recent studies have been located in which psychoeducational interventions did not appear to be helpful with 39 women whose pregnancies had ended in miscarriages. Lee, Slade, and Lygo (1996) found no significant differences between their experimental and control groups in measures of anxiety, depression, intrusion, or avoidance 4 months after the miscarriage.

A 10-session cognitive psychotherapy program designed to reduce the 1-year recurrence rate of duodenal ulcer by helping patients cope with anxiety and dependence failed to achieve its objective in a study reported by Wilhelmsen, Haug, Ursin, and Berstad (1994).

POSTTRAUMATIC STRESS DISORDERS

Investigation of brief approaches to the treatment of posttraumatic stress disorder (PTSD) has, until recently, been largely confined to the study of war-related traumas and natural or man-made disasters. In recent years, attention has also been directed to the treatment of victims of sexual assaults, terrorist attacks, vehicular accidents, gunshot injuries, violent crimes, and other traumas (Austin & Godleski, 1999; Choy & de Bosset, 1992; Foa & Meadows, 1997). Study of the psychological consequences of such events has a special appeal because, in contrast to most psychiatric disorders, there is a recognized and unequivocal precipitating event.

Principal symptoms of PTSD include pervasive anxiety, reexperiencing, avoidance, and hyperarousal following exposure to a traumatic event. The development of PTSD involves both psychological and biological components and can produce enduring neurohormonal changes and serious long-term morbidity. Accordingly, it is generally agreed that prompt and effective treatments are urgently needed.

Most brief treatment programs that have been reported were cognitive and behavioral in nature and included some combination of psychological debriefing, education, and imagery rehearsal. Both individual and group approaches have been studied, and programs have been evaluated that involved children as well as adults.

Rose, Brewin, Andrews, and Kirk (1999) conducted a randomized controlled trial of two brief individual approaches to crisis intervention—educational and psychological debriefing—in a sample of 157 adults who had been victims of violent crimes within the past month. The educational intervention had an average duration of 30 minutes, and the debriefing intervention lasted about 1 hour. One third of the sample served as a no-treatment control in that they participated in the assessment procedures but received no specific additional intervention. Follow-up assessments were conducted for the entire sample 6 months after the intervention and for about two thirds of the sample 5 months later.

The authors reported that all three groups improved over time but that there were no significant between-group differences. Based on their analysis of their own as well as prior studies, the authors suggest that somewhat more intensive interventions that allow for the recasting or restructuring of the traumatic experience to attribute new meanings to the event may be necessary.

The effectiveness of a brief psychotherapeutic approach in the management of PTSD was examined by Gersons, Carlier, Lamberts, and van der Kolk (2000) in a sample of 42 Dutch police officers randomly divided into a treatment group and a waitlist control (subsequently treated). All officers met the diagnostic criteria for PTSD. None exhibited evidence of organic mental disorders, substance abuse, psychoses, or severe depression, and all had been medication-free for at least 6 months prior to the start of treatment. Treatment consisted of 16 1-hour sessions of brief eclectic psychotherapy (BEP) with five elements: psychoeducation, imagery guidance, writing assignments, meaning and integration, and a farewell ritual.

Blind psychometric assessments were conducted 1 week before the start of treatment, after four sessions, at termination of treatment, and 3 months after termination. No significant differences between the two groups were found at the pretest or at the end of the fourth treatment session. In contrast, at the end of treatment and at the follow-up assessment, the BEP group demonstrated significant improvement in PTSD, in work resumption, and in some comorbid conditions, notably, phobic anxiety, depression, obsessive-compulsive symptoms, and sleeping problems. Symptom checklist scores were significantly above the norm at the pretest and after the fourth treatment session for both the treated and the waitlist groups. Waitlisted police officers remained significantly above the norm on all symptom checklist scores throughout the study, while treated officers' scores dropped to normative levels at the time of treatment termination and follow-up assessment.

A psychological debriefing technique thought to be particularly useful in working with new war zone cases has been reported by Busuttil et al. (1995; see also Choy & de Bosset, 1992) using a group therapy format. Psychological debriefing was originally proposed to help groups of military personnel who had undergone the same traumatic event to process their experiences together, usually within 48 hours of the event itself. Busuttil et al. (1995) used this general strategy in working with 34 cases of posttraumatic stress disorder in a 12-day residential treatment program, followed by group outpatient sessions for up to 1 year, and found it to be remarkably effective as assessed at the time of treatment termination, as well as at 6 weeks, 6 months, and 1 year during the follow-up period.

Debriefing involved (a) initial group formation; (b) detailed descriptions of the facts, emotions, and sensory perceptions associated with the traumatic events; (c) didactic presentations regarding stress and stress management, drugs commonly used in the treatment program, supplemented by relaxation exercises to reduce stress; (d) problem solving; and (e) family reintegration. Most of the improvement occurred within the first 2 months of treatment.

The use of imagery rehearsal therapy (IRT) in the treatment of chronic nightmares in the case of sexual assault survivors with posttraumatic stress disorders was examined by Krakow et al. (2001). The patients were 168 women who had suffered rape, other sexual assaults, or repeated exposure to sexual abuse in childhood or adolescence and who were divided randomly into a treatment or a waitlist control group.

The IRT consisted of two 3-hour group sessions 1 week apart, followed by a 1-hour follow-up session 3 weeks later. At the first session, after some didactic material was presented about nightmares, their causes, functions, and control, and how imagery rehearsal can help eliminate nightmares, participants were given the opportunity to learn cognitive-behavioral tools for dealing with unpleasant images and for practicing pleasant imagery. At the second session, participants were taught how to use IRT to modify a single, self-selected nightmare and to rehearse the "new dream." At the follow-up session, the group discussed progress, shared experiences, and raised questions.

Small, nonsignificant reductions in the control group were found in frequency of nightmares, sleep disturbances, and symptoms associated with the diagnosis of PTSD. In contrast, highly significant reductions in these and other related symptoms were found in the treated group, including nightmare severity and frequency, sleep quality disturbances, and PTSD symptoms. Improvement occurred during the first 3 months after the start of the treatment program and was maintained during the next 3 months. There was no difference in degree of improvement as a function of use of psychotropic medication.

Three controlled studies of brief interventions for children and adolescents with PTSD diagnoses have been located. The effectiveness of a group-based cognitive-behavioral psychotherapy treatment program was examined in a sample of 17 children and adolescents diagnosed with PTSD by March, Amaya-Jackson, Murray, and Schulte (1998). The weekly treatment program was 18 weeks in length, and PTSD, anxiety, depression, anger, locus of control, and disruptive behavior were assessed at baseline, the end of treatment, and at a 6-month follow-up.

The treatment program included anxiety management training, muscle relaxation training, interpersonal problem solving as a way of dealing with anger, positive self-talk, cognitive training, development of an individually tailored stimulus hierarchy, narrative sharing, and graded in vivo exposure. Two groups were formed, and the second group began 4 weeks after the first group had started. Precipitating events in the development of PTSD included automobile accidents, severe illness, gunshot injuries, fires, and death of a loved one by means of criminal assault, illness, car accidents, fire, or gunshot injury.

Fourteen of the 17 children completed the treatment program. Results were significant on virtually all measures at the end of treatment and at the 6-month follow-up evaluation. Continued work by this group has resulted in revision and shortening of the treatment program with no apparent loss of program effectiveness.

A number of studies described brief trauma-related treatment following the 1988 Armenian earthquake that resulted in the deaths of some 25,000 inhabitants. The program, completed within a 6-week period, comprising both group and individual psychotherapy, was instituted 18 months after the earthquake.

Five components were incorporated into the program: discussion of the trauma event and its resulting effects, reminders of the traumatic event, postdisaster stresses, bereavement, and developmental impact. The individual sessions provided an opportunity for more in-depth explorations of trauma and its effects.

A total of 64 early adolescents who lived in Gyumri and who were significantly affected by the quake were divided into two groups: a treatment group of 35 children and an untreated group of 29 children. Eighteen months after the treatment program was completed, all children were reevaluated. Measures of PTSD reaction and of its components—intrusion, avoidance, and arousal—and a measure of depression were completed at the start of the intervention program and again 18 months later.

Analysis of the data revealed significant improvement in the treated group and significant deterioration in the untreated group in PTSD reaction scores on all three PTSD components. As to the depression scores, there was no significant change in the treated group, while the untreated group demonstrated a significant increase in depression. The treatment program appeared to have helped prevent the worsening course of PTSD and comorbid depression.

Two brief individual therapy interventions for sexually abused girls and their nonoffending female caretakers were compared by Celano, Hazzard, Webb, and McCall (1996). A total of 32 girls, aged 8 to 13, and their nonoffending female caretakers (primarily but not always mothers) were randomly assigned to either an 8-week 1 hour per week, theoretically based, structured experimental treatment program (focused on self-blame/stigmatization, betrayal, traumatic sexualization, and powerlessness) or to a relatively unstructured supportive psychotherapy program of the same length. Approximately equal time was spent with the girls and with their caretakers. Measures provided by both children and their nonoffending caretakers were obtained before and after treatment, as well as assessments by a clinician blind to the treatment condition.

Both treatment programs yielded improvement in posttraumatic stress disorder symptoms and reductions in self-blame and in powerlessness, as well as increases in overall psychosocial functioning of the child. The experimental program appeared to produce greater parental support, reduced self-blame, and reduced expectations of a negative impact of abuse on the child.

Because PTSD involves a known precipitating event, psychological debriefing constitutes a significant component of virtually all psychotherapeutic approaches to its treatment. The outcome literature suggests that this debriefing is a valuable aspect of the treatment.

CONCLUDING REMARKS

The outcome studies reviewed in this chapter suggest that psychological approaches to the treatment of anxiety disorders are remarkably effective in their own right, adding significant components to the effectiveness of pharmacological approaches. While controlled studies are not common, there is increasing interest in identifying and refining best practice psychotherapeutic treatments for anxiety disorders. It is important to note that brief psychotherapeutic treatments were found to be no less effective than long-term treatments.

Brief cognitive-behavioral therapy generally seems to be more efficacious than brief psychodynamic therapy, support psychotherapy, or nondirective therapy. Brief cognitive-behavioral psychotherapeutic treatment has been provided in both group and individual formats, and outcome studies indicate that directed programs are usually superior to other formats.

Finally, there is consistent evidence of successfully augmenting physician treatment of anxiety disorders related to generalized medical conditions through the addition of a psychotherapeutic component. If these positive findings regarding the effectiveness of brief psychological treatments for anxiety disorders are corroborated by additional controlled outcome studies, one could safely conclude that psychotherapeutic approaches should become an integrated component within the treatment of each of these conditions.

References

American Psychiatric Association. (1994). *Diagnostic and statistical manual of mental disorders* (4th ed.). Washington, DC: Author.

Austin, L. S., & Godleski, L. S. (1999). Therapeutic approaches for survivors of disaster. *Psychiatric Clinics of North America, 22,* 897–910.

Baldoni, F., Baldaro, B., & Trombini, G. (1995). Psychotherapeutic perspectives in urethral syndrome. *Stress Medicine, 11,* 79–84.

Ball, S. G., & Otto, M. W. (1994). Cognitive-behavioral treatment of choking phobia: Three case studies. *Psychotherapy and Psychosomatics, 62,* 207–211.

Ballenger, J. C. (1999). Current treatments of the anxiety disorders in adults. *Biological Psychiatry, 46,* 1579–1594.

Barlow, D. H., Esler, J. L., & Vitali, A. E. (1998). Psychosocial treatments for panic disorders, phobias, and generalized anxiety disorder. In P. E. Nathan & J. M. Gorman (Eds.), *A guide to treatments that work* (pp. 288–318). New York: Oxford University Press.

Beck, A. T., Sokol, L., Clark, D. A., Berchick, R., & Wright, F. (1992). A crossover study of focused cognitive therapy for panic disorder. *American Journal of Psychiatry, 149,* 778–783.

Busuttil, W., Turnbull, G. J., Neal, L. A., Rollins, J., West, A. G., Blanch, N., et al. (1995). Incorporating psychological debriefing techniques within a brief group psychotherapy programme for the treatment of post-traumatic stress disorder. *British Journal of Psychiatry, 167,* 495–502.

Catalan, J., Gath, D. H., Anastasiades, P., Bond, S. A. K., Day, A., & Hall, L. (1991). Evaluation of a brief psychological treatment for emotional disorders in primary care. *Psychological Medicine, 21,* 1013–1018.

Celano, M., Hazzard, A., Webb, C., & McCall, C. (1996). Treatment of traumagenic beliefs among sexually abused girls and their mothers: An evaluation study. *Journal of Abnormal Child Psychology, 24,* 1–17.

Choy, T., & de Bosset, F. (1992). Post-traumatic stress disorder: An overview. *Canadian Journal of Psychiatry, 37,* 578–583.

Clark, D. M., Salkovskis, P. M., Hackmann, A., Wells, A., Ludgate, J., & Gelder, M. (1999). Brief cognitive therapy for panic disorder: A randomized controlled trial. *Journal of Consulting and Clinical Psychology, 67,* 583–589.

Craske, M. G., Maidenberg, E., & Bystritsky, A. (1995). Brief cognitive-behavioral versus nondirective therapy for panic disorder. *Journal of Behavior Therapy and Experimental Psychiatry, 26,* 113–120.

Crits-Christoph, P., Connolly, M. B., Azarian, K., Crits-Christoph, K., & Shappell, S. (1996). An open trial of brief supportive-expressive psychotherapy in the treatment of generalized anxiety disorder. *Psychotherapy, 33,* 418–430.

De Jongh, A., Muris, P., ter Horst, G., van Zuuren, F., Schoenmakers, N., & Makkes, P. (1995). One-session cognitive treatment of dental phobia: Preparing dental phobics for treatment by restructuring negative cognitions. *Behaviour Research & Therapy, 33,* 947–954.

Durham, R. C., Murphy, T., Allan, T., Richard, K., Treliving, L. R., & Fenton, G. W. (1994). Cognitive therapy, analytic psychotherapy and anxiety management training for generalised anxiety disorder. *British Journal of Psychiatry, 165,* 315–323.

Foa, E. B., & Meadows, E. A. (1997). Psychosocial treatments for posttraumatic stress disorder: A critical review. *Annual Review of Psychology, 48,* 449–480.

Franklin, M. E., Foa, E. B., & Kozak, M. J. (1999). Time-limited cognitive-behavioral therapy and pharmacotherapy of obsessive-compulsive disorder. *Crisis Intervention and Time-Limited Treatment, 5,* 37–57.

Gatz, M., Fiske, A., Fox, L. S., Kaskie, B., Kasl-Godley, J. E., McCallum, T. J., et al. (1998). Empirically validated psychological treatments for older adults. *Journal of Mental Health and Aging, 4,* 9–46.

Gersons, B. P. R., Carlier, I. V. E., Lamberts, R. D., & van der Kolk, B. A. (2000). Randomized clinical trial of brief eclectic psychotherapy for police officers with posttraumatic stress disorder. *Journal of Traumatic Stress, 13,* 333–347.

Greer, S., Moorey, S., Baruch, J. D. R., Watson, M., Robertson, B. M., Mason, A., et al. (1992). Adjuvant psychological therapy for patients with cancer: A prospective randomised trial. *British Medical Journal, 304,* 675–680.

Gross, D. A., & Rosen, A. (1997). The managed care of anxiety disorders. In S. R. Sauber (Ed.), *Managed mental health care: Major diagnostic and treatment approaches* (pp. 279–296). Bristol, PA: Brunner/Mazel.

Harrison, S., Watson, M., & Feinmann, C. (1997). Does short-term group therapy affect unexplained medical symptoms? *Journal of Psychosomatic Research, 43,* 399–404.

Harvey, A. G., & Rapee, R. M. (1995). Cognitive-behavior therapy for generalized anxiety disorder. *Psychiatric Clinics of North America, 18,* 859–870.

Hellstrom, K., & Öst, L.-G. (1995). One-session therapist directed exposure vs. two forms of manual directed self-exposure in the treatment of spider phobia. *Behavior Research and Therapy, 33,* 959–965.

Hersen, M., & Biaggio, M. (Eds.). (2000). *Effective brief therapies: A clinician's guide.* San Diego: Academic Press.

Juster, H. R., & Heimberg, R. G. (1995). Social phobia: Longitudinal course and long-term outcome of cognitive-behavioral treatment. *Psychiatric Clinics of North America, 18,* 821–842.

Kelly, J. A., Murphy, D. A., Bahr, G. R., Kalichman, S. C., Morgan, M. G., Stevenson, Y., et al. (1993). Outcome of cognitive-behavioral and support group brief therapies for depressed, HIV-infected persons. *American Journal of Psychiatry, 150,* 1679–1686.

Krakow, B., Hollifield, M. D., Johnston, L., Koss, M., Schrader, R., Warner, T. D., et al. (2001). Imagery rehearsal therapy for chronic nightmares in sexual assaults survivors with posttraumatic stress disorder. *Journal of the American Medical Association, 286,* 537–545.

Kush, F. R., & Fleming, L. M. (2000). An innovative approach to short term group cognitive therapy in the combined treatment of anxiety and de-

pression. *Group Dynamics: Theory, Research and Practice, 4,* 176–183.

Lane, J. B. (2000). Overview of assessment and treatment issues. In M. Hersen & M. Biaggio (Eds.), *Effective brief therapies: A clinician's guide* (pp. 3–15). San Diego: Academic Press.

Lee, C., Slade, P., & Lygo, V. (1996). The influence of psychological debriefing on emotional adaptation in women following early miscarriage: A preliminary study. *British Journal of Medical Psychology, 69,* 47–58.

March, J. S., Amaya-Jackson, L. A., Murray, M. C., & Schulte, A. (1998). Cognitive-behavioral psychotherapy for children and adolescents with posttraumatic stress disorder after a single-incident stressor. *Journal of the American Academy of Child and Adolescent Psychiatry, 37,* 585–593.

Marks, I. M. (1990). Psychotherapie comportementale des troubles obsessionnels-compulsifs. *Encephale, 16,* 341–346.

Marmar, C. R. (1991). Brief dynamic psychotherapy of post-traumatic stress disorder. *Psychiatric Annals, 21,* 405–414.

McCullough, L. (2000). Short-term therapy for character change. In J. Carlson & L. Sperry (Eds.), *Brief therapy with individuals and couples* (pp. 127–160). Phoenix, AZ: Zeig, Tucker & Theisen.

Newman, M. G. (2000). Generalized anxiety disorder. In M. Hersen & M. Biaggio (Eds.), *Effective brief therapies: A clinician's guide* (pp. 157–178). San Diego: Academic Press.

Öst, L.-G. (1989). One-session treatment for specific phobias. *Behaviour Research and Therapy, 27,* 1–7.

Otto, M. W., & Whittal, M. L. (1995). Cognitive-behavior therapy and the longitudinal course of panic disorder. *Psychiatric Clinics of North America, 18,* 803–820.

Pollack, M. H., & Smoller, J. W. (1995). The longitudinal course and outcome of panic disorder. *Psychiatric Clinics of North America, 18,* 785–801.

Rose, S., Brewin, C. R., Andrews, B., & Kirk, M. (1999). A randomized controlled trial of individual psychological debriefing for victims of violent crime. *Psychological Medicine, 29,* 793–799.

Schmidt, N. B., & Harrington, P. (1995). Cognitive-behavioral treatment of body dysmorphic disorder: A case report. *Journal of Behavior Therapy and Experimental Psychiatry, 26,* 161–167.

Shear, M. K. (1995). Psychotherapeutic issues in long-term treatment of anxiety disorder patients. *Psychiatric Clinics of North America, 18,* 885–894.

Sifneos, P. E. (1985). Short-term dynamic psychotherapy of phobic and mildly obsessive-compulsive patients. *American Journal of Psychotherapy, 39,* 314–322.

Stanley, M. A., & Averill, P. M. (1999). Strategies for treating generalized anxiety in the elderly. In M.

Duffy (Ed.), *Handbook of counseling and psychotherapy with older adults* (pp. 511–525). New York: Wiley.

Starcevic, V., & Durdic, S. (1993). Post-traumatic stress disorder: Current conceptualization, an overview of research and treatment. *Psihijatrija Danas, 25,* 9–31.

Sutherland, S. M., Tupler, L. A., Colket, J. T., & Davidson, J. R. (1996). A 2-year follow-up of social phobia: Status after a brief medication trial. *Journal of Nervous and Mental Disease, 184,* 731–738.

Walley, E. J., Beebe, D. K., & Clark, J. L. (1994). Management of common anxiety disorders. *American Family Physician, 50,* 1745–1753.

Warneke, L. B. (1985). Intravenous chlorimipramine in the treatment of obsessional disorder in adolescence: Case report. *Journal of Clinical Psychiatry, 46,* 100–103.

Weiss, D. S., & Marmar, C. R. (1993). Teaching time-limited dynamic psychotherapy for post-traumatic stress disorder and pathological grief. *Psychotherapy, 30,* 587–591.

Westling, B. E., & Öst, L.-G. (1999). Brief cognitive behaviour therapy of panic disorder. *Scandinavian Journal of Behaviour Therapy, 28,* 49–57.

Wiborg, I. M., & Dahl, A. A. (1996). Does brief dynamic psychotherapy reduce the relapse rate of panic disorder? *Archives of General Psychiatry, 53,* 689–694.

Wilhelmsen, I., Haug, T. T., Ursin, H., & Berstad, A. (1994). Effect of short-term cognitive psychotherapy on recurrence of duodenal ulcer: A prospective randomized trial. *Psychosomatic Medicine, 56,* 440–448.

Wright, J. H., & Borden, J. (1991). Cognitive therapy of depression and anxiety. *Psychiatric Annals, 21,* 424–428.

COGNITIVE-BEHAVIORAL THERAPY WITH POSTTRAUMATIC STRESS DISORDER

31

An Evidence-Based Approach

M. Elizabeth Vonk, Patrick Bordnick, & Ken Graap

Posttraumatic stress disorder (PTSD) occurs worldwide among people of all ages who experience traumatic events. The events, in which severe injury or threat of injury and death occur, may be natural disasters, such as earthquakes, or man-made, including war, automobile accidents, and crime. While most people are likely to experience some form of traumatic experience in their lifetimes, not all go on to develop PTSD. In fact, estimates of the lifetime prevalence vary widely, from 9% of the general population to 30% or more of those exposed to particular traumas such as rape, combat, or disaster (Keane & Kaloupek, 2002). In addition, several conditions are often comorbid with PTSD, including depressive and other anxiety disorders and substance abuse. Several risk factors for the development of PTSD have been identified, including female gender, history of prior psychiatric problems or abuse, and unavailability of social support (Brewin, Andrews, & Valentine, 2000). Furthermore, characteristics of the trauma itself—the severity of the trauma, the person's sense of control over the outcome and extent of injury, and the degree of actual loss—may increase the rate of PTSD development. In general, men are more likely to be exposed to trauma related to war, and women's exposure is more likely to be related to rape or assault.

Posttraumatic stress disorder involves symptoms that are organized (American Psychiatric Association, 2000) into three clusters. The reexperiencing cluster involves persistent reexperiencing of the traumatic event, including such things as intrusive images, persistent thoughts, or vivid dreams of the event. The arousal cluster includes sleep difficulties, irritability, decreased ability to concentrate, and increased startle response. The avoidance cluster includes efforts to avoid thoughts, feelings, activities, places, or persons that are reminders of the event. In addition, the person with PTSD may experience a sense of detachment or numbing.

Although trauma survivors may not meet all of the *DSM-IV* criteria for PTSD, they may still experience severe distress and trauma-related symptoms. For example, a client may appear to be experiencing PTSD related to an event that does not reach the threshold of the *DSM-IV* definition; that is, the event was not directly life-threatening. While it is not thoroughly understood why some people appear to develop PTSD symptoms related to subthreshold events, they nonetheless require specific treatment.

Fortunately, there is an available and growing evidence base for the treatment of PTSD, including systematic reviews, practice guidelines, and expert consensus guidelines. Despite the time constraints of clinical practice, there are sources available from which, with a modest time investment, social workers may find the most current reviews of treatment effectiveness research related to PTSD. Each of the sources listed in Table 31.1 helps to bridge the gap between research and practice in that they give the practitioner ready access to systematic reviews or summaries of the most recent empirical research. Practice guidelines are also useful in that they often provide more detailed instructions about particular interventions, as well as guidance for common clinical issues. For example, while a systemic review may reveal the effectiveness of exposure therapy for intrusive symptoms of PTSD, practice guidelines may help inform timing of the intervention in relation to engagement with the client, comorbidity, and other unique client characteristics. In other words, research reviews tell us "what" intervention to use with PTSD, and practice guidelines tell us "how to" apply the intervention. The guidelines are often thought to be more "user-friendly" to the practitioner, but both pieces are

TABLE 31.1 Sources of Information for Evidence-Based Practice with PTSD

Source	Web Site Address	Availability
PILOTS Database	www.ncptsd.org/publications/pilots/	Electronic searchable database of traumatic stress literature; abstracts
MedScape (from WebMD)	www.medscape.com	Summary articles of EBP; references
National Center for PTSD	www.ncptsd.org	Summary articles of EBP; references; abstracts; info about assessment tools
Expert Consensus Guidelines	www.psychguides.com	Full-text expert consensus guidelines for PTSD (and other mental disorders)
Journal of Clinical Psychiatry	www.psychiatrist.com/supplenet/	Abstracts and some full-text systematic reviews of EBP for various disorders
Journal of Clinical Psychology	http://www3.interscience.wiley.com/cgi-bin/jtoc?ID=31171	Abstracts of and references for systematic reviews of EBP

TABLE 31.2 Current Systematic Reviews and Practice Guidelines for EBP with PTSD

Year	Author	Title	Source	Type
2002	Yehuda, R. (Ed.)	*Treating Trauma Survivors with PTSD*	Book	Guidelines
2000	Foa, E. B., et al. (Eds.)	*Effective Treatments for PTSD: Practice Guidelines*	Book	Guidelines
2002	Vonk, M. E.	Assessment and treatment of PTSD in *Social Workers' Desk Reference*	Book chapter	Guidelines
2000	Foa, E. B.	Psychosocial treatment of PTSD	*Journal of Clinical Psychiatry*	Review
2002	Schnurr, P. P., et al.	Research on PTSD: Epidemiology, pathophysiology, and assessment	*Journal of Clinical Psychology*	Review
2002	Solomon & Johnson	Psychosocial treatment of PTSD: A practice-friendly review of outcome research	*Journal of Clinical Psychology*	Review
2002	Korn, M. L.	Recent developments in the science and treatment of PTSD	MedScape	Review
1999	E. B. Foa, et al.	Treatment of PTSD	*Journal of Clinical Psychology*	Expert consensus
2003	NCPTSD	Treatment of PTSD: A National Center for PTSD fact sheet	http://www.ncptsd.org	Overview of treatment

needed because our knowledge base is expanding so rapidly. The most up-to-date and readily available systematic reviews and practice guidelines for the assessment and treatment of PTSD at this time are listed in Table 31.2.

In order to apply evidence-based practice (EBP) in the treatment setting, Corcoran and Vandiver (Chapter 2 in this book) suggest seven steps: (a) biopsychosocial assessment, (b) accurate five-axis *DSM* diagnosis, (c) valid description of the identifying problem(s) and focus of treatment, (d) description of goals and specific target(s) of change, (e) selection of a specific evidence-based treatment plan, (f) selection of outcome measures, and (g) evaluation of progress and outcome. Here a case involving rape trauma illustrates application of these steps for EBP with PTSD.

CASE EXAMPLE: JEN

Jen is a 23-year-old European American female who is an account manager with a highly regarded financial corporation. She experienced a rape at gunpoint 4 months previously and has been referred to treatment by the employee assistance program, where she had gone at the urging of her fiancé. Since the rape, Jen has coped by "not thinking about it." Although she has had to change some of her daily routines, she makes efforts to stay away from the part of town where the attack took place. Jen has become unable to concentrate at meetings or to feel connected to her friends in social settings. She frequently wonders whether she should have done more to prevent the rape from occurring. Even more disturbing to her, Jen has frequent nightmares that interfere with her sleep. On a few occasions, she has suddenly "remembered" frightening aspects of the attack while working at her desk. In addition, while she expected to experience difficulties for a week or so following the attack, she feels disappointed and angry with herself about being unable to "just get over it" now that 4 months have passed. She worries that her fiancé will be unable to tolerate her continued avoidance of physical intimacy. More than anything, she wants to return to her former high level of functioning at work, with her fiancé, and with friends. Jen reported no pre-vious trauma, has had no medical complications, and is maintaining medical follow-up.

Assessment and Diagnosis

Hoping to help Jen as effectively and efficiently as possible, the social worker wanted to choose interventions that were supported by the evi-dence base. Following the recommendation of Corcoran and Vandiver (Chapter 2 in this book), she began with a thorough biopsychosocial as-sessment. Through a clinical interview, the social worker allowed Jen to tell her story about the rape and its aftermath. Following suggestions by McFarlane, Golier, and Yehuda (2002) regarding initial evaluation, she was careful not to press Jen for details, but rather to lay the groundwork for future in-depth exploration of the assault, as well as to begin to tie the current difficulties to the trauma-related stress. She also explored Jen's pretrauma functioning, family history, current living situation, current methods of cop-ing, support system, previous traumatic life events, and expectations of therapy (Vonk, 2002). The social worker also paid close attention to Jen's thoughts about the rape, noting any in-dications of self-blame or guilt about the assault or about how she is handling the aftermath. In addition, the social worker listened for signs and symptoms of psychiatric problems that often co-occur with PTSD, including depression, anxiety, substance abuse, and somatic complaints.

To augment her assessment and prepare for future outcome measurement, the social worker decided to use a self-report measure. After re-viewing the self-report inventories described both by Keane and Kaloupek (2002) and on the Web site of the National Center for PTSD (http://www.ncptsd.org/publications/assessment/adult_self_report.html), she chose the Posttrau-matic Diagnostic Scale (PTDS) (Foa et al., 1997). The PTDS is a 17-item Likert-scale instrument that measures the presence and severity of each of the 17 symptoms in the three clusters of *DSM-IV* criteria for PTSD. This provides valu-able information to the social worker about Jen's particular constellation of symptoms and their severity. The PTDS also allows the client to rate her level of impairment in nine areas of life functioning (i.e., work, household duties, friend-ships, leisure, school, family relationships, sex life, general life satisfaction, and overall func-tioning). In addition, it provides a checklist of traumatic events and asks the client to endorse any to which she has been exposed and the one that is causing the greatest concern. The instru-ment is psychometrically sound; has been tested with men and women who have experienced a broad range of traumas, including sexual assault; and requires only a few minutes to complete. This self-report instrument was chosen over a psychometrically sound structured clinical inter-view such as the Clinician Administered PTSD Scale (CAPS) (Blake et al., 1995) in the interest of time.

Based on the clinical interview and the results of the PTDS, the social worker diagnosed Jen as follows:

Axis I: 309.81 Posttraumatic Stress Disorder (Chronic)
Axis II: V71.09 No Diagnosis
Axis III: None
Axis IV: Problems related to crime
Axis V: GAF = 55 (current)

Identification of Treatment Focus and Goals

The focus and goals of treatment follow directly from the results of the assessment and diagnosis. Jen presented with symptoms of reexperiencing, increased arousal, numbing, and avoidance. In addition, she reported feelings of guilt and self-blame for the rape. Among all of her symptoms, Jen reported that nightmares and intrusive thoughts of the rape were most disturbing to her. Before beginning to treat the PTSD directly, the social worker provided Jen with education about the symptoms and available treatments for PTSD. In the process, she helped Jen nor-malize her reactions and provided reassurance about the potential for recovery. She also en-couraged Jen to share psychoeducational mate-rials with her fiancé. (See Foa et al., 1999, pp. 69–77, for a printable handout for patient or family.) By working together, the following mu-tually defined, positive, feasible, and well-defined goals were established:

1. Increase Jen's ability to actively manage her anxiety at work and in social settings at least 75% of the time.
   a. Jen will increase her ability to concen-trate at work.
   b. Jen will increase her enjoyment in social settings.

2. Increase Jen's ability to tolerate exposure to places, thoughts, feelings, and conversations that are reminders of the assault.
   a. Jen will be able to shop for groceries and run errands near the location of the assault.
   b. Jen will be able to share her experience, its aftermath, and her ongoing progress toward recovery with her fiancé and best friend.
   c. Jen will be able to gradually increase her enjoyment of physical intimacy with her fiancé.
3. Decrease the frequency of Jen's nightmares and intrusive thoughts of the assault.
   a. Modify Jen's beliefs about the assault that are associated with disturbing emotions.
   b. Jen will modify her belief that she is somehow to blame for the assault.
   c. Jen will identify and modify other disturbing thoughts about herself, others, and the world in relation to the assault.

Jen and the social worker agreed to work toward these goals with weekly meetings for a period of 3 months, at which time they would reassess to see what additional work might be needed. In addition, Jen agreed to follow through with a referral for a medication evaluation with a psychiatrist.

Overview of Evidence Base and Selection of Intervention

While already aware of several effective interventions, the social worker wanted to make sure she had the most up-to-date information available on which to base her treatment decisions. Following Corcoran and Vandiver's (Chapter 2 in this book) suggestions for implementing evidence-based knowledge in practice, the social worker looked to credible sources of knowledge, including systematic reviews (e.g., Solomon & Johnson, 2002), practice guidelines (e.g., Yehuda, 2002), and expert consensus (e.g., Foa et al., 1999). In addition, she quickly went to the National Center for PTSD Web site (http://www.ncptsd.org) to examine the treatment fact sheet to see if there have been recent notable developments. From these sources, the social worker learned the following about intervention with PTSD.

Empirical research has supported the effec-

tiveness of several interventions for the treatment of rape-related PTSD. The literature most clearly supports exposure therapy, cognitive therapy, and anxiety management techniques. Eye movement desensitization and reprocessing (EMDR) and insight-oriented treatments are supported, although less conclusively than the cognitive-behavioral interventions because of the methodological rigor with which they have been studied (Rothbaum, Meadows, Resick, & Foy, 2000; Solomon & Johnson, 2002). In addition, there is growing support for the use of psychopharmacological treatment, especially with sexual assault survivors (Mellman, 2002). Expert consensus suggests that particular psychosocial interventions appear to be more effective in treating specific clusters of symptoms (Foa et al., 1999). For instance, intrusive symptoms respond particularly well to exposure techniques; avoidance symptoms respond well to exposure and cognitive therapy; numbing, guilt, and shame to cognitive therapy; and increased arousal symptoms to exposure and anxiety management.

Exposure Therapy

Exposure therapy is a behavioral intervention involving affective and cognitive activation of the trauma by using associated memories and cues. The cues may be either imaginal, such as retelling the experience of the assault, or in vivo, such as returning to a place that is a reminder of the assault. The exposure must be of significant duration to allow the client's anxiety level to substantially subside in the presence of the feared but harmless cue. Exposure therapies are effective in at least four ways (Foa & Cahill, 2002). First, they help to decrease anxiety related to the trauma. Next, they help survivors learn that thinking about the traumatic experience is not in itself dangerous. They also help survivors differentiate between the traumatic experience and other situations that may be safe, although similar in some ways. Finally, confronting through exposure rather than avoiding memories and cues of the assault helps survivors develop a sense of mastery. Because the idea of confronting or reliving the assault is frightening, survivors need to have a clear rationale and understanding of how exposure therapies work in order to be informed participants in the intervention. In addition, the development and maintenance of a trusting therapeutic relationship seems to be essential for successful completion of exposure therapies. A description of exposure therapy designed for use with sexual assault survivors can be found in Foa and Rothbaum (1998).

Cognitive Therapy

Cognitive therapy (CT) (Beck, 1995) has long been recognized as an effective treatment for anxiety and depression. The basic idea of CT is that the way one thinks about the world, others, and self influences one's interpretation of events. In turn, the interpretation influences subsequent feelings and actions. Dysfunctional beliefs following sexual assault vary, but several themes are common, including overgeneralizations about danger in the world and one's personal vulnerability, unrealistic self-blame and guilt about the rape or inability to prevent its occurrence, loss of meaning for one's life, and broken trust in others and self (Solomon & Johnson, 2002; Vonk, 2002). The goal of CT is to learn to identify specific thoughts that are causing negative emotional reactions and behaviors and then to challenge the thoughts through a process of logical examination of the veracity or functionality of the thoughts, followed by replacement of those that are dysfunctional with more reasonable ones. Cognitive restructuring in the treatment of PTSD is described by Meichenbaum (1994).

Anxiety Management

The most widely studied of anxiety management programs, stress inoculation training (SIT) was originally developed by Meichenbaum (1994) to treat a variety of anxiety disorders, including PTSD. SIT aims to help clients manage and reduce anxiety through the development of coping skills such as relaxation and breathing techniques, cognitive restructuring, guided self-dialogue, thought-stopping, and role playing. The treatment takes place in three phases. First, the client is educated about responses to trauma and PTSD. Next, the coping skills are taught to and rehearsed by the client. Finally, the newly developed skills are applied through graduated exposure to stressful cues and memories associated with the rape. Although not as well studied as exposure therapies, SIT has been studied both with groups of clients and with individuals. Foa's (2000) summary of those studies suggests that SIT is more effective when administered to in-dividuals rather than in group treatment settings.

Eye Movement Desensitization and Reprocessing

Eye movement desensitization and reprocessing (EMDR) is a relatively new treatment that combines aspects of cognitive reappraisal and exposure techniques with guided eye movement in a specified protocol (Shapiro, 1995). Many experts remain skeptical of EMDR because of the mixed results of its effectiveness and because of questions concerning its theoretical foundation. Summaries of the results of recent effectiveness studies (Chemtob, Tolin, van der Kolk, & Pitman, 2000; Solomon & Johnson, 2002) still provide mixed results. Some studies suggest that the effectiveness of EMDR is comparable to cognitive-behavioral interventions. However, when EMDR was compared with a well-established cognitive-behavioral technique (Devilly & Spence, 1999), EMDR was not as effective in reducing PTSD symptoms either immediately following treatment or at a 3-month follow-up. In addition, the results of dismantling research spread doubt on the necessity of eye movements, without which EMDR appears to be a variation of a cognitive-behavioral intervention.

Short-Term Psychodynamic Therapy

As described by Solomon and Johnson (2002), psychodynamic treatment for PTSD was developed by Horowitz, who conceptualized trauma response in two phases: denial, in which the avoidance and numbing symptoms are prominent, and intrusive, in which the intrusive and arousal symptoms are prominent. The brief psychoanalytic treatment is geared to fit the client's phase of response. In the intrusive phase, the client is encouraged to avoid upsetting memories and to manage anxiety through the use of therapeutic relationship and other coping skills, sometimes including medication. The client in the denial phase is encouraged to confront memories until affect has subsided, at which time the client can focus on the meaning of the trauma and symptoms in order to integrate the experience into a revised sense of self, life meaning, and world image. The limited amount of research available on psychodynamic treatment of PTSD suggests that it may be more effective at reducing avoidance than intrusive symptoms; more research is needed.

Medication

While social workers and others who provide psychosocial intervention are generally not qualified to prescribe psychotropic medication, it is important to be informed of available treatments and issues related to integration of medication treatment with psychosocial intervention. Noting several limitations in the available evidence-based knowledge about medication effectiveness for PTSD, Mellman (2002) describes clear empirical support for the use of selective serotonin reuptake inhibitors (SSRIs) in the treatment of women with assault-related PTSD. He goes on to describe issues related to integrating medical and psychosocial interventions. First, he notes the importance of discussing a clear rationale for medication with the client. In some cases, it may be appropriate to augment treatment with medication following a partial response to the initial psychosocial intervention. In other cases, however, it may be appropriate to complement psychosocial intervention with medication from the outset, particularly if there are comorbid psychiatric disorders or severe symptomatology that would interfere with the progress of psychosocial treatment. Regardless of the chosen method, the client, primary therapist, and prescribing physician must maintain a close collaboration in the service of the client's recovery from PTSD.

After sharing information with Jen about the various effective interventions, the social worker and Jen decided to proceed with a combination of exposure and cognitive therapy. Both Jen and the consulting psychiatrist decided on an augmentation approach to medication, asking that the social worker monitor Jen's progress to assess the need for medication in the future.

Implementation of Treatment

Having decided on treatment goals and preferred interventions, Jen indicated that she would like to start with prolonged exposure (Foa & Rothbaum, 1998) because of its success at decreasing symptoms in all three clusters. She very much wanted to stop having nightmares, and from the information about the various interventions, Jen thought exposure would provide relief most efficiently. Knowing that the success of exposure relies on a good therapeutic relationship, the so-cial worker spent time preparing Jen for the intervention. She carefully explained the intervention, including the potential for a temporary increase in Jen's level of distress and the potential need for sessions longer than 1 hour. Jen was encouraged to ask her fiancé and best friend for support between sessions.

Only when the social worker was confident that Jen understood the intervention thoroughly did she proceed with exposure. The first two sessions in which exposure was used were 90 minutes long; the extra time was required for Jen's anxiety to subside. In each of the following five sessions, exposure required less and less time as Jen was increasingly more able to recount the event with a more manageable level of anxiety. Between sessions, Jen was asked to listen to a tape recording of her recounting of the assault, as well as to confront concrete reminders of the assault by going back to the neighborhood where the assault took place. The social worker gave Jen lots of encouragement to do her "homework," and although she was not able to follow through the first week, Jen started listening to the tape and, accompanied by her fiancé, driving into her old neighborhood after the second session of exposure.

During the course of exposure intervention, the social worker listened carefully to Jen's narrative in order to identify beliefs about the rape, the world, others, and herself that were causing Jen pain, particularly those that indicated guilt or self-blame. Two cognitive themes emerged. First, Jen had come to believe that she was to blame for the rape, in part because she did not "fight back." Second, she had come to the conclusion that she could not trust herself to distinguish between safe and dangerous men because she had accepted the perpetrator's offer to help her with some heavy packages, providing him the opportunity to isolate and then assault her. After teaching Jen the basics of cognitive therapy (Beck, 1995), the social worker and Jen began to work toward modifying her self-blaming and other dysfunctional beliefs related to the assault.

At the end of 3 months, Jen was pleased with her progress with the presenting problems of intrusive and avoidance symptoms, but she was still experiencing more difficulty with concentration than she would like. The social worker reviewed options with Jen, including continuing with cognitive therapy, adding some education in anxiety management, or augmenting treat-

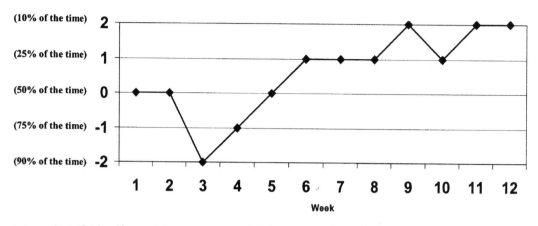

FIGURE 31.1 GAS self-report for occurrence of nightmares each week

ment with medication. Jen preferred to learn some anxiety management techniques (Meichenbaum, 1994) and to continue with cognitive work. The social worker taught Jen how to use thought-stopping, deep breathing, and guided self-dialogue techniques.

As Jen continued to make progress with her goals, the social worker increased the time between sessions. During the last session, Jen reported that she felt ready to stop treatment. She went on to describe her current thinking about being a rape survivor. Like many survivors of trauma, she was able to acknowledge personal growth along with the difficulties related to her assault (Calhoun & Tedeschi, 1999). Although she still experienced sadness, moments of anxiety, and anger that she had been victimized, Jen believed that she was a "very strong person" to have managed the aftermath of her traumatic experience. She and her fiancé had reevaluated the importance of their relationship to one another and were actively planning their wedding rather than remaining engaged without a specific date in mind. She was also reevaluating her choice of careers and was looking into taking the steps necessary to become a physical therapist, a strong interest she had set aside a few years earlier at the urging of her parents.

Ongoing Evaluation of Treatment

Throughout treatment, the social worker monitored Jen's progress, relying both on Jen's report and on clinical judgment. In addition, however, she utilized two quantitative methods. First, she utilized goal attainment scaling (GAS) (Pike,

2002). GAS is a useful tool for monitoring progress because the scales can be tailored to the individual's goals, are easy to administer, can be administered repeatedly, and can be weighted according to the relative importance of each of the goals. A 5-point goal attainment scale was developed for each of Jen's goals as they were defined in treatment, and at the start of each session, the social worker asked Jen to rate her progress on each of them. The use of the GAS method is illustrated in Figure 31.1, showing Jen's progress on the goal of decreasing the frequency of her nightmares. Finally, the PTDS (Foa et al., 1997), administered at the outset of treatment, was readministered at the close of treatment. Jen no longer qualified for the diagnosis of PTSD by the end of treatment, although she had not reached a satisfactory level of enjoyment with physical intimacy, nor could she concentrate at work at least 75% of the time. She planned to continue working toward those goals by applying the skills learned in treatment.

CONCLUSION

The evidence base for practice with clients suffering from PTSD related to rape and other traumas is still growing. To date, the cognitive-behavioral interventions, including exposure, cognitive restructuring, and anxiety management, appear to be the most effective (Solomon & Johnson, 2002). Research on psychotropic medications has also yielded support for several drugs, including the class of drugs known as SSRIs. Yet, there are many unanswered questions regarding treatment of PTSD. Among them is the question of effective matching of a particular treatment to a particular problem or client characteristic. Another is the question of whether or when it is effective to combine psychosocial interventions. While it seems logical that two effective interventions such as exposure and cognitive therapy would complement each other to enhance treatment, some of the existing research appears to contradict this logic (Foa, 2000). In addition, more knowledge is needed about the effectiveness of psychosocial interventions in combination with psychotropic medicine (Mellman, 2002).

While the treatment of real people who suffer from PTSD is rarely as clear-cut as the case of "Jen," effective treatment is more likely when the steps of evidence-based practice are followed, from thorough biopsychosocial assessment to evaluation of outcomes. Any who fear that these steps will create a mechanized therapeutic process can rest assured that individual differences among clients will always require the use of clinical judgment; relationship-building skills to ensure engagement and continuation in treatment; and the ability to convey trustworthiness, warmth, and caring. Evidence-based practice may indeed increase the practitioner's ability to instill hope in clients with the confidence that comes from knowing that the service being offered is well supported in theory and in practice.

References

American Psychiatric Association. (2000). *Diagnostic and statistical manual of mental disorders* (4th ed., text rev.). Washington, DC: Author.

Beck, J. S. (1995). *Cognitive therapy: Basics and beyond.* New York: Guilford.

Blake, D. D., Weathers, F. W., Magy, L. M., Kaloupek, D. G., Gusman, F. D., Charney, D. S., et al. (1995). The development of a clinician-administered PTSD scale. *Journal of Traumatic Stress, 8,* 75–90.

Brewin, C. R., Andrews, B., & Valentine, J. D. (2000). Meta-analysis of risk factors for PTSD in trauma-exposed adults. *Journal of Consulting and Clinical Psychology, 68,* 748–766.

Calhoun, L. G., & Tedeschi, R. G. (1999). *Facilitating posttraumatic growth.* Mahwah, NJ: Lawrence Erlbaum.

Chemtob, C. M., Tolin, D. F., van der Kolk, B. A., & Pitman, R. K. (2000). Eye-movement desensitization and reprocessing. In E. B. Foa, T. Keane, & M. Friedman (Eds.), *Effective treatments for PTSD* (pp. 139–154). New York: Guilford.

Devilly, G. J., & Spence, S. H. (1999). The relative efficacy and treatment distress of EMDR and a cognitive behavioral trauma treatment protocol in the amelioration of PTSD. *Journal of Anxiety Disorders, 13,* 131–158.

Foa, E. B. (2000). Psychosocial treatment of PTSD. *Journal of Clinical Psychiatry, 61*(Suppl. 5), 43–48.

Foa, E. B., & Cahill, S. P. (2002). Specialized treatment for PTSD: Matching survivors to the appropriate modality. In R. Yehuda (Ed.), *Treating trauma survivors with PTSD* (pp. 43–62). Washington, DC: American Psychiatric Publishing.

Foa, E. B., Cashman, L., Jaycox, L., et al. (1997). The validation of a self-report measure of PTSD: The Posttraumatic Diagnostic Scale. *Psychological Assessment, 9,* 445–451.

Foa, E. B., Davidson, J. R. T., & Frances, A. (1999). The expert consensus guideline series: Treatment of PTSD. *Journal of Clinical Psychiatry, 60*(Suppl. 16), 4–32.

Foa, E. B., Keane, T., & Friedman, M. (Eds.). (2000). *Effective treatments for PTSD: Practice guidelines.* New York: Guilford.

Foa, E. B., & Rothbaum, B. O. (1998). *Treating the trauma of rape.* New York: Guilford.

Keane, T. M., & Kaloupek, D. G. (2002). In R. Yehuda (Ed.), *Treating trauma survivors with PTSD* (pp. 21–42). Washington, DC: American Psychiatric Publishing.

Korn, M. L. (n.d.). Recent developments in the science and treatment of PTSD. Retrieved April 14, 2003, from http://www.medscape.com/viewarticle/436398

McFarlane, A. C., Golier, J., & Yehuda, R. (2002). Treatment planning for trauma survivors with PTSD. In R. Yehuda (Ed.), *Treating trauma survivors with PTSD* (pp. 1–20). Washington, DC: American Psychiatric Publishing.

Meichenbaum, D. (1994). *A clinical handbook/practical therapist manual for assessing and treating adults with PTSD.* Waterloo, Ontario: Institute Press.

Mellman, T. A. (2002). Rationale and role for medication in the comprehensive treatment of PTSD. In R. Yehuda (Ed.), *Treating trauma survivors with PTSD* (pp. 63–74). Washington, DC: American Psychiatric Publishing.

Pike, C. K. (2002) Developing client-focused measures. In A. Roberts & G. Greene (Eds.), *The social worker's desk reference* (pp. 189–193). New York: Oxford University Press.

Rothbaum, B. O., Meadows, E. A., Resick, P., & Foy, D. W. (2000). In E. B. Foa, T. Keane, & M. Friedman (Eds.), *Effective treatments for PTSD* (pp. 60–83). New York: Guilford.

Schnurr, P. P., Friedman, M. J., & Bernardy, N. C. (2002). Research on PTSD: Epidemiology, pathophysiology, and assessment. *Journal of Clinical Psychology, 58*(8), 877–889.

Shapiro, F. (1995). *Eye movement desensitization and reprocessing.* New York: Guilford.

Solomon, S. D., & Johnson, D. M. (2002). Psychosocial treatment of PTSD: A practice-friendly review of outcome research. *Journal of Clinical Psychology, 58*(8), 947–959.

Vonk, M. E. (2002). The assessment and treatment of PTSD. In A. Roberts & G. Greene (Eds.), *The social worker's desk reference* (pp. 356–359). New York: Oxford University Press.

Yehuda, R. (Ed.). (2002). *Treating trauma survivors with PTSD.* Washington, DC: American Psychiatric Publishing.

32 EVIDENCE-BASED LIFE SKILLS INTERVENTIONS FOR PREGNANT ADOLESCENTS IN SCHOOL SETTINGS

Mary Beth Harris & Cynthia Franklin

Practitioners working with adolescents in schools are confronted with many problems that these youths face. Common difficulties encountered by practitioners include violence, behavioral problems, substance abuse, HIV infection, pregnancy, and homelessness. Practice guidelines and interventions that facilitate change or that can counter or reverse these life trends are needed. This chapter examines current practice trends and guidelines for cognitive-behavioral life skills interventions—a type of cognitive-behavioral group intervention—that are being delivered to adolescents in a school setting. This chapter also offers guidance to practitioners for developing and using evidence-based, cognitive-behavioral life skills interventions in schools. Considerations for program interventions in school settings are discussed, including points that apply to psychiatric and behavioral settings, court systems, and other youth-serving institutions. Finally, the chapter presents an example of a life skills intervention that was developed in

a school setting. The intervention discussed is the school-based group for adolescent mothers known as the Taking Charge curriculum. Discussion of the intervention in this chapter includes the theoretical frame, curriculum content, and evaluation. This curriculum serves as one example of an evidence-based, cognitive-behavioral intervention that is being developed for at-risk student populations in schools.

AT-RISK ADOLESCENT POPULATIONS IN SCHOOLS

Today's adolescents are under extreme stressors from the erosion of family and community supports. The Children's Defense Fund reports (2000), for example, reports that in 1998 one of every five children lived in poverty and that almost half of these lived in single-parent homes with mothers who were three times more likely to be poor than other adults raising children.

The current poverty rate for children and adolescents in some states is as high as 27% (Annie E. Casey Foundation, 2002). Poverty is an ever-present burden for innumerable youth and has been repeatedly established as a mediating factor for multiple negative outcomes for adolescents (Bolger, Patterson, Thompson, & Kupersmidt, 1995; Franklin, Corcoran, & Harris, in press). For example, Rosenthal (1995) reported low socioeconomic status as one of the most critical variables associated with school dropout, and Males (1994) reported a correlation of .81 between poverty and adolescent parenting.

Vulnerability and Psychosocial Stress

An overriding factor that places many adolescents in the at-risk student population is the adolescent's vulnerable stage of development, coupled with complex psychosocial stressors. Between the ages of 13 and 20, adolescents have the task of moving out of childhood and establishing a functional identity and role in the adult community. In a relatively accommodating or enriched environment, most adolescents can successfully accomplish this process, supported early by family and later by individuals and systems in the larger community. However, with increasing frequency, the passage between childhood and adulthood is a treacherous crossing that ends with vastly diminished life potential. Important social phenomena in recent decades have distorted this developmental transition for numerous groups of the country's youths. Withdrawal of economic and social resources from communities has brought adverse consequences for youths and their families (Carlson, Clark, & Marx, 1992). Violent crime has increased in both urban and rural communities to the point that violence is associated with a growing sense of hopelessness and antisocial behavior in youths (Eamon, 2001; Fick & Thomas, 1995; Garbarino, DuBrow, Kostelny, & Pardo, 1992). Disengagement from the neighborhood out of fear has become the norm for many urban dwellers (Bowen & Van Dorn, 2002).

Problems in Behavioral and Academic Functioning

The result of these and other societal patterns is that adolescents are at greater risk for problems in their behavioral and social functioning and ac-ademic achievement. Every year one in five youths experiences symptoms of a *DSM-IV* disorder (Mental Health, 2002). Suicide is the third leading cause of death for adolescents, and AIDS is the sixth leading cause of death among people ages 15 to 24 (Natasi, 1998). Fifty-four percent of high school seniors report using illicit drugs as well as alcohol (Johnston, Bachman, & O'Malley, 1996). Thirty-seven percent of high school students report being involved in school violence (Kann et al., 1997), and U.S. cities report an estimated 31,000 adolescent gangs (Moore & Terrett, 1998), with gang presence in schools increasing from 15% in 1989 to 28% in 1995 (Thornberry & Burch, 1997).

The overall adolescent birth rate has fallen since the 1950s. There was a sharp increase in the birth rate in the 1980s, followed by a continuous decrease in the 1990s. Statistical data from the Center for Health Statistics indicate that birth rates for adolescents were at a historic low in 2001 (Centers for Disease Control, 2003). There were 45.3 births per 1,000 women ages 15 to 19, down 5% since 2000 and 24% lower than in 1990. For girls ages 10 to 14, the rate per 1,000 was 0.8, and that figure was 8% lower than in 2000 and 34% lower than in 1990. The pregnancy rates for 18- and 19-year-olds were 76.1 per 1,000, and this figure was down 3% from 2000 and 14% from 1990. The U.S. teen birth rate, however, remains the highest among developed countries. Births to adolescents also vary a great amount based on race and ethnicity. Non-Hispanic Whites had a birth rate of 30.3 per 1,000 in 2001, non-Hispanic Blacks had a birth rate of 73.5 per 1,000, American Indians were at 56.3, Asian Pacific Islanders were at 19.8, and Hispanics were at 86.4. Hispanics as a group clearly have the highest birth rates.

Despite the fact that the overall birth rates of adolescent women have decreased for 50 years, the proportion of adolescents with children who are unmarried has continued to rise, from 14% in 1940 to 67% in 1990 and 79% in 2000 (Centers for Disease Control, 2001). These data are keeping alive an ongoing public debate about the unacceptability and the social problem of adolescent childbearing. Recent data from Child Trends (2000) indicate that 22% of births to unmarried adolescents are repeat (second or subsequent) childbirths.

Pregnancy is not a disease to be prevented but a normal condition for females of childbearing ages who are sexually active and do not use contraceptives (Franklin, Corcoran, & Harris, in press). Adolescent pregnancy would not be a problem except that a woman's pregnancy occurs in a certain social and developmental context that produces harmful or unwanted outcomes for herself and others. The social and developmental context of adolescent pregnancy, for example, is usually believed to be accompanied by negative and adverse health, social, and economic consequences for the young woman and her child. Many of these consequences, however, are intricately intertwined with the social and economic circumstances of adolescent women who are poor. Poverty causes some researchers to question the social and economic validity of the core issues that are discussed as problems produced by adolescent pregnancy. It is believed, for example, that the health, social, and economic problems associated with adolescent pregnancy would exist for these young women even if they were not pregnant, because they are poor and lack education, resources, and skills. Poverty serves as a key factor in the social and behavioral difficulties of today's youths (Burns, 2002).

Immigrants, Refugees, and Other Stigmatized Groups

A growing number of adolescents are immigrants and refugees, homeless youth, or those with HIV, and these youths often suffer stigma or isolation that can render clients difficult to reach. The needs of at-risk populations, such as adolescent parents (Kelly, 1996) or gay and lesbian youth (Elia, 1993), are often politically stigmatized and fall outside prevalent funding guidelines. Changing proportions of race and culture pose challenges of language and acculturation for increasing numbers of immigrant and refugee youth (Rosenberg, 1991) for schools and other institutions that serve these populations. Twenty-nine percent of Hispanic youth drop out of school, as do a staggering 44% of those born outside the United States (National Center for Education Statistics, 1999).

Many of these at-risk adolescent populations are accessed only through institutions such as public schools, the criminal justice system, or health care organizations. Of these organizations, public schools appear to offer one of the best points for intervention because the majority of at-risk youths have contact with these institutions. Providing the best services for these at-risk adolescent populations in schools is important. The challenges of helping at-risk youths indicate a need for school-based practitioners to use well-designed and empirically robust interventions and methodology if they are to have a chance at making an impact on these youths' outcomes. The following section discusses some current practices in the area of cognitive-behavioral life skills interventions. These practice methods with adolescents are supported with numerous outcome studies concerning their effectiveness in schools with special adolescent populations.

COGNITIVE-BEHAVIORAL SKILLS TRAINING APPROACHES

Cognitive-behavioral therapies that use skills-building interventions and cognitive restructuring and that focus on mastery and self-management are reported with high efficacy across the social and educational literatures (e.g., Jemmont, Jemmont, Fong, & McCaffree, 1999; Kendall, 2002; McWhirter & Page, 1999; Vallerand, Fortier, & Guay, 1997). Earlier studies of special adolescent populations, such as youth with depression (Clarke, 1992), those at risk for delinquency (Hawkins, Jenson, Catalano, & Wells, 1991), and youth in residential treatment (Foxx et al., 1989), concluded that interventions with social skills–building components would be effective for these populations. This suggests that the current skills-based practice trend was initiated with evidence identified in prior studies with adolescents.

Current interventions are based on cognitive-behavioral theories and utilize solution-focused, problem-solving, skills training and acquisition, and task-centered treatment models (e.g., Corcoran, 2002; de Anda, 1998; Forman, Linney, & Brondino, 1990; Harris & Franklin, 2002). The approach seeks to help adolescents compensate for a range of life challenges through the strengthening of cognitive and behavioral skills such as coping with stress, goal setting, and rational problem solving (Dupper, 1998; Forman et al., 1990; Rice & Meyer, 1994). Enhancing locus of control, a cognitive concept referring to one's sense of competence in affecting personal outcomes, is theoretically bound to coping and problem-solving skills and is often an outcome variable in studies of skills-building interventions (e.g., McWhirter & Page, 1999; Rice &

Meyer, 1994). Most such interventions include strategies for mastery of behaviors specifically associated with life outcome predictors, such as education, employment, social relationships, and health (e.g., Griffin, 1998; Harris & Franklin, in press; Jemmont et al., 1999).

COGNITIVE-BEHAVIORAL INTERVENTIONS IN SCHOOLS

Life skills–building interventions with a cognitive-behavioral frame are gaining more and more evidence as effective for a growing number of adolescent issues (Harris & Franklin, in press). In a meta-analysis of programs and practices for adolescent pregnancy prevention, for example, Franklin, Grant, Corcoran, O'Dell, and Bultman (1997) identified skills building associated with mastery experiences and the processing of logical consequences as an important component for pregnancy prevention programs. Although this analysis indicated that community-based programs were perhaps more effective than school-based programs for preventing adolescent pregnancy, the authors noted that schools were often prevented for political reasons from delivering effective interventions such as the mastery of contraceptive knowledge building and learning how to effectively use contraceptives. Several evidence-based curricula offered in schools for preventing adolescent pregnancy, however, use a skills-building orientation, emphasizing the need to move beyond changes in knowledge and attitudes to application of the knowledge learned. Pregnancy curricula have clearly written manuals and materials and have been found to be effective in one or more experimental and quasi-experimental studies on pregnancy prevention. See Corcoran and Franklin (2001) and Franklin and Corcoran (1999) for a summary of these curricula and for more information on obtaining these materials.

Cognitive-behavioral interventions are found to be effective for other adolescent issues as well, such as depression (Barth, 1985; Clarke, 1992; Clarke et al., 1995), problem school behavior (Bennett & Gibbons, 2000; Dupper, 1998), and anger management (St. Lawrence, Crosby, Belcher, Yazdani, & Brasfield, 1999). In a National Institute of Mental Health study, Webster-Stratton (1996) conducted a series of clinical trials in a school setting that showed the progressive effectiveness of a cognitive-behavioral intervention program for children with behavioral problems. A meta-analysis completed by Tobler (1986) of 143 studies demonstrated that skills building is the most helpful intervention for preventing adolescent substance abuse. Hoagwood and Erwin (1997) reviewed the evidence-based literature on the effectiveness of mental health services in the schools from 1985 to 1995. Of the 16 studies identified that had acceptable research designs, two basic types of interventions were represented, cognitive-behavioral approaches, including social skills training, and teacher consultation. Cognitive-behavioral and skills-building interventions clearly showed the most promise when applied to mental health interventions conducted in school settings.

Finally, Rones and Hoagwood (2000) conducted a synthetic review of the evidence-based school mental health literature between 1985 and 1999 and identified several cognitive-behavioral programs offered within multicomponent treatment packages that were effective in treating mental health problems in a school context. It is important to point out, however, that the authors also found an amazing lack of efficacy and effectiveness studies on school-based mental health services. Of 337 program evaluations, for example, they found only 47 studies that met even minimum requirements for intervention research, 36 randomized experiments, 9 quasi-experimental designs, and 2 multiple-baseline designs. This leads one to conclude that even though there is considerable evidence for the efficacy of the cognitive-behavioral skills-building interventions across child psychotherapy populations (Weisz & Jenson, 1999), there is a need for researchers to continue to work with school practitioners to test and perfect these interventions in school settings.

THEORETICAL UNDERPINNINGS OF COGNITIVE-BEHAVIORAL SKILLS-BUILDING APPROACHES

For the skills-building approach, one well-established theory is Lazarus and Folkman's (1984) model of transactional coping. This theory provides the constructs of active and palliative modes of coping, where the coping mode is hypothesized to explain outcome variability, even when the stressors are basically the same. Research results showed only a small association between stressor event and outcome, suggesting that the mode of coping may be more important than the frequency and severity of the stressor (Zeidner & Hammer, 1990). Endler and Parker (1990) developed a model, researched in recent studies, which identifies three coping dimensions: task- or problem-focused, emotion-focused, and avoidance. Task-focused or problem-focused coping, which refers to active efforts to change or reduce the external stress, has been demonstrated to produce more positive outcomes for adolescents than emotion-focused coping or avoidance, neither of which seeks to influence the stressor. An effort to increase skills in the problem-focused dimension has been a primary goal of skills-building treatment models with adolescents over the past decade.

PROBLEM-SOLVING MODELS

Problem-solving models, such as the one developed by D'Zurilla and Nezu (1982), and Bandura's (1997) social learning constructs are also important theoretical cornerstones for the skills approach. The primary objective in a treatment that seeks to strengthen problem-focused coping is to enhance cognition and skills that most strongly enforce problem-focused as the preferred coping strategy. It is logical to assume that problem-solving skills are paramount to enhancing problem-focused behavior. D'Zurilla and Nezu's (1982) social problem–solving model, a step-by-step process for social problem solving, was developed as a clinical application of transactional coping theory. It was initially used with depressed individuals and has subsequently been demonstrated effective with numerous other problems, such as anxiety, weight loss, delinquent behavior, and academic competence (e.g., Black, 1987; Cormier, Otani, & Cormier, 1986; D'Zurilla & Sheedy, 1992; Wege & Moller, 1995).

In this approach to problem solving, *problem* is defined as a life situation that demands a response for effective or adaptive functioning, but for which no effective or adaptive response is immediately apparent or available to the individual confronted with the situation. *Social problem solving* is defined by the model as a cognitive-behavioral process through which an individual attempts to identify, discover, or invent effective means of coping with problems encountered in everyday living (D'Zurilla & Nezu, 1982).

A related benefit is that a sense of *mastery*, a concept that Bandura (1997) describes as essential to self-management, is also likely to enhance problem-solving skills. Mastery positively impacts self-appraisal of one's ability and is demonstrated to increase problem-focused thinking.

GROUP MODALITY

With few exceptions, current skills-building interventions utilize group modality. In fact, across the adolescent literature, group intervention dominates as the modality of choice (Glodich & Allen, 1998). Group modality studies (e.g., Chaffin, Bonner, Worley, & Lawson, 1996; Glodich & Allen, 1995) identify a number of considerations that support the use of groups for adolescents: (a) Adolescents accept feedback more readily from peers than from adults, (b) groups offer the advantage of peer interactions and accentuate the importance of relationships, (c) group norms can be powerfully socializing, (d) members can benefit vicariously from the work done by others, and (e) groups give opportunities for listening without demanding immediate participation.

Groups have been demonstrated effective for a variety of adolescent problems, such as school dropout (Taub, 1998), depression (Rice & Meyer, 1994), sexual abuse (Cornman, 1989), violence and physical abuse (Glodich & Allen, 1998), and behavioral disorders (Hawkins et al., 1991).

BRIEF TREATMENT MODELS

The evidence for benefits of short-term versus longer-term treatment with adolescents is inconclusive. Some studies suggest that adolescents benefit most from comprehensive intervention programs in which they participate for 6 months or more. Program evaluations by Lie and Moroney (1992); Opuni, Smith, Arvey, and Solomon (1994); and Wassef, Mason, Collins, VanHaalen, and Ingham (1998) support such a position. Other studies with adolescents have found significant results within 10 weeks (e.g., de Anda, 1998; Dupper, 1998). Although a few well-funded programs in the past have offered adolescents participation for up to 2 years (e.g., Lie & Moroney, 1992; Quint, 1991), current programs in schools, juvenile justice programs, and residential treatment programs primarily limit participants to time periods of 1 to 3 months (e.g., Seitz & Apfel, 1993). This would suggest that using short-term intervention is essential in most program settings.

In support of the viability of short-term interventions, most outcome studies with adolescent groups across the behavioral science literature are brief, from 5 to 12 weeks (e.g., de Anda, 1998; Harris & Franklin, in press; St. Lawrence et al., 1999; Wege & Moller, 1995). Most are well-designed experimental studies with only negligible or minor problems, providing substantial credibility for the results. For example, de Anda's (1998) randomized study of a 10-week stress management program for middle school adolescents found a significantly lower degree of stress in the group ($N = 36$) who received the treatment than in the control group ($N = 18$). Dupper's (1998) randomized study of a 10-week intervention for middle school youths with behavior problems also reported significant differences in locus of control between the experimental ($N = 46$) and control ($N = 36$) groups, which were maintained at a 4-week follow-up.

INTEGRATING COGNITIVE-BEHAVIORAL SKILLS TRAINING AND EFFECTIVE SERVICE DELIVERY COMPONENTS FOR THE PURPOSES OF BUILDING EVIDENCE-BASED SCHOOL INTERVENTIONS

The literature reviewed indicates that in order to build effective interventions for adolescents in a school setting, cognitive-behavioral technologies should be combined with other service delivery components, such as group modalities, structured curricula, and brief, time-limited classroom formats that match the school structure. The interventions should also be purposeful and very focused, targeting a specific problem of the adolescents who are participating (e.g., depression, anxiety, substance abuse, adolescent pregnancy prevention). At the same time, however, effective school programs may also be multicomponent and target more than one risk factor for that behavior or systematically teach more

than one set of cognitive and behavioral skills that will help prevent or stop the behavior. School programs also take into the consideration the context and ecological environment in which problems exist. The cognitive-behavioral change technologies, however, still remain very systematic as they target differing risk factors. Youths learn new skills for thinking, behaving, coping, and interacting and rehearse those skills with coaching and feedback. They subsequently practice those skills in their real-world environments, followed by immediate rewards (social and tangible) for mastery of the new skills.

Rones and Hoagwood (2000) provide additional suggestions for how to implement effective school-based mental health interventions. Among their cadre of effective methods is the fact that the programs themselves may be hampered by school climate and school organizational variables. Practitioners working in schools must first and foremost learn to effectively engage and work collaboratively with teachers, parents, and other school personnel to implement cognitive-behavioral skills training programs in schools.

TAKING CHARGE: A COGNITIVE-BEHAVIORAL LIFE SKILLS CURRICULUM FOR ADOLESCENT MOTHERS

It is clear from this discussion of outcome research that a cognitive-behavioral approach to building skills for self-management and autonomy is effective with adolescent populations. The social skills–building approach used with other adolescent problems has addressed many issues that are also salient to adolescent mothers. This section presents a school-based intervention developed and tested by Harris and Franklin (in press) for adolescent mothers, conceived from outcome studies of social skills–building treatments with similar adolescent groups. Harris and Franklin developed this curriculum because they saw the challenge of educating adolescent pregnant and parenting mothers, who are often dependent and lack competencies and skills for independence and self-sufficiency. Most existing curricula for adolescent pregnancy are child-centered and focus the mother on child development, parenting skills, or prevention of a second pregnancy. The curricula are obsessed with the mothers becoming good mothers and lack adequate cultural and strengths-based orientations. They do not adequately address a developmental framework for adolescent development nor address how these mothers can work toward developing into competent, self-sufficient adults. The Taking Charge curriculum is strengths-focused and, contrary to some other curricula, it nurtures the mother and her problem-solving capacities while giving full respect to her goals and cultural beliefs.

A review of relevant literature on pregnant and parenting adolescent girls reveals four domains of life outcome prediction that inform school-based intervention toward self-sufficiency for this population: (a) education, (b) employment, (c) social relationships, and (d) parenting. The four correlate strongly to life quality for parent and child, and each requires exceptional problem-solving and coping skills for young mothers. For this reason, Harris and Franklin concluded that a social problem–solving process like the one developed by D'Zurilla and Nezu (1982), combined with other social learning skills, might help adolescent mothers increase their self-efficacy in areas of education, employment, social relationships, and parenting. The authors believed this to be the case because of the developmental stage of the adolescent women. Most youths at this stage, for example, had not developed such life management skills, and these mothers were being asked to do something extraordinary. What they needed was a "foundation mindset" that would build self-efficacy and help them acquire all the other skills they needed to master all these developmental challenges that had been thrust upon them because of early pregnancy. Harris and Franklin believed that the social problem–solving process would be an effective way to help them if it was delivered in a task-centered group format where the adolescent mothers could receive emotional support and at the same time practice resolving their personal problems in the main life areas.

Harris and Franklin also believed that education is the most immediate problem area, as well as the best researched predictor of long-term economic self-sufficiency for the adolescent mother (Chase-Lansdale, Brooks-Gunn, & Paikoff, 1992; Duncan, Harris, & Boisjoly, 1997). So, it was most important have a positive impact on the women's education. For this reason, the intervention was tailored toward and delivered in a school setting.

Outcome Goals

Issues confronting adolescent mothers, including low school achievement and high dropout rates, are similar to those of other adolescent groups who have responded positively to a life skills–building approach. It is reasonable to conclude that a social skills–building and mastery intervention with adolescent mothers is likely to be effective. Therefore, the three outcome goals are each concerned with behavioral skills. The first goal is to increase problem-focused coping. In testing the effectiveness of the intervention, this outcome was measured with subscales from the Adolescent Coping Orientation for Problem Experiences (A-COPE) (Patterson & McCubbin, 1983). The second goal is to increase social problem–solving skills. In testing the intervention, this outcome was measured with D'Zurilla's (1993) Social Problem-Solving Inventory–Revised Short Form (SPSI-R). The third outcome goal is to increase school achievement, defined by attendance and grade point average. These outcomes were measured with school attendance data and periodic grade reports.

Intervention Structure

The intervention uses a group format designed for 8 to 12 participants. It is a curriculum for 8 weekly sessions that can be easily adapted to 12 weeks by allotting two sessions rather than one for each goal. The group was designed to be facilitated by two group leaders, although it has been facilitated effectively with one leader. To minimize classroom interruption, the group is planned for the students' lunch period, when they ordinarily have a block of unscheduled time.

Treatment Manual

One of the most important aspects of this curriculum is a treatment manual that contains step-by-step instructions for group leaders. The manual includes objectives and activities for each session, physical setup, a supply list, forms for record maintenance, handouts for participants, and actual dialogue for teaching and facilitating the content.

Having a treatment manual is valuable in several ways. First, specific and comprehensive instructions allow a variety of school-based staff or volunteers to successfully lead the group. Personnel resources for adolescent parents are limited in many schools, which can limit programs to few services beyond case management. This group has been led effectively by MSW and BSW social workers and graduate students, special education teachers, school nurses, counselors, and volunteers who use the treatment manual after a few hours of training,

The manual provides clear guidelines that maintain the integrity of the treatment. Avoiding professional jargon, it gives facilitators an understanding of the rationale for the group and explains the importance of maintaining the curriculum as directed in the manual.

Eight-Session Content

The eight-session curriculum was based on D'Zurilla and Nezu's (1982) six-step social problem–solving model, using a task-centered group format. The curriculum objectives are (a) for participants to learn the problem-solving model, (b) for participants to relate the problem-solving steps to themselves, and (c) for participants to identify goals and apply the problem-solving model in four areas of their lives: school, parenting, personal relationships, and career planning.

The first three sessions are concerned with establishing the group's purpose and teaching participants the social problem–solving process. Handouts in the treatment manual are used in this process and throughout the intervention.

In session four, participants identify an education goal. They work through the problem-solving steps until they identify two tasks that they can complete during the coming week toward achieving the goal. It is essential to this process that participants identify their own goals and tasks with minimal input from group leaders. Mastering the problem-solving process and developing a problem-focused mode of coping are the desired outcomes for participants, and their specific goals and tasks while learning these skills are of less importance. Prior group participants identified goals that generally relate to improved academic performance or graduating from high school, although some used this goal for planning alternatives, such as a GED, or for entering college or vocational training. Favored tasks among participants have included arranging for childcare, spending time in the library or doing homework, and problem solving with teachers, parents, and academic counselors.

Sessions five through seven repeat the process of session four, with goals around parenting, personal relationships, and career planning. These sessions include time to process and perhaps replan tasks from the previous week. Achievements are reviewed in session eight and plans made for continued work outside the group.

Incentives

To increase the likelihood that participants will receive the full benefit of the group, incentives are included. This is explained by Bandura's (1997) social learning construct of self-mastery, which assumes the capacity to shape and regulate one's environment to fit a desired outcome. It is anticipated that participants can conceptualize the satisfaction of receiving rewards and can self-regulate their behavior toward ensuring that they will receive these benefits. Incentives include lunch or a snack at each session, small gifts, and a system where participants can earn points for school and group attendance, task completion, homework, and extra-credit assignments toward an award at the end of the group series. Group leaders tally points and inform participants of their weekly progress. Awards have included gift certificates, field trips, and special school privileges.

Outcomes of Effectiveness Study

Taking Charge was tested in five high schools with 78 adolescent mothers. Thirty-eight study participants were randomly assigned to receive the intervention, and 40 were randomly assigned to the control group. While the two groups were found to be equivalent on all outcome variables at pretest, there was a significant overall difference between groups on the posttests, with pretests as covariates ($F = 7.20$; $df = 4$, 58; $p < 000$). A separate analysis of covariance on each outcome variable also found significant difference at the .01 level or greater.

The clinical significance for school-related outcomes is especially meaningful when examining the groups' actual grades and school attendance. Both groups began the study with a high C grade average (77.8 and 77.5). At the end of the semester, the treatment group mean had achieved a low B (79.7), while the control group mean had dropped to a low D (71.6), just above passing. Both groups began the study with .83

school attendance. At the end of the intervention, the treatment group attendance was .90, while the control group attendance was still at .83. At the end of the semester 6 weeks later, the control group attendance had dropped to .75, while the treatment group maintained at .87. Considering the importance of skills that support high school graduation for adolescent mothers, outcomes such as these are extremely important for interventions with this population.

Considerations for Use in a School Setting

Taking Charge is an intervention that places minimal strain on resources and the day-to-day program environment of most school-based teen pregnancy programs. It utilizes staff, facilities, and supplies found in most programs across the country, suggesting that it can be used relatively well with existing budgets. As well, its duration fits well into the calendar of the school year.

The intervention is among the least controversial of programs relevant to pregnant and parenting adolescents. It appeals to social workers and educators as well as community stakeholders around common concerns for school achievement and economic self-sufficiency. As a result, teen parent programs in school settings may find enhanced support from school staff and the community in offering the intervention.

Although Taking Charge has a social work orientation, it can be led effectively by other pupil-services staff. Teachers, nurses, counselors, and social workers have required minimal training to facilitate the intervention, and volunteers have served well as cofacilitators.

CONCLUSIONS

This chapter has discussed the special needs and vulnerability of adolescent populations in school settings, which enhance the need for evidence-based, cognitive-behavioral skills-building programs. Four empirically supported practice trends have been discussed that can serve as guides for selecting, adapting, and developing school-based interventions.

1. Numerous outcome studies demonstrate that a skills-building curriculum is an effective tool for change in schools with adoles-

cent populations, even though much more research on these interventions in school settings is still needed before we will have a truly evidence-based knowledge base for school mental health practices.

2. Several cognitive-behavioral theories, such as Lazarus and Folkman's (1984) stress and coping theory, Bandura's (1997) social learning constructs, and D'Zurilla and Nezu's (1982) problem-solving model, provide empirical grounding for social skills building. In the absence of evidence-based curricula and interventions, practitioners may work to combine these models into interventions that may prove to be effective with school-based populations.

3. The use of the group modality with special adolescent populations in schools is demonstrated to be more effective in promoting change than other modalities.

4. Numerous brief treatments of 5 to 12 weeks with adolescents are demonstrated to be effective, and these types of interventions are also found to be compatible with service delivery in school settings.

5. This chapter also provides some guidance on how to develop and test interventions in a school setting. First, practitioners should seek to ground their interventions in evidence-based theories for changing human behaviors such as problem solving, learning theories, risk reduction, and protection. Second, practitioners should develop specific interventions that target specific behaviors that are tailored to specific settings such as schools. Third, interventions should be written down with clear guidelines, philosophy, and implementation procedures in intervention or training manuals. Fourth, practitioners should work with researchers to test those interventions by using acceptable experimental designs, measurement systems, and the best accountability tools. Fifth, results of these tests should be disseminated so that other practitioners and researchers can evaluate those findings, and those results can be included in the knowledge base for school-based practices.

The chapter has presented how Taking Charge, one example of a cognitive-behavioral group intervention for an adolescent population, was developed along these evidence-based guidelines. From this chapter, practitioners who work with a number of adolescent populations can find guidance for developing and applying current evidence-based, cognitive-behavioral skills interventions with at-risk youths in schools.

References

Annie E. Casey Foundation. (2002). *Kids count data book: 2002.* Baltimore, MD: Author.

Bandura, A. (1997). *Self-efficacy: The exercise of control.* New York: W. H. Freeman.

Barth, R. P. (1985). Beating the blues: Cognitive-behavioral treatment for depression in child-maltreating young mothers. *Clinical Social Work Journal, 13*(4), 317–328.

Bennett, D., & Gibbons, T. (2000). Efficacy of child cognitive-behavioral interventions for anti-social behavior: A meta-analysis. *Child and Family Behavior Therapy, 22,* 1–15.

Black, D. R. (1987). A minimal intervention program and a problem-solving program for weight control. *Cognitive Therapy and Research, 11,* 107–120.

Bolger, K. E., Patterson, C. J., Thompson, W. W., & Kupersmidt, J. B. (1995). Psychosocial adjustment among children experiencing persistent and intermittent family economic hardship. *Child Development, 66,* 1107–1129.

Bowen, G. L., & Van Dorn, R. A. (2002). Community and violent crime rates and school danger. *Children in Schools, 24,* 90–104.

Burns, B. J. (2002). Reasons for hope for children and families: A perspective and overview. In B. J. Burns & K. Hoagwood (Eds.), *Community treatment for youth* (pp. 1–15). New York: Oxford University Press.

Carlson, S., Clark, J. P., & Marx, D. (1992). *School and community resource collaboration: A position paper.* The Midwest School Social Work Council.

Centers for Disease Control and Prevention (CDC). (2001). Births to teenagers in the United States, 1940–2000. *National Vital Statistics Reports (NVSR), 49*(10).

Centers for Disease Control and Prevention (CDC). (2003). Revised birth and fertility rates for the United States in 2000–2001. *National Vital Statistics Reports (NVSS), 51*(4), 1–24.

Chaffin, M., Bonner, B., Worley, K., & Lawson, L. (1996). Treating abused adolescents. In J. Briere, L. Berliner, J. Bulkley, C. Jenny, & T. Reid (Eds.), *The APSAC handbook on child maltreatment* (pp. 119–139). Thousand Oaks, CA: Sage.

Chase-Lansdale, P. L., Brooks-Gunn, J., & Paikoff, R. L. (1992). Research and programs for adolescent mothers. *American Behavioral Scientist, 35*(3), 290–312.

Child Trends. (2001). Facts at a glance, 12/99 overview. http://www.childtrends.org/.8

Clarke, G. (1992). Cognitive-behavioral group treatment of adolescent depression: Prediction of outcome. *Behavior Therapy, 23,* 341–354.

Clarke, G., Hawkins, W., Murphy, M., Sheeber, L., Lewinsohn, P., & Seely, J. (1995). Targeted prevention of unipolar depressive disorder in an at-risk sample of high school adolescents: A randomized trial of a group cognitive intervention. *Journal of the American Academy of Child and Adolescent Psychiatry, 34,* 312–321.

Corcoran, J. (2002). Evidenced-based treatments for adolescents with externalizing disorders. In A. R. Roberts & G. J. Greene (Eds.), *Social Workers' Desk Reference* (pp. 793–797). New York: Oxford University Press.

Cormier, W. H., Otani, A., & Cormier, L. S. (1986). The effects of problem-solving training on two problem-solving tasks. *Cognitive Therapy and Research, 10,* 95–108.

Cornman, B. (1989). Group treatment for female adolescent sexual abuse victims. *Issues in Mental Health Nursing, 10,* 261–271.

De Anda, D. (1998). The evaluation of a stress management program for middle school adolescents. *Child and Adolescent Social Work Journal, 15*(1), 73–85.

Duncan, G. J., Harris, K. M., & Boisjoly, J. (1997). *Time limits and welfare reform: New estimate of the number and characteristics of affected families.* Chicago: Northwestern University—University of Chicago Joint Center for Poverty Research.

Dupper, D. R. (1998). An alternative to suspension for middle school youths behavior problems: Findings from a "school survival" group. *Research on Social Work Practice, 8*(3), 354–366.

D'Zurilla, T. J., & Nezu, A. (1982). Social problem-solving in adults. In P. C. Kendall (Ed.), *Advances in cognitive-behavioral research and therapy* (pp. 202–269). New York: Academic Press.

D'Zurilla, T. J., & Nezu, A. (2000). Social problem-solving inventory [SPSI]. In K. Corcoran & J. Fischer (Eds.), *Measures for clinical practice: A sourcebook: Vol. 2* (3rd ed., pp. 772–779). New York: Free Press.

D'Zurilla, T. J., & Sheedy, C. F. (1991). Relation between social problem-solving ability and subsequent level of psychological stress in college students. *Journal of Personality and Social Psychology, 61,* 841–846.

Eamon, M. K. (2001). Poverty, parenting, peer, and neighborhood influences on young adolescent antisocial behavior. *Journal of Social Service Research, 28*(1), 1–23.

Elia, J. P. (1993). Homophobia in the high school: A problem in need of a resolution. *The High School Journal, 77,* 177–185.

Endler, N. S., & Parker, J. (1990). Multidimensional

assessment of coping: A critical review. *Journal of Personality and Social Psychology, 58,* 844–854.

Fick, A. C., & Thomas, S. M. (1995). Growing up in a violent environment: Relationship to health-related beliefs and behaviors. *Youth and Society, 27*(2), 136–147.

Forman, S. G., Linney, J. A., & Brondino, M. J. (1990). Effects of coping skills training on adolescents at risk for substance abuse. *Psychology of Addictive Behaviors, 4*(2), 67–76.

Franklin, C. & Corcoran, J. (1999). Preventing adolescent pregnancy: A review of programs and practices. *Social Work, 45*(1), 40–52.

Franklin, C., Corcoran, J., & Harris, M. B. (in press). Risk, protective factors, and effective interventions for adolescent pregnancy. In M. W. Fraser (Ed.), *Risk and resiliency in childhood and adolescents* (2nd ed.). Washington, DC: NASW Press.

Franklin, C., Grant, D., Corcoran, J., O'Dell, P., & Bultman, L. (1997). Effectiveness of prevention programs for adolescent pregnancy: A meta-analysis. *Journal of Marriage and the Family, 59*(3), 551–567.

Franklin, C., McNeil, J. A., & Wright, R. (1991). The effectiveness of social work in an alternative school for high school dropouts. *Social work with Groups, 14*(2), 59–73.

Fulton, A. M., Murphy, K. R., & Anderson, S. L. (1991). Increasing adolescent mothers' knowledge of child development: An intervention program. *Adolescence, 26*(101), 73–81.

Garbarino, J., DuBrow, N., Kostelny, K., & Pardo, C. (1992). *Children in danger: Coping with the consequences of community violence.* San Francisco: Jossey-Bass.

Gibbs, L., & Gambrill, E. (2002). Evidence-based practice: Counterarguments to objections. *Research on Social Work Practice, 12*(9), 452–477.

Glodich, A., & Allen, J. G. (1998). Adolescents exposed to violence and abuse: A review of the group therapy literature with an emphasis on preventing trauma reenactment. *Journal of Child and Adolescent Group Therapy, 8*(3), 135–153.

Griffin, N. C. (1998). Cultivating self-efficacy in adolescent mothers: A collaborative approach. *Professional School Counseling, 1*(4), 53–58.

Harris, M. B., & Franklin, C., (in press-a). The design of social work services. In P. Allen-Meares (Ed.), *Social work services in schools* (4th ed.). Boston: Allen & Bacon.

Harris, M. B., & Franklin, C. (in press-b). Effects of a cognitive-behavioral, school-based, group intervention with Mexican-American pregnant and parenting mothers. *Social Work Research.*

Hawkins, J. D., Jenson, J. M., Catalano, R. F., & Wells, E. A. (1991). Effects of a skills training interven-tion with juvenile delinquents. *Research on Social Work Practice, 1*(2), 107–121.

Herie, M., & Martin, G. W. (2002). Knowledge diffusion in social work: A new approach to bridging the gap. *Social Work, 47*(1), 85–104.

Hudson, W. (1996). *Multidimensional adolescent assessment scale (MAAS).* Tallahassee, FL: WAL-MYR Publishing.

Jemmont, J. B., Jemmont, L. S., Fong, G. T., & Mc-Caffree, K. (1999). Reducing HIV risk–associated sexual behavior among African American adolescents: Testing the generality of intervention effects. *American Journal of Community Psychology, 27*(2), 161–187.

Johnston, L., Bachman, J., & O'Malley, P. (1996). *Monitoring the future: Questionnaire responses from the nation's high school seniors, 1995.* Ann Arbor, MI: Institute for Social Research, University of Michigan.

Kann, L., Kinchen, S., Williams, B., Ross, J., Lowry, R., Hill, C., et al. (1998). Youth risk behavior surveillance: United States, 1997. *Morbidity and Mortality Weekly Report, 47*(SS-3), 1–89.

Kelly, D. M. (1996). Stigma stories: Four discourses about teen mothers, welfare, and poverty. *Education and Urban Society, 27*(4), 421–449.

Kendall, P. C. (Ed.). (2000). *Child and adolescent therapy. Cognitive behavioral procedures* (2nd ed.). New York: Guilford.

Lazarus, R. S., & Folkman, S. (1984). *Stress, appraisal and coping.* New York: Springer.

Lie, G. Y., & Moroney, R. M. (1992). A controlled evaluation of comprehensive social services provided to teenage mothers receiving AFDC. *Research on Social Work Practice, 2*(4), 429–447.

Males, M. (1994). Poverty, rape, adult/teen sex: Why pregnancy prevention programs don't work. *Phi Delta Kappan, 54,* 407–410.

Maynard, R. (1997). *Kids having kids: Economic costs and social consequences of teen pregnancy.* Washington, DC: Urban Institute Press.

McWhirter, B. T., & Page, G. L. (1999). Effects of anger management and goal setting group interventions on state-trait anger and self-efficacy beliefs among high risk adolescents. *Current Psychology: Developmental, Learning, Personality, Social, 18*(2), 223–237.

Mental health: A report of the Surgeon General, chapter 3. Retrieved April 15, 2002, from http://www.surgeongeneral.gov/library/mentalhealth/chapter3/sec1.html

Moore, P., & Terrett, C. (1998). Highlights of the 1996 National Youth Gang Survey. *OJJDP fact sheet* (#86). Washington, DC: Office of Juvenile Justice and Delinquency Prevention.

Natasi, B. K. (1998). A model for mental health programming in schools and communities: Introduction to the mini-series. *The School Psychology Review, 27*(2), 165–174.

National Center for Education Statistics. (1999). *Dropout statistics.* Washington, DC: Author.

Opuni, K. A., Smith, P. B., Arvey, H., & Solomon, C. (1994). The Northeast Adolescent Project: A collaborative effort to address teen-age pregnancy in Houston, Texas. *Journal of School Health, 64*(5), 212–215.

Patterson, J., & McCubbin, H. I. (1983). Adolescent coping orientation for problem experiences (A-COPE). In H. I. McCubbin, A. I. Thompson, & M. A. McCubbin (Eds.), (1996). *Family assessment and resiliency, coping, and adaptation: Inventories for research and practice* (pp. 537–583). Madison: University of Wisconsin System.

Quint, J. (1991). Project Redirection: Making and measuring a difference. *Evaluation and Program Planning, 14*(1–2), 75–86.

Rice, K. G., & Meyer, A. L. (1994). Preventing depression among young adolescents: Preliminary process results of a psycho-educational intervention program. *Journal of Counseling and Development, 73,* 145–152.

Rones, M., & Hoagwood, K. (2000). School-based mental health services: A research review. *Clinical Child and Family Psychology Review, 4,* 223–241.

Rosenberg, D. E. (1991, Winter). Serving America's newcomers: States and localities taking the lead in the absence of a comprehensive national policy. *Public Welfare,* 28–37.

Rosenthal, B. (1995). The influence of social support on school completion among Haitians. *Social Work in Education, 17,* 30–39.

Snyder, H. N., & Sickmund, M. (1999). Juvenile offenders and victims: 1999 national report, National Center for Juvenile Justice. Washington, DC: Office of Juvenile Justice and Delinquency Prevention.

St. Lawrence, J. S., Crosby, R. A., Belcher, L., Yazdani, N., & Brasfield, T. L. (1999). *Journal of Sex Education & Therapy, 24*(1-2), 9–17.

Thornberry, T., & Burch, J. (1997). Gang members and delinquent behavior. In *OJJDP Juvenile Justice Bulletin.* Washington, DC: Office of Juvenile Justice and Delinquency Prevention.

Tobler, N. (1986). Meta-analysis of 143 adolescent drug prevention programs: Quantitative outcome results for program participants compared to control or comparison group. *Journal of Drug Issues, 16,* 537–567.

Vallerand, R. J., Fortier, M. S., & Guay, F. (1997). Self-determination in a real-life setting: Toward a motivational model of high school dropout. *Journal of Personality and Social Psychology, 72*(5), 1161–1176.

Wassef, A., Mason, G., Collins, M. L., VanHaalen, J., & Ingham, D. (1998). Effectiveness of one-year participation in school-based volunteer-facilitated peer support groups. *Adolescence, 33*(129), 91–97.

Wege, J. W., & Moller, A. T. (1995). Effectiveness of a problem-solving training program. *Psychological Reports, 76,* 507–514.

Zeidner, M., & Hammer, A. L. (1990). Life events and coping resources as predictors stress symptoms in adolescents. *Personality and Individual Differences, 11,* 693–703.

Zlotnik, J. L., Biegel, D. E., & Solt, B. E. (2002). The Institute for the Advancement of Social Work Research: Strengthening social work research in practice and policy. *Research on Social Work Practice, 12*(2), 318–337.

EVIDENCE-BASED PRACTICE WITH EYE MOVEMENT DESENSITIZATION AND REPROCESSING

Karen S. Knox

The development of treatment models that have empirically based protocols has coincided with the emphasis on evidence-based practice in professional counseling and social work. One such model is eye movement desensitization and reprocessing (EMDR), which was developed in 1987 by Francine Shapiro to relieve posttraumatic stress symptoms. This therapy approach uses bilateral eye movement to desensitize the distressing memories, feelings, and cognitions associated with the traumatic incident(s) and to enhance the reprocessing and replacement of negative cognitions with more positive ones (Rubin, 2002). Using EMDR with a woman who has been sexually assaulted, the therapist would target any PTSD symptoms, as well as any negative cognitions, such as blaming herself for the rape or believing that she could have prevented the assault in some way.

This chapter begins with a discussion of the concepts and process of evidence-based practice, along with operational definitions and steps to follow as a guide for practitioners. Then, the steps of evidence-based practice are applied to EMDR, with an overview of the major principles and treatment protocol of EMDR. A case application illustrates how this therapy approach is used in evidence-based practice to evaluate EMDR's effectiveness in minimizing the maladaptive and negative reactions from recent trauma experiences, such as sexual assault.

The purpose of this chapter is to give the reader a clear idea of how to apply evidence-based practice steps when working with clients who may benefit from EMDR. The advantages of using this process are presented with the ob-jective of encouraging readers to apply these steps in their own practice. Evidence-based practice techniques can be used to provide empirical results of practice effectiveness with different theoretical models and fields of practice.

EVIDENCE-BASED PRACTICE

During the 1990s, the term *evidence-based practice* began to appear in the medical professional literature, initially by the Evidence-Based Medicine Working Group (1992) at McMaster University in Canada (Gambrill, 1999; Gibbs, 2003; Sackett, Rosenberg, Gray, Haynes, & Richardson, 1996). As applied by the medical field, this term means to use the current best evidence in making decisions about patient care. Current best evidence is based on empirical evidence from research studies that are published in the professional literature. This implies that the practitioner must be motivated to read and use the current best evidence as a continued educational process of professional development.

As applied to the helping professions, evidence-based practice is lifelong problem-based learning to keep up-to-date and improve clinical practice and treatment outcomes. Evidence-based practice means that practitioners use theories and interventions based on the empirical evidence of their effectiveness, apply approaches appropriate to the client and setting, and evaluate their own practice effectiveness (Rosen & Proctor, 2002; Thyer, 2002; Vandiver, 2002).

An operational definition of evidence-based practice would include the steps of the process, which start with being motivated to use it (Gibbs, 2003). Motivations can range from professional values such as do no harm, provide the best possible practice, and the client's best interests to professional development issues such as clinical expertise, continued education and licensing, and practice effectiveness. Clinicians must also know where to locate and how to use the current best evidence in their field of practice.

The next step is associated with the assessment and diagnosis phase of treatment, with the practitioner using data and information to identify the problems and targets for work (Gibbs, 2003; Vandiver, 2002). This requires the use of diagnostic criteria and instruments to develop a clinical assessment and treatment plan. The practitioner must know how to find current research and scholarship in a particular field of practice and how to apply those findings to a particular client. The main resources for professional literature are public and university libraries and Web sites, professional journals and books, Internet Web sites and search engines, and doctoral dissertations. Electronic technology has made the task of keeping up with the research much easier and more accessible.

In the third step, the practitioner must be able to critically appraise the current best evidence, as to the quality of the research or study, the methodology used, and the significance of the results or findings. To be effective consumers of research, clinicians must know how to read and critique professional literature that is empirically based, which requires knowledge of research methods, designs, and analysis.

Applying the results of this evidence search is the fourth step. This starts with the development of an intervention plan with the client based on the current best evidence that identifies the targets and goals of treatment, the roles of those involved, the intervention techniques being applied, and the outcome measures. The targets, goals, and outcomes must be operationally defined and measurable. The clinician and client must both be motivated to use monitoring and measurement strategies to evaluate the effectiveness of the treatment.

Evaluating practice effectiveness is the fifth step. The client and the practitioner review measurable outcomes and evidence to determine whether the goals of treatment are being achieved. Having objective measures of improvement or change can also motivate the client

and practitioner to continue or maintain progress. If there is no documented effectiveness, then that allows the client and clinician to reevaluate the treatment model or plan and adjust appropriately.

The last step in evidence-based practice is to advocate and teach others to use it. With managed care and funding requirements, most agencies and practitioners have to document services and results, and this process lends itself easily to those requirements. The primary motivations for teaching and advocating this process are to improve the knowledge base of the professional disciplines and to ensure the best practice standards for clients. These standards can be developed into practice guidelines that provide synthesized and organized knowledge about interventions based on empirical evidence (Rosen & Proctor, 2002).

APPLICATION OF EVIDENCE-BASED PRACTICE STEPS TO EMDR

Step 1: Motivation to Use

This therapy model is a specialized treatment protocol that requires formal education and training through workshops, classes, and conferences sponsored by the EMDR Institute. Information about the EMDR Institute's training and certification process can be found at the Internet Web site http://www.emdr.org. To provide ethical and effective therapy, the therapist or social worker must be certified and experienced in using EMDR, as well as knowledgeable and competent in the respective field of practice or client population. Therefore, the practitioner must be motivated to make the time and effort to investigate and participate in the formal training required with EMDR.

What possible motivations are there for clinicians working with sexual assault victims to take these steps? I had more than 10 years of clinical experience working with both child and adult survivors of sexual assault before learning about EMDR through professional colleagues and the literature in the early 1990s. Intrigued by the success of this model with clients with PTSD, I developed an interest in investigating the current best evidence. My primary motivation for learning about EMDR was to be more effective in clinical practice and to keep current with innovations in treatment with clients experiencing PTSD and survivors of sexual assault.

Step 2: Current Best Evidence

To learn more about this theory, I attended Level II training, which was a 3-day seminar conducted by the EMDR Institute. The training consisted of didactic workshops with experiential exercises for the participants to develop and experience the treatment techniques. The facilitators had experience in clinical settings with the model and had conducted research to substantiate its effectiveness with clients. The conference participants are required to experience the techniques both as a recipient and as a provider to have firsthand knowledge about its effects.

I also gained experience with the techniques and process of EMDR as a clinical researcher in a study (Edmond, Rubin, & Wambach, 1999) conducted with childhood survivors of sexual assault. This experimental study of 59 women, who were randomly assigned to one of three groups—(a) individual EMDR sessions (6), (b) traditional individual treatment sessions (6), and (c) delayed treatment group—found that the EMDR participants scored significantly better on two of the four measures than routine individual treatment participants at 3-month follow-up. I have continued to use EMDR in private practice with victims and family survivors of trauma, including sexual assault, homicide, and child abuse. I developed these areas of expertise through other training, workshops, education, and professional experience at Child Protective Services, the Victim Services Division of the Austin Police Department, the Victim Advocacy Unit of the Travis County District Attorney's Office, and the Austin Rape Crisis Center.

A review of the literature at that time revealed research studies indicating EMDR's effectiveness with a variety of client populations experiencing PTSD, including Vietnam War veterans, burn victims, and individuals with phobias (Jenson, 1994; McCann, 1992; Sanderson & Carpenter, 1992; Wilson, Becker, & Tinker, 1995). A current literature search using the database PsychINFO indicates that more than 300 professional journal articles have been published on EMDR since 1990. Clearly, interest and investigation into this theory have increased over the past decade. By 1999, both the International Society for Traumatic Stress Studies and Division 12 (Clinical Psychology) of the American Psychological Association supported the efficacy of EMDR as an effective and empirically validated treatment approach for PTSD (Rubin, 2002).

Step 3: Critical Consumer of Research

While most of the earlier studies had methodological limitations or lacked true experimental designs, subsequent research that is more empirically sound has documented the effectiveness of EMDR (Edmond et al., 1999; Rubin, 2002). Other studies have argued that EMDR is no more effective than validated cognitive-behavioral techniques, such as systematic desensitization, flooding, and covert rehearsal (Edmond et al., 1999; Rosen, 1999; Rubin, 2002). Other limitations of EMDR are associated with clients who have dissociative disorders or psychoses and those who are experiencing ongoing abuse (Paulsen, 1995; Rubin, 2002).

Over the past decade, there have been refinements and changes in the techniques of EMDR but not in the basic principles and process of the model. Most of the current literature examines the model's effectiveness with specific client populations or clinical areas, including social anxiety disorder, phobias, eating disorders, chronic pain, and complex PTSD, and there is more evidence as to its use with children (Alto, 2001; Chemtob, Nakashima, & Carlson, 2002; DeJongh, van den Oord, & ten Broeke, 2002; Dziegielewski & Wolfe, 2000; Grant & Threlfo, 2002; Gross & Ratner, 2002; Korn & Leeds, 2002; Largo-Marsh & Spates, 2002; Lipsitz & Marshall, 2001; Soberman, Greenwald, & Rule, 2002; Sprang, 2001; Taylor, 2002; Taylor et al., 2003). There are two special issues of the *Journal of Clinical Psychology* (issues 1 and 12 of volume 58, 2002) that are devoted to EMDR that would be excellent resources for those who want to review the current research. Additionally, there are several books and a video that would be helpful for learning this model (Dawkins, 1999; Manfield, 1998; Shapiro, 1995; Shapiro & Forrest, 1997; Tinker & Wilson, 1999).

Step 4: Applying the Current Best Evidence

This step first requires a presentation of the major principles and the treatment process of EMDR so the reader can understand how the treatment protocol is compatible with evidence-based practice. The EMDR model is based on the hypothesis that traumatization produces neural networking that processes those memories and experiences either incompletely, because of their raw, affect-laden nature, or are dissociated from conscious awareness altogether (Shapiro, 1994). Additionally, the raw affect interferes with successful processing, because it inhibits accessing, verbalizing, and expressing emotions and reactions associated with the trauma, which are too sensitive, anxiety provoking, and threatening to the client (Knox, 2002). The rapid eye movement technique developed by Shapiro (1995) facilitates accessing, desensitizing, and reprocessing trauma memories and feelings by accessing the full information-processing system, which results in diffusing the traumatic imagery, cognitive restructuring, and neutralizing negative affect.

The EMDR process begins with establishing rapport and conducting a client history and intake screening. Survivors of trauma may question their own safety and vulnerability, and they may have difficulty in establishing trust at this time. Therefore, active listening and empathic communication skills are essential to establishing rapport and engaging the client. Empathic communication skills include minimal encouragers, attending to nonverbal behaviors and communication, reflection, and being genuine (Knox, 2002).

Trust is also facilitated in the second stage, when the client is educated about the EMDR procedures and any possible negative reactions to it (Rubin, 2002). The client should be able to choose whether to use EMDR or more traditional therapies, which requires that the therapist have expertise in a repertoire of theoretical approaches. The therapist also addresses any fears or safety concerns and discusses client goals and expectations during this stage.

The third stage requires an assessment and identification of the target issues, such as the presenting problem(s), and the associated memories by having the client select a target image that represents the trauma. The counselor then asks the client to measure the cognitions and affect associated with the target image through the subjective units of disturbance (SUDS) and the validity of cognition (VOC) instruments. These rank the client's scores from 0 to 10 on a scale of severity and are done pretest and posttest for each counseling session to evaluate changes in those thoughts and feelings. The use of preintervention and postintervention testing gives immediate feedback to the client and the therapist to measure the effectiveness of treatment.

The desensitization phase (fourth stage) involves using bilateral eye movements to activate the neural network, which typically results in the client recalling the target image and experiencing a sequence of emotions. In this phase, EMDR can be effective in minimizing or eliminating the blockage experienced through the client's traumatized neural networking system. A nondirective approach is used, with the counselor avoiding any interpretation or reframing of those images, thoughts, or feelings, thereby enabling the client to reprocess those reactions in his or her own way (Knox, 2002).

The fifth stage is the installation phase that serves to close down this catalytic process and install more desired cognitive and affective responses. These positive, adaptive responses are elicited from the client and illustrate how the client would prefer to think or feel about the trauma event or memory. Clients are asked to rank the validity of the new cognition as to how true it feels until it has been successfully installed.

In the sixth stage, a body scan is conducted to assess if any residual target issues are unresolved, and stages four and five are repeated as needed. One of the principles of EMDR is that this technique taps into related nodes of memories or unresolved issues, which may require work as well. The seventh stage involves closure by using relaxation techniques with the client at the end of the session. The therapist also recommends that the client keep a journal of any intrusive thoughts or distressing feelings experienced, as it is common that reprocessing continues between sessions. The last stage evaluates whether the targeted trauma is resolved successfully, and if there is any need to continue further reprocessing (Rubin, 2002).

Typically, the EMDR process is completed within a brief time frame of four to six sessions, which typically last from 60 to 90 minutes each. The immediate effects of the treatment should allow the client to move toward a higher level of pretrauma functioning. Trauma survivors may also gain a more positive future orientation as well, with an understanding that they can overcome current problems and hope that change can occur (Roberts, 1996). When the client is able to process and ventilate her or his feelings and reactions to the trauma, the release is energizing and enables the client to work through the grief process. After the EMDR intervention process is completed, the client may want to follow up on referrals for other services and programs, such as support groups, advocacy groups, relief organizations, or charitable and volunteer programs.

Case Application

Debbie wanted to go out with her girlfriends to celebrate a birthday, but her fiancé told her not to because he was out of town. She decided to go anyway, and at the nightclub she met a man who offered her drugs. They went to her apartment, where he sexually assaulted her before leaving. She had resisted, told him no during the rape, and called the police to report it. She also went to the hospital for a rape exam, where she disclosed her drug use, despite her concerns about how the police would react. She was reluctant to tell her fiancé about the rape, because she felt that he would get angry at her for going out after he told her not to go.

Initial services were provided to the rape victim by the police department victim services counselor, who provided crisis intervention and referral services. The counselor referred the client to me for clinical treatment of the sexual assault and also referred the case to the district attorney office's victim's advocate for services during the court process. The presenting problems for the client were PTSD symptoms of anxiety and recurring intrusive thoughts about the rape. She evidenced self-blame and guilt about the rape, which was reinforced by her fiancé (who was out of town at the time of the rape), who had told her not to go out with her girlfriends that night. An intake and assessment was conducted in the first session with the client, and the therapist explained her options for traditional individual sessions, EMDR individual sessions, and group treatment. The client expressed interest in trying EMDR with the goals of reducing PTSD symptoms and negative self-thoughts and feelings associated with the rape. The client was seen over a 3-week period for a total of three sessions, with one of the sessions lasting 2 hours and the other two lasting 90 minutes each.

By this time, the client had disclosed the rape to her fiancé, who had reacted as she suspected. This led to arguments and emotional abuse, which contributed to her anxiety levels and intrusive thoughts. During the initial assessment, the client described her current subjective units

of disturbance (SUDS) as a 9 (on a scale of 0 to 10, with 10 being the most severe), and the validity of cognition (VOC) that she could have prevented the rape ranked as a 10 (on a scale of 0 to 10, with 10 feeling true to me). Using the bilateral eye movement technique, the client described the process as similar to "watching a videotape of the rape on slow rewind." She visualized the rape scenes from the end to the beginning, and by the end of that session, her VOC had changed considerably. She began by believing that she could have prevented the rape somehow—by obeying her fiancé, by not asking the man for drugs or taking him to her apartment—and that she had made bad decisions that put her at risk. That belief changed to her realization that he was in control throughout the incident and that she could not have controlled the situation as she had previously thought. She ranked her feelings that the new belief was true at a 5.

Her SUDS level lowered to a 6 at the end of the session, and she expressed relief at feeling less self-blame and guilt over the sexual assault. The therapist asked her to note and record any thoughts and feelings associated with the rape or session during the week, to monitor the number of intrusive thoughts and her anxiety levels, and to bring her journal to the next session. At that session, the client disclosed that her VOC and SUDS levels had changed during the week, with the VOC at a 10 and the SUDS at a 3. She stated that her anxiety level and number of intrusive thoughts had also decreased.

She also revealed that related nodes of control and emotional abuse issues were triggered. She described having past relationships with controlling men who were both emotionally and physically abusive, and she expressed anger at the way her fiancé had reacted to her rape. She related that he had blamed her, yelled at her, and was not supportive about her feelings or reactions to the rape. She discussed whether she wanted to continue this pattern of abusive, controlling relationships or to reevaluate her upcoming nuptials. We continued the EMDR techniques, focusing on these related nodes and issues, rather than the sexual assault, as she requested. Her VOC at the beginning of the session was that she sought out controlling relationships because of her own weaknesses (8 on a 10-point scale), and that was replaced with the belief that she could have a happier life without men telling her what to do (8 on a 10-point scale). Her SUDS level went from a 10, described as very agitated and angry, to a 7, and she expressed more confidence in herself and her decision-making skills at the end of the session.

By the third and last session, the client appeared to be much more confident and happy. She disclosed that she had ended her engagement and relationship with her fiancé and had already moved to another apartment with a girlfriend. She said that she was having very few anxious or intrusive thoughts about the rape, mostly in connection with the court process. She agreed to follow through with the victim advocate at the prosecutor's office and to contact me if additional sessions were needed during this process. She described herself as being very happy with her decisions SUDS-1 and felt she had gained insight into a destructive pattern in her life that she wanted to discontinue VOC-2. The therapist also referred her to a support group for sexual assault survivors, in case she needed any additional long-term therapy. The client expressed satisfaction with the EMDR treatment and felt that she didn't need any more individual sessions at that time, nor did she want to follow up with the group, but she did take the contact information for the future if needed. EMDR techniques were implemented to address any residual effects of the sessions, and a body scan and relaxation exercises finished the session.

Step 5: Evaluating Practice Effectiveness

This particular case resulted in successful completion of the client's goals for therapy. She made remarkable progress in only three sessions, which reflects one of the basic principles of EMDR: that resolution of the trauma can happen as immediately as the trauma effects were instilled at the time of the incident(s). This challenges the traditional beliefs that it takes time to grieve and mourn and that healing and resolution take many years.

On a subsequent follow-up phone call to the client, she stated that she was doing great, not dating any one seriously, and being more selective about her choices in men. She related having more confidence in herself and her decisions and liked the direction her life was going, both professionally and personally. She did not feel the need for any continuing clinical treatment and had worked with the victim advocate during the court proceedings. The offender had taken a plea bargain so she did not have to testify at the hearing, which was a relief for her.

I have experienced the effects of EMDR myself as the client in the experiential exercises in the Level II training and as the therapist with clients in private practice. Some of my clients have benefited from EMDR, and others did not like it or find it helpful. In my experience, clients who have direct, clear memories and can visualize well are more receptive to the process and techniques. Of course, one must always be critical of client self-reports with issues of social desirability and bias.

Step 6: Advocating and Teaching Others

The last step in evidence-based practice is to advocate and teach others, which I have done by publishing scholarly literature about EMDR and by informing graduate students of the model in social work direct practice classes. I hope that through dissemination of the research, professional literature, and continuing educational opportunities about EMDR, more social workers and professional counselors will learn the model and incorporate it in their practice when appropriate. I also hope that this chapter has interested the reader in further exploration and learning of EMDR through the resources discussed here.

CONCLUSION

This chapter has presented the principles and steps of evidence-based practice in an attempt to convey to the reader the importance of critically analyzing and implementing the current best evidence for treatment effectiveness and to continue to develop one's clinical skills.

The motivation to lifelong learning remains the challenge, since complacency with one's expertise may lull one into thinking there is no more to learn. With the advances and changes in our world, the potential for contributing to the knowledge base of clinical practice reaches far beyond the university classroom to the practice community, where the integration of theories and skills emerges. Leadership in developing and promoting evidence-based practice must come from those who are committed to continuing professional development based on empirical evidence. Commitment to evidence-based practice requires courage and effort, combined with an inner sense of purpose that guides professional excellence—that is the challenge to the helping professional.

References

Alto, C. (2001). Meta-analysis of eye movement desensitization and reprocessing efficacy studies in the treatment of PTSD. *Dissertation Abstracts International: Section B: The Sciences and Engineering, 62*(5-B), 2474.

Chemtob, C. M., Nakashima, J., & Carlson, J. G. (2002). Brief treatment for elementary school children with disaster-related posttraumatic stress disorder: A field study. *Journal of Clinical Psychology, 58*(1), 99–112.

Dawkins, K. (Producer/Director). (1999). *EMDR: A closer look* [Videorecording]. New York: Guilford.

DeJongh, A., vandenOord, H. J. M., & ten Broeke, E. (2002). Efficacy of eye movement desensitization and reprocessing in the treatment of specific phobia: Four single-case studies on dental phobia. *Journal of Clinical Psychology, 57*(12), 1489–1503.

Dziegielewski, S. F., & Wolfe, P. (2000). Eye movement desensitization and reprocessing (EMDR) as a time-limited treatment intervention for body image disturbance and self-esteem: A single subject case design study. *Journal of Psychotherapy in Independent Practice, 1*(3), 1–16.

Edmond, T., Rubin, A., & Wambach, K. G. (1999). The effectiveness of EMDR with adult female survivors of childhood sexual abuse. *Social Work Research, 23*(2), 103–116.

Evidence-Based Medicine Working Group. (1992). Evidence-based medicine: A new approach to teaching the practice of medicine. *Journal of the American Medical Association, 268*(17), 2420–2425.

Gambrill, E. (1999). Evidence-based practice: An alternative to authority-based practice. *Families in Society: Journal of Contemporary Human Services, 80*(4), 341–350.

Gibbs, L. (2003). *Evidence-based practice for the helping professions: A practical guide with integrated multimedia.* Pacific Grove, CA: Brooks/Cole–Thompson Learning.

Grant, M., & Threlfo, C. (2002). EMDR in the treatment of chronic pain. *Journal of Clinical Psychology, 58*(12), 1505–1520.

Gross, L., & Ratner, H. (2002). The use of hypnosis and EMDR combined with energy therapies in the treatment of phobias, and dissociative, posttraumatic stress, and eating disorders. In F. R. Gallo (Ed.), *Energy psychology in psychotherapy: A comprehensive sourcebook* (pp. 219–231). New York: W. W. Norton.

Knox, K. S. (2002). Case application of EMDR in trauma work. *Brief Treatment and Crisis Intervention, 2*(1), 49–53.

Korn, D. L., & Leeds, A. M. (2002). Preliminary evidence of efficacy for EMDR resource development and installation in the stabilization phase of treatment of complex posttraumatic stress disorder. *Journal of Clinical Psychology, 58*(12), 1465–1487.

Largo-Marsh, L., & Spates, C. R. (2002). The effects of writing therapy in comparison to EMDR on traumatic stress: The relationship between hypnotizability and client expectancy to outcome. *Professional Psychology: Research and Practice, 33*(6), 581–586.

Lipsitz, J. D., & Marshall, R. D. (2001). Alternative psychotherapy approaches for social anxiety disorder. *Psychiatric Clinics of America, 24*(4), 817–829.

Manfield, P. (Ed.). (1998). *Extending EMDR: A casebook of innovative applications.* New York: W. W. Norton.

McCann, D. (1992). Post-traumatic stress disorder due to devastating burns overcome by a single session of eye movement desensitization. *Journal of Behavior Therapy and Experimental Psychiatry, 23*, 319–323.

Paulsen, S. (1995). Eye movement desensitization and reprocessing: Its cautious use in dissociative disorders. *Dissociation, 8*(1), 3–44.

Roberts, A. (1996). Epidemiology and definitions of acute crisis in American society. In A. Roberts (Ed.), *Crisis management and brief treatment: Theory, techniques, and application* (pp. 16–33). Chicago: Nelson-Hall.

Rosen, A., & Proctor, E. K. (2002). Standards for evidence-based social work practice: The role of replicable and appropriate interventions, outcomes, and practice guidelines. In A. R. Roberts & G. J. Greene (Eds.), *Social workers' desk reference* (pp. 743–747). New York: Oxford University Press.

Rosen, G. (1999). Treatment fidelity and research on eye movement desensitization and reprocessing (EMDR). *Journal of Anxiety Disorders, 13*, 173–184.

Rubin, A. (2002). Eye movement desensitization and reprocessing. In A. R. Roberts & G. J. Greene (Eds.), *Social workers' desk reference* (pp. 412–417). New York: Oxford University Press.

Sackett, D. L., Rosenberg, W. M., Gray, J. A. M.,

Haynes, R. B., & Richardson W. S. (1996). Evidence-based medicine: What it is and isn't. *British Medical Journal, 312*, 71–72.

Sanderson, A., & Carpenter, R. (1992). Eye movement desensitization versus image confrontation: A single-session crossover study of 58 phobic subjects. *Journal of Behavior Therapy and Experimental Psychiatry, 23*, 269–275.

Shapiro, F. (1994). *Eye movement desensitization and reprocessing: Level I training manual.* Pacific Grove, CA: EMDR Institute.

Shapiro, F. (1995). *Eye movement desensitization and reprocessing: Basic principles, protocols, and procedures.* New York: Guilford.

Shapiro, F., & Forrest, M. S. (1997). *EMDR: The breakthrough therapy for overcoming anxiety, stress, and trauma.* New York: Basic Books.

Soberman, G. B., Greenwald, R., & Rule, D. L. (2002). A controlled study of eye movement desensitization and reprocessing (EMDR) for boys with conduct problems. *Journal of Aggression, Maltreatment and Trauma, 6*(1), 217–236.

Sprang, G. (2001). The use of eye movement desensitization and reprocessing (EMDR) in the treatment of traumatic stress and complicated mourning: Psychological and behavioral outcomes. *Research on Social Work Practice, 11*(3), 300–320.

Taylor, R. J. (2002). Family reunification with reactive attachment disorder children: A brief treatment. *Contemporary Family Therapy, 24*(3), 475–481.

Taylor, S., Thordarson, D. S., Maxfield, L., Fedoroff, I. C., Lovell, K., & Ogrodniczuk, J. (2003). Comparative efficacy, speed, and adverse effects of three PTSD treatments: Exposure therapy, EMDR, and relaxation training. *Journal of Consulting and Clinical Psychology, 7*(2), 330–338.

Thyer, B. A. (2002). Principles of evidence-based practice and treatment development. In A. R. Roberts & G. J. Greene (Eds.), *Social workers' desk reference* (pp. 739–742). New York: Oxford University Press.

Tinker, R., & Wilson, S. (1999). *Through the eyes of a child: EMDR with children.* New York: W. W. Norton.

Vandiver, V. L. (2002). Step-by-step practice guidelines for using evidence-based practice and expert consensus in mental health settings. In A. R. Roberts & G. J. Greene (Eds.), *Social workers' desk reference,* (pp. 731–738). New York: Oxford University Press.

Wilson, S., Becker, L., & Tinker, R. (1995). Eye movement desensitization and reprocessing (EMDR) treatment for psychologically traumatized individuals. *Journal of Consulting and Clinical Psychology, 63*(6), 928–937.

34

DYSTHYMIC DISORDER AND THE COLLEGE STUDENT

Evidence-Based Mental Health Approach

Joseph Walsh & Jacqueline Corcoran

This chapter describes the efforts of a clinical social worker to provide evidence-based interventions to a female college student with dysthymic disorder. This disorder is a relatively chronic (at least 2 years) low-grade depression that afflicts between 3% and 6% of the population (American Psychiatric Association [APA], 2000). Women are two to three times more likely to suffer from dysthymic disorder than men (APA, 2000). The disorder usually emerges in adolescence or young adulthood, although it can begin in middle age. Comorbidity is a significant issue for those suffering from the disorder, with three quarters having another medical or psychiatric problem. Common comorbid diagnoses include anxiety disorder (such as panic disorder and social phobia) and alcohol use disorders, but the most prevalent is major depressive disorder (Brunello et al., 1999).

Despite the prevalence and negative impact of dysthymic disorder, it tends to be underdiagnosed and go untreated (Division of Psychopharmacology, 1997). People with the disorder may not see themselves as depressed. They may present only to their general practitioners, who may not recognize and classify the symptoms correctly, especially if medical problems are the main complaint. Dysthymic disorder results in significant impairment, however, and can put people at risk for major depression, according to a review by Schmaling, Dimidjian, Katon, and Sullivan (2002). Therefore, accurate diagnosis and appropriate treatment by clinical social workers are critical for its resolution.

EVIDENCE-BASED PRACTICE

Evidence-based practice is a process of locating research findings through electronic searches in a particular problem area to decide the intervention that has the best available support. To promote confidence in one approach over another for a defined problem, priority is given to studies using experimental designs (randomization to treatment conditions and a control group, pretest–posttest follow-up, data collection with standardized measures), followed by comparison-group studies (with randomization to treatment conditions and then comparison group designs with nonrandomization), and finally pretest–posttest designs. (For discussions of evidence-based practice, see Chambless & Hollon, 1998; Cournoyer & Powers, 2002; Gambrill, 1999; Sackett, Robinson, Rosenberg, & Haynes, 1997; Thyer, 2002.)

STEPS FOR USING PRACTICE GUIDELINES

Vandiver (2002) provides one example of a structured process to guide evidence-based clinical social work with practice guidelines:

1. Conduct a thorough assessment to serve as a guide for selecting a diagnosis.
2. Arrive at a five-axis diagnosis and, if available, select diagnosis-specific practice guidelines.
3. Use the practice guidelines or expert consensus literature for assistance with identi-

fying and articulating the presenting problem and for strategies to track client change.

4. Develop clear goals.
5. Use practice guidelines to develop an intervention plan.
6. Use practice guidelines to establish appropriate outcome measures.
7. Evaluate the intervention.

The remainder of this chapter, which describes an intervention conducted by a male social worker with a female client, is organized in accordance with this outline.

CASE ILLUSTRATION

The Agency

The Student Counseling Center (SCC) provides individual and group mental health counseling services at a university located in a large urban environment. The center is staffed by professionals from the fields of psychology and social work and also includes dozens of graduate students in training and newly graduated practitioners in residency. Students and residents participate intensively in educational programs while at SCC, and clinical supervision is extensive. The agency has not formally embraced a strict evidence-based approach to practice, but because it is a university setting staff and students tend to be well informed about the most recent clinical research.

The Assessment

Consuela (who preferred to be called Connie) was a self-referred 21-year-old single psychology major in her senior year who also worked 30 hours per week as a retail makeup artist. She arrived for her initial interview in casual dress, well groomed and healthy in appearance. She maintained excellent eye contact, was highly verbal, and demonstrated an appropriate range of facial expressions. She lived locally with her mother. Both of her parents were born in Puerto Rico, and Connie was born and raised in Spanish Harlem, New York City.

Connie shared concerns about having a "pessimistic outlook," a lack of trust in other people, and general feelings of negativity. She said that these feelings were intensified by a romantic relationship that was "going bad." Connie described herself, however, as being generally unhappy and said that she "worried way too much about a lot of things." She admitted to chronic fears about unfaithfulness and jealousy in all of her relationships and to frequent angry outbursts when feeling threatened. The client often resorted to sarcastic comments toward people close to her, describing her behavior at those times as "hyperemotional" and admitting that it had driven away many of her friends. Connie also reported excessive worrying about tuition debt and school performance, although these were not primary concerns (she was passing all of her courses).

The client explained that her unhappiness became worse after seeing her boyfriend casually talking with another woman at a party. She and her boyfriend (also of Puerto Rican heritage) had been seeing each other exclusively for 4 months, and she described the relationship in mostly positive terms. She was unsure whether there was any factual basis for her feelings of jealousy. Connie felt that this episode represented a recurring pattern in her life that needed to be addressed in counseling.

Connie had received counseling on two previous occasions. One year ago she had seen a social worker in private practice approximately four times, in connection with another boyfriend problem. She quickly felt better and discontinued that intervention. Further, when her parents divorced 13 years ago, Connie was referred to a school-based group for children of divorced parents. She attended "a couple of times" but had no recollection of issues discussed there.

Connie was an only child. Her parents were married for 14 years before divorcing when Connie was 8 years old. Her mother had already moved to their current city of residence, however, 3 years prior to the divorce. Connie remained in the custody of her father, now 48, who worked as a computer programmer in New York City. Although Connie lived with her father until finishing high school, she described their relationship as "not good." She said that he was not affectionate toward her and was still bitter about the divorce. She said, "He sees me as an obligation," "has no feelings of love toward me," and had not offered any financial support for her schooling. She described him as having a problem with alcohol and added that several members of her extended family had substance abuse problems. Connie's mother, 46, with whom she got along well, worked full-time as an aide for a city councilman. She had never remarried. Connie's grandparents were deceased, but she had an extensive network of aunts, uncles, and cousins in New York City with whom she remained in regular contact.

School and her job occupied most of Connie's time (she was on schedule to graduate in 3 months), but she maintained an active social life. She reported knowing "a lot of people" but had only two close friends, one male and one female, besides her boyfriend. She liked to shop, dance, work, go to movies, and visit parks. Her strengths included a strong work ethic, great talent in cosmetic work, intelligence, social skills, and the ability to take care of herself.

Connie had no health or medical problems and did not take any medications. She admitted to smoking marijuana every few weeks and to smoking cigarettes and drinking alcohol socially "during weekends." She said that she was cautious about how she drank because of the alcohol problems in her family. Interestingly, she added that she would not consider using medications to deal with her problems. She felt strongly that people should be able to learn to overcome their problems without using drugs of any type.

Diagnosis

Based on her presenting symptoms, the social worker diagnosed Connie on Axis I with dysthymic disorder, early onset, and a partner relational problem. She had felt depressed most of the day, for most days, since mid-adolescence. Her primary symptoms included low self-esteem (feeling inferior to and detached from her friends and peers), difficulty in making decisions to a degree that she regularly felt anxious and overwhelmed, overeating, and feelings of hopelessness with occasional ruminations about self-harm. The relationship between her and her boyfriend was characterized by many arguments. The social worker made no diagnoses on either Axis II or Axis III. On Axis IV he noted problems with the primary support group (her father and her boyfriend). He scored her global assessment of functioning at 60, because of her moderate symptoms and ability to generally function well in school and at work.

Articulation of the Problem for Work

The social worker was trained in both ego psychology and cognitive therapy but was inclined to use the latter perspective in this case because of the client's observed habit of ruminating about her problems rather than acting on them. He conceptualized her as a young adult whose negative core beliefs regarding her self-worth and lovability were contributing to her present relationship problems. He looked to the literature for any support for interventions related to cognitive theory.

EMPIRICAL BASIS FOR INTERVENTION

A review of the literature was conducted in PsychInfo for the last 5 years using the term *dysthymia*. This yielded 375 studies. A meta-analysis of 15 studies involving antidepressants versus placebo found antidepressants to be efficacious in the treatment of dysthymia. No differences emerged between and within classes of drugs (Lima & Moncrieff, 2002). In individual studies, cognitive-behavioral therapy, most often problem-solving therapy, was compared against medication and placebo, and few differences were found between conditions, with all showing improvement (Barret et al., 2001; Ravindran et al., 1999). Findings were mixed as to whether adding cognitive-behavioral therapy to medication improves outcomes (Hellerstein et al., 2001; Ravindran et al., 1999).

A related literature review on depression was conducted to examine the treatment of major depressive disorder. Substantial empirical evidence developed from randomized comparison group and control group designs and meta-analyses have indicated support for cognitive therapy for this disorder (DeRubeis & Crits-Cristoph, 1998; Dobson, 1989; Gaffan, Tsaousis, & Kemp-Wheeler, 1995; Young, Weinberger, & Beck, 2001). The social worker determined that he could use several nonmedication intervention techniques described in the literature that were found to be effective in treating clients with dysthymic disorder and major depression.

CONCEPTS USED TO GUIDE THE INTERVENTION

In evidence-based practice, concepts used for articulating outcomes (conditions that an intervention is intended to affect) and interventions (the activities undertaken by the practitioner to achieve the desired outcomes) must be operationally defined (Rosen & Proctor, 2002).

Goals

During the assessment, Connie articulated three goals for her counseling: improving her ability to cope with negative feelings, developing a more positive outlook on her life, and understanding the root causes of her relationship patterns so that she could manage them more satisfactorily. The social worker did not question or fundamentally change any of these, but he helped the client articulate them in a manner that would more clearly suggest intervention strategies and outcome indicators. Connie's goals remained somewhat abstract, but concrete indicators were attached to them, as follows:

- I will resolve the status of my current romantic relationship as evidenced by my self-report of satisfaction with the manner in which my boyfriend and I are relating to one another (this includes the possibility of our relationship ending).
- I will develop a positive sense of self-worth as evidenced by making positive statements to my social worker about my actions when reviewing interpersonal events of significance.
- I will develop improved relationship patterns as evidenced by (a) spending more time with people other than my boyfriend and two close friends and (b) arguing less with all of my friends.
- I will clarify the nature of my relationship with my father as evidenced by (a) sharing my feelings about our relationship with him and (b) attempting to reach a mutual agreement about how we will organize our relationship for the future.
- The client agreed with the social worker's suggestion that they monitor her progress during each session by rating her self-reports regarding each goal on a scale of 1 to 10, with the higher number indicating positive change. The use of such individualized rating scales has been shown to be an effective means of evaluating progress in clinical intervention (Bloom, Fischer, & Orme, 1995).

The Intervention Plan

The intervention plan was constructed collaboratively between social worker and client during their first session. Based on the social worker's awareness of the literature on effective practice, he recommended the following procedures: The social worker and client would meet once per week for 1 hour of individual counseling. Connie was opposed to group counseling, stating that the format would inhibit her participation. They agreed to six sessions (the social worker's standard approach), after which they would formally review Connie's progress and decide whether to meet further, based on the client's perceptions of her gains. The social worker introduced Connie to his philosophy of cognitive therapy and its rationale. Orienting clients to the theory and general procedures has been shown to enhance its effectiveness (Beck, 1995). The social worker shared his concern with Connie that she was so obsessively self-analytical that exclusively reflective interventions might be detrimental to her. He did not describe the specific techniques he planned to use with her, but they included relaxation techniques for anxiety management, self-talk, thought stopping, and point-counterpoint. All of these have been shown to be effective in treating dysthymic disorder (Jacobson et al., 1996). He would also expect Connie to perform tasks between sessions as "homework" (Niemeyer & Fleixas, 1990).

Part of researching practice guidelines is learning about the characteristics of the ethnic group of which the client is a member when it differs from the practitioner's own. Members of ethnic groups often have unique perspectives on themselves, the world, and the nature of clinical intervention. The social worker, a middle-aged Caucasian male from a small Midwestern city, reviewed two textbooks for information about persons from Puerto Rico (Fong & Furuto, 2001; Green, 1999). He learned that Puerto Ricans are the second-largest Latino subgroup in the United States. Their culture emphasizes spirituality (sometimes out of the frame of formal religion), the importance of extended and cross-generational family, and the values of community, children, respect, and cooperation. Interestingly, and significant to Connie's presentation, Latino children tend to have a heightened sensitivity to the nonverbal behaviors of others. Latino people also value personalism in relationships—informality and warmth rather than observances of formal roles.

THE INTERVENTION PROCESS

The social worker met with Connie eight times. During their second session, Connie shared many more details of her background. The social worker observed that Connie was insecure and continuously self-critical, and she assumed that she was not attractive to others. He presented Connie with three strategies that she could use to gain a sense of control over her environment and combat her tendencies to ruminate over negative possibilities. He described the first, deep breathing, as a means for her to relax before entering any potentially anxiety-provoking interpersonal situations (Davis, Eschelman, & McKay, 1995). Through thought stopping (Peden, Rayens, Hall, & Beebe, 2001), Connie could interrupt her negative interpretations of the behaviors of significant others with images that were more pleasing to her. The point-counterpoint technique (Leahy, 1996) would require Connie at the end of each day to review events of concern and list on a sheet of paper the evidence for and against her interpretations. Connie responded positively to these ideas, which represented new strategies for her. She practiced them with the social worker and further agreed to practice the breathing and thought-stopping techniques for 15 minutes each day to gain facility in their use.

During the third session, they continued to focus on Connie's cognitive patterns and her capacity to reevaluate the external evidence for her beliefs. The social worker noted that Connie had made improvements in her ability to control negative thoughts with the application of the techniques introduced the previous week. To support his observations, the social worker (during this and every subsequent meeting) asked Connie to chart her movement toward each goal on the informally created scales discussed earlier. Their discussion then focused on Connie's fears of losing friends by driving them away with her complaints. The social worker suggested an additional behavioral strategy in which the client would limit the amount of time she talks about her worries with those close to her (Richey, 1994). She agreed and decided herself that she would carry a watch and limit herself to 5 minutes per interaction. Toward the end of the hour, the social worker affirmed her progress in therapy and used their relationship to illustrate how her habits of seeing herself through the eyes of others may be skewed toward a negative end. That is, Connie had been playing out her relationship problems with the social worker, wondering openly at times if he cared about her. The social worker used these instances to practice the point-counterpoint technique with her.

At the next session, Connie continued to demonstrate progress. She had developed insight into her unrealistic suspiciousness and jealousy, thus making quick progress in her feelings about herself and others. The social worker praised the client's accomplishments. Despite this, she continued to perceive rejection frequently. In fact, she again admitted to distrusting the social worker's interest in her. He had noted in the beginning of their work that she was sensitive to nonverbal cues (a characteristic of many Puerto Rican people) and had been vigilant in this regard. Still, he was tired on this particular morning, and the client interpreted his affect as boredom. The social worker was careful to reassure the client by listening actively, conveying an attitude of goodwill, and expressing confidence in her.

The client canceled her next session because of a work conflict. One week later she returned and announced that she had broken up with her boyfriend. She felt it was the right decision but was having difficulty maintaining boundaries with her boyfriend since the event. Connie had been calling him five or more times per day to check on his whereabouts and mood. He processed this behavior with Connie and suggested she set limits on her extent of phone and in-person contact for at least 2 weeks so that she could make the transition out of the relationship. She was agreeable to limiting her calls to no more than two per day.

The following week, the client showed more confidence than the social worker had yet seen. For the first time, Connie appeared calm. She reported that the relationship with her boyfriend was over and they were having no further contact. Connie felt good about her decision and was regaining a sense of independence. The social worker guided her through a discussion about what she had learned from the boyfriend experience and from therapy thus far. This became their "review and renegotiation" session, 1 week early. Connie expressed her awareness that she could not control the behavior of others and that she needed to accept herself without so much external reassurance. It appeared that she had met her most immediate goals, but Connie wanted to spend more time in counseling to see if her changing attitudes would persist. The social worker and client agreed to meet for another 3 weeks to monitor her progress and begin to address the family issues that concerned her. The social worker reminded her to continue implementing the strategies they had rehearsed.

One week later, Connie was continuing to function well. She described several recent stressful scenarios involving family and friends and processed them with the social worker for his input about the "reality basis" of her thoughts, feelings, and behaviors. Connie spoke at length about her parents, particularly her father. She hoped that she could share her concerns about their relationship more openly with him now that her confidence was higher. The social worker knew that Connie would be having contact with him during the coming week and engaged her in several role plays, so that she could practice her communications and test how she might react to his behavior. Role plays are effective in both cognitive and behavioral therapy for helping dysthymic clients test out and refine new interaction strategies (Nurius & Berlin, 1994).

Ending and Evaluating the Intervention

The next week, Connie announced that this would be her final session. While earlier than expected, the decision seemed appropriate to the social worker. Connie's college graduation would take place in 3 weeks, and she wanted to focus her energies on that event, including arranging for several extended family members to join her at school. Once again the social worker and client reviewed her progress in therapy. Connie recorded her progress toward goal achievement on the rating scales, and the social worker emphasized her steady positive movement in all four areas over the past 7 weeks. The client had resolved her presenting problems, and her gains had persisted for several weeks. She no longer met the criteria for dysthymic disorder, but the social worker reminded Connie that she should self-monitor her mood for several more months, perhaps using the same scales, as a precaution against backsliding. They next reviewed her activities over the past week and her plans for the near future. The social worker was engaging Connie in a process of anticipatory guidance, a technique that helps clients maintain their therapy gains (Ludgate, 1995). He described a number of possible scenarios in the immediate future regarding her father and friends that might threaten Connie's progress and then helped her formulate adaptive responses for those scenarios. Since dysthymia tends to be a chronic, relapsing disorder and life stress events can bring about major depressive disorder (Moerk & Klein,

2000), continuation with treatment or maintenance of treatment gains is critically important (Oxman et al., 2001). As they ended, the social worker invited Connie to return if she so desired (she would retain service eligibility for 2 months after graduation), but he did not hear from her again.

LIMITATIONS OF THE PROCESS

Efforts to identify evidence-based practice models have been controversial among human service professionals (Beutler & Baker, 1998; Chambless, 1998; Elkin, 1999; Goldfried & Wolfe, 1998). In working with Connie, the social worker noted the following limitations of attempting to follow prescribed approaches:

- The literature on practice guidelines and expert consensus does not adequately address relationship factors in therapy. The social worker in this case continuously made quick decisions about how to interact with the client based on her changing and unpredictable thoughts, moods, and actions. These decisions reflected his experience rather than strict adherence to a particular intervention approach.
- In reading about practice guidelines, it seemed to the social worker that the personal characteristics of the practitioner were often overlooked, such as his or her experience with particular problem areas and interventions.
- Related to those points, efforts to use structured intervention manuals may unduly limit the natural responsiveness of practitioners in clinical situations. The social worker's choices about techniques in this case were based on what he found in the literature, but he adapted these to his own preferences and to the clinical situation as it unfolded.
- Diagnostic categories are rarely precise in capturing the essence of a clinical condition. Researchers tend not to be sensitive to differences among clients who share the same diagnosis. Variables such as social support, socioeconomic status, distress level, motivation, and intelligence may be more important predictors of client response to a model of intervention than diagnosis.

Clinical social workers, perhaps in collaboration with researchers, can disentangle the practitioner versus intervention strategy "confound" by assessing the practitioner's personal characteristics. Monitoring the clinical relationship might be a productive way to take this variable into account. Horvath's (1994) Working Alliance Inventory provides one example of doing so. The client and social worker complete the 36-item instrument at various intervals to provide comparison data on their perceptions of bonding, goal orientation, and task focus.

Focusing research on client characteristics that dictate therapeutic strategy might be a productive means of elaborating on the diagnosis–intervention connection (Beutler & Baker, 1998). Connie experienced dysthymic disorder, but the social worker felt that her progress was a function of her personal characteristics as much as his particular intervention strategies. She was an intelligent, motivated young woman with good social skills and the capacity to successfully manage a busy school and work life. Another client with different characteristics and a lower level of motivation may not have responded to the same techniques offered by this social worker.

Interestingly, Connie displayed some personality characteristics that were different from what might be expected of a woman with a strong Puerto Rican ethnic background. She certainly was sensitive to nonverbal behaviors and maintained an informal relationship with the social worker, but on the other hand her family background featured conflict and splintering rather than the close ties that are attributed to Puerto Rican families. Connie had also moved far away from her extended family, and she was willing to seek mental health treatment, when it is often described that those with Puerto Rican origins are more likely to get help from spiritual advisors or medical doctors (Garcia-Preto, 1996). Further, the client did not seem guided by a spiritual frame of reference. Thus, while understanding a client's unique cultural background is important, the social worker must be careful not to use this information to stereotype the client.

CONCLUSION

This chapter describes one social worker's process of applying evidence-based practice to the mental health problem of dysthymic disorder. His diagnosis, assessment, gathering of evidence on research-based treatments, collaborative implementation of techniques based on client char-

acteristics and cultural background, and evaluation of the effects of the intervention were demonstrated with a client seen in a university counseling center. Although dysthymic disorder has been discussed in this chapter as a mental health problem to which evidence-based practice can be applied, the process can be flexibly adapted to other mental health disorders for which people commonly seek help.

References

American Psychiatric Association. (2000). *Diagnostic and statistical manual of mental disorders* (4th ed., text revision). Washington, DC: Author.

Barret, J., Williams, J., Oxman, T., Frank, E., Katon, W., Sullivan, M., et al. (2001). Treatment of dysthymia and minor depression in primary care: A randomized trial in patients aged 18 to 59 years. *Journal of Family Practice, 50,* 405–412.

Beck, J. S. (1995). *Cognitive therapy: Basics and beyond.* New York: Guilford.

Beutler, L. E., & Baker, M. (1998). The movement toward empirical validation: At what level should we analyze, and who are the consumers? In K. S. Dobson, & K. D. Craig, (Eds.), *Empirically supported therapies: Best practice in professional psychology* (pp. 43–65). Thousand Oaks, CA: Sage.

Bloom, M., Fischer, J., & Orme, J. G. (1995). *Evaluating practice: Guidelines for the accountable professional* (2nd ed.). Needham Heights, MA: Allyn & Bacon.

Brunello, N., Akiskal, H., Boyer, P., Gessa, G. L., Howland, R. H., Langer, S. Z., et al. (1999). Dysthymia: Clinical picture, extent of overlap with chronic fatigue syndrome, neuropharmacological considerations, and new therapeutic vistas. *Journal of Affective Disorders, 52*(1–3), 275–290.

Chambless, D. L. (1998). Empirically validated treatments. In G. P. Koocher, J. C. Norcross, & S. S. Hill (Eds.), *Psychologists' desk reference* (pp. 209–219). New York: Oxford University Press.

Chambless, D. L., & Hollon, S. D. (1998). Defining empirically supported therapies. *Journal of Consulting and Clinical Psychology, 66,* 7–18.

Cournoyer, B., & Powers, G. (2002). Evidence-based social work: The quiet revolution. In A. Roberts & G. Greene (Eds.), *Social workers' desk reference* (pp. 798–807). New York: Oxford University Press.

Davis, M., Eschelman, E. R., & McKay, M. (1995). *The relaxation and stress reduction workbook.* New York: New Harbinger.

DeRubeis, R., & Crits-Cristoph, P. (1998). Empirically supported individual and group psychological treatments for adult mental disorders. *Journal of Consulting and Clinical Psychology, 66,* 37–52.

Division of Psychopharmacology, Vanderbilt University Medical Center. (1997). The undertreatment of dysthymia. *Journal of Clinical Psychiatry, 58,* 59–65.

Dobson, K. S. (1989). A meta-analysis of the efficacy of cognitive therapy for depression. *Journal of Consulting and Clinical Psychology, 57,* 414–419.

Elkin, I. (1999). A major dilemma in psychotherapy outcome research: Disentangling therapists from therapies. *Clinical Psychology Science and Practice, 6*(1), 10–32.

Fong, R., & Furuto, S. (Eds.). (2001). *Culturally competent practice: Skills interventions, and evaluations.* Boston: Allyn & Bacon.

Gaffan, E., Tsaousis, I., & Kemp-Wheeler, S. (1995). Researcher allegiance and meta-analysis: The case of cognitive therapy for depression. *Journal of Consulting and Clinical Psychology, 63,* 966–980.

Gambrill, E. (1999). Evidence-based practice: An alternative to authority-based practice. *Families in Society, 80,* 341–350.

Garcia-Preto, N. (1996). Puerto Rican families. In M. McGoldrick, J. Giordano, & J. Pearce (Eds.), *Ethnicity and family therapy* (2nd ed.). New York: Guilford.

Goldfried, M. R., & Wolfe, B. E. (1998). Toward a more clinically valid approach to therapy research. *Journal of Consulting and Clinical Psychology, 66*(1), 143–150.

Green, J. W. (1999). *Cultural awareness in the human services: A multi-ethnic approach* (3rd ed.). Boston: Allyn & Bacon.

Hellerstein, D., Little, S., Samstag, L., Batcheler, S., Muran, J., Fedak, M., et al. (2001). Adding group psychotherapy to medication treatment in dysthymia: A randomized prospective pilot study. *Journal of Psychotherapy Practice and Research, 10,* 93–103.

Horvath, A. O. (1994). Research on the alliance. In A. O. Horvath & L. S. Greenberg (Eds.), *The working alliance: Theory, research, and practice* (pp. 259–286). New York: Wiley.

Jacobson, N. S., Dobson, K. S., Truax, P. A., Addis, M. E., Koerner, K., Gollan, J. K., et al. (1996). A component analysis of cognitive-behavioral treatment of depression. *Journal of Consulting and Clinical Psychology, 64,* 295–304.

Katon, W., Russo, J., Frank, E., Barrett, J., Williams, J., Oxman, T., et al. (2002). Predictors of nonresponse to treatment in primary care patients with dysthymia. *General Hospital Psychiatry, 24,* 20–27.

Leahy, R. L. (1996). *Cognitive therapy: Basic principles and applications.* Northvale, NJ: Jason Aronson.

Lima, M., & Moncrieff, J. (2002). Drugs versus placebo for dysthymia (Cochrane Review). In *The Cochrane library, 4.* Oxford: Update Software.

Ludgate, J. L. (1995). *Maximizing psychotherapeutic gains and preventing relapse in emotionally distressed clients.* Sarasota, FL: Professional Resource Press.

Moerk, K., & Klein, D. (2000). The development of major depressive episodes during the course of dysthymic and episodic major depressive disorders: A retrospective examination of life events. *Journal of Affective Disorders, 58,* 117–123.

Neimeyer, R. A., & Fleixas, G. (1990). The role of homework and skill acquisition in the outcome of group cognitive therapy for depression. *Behavior Therapy, 21* (3), 281–292.

Nurius, P. S., & Berlin, S. B. (1994). Treatment of negative self-concept and depression. In D. K. Granvold (Ed.), *Cognitive and behavioral treatment: Methods and applications* (pp. 249–271). Pacific Grove, CA: Brooks/Cole.

Oxman, T. E., Barrett, J. E., Sengupta, A., Katon, W., Williams, J. W., Frank, E., et al. (2001). Status of minor depression or dysthymia in primary care following a randomized controlled treatment. *General Hospital Psychiatry, 23*(6), 301–310.

Peden, A. R., Rayens, M. K., Hall, L. A., & Beebe, L. H. (2001). Preventing depression in high-risk college women: A report of an 18-month follow-up. *Journal of American College Health, 49*(6), 299–306.

Ravindran, A., Anisman, H., Merali, Z., Charbonneau, Y., Telner, J., Bialik, R., et al. (1999). Treatment of primary dysthymia with group cognitive therapy and pharmacotherapy: Clinical symptoms and functional impairments. *American Journal of Psychiatry, 156,* 1273–1289.

Richey, C. A. (1994). Social support skill training. In D. K. Granvold (Ed.), *Cognitive and behavioral treatment: Methods and applications* (pp. 299–338). Pacific Grove, CA: Brooks/Cole.

Rosen, A., & Proctor, E. K. (2002). Standards for evidence-based social work practice: The role of replicable and appropriate interventions, outcomes, and practice guidelines. In A. R. Roberts & G. J. Greene (Eds.), *Social workers' desk reference* (pp. 743–747). New York: Oxford University Press.

Sackett, D., Robinson, W., Rosenberg, W., & Haynes, R. (1997). *Evidence-based medicine: How to practice and teach EBM.* New York: Churchill Livingston.

Schmaling, K., Dimidjian, S., Katon, W., & Sullivan, M. (2002). Response styles among patients with minor depression and dysthymia in primary care. *Journal of Abnormal Psychology, 111,* 350–356.

Thyer, B. A. (2002). Principles of evidence-based practice and treatment development. In A. R. Roberts & G. J. Greene (Eds.), *Social workers' desk ref-*

erence (pp. 739–742). New York: Oxford University Press.

Vandiver, V. L. (2002). Step-by-step practice guidelines for using evidence-based practice and expert consensus in mental health settings. In A. R. Roberts & G. J. Greene (Eds.), *Social workers'*

desk reference (pp. 731–738). New York: Oxford University Press.

Young, J., Weinberger, A., & Beck, A. (2001). Depression. In D. Barlow (Ed.), *Clinical handbook of psychological disorders: A step-by-step treatment manual* (3rd ed.). New York: Guilford.

35   IMPLEMENTING EVIDENCE-BASED PRACTICES IN OPIOID AGONIST THERAPY CLINICS

Mark L. Willenbring & Hildi Hagedorn

Opioid agonist therapy (OAT) is a form of treatment for opioid (mainly heroin) dependence, in which counseling and other psychosocial services are coupled with provision of a daily dose of an opioid agonist medication. Currently, three agonist medications are available: methadone, levo-alpha acetyl methadol (LAAM), and buprenorphine. Opioid addicts often have persistent dysphoria and craving after withdrawal from opioids, so providing a daily dose of a long-acting opioid medication reduces or eliminates craving and illicit drug use. Unfortunately, rehabilitation treatments with goals of abstinence from both illicit opioids (such as heroin) and prescribed opioids (such as methadone) are effective for only a small percentage of addicted persons (Magura & Rosenblum, 2001; Sees et al., 2000). In contrast, compelling evidence accumulated over three decades demonstrates that OAT is the most effective treatment for opioid dependence, leading to improved patient outcomes, including reduced drug and alcohol use, fewer psychiatric symptoms and medical problems (e.g., reduced prevalence of HIV infection, AIDS, tuberculosis, and hepatitis C), less involvement in criminal activity, improved psychosocial functioning, a higher likelihood of employment, and reduced premature mortality (Ball & Ross, 1991; Ling et al., 1998; Marsch, 1998; McLellan, Arndt, Metzger, Woody, & O'Brien, 1993; Newman & Whitehill, 1979; Sees et al., 2000; Zaric, Barnett, & Brandeau, 2000).

In addition to research into the effectiveness of OAT in general, there is a growing body of work demonstrating that OAT program characteristics, in interaction with each other and with client characteristics, are related to such outcomes as program retention and reduction in drug use (Chou, Hser, & Anglin, 1998; Joe, Simpson, & Broome, 1999). Such work has shown that program characteristics are stronger predictors of outcome than client characteristics (Magura, Nwakeze, & Demsky, 1998). Four individual elements of OAT programs have been particularly well studied.

Dose of opioid agonist (methadone or LAAM):
    Higher doses of methadone are associated

with decreased use of illicit opioids (Caplehorn, Dalton, Cluff, & Petrenas, 1994; del Rio, Mino, & Perneger, 1997; D'Ippoliti, Davoli, Perucci, Pasqualini, & Bargagli, 1998; Eissenberg et al., 1997; Hartel et al., 1995; Ling et al., 1998; McGlothlin & Anglin, 1981; Rhoades, Creson, Elk, Schmitz, & Grabowski, 1998) and improved program retention (Caplehorn & Bell, 1991; Caplehorn et al., 1994; del Rio et al., 1997; D'Ippoliti et al., 1998; McGlothlin & Anglin, 1981; Rhoades et al., 1998; Strain, Bigelow, Liebson, & Stitzer, 1999). Current guidelines call for doses of 60 mg per day of methadone or more (or its equivalent in LAAM) (del Rio et al., 1997; McGlothlin & Anglin, 1981; Strain et al., 1999). Some patients require much higher doses than that, and for most patients, methadone equivalent doses of 80 mg or more result in the least illicit opioid use (Caplehorn & Bell, 1991; Caplehorn et al., 1994; Maremmani et al., 2000).

Counseling: Although provision of an opioid agonist alone results in improvement in some patients, counseling is a necessary component for most (Broome, Simpson, & Joe, 1999; Hser, Grella, Hsieh, Anglin, & Brown, 1999; Joe et al., 1999; Magura et al., 1998). Counseling provided weekly for the first month of OAT, followed by an average of two visits per month, is adequate (McLellan et al., 1993). Increasing psychosocial services results in additional improvement in outcomes but may not be as cost-effective (Kraft, Roghbard, Hadley, McLellan, & Asch, 1997).

Maintenance (versus detoxification) orientation: Indefinite provision of OAT continues to be a subject of controversy because of a concern about "substituting one addiction for another." However, long-term maintenance has been supported by more than 30 years of research and leads to superior outcomes compared with detoxification, even when detoxification is combined with enhanced psychosocial services (Sees et al., 2000). A detoxification orientation is expressed in restrictive clinic policies and attitudes, such as placing an arbitrary limit on dose, encouraging patients to detoxify early in treatment, discouraging patient participation in decisions about dose of agonist, restrictive policies on take-home privileges, and excessively punitive policies about any illicit substance use (Caplehorn, 1994). Detoxification orientation among physicians and other staff members results in lower agonist doses, increased dropouts, and increased drug use among patients (Caplehorn, Irwig, & Saunders, 1996; Caplehorn, Lumley, & Irwig, 1998; Caplehorn, McNeil, & Kleinbaum, 1993; D'Ippoliti et al., 1998).

Contingency Management (CM): CM involves a system of incentives and disincentives that enhance motivation to reduce or eliminate drug use (Griffith, Rowan-Szal, Roark, & Simpson, 2000; Stitzer, Iguchi, & Felch, 1992). Randomized controlled trials have demonstrated that incentive systems produce reductions in illicit drug use and improve compliance with counseling and other therapeutic activities (Kidorf & Stitzer, 1999; Petry, 2000). The most effective incentive in the context of OAT is access to take-home doses (so patients do not have to come to the clinic every day). Our experience indicates that many OAT clinics reward clients with take-home doses contingent on abstinence from illicit substances. However, the rewards tend to occur too long after the contingent event (e.g., 90 days abstinence). CM research has shown the benefits of providing a reward for as little as two weeks of abstinence (Stitzer et al., 1992).

Refer to Table 35.1 for a summary of findings and references related to each of the four practice areas.

THE OPIOID AGONIST THERAPY EFFECTIVENESS (OPIATE) INITIATIVE

The OpiATE Initiative is a part of the Quality Enhancement Research Initiative (QUERI), a large-scale translational research program of the Veterans Affairs (VA) Health Services Research and Development Service (Demakis, McQueen, Kitzer, & Feussner, 2000; Finney, Willenbring, & Moos, 2000). One goal of the OpiATE Initiative is to develop and test methods for improving the quality of OAT services by implementing evidence-based practices.

Development of the Implementation Tool Kit

Few clinicians have time to keep up-to-date on new developments published in the professional

TABLE 35.1 Four Specific Clinical OAT Practices That Have a Strong Evidence Base

OAT Practice	Findings	Key References
Dose of opioid agonist (methadone, LAAM, buprenorphine)	• Most patients require at least 60 mg of daily methadone or equivalent doses of other agonists • Doses of 80 mg or more methadone equivalents improve outcomes	• Caplehorn & Bell, 1991 • McGlothlin & Anglin, 1981 • Rhoades et al., 1998 • Strain et al., 1999
Level of counseling support	• Minimum counseling (weekly × 4 weeks then twice monthly on average) most cost-effective • Additional psychosocial services improve outcomes	• Broome et al., 1999 • Kraft et al., 1997 • Magura et al., 1998 • McLellan et al., 1993
Goal orientation	• Indefinite maintenance orientation improves outcomes • Goal of "abstinence" (discontinuation of OAT) increases dropouts and illicit drug use	• Caplehorn, 1994 • Caplehorn et al., 1993 • Magura & Rosenblum, 2001 • Sees et al., 2000
Contingency management	• Using take-home doses as contingent incentives improves outcomes when done correctly	• Griffith et al., 2000 • Kidorf & Stitzer, 1999 • Petry, 2000 • Stitzer et al., 1992

literature. Even awareness of study results does not translate easily into an understanding of how this research should be applied. Clinicians need to have information presented to them in a way that is convincing and thorough yet facilitates rapid implementation. In other words, research needs to be interpreted and adapted to a real-world clinical environment.

Two tools were developed to address these concerns. First, brief summaries of evidence were created for each of the four practices. These summaries were complete but emphasized practical conclusions applicable to clinical work. Second, a tool was needed to assist physicians to individualize agonist dose. This is necessary because although guidelines call for most patients to receive a minimum of 60 mg methadone equivalents, some patients do well on lower doses. An expert consensus panel was convened to develop a specific strategy, which was summarized in a dosing consensus statement. A dosing algorithm was then developed that provides a stepwise decision process for determining the proper dose of agonist. A dose review form provided a way to document the individualized review of agonist dose for all patients receiving

less than 60 mg methadone equivalents using the dosing algorithm.

Another key challenge facing those wanting to implement evidence-based practices is to overcome clinician resistance. Especially in today's health care systems, most clinicians feel at least very busy, if not overwhelmed. The idea of adding any new activity or practice may seem impossible. Another staff-based barrier is that most clinicians feel that they are doing the right thing already (Noe & Markson, 1998), and they may be unaware of how their practices relate to evidence-based practice guidelines.

To meet this challenge, a log form was developed, on which staff can record patient-level data in less than two minutes per patient per month. The log provides information about agonist dose and counseling frequency. For the research demonstration project, completed forms were faxed to study staff, who entered the data and produced graphic feedback concerning each practice, which were then mailed to the program leaders. Feedback was given for the program as a whole and for individual clinicians. Programs were also given mean values from all participating sites to which they could compare their own data. A version of this log in which clinics can enter and analyze their own data is under development. Figure 35.1 provides an example of the log form.

Addressing program orientation (maintenance versus detoxification) involves analysis of clinic policies and assessment of clinician attitudes. The Abstinence Orientation Scale (Caplehorn et al., 1996, 1998) measures these attitudes that have previously been shown to predict program retention and illicit drug use (Caplehorn, 1994; Caplehorn et al., 1993). The Abstinence Orientation Scale includes 14 items scored on a 5-point Likert scale: 1 = strongly disagree to 5 = strongly agree. Scores are calculated by dividing the total for the scale by the number of questions answered. Higher scores represent a greater endorsement of abstinence-oriented attitudes. Representative statements include "Methadone maintenance patients who continue to use illicit opiates should have their dose of methadone reduced," "Maintenance patients who ignore repeated warnings to stop using illicit opiates should be gradually withdrawn off methadone," and "Methadone should be gradually withdrawn once a maintenance patient has ceased using illicit opiates." For a complete copy of all 14 Abstinence Orientation Scale items, see Caplehorn et al., 1998. In addition to this instrument, the study translation facilitator conducted a policy analysis with clinic leadership.

Finally, CM tools were developed to assist clinicians with implementation. In addition to the evidence summary, tools included an example CM policy, a guide for team discussion for tailoring the policy to the specific clinic, and a template for a patient CM contract.

The resulting tool kit, including evidence summaries, practice-monitoring forms, and specific quality improvement tools, is referred to as the OpiATE Monitoring System (OMS). Table 35.2 provides a summary of the components of the OMS for each of the four practice areas.

Implementing Quality Improvement

Site Recruitment

Nine sites were recruited by initially selecting a sample from available VA OAT programs. The sites included large and small clinics from diverse areas of the country. Of note is that the essentials of the tool kit had to be developed prior to site recruitment, because sites would not commit to participation unless they could have a concrete idea of exactly what would be required. This reflected anticipated concerns about perceptions of how busy clinicians were and how well received a new quality improvement (QI) initiative would be.

Baseline Assessment

The translation facilitator visited each facility for about 1.5 days. At this visit, staff were educated about evidence-based OAT practices and instructed in the use of the OMS. The translation facilitator also completed a policy review with clinic leadership. Following the site visit, staff completed the OMS baseline assessments and sent completed forms to the study center. The translation facilitator then reviewed the results of the baseline assessment with clinic leaders by telephone.

Goal Development

Using the information from the baseline assessment, the translation facilitator helped clinic

FORM 2. Baseline Case Management Log									
Clinic ID: 02						Begin date: ___ / ___ / ___		End date: ___ / ___ / ___	
Counselor ID: 02 - 01									
				TREATMENT PLAN				*OUTCOMES in Past 30 Days*	
Patient ID	Pt. birth month and day	Meth or LAAM? (circle)	Current dose* (mg/day)	Pt. treatment goal (circle one)	# of take-homes per week	# counsel. visits, past 30 days**	# utox screens, past 30 days***	# urines pos. for OPIOIDS, past 30 days**	# urines pos. for non-opioids, past 30 days** (EXCEPT cannabinoids)
0400	___ / ___	M L		detox maint					
0401	___ / ___	M L		detox maint					
0402	___ / ___	M L		detox maint					

FIGURE 35.1 OMS log form example

TABLE 35.2 Components of the OpiATE Monitoring System (OMS)

Evidence-Based Practice	Purpose	Tool
Prescribe adequate dose of opioid agonist	• Educate about evidence base and current guidelines • Determine current dosing pattern and compare with best practices • Provide guidance for individualizing dose	• Evidence summary • OMS log • Dosing algorithm • Dose review form
Provide adequate counseling	• Educate about evidence base and current guidelines • Determine current visit frequency and compare with best practices	• Evidence summary • OMS log
Approach OAT with maintenance orientation	• Educate about evidence base and current guidelines • Examine current clinic policies to determine concordance with best practices • Determine current staff orientation and compare with best practices	• Evidence summary • Policy review • Abstinence Orientation Scale
Optimal use of contingent incentives (contingency management)	• Educate about evidence base and current guidelines • Determine current use of contingency management and compare with best practices • Implement optimal contingency management practices	• Evidence summary • Policy review • Contingency management sample plan • Team discussion guide • Example patient contract

leaders develop specific goals for their program and at least a tentative strategy for achieving their goals. The first practice assessed and addressed is almost always dose. The rate of concordance with best practices is not clear until completion of the dose review for every patient receiving less than 60 mg of methadone equivalents. Although initial rates of concordance may vary considerably, all clinics using the system so far have determined that at least a few patients were receiving nonconcordant doses. For some clinics, nonconcordance with dose is a major concern, and considerable effort may be required to change staff beliefs and practices erroneously supporting the use of low doses.

Program orientation or philosophy is the second most common area of focus, and this focus has usually occurred simultaneously with the dose review. Detoxification orientation is associated with a low-dose approach (Caplehorn et al., 1993), and both are associated with poor retention and higher levels of illicit drug use (Caplehorn, 1994; Caplehorn et al., 1998; Mc-

Glothlin & Anglin, 1981; Strain et al., 1999). Clinics may also have policies that place an arbitrary upper limit on dose. Program orientation is also related to use of contingent incentives, one of the most common policy areas nonconcordant with best practices. Clinics most often use punishment such as revocation of take-home doses and dose reduction as ways to discourage illicit drug use and other unhealthy behaviors. Furthermore, lengthy periods of improvement such as three months are often required in order to start earning privileges. Providing the tools to implement more optimal and effective use of contingent incentives has been helpful to programs wishing to change punitive policies, such as administrative discharge for illicit drug use.

At times, intermediate goals are adopted in order to make implementation of the best practices possible. For example, clinics may have to increase their use of urine drug screens in order to implement CM principles. Finally, the process of goal development is not static. New goals are selected as initial goals are met.

Implementation and Change

Programs implemented strategies to achieve goals and were assisted in doing so by monthly telephone consultations with the translation facilitator and by a regularly scheduled conference call that included clinic leaders at each involved site.

Reevaluation

Clinic staff filled out the OMS log on a monthly basis. Reassessment of program orientation using the Abstinence Orientation Scale was recommended every three to six months.

Experience to Date with the OMS

OpiATE Initiative staff members have been working intensively with nine VA OAT clinics on refinement, implementation, and evaluation of the OMS. These nine clinics have been working on QI using the OMS for varying amounts of time (8 months to 1 year). Response to the OMS system has been highly positive. Clinic leaders report that the amount of time that staff are required to spend collecting necessary data is well worth the quality of feedback received. They also report that having well-defined QI goals, with regular feedback to track progress on these goals, has been positively received by Joint Commission on Accreditation of Healthcare Organizations reviewers.

All nine clinics have completed a baseline assessment and have prioritized their QI goals. Counseling was adequate in all of the nine clinics at the time of the baseline assessment. Dose reviews revealed variation from dosing recommendations for five of the nine clinics. All of these five clinics have demonstrated increases in their dose concordance. Increases in the percentage of patients receiving doses of 60 mg or more range from 3% to 15%, depending on how long the clinic has been using the OMS system and the level of concordance with dose recommendations at baseline. Two of the five clinics are now in concordance with dosing recommendations and have shifted focus to CM goals. The other three clinics continue to use monthly dose reviews to increase concordance. Of the remaining four clinics, two identified both program philosophy and CM as areas of QI, and two were strong on concordance with recommendations regarding program philosophy and are focusing on establishing or refining CM protocols. Qualitative data from monthly consultation and research evaluation calls with clinic leadership have documented changes in clinic policies that have increased concordance with best-practice recommendations in these areas.

The most important lesson learned from experience with these nine OAT clinics is that substantial prompting is necessary to create and sustain momentum for change. Participation in this intervention was often viewed as an additional burden for both clinic leadership and staff. Feedback from participating clinics indicated that continuing contact with the OpiATE Initiative staff was vital to establishing and maintaining momentum. Through monthly facilitation calls, conference calls, and research calls, clinic leaders were constantly reminded of their identified goals and the steps that they had committed to making in pursuit of their goals. Even with this high level of contact, circumstances arose that forced leadership and staff to divert their attention to other pressing issues, and progress with QI goals would stagnate for a month or more. Feedback from participating clinics indicated that without continuing contact with the OpiATE Initiative staff, it would be unlikely that the clinic would return to a QI focus after such a period of stagnation.

For clinics that choose to implement the OMS independently, a high level of commitment to the process on the part of clinic leadership is necessary, as implementation will require staff time and clinic resources. It is absolutely essential that someone is designated to be responsible for maintaining the QI focus. Volunteers are preferable for this role to ensure that they are motivated and excited about taking on this challenging task. This person's duties will include assuring that clinic staff turn in all necessary data, that feedback is provided in a timely manner, that baseline data are reviewed and QI goals selected, and that appropriate QI strategies are identified and implemented. This person should be a clinic leader or have the full support of clinic leadership in order to have the power to request necessary materials from other staff members and instruct other staff on policy changes. Freeing up some portion of the responsible person's time to devote to this process is preferable.

In summary, practice change in the context

of providing a treatment as complex as OAT is a difficult undertaking. We have developed a system that provides fast and easy assessment of clinic practices and outcomes, that allows tailoring of the QI process to the individual clinic's needs, and that provides educational materials and QI tools to assist in making the process as simple as possible. Clinics currently using the OMS perceive that the value of implementation is worth the effort required. Data provided by the system have documented changes in clinical practices directly and immediately resulting from its use, as well as continuing efforts to change. At the completion of the OpiATE Initiative, future clinics that undertake this challenging process will be able to produce evidence demonstrating a positive change in clinic practices and will have the knowledge that they are providing the best possible care to a group of patients badly in need of it.

Note

For copies of OpiATE Monitoring System forms and tools referenced in the text, contact Hildi Hagedorn at 612-467-3875 or hildi.hagedorn@med.va.gov.

References

Ball, J. C., & Ross, A. (1991). *The effectiveness of methadone maintenance treatment.* New York: Springer Verlag.

Broome, K. M., Simpson, D. D., & Joe, G. W. (1999). Patient and program attributes related to treatment process indicators in DATOS. *Drug and Alcohol Dependence, 57,* 127–135.

Caplehorn, J. R. (1994). A comparison of abstinence-oriented and indefinite methadone maintenance treatment. *The International Journal of the Addictions, 29*(11), 1361–1375.

Caplehorn, J. R., & Bell, J. (1991). Methadone dosage and retention of patients in maintenance treatment. *The Medical Journal of Australia, 154,* 195–199.

Caplehorn, J. R., Dalton, M. S., Cluff, M. C., & Petrenas, A. (1994). Retention in methadone maintenance and heroin addicts' risk of death. *Addiction, 89,* 203–207.

Caplehorn, J. R., Irwig, L., & Saunders, J. B. (1996). Physicians' attitudes and retention of patients in their methadone maintenance programs. *Substance Use and Misuse, 31*(6), 663–677.

Caplehorn, J. R., Lumley, T. S., & Irwig, L. (1998). Staff attitudes and retention of patients in methadone maintenance programs. *Drug and Alcohol Dependence, 52,* 57–61.

Caplehorn, J. R., McNeil, D. R., & Kleinbaum, D. G.

(1993). Clinic policy and retention in methadone maintenance. *The International Journal of the Addictions, 28*(1), 73–89.

Chou, C. P., Hser, Y. I., & Anglin, M. D. (1998). Interaction effects of client and treatment program characteristics on retention: An exploratory analysis using hierarchical linear models. *Substance Use and Misuse, 33*(11), 2281–2301.

Del Rio, M., Mino, A., & Perneger, T. V. (1997). Predictors of patient retention in a newly established methadone maintenance treatment program. *Addiction, 92*(10), 1353–1360.

Demakis, J. G., McQueen, L., Kitzer, K. W., & Feussner, J. R. (2000). Quality Enhancement Research Initiative (QUERI): A collaboration between research and clinical practice. *Medical Care, 38*(6 Suppl 1), I17–I25.

D'Ippoliti, D., Davoli, M., Perucci, C. A., Pasqualini, F., & Bargagli, A. M. (1998). Retention in treatment of heroin users in Italy: The role of treatment type and of methadone maintenance dosage. *Drug and Alcohol Dependence, 52*(2), 167–171.

Eissenberg, T., Bigelow, G. E., Strain, E. C., Walsh, S. L., Brooner, R. K., Stitzer, M. L., et al. (1997). Dose-related efficacy of levomethadyl acetate for treatment of opioid dependence. *Journal of the American Medical Association, 277*(24), 1945–1951.

Finney, J. W., Willenbring, M. L., & Moos, R. H. (2000). Improving the quality of VA care for patients with substance use disorders: The Quality Enhancement Research Initiative (QUERI) substance abuse module. *Medical Care, 38*(6 Suppl 1), I105–I113.

Griffith, J. D., Rowan-Szal, G. A., Roark, R. R., & Simpson, D. D. (2000). Contingency management in outpatient methadone treatment: A meta-analysis. *Drug and Alcohol Dependence, 58,* 55–66.

Hartel, D. M., Schoenbaum, E. E., Selwyn, P. A., Kline, J., Davenny, K., Klein, R. S., et al. (1995). Heroin use during methadone maintenance treatment: The importance of methadone dose and cocaine use. *American Journal of Public Health, 85*(1), 83–88.

Hser, Y. I., Grella, C. E., Hsieh, S., Anglin, M. D., & Brown, B. S. (1999). Prior treatment experience related to process and outcomes in DATOS. *Drug and Alcohol Dependence, 57,* 138–150.

Joe, G. W., Simpson, D. D., & Broome, K. M. (1999). Retention and patient engagement models for different treatment modalities in DATOS. *Drug and Alcohol Dependence, 57,* 113–125.

Kidorf, M., & Stitzer, M. L. (1999). Contingent access to clinical privileges reduces drug abuse in methadone maintenance patients. In S. T. Higgins & K. Silverman (Eds.), *Motivating behavior change among illicit-drug abusers: Research on contin-*

gency management interventions (pp. 221–241). Washington, DC: American Psychological Association.

Kraft, M. K., Roghbard, A. B., Hadley, T. R., McLellan, A. T., & Asch, D. A. (1997). Are supplementary services provided during methadone maintenance really cost-effective? *American Journal of Psychiatry, 154*(9), 1214–1219.

Ling, W., Charuvastra, C., Collins, J. F., Batki, S., Brown Jr., L. S., Kintaudi, P., et al. (1998). Buprenorphine maintenance treatment of opiate dependence: A multicenter, randomized clinical trial. *Addiction, 93*(4), 475–486.

Magura, S., Nwakeze, P. C., & Demsky, S. Y. (1998). Pre- and in-treatment predictors of retention in methadone treatment using survival analysis. *Addiction, 93*(1), 51–60.

Magura, S., & Rosenblum, A. (2001). Leaving methadone treatment: Lessons learned, lessons forgotten, lessons ignored. *Mount Sinai Journal of Medicine, 68*(1), 62–74.

Maremmani, I., Zolesi, O., Aglietti, M., Marini, G., Tagliamonte, M., Shinderman, M., et al. (2000). Methadone dose and retention during treatment of heroin addicts with Axis I psychiatric comorbidity. *Journal of Addictive Diseases, 19*(2), 29–41.

Marsch, L. A. (1998). The efficacy of methadone maintenance interventions in reducing illicit opiate use, HIV risk behavior, and criminality: A meta-analysis. *Addiction, 93*, 515–532.

McGlothlin, W. H., & Anglin, D. (1981). Long-term follow-up of clients of high- and low-dose methadone programs. *Archives of General Psychiatry, 38*, 1055–1063.

McLellan, A. T., Arndt, I. O., Metzger, D. S., Woody, G. E., & O'Brien, C. P. (1993). The effects of psychosocial services in substance abuse treatment. *Journal of the American Medical Association, 269*(15), 1953–1959.

Newman, R. G., & Whitehill, W. B. (1979). Double-blind comparisons of methadone and placebo maintenance treatments of narcotic addicts. *Lancet, 8141*, 485–488.

Noe, C. A., & Markson, L. J. (1998). Pneumococcal vaccination: Perceptions of primary care physicians. *Preventive Medicine, 27*(6), 767–772.

Petry, N. M. (2000). A comprehensive guide to the application of contingency management procedures in clinical setting. *Drug and Alcohol Dependence, 58*, 9–25.

Rhoades, H. M., Creson, D., Elk, R., Schmitz, J., & Grabowski, J. (1998). Retention, HIV risk, and illicit drug use during treatment: Methadone dose and visit frequency. *American Journal of Public Health, 88*(1), 34–39.

Sees, K. L., Delucchi, K. L., Masson, C., Rosen, A., Clark, H. W., Robillard, H., et al. (2000). Methadone maintenance vs. 180-day psychosocially enriched detoxification for treatment of opioid dependence: A randomized controlled trial. *Journal of the American Medical Association, 283*(10), 1303–1310.

Stitzer, M. L., Iguchi, M. Y., & Felch, L. J. (1992). Contingent take-home incentive: Effects on drug use of methadone maintenance patients. *Journal of Consulting and Clinical Psychology, 60*(6), 927–934.

Strain, E. C., Bigelow, G. E., Liebson, I. A., & Stitzer, M. L. (1999). Moderate- vs. high-dose methadone in the treatment of opioid dependence: A randomized trial. *Journal of the American Medical Association, 281*(11), 1000–1005.

Zaric, G. S., Barnett, P., & Brandeau, M. (2000). HIV transmission and the cost-effectiveness of methadone maintenance. *American Journal of Public Health, 90*, 1100–1111.

36

EVIDENCE-BASED COUPLES THERAPY WITH DEPRESSED CLIENTS

Jacqueline Corcoran

Evidence-based involves a process of comprehensively gathering and then synthesizing treatment outcome studies in a particular problem area or with a certain population in order to find the treatment with the best available empirical support. A second aspect to evidence-based practice involves the quantitative assessment and evaluation of the individual client's progress in response to the treatment chosen (Cournoyer & Powers, 2002). Following an evidence-based approach, this chapter explores the treatments designed and tested for patients whose depression and marital problems co-occur. Available outcome studies are reviewed, and cognitive-behavioral marital therapy is presented, along with a case illustration.[1]

STATEMENT OF THE PROBLEM

According to the National Institute of Mental Health (NIMH, 2001), in any 1-year period, almost a tenth (9.5%) of the U.S. population, translating into 18.8 million adults, experience depression. Depression is often associated with marital problems (Beach, Fincham, & Katz, 1998; O'Leary, Christian, & Mendell, 1994; Weissman, 1987). Indeed, a review of the literature indicates that 40% to 50% of individuals suffering with depression also present with significant marital discord (Prince & Jacobson, 1995). The relationship seems to be reciprocal in nature in that marital problems can lead to depression (Beach, Harwood, Horan, et al., 1995, cited in Beach et al., 1998; Fincham, Beach, Harold, & Osborne, 1997) and depression can result in marital problems (Prince & Jacobson, 1995).

While individual therapy is often selected for individuals who are depressed, Beach and Whitman (1994) estimate that possibly 40% of those who have a diagnosis of major depression are suitable candidates for a conjoint intervention. To determine whether individual or couples treatment is more appropriate for an individual with depression, see the guidelines in Table 36.1.

EVIDENCE BASIS

A small body of literature has accumulated on the use of conjoint therapy to treat depression when marital discord is also present. See Table 36.2 for a detailing of studies. Despite the limitations of the studies, including small sample size and a reliance on white, middle-class samples, overall, it appears that when couples report marital distress and when the depressed partner views the depression as connected to marital problems, then conjoint therapy is the treatment of choice. While marital and individual therapy, no matter the theoretical framework—cognitive-behavioral or interpersonal therapy—produce equally effective results in terms of reducing depression, marital interventions are superior for positively impacting the couple relationship. These results seem to hold for individuals seeking treatment in outpatient settings; the one study on hospitalized individuals did not find an advantage for marital therapy over individual supportive psychotherapy for either the individual or the couple. More studies looked at women exclusively (Jacobson et al., 1991; O'Leary & Beach, 1990; Waring, 1994) than at both men and women (Emanuels-Zuurveen & Emmel-

TABLE 36.1 Individual or Couples for the
Treatment of Depression?

Individual is indicated if:

- Client is suicidal.
- The individual sees the depression as arising
  before relationship problems or as unrelated
  to the relationship.
- Client wants to attend to a lot of personal is-
  sues.
- Marital violence is present.
- There is lack of commitment to the relation-
  ship.
- A partner is having an affair.

Conjoint therapy is indicated if:

- Individual perceives the depression as caused
  by relationship problems (Addis & Jacobson,
  1996; Beach & O'Leary, 1992; O'Leary,
  Risso, & Beach, 1990).
- A moderate rather than severe level of conflict exists in the relationship.
- The woman in the relationship is depressed.
  (More studies have been conducted with
  women, although men should also benefit.)

COGNITIVE-BEHAVIORAL CONJOINT TREATMENT

kamp, 1996; Foley et al., 1989), although men
also benefit.

While there are varying formats for conjoint
therapy for the treatment of depression, Beach,
Sandeen, and O'Leary (1990) have done extensive research and writing on the topic, and
therefore, their marital therapy format will be
presented here. Cognitive-behavioral marital
therapy is a skill-building approach following
the principles of social learning, cognitive techniques, and behavioral exchange. Skills are
taught to enhance marital support and intimacy
and to reduce marital stress and negative expectancies. Behavioral methods of change are used
to teach skills. The therapist models and then
acts as surrogate partner for each person so that
skills are rehearsed. Feedback is provided, keeping in mind that depressed individuals might
personalize and globalize statements. Only when

behavior is successfully performed in session
should clients be assigned it as homework. Practice of skills at home is critical to the model's
success.

Application

In the upcoming sections, the different stages of
cognitive-behavioral marital therapy are illustrated in a case study. Assessment of the depression, engagement of the spouse, and the
three stages described by Beach et al. (1990) in
their cognitive-behavioral format are discussed
and applied. In the first stage, couple cohesion,
caring, and companionship are enhanced, while
negative patterns, such as criticism and blame,
lack of time spent together, and threats to terminate the relationship, are addressed. The second stage is more flexible and individualized to
a couple's needs, although structuring communication and teaching problem-solving skills are
major focuses. The third stage is geared toward
helping couples maintain their changes and preventing relapse of couple distress and depression
(Beach et al., 1990).

CASE STUDY

Gloria Herbert sought the help of a therapist at
the suggestion of her 2-year-old daughter's pe-
diatrician. Gloria's daughter had suffered from
repeated colds and flu, and Gloria was crying at
the doctor's office about feeling overwhelmed by
taking care of her three children (ages 1, 2, and
4) without any support from her husband, Jim.
Jim worked long hours as a bricklayer and often
spent time after work socializing with the other
men at the job site. When he got home, Gloria
was sick of staying home with the children all
day long and resentful that her husband did not
spend more time with his family, help around
the house, and give her a break from the children. They would invariably argue about this
during the evenings. Jim wanted to be responsible for working and making money; her responsibility was to look after the children. Gloria
said she wouldn't mind working again because
she missed the camaraderie at the office where
she used to hold the position of receptionist. Jim
said her job didn't pay enough and that it would
end up costing them more in childcare to have
her working than the money she would earn.

TABLE 36.2 Studies Involving the Treatment of Depression and Marital Discord

Author and Therapy	Design and Sample	Findings	Limitations
Emanuels-Zuurveen & Emmelkamp (1996) Skills-building marital therapy 16 sessions	Random assignment to individual cognitive-behavioral or marital therapy N = 27 men and women experiencing marital distress	Individual and marital therapy were equally effective in reducing depression; while there were positive effects from both treatments on the marital relationship, the marital condition produced a significantly greater impact.	Small sample size; lack of follow-up
Foley et al. (1989) Interpersonal therapy	Random assignment to either individual or conjoint interpersonal therapy N = 18 married men and women; all couples reported marital distress	Both individual and conjoint conditions demonstrated amelioration of depression; the conjoint condition was somewhat more effective at positively impacting the marital relationship.	Small sample size; lack of follow-up
Jacobson et al. (1991, 1993) Behavioral couple therapy	Random assignment to behavioral couple therapy, individual cognitive-behavioral therapy, and combined couple and individual therapy N = 60 married women with major depression (did not screen for marital dissatisfaction)	For people who were distressed but without marital discord, individual or combined couple and individual reduced depression; for couples in which at least one spouse reported marital distress, individual and couple therapy were equally effective in reducing depression but only the couple condition produced positive effects on the marital relationship. Relapse rates for depression were not significantly different between groups at 6- and 12-month follow-ups.	Small sample size
O'Leary, Riso, & Beach (1990); Beach & O'Leary (1992) Behavioral marital therapy 15 sessions	Random assignment to behavioral marital therapy, individual cognitive therapy, or waitlist control N = 45 couples in which both partners complained of marital discord and the wife had either major depression or dysthmia	Marital therapy and individual therapy were equally effective in reducing depressive symptoms over the control group; marital therapy was more effective in improving marital adjustment over individual therapy and waitlist control. These results were found at both posttest and 1-year follow-up.	Small sample size

Author and Therapy	Design and Sample	Findings	Limitations
Waring (1988); Waring (1994) Marital therapy focusing on self-disclosure between partners 10 sessions	*Study I*: Random assignment to marital therapy + antidepressant medication or supportive psychotherapy + antidepressant medication *N* = 27 married women who were hospitalized for depression	*Study I*: Marital therapy performed significantly less well than the control group on lowering depression scores.	High attrition rate; small sample size; lack of follow-up
	Study II: Random assignment to antidepressant or placebo and then random assignment to either marital therapy or supportive psychiatrist–couple contact *N* = 29 married women with depression seen on an outpatient basis	*Study II*: Marital therapy did not produce significantly greater reductions in depression than the support condition but did show improvements in sexuality scores for the couple over the support condition.	
	Study III: Random assignment to marital therapy or waitlist control *N* = 17 married women, seen in an outpatient setting, who attributed their depression to marital problems	*Study III*: Marital therapy significantly reduced depression in comparison with the control group; pretest to posttest, there were significant improvements on some aspects of marital intimacy for the marital therapy group.	

He was critical that she was not able to manage her responsibilities better; they had only three children, whereas they had both come from large families, and their mothers had done just fine. Gloria would then point out that her own mother had a drinking problem. She also resented her mother-in-law for being judgmental of Gloria for not cooking meals for Jim and for not being a better disciplinarian of her children. Jim would subsequently become defensive on behalf of his mother.

Gloria further described difficulties in getting up in the morning, crying spells throughout the day, and irritability with her children. She admitted that she fluctuated in her treatment of them: Sometimes she yelled at them harshly, and other times she would let them get away with the same infraction. She also felt disgusted

with herself for the weight she had gained during her pregnancies and had not lost. She said it didn't help that her husband would tease her about it and compare her unfavorably with his own sister, who had managed to maintain her figure despite childrearing.

Jim complained that their sex life had not returned to normal after the birth of her last child. Gloria said she felt uncomfortable with all the weight she had failed to lose, especially when he teased her. She also admitted that her resentment at him had undercut her desire. Gloria said she sometimes felt like running away and hated what her life had become, but she did not consider hurting herself.

When asked about her sources of support, Gloria said she didn't have much in common anymore with her former work mates and hadn't developed other friendships since she was "always stuck in the house." As described, her mother was an inconsistent support because of a drinking problem. Gloria also had a sister; however, she had children of her own and worked outside the home, so they didn't see each other often. In addition, Gloria's sister and husband were doing better financially than Gloria and her husband, so contact made Gloria feel jealous and even worse about herself.

During the assessment, the therapist administered the Beck Depression Inventory to Gloria. Results indicated that Gloria was experiencing a moderate level of depression. Gloria attributed her depression to her marital problems. Since the best determinant of the appropriateness of conjoint therapy is the individual's perception of a causal relationship between marital distress and depression rather than a score on a standardized measure (Foley, Rounsaville, & Weissman, 1989; O'Leary & Beach, 1990), the therapist posed the option of marital counseling.

Jim agreed to attend, if it could help Gloria feel better. In the first conjoint session, Jim said he and his wife didn't have marital problems; the only problem they had was Gloria's dissatisfaction with her life. The therapist gave Jim a publication from NIMH (2001), which provided some information for family members of people with depression. The therapist also educated him that many of the symptoms his wife was experiencing—tearfulness, irritability, dissatisfaction, lack of enjoyment, weight gain—could be attributed to depression, which, with treatment, would in all likelihood lift.

Stage One

The marital therapy started in stage one with alleviating the negative patterns that had developed in the marriage, such as criticism and blame, and the fact that Gloria felt stuck at home with young children. The therapist posed deductive questions about the effects of their criticism and blaming on each other: "Gloria, how do you feel when he compares you with his sister?" "Jim, how do you feel when you come home and she starts yelling at you?" "Does that get you what you want?" "How is that improving the closeness in your marriage?" Both partners could see the destructive effects such communication had in terms of feelings of defensiveness and then counterattacks. However, the cou-

ple found such behaviors difficult to stop. The therapist continued to block this pattern as it arose in sessions and redirect the couple to deductive questioning to get them to examine their behaviors and be willing to take different actions.

The other destructive pattern in the relationship was that Gloria was isolated at home with young children. The therapist explored various options about what Gloria could do to experience some relief from childcare. This was also in alignment with the goal of increasing individual activities, since a typical expectation from individuals with depression is that their partner should be their primary source of satisfaction in terms of companionship and activities. However, this places a significant burden on spouses, decreasing couple cohesion.

Gloria said that a few women in her neighborhood were licensed daycare providers. Jim had not wanted to spend money on childcare before because "that was what his wife was for." But when he understood the necessity of her getting some respite, he realized that it was money well spent, ruefully admitting that the cost might not be much more than what he spent on the six-packs he bought for the guys at work.[2]

Once some of the couple's negative patterns were addressed, the therapist turned toward increasing satisfaction in the relationship. One way to achieve this aim was through helping them schedule pleasant events, so that the relationship became associated with enjoyment and pleasure rather than coercion and dissatisfaction (Beach et al., 1990). The Herberts agreed to go dancing, an activity they used to enjoy before the birth of their second child. They also agreed to have an outing each week as a family—to a park or a playground.

During stage one, partners are also trained on complimenting, how to positively track and reinforce a partner's behaviors by communicating verbally their appreciation the other's behaviors or qualities (Beach et al., 1990). The therapist modeled and then rehearsed with each partner how to both give and receive compliments. With feedback and prompting, Gloria was able to tell Jim that she liked his body, compliment him on his ability to work hard and provide for the family, and express appreciation for his participation in counseling. Jim told Gloria that he liked how she fixed her hair, that she was taking care of the children, and that she was addressing her problems through counseling so that she could be a better mother.

Because the couple appeared to have difficulty following through with complimenting outside the sessions, the therapist questioned them about the barriers involved. Both partners said that complimenting each other seemed artificial. The therapist asked them to remember back to the beginning of the relationship. Gloria and Jim recalled that compliments had been abundant initially, when the relationship had been more positive overall. The therapist urged them to return to this pattern, reiterating her original explanation of complimenting, which was that it helped build positive feelings and let the partner know what behaviors to continue. She asked them how it felt when they received compliments: Jim said he already knew how Gloria felt without her having to say anything; Gloria said that compliments made her feel uncomfortable, like she didn't deserve them.

The therapist went on to address the couple's beliefs. First, she asked Jim if he could always read Gloria accurately, and he admitted he didn't. The therapist talked about some of the dangers of "mind reading," which tends to be negatively biased for people with depression and for couples who were experiencing marital discord. The therapist then discussed Gloria's belief that she didn't deserve compliments and that this type of thinking might be leading to depression. The therapist taught the process of cognitive restructuring in which negative and irrational thoughts were recognized, debunked, and then replaced with positive thoughts.

Another way the therapist built marital cohesion was through behavior exchange, increasing the number of day-to-day caring gestures (Beach et al., 1990). (For the process of assigning behavior exchange, see Table 36.3.) Jim wanted meals prepared when he got home from work, which he said would motivate him to come home earlier. He also requested more sex ("at least once a week"). Gloria asked Jim for more time spent alone with her after the children had gone to bed without him falling asleep on the couch watching TV. She also wanted him to take the children out once a week so that she could have time for herself.

Stage Two

Stage two of the therapy process is more individualized, addressing the particular concerns of

TABLE 36.3 Guidelines for Behavior Exchange (Wheeler et al., 2001)

1. Each partner is instructed to compile a list of activities that each can do to improve the other person's satisfaction with the relationship.

2. The activities on the list should involve:
   - small and concrete units of behavior that are already part of the other person's repertoire
   - increased positive behavior rather than decreased negative behavior
   - the potential for frequent performance
   - being under the giver's total control
   - no monetary expenditure attached to them

3. Lists are discussed in session.

4. Each partner is assigned to do one of the activities on the list each day (Beach et al., 1990) to once a week (Wheeler et al., 2001) without waiting until the other person has acted before implementing the spouse's desired activities.

5. When a caring gesture has been performed, the receiver should provide recognition in terms of complimenting, displaying a pleased facial expression, and attending physically to the partner simultaneously.

6. Each person should track his or her own caring gestures in a place the spouse can access (Cordova & Jacobson, 1993). In this way, spouses are trained to notice the other partner's positive actions, which helps to emphasize individual responsibility for the change process.

7. In the next session, partners are asked to evaluate the caring gestures they performed and what effect they had on the partner.

the couple, although it should contain communication and problem-solving training. In the first part of communication training, couples are taught the necessity of talking about their own feelings and revealing their vulnerabilities in the relationship rather than accusing and blaming the other person. After building this rationale, the practitioner provided the basic format for giving "I" messages: I feel (the reaction) to what happened (a specific activating event). For example, Gloria was able to say: "Jim, I feel sad when you spend time with the guys after work instead of coming straight home to be with me and the kids." The couple was also taught reflective listening so that the speaker's perspective is understood by the partner. It prevents partners' tendency to draw conclusions about the intentions and meaning of a partner's statement (i.e., "mind reading") (Wheeler, Christensen, & Jacobson, 2001). For example, Jim, in response to Gloria's message, said: "You feel sad when it seems like I don't want to spend time with you."

As part of communication skills training, couples are further trained on how to make specific behavior requests. People with depression often have difficulty with specifics and clarity, often seeing others or life circumstances in absolutist and negative terms ("Why even bother? Nothing's going to change"). Several guidelines are offered for making requests more effective, including that they should be specific, measurable, and stated as the presence of positive behaviors rather than the absence of negative behaviors. With the therapist's help, Gloria was able to formulate the following request to Jim: "I'd like you to spend 5 minutes playing with the children each night, and I would like you to talk to me for 15 minutes each night."

Gloria was also guilty of some unproductive communication patterns that are often characteristic of people with depression: seeking constant reassurance ("Do you still love me?" "Do you still think I'm pretty?" "Do you think I'm fat?") and negative verification ("I've gained a lot of weight, haven't I?" "Your sister looks better than me after having kids, doesn't she?"). Rather than Jim's current response, which was to react angrily to Gloria's attempts to engage him in these patterns, the therapist trained him how provide support at a general level without encouraging her to seek reassurance or negative feedback. Beach (personal communication, January 16, 2002) offers the following statement for spouses: "I am very committed to making our relationship work well and to helping you feel better. I would answer your question if I didn't think it would work against both those goals. I think it will be better if I show you over time instead of answering this question. Is that O.K.?" Just as important, Gloria was trained to notice that she had drifted into the reassurance-seeking pattern and to respond with the following: "Even though I really want to press you for an answer right now, I won't. I know you are doing what you think will help our relationship

the most in the long run." In this way, both partners act to help the couple exit from a counterproductive pattern.

Both partners found the communication skills training they received to be applicable to individual issues as well. For instance, in session, Jim practiced how he would address his mother about her tendency to criticize Gloria. Gloria used the new pattern of communicating to set limits on her mother's being around Gloria's children when she was drinking.

When communicating concerns fails to resolve a disagreement, problem-solving training is used to instruct couples on strategies they can use for managing problems of everyday life (Beach et al., 1990). The format for problem solving involves defining the problem, brainstorming, examining possible options, deciding on an option, implementing an option, and evaluating the implementation. As an example, the Herberts problem-solved about how to keep the house more organized. They brainstormed the following options: (a) training the children to put away their own toys and make their beds; (b) purchasing baskets for toys, mail, and other sundry items that accumulated around the house; (c) Jim taking on more responsibility for cleaning the house; (d) Gloria cleaning a different room in the house each day rather than feeling like she had to tackle it all at once and feeling overwhelmed; (e) hiring a teenager in the neighborhood to help clean; and (f) Gloria cleaning the house when the children were at childcare. Upon evaluation, all options seemed viable; the therapist then worked with the couple on exactly how each option could be implemented.

Stage Three

The ending stage of therapy involves slowly fading out the role of the therapist so that he or she is less involved in directing the activity of the session. Gains are highlighted and potential trouble spots are identified. The couple can be directed to use their problem-solving skills to examine how best to avoid possible pitfalls. The practitioner reinforces the skills the couple developed to manage depressive moods or relationship conflicts as they emerge. Booster sessions can also be scheduled so couples are reassured that they can fall back on the therapist if they are unable to extricate themselves from old patterns. After 16 weeks of therapy, the Herberts reported that they were "back on course" as a couple and now had some tools to help themselves "stay on course." Gloria retook the Beck Depression Inventory and scored in the nondepressed range. She reported that she had started playing tennis and walking with a neighbor on her half-day off, which resulted in some weight loss and increased feelings of well-being. She had also begun attending a parenting class, which offered support and instruction on how to better manage her children's behavior.

CONCLUSION

Following guidelines for evidence-based practice, this chapter has explored the treatment of depression when marital problems are also a significant issue, as they often are with depression. Cognitive-behavioral marital therapy offers promise for the alleviation of both problems in a relatively short-term treatment format. Beach et al.'s (1990) cognitive-behavioral format has been chosen specifically since a manual has been developed for its application, although the format shares components with other marital therapies used with depression. A case illustration demonstrated how the model can be applied in practice, with guidelines also offered for the evaluation of progress in treatment.

Notes

1. Parts of this chapter have been adapted from Corcoran's (2003) *Clinical Applications of Evidence-Based Family Intervention.*

2. As part of the assessment, Jim's drinking was examined, and both partners agreed that drinking was not an issue since Jim limited himself to two beers after work.

References

Addis, M., & Jacobson, N. (1991). Integration of cognitive therapy and behavioral marital therapy for depression. *Journal of Psychology Integration, 1,* 249–264.

Beach, S., Fincham, F., & Katz, J. (1998). Marital therapy in the treatment of depression: Toward a third generation of therapy and research. *Clinical Psychological Review, 18,* 635–661.

Beach, S., & O'Leary, K. (1992). Treating depression in the context of marital discord: Outcome and predictors of response of marital therapy versus cognitive therapy. *Behavior Therapy, 22,* 507–528.

Beach, S., Sandeen, E., & O'Leary, K. (1990). *Depression in marriage: A model for etiology and treatment.* New York: Guilford.

Beach, S., & Whitman, M. (1994). Marital therapy for depression: Theoretical foundation, current status, and future directions. *Behavior Therapy, 25,* 345–371.

Christensen, A., Jacobson, N., & Babcock, J. (1995). Integrative behavioral couple therapy. In N. S. Jacobson & A. S. Gurman (Eds.), *Clinical handbook of couple therapy* (pp. 31–64). New York: Guilford.

Corcoran, J. (2003). *Clinical applications of evidence-based family interventions.* New York: Oxford University Press.

Cordova, J., & Jacobson, N. (1993). *Couple distress* (pp. 481–512). New York: Guilford.

Cournoyer, B., & Powers, G. (2002) Evidence-based social work: The quiet revolution continues. In A. Roberts & G. Greene (Eds.), *Social workers' desk reference* (pp. 798–807). New York: Oxford University Press.

Emanuels-Zuurveen, L., & Emmelkamp. P. (1996). Individual behavioural-cognitive therapy v. marital therapy for depression in maritally distressed couples. *British Journal of Psychiatry, 169,* 181–188.

Fincham, F., Beach, S., Harold, G., & Osborne, L. (1997) Marital satisfaction and depression. *American Psychological Society, 8,* 351–357.

Foley, S., Rounsaville, B., Weissman, M., Sholomaskas, D., & Chevron, E. (1989). Individual versus conjoint interpersonal psychotherapy for depressed patients with marital disputes. *International Journal of Family Psychiatry, 10,* 29–42.

Gotlib, I., & Beach, S. (1995). A marital/family discord model of depression: Implications for therapeutic intervention. In N. S. Jacobson & A. S. Gurman (Eds.), *Clinical handbook of couple therapy* (pp. 411–436). New York: Guilford.

Jacobson, N. S., Dobson, K., Fruzzetti, A., Schmaling, K. B., & Salusky, S. (1991). Marital therapy as a treatment for depression. *Journal of Consulting and Clinical Psychology, 59,* 547–557.

Jacobson, N., Fruzzetti, A., Dobson, K., Whisman, M., & Hops, H. (1993). Couple therapy as a treatment for depression: II. The effects of relationship quality and therapy on depressive relapse. *Journal of Consulting and Clinical Psychology, 61,* 516–519.

Kung, W. (2000). The intertwined relationship between depression and marital distress: Elements of marital therapy conducive to effective treatment outcome. *Journal of Marital and Family Therapy, 26,* 51–63.

National Institute of Mental Health (NIMH). (2001). *Depression* (NIH Publication No. 00-3561). Retrieved January 16, 2002, from http://www.nimh.nih.gov/

O'Leary, K. D., Riso, L., & Beach, S. (1990). Attributions about the marital discord/depression link and therapy outcome. *Behavior Therapy, 21,* 413–422.

Prince, S., & Jacobson, N. (1995). A review and evaluation of marital and family therapies for affective disorders. *Journal of Marital and Family Therapy, 21,* 377–401.

Waring, E. (1998). *Enhancing marital therapy through cognitive self-disclosure.* New York: Brunner/Mazel.

Waring, E. (1994). The role of marital therapy in the treatment of depressed married women. *Canadian Journal of Psychiatry, 39,* 568–571.

Wheeler, Christensen, A., & Jacobson, N. (2001). Couple distress. In D. Barlow (Ed.), *Clinical handbook of psychological disorders: A step-by-step treatment manual* (3rd ed.). New York: Guilford.

SECTION IV

Epidemiological and Public Health Research

37 EPIDEMIOLOGY BASICS AND FOUNDATION SKILLS

David L. Streiner

No, you have not inadvertently picked up the wrong book; this is not (as some people might believe) a chapter on skin diseases. In fact, the root of the word *epidemiology* is *epidemic*, not *epidermis*. The full derivation is from the Greek *epi*, meaning "among," and *demos*, meaning "the people." Last's *Dictionary of Epidemiology* (2001) defines it as "the study of the distribution and determinants of health-related states or events in specified populations, and the application of this study to control of health problems" (p. 62), which really does not help too much in explaining the term. Somewhat more useful is Alderson's (1983) description of three types of studies used in epidemiological research.

Descriptive studies address questions such as "Who is most likely to develop a certain disorder?" (e.g., AIDS, schizophrenia, coronary heart disease), or "Is there any association between a putative risk factor and an outcome?" (e.g., early loss of a parent and suicide, or sexual abuse and dissociative reactions), or "What accounts for the sudden outbreak of a health problem?" (salmonella poisoning, Severe Acute Respiratory Syndrome (SARS), or "mass hysteria" in a boarding school). This type of research (a) looks at the world without trying to change it, (b) relies on existing databases such as census or medical insurance claims data, or (c) is based on surveys of large groups of people used to collect the information.

Once we have (or think we have) some idea of what factors are related to each other, we can ask more specific questions and move to the second type of epidemiological study, which involves *hypothesis testing*. For example, if we found in a large survey that people with a depressive disorder were more likely to have reported that they were orphaned at an early age, we can deliberately sample from one group of people who lost their parents when they were young and from another group whose parents are still alive to see if the prevalence of depression is higher in the first group. Again, the researcher is largely leaving the world as it is and simply gathering either more focused information or data from more specific groups—data that can either support or refute the hypothesis.

If the hypothesis survives its encounter with data (and it is amazing how few actually do; witness the demise of hypotheses linking high tension wires to leukemia, silicone breast implants to lupus, or ulcers to stress), we can move on to *intervention studies*. Now we have an opportunity to change things. Continuing with our example, we may design a study so that some children who suffered the loss of a parent get therapy and others are simply followed over time to see if the intervention results in a lower incidence of depression later in life. (Needless to say, with such a long time between the intervention and the outcome papers, a study such as this should only be undertaken by someone with tenure.) In the health care community, the intervention studies field is also called *clinical epidemiology*, whereas the first two types of research are referred to as *classical epidemiology* or *big-E epidemiology*.

Thus, epidemiology covers a broad spectrum, overlapping with demography at one end, survey research in the middle, and experimentation at the other end. The common thread is the focus on groups of people rather than on individuals, molecules, cells, or mice.

No self-respecting field can call itself a discipline unless it develops its own set of arcane words, and epidemiology is no exception. The next sections will introduce some of these terms and explain their meanings.

RESEARCH METHODS

There are many different types of designs used in research, each with its own strengths and weaknesses. Before discussing them, however, it is necessary to go over some of the elements common to all of them.

Design Elements

Observational or Experimental Studies

In *experimental studies*, the intervention is under the researcher's control. He or she determines which people receive a novel treatment, for example, and which receive treatment as usual or a placebo. The aim is to discover how the *independent variable*—the one under the researcher's control—affects the outcomes, or *dependent variables*. Observational studies, by contrast, are "experiments in nature." That is, by chance or choice some people in the community have been exposed to some risk factor (such as physical abuse, cigarette smoking, or being male) and others haven't been; and within each group, some have experienced the outcome of interest (psychological problems, lung cancer, or coronary heart disease) and others have not. The issue again is whether the outcome is more frequent in one group than the other. While experimental studies give us more definitive answers regarding causation (for reasons I will discuss later), they may be infeasible or unethical in many cases; for example, it would be hard for an ethics committee to approve a study that forced some people to smoke to see if smoking is associated with lung cancer later in life.

Direction of Data Gathering

Data can be gathered in one of two ways: (1) by looking forward in time and gathering them during the course of the study, or (2) by looking backward and using data that have already been collected. One advantage of *prospective* data collection is that the type of information, the definition of the disorder, and other matters can be worked out ahead of time and are therefore constant for all people in the study. Another major advantage is that a prospective design gives better information about the *directionality* between variables—which ones occurred before others, which strengthens the case if we want to say anything about causality. Studies that use *retrospective* data rely on existing databases or the participants' (fallible) memory. The advantage of retrospective data collection is that it is relatively cheap; the downside is that definitions of a disorder or diagnostic practices may have changed over the interval being studied, and the data were rarely gathered with researchers in mind, so important information may be missing.

Comparison Groups

It is not enough to know that 9% of children whose birth weight was less than 1,000 grams needed special assistance at school (Saigal, Hoult, Streiner, Stoskopf, & Rosenbaum, 2000) because we have nothing to which to compare this number. Is this figure higher, lower, or the same as the proportion for normal-birth-weight children? In order to answer this, we need a *comparison group*. Comparison groups can either be *historical*, meaning that data for them already exist; or *concurrent*, in which case they are enrolled in the study at the same time as the group under investigation. In this example a historical comparison group could have been gathered from school records whereas a concurrent group would be followed prospectively, alongside the study group. In experimental studies, the comparison group is often referred to as a *control group*.

Sampling

If we were interested in the relationship between parental loss and later depression, our *population* would be everyone who lost a parent before a certain age. It is obviously impossible to include all such people, if for no other reason than that no agency would pay us to travel all around the country (naturally visiting Hawaii in the winter and Ontario in the fall). Furthermore, statistics tell us that it is not necessary to measure everybody in the population that we are studying; we can look at a *sample*, or subset, of them. In a *random* sample every member of the population has an equal chance of being included; this is the technique used in most survey research and polls. However, sometimes random sampling may result in having too few people in certain groups, such as those over 80 years of age or belonging to a minority group. In this case it is necessary to use *stratified random sampling* in which the population is divided into strata (in this case, based on people's ages or ethnic backgrounds) and then randomly sampled within each stratum. This ensures that we will have a sufficient sample size in each stratum. Because we know how the strata deviate from a strictly random sample, we can correct for this during the analyses.

All too often studies use *haphazard sampling* in which people are selected simply because they are available. Doing a telephone survey during the day is easier than staffing the phones 24 hours a day but will result in a sample that is disproportionately composed of housewives, the unemployed, or shift workers. Most health care researchers are based at tertiary care teaching hospitals and draw their samples from these hospitals because of convenience. However, these hospitals tend to have more patients with serious problems than do community hospitals. The problem with haphazard sampling is that the people who are included likely differ in significant ways from the population at large.

Research Designs

I have alluded to the fact that there are many different ways to conduct a study based on the nature of the question, the availability of the data, and other issues. In this section, I will discuss the various designs in more detail. So that the reader can see how the same question can be approached from a number of different perspectives, I will use the same one throughout: whether there is an association between early parental loss and depression.

Cross-Sectional Survey

This design is used most often in conducting surveys. At one particular time people are interviewed to determine the presence or absence of both the risk factors (i.e., parental loss) and the outcomes (for example, depression, psychiatric hospitalization, or suicidal ideation). The advan-

tage of this design is that it is relatively cheap and simple to carry out. However, because information about the exposure and the outcome are gathered at the same time, it is impossible to determine causation; what the person being surveyed remembers as having occurred first may be distorted through recall bias (i.e., the depression may have been present before the parent died but not recognized until afterward). Also, this design fails to count people who may have died from the disorder and may miss those who have recovered.

Longitudinal Survey

One research design that helps solve the issue of whether the risk factor did in fact occur before the outcome is the *longitudinal survey*. This is basically a series of cross-sectional surveys carried out over a period of time and following the same people. This allows the researcher to select a subsample of people who did not have the outcome when they were interviewed during one wave of the study but developed it by the time a later wave was conducted. This strategy was used successfully in the Ontario Child Health Survey (Boyle et al., 1987) to identify risk factors for childhood psychological problems. The major problems associated with the longitudinal survey, naturally, are the cost and the fact that some participants are lost from one assessment wave to the next because they move, die, or become tired of being in the study.

Case-Control Study

In a *case-control study* people are identified on the basis of the *outcome*, and the search for the exposure is done retrospectively. For example, we would identify two groups, one depressed and one nondepressed, and then see if the proportion of participants who had lost one or both parents is higher in the first group than in the second. The advantages of case-control studies are their low cost and that they may offer the only feasible design when studying rare conditions. The disadvantages are many. The first disadvantage, as with cross-sectional surveys, is the reliance on recall. The major shortcoming of this type of study is the fact that the exposure may have been caused by some other factor that is correlated with the outcome—a problem called *confounding*. For example, low socioeconomic status is related both to premature death (which affects the parent) and to psychological problems (which affect the offspring), so it would be wrong to say that parental loss "causes" the depression; both may simply be markers of poorer economic circumstances.

Cohort Study

In a *cohort study* people are identified on the basis of the exposure and then followed to see whether those in the exposed group have a higher rate of the outcome than people in the comparison group. This type of study can be either prospective (e.g., people who have and have not lost their parents are identified now and followed for the next 10 to 15 years) or retrospective (through death records we identify people who were orphaned or not orphaned 10 to 15 years ago and see how many are depressed today). This is a more powerful design than the case-control one because people in the two groups can be matched for other factors, such as socioeconomic status, that may affect the outcome, and it establishes the timing and directionality of events. However, if the exposure is a popular treatment, it may be difficult to find a comparison group, and confounding may again be present in that the exposure itself may be related to some other unknown factors that are correlated with the outcome.

Randomized Controlled Trial

The *randomized controlled trial* (RCT) is a true experimental design in that the researcher has full control over who does and does not receive the intervention, and participants are randomly assigned to the groups. The major advantage of the RCT is that the groups studied will tend to be similar because possible confounding variables are balanced out by the randomization; for example, people from different socioeconomic strata should be equally represented in both groups. Its major problems are that (a) RCTs tend to be very expensive and time consuming; (b) those who volunteer are not likely to be representative of patients in general; (c) a potentially helpful treatment is withheld from half of the patients (or conversely, half are exposed to a potentially dangerous treatment); (d) the results may not be available for many years; and (e) randomization makes the groups equivalent only if the study has a very large number of

participants. Despite these drawbacks, however, the RCT remains the "gold standard" for establishing the effectiveness of a treatment or program.

Threats to Validity

The purpose of any study is to tell us what is really happening in the world: is depression related to early loss, or is cognitive behavioral therapy effective for patients with personality disorders, or is extremely low birth weight associated with later learning difficulties? We hope that the results from our sample can be generalized to the population at large so that our findings also hold true for similar people. Consequently, it is disconcerting, to say the least, to find different studies coming to opposite conclusions. For example, of the 27 articles that reported the relationship between obesity and socioeconomic status in men, 12 found a positive correlation, 12 found a negative one, and 3 reported no relationship (Sobal & Stunkard, 1989). The major reason for differences among studies is that all have flaws involving (a) the definition of the disorder or the phenomenon of interest, (b) the selection of subjects, or (c) the design or execution of the study itself. Cook and Campbell (1979) call these flaws *threats to validity*. In this section, I will discuss a few of them.

Healthy Worker Bias

Random sampling does not help us if the group from which the sample is drawn is unrepresentative of the population to which we want to generalize. Any study that draws its sample from working people—for example, using data from a company's medical claims database—is subject to the *healthy worker bias*. People who work are healthier than the population as a whole. The entire adult population consists of people who are working, those who are able to work but do not for one reason or another, and those who cannot work because of health problems. Any group of workers, by definition, does not include this last category of people, whose inclusion tends to lower the overall health status of the population. This selection bias operates even more strongly when the job applicants to a particular company or industry have to pass a physical examination, as in the armed forces or certain labor-intensive or highly critical jobs (e.g., airline pilots). Seltzer and Jablon (1974), for example, found lower morbidity rates among people discharged from the army than among people of similar ages in the general population. This effect was seen even 23 years after the men had been discharged. (Some have hypothesized that this is caused by army food killing off the less fit before they can be discharged.)

Incidence-Prevalence (Neyman) Bias

If a group is investigated a significant amount of time after exposure has occurred or after a condition has already developed, those who have died and those who have recovered will be missed. For example, a cross-sectional survey of women currently receiving Aid for Families with Dependent Children (AFDC) found that 65% of them were on it for more than seven years. However, when looking at women who have *ever* received AFDC, they found that only 30% had been on it more than seven years (Duncan, Hill, & Hoffman, 1988). The reason for the disparity is that a cross-sectional survey is more likely to pick up long-term recipients than people who are on AFDC for a short period. The same phenomenon exists in samples drawn from hospitals; more chronic cases are disproportionately represented, which may lead to overly pessimistic estimates of the natural history of a disorder.

Volunteer Bias

Because of ethical and practical considerations, all studies that involve direct contact with participants must allow them the opportunity to decline to participate or drop out. The problem is that there are systematic differences between those who agree to participate and those who do not. For example, the National Diet-Heart Study (American Heart Association, 1980) found that, compared to nonvolunteers, volunteers more often (a) were nonsmokers, (b) were concerned about health matters, (c) had a higher level of education, (d) were employed in professional and skilled jobs, (e) were Protestant or Jewish, (f) were living in a household with children, and (g) were active in community affairs. A related effect is the *compliance bias*. In one arm of the Coronary Drug Project (1980) the five-year mortality rate for compliers (those who took 80% or more of their medication) was 15.1%.

It was almost twice as high among noncompliers (28.2%), even though the "medication" they were taking was placebo. The lesson is that those people who are compliant—either in terms of enrolling in a study or adhering to treatment—are different from those who are not.

Hawthorne Effect

According to legend, worker productivity improved at the Hawthorne plant of Western Electric not only when the interior illumination was increased a number of times but also when it was later decreased. The reason for this was purported to be the attention that the researchers paid to the workers and not the lighting itself. Although later studies showed that the increase in productivity probably resulted from other factors (e.g., Bramel & Friend, 1981; Parsons, 1974), the term *Hawthorne effect* is still used to explain the phenomenon that occurs when a participant's performance changes simply because he or she is being studied. For example, Frank (1961) reported that the introduction of a research project on the back wards of a psychiatric hospital was followed by considerable behavioral improvement in the patients, even though the project did not involve medication or a novel treatment. In order to account for this effect, in designing research studies it is often necessary to use an *attention control group*, which is treated exactly the same way as the experimental group—filling out questionnaires, being interviewed, and so forth—except for the active treatment itself.

Blinding

One effect of the attention control group is to *blind* the participants (figuratively only, mind you) so that they are unaware of which group they belong to. The purpose is to prevent various biases such as the *placebo effect* from influencing the results. A placebo effect occurs when people know (or think they know) that they are receiving an active treatment. For example, while 80% to 85% of patients responded positively to various medications for headache, more than 50% of the patients in the placebo group did, too (Beecher, 1955). In a *double-blind* study neither the participants nor the researcher know who is in which group. This is to minimize *expectation bias* in the investigator, who may observe what he or she wants to observe, irrespective of whether it actually occurred (e.g., Rosenthal, 1966).

Surrogate End Points

Returning for a moment to our example of parental loss and depression, one possible outcome a researcher may be interested in is suicide. Because this is (thankfully) a relatively rare event, the investigator may use a suicidal ideation scale as an end point. Bear in mind, however, that this is a *surrogate* measure; that is, the researcher is not really interested in a score on a test (the suicidal ideation scale), except to the degree to which it is highly correlated with the actual behaviour (suicide). Similarly, measuring CD4+ cell counts in people with AIDS or blood pressure in people at risk for stroke are surrogates for what we are really interested in: AIDS or a disabling stroke. If the surrogate measure is not strongly related to the outcome, we may be deluding ourselves into thinking that the intervention was successful. For example, the ultimate aim of the Cardiac Arrhythmia Suppression Trial (Strandberg, Salomaa, & Naukkarinen, 1991) was to reduce deaths from heart attacks. Because this is also a relatively rare event, they measured the frequency of premature ventricular contractions (PVCs), which are supposedly linked to heart attacks. The good news is that the drugs did in fact suppress PVCs; the bad news is that these patients died at a rate two and a half times higher than that of the control group. The moral of the story is to be wary of surrogate end points.

Regression Toward the Mean

Regression toward the mean does not mean reverting to an earlier, sadistic stage in life. Rather, it refers to the phenomenon that if people are selected to be in a study because their scores on a test are higher (or lower) than average, then their scores will be closer to the mean when they are retested, even if there were no intervention (Streiner, 2001). This is an inescapable fact, resulting from the unreliability of the test. Because no test is perfectly reliable—whether it is a paper-and-pencil questionnaire, an interview, or a physical measurement (Streiner & Norman, 2004)—all studies that select people because of extreme scores will be subject to this bias. The solutions are to (a) use tests that are as reliable

as possible, and (b) base entry into the study on multiple test scores, rather than just one.

MEASURES OF OUTCOMES

One of the major challenges in epidemiological research, especially for descriptive studies, is how to count and measure the variables of interest. In this section, I will examine a few of these indices (other indices can be found in Kleinbaum, Kupper, & Morgenstern, 1982; Streiner, 1998). As an example, we will use a dread disease previously unknown to Western science (or Eastern, Northern, or Southern, for that matter)—Somali Camelbite Fever (SCF)—that Geoff Norman and I introduced in a previous book (Norman & Streiner, 2003). Imagine that we surveyed a small town of 200 people for one year, recording all people who contracted SCF and what the outcome was. The results are shown in Figure 37.1 for the 12 people who had the disease at some time during the year. Lines that start at the left edge indicate that those people had SCF when the survey began, and those that extend to the right edge indicate that the person with SCF was still alive when the study ended.

The *incidence* of SCF is defined as follows:

$$[1] \quad \text{Incidence} = \frac{\text{Number of new cases in a given period}}{\text{Number of people at risk}}$$

In this case, the *annual incidence* is 8 / 196 = 0.0408 cases per year. Two questions immediately arise: why is the numerator 8 rather than 12, and why is the denominator 196 rather than 200? The reason is that four people (numbers 1, 3, 4, and 7) already had the disease, so they are neither new cases nor at risk for contracting it. In order to make the results more understandable the incidence is sometimes expressed as cases per 1,000 or 10,000 people in the time period (or even per million a year for rare disorders); in this example there are 40.8 cases per 1,000 people per year.

If we are interested in establishing health care services, we are more concerned with how many people have the disorder at any one time; this is called the *point prevalence* of a disorder:

$$[2] \quad \frac{\text{Point}}{\text{Prevalence}} = \frac{\text{Number of people with the disorder at time } t}{\text{Number of people at risk}}$$

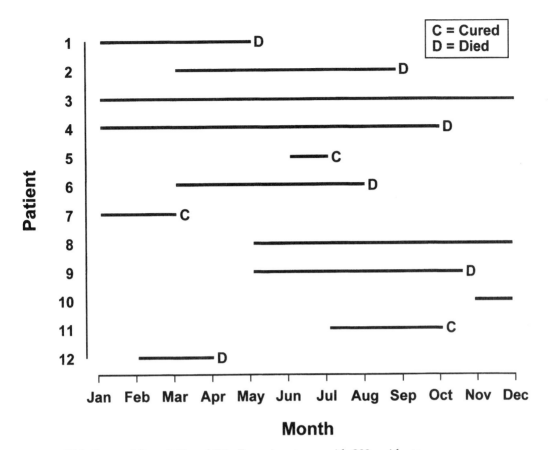

FIGURE 37.1 Cases of Somali Camel Bite Fever in a town with 200 residents

In contrast to incidence, point prevalence, as its name implies, is determined at a single point in time, which we denote by *t*. If we look at July, six people had SCF (numbers 2, 3, 4, 6, 8, and 9); number 5 was cured some time during the month and would therefore also be counted as of July 1, whereas number 11 was diagnosed during the month and would not be included. Therefore, the numerator is seven. The denominator again is not 200 because two people (1 and 12) died before July 1 and thus were highly unlikely to contract SCF again. The point prevalence as of July 1 is therefore 7 / 198 = 0.0354, or 35.4 per 1,000.

In order to determine point prevalence the disorder being studied must have a rapid and identifiable onset, and the data must be gathered in a short period of time. In the mental health field neither criterion obtains; the onset of disorders such as anxiety, depression, and schizophrenia is slow and insidious, and surveys often extend over months. For these reasons, it is more common to determine the *period prevalence*, which counts the number of people with the disorder during a defined time (usually six months or a year):

$$[3] \quad \frac{\text{Period}}{\text{Prevalence}} = \frac{\begin{array}{c}\text{Number of people with the}\\\text{disorder during the interval}\end{array}}{\begin{array}{c}\text{Number of people at}\\\text{risk during the interval}\end{array}}$$

which in this case is 12 / 200 = 0.06 for the year, or 60 per 1,000.

The relationship between incidence and prevalence can be described by the following formula:

$$[4] \quad \text{Prevalence} = \frac{\text{Incidence}}{\text{Duration}}$$

For chronic conditions such as schizophrenia, where the duration is much longer than the time during which prevalence is measured, the prevalence is higher than the incidence. For very brief disorders such as the common cold, the number of new cases in a year (the incidence) is much larger than the number of people who have the disorder at any given time (the prevalence). We can also manipulate this equation just like any algebraic expression, so that

$$[5] \quad \text{Incidence} = \frac{\text{Prevalence}}{\text{Duration}}$$

Unfortunately for the people, but luckily for expository purposes, some people die of SCF, leading to two other indices. The *mortality rate* is

$$[6] \quad \frac{\text{Mortality}}{\text{Rate}} = \frac{\begin{array}{c}\text{Number of deaths from the} \\ \text{disorder in the time period}\end{array}}{\text{Number of people at risk}}$$

which is 6 / 200 = 0.03 per year in this example, or 30 per 1,000. (When the time period is one year, this number is also called the *annual mortality rate*.)

A related number is the *case fatality rate*, which focuses only on those people who have the disorder:

$$[7] \quad \frac{\begin{array}{c}\text{Case} \\ \text{Fatality} \\ \text{Rate}\end{array}}{} = \frac{\begin{array}{c}\text{Number of deaths from the} \\ \text{disorder in the time period}\end{array}}{\text{Number of people with the disorder}}$$

Naturally, this rate is much higher than the mortality rate; in this case, it is 6 / 12 = 50% per year.

One question that arises is how serious SCF is in relation to other, potentially life-threatening disorders. To determine this, we calculate the *proportional mortality rate* (PMR) for each disease:

$$[8] \quad \text{PMR} = \frac{\begin{array}{c}\text{Number of deaths from} \\ \text{a particular cause}\end{array}}{\text{Total number of deaths}}$$

However, this number can be tricky to interpret in isolation. It is not unusual for the morning headlines to proclaim that more people are dying of disease X than ever before. This *may* be due to the fact that more people are contracting X or that it is becoming more deadly over time. A more reasonable explanation is that fewer people are dying from diseases Y and Z. The sad fact is that, in the long run, the probability that a person will die of something is 100% (despite the belief in Southern California and elsewhere that if we jog enough, drink plenty of bottled water, and eat raw fish and granola bars, we will live

forever). As we get better at reducing the death rate from heart disease and infectious disorders, the PMRs for other disorders such as cancer *must* rise.

Sometimes, even looking at "simple" statistics such as the annual mortality rate can be somewhat misleading. If we are to believe the data, the mortality rate in Florida from heart disease is 328.3 per 100,000 people, compared to a national average of 258.2 per 100,000; and the mortality rate for Alzheimer's disease is 21.3 versus the national average of 18.0 (Miniño, Arias, Kochanek, Murphy, & Smith, 2002). Does this mean that living in Florida rots your brain and kills you, or is something else going on? Despite the opinions of some Northerners, the real answer is that there is another phenomenon at work here; many people go to Florida when they retire, so the proportion of elderly people is higher there than in the United States as a whole. To compensate for this, we can calculate *standardized mortality rates*. This is a relatively laborious procedure (although not a difficult one) and requires us to have fairly detailed information about age-related death rates in both the region we are interested in (Florida, in this case) and the country as a whole. The first step is to calculate the *age-specific mortality rate* for the disease we are examining:

$$[9] \quad \frac{\begin{array}{c}\text{Age-Specific} \\ \text{Mortality Rate}\end{array}}{} = \frac{\begin{array}{c}\text{Number of deaths from} \\ \text{disease X in age range Y}\end{array}}{\begin{array}{c}\text{Total number of} \\ \text{deaths in age range Y}\end{array}}$$

That is, the age-specific mortality rate is very similar to the proportional mortality rate, except that it is broken down by age. The second step is that, for each age range, we compare the number of people in Florida to the comparison group, which is the total population of the United States. So, for example, if we get an answer of 1.0 for the age range 10–14, that would mean that Florida's proportion of people of this age is the same as that of the entire country; a number greater than 1.0 means that the proportion in this age range is higher, and a number less than 1.0 means it is lower. Finally, for each age stratum, we multiply the age-specific mortality rate by the proportion of people and add up the results across strata. What we end up with is the mortality rate, standardized (hence the name) to the comparison group. When we do this, we find that the age-adjusted (or standardized) mortality rate for Alzheimer's disease in Florida is 15.1, and the rate for heart disease is 243.5, both of which are *below* the national average.

Primary prevention programs are predicated on the belief that if we can reduce the risk factors for a disorder, we will therefore reduce the prevalence of the disorder itself. This is the basis for public health campaigns aimed at lowering blood pressure, lowering "bad" cholesterol, and increasing physical activity levels to reduce the risk of stroke and heart disease (although not at changing men's sex, which is the major risk factor). The problem is that not all cases occur as a result of these risk factors. Let us return to our example of early parental loss and depression. Even if we were able to enroll all children who suffered a loss in an effective therapy program, we would not totally eliminate depression because there are also other causes of the disorder. As a result, we first have to determine the proportion of cases that occur due to parental loss. This figure goes by a number of names—the *attributable risk*, the *attributable fraction*, or the *etiological fraction* (EF)—and is defined as

$$[10] \quad EF = \frac{\{\text{Number of new cases during the period attributable to the risk factor}\}}{\{\text{Total number of new cases during the period}\}}$$

If it turns out that the EF is 0.10, for example, then that means that only 10% of all cases of depression are a result of parental loss. This then puts an upper limit on the possible effectiveness of the intervention; even if all children could be enrolled in such a program, and even if it were 100% successful in preventing later depression (both highly questionable assumptions), 90% of depressions would not be prevented. This puts us in a better position to determine whether the cost of such a program is justified in light of its expected success rate.

SUMMARY

Epidemiology is a broad field, covering studies of prevalence to hypothesis testing to intervention trials. Even a basic knowledge of its principles enables the researcher to be aware of possible biases that may lead to erroneous conclusions and to design better studies. As an added bonus, it can be a source of new terms that can be used to impress friends at cocktail parties.

ACKNOWLEDGMENT Portions of this paper were modified and thoroughly updated from Streiner and Norman, 1996, with the permission of B. C. Decker, Inc.

References

Alderson, M. (1983). *An introduction to epidemiology* (2nd ed.). London: Macmillan Press.

American Heart Association. (1980). The National Diet-Heart Study: Final report. *American Heart Association Monograph No. 18.* New York: Author.

Beecher, H. K. (1955). The powerful placebo. *Journal of the American Medical Association, 159,* 1602–1606.

Boyle, M. H., Offord, D. R., Hoffman, H. G., Catlin, G. P., Byles, J. A., Cadman, D. T., et al. (1987). Ontario Child Health Survey: Part I. Methodology. *Archives of General Psychiatry, 44,* 826–831.

Bramel, D., & Friend, R. (1981). Hawthorne: The myth of the docile worker and class bias in psychology. *American Psychologist, 36,* 867–878.

Cook, T. D., & Campbell, D. T. (1979). *Quasi-experimentation: Design issues for field settings.* Chicago: Rand McNally.

Coronary Drug Project Research Group. (1980). Influence of adherence to treatment and response to cholesterol on mortality in the Coronary Drug Project. *New England Journal of Medicine, 303,* 1038–1041.

Duncan, G. J., Hill, M. S., & Hoffman, S. D. (1988). Welfare dependence within and across generations. *Science, 239,* 467–471.

Frank, J. D. (1961). *Persuasion and healing.* Baltimore: Johns Hopkins Press.

Kleinbaum, D. G., Kupper, L. L., & Morgenstern, H. (1982). *Epidemiologic research: Principles and quantitative methods.* Belmont, CA: Lifetime Learning Publications.

Last, J. M. (2001). *A dictionary of epidemiology* (4th ed.). Oxford: Oxford University Press.

Miniño, A. M., Arias, E., Kochanek, K. D., Murphy, S. L., & Smith, B. L. (2002). Deaths: Final data for 2000. *National Vital Statistics Reports, 50*(15). Hyattsville, MD: National Center for Health Statistics.

Norman, G. R., & Streiner, D. L. (2003). *PDQ statistics* (3rd ed.). Toronto: B. C. Decker.

Parsons, H. M. (1974). What happened at Hawthorne? *Science, 183,* 922–932.

Rosenthal, R. (1966). *Experimenter effects in behavioral research.* New York: Appleton-Century-Crofts.

Saigal, S., Hoult, L. A., Streiner, D. L., Stoskopf, B. L., & Rosenbaum, P. L. (2000). School difficulties at adolescence in a regional cohort of children who were extremely low birth weight. *Pediatrics, 105,* 325–331.

Seltzer, C. C., & Jablon, S. (1974). Effects of selection on mortality. *American Journal of Epidemiology, 100,* 367–372.

Sobal, J., & Stunkard, A. J. (1989). Socioeconomic status and obesity: A review of the literature. *Psychological Bulletin, 105,* 260–275.

Strandberg, T. E., Salomaa, V. V., & Naukkarinen, V. A. (1991). Long-term mortality after 5-year multifactorial primary prevention of cardiovascular diseases in middle-aged men. *Journal of the American Medical Association, 266,* 1225–1229.

Streiner, D. L. (1998). Let me count the ways: Measuring incidence, prevalence, and impact in epidemiological studies. *Canadian Journal of Psychiatry, 43,* 173–179.

Streiner, D. L. (2001). Regression toward the mean: Its etiology, diagnosis, and treatment. *Canadian Journal of Psychiatry, 46,* 72–76.

Streiner, D. L., & Norman, G. R. (2004). *Health measurement scales: A practical guide to their development and use* (3rd ed.). Oxford: Oxford University Press.

38

APPLICATION OF REMOTE SENSING FOR DISEASE SURVEILLANCE IN URBAN AND SUBURBAN AREAS

Annelise Tran, Jacques Gardon, & Laurent Polidori

For 30 years the use of remotely sensed data (satellite images, aerial photographs, etc.) in epidemiological studies has become more and more frequent (Boone, McGwire, Otteson, et al., 2000; Cline, 1970). Indeed, because it provides information on the environment, remote sensing offers an important potential for the study of diseases related to environmental conditions (Curran, Atkinson, Foody, et al., 2000). In particular, remote sensing is of particular relevance for the comprehension and modeling of vector-borne diseases, the spatial distribution of which is related to the vector habitat (Linthicum, Anyamba, Tucker, et al., 1999; Thomson, Connor, Milligan, et al., 1997). The main difficulty with the use of this kind of data is in establishing successive links between the information contained in the remotely sensed image and the risk of disease. This relationship is particularly dif-

ficult to clarify in urban or suburban areas, where the application of remote sensing is limited by the satellite images' spatial resolution and landscape complexity (Beck, Lobitz, & Wood, 2000).

In this chapter, we present a brief review of the methods usually adopted to include remotely sensed data in an epidemiological study (see section 2). This exploration highlights the underuse of remote sensing to describe the "human" environment and map urban, social, or demographic parameters that could be relevant to epidemiological studies (see section 3). In section 4, we describe a method for mapping disease incidence at a regional scale using a satellite image. We conclude the chapter with a description of an operational monitoring system that includes new technologies such as remote sensing and Geographic Information Systems (GIS).

1. APPLICATION OF REMOTE SENSING TO EPIDEMIOLOGY: A BRIEF SUMMARY

Many review articles list the investigations that have used remote sensing techniques for the study of diseases (Hay, Packer, & Rogers, 1997; Kitron, 1998; Washino & Wood, 1994). Generally the examples of such investigations are classified according to disease. In this chapter we present a general approach that emerges from related studies in the literature.

Hypotheses

The main goals of using remote sensing in epidemiology are to map risk areas and identify risk periods in order to improve disease surveillance. The underlying hypothesis of this remote sensing application is that the disease is linked to the environment, which can be characterized using remotely sensed data (Curran et al., 2000; Hay et al., 1997).

General Approach

Different approaches can be distinguished according to the degree of knowledge of the disease characteristics. When the disease characteristics are well documented, remote sensing is used as a cartographic tool. Indeed, the use of satellite images is particularly relevant for the follow-up of a changing landscape or in a regional context where the cartography is incomplete or obsolete. The most frequent example of such a use in the literature is the mapping of areas favorable to the proliferation of vectors with a known habitat: flooded areas (Hayes, Maxwell, Mitchell, et al., 1985; Pope, Sheffner, Linthicum, et al., 1992), swamps (Rejmankova, Roberts, Pawley, et al., 1995), rice fields (Wood, Beck, Washino, et al., 1992), and so on.

However, when the understanding of the disease is incomplete, remote sensing constitutes an additional information source for better comprehension of the transmission mechanisms, in particular clarifying the link between environment and disease. In such cases environmental parameters are derived from the images, and a statistical analysis is performed in order to test the parameters' relationship with epidemiological or entomological field data. This approach allows researchers to identify risk factors and therefore improve the understanding of the disease. The inversion of the statistical relationship leads to the establishment of a statistical model of the disease occurrence risk. Various examples of this type of approach are reported in the literature, linking remotely sensed data with disease occurrence (Daniel, Kolar, Zeman, et al., 1999; Hay, Snow, & Rogers, 1998; Linthicum et al., 1999; Lobitz, Beck, Huq, et al., 2000; Malone, Huh, Fehler, et al., 1994) or vector distribution (Beck, Rodriguez, Dister, et al., 1994; Dister, Fish, Bros, et al., 1997; Estrada-Peña, 1999; Rogers, Hay, & Packer, 1996).

Environmental Parameters Derived From Remote Sensing Data

Several review papers present the variables of particular relevance to epidemiology that can be derived from remotely sensed data (Curran et al., 2000; Goetz, Prince, & Small, 2000; Hay, 2000). These variables are mostly related to the natural environment: landscape structure, vegetation cover and type (Daniel et al., 1999; Beck et al., 1994; Dister et al., 1997), land (Malone et al., 1994; Estrada-Peña, 1999) and sea (Lobitz et al., 2000; Linthicum et al., 1999) surface temperature, rainfall indices (Hay et al., 1998; Linthicum et al., 1999), sea surface height (Lobitz et al., 2000), and water bodies. Although urban features detection could be relevant for epidemiological studies (Beck et al., 2000), very few investigations have explored the potential of remote sensing for human habitat characterization and social or demographic parameters calculation (Barbazan, Amrehn, Dilokwanich, et al., 2000; Lointier, Truc, Drapeau, et al., 2001).

Sensors

The sensor type is naturally chosen depending on the study's spatial scale (local, regional, national, continental) and temporal scale (daily, monthly, annual follow-up). Choosing the sensor type requires a good understanding of sensor characteristics and image processing (Curran et al., 2000; Hay, 2000) and, even better, a multi- and interdisciplinary approach.

Limitations

While a number of remote sensing demonstrations are reported in the literature, the application of remote sensing to the health domain for actual disease control still must be proven effective (Barinaga, 1993). Indeed, because of the difficulty in establishing a solid relationship between disease risk and remotely sensed data, the implementation of a generic methodology is limited by the diseases' local specificities; also, the human factor is seldom taken into account in remote sensing–based models for predicting disease risk. Finally, very few remote sensing models are evaluated (Beck, Rodriguez, Dister, et al., 1997) and integrated into an operational disease surveillance system.

2. THE CONTRIBUTION OF REMOTE SENSING FOR DISEASE SURVEILLANCE IN URBAN AND SUBURBAN AREAS

Geographically, the most important need for the use of remote sensing techniques in the health domain is in intertropical area countries, where diseases closely linked to the environment, such as malaria, are most prevalent (Hay, Packer, & Rogers, 1997). Moreover, infectious diseases often occur in areas where environmental changes are important. Those changes, either natural or anthropogenic, may determine epidemic emergence. This is generally the case in tropical areas.

In such areas, field access difficulties, landscape change, and the lack of maps make remote sensing a suitable tool for environmental and epidemiological monitoring. Indeed, in spite of the severe difficulties inherent in these regions (the natural and urban landscape complexity, cloud cover that limits optical image acquisition to a short period, operational constraints), remote sensing could provide rapidly acquired, low-cost information on land cover, which is needed for landscape changes monitoring (urban growth, deforestation, etc.). In particular, high spatial resolution sensors can yield images allowing the detection of urban features required for the measurement and monitoring of urban spatial growth (Gar-On Yeh & Li, 2001; Yang, 2002), mapping of urban/suburban infrastructure and socioeconomic attributes (Shaban & Dikshit, 2001), and population estimation (Harvey, 2002).

However, a review of the remote sensing applications to the health domain shows that the potential of remotely sensed data for the mapping of urban parameters has been rarely ex-

ploited in epidemiological studies. Such parameters could include housing quality, urban space structure, road network, population density, and so on.

In particular, remotely sensed data could be processed in order to provide population densities maps, which are of interest for the calculation of disease incidence rates (Tran, Gardon, Weber, et al., 2002). Indeed, during an epidemiological survey, disease incidence estimation is the first requirement in order to concentrate the investigation on high-incidence areas, determine risk factors, and take preventive measures. It involves the estimation of both the number of cases and the number of susceptible persons. In many cases the census of the risk population amounts to the estimation of the number of people living in the target area. This requires population census data that are classically obtained from ground-based surveys. The problem is that these data are often expensive to acquire, difficult to obtain in a short time, and in some cases are incomplete or obsolete, particularly in developing countries with a high and unplanned population growth rate.

Because of these limitations, methods using remotely sensed data have been developed in order to provide urban planners with a low-cost and regularly updated tool for population estimation (Adeniyi, 1983; Harvey, 2002). Most models are based on the detection of homogeneous urbanization areas, which are linked with real population densities (Dureau, 1997; Olorunfemi, 1984; Sabine, 1999) or directly based on the reflectance values measured by the satellite optical sensors (Iisaka & Hegedus, 1982). The existing models are limited for use in accurate demographic surveys by the complexity of urban morphology, particularly at the extremes of population density (in low-density and high-density population areas) (Harvey, 2002). Nevertheless, as far as epidemiological surveys actually do not require an absolute accuracy in the population estimation but do require discrimination between low- and high-population density areas, the use of remote sensing for the characterization of population densities could provide sufficient information for epidemiologists to estimate the incidence heterogeneity in a region.

In the next two sections, a simple method for mapping disease incidence using remotely sensed data is presented and evaluated by comparison with an incidence map derived from ground-based population census data. The results show that remote sensing could also provide epidemiologists with an interesting tool for the study of diseases in an urban context.

3. MAPPING DISEASE INCIDENCE IN SUBURBAN AREAS USING REMOTE SENSING DATA

The method presented in this section demonstrates remote sensing's potential as a new tool for the characterization and mapping of high-incidence areas (see Tran et al., 2002). In the target area, the incidence rate is computed alternatively with census data used as the denominator and with a population estimation derived from a SPOT (Satellite Pour l'Observation de la Terre) multispectral image. Although this method has been developed for the case of a Q fever outbreak investigation in Cayenne, French Guiana, and its suburbs (Gardon, Héraud, Laventure, et al., 2001), it can be applied to the regional scale incidence mapping of other diseases. The process involves the following steps: (a) case location, (b) landscape map generation, (c) calculation of a population density index, and (d) incidence index mapping.

Case Location

The definition of case location is not obvious. In most studies that include a spatial component in the analysis, patients are located at their residential addresses. This implies that they have contracted the disease at home; this hypothesis is often based on practical constraints (because the location at the residential address is the easiest implementation of a location criterion) and on the fact that people spend most of their daily time at home. Thus, the case location should be questioned, chosen according to the study's objectives, and taken into account in the results analysis and discussion.

In practice, the geographic coordinates of each case can be obtained via an address georeferencing system, if such a system exists in the target area, or via Global Positioning System (GPS). In our study, 140 cases of Q fever have been reported in Cayenne and its suburbs over the 1996–2000 period. Among them, 112 have been accurately located at their residential address via GPS. A first interpretation of the disease's spa-

tial distribution shows an apparent homogeneity: cases are present in the town center as well as in the suburbs (Figure 38.1).

Landscape Map Generation

The remote sensing image used for the characterization of an area should be chosen according to the spatial and temporal scales required for the study (Hay, 2000). On a regional scale multispectral images such as those provided by the optical sensors onboard SPOT and Landsat satellites are appropriate for mapping landscape elements.

Our study area encompasses the city of Cayenne and two adjacent towns, Rémire-Montjoly and Matoury, representing around 80,000 inhabitants. The landscape includes housing areas surrounded by wooded hills and coastal wetlands. People mainly live in individual houses and small buildings (Gardel, 2001). A first interpretation of a SPOT XS (XS: multispectral mode) scene allows us to discriminate between different types of land cover: housing areas, forests, swamp, free water. For this image, the pixel size, corresponding to the smallest area for which the sensor can record data, is 20 m

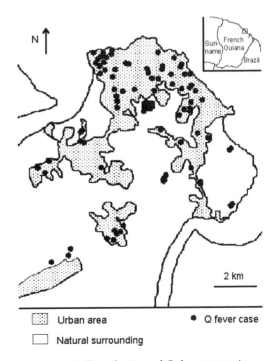

FIGURE 38.1 Distribution of Q fever cases in Cayenne, French Guiana, 1996–2000.

× 20 m. The satellite image has to be geometrically processed to be compatible with GPS data.

Because of the link between an object's characteristics and its spectral properties, spectral information given by the multispectral sensors allows researchers to differentiate objects having different spectral responses. The process used to discriminate and map different types of land cover is called image classification; it merges into the same class pixels with similar spectral responses.

The high resolution visible and infrared (HRVIR) sensor onboard the SPOT-4 satellite measures the intensity of solar radiation reflected by objects on the Earth in four spectral channels: green, red, near infrared, and middle infrared. A classification based on the four channels using a Bayesian process called *maximum likelihood classification* (IMAGINE, 1998; Richards, 1994) allows the mapping of 11 landscape elements: dense urban areas, suburban areas, mangrove areas, dense secondary forest, sparse secondary forest, swamp, sand, bare soils, roads, free water, and a miscellaneous nonlandscape class (clouds, cloud shadows).

Calculation of a Population Density Index

Assuming that population density is statistically related to the presence of urban elements such as roads, buildings, houses, and so on, a population density map can be derived from the landscape classification result from SPOT imaging. Because the classification of the Cayenne SPOT image allows the researcher to discriminate between urban areas (dense urban areas, suburban areas, bare soils, roads) and natural areas (mangrove areas, dense secondary forest, sparse secondary forest, swamp, sand, and free water), the different landscape elements can be merged into two classes: urban and nonurban. Figure 38.2 shows the map of all urban elements.

Next a population density index map is computed by calculating for each pixel the proportion of neighboring pixels belonging to the urban class, within 200 m of the central pixel boundary (Figure 38.3). This boundary size was the most adapted size in our study (Tran et al., 2002). The population density index map derived this way from the SPOT data is represen-

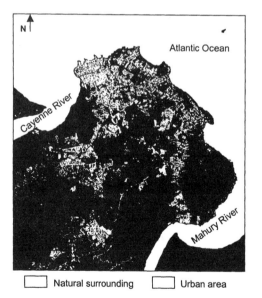

FIGURE 38.2 Map of the urban elements (buildings, houses, roads) derived from the SPOT XS classification in the region of Cayenne, French Guiana. Natural areas are in black, urban areas are in white.

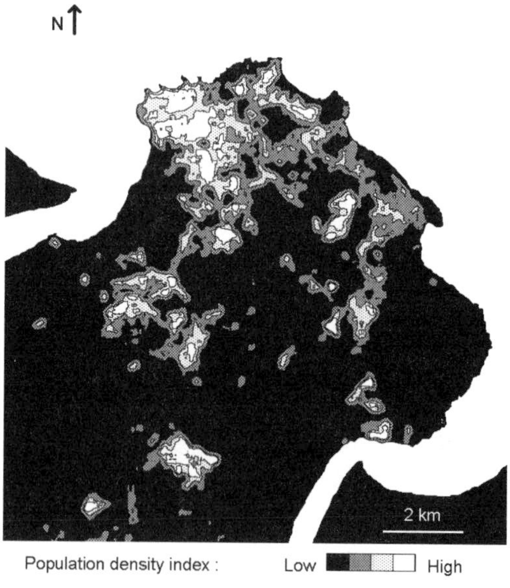

FIGURE 38.3 Population density in Cayenne, French Guiana, according to a population density index derived from SPOT data. Areas in white correspond to high urban elements (buildings, roads, . . .) density areas. Lower urban density areas are in dark.

tative of the different types of urbanization in Cayenne and its surroundings.

Incidence Index Mapping

A disease incidence index can be defined for each pixel as the ratio between the number of cases and the population density index. The final disease incidence map is obtained by the spatial interpolation of the resulting values taken for each disease case (Figure 38.4).

In the case of the Q fever investigation in the Cayenne region the incidence index map highlighted several incidence areas with high Q fever incidence rates (Camp du Tigre, Rorota, Prison, etc.), so the apparent homogeneity in the distribution of Q fever cases in Cayenne and its surroundings disappeared when population density was taken into account. The identification of these high incidence spots will aid in the research on the risk factors for Q fever and the identification of the reservoir of the bacterium *Coxiella burnetii*.

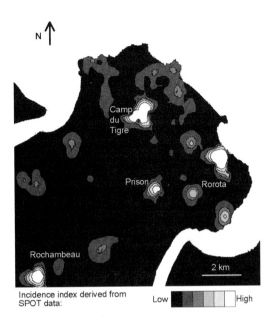

FIGURE 38.4 Map of Q fever incidence in Cayenne, French Guiana (disease incidence index map), obtained using satellite data.

4. VALIDATION

In order to validate remote sensing's use in population estimation and mapping disease incidence, ground-based population census data are required. Nevertheless, because the population census data are only available at a much lower spatial resolution than the remote sensing data, the comparison and evaluation of the results are not easy (Harvey, 2002).

In the Cayenne region the French National Institute of Statistics and Economic Studies (Institut National de la Statistique et des Etudes Economiques) provides population census data for 35 districts called statistical block groups (IRIS: Ilots Regroupés pour l'Information Statistique) with a mean surface area of 6.2 km² (Figure 38.5) (*Recensement de la population*, 1999).

Qualitative Validation

For each district, the real incidence value can be computed by dividing the number of cases in the district by the number of inhabitants. The resulting map is an accurate incidence map but with a low spatial resolution corresponding to the census district size. To visually compare two

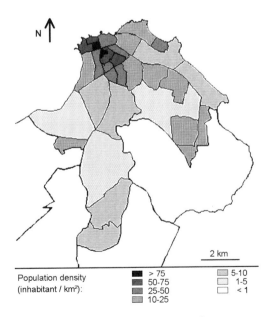

FIGURE 38.5 Population density in Cayenne, French Guiana, according to 1999 population census data from the Institut National de la Statistique et des Etudes Economiques.

maps with the same spatial resolution, the incidence values taken for each Q fever case were interpolated within a 20 m grid, corresponding to the SPOT pixel size (Figure 38.6).

A strong concordance exists between the high incidence spots highlighted in the disease incidence map derived from SPOT data (Figure 38.4) and those observed in the incidence map derived from population census data (Figure 38.6). This shows that the incidence index map derived from satellite data is relevant for epidemiological study as long as absolute values are not needed. Indeed, epidemiological investigation based on this map would concentrate on the same strong incidence areas as surveys using the real incidence map obtained with population census data.

Quantitative Validation

The average population density index derived from the SPOT data was computed for each population census district and compared with the population density value generated by the census. We performed a logarithmic transformation in order to reduce the saturation of the population density index from the SPOT data for high population densities. The result is then correlated with the real density given by the population census with a high correlation coefficient ($r = 0.91; p < 10^{-5}$) (Figure 38.7). This correlation confirms the validity of our hypothesis that population density is related to the presence of urban elements and thus can be roughly estimated and mapped using remote sensing images.

Method Extrapolation

The method implemented in Cayenne for population estimation using remote sensing data has recently been tested in the region of Belém, Pará, Brazil (Faure, Tran, Gardel, et al., 2003). With 1.8 million inhabitants, the region of Belém is very different from Cayenne, where urban landscape corresponds to a suburban area rather than dense urban area. The same methodology was implemented in Belém using a Thematic Mapper (TM) image from the Landsat satellite (6 optical channels, pixel size = 30 m). The results were evaluated using ground-based population census data from the Brazilian Institute of Geography and Statistics (IBGE: Instituto Brasileiro de Geografia e Estatísticas). The eval-

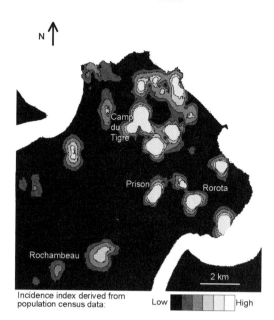

FIGURE 38.6 Map of Q fever incidence in Cayenne, French Guiana, obtained using 1999 population census data from the Institut National de la Statistique et des Etudes Economiques.

uation shows that there is also a strong correlation between population estimation derived from the TM data and the census population. This demonstrates the method's potential for population estimation in other sites that present different urban morphologies.

5. CONCLUSIONS AND PERSPECTIVES

Research Perspectives

A review of the current applications of remote sensing in epidemiology shows the important potential of remote sensing technology in the surveillance of diseases related to the environment. It also highlights the fact that until now, although remotely sensed data have been widely used in the health domain to describe the natural environment, they were rarely used to provide information on the urban or suburban environment. In this chapter, we described a method for mapping disease incidence using multispectral data and detailed its evaluation. The positive results show a new possible development of using

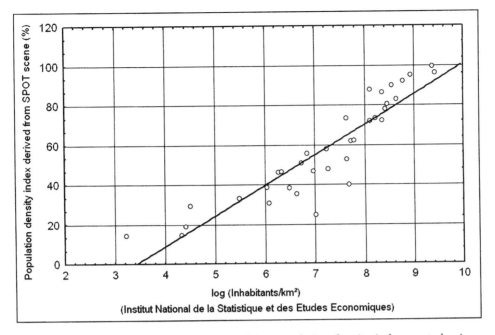

FIGURE 38.7 Bidimensional representation of the population density index created using multispectral data from the Satellite Pour l'Observation de la Terre (SPOT) versus the logarithm of real population density in Cayenne, French Guiana. The circles show the population density values derived from the SPOT data, and the solid line is the regression line.

remote sensing in epidemiology through the use of satellite images for characterization and mapping of parameters related to human activities. Remote sensing could therefore be used to characterize the two risk components: the hazard, which is linked to natural environmental conditions (for example, vector abundance), and population vulnerability, which corresponds to demographic, social, and cultural characteristics. Further research is needed to more fully explore this double potential.

Practice Implications

In practice several conditions are required for the integration of remote sensing data into an operational disease control and surveillance system. Above all, remote sensing's contribution should be evaluated by researchers of the different domains involved. Then all disease- and environment-related data should be collected in a shared georeferenced database with an efficient location system. Because it allows the storage, analysis, and display of heterogeneous spatially

referenced data, a GIS should constitute this central database. Finally, results of remotely sensed data analysis and risk modeling should be communicated in real-time to the health stakeholders through the GIS in order to improve disease control.

Such a surveillance system is being deployed for dengue fever surveillance in French Guiana. A research program called S2 Dengue (Spatial Surveillance of Dengue) connects the different health stakeholders for the real-time collection of all dengue-related information (suspected and confirmed cases, vector densities, etc.) (Tran, Deparis, Dussart, et al., 2003). The project's first objective is to provide all participants with weekly maps of dengue incidence in order to improve prevention measures. The second objective is to link this information with relevant environmental factors derived from remote sensing images and establish a model of the epidemic dynamic (Figure 38.8). This program will aid in the comprehension of dengue transmission mechanisms and precisely evaluate the potential

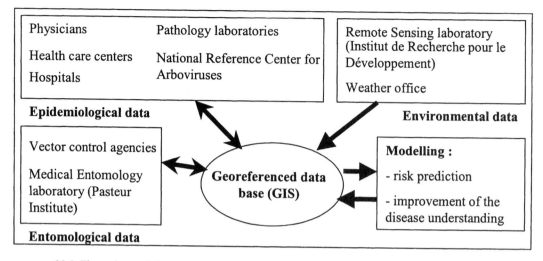

FIGURE 38.8 Flow chart of the research program S2 Dengue (Spatial Surveillance of Dengue fever) deployed for dengue fever surveillance in French Guiana.

of integrating GIS and remotely sensed data for disease surveillance at a national level.

GLOSSARY TERMS

Q fever: a zoonosis caused by the bacterium *Coxiella burnetii*. People become infected mainly by inhaling aerosols generated during parturition of contaminated animals. In French Guiana, a French administrative unit located between Suriname and Brazil, Q fever incidence has significantly increased since 1996 (Gardon et al., 2001). This original epidemic remains an enigma because the reservoir responsible for transmission has not yet been identified. In addition, several facts make this epidemic different from the usual case: First, it occurs in the Cayenne region, the main urban area of the country although Q fever is generally considered to be a rural disease. Also, many facts strengthen the hypothesis that there exists a wild reservoir for the bacteria even though it is usually found in domestic ungulates. The main goal in analyzing the spatial distribution of the disease data was to identify high-incidence areas in order to concentrate the investigation on these risk areas for the identification of Q fever risk factors.

Remote sensing: the process of acquiring information about an object from a distance. This broad definition includes Earth observation using airborne and spaceborne sensors, which measure the electromagnetic radiation reflected or radiated from the earth's surface and store the measurements in two-dimensional images.

There is a wide range of remote sensing sensors that provide information about sea and land surfaces. Distinctions are usually made between passive (which respond to the natural radiation incident on the instrument) and active (which generate their own radiation and measure the reflected signal) sensors; between high spatial resolution (resolution < 100 m) and low spatial resolution (resolution around 1 km) sensors; and between imaging and nonimaging instruments. Remote sensing systems can also be categorized according to the range of wavelengths in which they are operating: visible and near-infrared sensors, thermal-infrared sensors, microwave sensors.

Spaceborne remote sensing: satellite remote sensing dates back to the early 1970s, when images provided by spaceborne sensors began to be used for environmental monitoring, either with wide-field (e.g. NOAA AVHRR) or medium to high resolution (Landsat TM). Nowadays, wide-field sensors with resolution of around 1 km generally have been designed for specific application, for example, SeaWiFS or MeRIS for ocean color, AATSR for sea surface temperature, or SPOT-Vegetation for biosphere monitoring. High-resolution sensors have reached performances comparable to those classically obtained with airborne sensors, that is, resolution of 1–3 m (SPOT-5, IKONOS, QuickBird).

Geographic Information System (GIS): a computer system that facilitates collection, storage, integration, analysis, and display of spatially referenced data.

Global Positioning System (GPS): a satellite constellation that allows users equipped with a GPS receiver to determine their location anywhere on Earth in real-time, with an accuracy ranging from a few millimetres to several meters.

ACKNOWLEDGMENTS The research reported in this chapter was carried out within a wider research program on remote sensing and epidemiology funded by the European Commission (FEDER funds), the French Ministry of Research (RNTS network funds), and the Regional Council of French Guiana. The authors thank Jean-François Faure of the Nucleus of Higher Amazonian Studies, Pará University, and Antoine Gardel from the Laboratoire Régional de Télédétection, IRD-Guyane, for helpful discussion on remote sensing and urbanization; M. Guillemet from the Institut National de la Statistique et des Etudes Economiques for 1999 census data; the Programme National d'Environnement Côtier and the Centre National d'Etudes Spatiales (isis programme) for the 2001 SPOT image; and Thierry Tran of Nottingham University for his assistance in the manuscript revision.

References

Adeniyi, P. O. (1983). An aerial photographic method for estimating urban population. *Photogrammetric Engineering and Remote Sensing, 49,* 545–560.

Barbazan, P., Amrehn, J., Dilokwanich, S., et al. (2000). Dengue haemorrhagic fever (DHF) in the central plain of Thailand: Remote sensing and GIS to identify factors and indicators related to dengue transmission. In *The Chao Phraya delta: Historical development, dynamics, and challenges of Thailand's rice bowl* (pp. 141–151). Bangkok: Kasetsart University.

Barinaga, M. (1993). Satellite data rocket disease control efforts into orbit. *Science, 261,* 31–32.

Beck, L. R., Lobitz, B. M., & Wood, B. L. (2000). Remote sensing and human health: New sensors and new opportunities. *Emerging Infectious Diseases, 6,* 217–226.

Beck, L. R., Rodriguez, M. H., Dister, S. W., et al. (1994). Remote sensing as a landscape epidemiologic tool

to identify villages at high risk for malaria transmission. *American Journal of Tropical Medicine and Hygiene, 51,* 271–280.

Beck, L. R., Rodriguez, M. H., Dister, S. W., et al. (1997). Assessment of a remote sensing–based model for predicting malaria transmission risk in villages of Chiapas, Mexico. *American Journal of Tropical Medicine and Hygiene, 56,* 99–106.

Boone, J. D., McGwire, K. C., Otteson, E. W., et al. Remote sensing and geographic information systems: Charting *sin nombre* virus infections in deer mice. *Emerging Infectious Diseases, 6,* 248–258.

Cline, B. L. (1970). New eyes for the epidemiologists: Aerial photography and other remote sensing techniques. *American Journal of Epidemiology, 92,* 85–89.

Curran, P. J., Atkinson, P. M., Foody, G. M., et al. (2000). Linking remote sensing, land cover and disease. *Advances in Parasitology, 47,* 37–80.

Daniel, M., Kolar, J., Zeman, P., et al. (1999). Tick-borne encephalitis and Lyme borreliosis: Comparison of habitat risk assessments using satellite data (an experience from the central Bohemian region of the Czech Republic). *Central European Journal of Public Health, 7,* 35–39.

Dister, S. W., Fish, D., Bros, S. M., et al. (1997). Landscape characterization of peridomestic risk for Lyme disease using satellite imagery. *American Journal of Tropical Medicine and Hygiene, 57,* 687–692.

Dureau, F. (1997). La production rapide d'informations démographiques et économiques par sondage aréolaire sur une image satellitaire: Application à trois villes de pays en développement (Quito, Bogotá et Yaoundé). In J.-M. Dubois, J.-P. Donnay, A. Ozer, F. Boivin, & A. Lavoie (Eds.), *Télédétection des milieux urbains et périurbains* (pp. 215–224). Montreal: AUPELF-UREF.

Estrada-Peña, A. (1999). Geostatistics and remote sensing using NOAA-AVHRR satellite imagery as predictive tools in tick distribution and habitat suitability estimations for *Boophilus microplus* (Acari: *Ixodae*) in South America. *Veterinary Parasitology, 81,* 73–82.

Faure, J.-F., Tran, A., Gardel, A., et al. (2003, April). Sensoriamento remoto das formas de urbanização em aglomerações do litoral amazônico: Elaboração de um índice de densidade populacional. Paper presented at the Proc XIe Simpósio Brasileiro de Sensoriamento Remoto, Belo Horizonte, Brazil.

Gardel, A. (2001). Les paysages urbains de l'île de Cayenne. *Mappemonde, 63,* 16–22.

Gardon, J., Héraud, J.-M., Laventure, S., et al. (2001). Suburban transmission of Q fever in French Guiana: Evidence of a wild reservoir. *Journal of Infectious Diseases, 184,* 278–284.

Gar-On Yeh, A., & Li, X. (2001). Measurement and monitoring of urban sprawl in a rapidly growing region using entropy. *Photogrammetric Engineering and Remote Sensing, 67*, 83–90.

Goetz, S. J., Prince, S. D., & Small, J. (2000). Advances in satellite remote sensing of environmental variables for epidemiological applications. *Advances in Parasitology, 47*, 289–304.

Harvey, J. T. (2002). Estimating census district populations from satellite imagery: Some approaches and limitations. *International Journal of Remote Sensing, 23*, 2071–2095.

Hay, S. I. (2000). An overview of remote sensing and geodesy for epidemiology and public health application. *Advances in Parasitology, 47*, 1–35.

Hay, S. I., Packer, M. J., & Rogers, D. J. (1997). The impact of remote sensing on the study and control of invertebrate intermediate hosts and vectors of disease. *International Journal of Remote Sensing, 18*, 2899–2930.

Hay, S. I., Snow, R. W., & Rogers, D. J. (1998). Predicting malaria seasons in Kenya using multitemporal meteorological satellite sensor data. *Transactions of the Royal Society of Tropical Medicine and Hygiene, 92*, 12–20.

Hayes, R. O., Maxwell, E. L., Mitchell, C. J., et al. (1985). Detection, identification, and classification of mosquito larval habitats using remote sensing scanners in earth-orbiting satellites. *Bulletin of the World Health Organization, 63*, 361–374.

Iisaka, J., & Hegedus, E. (1982). Population estimation from Landsat imagery. *Remote Sensing of Environment, 12*, 259–272.

IMAGINE Software, version 8.3.1. (1998). Atlanta, GA: ERDAS.

Kitron, U. (1998). Landscape ecology and epidemiology of vector-borne diseases: Tools for spatial analysis. *Entomological Society of America, 35*, 435–445.

Linthicum, K. J., Anyamba, A., Tucker, C. J., et al. (1999). Climate and satellite indicators to forecast RVF epidemics in Kenya. *Science, 285*, 397–400.

Lobitz, B., Beck, L., Huq, B., et al. (2000). Climate and infectious disease: Use of remote sensing for detection of *Vibrio cholerae* by indirect measurement. *Proceedings of the National Academy of Sciences, 97*, 1438–1443.

Lointier, M., Truc, P., Drapeau, L., et al. (2001). Méthodologie de détermination de zones à risque de maladie du sommeil en Côte d'Ivoire par approche spatialisée. *Médecine Tropicale, 61*, 390–396.

Malone, J. B., Huh, O. K., Fehler, D. P., et al. (1994). Temperature data from satellite imagery and the distribution of schistosomiasis in Egypt. *American Journal of Tropical Medicine and Hygiene, 51*, 714–722.

Olorunfemi, J. F. (1984). Land use and population: A linking model. *Photogrammetric Engineering and Remote Sensing, 50*, 221–227.

Pope, K. O., Sheffner, E. J., Linthicum, K. J., et al. (1992). Identification of central Kenyan rift valley virus vector habitats with Landsat TM and evaluation of their flooding status with airborne imaging radar. *Remote Sensing of Environment, 40*, 185–196.

Recensement de la population: March 1999—Exploitation principale [CD-ROM]. Paris: Institut National de la Statistique et des Etudes Economiques.

Rejmankova, E., Roberts, D. R., Pawley, A., et al. (1995). Predictions of adult *Anopheles albimanus* densities in villages based on distances to remotely sensed larval habitats. *American Journal of Tropical Medicine and Hygiene, 53*, 482–488.

Richards, J. A. (1994). *Remote sensing digital image analysis.* Berlin: Springer-Verlag.

Rogers, D. J., Hay, S. I., & Packer, M. J. (1996). Predicting the distribution of tsetse flies in West Africa using temporal Fourier processed meteorological satellite data. *Annals of Tropical Medicine and Parasitology, 90*, 225–241.

Sabine, H. (1999). Le couplage d'une image satellitaire à des photographies aériennes obliques pour l'étude de la croissance démographique d'une ville du Monde arabe à partir du lien entre le bâti et la population: Application au cas de Marrakech. *Télédétection, 1*, 71–94.

Shaban, M. A., & Dikshit, O. (2001). Improvement of classification in urban areas by the use of textural features: The case study of Lucknow City, Uttar Pradesh. *International Journal of Remote Sensing, 22*, 565–593.

Thomson, M. C., Connor, S. J., Milligan, P.J.M., et al. (1997). Mapping malaria risk in Africa: What can satellite data contribute? *Parasitology Today, 13*, 313–318.

Tran, A., Deparis, X., Dussart, P., et al. (2003). *Analysis of dengue spatial and temporal patterns using a Geographic Information System: Case of an outbreak in Iracoubo, French Guiana, 2001.* Manuscript submitted for publication.

Tran, A., Gardon, J., Weber, S., et al. (2002). Mapping disease incidence in suburban areas using remotely sensed data. *American Journal of Epidemiology, 156*, 662–668.

Washino, R. K., & Wood, B. L. (1994). Application of remote sensing to arthropod vector surveillance and control. *American Journal of Tropical Medicine and Hygiene, 50*, 134–144.

Wood, B. L., Beck, L. R., Washino, R. K., et al. (1992). Estimating high-mosquito-producing rice fields using spectral and spatial data. *International Journal of Remote Sensing, 13*, 2813–2826.

Yang, X. (2002). Satellite monitoring of urban spatial growth in the Atlanta metropolitan area. *Photogrammetric Engineering and Remote Sensing, 68*, 725–734.

39

ESTABLISHING COLLABORATIONS THAT ENGENDER TRUST IN THE PREVENTION OF SEXUALLY TRANSMITTED DISEASES

James C. Thomas, Eugenia Eng, Sara Ackerman, Jo Anne Earp, Hattie Ellis, & Colleen Carpenter

A small proportion of any given community bears the burden of the majority of sexually transmitted disease (STD) infection. This subpopulation has been termed the "core" of transmission. Definitions of the core vary. They include people repeatedly infected, people who infect more than one other person, sex workers, and people who reside in a particular geographical area (Thomas & Tucker, 1995).

Preventing infections and transmission among the core is viewed as a strategic way to limit infections for the entire community (Over & Piot, 1993). However, people in the core, by whatever definition, are often marginalized in society because of their infections. Conversely, their infections are partially a reflection of their marginalization on the basis of other factors such as race and class. Marginalization breeds distrust of people in the establishment and engenders a lack of cooperation with the establishment's interventions. This vicious cycle creates a formidable barrier to health care providers who want to target the core for disease reduction. The administration of hepatitis B vaccine provides an example. Initially, the national immunization strategy focused on people most at risk, including users of illicit injection drugs. High immunization coverage could not be achieved among marginalized populations, however, so care providers changed to a strategy of immunizing all children (Centers for Disease Control and Prevention, 1990, 1991).

However, hepatitis B is the only sexually transmissible infection that can be prevented through a childhood vaccine. To prevent and control the transmission of other infections, STD care providers must design behavior change interventions that are appropriate to the age at disease acquisition and can effectively reach the core as defined for the providers' purposes. In describing the application of their theory of diffusion to HIV prevention Dearing, Meyer, and Rogers (1994) highlight the special circumstances of introducing innovations to socially marginalized groups, such as low-income African Americans, to reduce socially stigmatizing problems such as AIDS. They argue that, due to distrust of people outside their group such as professional health care providers, people in marginalized groups are more likely to adopt new ideas and skills presented by people they know, who are more like themselves and who they therefore trust. The influence of outside opinion leaders (i.e., prominent people) is displaced by marginalized groups' need for trust and interpersonal familiarity.

Lay health advisor (LHA) interventions are based on a natural helping model informed by the concepts of social support and social networks. People who are recognized as natural helpers by members of their community are trusted to provide reliable and confidential information, referrals, emotional support, and tangible assistance. Natural helpers, identified and recruited for LHA interventions, participate as volunteers rather than serving as paid outreach workers for a health and human service agency. In this way LHA interventions enable natural helpers to maintain their primary allegiance, credibility, and effectiveness with the people and groups in their natural helping networks. Furthermore, LHAs differ from peer advisor and outreach workers who often interact with people they do not know.

From 1995 to 1999 researchers from the University of North Carolina School of Public Health collaborated with community members of a rural county in eastern North Carolina to implement an LHA intervention to alter behaviors affecting the transmission of STDs among low-income African American women, ages 18–34 years, residing in a cluster of contiguous neighborhoods with the highest rates of syphilis and gonorrhea in the county. The collaboration was called the Sexually Transmitted Epidemic Prevention (STEP) Project; we refer to the county in which it occurred as Step County. The project was based on theories of diffusion and empowerment. The ability to achieve the disease prevention goals depended on the development of trusting relationships between the researchers and community members. The researchers included two white males, one white female, one Asian American female, and one African American female. Their interactions with the community were principally with African Americans. In this chapter we describe how a research collaboration that included trust was established. To set the context we briefly describe aspects of the study that have been reported in more detail elsewhere (Blumenthal, Eng, & Thomas, 1999; Thach, Eng, & Thomas, 2002; Thomas, Earp, & Eng, 2000; Thomas, Eng, Clark, Robinson, & Blumenthal, 1998; Thomas, Schoenbach, Eng. & McDonald, 1996).

THE COLLABORATION

Step County lies in the rural tobacco-growing area of eastern North Carolina, about an hour and a half driving time from Chapel Hill. In 1990 its population was about 67,000, of which 38% were African American. The county's central town, where the LHA program was implemented, had a population of 37,000. Although not officially segregated today, the county ranked very high in residential isolation, a measure of de facto segregation. The Step County score was 15 standard errors above the state

mean (Thomas & Thomas, 1999). This isolation is manifested in the fact that low-income African American neighborhoods clustered almost completely on one side of the railroad tracks that transect the town. The rate of reported gonorrhea infection in these neighborhoods in 1993 was 1,746 cases per 100,000 person-years (based on 516 cases), a rate as high as those experienced by large U.S. cities with the highest rates in the same year (Thomas et al., 1996).

During years of observational research preceding the LHA intervention (1991–1995), the researchers sought out community residents and STD care providers who could inform and advise them about community life and which groups would collaborate on the design and conduct of the study. The investigators began by asking staff in the county health department and representatives from a variety of other community service agencies for the names of people influential among local African Americans. Once identified, these individuals then informed the researchers of others less recognized who could also provide key perspectives on community life. Eventually 14 members for STEP's community advisory group were identified. They ranged from a Ministerial Alliance pastor and an undercover police officer to a transgender party host and an ex–drug abuser. It was readily evident that several advisors would not be comfortable in the presence of the others. Thus, rather than convene them as a group, their perspectives and advice were sought individually. The advisors informed the researchers about the community's dynamics and history and assisted in identifying potential groups to guide the design and conduct of STEP's intervention phase based on their firsthand knowledge and the findings from the formative phase.

At the conclusion of the preliminary research period the community advisory group was reconstituted to assist in designing the intervention. Some of the people left their advisory role because they felt they had less to offer at this point in the project while others with links to various community organizations were identified as new advisors. All of the advisors were African American. The group was actively engaged in all aspects of the intervention: its design, implementation, and evaluation. Because the resources they brought to the effort went beyond advice, they chose to be referred to as the community resource group (CRG). This group met together with the university investigators. Meetings were convened by STEP's community outreach specialist (COS) every 2–3 months, usually during lunchtime on a weekday. STEP researchers provided lunch, and local agencies provided meeting rooms.

The COS was the member of the university research team who served as the connecting point to Step County agencies and the African American community. Stationed in Step County, she maintained contact with the members of the CRG, the researchers, the LHAs, staff of the local health care agencies, and other groups in the community. Two women served sequentially in this role. The first COS was an African American woman who lived outside of Step County but who was well integrated into the community. She placed her children in Step County day-care and preschool programs, did some shopping in the county (at times encountering people associated with the STEP project), and visited members of the CRG and LHAs in their homes and workplaces. She was the COS for all but one year of the project. Following her for the last year of the project was an African American woman who lived in Step County. She worked half-time for the health department as a health educator and half-time for the STEP project.

The researchers and the CRG sought to base the intervention on community strengths, not community liabilities. During the years of observational study, the researchers had identified a strong natural helping network of mutual assistance among low-income and younger African American women. This network appeared to have formed, in part, because many of the women were single mothers and relied on help from other women for basic needs with child care, housing, and food. Because of this naturally occurring helping network, and because the collaborators wanted to effect changes in sensitive behaviors among a socially disenfranchised group, the CRG and researchers chose to use a method of disseminating information, attitudes, and skills through existing trust-based relationships (Thomas et al., 1998). The behaviors to be influenced were seeking care for known or potential STDs and condom use with main sexual partners. The intervention was therefore designed to enhance low-income African Americans' capacity to communicate their concerns about STD prevention and treatment in discussions within their own social networks and with local health care agencies. The relationships between the component parts of the intervention are diagrammed in Figure 39.1.

Meetings with the CRG were led by the COS rather than the university researchers, helping reduce the power inequity between the researchers and community members as meeting participants. The group agreed that all discussions of the CRG would be confidential, thereby freeing people to speak candidly. Critical comments on the project were actively sought, and researchers usually acted quickly on advice given by the community members.

One of the CRG's early tasks was to identify potential LHAs. They worked with the university researchers to identify the desired characteristics of an LHA. The criteria included being an African American woman who was trusted and sought out for advice about relationships,

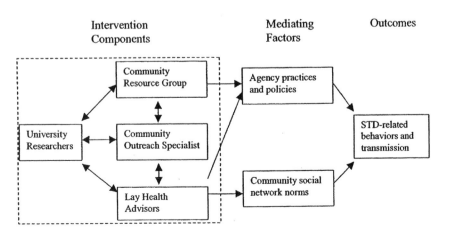

FIGURE 39.1 Conceptual model of the lay health advisor intervention

sex, and STDs. Each of the CRG members then wrote down the names of people whom they felt met the criteria. The COS contacted those women who were named by more than one CRG member to confirm their fit for the role and explain the project to them. The LHAs were not reimbursed, yet all 21 women who were invited to become an LHA accepted. They included single parents in public housing, lay ministers, students at a vocational school, and employees of a community clinic, a factory, the Department of Social Services, and the local health department.

Training to become an LHA was organized by the COS and conducted by a university graduate student and a STEP investigator. Over a five-week period, 15 hours of training ensued, most of it on Saturdays to accommodate the LHAs with jobs. The training modules were designed with much input from the CRG. The training techniques were based on popular education methodology (Freire, 1970) and focused on information about STD prevention, when to use STD services, negotiating condom use, and listening and advising skills.

Representatives from local health care agencies led a number of training sessions. For example, a nurse from the county STD clinic spoke about the clinic and answered the LHAs' questions. However, the information conveyed to the LHAs was only a secondary objective of the sessions involving local care providers. The primary objectives were to enable the care providers to become familiar with the LHAs and become invested in the project and for the LHAs to become familiar with some people working in the health care agencies, with the hope that this would decrease barriers for the LHAs to communicate their needs and desires to the agencies.

Relationships between the LHAs, the researchers, and the community continued to grow as the LHAs completed their training and became active in the community. Their training graduation was a public event that the mayor attended and at which the director of the Step County Health Department presented the LHAs with their certificates. The LHAs sponsored several other public events such as an AIDS vigil, which the researchers usually attended.

OUTCOME EVALUATION

We evaluated the first 18 months of LHA activity. The time period was chosen solely as a func-

tion of the project's funding duration. The outcome evaluation consisted principally of standardized face-to-face interviews administered before and after the intervention to African American women aged 18–34 living in the high-incidence neighborhoods. The baseline and follow-up questionnaires each consisted of about 265 items pertaining to the frequency of the targeted behaviors; attitudes toward the behaviors, including future intentions; peer norms and barriers to the behaviors; variation in sexual behaviors with different partner types; drug use; and sociodemographics. The follow-up questionnaire also asked about interactions with acquaintances who talked with them about STD treatment or prevention. Pictures of the individual LHAs and a few other women (as controls) were shown to the respondents. They were asked if they had spoken with any of the women about STDs.

Because this was a community-level intervention, the unit of analysis was the community rather than the individual. The study thus represented a sample of one and was regarded as a demonstration project. Statistical tests were not applied to the differences in various proportions measured before and after the intervention (Thomas et al., 2000).

In the household surveys the number of households with an eligible respondent was 450 at baseline and 512 at follow-up. Of these, 217 (48%) at baseline and 258 (50%) at follow-up agreed to an interview. The respondents in the two samples were similar in age, age at first sexual encounter, church attendance, and in the proportions raised in Step County. After 18 months of the intervention 18% of the female African American respondents aged 18–34 years participating in the household survey identified an LHA from a page of individual photos as someone who had spoken to them about STDs within the last year. One-third (32%) of the respondents to the follow-up questionnaire reported having talked to a female acquaintance or another woman "like yourself" about STDs in the last three months. These may have been LHAs or women who were further disseminating information that they themselves received from the LHAs; we were not able to determine the exact source with our research methods. Each of the three targeted behaviors improved during the 18-month intervention period we evaluated. Consistent condom use increased by 23%. Seeking care for an STD within three days of symptoms increased by 60%. Seeking screening for an STD by those who suspected exposure increased by 26% (Thomas et al., 2000).

PROCESS EVALUATION: DEVELOPING TRUST

The process evaluation included interviews with the LHAs about their project-related activities, field notes written by the university researchers, an activity log maintained by the COS, and interviews with the CRG after the intervention ended to evaluate whether they would change anything about the process of selecting people to train as LHAs. The findings from these components of the evaluation have been reported elsewhere (Blumenthal et al., 1999; Thach et al., 2002; Thomas et al., 1998; Thomas et al., 2000). In this chapter we focus on another aspect: the essential elements for developing a research partnership that includes trust among the university researchers, the COS, and the CRG. One year after the STEP project's funding period ended, the researchers obtained a small grant to study this question.

Semistructured interviews were completed with the COS, two university investigators, and nine CRG members who were the most active (the total number in the CRG varied over time but was usually 10–12 people). The interviews, each lasting about an hour, addressed the nature of the interactions between the researchers and the CRG. The researchers and the COS were interviewed together and were asked to describe the history of STEP, how STEP gained entrée in the community, the formation of advisory groups, the role of local and state-level institutions, challenges and lessons learned during the course of the project about building trust, and community and individual-level changes that took place as a result of STEP.

CRG members who were interviewed were asked to describe what it was like to work with STEP researchers and how the researchers interacted with community members and local health agencies; reflect on the CRG's collaborative and decision-making power within STEP; identify the researchers' successes and mistakes; evaluate how STEP's research and intervention approach was similar to or different from that of other local health organizations; and comment on the overall impact of STEP on the local community. Interviews were audio recorded and then transcribed verbatim for analysis with text analysis

software (Atlas.ti, version 4.2). The interviews were conducted by two graduate students; both had skills and experience in qualitative research. One had not been part of the STEP project while the other had contributed to the project but interacted with the CRG members only infrequently. To ensure confidentiality of responses, only the interviewers had access to the verbatim transcripts for analysis. They coded and retrieved responses using a text analysis software program and identified generative themes from response text that were assigned the same code. The study's procedures were approved by the institutional review board at the University of North Carolina at Chapel Hill.

This rest of this chapter reports on the themes generated from the analysis of the 12 interview transcripts (from the COS, two university researchers, and nine CRG members). We focus on respondents' comments that shed light on how trust developed between the researchers and the CRG. We identified five interrelated elements that helped build trust: valuing the community, sharing decision-making power, being genuine, being trustworthy, and mutual learning. Examples of these elements are summarized in Table 39.1. In the following sections we provide more detail on the findings, including illustrative quotes from the respondents.

Valuing the Community

Respondents noted that, unlike the county health department, the STEP project "really went out into the community" by investing in the unique expertise of CRG members and LHAs to act and lead in their community. As expressed by a CRG member, seeking out a wide range of groups as potential collaborators was important:

I mean they tried to include people from—representatives of all walks of the community. . . . They went about that perfectly, as far as involving different segments of the population—of the community, and definitely within the health—health, um, facilities. That part was strong to me, in my opinion. Very strong.

Moreover, respondents commented on the COS and investigators' participating in the everyday life of their community beyond what the research required. For example, the COS entrusted a local day-care center with the daily care

TABLE 39.1 The Means of Establishing Trust Between the Researchers and the Community Resource Group

Element of trust	Examples from the project
Valuing the community	• The intervention went deep into the community. • The intervention was based on community members and invested in them. • The researchers spent time in the community beyond just conducting the research.
Sharing decision-making power	• There were real opportunities for the advisors to make decisions. • The researchers encouraged the advisors to disagree with the researchers. • Input from the advisors was actually used.
Being genuine	• There were egalitarian interactions between the researchers and the community members. • The researchers were "down-to-earth."
Being trustworthy	• Confidentiality was maintained. • The researchers showed up for community events. • Input from the advisors was actually used.
Mutual learning	• The researchers provided an opportunity for learning that was valued by the community collaborators. • The LHAs felt truly empowered by the project.

of her two young daughters. She and the investigators attended evening and weekend events such as revivals, holiday celebrations, and open houses sponsored by local churches and other organizations.

Sharing Decision-Making Power

CRG members described the decision-making process as being transparent and in need of their

expertise. They noted, for example, that the COS facilitated regularly scheduled meetings of the CRG and investigators; prepared an agenda of issues relevant to the particular phase of the study at that time; reported on actions from decisions made earlier by the CRG; and for the issues at hand, encouraged differing opinions and ideas. As expressed by a CRG member, the structure and process of these meetings were fundamental to shared decision-making power:

I mean, she didn't say, "Well I'm in charge" or whatever; she let us help out. So that kind of worked out pretty good. Which I think that's the way it was planned, that's the way it should have been, 'cause you had the community involved, as far as the program instead of just, she just dictating or whatever.

Being Genuine

In addition to noting how the researchers shared power, some CRG members mentioned how the researchers did not fit the stereotype of arrogant or ivory-tower professors. Instead, they observed that

their presence was here, enough for people to get to know them, and to see them as friends, you know, was very important, because I think if that part of it was not there, then [CRG/LHAs] would have not looked at it as being as important as I think they really came to feel about it . . . so without that presence I don't think it . . . would have been as successful.

[The researchers] were beautiful—always so warm and we just had a good time, just lighthearted. Everybody was comfortable; you didn't feel any pressure; you didn't feel uncomfortable; you could talk about anything.

Being Trustworthy

Closely related to the essential elements already discussed, the COS and investigators established trust with the community in part by following through on decisions and commitments made with the CRG. As noted earlier, they showed up for events initiated by the LHAs. This entailed a three-hour round trip, often on a weekend.

CRG respondents remarked that they felt that their input was actually used. Of particular significance was the fact that the COS and investigators maintained the confidentiality of CRG discussions. For example, one CRG member said she felt safer expressing herself at STEP meetings than she did at her church, and another expressed the following about one of the investigators: "She wanted to make sure nobody was exploited, you know. She went overboard to ensure that no matter what we said, it was confidential, you know, and I, and I felt good about that."

Mutual Learning

Another essential element related to sharing decision-making power was the benefit to the community of gaining new knowledge through collaboration in the project. The mutual learning gained by LHAs and the researchers, for example, was cited as an important benefit:

I think what the impact the STEP project had was, is that, it really did educate the lay health advisors where they were really able to go out and advocate in the community and be able to educate their families, their friends, and their loved ones. . . . I think that the women, that the lay health advisors, truly became empowered. I think that they learned about, a lot about themselves; that they were—you're talking about low-income women—that they were capable, that they were worth something. I think it gave them a lot of self-esteem.

In addition, the mutual learning gained by CRG members and the researchers was cited as a motivating force for sustaining involvement despite the constant pull from other commitments:

I would say, "Well, I just don't have time," and then I would go to a [STEP] meeting and I would say, "Boy, I can't give this up," you know? Cause one thing—you—I learned so much that I could—could bring back to my church! I mean, when I took it back to the church, they said, "Yes! Yes! Yes! I want to serve; I want to be there; I want to be on that!"

These five elements for establishing trusting academic–community collaborations epitomize the interactions between the STEP project's CRG members, the COS, and the investigators. The interviews also revealed the researchers' shortcomings. For example, it was noted that they might have developed a stronger relationship with the state health department and communicated more effectively with the CRG and LHAs about the departure of the first COS and the end of the project. Space limitations prevent us from including here full discussion of these comments. Moreover, although the CRG members interviewed were encouraged to speak critically, we realize that the interviewers' affiliation with the researchers would be likely to temper some of the respondents' critical comments. Nonetheless, our confidence in the validity of the five elements we have identified stems from the fact that they were not reflected only in isolated comments but in observations shared by several respondents. In the next two sections we summarize the project's elements that both required and developed trust and the implications for other interventions and research.

DISCUSSION

Researchers are among those with privileged status, access to resources, and authority in American society. A key challenge to investigators aiming to decrease STD transmission among people disenfranchised by society is transcending these people's distrust of those with high social status. To overcome the community's distrust of the study, STEP's interactions with community groups addressed (a) who would conduct the research, that is, which groups would collaborate with the university to conduct the research; (b) how the research would be conducted; and (c) for whom the research would be conducted, that is, whose issues would be addressed.

During STEP's observational study phase, the 14 advisors represented a wide range of STD care agencies and at-risk populations in the community. They guided the collection and analysis of observational data. Based on findings about African American women's natural helping networks, members of the CRG represented the range of groups that assisted African American women at risk for STDs. The CRG members were recognized and trusted by the African American community. At the same time they were experienced in working in the wider society with individuals and groups in positions of authority. Because they were willing to develop trusting relationships with university researchers, CRG members were able to influence the direction and implementation of the intervention, as well as to identify and recruit people who were natural helpers in their community. The researchers could not have found these helpers had they worked on their own. Moreover, the women who were eventually trained as

LHAs trusted the intervention because they were nominated by CRG members whom they knew. Indeed, some of the CRG members even took part in the LHA training. The CRG was critical in bringing to the intervention representatives of the people most affected by the local negative social forces.

The LHAs carried the intervention even deeper into the local social networks. Like the CRG members, they were people trusted in the community, and the people who trusted them were their relatives, friends, and coworkers, the very people for whom the intervention was designed. Because it was the LHAs who disseminated information, attitudes, and skills about STDs and care-seeking among people they knew, the message they communicated was much more likely to be heard, believed, and put into practice than it would have been if carried by a stranger or an agency outreach worker who represented the power structure.

The intervention also overcame distrust through the new relationships that LHAs developed with local agency staff. LHAs gained a direct link to agency staff, sometimes by referring or escorting a friend to the clinic or by participating in an agency-sponsored event with clinic staff or serving on agency task forces. The LHAs also provided a community voice to begin shaping agencies' awareness of STD-related issues including AIDS.

The LHAs' training and work and the interactions with the CRG were all facilitated by the COS; she also held a key gatekeeper position. Unlike the researchers, she spent every working day in Step County. To the CRG, LHAs, and others in Step County her presence and skills represented a tangible investment in the community. To the researchers she was a direct link to everyday life in the county, able to inform the researchers of local news and rumors, strengths and opportunities.

The researchers, in turn, were able to document, translate, and disseminate the LHAs' work to public health practitioners and scholars. Within Step County the researchers used their university affiliation, which was held in high regard, to gain entry to local circles of power. One of the ways they did this was to make progress reports to elected officials and agency CEOs and their boards to help shape their awareness of community issues related to STDs. To move the public health field forward nationally STEP investigators used their credentials and professional networks to coauthor a large number of presentations and publications with CRG members and LHAs. For example, three LHAs presented on a panel at the annual meeting of the American Public Health Association, and another LHA addressed the plenary session of a national STD conference.

Each collaborator—whether a member of the CRG, the LHAs, the COS, or the university researchers—made unique, essential contributions. Without any one of them the intervention would not have been effective; indeed, it might not have occurred at all. The intervention not only achieved changes in targeted behaviors (Thomas et al., 2000) but also changed some aspects of the social dynamics in Step County, such as the interactions between African American clients at the county health department and the STD clinic staff, that underlie the high STD rates (Thomas, Eng, Earp, & Ellis, 2001).

IMPLICATIONS

Can this model can be replicated elsewhere? The STEP project was implemented in only one Southern community. As a demonstration project it showed that such a model *can* work. Our results do not provide enough information to judge whether it *will* work elsewhere. Findings from our process evaluation suggest, however, that there are aspects of the model that could be replicated and other aspects that would be inappropriate to assume would apply to another community.

We believe, however, that the five elements for establishing a research collaboration that includes trust are transferable to other settings. When the goal is to implement and have accepted a theory-based community intervention, or to thoroughly evaluate a community intervention, a collaborative relationship between researchers and community members is indispensable. The contributions each of our collaborators made to this project are summarized in Table 39.2.

Using a collaborative approach we were able to effectively address some of the needs and overcome, at least in part, some of the social barriers that underlie the disproportionately higher rates of STDs among African Americans in this community. In other communities where high STD rates are a concern the reasons behind the rates may be different from those found in Step

TABLE 39.2 Productive Elements of a Research Partnership Between Community Members and Academic Researchers in the Design, Implementation, and Evaluation of an Intervention to Influence STD-Related Behaviors

Study component	Contribution by the community resource group (CRG)	Contribution by the researchers
Intervention design		
Understanding the problem	Information on the local setting and advice on data collection prior to the intervention	Theory and prior experience with data collection and analysis; data collected to inform the intervention
Identifying an appropriate intervention	Insights into what would be feasible and well received in the community	Theory and prior experience with interventions
Implementation		
Accessing those most at risk	Identify natural helpers who could serve as LHAs	Assistance with identifying the characteristics of those most at risk
Credibility with community members	Personal relationships with community members	Prestige of the university
	Participation in the LHA training	Conducting the LHA training
Interactions with agencies	Knew people on staff at various agencies	Able to make suggestions to agencies that local residents could not make
Maintaining the intervention	Advice on interacting with local agencies to gain their support of the LHAs' work	Funding for the community outreach specialist (COS)
Evaluation		
Household survey	Guidance to researchers on interactions with households during the survey	Data collection, research design, and analysis expertise

County. For example, higher rates in an urban setting might be attributed to a greater number of commercial sex workers (not documented as a problem in Step County). In this case the desired qualities of an LHA to address this problem, as well as some of the knowledge and skills they would use and share with their social networks, would probably be different (perhaps they would be male clients of commercial sex workers). Community advisors (or, in our case, the CRG) must decide how to adjust the intervention to fit the assets and context of a particular community and be effective in that community. If advisors are in touch with the affected community and not just those community members most immediately accessed by researchers, they can provide invaluable guidance about the intervention's design and implementation. To gain such guidance it is incumbent upon the researchers to establish a relationship with their community advisors that is characterized by valuing community, sharing decision-making power, being trustworthy and genuine, and mutual learning. Without a collaborative relationship of this nature, the distrust of community research so often found among socially marginalized groups will continue to undermine STD prevention programs.

ACKNOWLEDGMENTS Components of this chapter were previously published in *Public Health Reports* (Thomas et al., 2001). The authors thank Jadis Robinson and Charlotte Williams for their roles as community outreach specialists in the project; the members of the STEP project community resource group; and the lay health advisors. The STEP project was supported by National Institute of Allergy and Infectious Disease grant U01-AI31496, with supplemental funds from Glaxo-Wellcome and the HIV/STD Control Branch of the North Carolina Department of Environment, Health, and Natural Resources.

References

Blumenthal, C., Eng, E., & Thomas, J. C. (1999). STEP sisters, sex, and STDs: A process evaluation of the recruitment of lay health advisors. *American Journal of Health Promotion, 14,* 4–6.

Centers for Disease Control and Prevention. (1991). Hepatitis B virus: A comprehensive strategy for eliminating transmission in the United States through universal childhood vaccination; recommendations of the Immunization Practices Advisory Committee (ACIP). *Morbidity and Mortality Weekly Report, 40*(RR-13), 1–25.

Centers for Disease Control and Prevention. (1990). Protection against viral hepatitis: Recommendations of the Immunization Practices Advisory Committee (ACIP). *Morbidity and Mortality Weekly Report, 39*(S-2), 1–76.

Dearing, J. W., Meyer, G., & Rogers, E. M. (1994). Diffusion theory and HIV risk behavior change. In R. J. DiClemente & J. L. Peterson (Eds.), *Preventing AIDS: Theories and methods of behavior interventions* (pp. 79–93). New York: Plenum Press.

Freire, P. (1970). *Pedagogy of the oppressed.* New York: Seabury Press.

Leaning, J., Eng, E., & Davis, E. (1998). STD prevention as a human rights obligation: The challenge to public health researchers and policy makers. Plenary session, National STD Prevention Conference, 1998, Dallas.

Over, M., & Piot, P. (1993). Health sector priorities review: HIV infection and sexually transmitted diseases. In D. T. Jamison & W. H. Mosley (Eds.), *Disease control priorities in developing countries* (pp. 455–527). New York: Oxford University Press for the World Bank.

Thach, S. B., Eng, E., & Thomas, J. C. (2002). Defining and assessing organizational competence in serving communities at risk for STDs. *Health Promotion Practice, 3,* 217–232.

Thomas, J. C., Earp, J. A., & Eng, E. (2000). Evaluation and lessons learned from a lay health advisor program to prevent sexually transmitted diseases. *International Journal of STD and AIDS, 11,* 812–818.

Thomas, J. C., Eng, E., Clark, M., Robinson, J., & Blumenthal, C. (1998). Lay health advisors: Sexually transmitted disease prevention through community involvement. *American Journal of Public Health, 88,* 1252–1253.

Thomas, J. C., Eng, E., Earp, J. A., & Ellis, H. (2001). Trust and collaboration in the prevention of sexually transmitted diseases. *Public Health Reports, 116,* 540–547.

Thomas, J. C., Schoenbach, V. J., Eng, G., & McDonald, M. A. (1996). Rural gonorrhea in the southeastern United States: A neglected epidemic? *American Journal of Epidemiology, 143,* 269–277.

Thomas, J. C., & Thomas, K. (1999). Things ain't what they ought to be: Social forces underlying high rates of sexually transmitted diseases in a rural North Carolina county. *Social Science and Medicine, 49,* 1075–1084.

Thomas, J. C., & Tucker, M. (1995). The development and use of the concept of a sexually transmitted disease core. *Journal of Infectious Diseases, 174*(Suppl. 2), S134–S143.

40 PREVALENCE OF SMOKING AND CESSATION AMONG NORTHERN PLAINS INDIANS

Greg Holzman, Todd Harwell, Dorothy Gohdes, & Steven Helgerson

Cigarette smoking is a leading behavioral cause of death in the United States (McGinnis & Foege, 1993). Although an estimated 23% of the general adult population smokes cigarettes (Centers for Disease Control and Prevention, 2002), the prevalence of this preventable cause of illness and death is much higher for some subgroups in the population, notably American Indians and Alaskan Natives (Bursac & Campbell, 2002; Denny & Holtzman, 1999; Kaplan, Lanier, Merritt, & Siegel, 1997) and specifically Northern Plains American Indians (Denny & Holtzman, 1999; Goldberg et al., 1991; Sugarman, Warren, Oge, & Helgerson, 1992; Welty et al., 1995). American Indians of the northern plains have higher cardiovascular and cancer mortality rates than American Indians from other regions of the United States (U.S. Indian Health Service, *Regional differences in Indian health: 1998–99*). This is likely associated with the higher prevalence of smoking in this group. Efficacious smoking cessation methods have been demonstrated (Fiore & U. S. Tobacco Use and Dependence Guideline Panel, 2000). Unfortunately, these evidence-based methods have not been systematically applied among American Indians in the northern plains. In this chapter we describe the extraordinarily high prevalence of smoking in this population, a variety of evidence-based smoking cessation steps, and the urgent need to apply and evaluate these steps in American Indian communities.

BACKGROUND

The association between cigarette smoking and lung cancer, first suspected in the early 20th century, was clearly documented by midcentury (Doll & Hill, 1950, 1952, 1954; Wynder & Graham, 1950). During the last half of the century evidence that smoking is the cause of a wide variety of cancers, a risk factor for cardiovascular disease, and a major contributor to morbidity from a variety of other severe diseases mounted, and the prevalence of cigarette smoking in U.S. adults aged 18 years or older declined from 43% in 1965 to 25% by 1997 (Centers for Disease Control and Prevention, 1999). Despite this overall decline, since 1995 the prevalence of smoking in some subgroups of the population has remained constant or increased, particularly in young adults, American Indians, and Alaskan Natives (Centers for Disease Control and Prevention, 1997, 2002).

Smoking among American Indians and Alaskan Natives drew little attention from medical and public health workers until the last two decades of the 20th century. There are at least two reasons for this. From the 1950s through the 1970s public health efforts focused primarily on maternal and child health issues and infectious diseases such as trachoma and tuberculosis. Also, smoking was uncommon among the Indians of the Southwest, where most Indian health studies were being generated (Gilliland, Mahler, & Davis, 1998; Mendlein et al., 1997; Sievers, 1968). In the 1960s and 1970s researchers did not present in the published literature the variability of cigarette usage between the different tribes. In the 1980s a few reports were published regarding the high prevalence of cigarette smoking among Alaskan Natives and Northern Plains Indians (Goldberg et al., 1991; Lanier, Bulkow, Novotny, Giovino, & Davis, 1990). Currently, cigarette smoking among American Indians and Alaskan Natives as a group is recognized as a major public health problem; this population has the highest race-specific smoking prevalence among U.S. adults, 36% (Centers for Disease Control and Prevention, 2002). Even this high prevalence estimate is deceptive: smoking rates among Alaskan Natives and Northern Plains Indians are markedly higher while the rates among the Indian populations of the Southwest are close to the national average (Centers for Disease Control and Prevention, 2000; Welty et al., 1995). Nevertheless, the contribution of smoking, including passive (secondhand) smoking (California Environmental Protection Agency, 1997; Cook & Strachan, 1999; U.S. Environmental Protection Agency, 1992) is a major concern for American Indian and Alaskan Native health (Rhodes, Rhoades, Jones, & Collins, 2000; Welty et al., 1995). Of particular concern is smoking's interaction with the diabetes epidemic in American Indian and Alaskan Native communities. Smoking is known to aggravate both microvascular and macrovascular complications of diabetes (Haire-Joshu, Glasgow, & Tibbs, 1999, 2003). Thus, smoking-related diseases are the leading killers of American Indians and Alaskan Natives (U.S. Indian Health Service, *Trends in Indian health: 1998–99*).

A recently published study of smoking behaviors among American Indians in Montana used an adapted Behavioral Risk Factor Surveillance System (BRFSS) survey to assess the prevalence of cigarette smoking in a large sample of adult American Indians on or near seven reservations in the state and compared the prevalence to the non-Indian population (Gohdes et al., 2002). There was a marked difference in smoking rates between the two groups: 38% of the American Indians were current smokers while 19% of the adult non-Indian population were smokers. In the American Indian population more current smokers had cardiovascular disease (CVD) risk factors (37%) than in the non-Indian population (17%). Interestingly, the prevalence

of smoking was about the same among adults known to have CVD in the two populations: 21% of the Indian population with a self-reported history of CVD smoked cigarettes compared to 27% of the non-Indian population with a similar CVD history. In addition, American Indian smokers were more likely to have tried to quit smoking over the past year than were non-Indian smokers: 67% compared to 43%. Nevertheless, the quit ratio, the proportion of smokers who successfully quit, greatly favored the non-Indian compared to the American Indian population.

Other studies conducted in the 1980s and 1990s also documented a high prevalence of smoking in Northern Plains Indians (see Table 40.1; Centers for Disease Control and Prevention, 2000). Smoking prevalence in Northern Plains Indians in these studies ranged from 38% to 62%. Based on the 2000 census, there were approximately 225,173 adult American Indians in the northern plains states of Indiana, Iowa, Michigan, Minnesota, Montana, Nebraska, North Dakota, South Dakota, Wisconsin, and Wyoming (U.S. Census Bureau, 2000). Using the minimum estimated cigarette smoking prevalence for Northern Plains Indians, the number of smokers would be approximately 101,000 (see Figure 40.1). An important, challenging opportunity to help many of these persons to stop smoking exists.

Total Population = 225,173

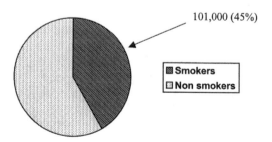

FIGURE 40.1 The number of American Indians aged ≥ 18 years in 10 northern plains states and the estimated number of current smokers, 2000

TABLE 40.1 Estimates of the Prevalence of Cigarette Smoking from Selected Population-Based Studies of Adult Northern Plains American Indians, 1985–1999

| | | | | Smoking prevalence (%) for | | | | |
| | | | | AI* | | Comparison prevalence | | |
Reference	Years	AI* population (state)	Age (years)	Total	Male/Female	Total	Male/Female	Comparison population (state)
Sugarman et al., 1992	1985–88	IA, MN, MT, NE, ND, SD, WI	+18	54	48/57	—	25/23	Whites in IA, MN, MT, NE, ND, SD, WI
Goldberg et al., 1991	1987	Urban MT	15–49	62	63/63	22	21/24	Whites in MT
Welty et al., 1995	1989–92	ND, SD	45–74	49	53/45	—	—	—
Centers for Disease Control and Prevention, 1996	1992–94	MN, WI	+25	52	51/52	—	—	—
U.S. Public Health Service et al., 2000	1995–98	IN, IA, MI, MN, MT, NE, ND, SD, WI, WY	+18	45	47/42	—	—	—
Harwell et al., 2001	1999	MT	+18	38	36/40	19	18/22	Non-Indians in MT

*AI = American Indian

TABLE 40.2 Strength of Evidence Classification Used to Rate Evidence-Based Recommendations

Strength of evidence classification	Criteria
A	Multiple well-designed, randomized clinical trials directly relevant to the recommendations yielded a consistent pattern of findings.
B	Some evidence from randomized clinical trials supported the recommendation, but the scientific support was not optimal.
C	Reserved for important clinical situations where the panel achieved consensus on the recommendation in the absence of relevant randomized controlled trials.

Modified from Fiore & U.S. Tobacco Use and Dependence Guideline Panel, 2000.

EFFICACIOUS SMOKING CESSATION METHODS

Fortunately for American Indian and Alaskan Native smokers the evidence for efficacious smoking cessation interventions is quite strong. These interventions have been described in two documents published by the U. S. Department of Health and Human Services: "Treating Tobacco Use and Dependence: Clinical Practice Guideline" (Fiore & U. S. Tobacco Use and Dependence Guideline Panel, 2000) and "Reducing Tobacco Use: A Report of the Surgeon General" (U. S. Public Health Service, Office of the Surgeon General, Centers for Disease Control and Prevention, National Center for Chronic Disease Prevention and Health Promotion, & U. S. Office on Smoking and Health, 2000; see also the end of this chapter for evidence-based smoking cessation resources on the Internet). The U. S. Public Health Service has evaluated the different interventions using specific criteria (see Table 40.2.). Based on this evaluation a number of provider–patient level interventions have been shown to be effective (Table 40.3). Smoking ces-

sation interventions at the community and health-system levels have also been shown to be effective (Table 40.4).

There are some distinct characteristics of the Northern Plains American Indian communities that may help or hinder widespread implementation of the much-needed community and health systems smoking cessation interventions. Many Northern Plains Indians live on or near reservations where communities are dealing not only with the high prevalence of cigarette smoking but also with high rates of unemployment and substance use. These conditions are likely to be barriers to successful community-based cessation efforts. With Northern Plains Indian smoking rates over 40% in adults (Centers for Disease Control and Prevention, 2000) it is likely that any smoker trying to quit will be exposed to other smokers in the home, and individual smoking cessation efforts may be impeded in these cases.

Nevertheless, the Northern Plains Indians have some unique opportunities that may assist in combating the smoking problem. Each federally recognized American Indian tribe is self-governing. This gives the individual tribal government or health system a unique opportunity to implement communitywide interventions that have been shown to contribute to successful smoking cessation (e.g., smoking bans). Traditional tobacco practices among Plains Indians have been used to help promote cessation efforts (Compact Disc University of Montana & Montana, 2001). Most American Indians in the northern plains are members of federally recognized tribes and are therefore entitled to health care through the Indian Health Service (IHS). Using health systems changes at IHS and tribal clinics to enhance smoking cessation efforts is an inviting strategy. In fact, IHS hospitals in the Southwest were among the first hospitals in the United States to eliminate smoking in the hospital setting (Centers for Disease Control and Prevention, 1987). Selected pharmaceuticals on local IHS formularies are provided free of charge to American Indians and Alaskan Natives. It is important to assure that appropriate pharmacologic agents, including over-the-counter medications, are available for all patients who want to use them to quit smoking, particularly in the relatively remote communities.

TABLE 40.3 Interventions Applied at the Provider–Patient Level

Intervention	Strength of evidence
Physician advice: Advice from a physician to quit smoking can increase smoking cessation rates.	A
Brief counseling: Cessation rates can be improved with brief person-to-person tobacco dependence counseling including individual or group sessions as well as counseling by telephone.	A
Intensity of counseling: A strong dose-response relationship has been observed between the time and intensity of tobacco dependence counseling and cessation rates.	A
Counseling and social support: Counseling that focuses on identifying social support systems, both within the health care system and in the patient's daily life, can improve cessation rates.	B
Counseling and behavior therapy: Behavior therapy that develops problem-solving skills and emphasizes skills training can improve cessation rates.	B
Medications: Unless there is a contraindication, every patient should be offered a pharmaceutical agent with proven effectiveness to assist the patient in the attempt to quit smoking.	A
Five first-line and two second-line pharmacotherapy agents have been identified to increase a patient's chance at success:	
First-line pharmaceutical agents	
Bupropion SR	A
Nicotine gum	A
Nicotine inhaler	A
Nicotine nasal spray	A
Nicotine patch	A
Second-line pharmaceutical agents	
Clonidine	A
Nortriptyline	B
Combination nicotine replacement: patch with either nicotine spray or gum	B

Source: Fiore & U.S. Tobacco Use and Dependence Guideline Panel, 2000.

MORE AGGRESSIVE APPLICATION OF EFFICACIOUS SMOKING CESSATION METHODS

Despite the availability of evidence-based smoking cessation methods, smoking rates for American Indians and Alaskan Natives remain high. There is little published evidence to suggest that the smoking cessation interventions have been applied systematically to American Indian and Alaskan Native populations. To date no practice-based research among the Northern Plains Indian population regarding effective smoking cessation has been published, and in fact, very little has been published regarding cessation in other American Indian and Alaskan Native populations (Hensel et al., 1995; Johnson, Lando, Schmid, & Solberg, 1997). All of the well-documented cessation strategies should be used to help control smoking-related morbidity and mortality among Northern Plains Indians.

Smoking cessation can have an important impact on the health of Indian communities. Recent studies in other populations have estimated

TABLE 40.4 Interventions Applied at the Community or Health-System Level

---

Community interventions: These interventions are communitywide and include

> smoking bans and restrictions.

> increasing the unit price for tobacco products.

> mass media education campaigns combined with other interventions.

> limiting young people's access to tobacco products.

Health care systems interventions: These interventions occur within health care settings and organizations and include

> provider reminders either alone or with provider education, with or without patient education.

> reducing patient's out-of-pocket costs for effective cessation therapies.

> support for patient cessation efforts.

> designing staff to provide smoking cessation assistance.

Sources: Fiore & U.S. Tobacco Use and Dependence Guideline Panel, 2000; Hopkins et al., 2001.

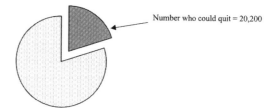

Total number of smokers = 101,000

Number who could quit = 20,200

FIGURE 40.2 Number of American Indian smokers aged ≥18 years in 10 northern plains states and the number who could quit if provided evidence-based smoking cessation (with 20% quit rate), 2000

There are many evidence-based interventions that have worked with other populations to decrease cigarette smoking rates. But to date there is little documented evidence that these strategies have been systematically applied and evaluated among the Northern Plains Indians. The need to provide effective strategies for both cessation and primary prevention is clear, and now is the time for action.

Evidence-based Smoking Cessation Resources on the Internet

Treating tobacco use and dependence—a systems approach: A guide for health care administrators, insurers, managed care organizations, and purchasers: http://www.surgeongeneral.gov/tobacco/systems.htm

Quick reference guide for clinicians treating tobacco use and dependence: http://www.surgeongeneral.gov/tobacco/tobaqrg.htm

References

Bursac, Z., & Campbell, J. E. (2002). Prevalence of current cigarette smoking among American Indians in Oklahoma: A comparison. *Journal of the Oklahoma State Medical Association, 95*(3), 155–158.

California Environmental Protection Agency. (1997). Health effects of exposure to environmental tobacco smoke. *Tobacco Control, 6*(4), 346–353.

Compact Disc University of Montana & Montana. (2001). Many voices, one message—Keep tobacco sacred: Tobacco use prevention program. University of Montana, Missoula, MT.

cessation rates of 20–25% with evidence-based counseling and pharmacotherapy (Katz, Muehlenbruch, Brown, Fiore, & Baker, 2002; U. S. Public Health Service et al., 2000). If 20% of the American Indian smokers quit by cessation methods that have been used in other populations, then approximately 20,200 Northern Plains American Indians would no longer smoke (Figure 40.2). These individuals would avoid premature death and preventable disabilities associated with smoking-related diseases. Tribal and IHS clinical sites would avoid substantial costs associated with treating smoking-related diseases (Centers for Disease Control and Prevention, 1994; Miller, Zhang, Rice, & Max, 1998). If the smoking prevalence for this population were reduced to the national average, more than 49,000 Northern Plains American Indians who currently smoke would be former smokers.

Cigarette smoking is at an epidemic level among American Indians of the northern plains.

Centers for Disease Control and Prevention. (1987). Indian Health Service facilities become smoke-free. *Morbidity and Mortality Weekly Report, 36*(22), 348–350.

Centers for Disease Control and Prevention. (1994). Medical care expenditures attributable to cigarette smoking—United States, 1993. *Morbidity and Mortality Weekly Report, 43*(26), 469–472.

Centers for Disease Control and Prevention. (1996). *Inter tribal heart project: Results from the Cardiovascular Health Survey*. Atlanta: Centers for Disease Control and Prevention.

Centers for Disease Control and Prevention. (1997). Cigarette smoking among adults—United States, 1995. *Morbidity and Mortality Weekly Report, 46*(51), 1217–1220.

Centers for Disease Control and Prevention. (1999). Tobacco use—United States, 1900–1999. *Morbidity and Mortality Weekly Report, 48*(43), 986–993.

Centers for Disease Control and Prevention. (2000). Prevalence of selected risk factors for chronic disease and injury among American Indians and Alaska Natives—United States, 1995–1998. *Morbidity and Mortality Weekly Report, 49*(4), 79–82, 91.

Centers for Disease Control and Prevention. (2002). Cigarette smoking among adults—United States, 2000. *Morbidity and Mortality Weekly Report, 51*(29), 642–645.

Cook, D. G., & Strachan, D. P. (1999). Health effects of passive smoking-10: Summary of effects of parental smoking on the respiratory health of children and implications for research. *Thorax, 54*(4), 357–366.

Denny, C., & Holtzman, D. (1999). Health behaviors of American Indians and Alaska Natives: Findings from the Behavioral Risk Factor Surveillance System, 1993–1996. Atlanta: U.S. Department of Health and Human Services, Centers for Disease Control.

Doll, R., & Hill, A. (1950). Smoking and carcinoma of the lung. *British Medical Journal, 2*(4682), 739–748.

Doll, R., & Hill, A. (1952). A study of the aetiology of carcinoma of the lung. *British Medical Journal, 2*, 1271–1286.

Doll, R., & Hill, A. (1954). The mortality of doctors in relation to their smoking habits: A preliminary report. *British Medical Journal, 1*, 1451–1455.

Fiore, M., & U. S. Tobacco Use and Dependence Guideline Panel. (2000). *Treating tobacco use and dependence*. Washington, DC: U.S. Department of Health and Human Services.

Gilliland, F. D., Mahler, R., & Davis, S. M. (1998). Non-ceremonial tobacco use among Southwestern rural American Indians: The New Mexico American Indian Behavioural Risk Factor Survey. *Tobacco Control, 7*(2), 156–160.

Gohdes, D., Harwell, T. S., Cummings, S., Moore, K. R., Smilie, J. G., & Helgerson, S. D. (2002). Smoking cessation and prevention: An urgent public health priority for American Indians in the Northern Plains. *Public Health Reports, 117*(3), 281–290.

Goldberg, H. I., Warren, C. W., Oge, L. L., Helgerson, S. D., Pepion, D. D., LaMere, E., et al. (1991). Prevalence of behavioral risk factors in two American Indian populations in Montana. *American Journal of Preventive Medicine, 7*(3), 155–160.

Haire-Joshu, D., Glasgow, R. E., & Tibbs, T. L. (1999). Smoking and diabetes. *Diabetes Care, 22*(11), 1887–1898.

Haire-Joshu, D., Glasgow, R. E., & Tibbs, T. L. (2003). Smoking and diabetes. *Diabetes Care, 26*(Suppl. 1), S89–90.

Harwell, T. S., Gohdes, D., Moore, K., McDowall, J. M., Smilie, J. G., & Helgerson, S. D. (2001). Cardiovascular disease and risk factors in Montana American Indians and non-Indians. *American Journal of Preventive Medicine, 20*(3), 196–201.

Hensel, M. R., Cavanagh, T., Lanier, A. P., Gleason, T., Bouwens, B., Tanttila, H., et al. (1995). Quit rates at one year follow-up of Alaska Native Medical Center Tobacco Cessation Program. *Alaska Medicine, 37*(2), 43–47.

Hopkins, D. P., Briss, P. A., Ricard, C. J., Husten, C. G., Carande-Kulis, V. G., Fielding, J. E., et al. (2001). Reviews of evidence regarding interventions to reduce tobacco use and exposure to environmental tobacco smoke. *American Journal of Preventive Medicine, 20*(Suppl. 2), 16–66.

Johnson, K. M., Lando, H. A., Schmid, L. S., & Solberg, L. I. (1997). The GAINS project: Outcome of smoking cessation strategies in four urban Native American clinics. *Addictive Behaviors, 22*(2), 207–218.

Kaplan, S. D., Lanier, A. P., Merritt, R. K., & Siegel, P. Z. (1997). Prevalence of tobacco use among Alaska Natives: A review. *Preventive Medicine, 26*(4), 460–465.

Katz, D. A., Muehlenbruch, D. R., Brown, R. B., Fiore, M. C., & Baker, T. B. (2002). Effectiveness of a clinic-based strategy for implementing the AHRQ Smoking Cessation Guideline in primary care. *Preventive Medicine, 35*(3), 293–301.

Lanier, A. P., Bulkow, L. R., Novotny, T. E., Giovino, G. A., & Davis, R. M. (1990). Tobacco use and its consequences in northern populations. *Arctic Medical Research, 49*(Suppl. 2), 17–22.

McGinnis, J. M., & Foege, W. H. (1993). Actual causes of death in the United States. *Journal of the American Medical Association, 270*(18), 2207–2212.

Mendlein, J. M., Freedman, D. S., Peter, D. G., Allen, B., Percy, C. A., Ballew, C., et al. (1997). Risk factors for coronary heart disease among Navajo Indians: Findings from the Navajo Health and Nutrition Survey. *Journal of Nutrition, 127*(Suppl. 10), 2099S–2105S.

Miller, L. S., Zhang, X., Rice, D. P., & Max, W. (1998). State estimates of total medical expenditures attributable to cigarette smoking, 1993. *Public Health Reports, 113*(5), 447–458.

Rhodes, D., Rhoades, E., Jones, C., & Collins, R. (2000). Tobacco use. In Everett Rhoades (Ed.), *American Indian health: Innovations in healthcare, promotion and policy*. Baltimore: The Johns Hopkins University Press.

Sievers, M. L. (1968). Cigarette and alcohol usage by Southwestern American Indians. *American Journal of Public Health and the Nation's Health, 58*(1), 71–82.

Sugarman, J. R., Warren, C. W., Oge, L., & Helgerson, S. D. (1992). Using the Behavioral Risk Factor Surveillance System to monitor year 2000 objectives among American Indians. *Public Health Reports, 107*(4), 449–456.

U.S. Census Bureau. (2000). *American FactFinder*. Retrieved March 2003 from http://factfinder. census.gov/servlet/BasicFactsServlet?_lang=en.

U.S. Environmental Protection Agency. (1992). *Respiratory health effects of passive smoking: Lung cancer and other disorders*. Washington, DC: U.S. Environmental Protection Agency, Office of Health and Environmental Assessment.

U.S. Indian Health Service. *Regional differences in Indian health: 1998–99*. Retrieved March 2003 from http://www.ihs.gov/PublicInfo/Publications/.

U.S. Indian Health Service. *Trends in Indian health: 1998–1999*. Retrieved March 2003 from http://www.ihs.gov/PublicInfo/Publications/.

U.S. Public Health Service, Office of the Surgeon General, Centers for Disease Control and Prevention, National Center for Chronic Disease Prevention and Health Promotion, & U.S. Office on Smoking and Health. (2000). Reducing tobacco use: A report of the Surgeon General Washington, DC: U.S. Department of Health and Human Services.

Welty, T. K., Lee, E. T., Yeh, J., Cowan, L. D., Go, O., Fabsitz, R. R., et al. (1995). Cardiovascular disease risk factors among American Indians: The Strong Heart Study. *American Journal of Epidemiology, 142*(3), 269–287.

Wynder, E., & Graham, E. (1950). Tobacco smoking as a possible etiologic factor in bronchiogenic carcinoma: A study of six hundred and eighty-four proved cases. *Journal of the American Medical Association, 143*(4), 329–336.

41 USING EVALUATION DATA AS THE BASIS FOR A LOCAL ORDINANCE TO CONTROL ALCOHOL AND TOBACCO BILLBOARDS IN CHICAGO

Diana P. Hackbarth, Daniel Schnopp-Wyatt, David Katz,
Janet Williams, Barbara Silvestri, & Michael Pfleger

Practice-based research that systematically evaluates the implementation and outcomes of health-related public policies can have a profound impact on society. Research findings based on practice can be used to validate existing policies, promote modification in policies, or justify abandoning current policies and seeking another course of action (Gerston, 1997). Methods are similar to those used to evaluate other types of health and social programs (Posavac & Carey, 2003). However, additional factors must be considered if the goal is to produce data that can serve as a catalyst for policy change at the community level. One important factor is the social, political, economic, and legal climate in which the evaluation is conducted. A second consideration is the possible uses of the data once the evaluation is completed. Sensitivity to these issues is essential when researchers from the advocacy community are scrutinizing the business practices of powerful special interests such as the alcohol, tobacco, or outdoor advertising industries (Bobo, Kendall, & Max, 2001; Meredith & Dunham, 1999).

Practice-based evaluation is often messy and not for the timid. Stakeholders with conflicting goals may seek to influence what questions are asked, control access to data sources, attempt to place their own spin on findings, or suppress or misuse results to accomplish policy goals. Practice-based research in this volatile arena is best accomplished in a coalition that brings together the expertise of academic researchers, the advocacy skills of health and community groups, existing data sources of government agencies, and support from affected communities that have a stake in the outcome. The goal is to leverage resources while maintaining the integrity of the research process. Data generated needs to be credible and in a format that is easily understood by policy makers, the press, community groups, and the public.

The case study on geographic placement of alcohol and tobacco billboards discussed in this chapter illustrates these principles. The evaluation study was conducted in 1997 and was a collaborative research and action project with the goal of policy change. The study's findings have been used to spark legislative action at the local level, influence discussions among state attorneys general and tobacco companies negotiating the Master Settlement Agreement (an agreement between states' attorneys general and the major tobacco companies, spelling out how much money the tobacco companies must reimburse states over 25 years for medical care of sick smokers and delineating changes in tobacco marketing practices in the United States), and as evidence for four years of federal court proceedings and appeals (Hackbarth et al., 2001). Lessons learned from this study can be applied to similar public health policies and other communities.

SOCIAL, ECONOMIC, POLITICAL, AND LEGAL CONTEXT

Alcohol and Tobacco Advertising

Alcohol and tobacco are among the most heavily advertised products in the United States. The six major tobacco companies spend more than $8.2 billion annually in the United States on advertising and promotion. Measured media for alcohol is almost $1.49 billion annually: beer, $971 million; liquor, $407 million; and wine, $115 million (Competitive Media Reporting/Adams Beverage Group, 2002). These figures include only magazine, newspaper, broadcast, and outdoor alcohol advertising. Including sponsorships and promotions would likely increase these numbers (Community Anti-Drug Coalitions of America). During the 1990s tobacco and alcohol companies still ranked among the top five advertisers in magazines and newspapers. Tobacco and alcohol long reigned as the most heavily advertised products in outdoor media, accounting for 58% of all outdoor advertising expenditures in 1979 (Outdoor Advertising Association of America). In the mid-1990s six of the top 10 outdoor advertisers were tobacco companies (*Standard Directory of Advertisers*, 2001).

In 1998 tobacco ranked as the number one product advertised on billboards, accounting for 9% of total billboard advertising expenditures (Outdoor Advertising Association of America). The percentage of tobacco billboard advertising expenditures has dropped dramatically since 1999 as a result of the Master Settlement Agreement (MSA) signed by the state attorneys general. Between 1995 and 1999 liquor and wine outdoor advertising expenditures increased while outdoor advertising expenditures for beer decreased (*Standard Directory of Advertisers*, 2001). In 2001, the most recent year for which data is available, beer companies spent $96.3 million, liquor $49 million, and wine $2.6 million on outdoor print advertising (Competitive Media Reporting/Adams Beverage Group, 2002). Currently three of the top five most heavily advertised brands in outdoor advertising are alcohol brands: Miller Beer, Anheuser-Busch, and Seagrams. Tobacco companies continue to advertise heavily in the print media but increasingly focus on event sponsorships, direct mailing, and special sales promotions. Tobacco advertising in the United States has actually increased since the Master Settlement Agreement,

despite the fact that the MSA includes tobacco advertising restrictions (Federal Trade Commission, 2001).

Outdoor Advertising of Age-Restricted Products

Outdoor advertising of age-restricted products is a form of advertising that raises both legal and public health concerns. Motorists and pedestrians, including nonsmokers, nondrinkers and children, cannot avoid exposure to outdoor advertising. Billboards are placed for maximum visibility in designated markets. Billboard ads are created to match the demographic makeup and socioeconomic characteristics of the market (Guthrie, 1994; Luke, Esmundo, & Bloom, 2000; Rossman, 1994; Schooler, Basil, & Altman, 1996). Advertisers have heavily saturated minority neighborhoods with outdoor advertising of tobacco and alcohol products (Altman, Schooler, & Basil, 1991; Hackbarth, Silvestri, & Cosper, 1995; Lee & Callcott, 1994; Mayberry & Price, 1993; Stoddard, Johnson, Sussman, Dent, & Boley-Cruz, 1998). Billboards advertising age-restricted products can be found near convenience stores, shopping centers, fast-food restaurants, homes, and day care centers; along major streets and expressways; on mass transit lines; and in sports stadiums, all places frequented by young people.

Industry "Voluntary Marketing Codes"

Historically, the billboard industry has exercised little restraint in ad placement. In 1991 the Outdoor Advertising Association of America (OAAA) responded to public criticism and adopted a voluntary "Code of Industry Principles for Billboards," which is supposed to assure that outdoor advertisements of products illegal for sale to minors are at least 500 feet from schools, playgrounds, and places of worship (Outdoor Advertising Association of America). Billboards near areas where children congregate are supposed to be voluntarily labeled with a placard representing the international symbol of a child, indicating that age-restricted products are not to be advertised on them. The code is also designed to set voluntary limits on the number of billboards in a market that advertise products that cannot legally be sold to minors. It also seeks to maintain diversification of customers who advertise in the outdoor medium. The Beer Institute (BI) and Distilled Spirits Council of the United States (DSCUS) also promulgate voluntary marketing codes that suggest that liquor ads should not be placed where most of the audience is below the legal drinking age (Beer Institute; Distilled Spirits Council of the United States; Evans & Kelly, 1999).

Health Disparities Related to Alcohol and Tobacco Use

The links between social conditions and health disparities are an increasing public health concern (Link & Phelan, 1995). Health disparities related to alcohol and tobacco are especially pronounced among the poor and minorities residing in inner-city communities targeted by alcohol and tobacco marketers. People with the lowest levels of educational attainment and lower socioeconomic status are more likely to smoke than those with more education and higher socioeconomic status (Kiefe et al., 2001). Alcohol use patterns also vary by gender, age, and race. Four of the five leading causes of death in the United States are related to tobacco use, and three of the remaining top 15 causes are related to either tobacco or alcohol abuse (Miniño, Arias, Kochanek, Murphy, & Smith, 2002).

Life expectancy for Whites continues to be about 5.7 years longer than for African Americans, although the gap is shrinking. Age-adjusted death rates for heart disease and stroke are declining nationally, due in part to declines in smoking rates, changes in diet, and better control of hypertension. However, persons in lower socioeconomic groups have higher mortality, morbidity, and risk factor levels for heart disease and stroke than those of higher socioeconomic status. Death rates for chronic liver disease and cirrhosis are higher among Hispanic males than White males. Age-adjusted death rates for African Americans compared to the White population are at least 1.3 times greater for the leading causes of death: 2.9 times higher for hypertension, 1.3 times higher for stroke, and 1.3 times higher for heart disease (Miniño et al., 2002). The age-adjusted death rate for African Americans is 53% higher than it is for Whites (Murphy, 2000). Lung cancer, of which 85% of cases are smoking induced, is the leading cause of cancer death for both sexes and all races. However, lung cancer accounts for a higher percentage of cancer deaths among African Ameri-

can males than among White males (American Lung Association, 2000). Alcohol and tobacco use clearly contribute to observed health disparities. Reducing alcohol and tobacco consumption among disadvantaged groups through community-level interventions is one way to remedy disparities.

TRIGGERS FOR THE PRACTICE-BASED EVALUATION

The collaborative research and action partnership between Loyola University Chicago (LUC), the American Lung Association of Metropolitan Chicago (ALAMC), and a grassroots community group began in the early 1990s. An activist priest and parishioners at St. Sabina's Church were concerned about drug and alcohol use in their community. An informal survey of the 10-block region surrounding the predominately African American church identified 118 billboards advertising alcohol and tobacco compared to only three billboards in a nearby White neighborhood. A comprehensive 1991 study revealed that there were five times as many alcohol billboards and three times as many tobacco billboards in predominately minority areas of the city compared to White areas (Hackbarth et al., 1995). Attempts were made over a six-year period to pass a local ordinance controlling alcohol and tobacco billboards, but were unsuccessful.

By 1997, public opinion was becoming increasingly critical of the tobacco industry. The Food and Drug Administration (FDA) was proposing tobacco advertising restrictions. States' attorneys general were banding together to sue the tobacco industry to recoup tax dollars spent on tobacco-related diseases. A citywide coalition against tobacco and alcohol billboards felt the time was right to push for a local billboard ordinance based on zoning rather than advertising content. Academic researchers from Loyola University Chicago School of Nursing partnered with ALAMC volunteers and community members to design a research study to provide the scientific basis for public policy initiatives. It was deemed necessary to evaluate the impact of the existing voluntary policy before the case could be made for government intervention (see Figure 41.1).

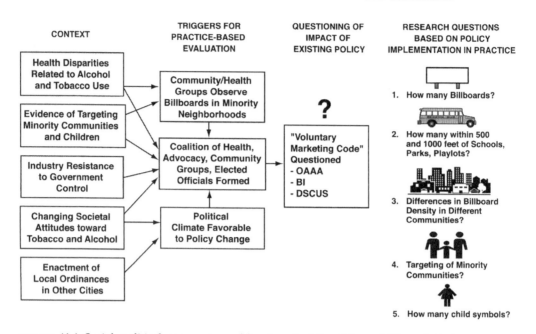

FIGURE 41.1 Social, political, economic, and legal context for Chicago billboard study

FORMULATION OF THE RESEARCH QUESTION

The study was designed to evaluate the effectiveness of the OAAA's voluntary code of principles in restricting the geographic placement of billboard advertisements for age-restricted products. The research questions flow directly from the OAAA code of principles (Outdoor Advertising Association of America). The goal was to see how implementation or lack of implementation of this voluntary code actually impacted Chicago communities. Table 41.1 outlines the research questions.

STUDY DESIGN AND SAMPLING PROCEDURES

The study was a descriptive, cross-sectional prevalence survey of all licensed billboards in Chicago. The unit of analysis for examining billboard prevalence was the Chicago ward. There are 50 wards in the city, which are the grassroots levels of local government. Zoning decisions concerning billboard licensing and geographic placement are made at the ward level. Ward boundaries are gerrymandered every 10 years to produce geographic areas that contain voting units of approximately 55,000 residents and a clear racial majority, ensuring that the city council will be racially diverse. In practice, Chicago remains a segregated city. Wards along the Lake Michigan lakefront are generally racially and socioeconomically diverse. Inner-city wards have high concentrations of either African American or Hispanic residents and are often economically depressed. Wards on the outer borders of the city are primarily White or racially mixed and are more affluent than the mostly minority wards. Based on ward maps produced after the 1990 census, there were 20 majority African American wards (55–99% African American; mean 85.8%), 18 majority White wards (57–94% White; mean 76%), 7 majority Hispanic wards (65–77% Hispanic; mean 71%), and 5 wards with no racial majority (Institute for Public Affairs, 1994). Wards in Chicago were stratified into four groups based on racial composition to create a sampling frame from which to select a representative sample of wards. Twenty-five of Chicago's 50 wards were included in the sample for visual inspection of billboards. However, all 4,278 licensed billboards in Chicago were geocoded into the database using the MapInfo program (MapInfo Professional 4.1, MapInfo Corp., 1997). Table 41.2 lists the data sources used in the study.

TABLE 41.1 Research Questions Emerging from the Code of Principles of the Outdoor Advertising Association of America (OAAA)

OAAA code of principles	Research questions
1. Establish exclusionary zones that prohibit outdoor advertising of age-restricted products within 500 feet of elementary and secondary schools, public playgrounds, and places of worship	1. How many total billboards are there in the city within 500 and 1,000 feet of schools, parks, and playlots? 2. How many of the billboards within 500 and 1,000 feet of schools, parks, and playlots in sample wards advertise tobacco or alcohol?
2. Establish reasonable limits on the total number of outdoor displays in a market that carry messages about products that are illegal for sale to minors	3. Is there a difference in the mean number of billboards in different markets defined by the racial makeup of communities? 4. Are there more billboards advertising alcohol and tobacco in minority markets compared to White markets, indicating racial targeting and market saturation?
3. Identify outdoor advertising displays in the exclusionary zone by attaching the international symbol of the child in a clearly visible location	5. Are there international child symbols on billboards near schools, parks, and playgrounds?

VISUAL SURVEY OF BILLBOARD CONTENT

The researchers developed a coding sheet that included the type of alcohol or tobacco product and brand advertised. A visual survey was conducted using ward maps with billboard addresses to obtain data on advertising content. Pairs of students and community volunteers were recruited and trained to collect data. One re-

TABLE 41.2 Data Sources for the Chicago Billboard Study

Existing data sources available to the researchers	Data not available to researchers
• Ward maps of 50 Chicago wards from the Chicago Board of Elections • Addresses of all 4,278 licensed billboards in Chicago from the Chicago Department of Buildings • OAAA definition of billboards (bulletins; 8-sheet posters; 30-sheet poster panels) from OAAA Web site and publications • Addresses of all public and private schools from the Chicago Board of Education • Addresses of all parks and playlots from the Chicago Park District • 1990 census data on ward population and race	• Addresses of places of worship • Addresses of unlicensed billboards • Outdoor advertising company data on monthly leases; names of leases or product advertised • Outdoor advertising company records identifying billboards marked with the international symbol of the child New evaluation data collected by the researchers • Advertising content (alcohol, tobacco, other) displayed on sample of 2,421 visually inspected billboards • Presence/absence of the international symbol of the child on sample of 2,421 visually inspected billboards

searcher drove slowly up and down each street while the other observed billboards and coded data on the products advertised. This methodology of coding billboards has been used in the past and shown to be effective (Hackbarth et al., 1995). Each ward was visited only once, and data was coded as of that day (point prevalence). These procedures resulted in information on billboard advertising content in the 25 sample wards. Content data was obtained for 2,421 billboards, approximately half of the licensed billboards in Chicago in the spring and summer of 1997. Presence or absence of the international symbol of the child on billboard structures was also noted (see Figure 41.2, which outlines the data collection steps). Table 41.3 outlines the data analysis steps. Table 41.4 is a summary of study findings.

LIMITATIONS OF THE STUDY

The study's limitations were as follows:

- The list of licensed billboards could have had errors or been incomplete, causing underreporting.
- Unlicensed billboards were not included, which could lead to underestimation of the total number of billboards and those within the 500- and 1,000-foot zones.

- The list of parks and schools was validated as accurate; the playlot list could not be verified.
- Churches, both established and storefront, were excluded from the study because no list was available. This exclusion could cause an underestimation of the number of billboards within the OAAA 500-foot exclusion zone.
- The sample of wards chosen for visual coding was purposive, not random. Hispanic wards were overrepresented. Wards of key aldermen were included because data from these wards was important to spur legislation. The sample included 50% of all wards and 50% of all billboards, so patterns are probably representative of the city as a whole.
- Visual coding of billboards can lead to ↑ or ↓ count or miscoding of content. Each ward was visited once with no recount. An earlier study included a 10% recount for reliability and found no statistical difference in recount (Hackbarth et al., 1995).
- Point prevalence was recorded on the day of survey. Data reflect advertising themes/campaigns in place on that particular day. The study lasted for 3 months. Advertising content is seasonal and could change in different months; alcohol ads peak in November–December around the holidays. This study was conducted in spring–summer of 1997. There could have been different results if a different 3-month time frame had been used.

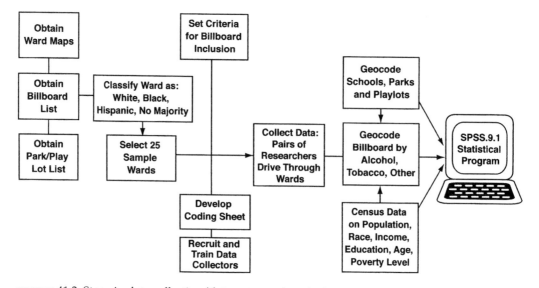

FIGURE 41.2 Steps in data collection/data entry and analysis

TABLE 41.3 Data Analysis Steps

1. Enter census data on wards using SPSS 9.1 statistical package

2. Use MapInfo program to create maps of all 50 wards showing ward boundaries and streets

3. Geocode locations of public and private schools by address

4. Geocode location of parks and playlots by address and map total geographic area within park boundary

5. Geocode location of licensed billboards by address

6. Identify advertising content of geocoded billboards as alcohol, tobacco, or other in 25 sample wards

7. Create and map 500- and 1,000-foot zones around each school, park, and playlot to represent OAAA voluntary child safe zone and proposed FDA 1,000-foot zone

8. Calculate the total number of billboards within the 500- and 1,000-foot zones; calculate the number of alcohol and tobacco billboards within the 500- and 1,000-foot zones

9. Compare total billboards and alcohol and tobacco billboards in African American, Hispanic, no ethnic majority, and White wards

10. Perform regression analysis with stepwise backward deletion to characterize demographic factors related to geographic billboard placement in wards

• Researchers only recorded international child symbols visible from the street on the front side of billboards. Other billboards could have been marked with the symbol in a location not visible to researchers in a moving vehicle.

IMPLICATIONS OF THE STUDY FINDINGS FOR POLICY CHANGE

The study demonstrated that the voluntary OAAA 500-foot zone around schools and play-grounds prohibiting advertising of age-restricted products is largely ignored. In African American wards 29.3% of all billboards advertising tobacco were near schools and parks. In Hispanic wards, 24.5% of all billboards advertising tobacco were near schools and parks. Fifteen percent of alcohol billboards in African American wards and 13.7% of alcohol billboards in Hispanic wards were similarly located near areas where children congregate. (See Table 41.4.)

A clear pattern of billboard saturation in minority communities was also evident. Minority communities contained both more total billboards and an excess number advertising alcohol and tobacco. There was a mean of 11 alcohol billboards in minority wards compared to 4 in White wards, an almost 3-to-1 ratio. When tobacco billboards were compared, there was a mean of 19 in minority wards compared to 5 in White wards, an almost 4-to-1 ratio. This phenomenon cannot be explained by zoning or density because all wards have similar zoning and population. Rather, demographic correlates of billboard placement were similar to recognized demographic correlates of poor health status: minority race, low levels of education, a high percentage of families living in poverty, and many residents under age 18 (see Table 41.4). Concerns that economically depressed minority communities are targeted with messages to smoke and drink were confirmed, as was the relationship between social conditions (billboard blight) and demographic correlates of poor health status.

A 500-foot versus 1,000-foot exclusionary zone also raises interesting questions. A 500-foot zone is quite small and probably offers little protection because children can easily view billboards from that distance. A 1,000-foot exclusionary zone, such as the one proposed but never adopted by the FDA, would have displaced 49% of billboards advertising alcohol and 54% advertising tobacco. A child walking to school in an African American or Hispanic area in Chicago had a 3-to-4-times greater chance of viewing an alcohol or tobacco billboard than a child residing in a White area of the city. Therefore, an even larger exclusionary zone eliminating billboards from all except manufacturing areas would better meet the objective of protecting children from advertisements for products that they cannot legally purchase. The study findings supported seeking relief through zoning of large ar-

TABLE 41.4 Summary of Study Findings

Question 1: How many billboards in the city are within 500 and 1,000 feet of schools, parks, and playlots?

4,278 licensed billboards in Chicago			
	0–500 feet	0–1,000 feet	Total
Number	845	2,167	4,278
Range per ward	1–59	6–115	13–213
Mean per ward	16.9	43.3	85.6
SD, per ward	13.11	27.94	38.49
Percent of total	19.75%	50.63%	100%

If OAAA code were followed, 20% of all billboards in Chicago would be off-limits to alcohol and tobacco ads.

If 1,000-foot exclusionary zone were established, 51% of all billboards in Chicago would be off-limits to alcohol and tobacco ads.

Question 2: How many of the billboards within 500 and 1,000 feet of schools, parks, and playlots in 25 sample wards advertise tobacco or alcohol?[1]

2,421 billboards visually surveyed		
	246 alcohol (10.2%)	404 tobacco (16.6%)
Range per ward	0–19	0–35
Mean per ward	9.8	16.2
% per ward	0–18%	0–57%
Mean % per ward	9.2%	20%

Percent of alcohol and tobacco billboards within OAAA 500-foot zone in sample wards		
	Alcohol	Tobacco
African American wards	15%	29.3%
Hispanic majority wards	13.7%	24.5%
No ethnic majority wards	3.3%	14%
White majority wards	6.6%	8.6%

Greater percent of alcohol and tobacco billboards are in 500-foot zone in minority wards than in White wards.

Question 3: Is there a difference in the mean number of billboards in communities with different racial makeup?

	Mean number billboards	SD
African American wards	110	45.66
Hispanic majority wards	104	34.87
No ethnic majority wards	50	41.48
White majority wards	59	30.59

Differences in mean billboards per ward by race are statistically significant; $F = 6.782$, $P = .001$.

Clear pattern of more billboards in minority wards exists.

Question 4: Are there more billboards advertising alcohol and tobacco in minority markets than in White markets, indicating racial targeting and market saturation? (11 African American, 6 Hispanic, and 3 no-ethnic-majority wards were combined to compare 20 "minority wards" to 5 White wards for this analysis.)

Comparison of number of alcohol billboards:
sample of 5 white and 20 minority wards

	White	Minority
Total number of alcohol billboards	19	227
Range per ward	0–12	0–19
Mean per ward	3.8	11.35
SD per ward	4.82	5.79

Comparison of number of tobacco billboards in
sample of 5 white and 20 minority wards

	White	Minority
Total number of alcohol billboards	25	377
Range per ward	1–9	2–33
Mean per ward	5.2	18.85
SD per ward	3.30	9.72

Demographic characteristics of wards associated with alcohol billboard placement

↑ percentage of African American residents;	$R = .594$	$(P = .002)$
—↓ median family income;	$R = .632$	$(P = .001)$
—↑ percentage families below poverty;	$R = .525$	$(P = .007)$
—↑ adults with < 12 years education;	$R = .673$	$(P = .001)$
—↑ percentage < age 18;	$R = .720$	$(P = .001)$
—↓ percentage of White residents;	$R = .799$	$(P = .001)$

Demographic characteristics of wards associated with tobacco billboard placement

—↑ percentage of African American residents;	$R = .663$	$(P = .001)$
—↑ percentage families below poverty line;	$R = .546$	$(P = .002)$
—↑ percentage adults < 12 years education;	$R = .544$	$(P = .002)$
—↑ percentage < age 18;	$R = .648$	$(P = .001)$

Multivariate analysis produced no definitive model because variables highly correlated. Best predictors of total billboards or alcohol or tobacco billboard placement is ↑ percentage of African American residents and ↓ educational attainment of adults.

Data confirm that poor and minority communities were targeted for outdoor advertising of alcohol and tobacco.

Question 5: Are there international child symbols on billboards near schools, parks, and playlots?

2,421 billboards visually surveyed

845 billboards within 500 feet and 10 child symbols identified	1,576 billboards beyond 500 feet and 0 child symbols identified

Only 10 symbols were visible from street, indicating that few billboards contain symbols that would restrict advertising content.

---

1. African American wards: $N = 11$
   Hispanic majority wards: $N = 6$
   No ethnic majority wards: $N = 3$
   White majority wards: $N = 5$

eas rather than a series of imaginary circles around schools and playgrounds, which would be difficult to delineate and monitor.

The international symbol of the child was rarely seen during the visual inspection of billboards. This symbol seems to be, in fact, a symbol used more for public relations purposes than to regulate billboard messages.

TRANSLATING COLLABORATIVE RESEARCH INTO COMMUNITY ACTION

The survey of Chicago billboards clearly documented that voluntary industry codes did not protect Chicago's children from messages encouraging them to use age-restricted products. In addition, mandating a 500- or 1,000-foot zone around schools and parks was shown to be of little practical significance because about half of alcohol and tobacco billboards would be unaffected. Members of the citywide coalition met with aldermen, city officials, and zoning experts to craft language for an ordinance that would be easy to understand and monitor and would maximize the geographic area where billboards advertising age-restricted products would be banned. The decision was made to restrict billboards advertising age-restricted products to manufacturing zones, which constitute about 20% of the city.

In the fall of 1997 a series of hearings on the billboard restrictions was held in the Chicago City Council. Press conferences about the restrictions included the St. Sabina community, LUC researchers, representatives from ALAMC, and aldermen who were cosponsors of the ordinance. Maps showing billboard placement and alcohol and tobacco ads in sample wards were shared with the press and aldermen. Members of the coalition offered expert testimony. The St. Sabina group took city officials and the press on neighborhood tours. Local radio and TV stations carried the story. Representatives of the alcohol industry and the trade group representing advertising interests in Chicago offered testimony opposing the ordinance. They argued that tobacco and alcohol are legal products and are not marketed to children and that advertisers do not place billboards in areas where children congregate. The representatives expressed surprise when one of the student researchers displayed pictures of an alcohol billboard adjacent to a schoolyard fence. Negotiations occurred between the major stakeholders with coalition members cast as the "little guys" challenging powerful special interests on behalf of the poor and minority communities.

The Chicago billboard ordinance passed in September 1997 with the mayor's approval. Outdoor advertising of age-restricted products was banned in all areas of the city except for manufacturing zones, where few children could be expected to see the signs. The city's ballparks were exempt. The ordinance placed approximately 80% of Chicago off-limits to tobacco and alcohol billboards. The ordinance allowed for existing advertising contracts to run their course. It also contained a 60-day grace period between passage and the implementation date when offending billboards had to be removed.

The tobacco and alcohol companies used the grace period as a loophole. They renegotiated long-term contracts, some for up to 20 years, making the ordinance unenforceable in many cases. A group of advertising organizations filed a lawsuit in federal court based on federal preemption of local tobacco advertising restrictions and commercial speech considerations (*Federated Advertising Industry Representatives v. City of Chicago*, 1998).

Public opinion was in favor of the ordinance. City officials were willing to risk a long and expensive federal lawsuit in defense of the ordinance. In February 1998 the City Council, angry with the tobacco and alcohol companies for renegotiating contracts, passed a substitute ordinance requiring the removal of all tobacco and alcohol billboards within 120 days regardless of existing contracts. However, a federal judge blocked implementation until a hearing could be held. Figure 41.3 summarizes the translation of the collaborative research process into practice, illustrating how data was used in the legislative and judicial arenas.

LEGAL BATTLES OVER BILLBOARD ORDINANCES

Legal and public policy issues surrounding outdoor advertising of age-restricted products are complex and controversial. Different federal circuit courts have rendered conflicting opinions (Garner, 1996). Several important legal issues are involved. In general, under the Constitution's Supremacy Clause, federal law takes pre-

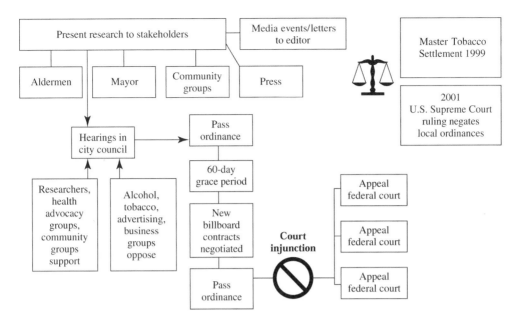

FIGURE 41.3 Translating practice-based collaborative research into practice

cedence over state laws or local regulations. The Federal Cigarette Labeling and Advertisement Act has been interpreted as preventing states and local governments from placing restrictions on tobacco advertising based on health concerns. Thus, only the federal government can mandate warning labels on cigarette packages or tobacco billboards.

The second legal issue is the First Amendment right to free speech, which also protects commercial speech, albeit with fewer protections than those provided for individual speech. The First Amendment does not protect commercial speech about unlawful activities, nor does it protect misleading speech (Garner & Whitney, 1997). When government regulates commercial speech, it must meet certain requirements established in *Central Hudson Gas and Electric v. Public Service Commission of New York* (1980). These requirements are that the government interest be directly and materially advanced by the advertising restrictions and that the speech restrictions be no more extensive than necessary to serve those interests. These principles have been explicated in *44 Liquormart, Inc. v. Rhode Island* (1996) and *Penn Advertising v. City of Baltimore* (1997).

In July 1998 a judge in the Chicago case ruled in favor of advertisers based on his interpretation of federal preemption. In his written opin-

ion the judge explained that although the stated purpose of the Chicago ordinance was to restrict advertising that encouraged minors to engage in illegal activities (tobacco and alcohol consumption), protecting health was the underlying intent of the ordinance (see *Federated Advertising Industry Representatives v. City of Chicago*, 1998). The judge found that the alcohol provisions were not severable from the tobacco provisions and stopped the city from enforcing the entire ordinance. Meanwhile, the billboard companies dropped the tobacco challenge from their complaint in the wake of the multistate tobacco settlement.

The City of Chicago appealed the judge's ruling, and the Seventh Circuit Court of Appeals in Chicago ruled that federal law did not preempt the Chicago regulations. The court did not review the commercial speech issue, which was sent back to district court (*Federated Advertising Industry Representatives v. City of Chicago*, 1998). Implementation of the ordinance was again delayed.

During this period, other cities and states, including New York and Massachusetts, enacted billboard bans based on advertising content and geographic placement (Petty, 1999). Tobacco and alcohol interests also challenged these laws. The U.S. Supreme Court declined to review the rulings of the appeals court in the Chicago and New

York cases but did agree to review the Massa-chusetts case.

In Chicago coalition activities continued while the ordinance was on hold awaiting a fed-eral court ruling. Action was taken to remove alcohol and tobacco advertisements from buses, trains, and transit shelters. In addition, an or-dinance was passed banning the sale of Bidis, an imported flavored cigarette favored by young smokers.

Supreme Court Rules on Tobacco Billboard Restrictions

In June 2001, the U.S. Supreme Court ruled on the State of Massachusetts's regulation of out-door and point-of-sale tobacco advertising in *Lorillard Tobacco Co. v. Reilly*. Those regula-tions included a ban on outdoor advertising of tobacco within 1,000 feet of schools and play-grounds, restrictions on in-store tobacco adver-tisements, and a ban on self-service displays of tobacco products. In a complex 5-4 decision, the Supreme Court acknowledged that the govern-ment's interest in preventing underage tobacco use is substantial. However, the Court struck down the 1,000-foot tobacco billboard ban, stat-ing that the outdoor advertising restrictions were too broad and not narrowly tailored, as re-quired by an earlier court ruling (*Central Hud-son Gas and Electric v. Public Service Commis-sion of New York*, 1980). The court let stand restrictions on self-service tobacco displays.

Future Actions

Lorillard Tobacco Co. v. Reilly (2001) dealt only with tobacco advertising, but the ruling affects many state and local laws governing outdoor ad-vertising of all types of age-restricted products, including alcohol. Federal law preempts state and local laws, and some local laws may be invali-dated or withdrawn in the wake of *Lorillard To-bacco Co. v. Reilly*. Although most tobacco bill-boards have been removed as a result of the Master Settlement Agreement, alcohol bill-boards remain prevalent and largely unregu-lated. Until the Supreme Court overturns its rul-ing, Congress removes federal preemption contained in the Cigarette Labeling and Adver-tising Act, or more creative legal theories can be fashioned by health advocates, laws restricting advertising of age-restricted products such as to-bacco and alcohol will be difficult to enact.

APPLICATION OF PRACTICE-BASED EVALUATION TO COMPREHENSIVE ALCOHOL AND TOBACCO CONTROL INTERVENTIONS

Practice-based evaluations are needed to validate the efficacy of policies and programs to reduce the detrimental health effects of tobacco use and alcohol abuse. These interventions could in-clude comprehensive school-, community-, and media-based prevention programs; smoking and alcohol cessation and treatment programs; in-creases in the price of tobacco and alcohol through excise taxes; reduced accessibility to age-restricted products by enforcement of youth access laws; monitoring of point-of-purchase ad-vertising of alcohol and tobacco products; and counteradvertising (Alcohol Policy Solutions, 2003; Mosher & Glenn, 2002; Tauras, O'Malley, & Johnson, 2001; Terry-McElrath et al., 2003). Limiting outdoor alcohol advertising will have to be accomplished through continual monitoring of billboard placement and public pressure to stop billboard saturation of poor and minority communities.

Practice-based research is needed to form the scientific basis for community-level inter-ventions and policy change. Community-level interventions, especially those that involve tax-ation, legislation, and regulation, cannot be achieved by any one group acting alone (Streicker, 2000). Partnerships that link acade-mia, community groups, the media, policy mak-ers, and public health practitioners and have broad public support are more likely to achieve desired policy goals.

References

Alcohol Policy Solutions. (2003). *Background infor-mation/table of prevention strategies*. Retrieved from www.alcoholpolicysolutions.net/bi-table -strat.htm.

Altman, D. G., Schooler, C., & Basil, M. D. (1991). Alcohol and cigarette advertising on billboards. *Health Education Research, 6*, 487–490.

American Lung Association. (2000). *Minority lung disease*. New York: American Lung Association.

Beer Institute. *Advertising and marketing code*. Re-trieved from www.beerinstitute.org/admarkcode .htm.

Bobo, K., Kendall, J., & Max, S. (2001). *Organizing for social change: Midwest academy manual for activists* (3rd ed.). Santa Ana, CA: Seven Locks Press.

Central Hudson Gas and Electric v. Public Service Commission of New York, 447 U.S. 557, 561 (1980).

Community Anti-Drug Coalitions of America. *Alcohol advertising: Its impact on communities, and what coalitions can do to lessen that impact.* Strategizer No. 32. Alexandria, VA: Center for Science in the Public Interest. Retrieved from www.cspinet.org/booze.

Competitive Media Reporting/Adams Beverage Group. (2002).

Distilled Spirits Council of the United States. *Code of good practice for distilled spirits advertising and marketing.* Retrieved from www.dscus.org/industry/code.

Evans, J. M., & Kelly, R. F. (1999). *Self-regulation of the alcohol industry: A review of industry efforts to avoid promoting alcohol to underage consumers.* Washington, DC: Federal Trade Commission.

Federated Advertising Industry Representatives v. City of Chicago, U.S. App. LEXIS 212267, 12 F. Supp. 2nd 844 (N.D. Ill. 1998, 7th Cir.).

Federal Trade Commission. (2001). *Federal Trade Commission cigarette report for 1999.* Washington, DC: Author.

44 Liquormart, Inc. v. Rhode Island, 517 U.S. 484 (1996).

Garner, D. (1996). Banning tobacco billboards: The case for municipal action. *Journal of the American Medical Association, 275,* 1263–1269.

Garner, D., & Whitney, R. J. (1997). Protecting children from Joe Camel and his friends: A new look at First Amendment and federal preemption analysis of tobacco billboard regulation. *Emory Law Journal, 46,* 479–585.

Gerston, L. N. (1997). *Public policy making: Process and principals.* Armonk, NY: M. E. Sharpe.

Guthrie, B. (1994). Tobacco advertising near schools. *British Medical Journal, 308,* 00–00.

Hackbarth, D. P., Schnopp-Wyatt, D., Katz, D., Williams, J., Silvestri, B., & Pfleger, M. (2001). Collaborative research and action to control the geographic placement of outdoor advertising of alcohol and tobacco products in Chicago. *Public Health Reports, 16,* 558–567.

Hackbarth, D. P., Silvestri, B., & Cosper, W. (1995). Tobacco and alcohol billboards in 50 Chicago neighborhoods: Market segmentation to sell dangerous products to the poor. *Journal of Public Health Policy, 16,* 213–230.

Institute for Public Affairs. (1994). *Metro Chicago political atlas.* Springfield, IL: Sangamon State University.

Kiefe, C. I., Williams, O. D., Lewis, C. E., Allison, J. J., Sekar, P., & Wagenknecht, L. E. (2001). Ten-year changes in smoking among young adults: Are racial differences explained by socio-economic factors in the CARDIA study? *American Journal of Pubic Health, 91,* 213–215.

Lee, W.-N., & Callcott, M. F. (1994). Billboard advertising: A comparison of vice products across ethnic groups. *Journal of Business Research, 30,* 85–94.

Link, B., & Phelan, J. (1995). Social conditions as fundamental causes of disease. *Journal of Health and Social Behavior,* extra issue, 88–94.

Lorillard Tobacco Co. et al. v. Reilly, Attorney General of Massachusetts, et al., certiorarie to the U.S. Court of Appeals for the First Circuit No. 00596 (2001).

Luke, D., Esmundo, E., & Bloom, Y. (2000). Smoke signs: Patterns of tobacco billboard advertising in a metropolitan region. *Tobacco Control, 9,* 16–23.

Mayberry, R.M., & Price, P. A. (1993). Targeting blacks in cigarette billboard advertising: Results from down south. *Health Values, 17,* 28–35.

Meredith, J., & Dunham, C. (1999). *Real clout.* Boston: Access Project.

Miniño, A. M., Arias, E., Kochanek, K. D., Murphy, S. L., & Smith, B. L. (2002). Deaths: Final data for 2000. *National Vital Statistics Reports, 50,* 00–00.

Mosher, J. F., & Glenn, P. *Partner or foe? The alcohol industry, youth alcohol problems and alcohol policy strategies.* Chicago: American Medical Association.

Murphy, S. L. (2000). Deaths: Final data for 1998. *National Vital Statistics Reports, 48,* 1–105.

Outdoor Advertising Association of America. Retrieved, from www.oaaa.org/government.

Penn Advertising v. City of Baltimore, 1996 101 F. 3rd 332 (4th Cir.) cert. denied, 117 S. Ct 1568 (1997), readopting 63 F. 3rd 1318 (4th Cir. 1995).

Petty, R. D. (1999). Tobacco marketing restrictions in the multistate attorneys general settlement: Is this good public policy? *Journal of Public Policy and Marketing, 18,* 249–257.

Posavac, E. J., & Carey, R. (2003). Program evaluation: Methods and case studies (6th ed.). Upper Saddle River, NJ: Prentice Hall.

Rossman, R. L. (1994). Multicultural marketing: Selling to a diverse America. New York: Amacom.

Schooler, C., Basil, M. P., & Altman, D. G. (1996). Alcohol and cigarette advertising on billboards: Targeting with social cues. *Journal of Health Communication, 8,* 109–129.

Standard directory of advertisers: Vol. 1. Business classifications. (2001). New Providence, NJ: National Publishing.

Stoddard, J. L., Johnson, C., Sussman, S., Dent, C., & Boley-Cruz, T. (1998). Tailoring outdoor tobacco advertising to minorities in LA country. *Journal of Health Communication, 3,* 137–146.

Streicker, J. (Ed.). (2000). *Case histories in alcohol policy.* San Francisco: Trauma Foundation.

Terry-McElrath, Y. M., Harwood, E. M., Wagner, A. C., Slater, S., Chaloupka, F. J., Brewer, R. D., et al. (2003). Point of purchase alcohol marketing and promotion by store type—United States 2000–2001. *Morbidity and Mortality Weekly Report, 52,* 310–313.

Tauras, J. A., O'Malley, P. M., & Johnson, L. D. (2001). *Effects of price and access laws on teenage smoking initiation: A national longitudinal analysis.* Retrieved from www.impacteen.org/imp_yes.htm.

42

USE OF RANDOM DIGIT DIALING TO RECRUIT REPRESENTATIVE POPULATION SAMPLES

Lynda F. Voigt

Random digit dialing (RDD) is a technique used to obtain a sample of the population that is representative of all households with telephones in a designated geographic area. It is used for scientific surveys and to obtain controls for epidemiologic case-control studies. Although this chapter focuses on the use of RDD to recruit controls for epidemiologic population-based case-control studies, the same basic principles apply to the use of RDD for scientific surveys.

The high proportion of households in the United States with telephones makes RDD an effective and relatively inexpensive method of obtaining a representative sample of U.S. households. Overall, 97.6% of U.S. households have telephones. Telephone ownership varies by state from 93.6% in Mississippi to 99.1% in Massachusetts ("Massachusetts Tops," 2003). Households with only cellular phone service and no landline telephone are generally excluded from RDD. Calling cellular telephones may violate federal regulations that prohibit calls to cellular phones without prior consent of the person called (Gillin, 2002). Recent data indicate that 2% of the U.S. population has only cellular service and no landline telephone ("Solely Cellular," 2001). This proportion seems to be increasing, particularly among young adults. Investigators contemplating the use of RDD should consider the potential impact of telephone ownership for a particular study because ownership of landline telephones varies by both geographic area and demographic characteristics.

Controls for epidemiologic case-control studies should come from the same population that gave rise to the cases (Wacholder, McLaughlin, Silverman, & Mandel, 1992). This principle requires that cases without residential landline telephones be excluded in studies that recruit controls by RDD. Case-control studies conducted by Fred Hutchinson Cancer Research Center in Seattle, Washington, in 2001 and 2002 excluded less than 2% of the eligible cases for these reasons.

Equal probability sampling methods give every residential telephone number in a defined geographic area an equal chance of selection. Two methods that accomplish this are simple random digit dialing and the Mitofsky–Waksberg modification of simple RDD. List-assisted RDD does not meet the criteria for equal probability sampling. Nevertheless, some list-assisted methods can provide samples of telephone numbers that have tolerable bias.

Once a method has been selected, investigators must decide whether or not to invest resources to develop their own RDD program or employ an experienced commercial firm. In either case the study investigators must understand the methodology well enough to assure that the random telephone numbers are selected and called in a manner that minimizes potential selection and response bias. Improperly conducted RDD can jeopardize the validity of the study or survey.

EXAMPLES OF TWO TYPES OF RDD METHODS

Equal Probability RDD

Selection of telephone numbers for simple RDD and the primary stage of Mitofsky–Waksberg RDD begins by random selection of an area code prefix combination from a list of all such combinations in the geographic area of interest and adding four random digits to create a telephone number. Electronic files of all working area code prefix combinations (prefixes are also called *exchanges*) in the United States can be purchased from Telcordia (New Jersey, USA). The files include place/city for each prefix and codes that identify prefixes used exclusively for directory assistance, paging, and mobile or cellular service. Prefix data should be updated at least twice a year so that new prefixes are included in the sampling process. Updates should be done more often in geographic areas that are growing rapidly. Prefix data can also be downloaded from the North American Numbering Plan Administration (NeuStar, Washington, DC; Web site: http://www.nanpa.com). Prefix assignments may overlap cities and counties, so researchers should take care to include all prefixes that are assigned in the geographic area of interest.

The Mitofsky–Waksberg method provides a two-stage, self-weighting sample. The second stage utilizes a fixed clustering factor designated as "k." A clustering factor of five is commonly used in the Epidemiology Program at Fred Hutchinson Cancer Research Center in Seattle, WA, because this minimizes the number of respondents in each cluster and nearly doubles the proportion of selected residential telephone numbers. The second calling stage should follow the primary stage closely in time to preserve the equal probability nature of the sample (Voigt, Davis, & Heuser, 1992). Figure 42.1 illustrates the general procedures for this method. The Mitofsky–Waksberg method saves RDD interviewer time by reducing the number of nonworking or business telephone numbers that must be called. The disadvantage of this method is that it is more complex and requires careful execution to avoid bias. This method is described in detail elsewhere (Casady & Lepkowski, 2000; Hartge et al., 1984; Olson, Kelsey, Pearson, & Levin, 1992; Pothoff, 1994; Waksberg, 1978; Waksberg, 2000).

List-Assisted RDD

The term *list-assisted RDD* includes a broad array of commercially available telephone number samples generated for marketing and survey use. Many samples generated using list-assisted RDD have limited use in scientific studies because they are derived from incomplete lists of telephone numbers. In addition, companies that focus on direct marketing clients may exclude telephone numbers that appear on "do not call" lists and telephone numbers that have been recently generated for other customers. Scientific research is specifically exempt from regulations regarding "do not call" lists.

One popular method of list-assisted sampling uses published directories to create a list of "banks" (area code, prefix, and next two digits of telephone numbers) that have at least one residential published number ("1+ banks"). A telephone number is created by selecting a bank at random and adding two random numbers. Residential telephone numbers in banks where none of the telephone numbers are directory-listed are excluded from these sampling methods. This occurs when telephone numbers are assigned in new prefixes that have been activated after directories have been pub

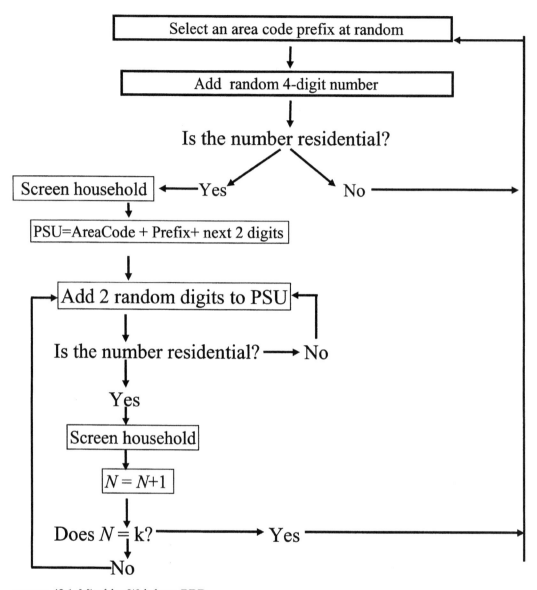

FIGURE 42.1 Mitofsky-Waksberg RDD

lished and when telephone customers request that their telephone number be unlisted. This 1+ bank sampling will be least biased in geographic areas that have low demand for new telephone service and a high percentage of directory-listed numbers. Approximately 90% of all residential telephone numbers in the northeastern and midwestern areas of the United States are published in directories whereas less than 50% of the telephone numbers in the far west are published (Edmondson, 1995). Studies have found that 2–4% of all U.S. residential telephone numbers are excluded from 1+ banks with variation by geographic area (Brick, Waksberg, Kulp, & Starer, 1995; Giesbrecht, Kulp, & Starer, 1996; Rizzo, DiGaetano, Cadell, & Kulp, 1995). The percentage of directory-listed numbers and residential growth of the study area should be considered when weighing the advantages and disadvantages of 1+ bank sampling. Cases with telephone numbers that are not included in 1+ banks should be excluded from case-control studies because cases and controls must arise from the same population. An ongoing case-control study in Connecticut is successfully using a commercial sample of random telephone numbers from 1+ banks. In that study, 99% of the case telephone numbers are included in banks with at least one listed telephone number (H. A. Risch, personal communication, March 18, 2003).

Supplementing samples from 1+ banks with a small percentage of telephone numbers selected from banks with no published numbers will produce samples of telephone numbers that are very close to equal probability samples (Tucker, Lepkowski, & Pierkarski, 2002). List-assisted samples of telephone numbers can be restricted to banks with higher minimum numbers of listed numbers (e.g., 5, 10, 20 listed numbers per bank), but the potential for bias will increase as more listed telephone numbers per bank are required.

Two other services offered by commercial vendors of telephone number samples are often used to decrease the number of nonresidential telephone numbers that must be called. Both introduce additional bias. One option deletes any selected telephone numbers that are listed as business numbers in directories. This procedure can potentially introduce a small amount of bias because published listings age rapidly, and telephone numbers that were formerly business numbers can be reassigned to residential service before a new directory is published. A second service is computerized prescreening of telephone numbers for working status. This is accomplished by using automated dialing software that is programmed to recognize the special "tritone" emitted when a nonworking or out-of-service telephone number is reached. Some systems can also identify fax and modem tones. One study found that 2.4% of the numbers classified as nonworking telephone numbers by an automated system were actually residential. This proportion varied by geographic area from 0–5% (Rizzo et al., 1995). Devices designed to reduce telemarketing calls by mimicking the nonworking tri-tone on home telephones were introduced after this study was completed.

Widespread use of these devices will increase the proportion of residential telephone numbers that are misclassified as nonworking by automated systems.

SPECIFIC PROCEDURES FOR SUCCESSFUL RDD

Generate Telephone Number Samples Frequently

Random telephone number samples should be generated every 3–4 months throughout the study so that new prefixes are included in the sample. Each set of generated telephone numbers is considered a "block" or "round." The number of telephone numbers generated in each RDD round can be increased or decreased according to the number of participants still needed.

Resolve Every Telephone Number in Each Round

Standard RDD protocols require nine or more calls to telephone numbers that are not answered, answered by machine, or answered by a person who requests to be called back. These calls must be made at different times of the day and evening and on different days of the week over a 2–3 week period before the telephone number is abandoned. Failure to pursue telephone numbers that are unanswered will result in a sample of only those people who are most easily reached by telephone. It is unlikely that such a sample will be representative of the population of interest. Studies have found significant differences in demographic characteristics between respondents recruited using only a single callback or few callbacks to unanswered or machine-answered numbers compared to those recruited after multiple callbacks (Curtin, Presser, & Singer, 2000; Keeter, Miller, Kohut, Groves, & Presser, 2000).

Screen for Eligibility

Studies generally have specific eligibility requirements. A conversational script that has been approved by the appropriate human-subjects board should be used to screen potential respondents for study eligibility. It may be helpful to include a statement in the script that the interviewer is not selling anything or asking for donations.

Select Respondent

Most studies require samples of individuals rather than households and select only one respondent per household if multiple household members are eligible. However, bias can be introduced if eligibility requirements are broad because individuals in households with more than one eligible person have a lower probability of inclusion in the study than do individuals in households with only one eligible person (Sudman, Sirken, & Cowan, 1988). An effective way to avoid this bias when both men and women are eligible for the study is to designate each telephone number for either men or women before it is called (Waksberg, 2000). For example, if the telephone number is designated "men only," the RDD interviewer screens only men in the household when that number is called and vice versa if the telephone number is designated "women only." The small increase in the number of RDD calls that this requires is well worth the substantial reduction of selection bias. Studies of children require similar measures to reduce selection bias (Greenberg, 1990).

Stratify by Frequency-Matching Variables

Epidemiologic studies usually frequency-match controls to the age distribution of the cases. Other variables such as race and geographic area are often also included as frequency-matching variables. Frequency matching during RDD is achieved using either one- or two-step stratification designs (Hartge et al., 1984). The one-step method screens and selects eligible respondents during the RDD contact (Harlow & Davis, 1988). Brief interviews may be completed at the time of screening, or the eligible participant can be contacted at a later date to arrange either a telephone or in-person interview. In two-step recruitment the RDD interviewer obtains a roster of all potentially eligible respondents. The required number of participants is selected randomly from each stratum after all numbers in a "round" have been completed (Hartge et al., 1984). One-step recruitment avoids losses that

occur by changes in telephone status between the two stages of recruitment and may improve response. The disadvantage of one-step methods is that there is more variation in the number of respondents selected for each stratum than for two-step methods.

Account for Households with Multiple Telephone Numbers

Households with multiple telephone numbers that are answered will have an increased probability of selection unless multiple telephone lines are accounted for. Screening should include a question about the number of separate telephone numbers that ring in the household. Telephone lines dedicated to computers or fax machines are not included in this number. The appropriate probabilities are easily programmed into computer-assisted telephone interviewing (CATI) systems. A simple way to reduce the probability of selecting a household with multiple telephones using paper RDD systems is to reject households with multiple telephone numbers if the last digit of the telephone number called is odd. This will reduce the probability of selection by one-half because the last digit of telephone numbers follows an approximately uniform distribution.

Record and Monitor RDD Effort

The RDD effort should be carefully monitored for adherence to detailed written protocol. Researchers should keep careful records of the calling effort so that screening response proportions can be completely and fairly reported (Olson, Voigt, Begg, & Weiss, 2002; Samet, 2002). Several commercial CATI systems are available that facilitate monitoring and automatically record screening results. A complete description of the RDD methods utilized should be included in published study reports.

Maintain High Response Proportions

Maintaining high response proportions is essential to recruiting a representative and unbiased sample. Hartge (1999) observed, "In practice, if response exceeds 90% the impact of nonresponse will be minimal, but response below, say, 50% offers little protection against bias" (p. 106). This is challenging because screening response proportions have been declining over time (Austin, Criqui, Barrett-Connor, & Holdbrook, 1981; Bates & Creighton, 2000; Olson, 2001). Procedures that increase screening response include multiple callbacks to unanswered numbers (Kristal et al., 1993), financial incentives (Slattery, Edwards, Caan, Kerber, & Potter, 1995; Strouse & Hall, 1994), recontact of those who initially refused screening or participation (Curtin et al., 2000; Kristal et al., 1993), recontact of numbers that were answered by machine on every attempt during the initial series of calls (Voigt, Koepsell, & Daling, 2003), and leaving messages on answering machines (Koepsell, McGuire, Longstreth, Nelson, & van Belle, 1996; Tuckel, 1997).

POTENTIAL BIAS IN RDD

Two studies have found that female respondents may not answer screening questions truthfully (Brogan et al., 2001; Glaser & Stearns, 2002). This misclassification can introduce bias into the selection process and should be considered in interpreting the results of studies that use RDD.

Characteristics of respondents who are more difficult to recruit or require more time to complete an interview differ from those of more easily interviewed respondents (Bates & Creighton, 2000; Cottler, Zipp, Robins, & Sptiznagel, 1987; Fitzgerald & Fuller, 1982; Voigt et al., 2003). Studies have also found differences between respondents who initially refuse but agree when recontacted and their more willing counterparts (Criqui, Barrett-Connor, & Austin, 1978; Lavrakas, Bauman, & Merkle, 1992; O'Neil, 1979; Triplett, Blair, Hamilton, & Kang, 1996).

Some colleagues and I conducted a study to compare study participants' characteristics according to the level of effort required for interview completion. A complete report of this study is published elsewhere (Voigt et al., 2003). We compared 4,404 respondents who were selected by RDD as controls for case-control studies of breast, endometrial, anogenital, thyroid, and oral cancer and rheumatoid arthritis. We grouped respondents by the level of effort required to obtain a completed interview. Respondents who delayed the interview for 2–6 months after initial contact ("intermediate responders"), delayed the interview for more than 6 months ("late responders"), and those who initially refused but agreed after recontact ("initial refusers") were compared to respondents who completed the interview within one month of first contact. Results are presented in Table 42.1. Late responders were younger, more likely to be nonwhite, less likely to have attended college, and more likely to be current smokers than early responders. Initial refusers were older, less likely to be currently married or have managerial occupations, had fewer lifetime sexual partners, and were more

TABLE 42.1. Characteristics (%) of Early Responders, Intermediate Responders, Late Responders, and Initial Refusers Among RDD Female Controls from Six Studies Conducted in Western Washington State, 1987–1998[a]

	Early responders	Intermediate responders[b]	Late responders[b]	Initial refusers[b]
	N = 2747	N = 837	N = 444	N = 376
Demographic characteristics				
Age (years) at reference date[c]				
≤ 30	7.6	11.5	9.2	7.7
30–39	25.1	26.2	23.0	22.3
40–49	19.6	21.3	21.8	20.7
50–59	20.7	19.7	22.5	20.2
≥ 60	27.1	21.4	23.4	29.0
Mean	48.6	46.2	47.6	49.7
p value		< .001*	0.056	0.54

(continued)

TABLE 4.1. (*continued*)

	Early responders	Intermediate responders[b]	Late responders[b]	Initial refusers[b]
Ever attended college[c]	58.0	54.7	48.0	51.3
p value		0.133	< .001*	0.003
Marital status[c]				
Not married	27.9	27.4	29.2	31.7
Currently married or living as married	72.1	72.6	70.8	68.3
p value		0.96	0.11	0.01
Race[c]				
Nonwhite	5.6	7.6	9.5	9.4
p value		0.03	0.008	0.007
Annual household income[c]				
< $45,000	70.1	68.5	66.9	69.7
≥ $45,000	29.9	31.5	33.1	30.3
p value		0.33	0.01	0.28
Occupation at reference date[d,e,f]				
Managerial, professional	22.2	23.1	19.2	12.9
p value				
Other occupation	36.1	38.4	39.0	49.3
p value		0.49	0.97	0.002
Retired	9.4	9.5	6.2	9.6
p value		0.25	0.07	0.31
Housewife, student	32.3	29.1	35.6	28.2
p value		0.18	0.84	0.05
Any first- or second-degree female relative with cancer[d,e,f]	59.9	54.8	56.5	51.0
p value		0.04	0.41	0.11
Reproductive characteristics				
No. of pregnancies[f,g]				
0	13.0	12.6	12.8	15.0
1 or 2	33.7	34.7	32.0	36.1
p value		0.50	0.94	0.77
>2	53.2	52.8	55.3	48.9
p value		0.66	0.48	0.13
Ever had an induced abortion among women who were ever pregnant[f,g]	16.7	14.9	12.9	15.6
p value		0.14	0.09	0.88
Ever used oral contraceptives[c]	62.3	61.3	59.8	61.6
p value		0.28	0.52	0.89
Ever had an infertility[f,g,h,]	11.7	9.3	7.6	9.7
p value		0.03	0.01	0.25
Lifetime no. of sexual partners[c]				
0	6.4	6.6	6.8	9.2
p value				
1	38.9	38.5	41.0	38.5
p value		0.58	0.58	0.49
2–4	32.5	32.1	33.1	33.6
p value		0.50	0.40	0.046
≥ 5	22.2	22.9	19.1	18.1
p value		0.42	0.095	0.04

	Early responders	Intermediate responders[b]	Late responders[b]	Initial refusers[b]
Health history				
Ever been diagnosed with hypertension[f,g]	23.1	23.4	23.8	22.4
p value		0.92	0.49	0.46
Ever had cancer[f,g]	8.6	8.9	9.3	8.1
p value		0.49	0.50	0.93
Ever been diagnosed with diabetes[c]	4.0	3.7	4.1	7.9
p value		0.31	0.55	0.51
Ever used noncontraceptive hormones among women aged ≥ 50 years[d,e,f]	60.1	61.0	52.6	51.9
p value		0.13	0.55	0.51
Body mass index[i] at reference date[b]				
< 25	66.5	65.7	66.3	64.0
p value				
25–29.9	20.9	20.9	22.0	23.7
p value		0.72	0.94	0.65
≥ 30	12.6	13.4	11.7	12.3
p value		0.45	0.59	0.53
Mean	24.3	24.2	24.2	24.5
Lifestyle factors				
Smoking history[c]				
Never smoked	50.7	48.2	46.9	48.1
Former smoker	26.4	25.7	23.2	29.1
p value		0.93	0.53	0.65
Current smoker	22.9	26.1	29.8	22.7
p value		0.07	0.001*	0.53
Ever drank alcohol[c]	79.9	82.7	75.8	80.6
p value		0.14	0.19	0.49
Regular exercise within 2 years of reference date [d,e,f]	51.2	51.2	42.6	46.1
p value		0.87	0.10	0.26

a. Voigt, Koepsell, & Daling, 2003; by permission of Oxford University Press.

b. Proportions for all variables except age were adjusted to the age distribution of early responders.

c. The p value was adjusted for all other variables in table except family history of cancer, number of pregnancies, induced abortion, infertility tests, hypertension, history of cancer, noncontraceptive hormone use, exercise, and occupation.

d. The p value was adjusted for all other variables in table.

e. This question was not asked in the anogenital cancer study.

f. This question was not asked in the oral cancer study.

g. The p value was adjusted for all other variables in table except occupation, family history of cancer, infertility tests, noncontraceptive hormone use, and exercise.

h. This question was added to the anogenital cancer interview after the study began.

i. Weight (kg)/height(m)^2.

*p value < .05 compared to early responders; adjusted for other variables and corrected for multiple comparisons using Bonferroni's correction (Fisher & van Belle, 1993).

likely to have a history of diabetes than early responders. The only variables that showed a consistent gradient according to difficulty of recruitment were education and race. Age differences between late and early responders and initial refusers and early responders were in opposite directions. These findings argue against the common assumption that the characteristics of respondents become more like those of refusers as the difficulty of recruiting them increases. The effort required to convert refusers into participants and delay interviews rather than accept refusal increases the likelihood that the sample will be representative of the population of interest.

SUMMARY

Random digit dialing is an effective tool for identifying representative population samples. Study investigators must understand RDD methodology well enough to select an appropriate method and assure that the selected telephone numbers are resolved in a manner that minimizes potential selection and response bias. Every effort should be made to screen and interview a high proportion of eligible potential participants because failure to do so may jeopardize the study's validity. A description of RDD methods and response statistics should be included in reports of scientific studies that use RDD.

References

Austin, M. A., Criqui, M. H., Barrett-Connor, E., & Holdbrook, M. J. (1981). The effect of response bias on the odds ratio. *American Journal of Epidemiology, 114*, 137–143.

Bates, N., & Creighton, K. (2000). The last five percent: What can we learn from difficult/late interviews? *Proceedings of the American Statistical Association Government Statistics Section*, 120–125.

Brick, J. M., Waksberg, J., Kulp, D., & Starer, A. (1995). Bias in list-assisted telephone samples. *Public Opinion Quarterly, 59*, 218–235.

Brogan, D. J., Denniston, M. M., Liff, J. M., Flagg, E. W., Coates, R. J., & Brinton, L. A. (2001). Comparison of telephone sampling and area sampling: Response rates and within-household coverage. *American Journal of Epidemiology 153*, 119–127.

Casady, R. J., & Lepkowski, J. M. (2000). Telephone sampling. In M. H. Gail & J. Benichou (Eds.), *Encyclopedia of Epidemiologic Methods* (pp. 908–920). New York: Wiley.

Cottler, L. B., Zipp, J. F., Robins, L. N., & Sptiznagel, E. L. (1987). Difficult-to-recruit respondents and their effect on prevalence estimates in an epidemiologic survey. *American Journal of Epidemiology, 125*, 329–339.

Criqui, M. H., Barrett-Connor, E., & Austin, M. (1978). Differences between respondents and non-respondents in a population-based cardiovascular disease study. *American Journal of Epidemiology, 108*, 367–372.

Curtin, R., Presser, S., & Singer, E. (2000). The effects of response rate changes on the index of consumer sentiment. *Public Opinion Quarterly, 64*, 413–428.

Edmondson, B. (1995). Unlisted America. *American Demographics, 17*, 60.

Fisher, L. D., & van Belle, G. (1993). *Biostatistics: A methodology for the health sciences*. New York: Wiley.

Fitzgerald, R., & Fuller, L. (1982). I hear you knocking but you can't come in. *Sociologic Methods and Research, 2*, 3–32.

Gillin, D. (2002, August). *Are you placing calls to cellular telephones? If you are—beware!* Council for Marketing and Opinion Research, Government Affairs News. Retrieved April 4, 2003, from http://www.cmor.org/govaffairs_news0802.htm.

Giesbrecht, L. H., Kulp, D. W., & Starer, A. W. (1996). Estimating coverage bias in RDD samples with current population survey (CPS) data. *Proceedings of the American Statistical Association, Survey Research Methods Section*, 503–508.

Glasser, S. L., & Stearns, C. B. (2002). Reliability of random digit dialing calls to enumerate an adult female population. *American Journal of Epidemiology, 155*, 972–975.

Greenberg, E. R. (1990). Random digit dialing for control selection: A review and a caution on its use in studies of childhood cancer. *American Journal of Epidemiology, 131*, 1–5.

Harlow, B. L., & Davis, S. (1988) Two one-step methods for household screening and interviewing using random digit dialing. *American Journal of Epidemiology, 127*, 857–863.

Hartge, P. (1999). Raising response rates: Getting to yes. *Epidemiology, 10*,105–106.

Hartge, B. L., Brinton, L. A., Rosenthal, J. F., Cahill, J. I., Hoover, R. N., & Waksberg, J. (1984). Random digit dialing in selecting a population-based control group. *American Journal of Epidemiology, 120*, 825–833.

Keeter, S., Miller, C., Kohut, A., Groves, R. M., & Presser, S. (2000). Consequences of reducing nonresponse in a national telephone survey. *Public Opinion Quarterly, 64*, 125–148.

Koepsell, T. D., McGuire, V., Longstreth, W. T., Nelson, L. M., & van Belle, G. (1996). Randomized trial of leaving messages on telephone answering machines for control recruitment in an epidemiologic study. *American Journal of Epidemiology*, 144, 704–706.

Kristal, A. R., White, E., Davis, J. R., Corycell, G., Raghunathan, T., Kinne, S., et al. (1993). Effects of enhanced calling efforts on response rates, estimates of health behavior, and costs in a telephone health survey using random-digit dialing. *Public Health Reports*, 108, 372–379.

Lavrakas, P. J., Bauman, S. L., & Merkle, D. M. (1992, May). *Refusal report forms (RRFs), refusal conversions, and non-response bias.* Paper presented at the meeting of the American Association for Public Opinion Research, St. Petersburg, FL.

Massachusetts tops telephone penetration at 99.1% (2003, March). *The Frame*. Retrieved April 4, 2003, from http://www.worldopinion.com/the_frame/2003/mar_2.html.

Olson, S. H. (2001). Reported participation in case-control studies: Changes over time. *American Journal of Epidemiology*, 154, 574–581.

Olson, S. H., Kelsey, J. L., Pearson, T. A., & Levin, B. (1992). Evaluation of random digit dialing as a method of control selection in case-control studies. *American Journal of Epidemiology*, 135, 210–222.

Olson, S. H., Voigt, L. F., Begg, C. B., & Weiss, N. S. (2002). Reporting participation in case-control studies. *Epidemiology*, 13, 123–126.

O'Neil, M. J. (1979). Estimating the nonresponse bias due to refusals in telephone surveys. *Public Opinion Quarterly*, 43, 218–232.

Pothoff, R. F. (1994). Telephone sampling in epidemiologic research: To reap the benefits, avoid the pitfalls. *American Journal of Epidemiology*, 139, 967–978.

Rizzo, L., DiGaetano, R., Cadell, D., & Kulp, D. W. (1995). The women's CARE study: The results of an experiment in new sampling designs for random digit dialing surveys. *Proceedings of the American Statistical Association*, Survey Research Methods Section, 644–649.

Samet, J. M. (2002). On revealing what we'd rather hide: The problem of describing study participation. *Epidemiology*, 13, 117.

Slattery, M. L., Edwards, S. L., Caan, B. J., Kerber, R. A., & Potter, J. D. (1995). Response rates among control subjects in case-control studies. *Annals of Epidemiology*, 5, 245–249.

Solely cellular phone usage only 2% (2001, December). *The Frame*. Retrieved April 4, 2003, from http://www.worldopinion.com/the_frame/2001/dec_5.html.

Strouse, R., & Hall, J. (1994, May). Effect of payments on response rates and data quality for a general population telephone survey. Paper presented at the meeting of the American Association for Public Opinion Research, Danvers, MA.

Sudman, S., Sirken, M. G., & Cowan, C. D. (1988). Sampling rare and elusive populations. *Science*, 240, 991–995.

Triplett, T., Blair, J., Hamilton, T., & Kang, Y. C. (1996). Initial cooperators vs. converted refusers: Are there response behavior differences? *Proceedings of the American Statistical Association*, Section on Survey Research Methods, 1038–1041.

Tuckel, P. (1997). The effect of different introductions and answering machine messages on response rates. *Proceedings of the American Statistical Association*, Survey Research Methods Section, 1047–1051.

Tucker C., Lepkowski J. M., & Piekarksi, L. (2002). The current efficiency of list-assisted telephone sampling designs. *Public Opinion Quarterly*, 66, 321–338.

Voigt, L. F., Davis, S., & Heuser, L. (1992). Random digit dialing: The potential effect on sample characteristics of the conversion of non-residential phone numbers. *American Journal of Epidemiology*, 136, 1393–1399.

Voigt, L. F., Koepsell, T. D., & Daling, J. R. (2003). Characteristics of telephone survey respondents according to willingness to participate. *American Journal of Epidemiology*, 157, 66–73.

Wacholder, S., McLaughlin, J. K., Silverman, D. T., & Mandel, J. S. (1992). Selection of controls in case-control studies. *American Journal of Epidemiology*, 135, 1019–1028.

Waksberg, J. (1978). Sampling methods for random digit dialing. *Journal of the American Statistical Association*, 73, 40–46.

Waksberg, J. (2000). Random digit dialing sampling for case-control studies. In M. H. Gail & J. Benichou (Eds.), *Encyclopedia of Epidemiologic Methods* (pp. 749–753). New York: Wiley.

SECTION V

Conceptualization, Operationalization, and Measurement

43

MEASURING AND EVALUATING EFFECTIVENESS OF SERVICES FOR FAMILIES AND CHILDREN

Charles L. Usher

Over the past decade, growing concern about the effectiveness of services to families and children has manifested itself in several ways. Most obvious are attempts to define and measure outcomes and to address questions about the extent to which improved outcomes may be attributable, at least in part, to the receipt of particular services. This has led to demands for accountability and related efforts by policy makers and human service professionals to put into place systems to monitor outcomes and to assess service effectiveness. As discussions along these lines have intensified, subtler issues have emerged, such as the complex interplay between formal services and the informal supports provided by extended family and others in the community. The result is that while few of the thorny issues in this area are fully resolved, we have a much better appreciation of important issues that must be addressed.

This chapter discusses three topics that are key to advancing our understanding of whether and how services to families and children improve the outcomes they experience. First, social intervention research has made researchers and practitioners more aware of the constrained role formal services play in the lives of many families and, concomitantly, how important informal supports are. This awareness forces us to con-

sider both the random and systematic ways in which services and supports interact to influence outcomes. This new sophistication is humbling for practitioners and challenging for researchers trying to evaluate new interventions.

Second, as we have become more sophisticated about the complexity of social interventions, we have been forced to acknowledge that the empirical foundation for them, or their evidence base, is far from definitive. Human services are not unique in this regard, but the challenges in building an evidence base in this particular area are daunting. In spite of the challenge, however, significant efforts are being made to correct past deficiencies in the design, delivery, and evaluation of services so that future interventions are more likely to be effective.

Third, the most promising developments in the effort to evaluate the effectiveness of services for families and children are investments in new data resources and changes in how we design and evaluate services. More data are now available, particularly longitudinal data, and new hardware, software, and analytic methods make it possible to explore issues that formerly were beyond our reach. Yet, data resources and technological advancements are only part of the promise. Equally important are changes in how researchers and human service practitioners perceive their roles relative to families and children in designing and testing new interventions. New collaborative approaches may yield approaches to service that will be both effective and more responsive to the needs and aspirations of those we seek to help.

This chapter is organized around these three broad and interrelated sets of issues. Our purposes are, first, to provide some perspective on the state of the art in this field and, second, to draw attention to areas of work that are likely to get more attention in coming years. We begin by outlining a broader conceptualization of services for families and children.

THE DEFINITION AND SCOPE OF "SERVICES"

Part of the tension that has always existed between evaluators and human service practitioners is the tendency toward reductionism among researchers—that is, the desire to isolate *the* critical factor or key ingredient in a service mix that determines success or failure. Practitioners' face-to-face interactions with families force them to recognize both the widely varying circumstances and characteristics of families and also what their clients fall back on when formal services are denied or are otherwise not available. They appreciate the unique characteristics of individual families, their children, and the communities in which they live, as well as the varied blends of formal services and informal supports upon which they draw.

One way that we now conceive of this is in terms of risk and resiliency (Fraser, 1997). This conveys the notion that each family and each child in a family has particular individual characteristics and that individuals and families exist in a constellation of forces, each of which either facilitates or impedes good outcomes. While they may follow certain patterns, different blends of these risks and protective factors determine short-term and, ultimately, longer term outcomes. Recognition of these factors is more likely to produce service strategies that seek to complement and build on protective factors and to respond to risk factors (Fraser, 1997).

Kinship care for children in child welfare custody is an example of a pronounced shift in service approach that explicitly draws on informal supports. Although national estimates are not entirely reliable and comparisons with earlier practice are difficult because of data limitations, more than 137,000 children or one fourth of the children in foster care in 2000 were living with relatives (Children's Bureau, 2002). While the level of financial support and types of nonfinancial supports for the families of these children vary widely by state (Ehrle & Geen, 2002), kinship care represents one of the most widely used forms of out-of-home care for children who have been abused or neglected. It is significant that this approach demonstrates an appreciation of the fact that risk and protective factors exist *within* families. More important, however, is that kinship care results in fewer placement moves for children in foster care, and they are more likely to retain ties to their families during and after foster care (Usher, Randolph, & Gogan, 1999).

In a similar way, experience in states and communities that have participated in the Family to Family initiative suggests that communities in which many risk factors are prevalent are also communities that have strengths on which to build. Sponsored by the Annie E. Casey Foundation and implemented in some of the nation's largest cities and other communities in 13 states, Family to Family seeks to build a partnership between child welfare agencies and the neighborhoods from which the greatest number of children enter out-of-home care (Annie E. Casey Foundation, n.d.). In almost every case, this process began with child welfare officials learning about community-based organizations and other resources in these communities that they had largely ignored in attempting to keep children safe and to provide them permanent homes. An evaluation of the initial phase of the initiative concluded that only by including families and community residents in decision making about out-of-home placements were officials able to demonstrate the sincerity of their commitment to the new partnership and, thus, to tap into these unused resources (Usher, Gibbs, Wildfire, & Gogan, 1997). Among the results have been reduced reliance on out-of-home care, fewer placement moves, and lower rates of reentry to care (Usher, Wildfire, & Gibbs, 1999).

Acknowledging the crucial role of informal supports in improving outcomes for families and children creates opportunities as well as challenges for both evaluators and human service practitioners. By definition, informal support from families, friends, and neighbors is often beyond the control (or perception) of evaluators.

The best that can be done is to assess its presence and to include measures of it in analyses of formal interventions, the availability of which may be controlled experimentally or quasi-experimentally. This becomes less of a problem, however, if the planning and development of interventions intentionally seek to incorporate informal supports into the design of the intervention. In effect, this requires a reconceptualization of interventions as an integrated bundle of services and supports that involves a wide range of providers—family and community resources as well as trained professionals.

BUILDING AN OUTCOME-ORIENTED EVIDENCE BASE

Efforts to promote evidence-based practice (EBP) in services for families and children can be traced to earlier efforts in health care. The Cochrane Collaboration in Great Britain began as a systematic effort to compile and assess the evidence base for practices in that field (Fowler, 2001), and the Agency for Healthcare Research and Quality (n.d.) is attempting to extend it through the establishment of evidence-based practice centers in the United States. Increasing references to EBP in the area of family and children's services indicate the growing influence of this perspective (Rosen, 2002; Tracy & Whittaker, 1987). The reality, however, is probably that the evidence base is not adequate to draw definitive conclusions about the effectiveness of particular services, even though this somewhat pessimistic assessment should not discourage rigorous and coordinated research on which future practices can rest.

In the United States, the movement toward EBP is one manifestation of demands for accountability that emerged during the 1990s in conjunction with the devolution of human services policy-making authority to state and local governments. The beginning of this transition was signaled by legislation replacing the Aid to Families with Dependent Children (AFDC) program with the Temporary Assistance to Needy Families (TANF) program in 1996. Just as changes in public assistance were preceded by state demonstration projects made possible by waivers of federal regulations, states are now experimenting with waivers of regulations based on Title IV-E of the Social Security Act, the legislation governing child welfare programs (Chil-

dren's Bureau, n.d.-b). The Bush Administration's proposal for the 2004 federal budget is that states may choose the option of operating under an alternative financing system that will relieve them of some regulatory constraints (Office of Management and Budget, 2003). However, the proposal also would require that states choosing this option undergo a "third-party evaluation" to ensure that they maintain or improve outcomes for children and families served in the child welfare system.

If the child welfare system undergoes a transformation similar to what has occurred in the public assistance system, the establishment of outcome-based accountability may be facilitated by a consensus on key outcomes that emerged in the late 1990s. Expressed in federal policy as well as in outcome frameworks developed in the private sector, outcomes are organized around the themes of safety, permanency, and family and child well-being (Children's Bureau, n.d.-c):

Safety

- Children are, first and foremost, protected from abuse and neglect.
- Children are safely maintained in their homes whenever possible and appropriate.

Permanency

- Children have permanency and stability in their living situations.
- The continuity of family relationships and connections is preserved for children.

Family and Child Well-Being

- Families have enhanced capacity to provide for their children's needs.
- Children receive appropriate services to meet their educational needs.
- Children receive adequate services to meet their physical and mental health needs.

The Child and Family Services Review (CFSR) process instituted by the federal government in fiscal year 2001 evaluates the performance of state child welfare agencies on the basis of indicators in all three areas (Children's Bureau, n.d.-a). The process relies on data from the Adoption and Foster Care Analysis and Reporting System (AFCARS), supplemented by findings from intensive on-site reviews of 50 cases and interviews with family members and other stakeholders.

Criticism of the CFSR review system has centered on the approach the Children's Bureau has taken in establishing national standards for performance with regard to six indicators within the broader outcome framework (Needell & Courtney, 2002; Usher, 2002):

- Recurrence of maltreatment
- Incidence of child abuse and/or neglect in foster care
- Foster care reentries
- Length of time to achieve reunification
- Length of time to achieve adoption
- Stability of foster care placement

A broad concern with regard to these indicators is that they fail to capture experiences of children and families that adequately reflect safety, permanency, and well-being outcomes. A more specific concern is that the nature of the data on which they are based and the manner in which they are measured produce biased and unreliable indicators. The underlying problem is that the measures are not based on the experiences of *all* children who enter the child welfare system but distinct segments of them, specifically a cross-section of children in care during a given review period or the group of children who happen to exit care during a particular period. As such, most of the resulting indicators are biased in one of two ways: (a) overrepresentation of the experience of children with long lengths of stay because of length-biased cross-sectional data or (b) underestimation of length of time to permanency outcomes because of the bias of exit-cohort samples toward children with shorter lengths of stay (Wulczyn, Kogan, & Dilts, 2001).

These measurement problems are compounded by the fact that the national standards were set at the 75th percentile, thereby guaranteeing that most states would fail to meet any single standard. Experience in the initial stages of the review process have been consistent with this design feature, with the result that no more than 4 of the 17 states reviewed in the first year were found to be in substantial conformity with any of the seven CFSR outcomes (Children's Bureau, n.d.-d) and all states have had to prepare a program improvement plan (Children's Bureau, 2000). Judged by these standards, the effectiveness of services for families and children directly involved with the child welfare system

in the United States would be highly questionable, if not scandalously ineffectual.

The situation with regard to the CFSR process serves to illustrate a fundamental challenge in assessing the effectiveness of services for families and children. The set of outcomes on which the system is based is consistent in many ways with others that have been proposed. Most notable is the approach developed in the Casey Outcomes and Decision Making Project organized by the American Humane Association and conducted in concert with the American Bar Association, the Annie E. Casey Foundation, the Casey Family Program, Casey Family Services, and the Institute for Human Services Management (American Humane Association, 1998). The key outcome "domains" in this framework are the same as those on which CFSR is based: safety, permanency, and well-being. The two approaches differ, however, with regard to the specific indicators and approaches to measurement that are recommended.

The problem posed by the CFSR measurement approach is illustrated by one of the state reviews done in the first year of the process. In evaluating this state's performance with regard to Outcome P1 (children have permanency and stability in their living situations), the review team found that this state did not meet national standards with regard to the length of time required to achieve reunification or adoption and that performance in a number of areas related to this outcome needed improvement (Region IV, 2001). This general conclusion stands in contrast to information developed in the state's own assessment and summarized in the report by the federal review team. For example, across four successive annual cohorts of children entering care in this state, the median length of stay declined from 425 days for the first cohort, to 401 days for the cohort entering in the next year, to 391 days for the next cohort, and finally to 369 days for the fourth cohort. During this period, the caseload declined from 6,982 in 1997 to 5,765 in 2000, and the rate of adoptions among all case terminations rose from 14.8% to 21.3%, an increase of nearly half (Region IV, 2001). The contrasting perspectives demonstrate that how outcomes are defined and measured can have a profound impact on conclusions about service effectiveness.

Child and family well-being is perhaps the most challenging outcome domain to define and measure, not only within CFSR but also in the field more generally. An issue of debate in child welfare is the extent to which a system that is intended to provide temporary care for children can be held responsible for aspects of well-being that are years in development. Only with the cooperation of other human service agencies and community supports is it possible for child welfare agencies to attend to the variety of needs that bear on child and family well-being. Yet, a growing number of child welfare practitioners now acknowledge responsibility in this area, particularly for that segment of children for whom permanency is an elusive goal.

Recent findings from the National Survey of America's Families (NSAF) reveal significant risks to the well-being of children in the child welfare system (Kortenkamp & Ehrle, 2002). Acknowledging that their data probably is skewed toward the experience of children who have longer stays in foster care, Kortenkamp and Ehrle provide a profile of children in foster care (or living with relatives after having been in foster care) that shows a high prevalence of behavioral and emotional problems. For example, 27% of the children in this subsample of NSAF families were found to have "high levels of behavioral and emotional problems," in contrast to 7% of children being cared for by their parents and 13% of children living in so-called high-risk parent care (low-income, single-parent families) (Kortenkamp & Ehrle, 2002). Similar proportions of children involved with the child welfare system were found to have problems in school, in extracurricular activities, and with physical, learning, or mental health conditions. While the data cannot support an assessment of the effectiveness of service being provided to these children to help them deal with these threats to their well-being, they do indicate that practitioners in the field must make efforts to promote child well-being among the children they are serving.

The findings of the NSAF survey also suggest that a substantial segment of children enter the child welfare system after other services and supports have failed them and their families. Awareness of the potential cost-effectiveness of prevention programs is another reason why our conception of "family and children's services" is now more expansive, encompassing a variety of supports and services, some targeted to children and others more broadly focused on families. Impetus for this perspective within child welfare can be traced to initial funding of the Promoting

Safe and Stable Families program in 1993, which now involves an annual allocation of more than $305 million to the states (Children's Bureau, n.d.-c).

As federal funding of family support programs has grown, concerns have arisen about the nature and effectiveness of supports and services provided under this rubric. This led to the National Evaluation of Family Support Programs, an effort that sought to compile and synthesize the findings of extant evaluations (Layzer, Goodson, Bernstein, & Price, 2001). A meta-analysis of evaluations of 260 programs led these researchers to conclude that family support services generally have a small but statistically significant impact on various outcomes for children and their parents. Their general conclusion was that these effects were commensurate with the typically small financial investments in these programs and that it was probably not reasonable to expect more pronounced effects, given the scale of effort. The researchers recommended caution in making more substantial investments without taking into account certain findings. For example, although most programs included education about parenting, the studies included in their review generally found only small improvements in parents' knowledge of child development and related issues. Indeed, they concluded that the only programs that appeared to enhance cognitive development and school readiness were those targeting children directly. Finally, the research team concluded from their review of the literature that programs involving professional services (in contrast to services by paraprofessionals) and group settings (e.g., hospitals rather than home visits to individual families) tended to be more effective.

PROMISING DEVELOPMENTS

Future efforts to evaluate services to families and children will be aided by the availability of new data resources and technological advances that will make it possible to pursue new and important lines of analysis. An important investment by the federal government involves its sponsorship of the National Survey of Child and Adolescent Well-Being (NSCAW Research Group, 2002). The study involves longitudinal tracking of the experiences of a national probability sample of more than 6,000 children who were reported as victims of abuse or neglect between October 1999 and December 2000. It also includes a separate national probability sample of children who had been in foster care for approximately 1 year when the survey entered the field.

Although not designed to provide the basis for an evaluation of services to families and children, NSCAW will yield important descriptive information about the receipt of services by sample members and the outcomes they experience. In addition to obtaining detailed data about child well-being from several sources, it seeks to answer several broader questions (National Data Archive on Child Abuse and Neglect, n.d.):

- What paths do children follow into and through the child welfare system?
- What factors affect investigation, services, placements, and length of involvement?
- What are the long- and short-term outcomes for children and families in the child welfare system in terms of safety, well-being, and permanence?

The Children's Bureau is making data from the survey available through the National Archive on Child Abuse and Neglect at Cornell University and attempting to expedite dissemination of the resulting database so that researchers will have ready access to it before the information becomes outdated. Complemented by longitudinal databases developed from state child welfare information systems (Needell et al., 2003; Usher, Locklin, Wildfire, & Harris, 2001; F. H. Wulczyn, Brunner, & Goerge, 1999), many of the questions outlined here can now be answered more fully and accurately.

Recent advances in analytic techniques and software will also facilitate evaluations of service effectiveness that take into account the fact that children are members of families, families are members of communities, and communities are components of urban and regional population centers. The landmark study that defined *collective efficacy* demonstrated the distinctive patterns of interaction within neighborhoods and how such neighborhood characteristics can influence the quality of life for families and children (Sampson, Raudenbush, & Earls, 1997). In the future, more studies will be designed to take into account the multiple levels of data required to address such complex issues and to apply recently developed analytic techniques that make

it possible to assess effects on outcomes across these different levels (Raudenbush & Bryk, 2002). Facilitating these analyses will be census and other geocoded data that provide richer and more accurate characterizations of neighborhoods and communities.

A final promising note concerning future evaluations of services for families and children has less to do with the nature of the data and the methods of analysis than with how the evaluations are planned and carried out. We now operate in a highly devolved system in which state and local governments have more discretion than ever to create new systems of supports and services for families and children. The scarcity of resources also dictates that informal supports be acknowledged and incorporated into service strategies. This can be accomplished only by tailoring interventions to the unique resources and needs of a community. Indeed, the strongest program effects found by the National Evaluation of Family Support Programs were confined to single sites, and no single program model was universally successful (Layzer et al., 2001).

This pattern of findings is instructive. Under such conditions, evaluators must be prepared to work more closely with the consumers and providers of supports and services in crafting and refining interventions that are tailored to local needs and that capitalize on local resources. New approaches to evaluation are being explored, and initial results are promising (Fetterman, 2001; Usher, 1995; Webster, Needell, & Wildfire, 2002). Also, as the National Evaluation of Family Support Programs demonstrated, meta-analysis provides a means of synthesizing what is being learned across various communities and drawing broader conclusions about the effectiveness of services to families and children. In this fashion, it may be possible to strike a satisfactory balance of interests among consumers, service providers, and researchers that is responsive both to local concerns and to the advancement of knowledge.

References

Agency for Healthcare Research and Quality. (n.d.). *Evidence-based practice centers: Overview.* Retrieved December 18, 2002, from http://www.ahcpr.gov/clinic/epc/

American Humane Association. (1998). *Assessing outcomes in child welfare services: Principles, concepts, and a framework of core outcome in-*

dicators. Englewood, CO: American Humane Association.

Annie E. Casey Foundation. (n.d.). *Overview of family to family*. Retrieved February 11, 2003, from http://www.aecf.org/initiatives/familytofamily/overview.htm

Children's Bureau. (2000). *Child and family services reviews: Procedures manual*. Washington, DC: Administration on Children, Youth and Families.

Children's Bureau. (2002). *The AFCARS report: Interim FY 2000 estimates as of August 2002*. Washington, DC: Administration for Children, Youth and Families.

Children's Bureau. (n.d.-a). *Background paper: Child and family services reviews national standards*. Retrieved February 11, 2003, from http://www.acf.hhs.gov/programs/cb/hotissues/background.htm

Children's Bureau. (n.d.-b). *IV-E waiver information*. Retrieved February 11, 2003, from http://www.acf.hhs.gov/programs/cb/initiatives/cwwaiver.htm

Children's Bureau. (n.d.-c). *Program assessment for child and family services reviews and title IV-E foster care eligibility reviews fact sheet*. Retrieved February 11, 2003, from http://www.acf.dhhs.gov/programs/cb/cwrp/geninfo/07200fsheet.htm

Children's Bureau. (n.d.-d). *Summary of the results of the 2001 and 2002 child and family services reviews*. Retrieved August 1, 2003, from http://www.acf.hhs.gov/programs/cb/cwrp/2002cfsrresults.pdf

Ehrle, J., & Geen, R. (2002). Kin and non-kin foster care-findings from a national survey. *Children and Youth Services Review, 24*(1–2), 15–35.

Fetterman, D. M. (2001). *Foundations of empowerment evaluation*. Thousand Oaks, CA: Sage.

Fowler, G. (2001). *Evidence-based practice: Tools and techniques*. Paper presented at the Systems, Settings, People: Workforce Development Challenges for the Alcohol and Other Drugs Field, Adelaide, AU.

Fraser, M. W. (1997). The ecology of childhood: A multisystems perspective. In M. W. Fraser (Ed.), *Risk and resilience in childhood: An ecological perspective*. Washington, DC: NASW Press.

Kortenkamp, K., & Ehrle, J. (2002). *The well-being of children involved with the child welfare system: A national overview* (No. Series B, No. B-43). Washington, DC: Urban Institute.

Layzer, J. I., Goodson, B. D., Bernstein, L., & Price, C. (2001). *National evaluation of family support programs: Final report*. Cambridge, MA: Abt Associates.

National Data Archive on Child Abuse and Neglect. (n.d.). *The national survey of child and adolescent well-being (NSCAW), wave 1*. Retrieved February 11, 2003, from http://www.ndacan.-cornell.edu/NDACAN/Datasets/Abstracts/DatasetAbstract_92_NSCAW.html

Needell, B., & Courtney, M. E. (2002, November 7–9). *National standards in the child and family service reviews: What do they really tell us?* Paper presented at the APPAM fall research conference, Dallas, TX.

Needell, B., Webster, D., Cuccaro-Alamin, S., Armijo, M., Lee, S., Brookhart, A., et al. (2003). *Child welfare services reports for California*. Retrieved February 11, 2003, from http://cssr.berkeley.edu/CWSCMSreports/

NSCAW Research Group. (2002). Methodological lessons from the national survey of child and adolescent well-being: The first three years of the USA's first national probability study of children and families investigated for abuse and neglect. *Children and Youth Services Review, 24*(6–7), 513–543.

Office of Management and Budget. (2003). *Budget of the United States government: Fiscal year 2004*. Washington, DC: Office of the President.

Raudenbush, S. W., & Bryk, A. S. (2002). *Hierarchical linear models: Applications and data analysis methods* (2nd ed.). Thousand Oaks, CA: Sage.

Region IV. (2001). *Child and family services review: Final assessment, North Carolina*. Atlanta, GA: Administration for Children and Families.

Rosen, A. (2002, January). *Evidence-based social work practice: Challenges and promise*. Paper presented at the annual meeting of the Society for Social Work and Research, San Diego, CA.

Sampson, R. J., Raudenbush, S. W., & Earls, F. (1997). Neighborhoods and violent crime: A multilevel study of collective efficacy. *Science, 277*(5328), 918–924.

Tracy, E. M., & Whittaker, J. K. (1987). The evidence base for social support interventions in child and family-practice: Emerging issues for research and practice. *Children and Youth Services Review, 9*(4), 249–270.

Usher, C. L. (1995). Improving evaluability through self-evaluation. *Evaluation Practice, 16*(1), 59–68.

Usher, C. L. (2002, November 7). *Measurement issues in the child and family service review process*. Paper presented at the annual meeting of the American Evaluation Association, Washington, DC.

Usher, C. L., Gibbs, D. A., Wildfire, J. B., & Gogan, H. C. (1997). *Evaluation of family to family*. Chapel Hill: University of North Carolina–Chapel Hill, Jordan Institute for Families.

Usher, C. L., Locklin, E., Wildfire, J. B., & Harris, C. C. (2001). Child welfare performance ratings: One state's approach. *Administration in Social Work, 25*(1), 35–51.

Usher, C. L., Randolph, K. A., & Gogan, H. C. (1999). Placement patterns in foster care. *Social Service Review, 73*(1), 22–36.

Usher, C. L., Wildfire, J. B., & Gibbs, D. A. (1999). Measuring performance in child welfare: Secondary effects of success. *Child Welfare*, 78(1), 31–51.

Webster, D., Needell, B., & Wildfire, J. (2002). Data are your friends: Child welfare agency self-evaluation in Los Angeles county with the family to family initiative. *Children and Youth Services Review*, 24(6–7), 471–484.

Wulczyn, F., Kogan, J., & Dilts, J. (2001). The effect of population dynamics on performance measurement. *Social Service Review*, 75(2), 292–317.

Wulczyn, F. H., Brunner, K., & Goerge, R. M. (1999). *Foster care dynamics 1983–1997: A report from the multistate foster care data archive*. Chicago: Chapin Hall Center for Children.

44

RISK-ADJUSTED MENTAL HEALTH OUTCOMES

Michael S. Hendryx

Donabedian (1980) defines a health care outcome as a "change in a patient's current and future health status that can be attributed to antecedent health care" (pp. 82–83). An outcome is the result of health care or, in other words, is *caused* by the health care that was received by the patient.

There continue to be intense and ongoing efforts to develop measures of health care outcomes. These efforts are in response to rising health care costs, capitation models of financing, and concerns with widespread variation in health care practices and outcomes across providers or settings (Iezzoni, 1997a; Kramer, Daniels, Zieman, Williams, & Dewan, 2000; Young, Sullivan, Burnam, & Brook, 1998). Measuring and reporting outcomes of care is an attempt to ensure that payers receive good value for their dollars and that patients receive high-quality care.

However, the measurement of outcome is influenced by other characteristics of the patient, in addition to health care. To measure an outcome accurately, we need to account for patients' risk of that outcome. Risk refers to the "confounding factors . . . that are causally related to the outcome under study" (Blumberg, 1986, p. 355). To account for these confounding factors and attempt to isolate the true effect of health care on the outcome, risk adjustment is necessary. As indicated by Iezzoni (1997a), "the goal of risk adjustment is to account for pertinent patient characteristics before making inferences about the effectiveness of care" (p. 4). Risk adjustment usually takes place in the context of comparing outcomes across groups, such as outcomes across providers, hospitals, or mental health centers. Accounting for risk is in effect like accounting for covariates in a quasi-experimental or nonexperimental design—accounting for those other pertinent variables that affect the measurement of the dependent variable aside from the independent variable. To take this analogy further, the independent variable is the mental health treatment that is received by people across different naturally occurring groups (e.g., treatment in mental health agency A versus B versus C), the dependent variable is the outcome, and in the absence of random assignment to treatment conditions, the risks are the covariates that must be measured and included in the statistical models of outcome. If we fail to account for these confounding influences, attempts to evaluate the effectiveness of care across groups may be misleading.

In the mental health services field, what are the outcomes, and what are the risks? There is no single, objective outcome indicator for mental health services. The types of outcomes that are most often assessed include measures of patient functioning, symptoms, recovery, quality of life, service use, and satisfaction with care. These outcomes may be assessed with a variety of instruments completed by patients themselves or by providers. A substantial effort has been made in the mental health services research field to identify and measure mental health treatment outcomes (e.g., Andreason, 1984; Corrigan et al., 1999; Cuffel, Fischer, Owen, & Smith, 1997; Eisen, Dill, & Grob, 1994; Overall & Gorham, 1962; Teague, Ganju, Hornik, Johnson, & Mc-Kinney, 1997; Zani, McFarland, Wachal, Barker, & Barron, 1999).

In contrast, the identification and measurement of risk variables for mental health treatment outcomes has not received the same level of attention (Dickey, Hermann, & Eisen, 1998). Research has been done to identify predictors or correlates of certain outcomes, for example, predictors of relapse in schizophrenia (Doering et al., 1998) or prognostic indicators for response to treatment for depression (Smith, Burnam, Burns, Clear, & Rost, 1998). However, this research has not been directed specifically to identifying risks for risk adjustment purposes.

This chapter summarizes challenges and possible solutions to developing risk-adjusted outcomes for mental health services. The emphasis is on the challenges faced by practice settings and on solutions that may be attempted within those settings to develop outcomes that appropriately account for risk.

CHALLENGES

To develop sound risk-adjusted outcomes for mental health treatment, a number of challenges must be addressed in the practice setting. These challenges are summarized, and potential solutions suggested, in the subsequent section. The challenges may be grouped into those concerning concept, data, analysis, and interpretation and uses.

Concept

Systematic efforts to build empirically grounded conceptual models of risk for mental health treatment outcomes have been lacking. An existing conceptual framework may be a useful starting point for developing mental health–specific models; Anderson's model (1995; Anderson & Newman, 1973) of health services utilization is one option, although it is designed to predict utilization, not mental health outcomes. Risks, under this model, would include predisposing, enabling, and need variables, which would have to be specified for each outcome and disease group (e.g., risks and outcomes for schizophrenia will not always be the same as for major depression). The major need variables are severity of illness and diagnosis. Predisposing variables include demographics and social prognostic indicators of treatment effectiveness, for example, age, gender, education, and marital status. Enabling variables are personal, family, or community characteristics that aid in access to care or benefit from care, for example, insurance coverage and levels of community poverty. To take a case example, imagine two people receiving the same form of treatment at the same agency. These people may have similar risks of a favorable outcome on some dimensions (e.g., diagnosis) but dissimilar risks on other dimensions. One person might be single or socially isolated or have a history of poor medication compliance, placing him or her at greater risk of poor treatment outcome than the second person, who has better social support and medication compliance. If there are systematic differences in the mix of treatment populations across agencies or providers (e.g., Agency A treats a riskier population than Agency B), outcomes could appear poorer in Agency A, even if they offer equally efficacious treatment.

Another conceptual framework comes from Iezzoni (1997a), who defines the dimensions of risk for health care outcomes in general, not specific to mental health care. Dimensions of risk include demographic variables, diagnosis and its severity, clinical stability, comorbidities, physical functioning and health status, psychosocial functioning, quality of life, patient attitudes and preferences, and cultural, ethnic, and socioeconomic factors. Table 44.1 summarizes these two conceptual models and provides examples of mental health risk variables that may correspond to each dimension.

Performance measurement tools focus on outcomes but give limited attention to risk variables. Performance measurement tools for mental health care include, for example, the Mental Health Statistics Improvement Program (MHSIP) consumer survey (Teague et al., 1997), the Multnomah Community Ability Scale (Zani et al., 1999), the Brief Psychiatric Rating Scale (BPRS) (Overall & Gorham, 1962), the Modified Scale for the Assessment of Negative Symptoms (MSANS) (Andreason, 1984), the BASIS-32 (Eisen et al., 1994), and a myriad of proprietary

TABLE 44.1 Conceptual Models of Mental Health Risk Variables. (Variables in parentheses are illustrative and not exhaustive.)

Dimension	Corresponding Iezzoni dimension and/or examples of mental health risk variables
Need	Diagnosis (Axis I, Axis II)
	Severity (Axis V, baseline Hamilton Depression score, baseline BPRS or MSANS)
	Clinical stability
	Comorbidities (co-occurring substance abuse)
	Physical functioning and health status (SF-36)
Predisposing	Demographics (age, sex)
	Cultural and ethnic factors (reliance on traditional healers)
	Preferences and attitudes
	Quality of life (California Quality of Life scale)
Enabling	Insurance coverage
	Community poverty
	Distance to treatment
	Socioeconomic status
	Social functioning

vendors' tools. Some vendor tools may claim to measure and adjust for risk, but the risk variables selected and the methods used for adjustment may not be clearly specified to the vendor's customers (i.e., persons working in the practice setting) and may not be justified empirically or conceptually.

Data

To the extent that risk adjustment is attempted in mental health practice settings, those attempts by and large rely on existing variables and data sets. Few special efforts are made to collect measures of risk. Existing mental health databases typically contain basic demographic information, perhaps diagnosis and limited clinical data, service utilization statistics, and payer information. These databases were developed to track utilization levels and costs, not to measure outcome risk. Therefore, it is not surprising that risk-adjusted mental health outcome models that use these data have had limited predictive power (e.g., Hendryx, Dyck & Srebnik, 1999; Hendryx et al., 2003).

The lack of appropriate risk variables is probably due primarily to lack of awareness of the problem, lack of information concerning what risk variables should be collected, and lack of adequate resources to collect the necessary data. Collecting data takes time for staff and patients, including time for staff to complete baseline assessments of patient status that include risk variables and then time to create the necessary database for subsequent analysis. Unless there is a clear understanding among staff of the benefits they can expect by collecting this information, it may not be viewed as a priority and so may not take place, given the severe resource constraints faced by many mental health practice settings.

Other data issues concern the logistics of measurement. The correct timing of outcomes and risk must be found; for example, response to mental health treatment may for some indicators be a function of state, as opposed to trait, variables and so may suggest, for some outcomes, the need for repeated risk and outcome assessment over fairly short intervals, even every few sessions, especially early in treatment (Howard, Lueger, Maling, & Martinovich, 1993). Another logistical issue is that if multiple treatment sites are to be compared, data must be collected uniformly across sites, using standardized and clearly explicated procedures.

Attrition and missing data are other problems to consider. Whereas some outcome measures may respond quickly to treatment, others may require longer periods, several months or more, before effects can be detected. To measure both risk and outcome under these conditions requires that patients be in treatment long enough for at least two measurement periods sufficiently spaced. But to the extent that patients receive treatment for brief periods only or discontinue treatment before outcomes can be measured, both data points will not be available. Patients who drop out do not do so randomly but may drop out because they have unusually mild or unusually severe risks relative to patients who continue in treatment. Risk-adjusted models may then not be representative of all patients.

Analysis

There is no single agreed method for conducting the actual risk adjustment statistical analysis. Risk adjustment work in other areas of health care suggests that linear and logistic multiple regression models are most commonly employed (e.g., Iezzoni, 1997a). But these may be supplemented by hierarchical regression models (Bryk & Raudenbush, 1992), repeated measures analysis of covariance models, recursive partitioning analysis, instrumental variable analysis (McClellan & Newhouse, 2000), propensity scores (Rubin, 1997), or stratification models (Banks, Pandiani, & Bramley, 2001). The use of one method of adjustment versus another can result in different conclusions about relative group performance (Hendryx, Moore, Leeper, Jackson, & Davis, 2001). Regression models offer a means to develop a standard approach that is commonly used in other areas of health care.

It may be the case, however, that the most appropriate method of analysis is not traditional regression but hierarchical regression (Bryk & Raudenbush, 1992). Hierarchical regression takes into account the fact that observations are not independent but clustered within treatment groups, and it results in more accurate model estimates than traditional regression. Little research has yet been reported on the practical advantage of using hierarchical modeling over traditional regression—that is, does it make a difference when drawing conclusions about group performance?—but some evidence suggests that hierarchical modeling does make a difference (Cuffel, 2003). The routine use of hier-

archical modeling may be beyond the current capacity of many mental health practice settings, but this may change as hierarchical modeling techniques become better understood in the general research field and become a mainstream tool in statistical software packages.

Interpretation and Uses

Once the data have been obtained and analyzed, they must be put to use. The risk adjustment per se is ultimately uninteresting; rather, we want to know what to do with the outcomes scores once they have been appropriately adjusted. Even a thorough risk adjustment may be imperfect and offers only a partial correction for the nonexperimental assignment of patients to groups (Iezzoni, 1997b). Furthermore, a thorough risk adjustment is not only imperfect but also limited: It gives us information only about group performance and may obscure important subgroup differences. If we "adjust away" the effects of diagnosis or symptom severity, for example, we cannot comment on the treatment effectiveness for that diagnostic or severity subgroup.

SOLUTIONS: HOW TO IMPLEMENT RISK ADJUSTMENT IN PRACTICE SETTINGS

Corresponding to the various challenges, solutions are suggested that must be undertaken if mature outcomes measurement systems are to be in place in mental health practice settings.

First and foremost, given the current underdeveloped state of risk measurement relative to outcome measurement, it is imperative that we begin to incorporate the selection of risk variables into performance measurement systems with the same care that is used to select the outcomes. The selection of risk variables should be based on strong conceptual and empirical foundations, as grounded in the literature, and ideally supplemented with local studies to identify risk variables for the outcomes and populations of interest. We need to figure out what risks we should be measuring and begin to measure them.

Once the candidate set of risk indicators is identified, they can be tested within practice-based research studies to confirm their importance or to eliminate them. One strategy is to test the available data against special studies of detailed data to see if available data are in fact adequate or inadequate. Alternative models can be tested for statistical strength (Hendryx et al., 2003) and for the practical difference they make in the conclusions we draw about group performance. The goal of these studies is to find the most parsimonious set of indicators, so that the burden of data collection and analysis can be minimized.

The problem of attrition and missing data can be addressed in part through conventional attempts to keep patients in treatment and to secure outcomes data from patients at time of last contact. However, consideration should be given to measuring early dropout as an outcome measure in itself. If the characteristics of early dropout indicate that people with serious illness are discontinuing treatment prematurely, this is a negative outcome measure that can be used as a performance indicator subject to risk adjustment.

In addition to studies to identify the best set of risk indicators, the statistical methods of adjustment can be tested to see if group level performance is sensitive to method. For example, one might compare regression, hierarchical, and stratification models to see if they lead to different conclusions; given the limited research to date, hierarchical models may be the best choice. By using the intercept and coefficient terms from either hierarchical or traditional regression models, each patient's expected outcome score based on her or his constellation of risk variables can be calculated. Then, the difference can be found between the average expected score for the agency as a whole and the average observed score to identify which agencies have statistically higher or lower risk-adjusted outcomes.

After risk-adjusted outcome scores are found, they may be used to identify other independent variables associated with adjusted performance. In other words, the risk-adjusted score becomes the new dependent variable, and independent variables are those that treatment agencies might change or improve. For example, does the new implementation of an evidence-based practice treatment protocol result in better risk-adjusted outcomes relative to standard care? Are better risk-adjusted outcomes associated with staffing variables such as education or caseloads or with program variables such as treatment modality? If so, staffing profiles or programs may be modified to improve outcomes. The risk-

adjusted scores thus become tools to use for quality improvement. They cannot serve as definitive performance scores but may be strongly suggestive of areas for improvement or benchmarks of top performance. Regarding benchmarks, agencies with the highest risk-adjusted outcomes can be used as models for other agencies to learn from.

Finally, use of risk-adjusted scores cannot be the sole method of performance measurement. They should, rather, be supplemented with other studies, such as those of subgroup performance. If we want to know which providers or treatment agencies are providing the best care for persons with co-occurring disorders, for patients in crisis, or for patients with more serious treatment histories, we have to study those risks separately and not simply include them as risks in a risk adjustment equation.

In summary, the idea that health care risks must be measured before outcomes can be fairly compared across groups is widely recognized (Iezzoni, 1997a), and that recognition is now extending to mental health care (Hendryx, Beigel, & Doucette, 2001). But before this recognition can be translated into practice, much work remains to be done. First, we need to do the critical conceptual and empirical work to identify the most parsimonious key set of risk variables corresponding to specific outcomes and treatment populations. And second, we need to develop the practical strategies for collecting and analyzing risk data in applied mental health treatment settings. Once we know what we should be measuring and how to measure it and begin to use risk-adjusted scores in the practice setting, we will have moved an important step closer to improving the quality of treatments for mental illness.

References

Anderson, R. (1995). Revisiting the behavioral model and access to medical care: Does it matter? *Journal of Health and Social Behavior, 36*, 1–10.

Anderson, R., & Newman, J. F. (1973). Societal and individual determinants of medical care utilization in the United States. *Milbank Memorial Fund Quarterly, 51*, 95–124.

Andreason, N. C. (1984.) Modified scale for the assessment of negative symptoms. Rockville, MD: National Institute of Mental Health.

Banks, S. M., Pandiani, J. A., & Bramley, J. (2001). Approaches to risk-adjusting outcome measures applied to criminal justice involvement after community service. *Journal of Behavioral Health Services and Research, 28,* 235–246.

Blumberg, M. S. (1986). Risk adjusting health care outcomes: A methodologic review. *Medical Care Review, 43,* 351–393.

Bryk, A. S., & Raudenbush, S. W. (1992). *Hierarchical linear models: Applications and data analysis methods.* Newbury Park, CA: Sage.

Corrigan, P. W., Giffort, D., Rashid, F., Leary, M., Okeke, I., & Lickey, S. (1999). Recovery as a psychological construct. *Community Mental Health Journal, 35,* 213–239.

Cuffel, B. J. (2003). Use of hierarchical linear modeling in the case mix adjustment of mental health provider profile scores. M. Hendryx (Ed.), *A toolkit for conducting risk adjustment of mental health performance indicators.* Cambridge, MA: The Evaluation Center at HSRI.

Cuffel, B. J., Fischer E. P., Owen, R. R., & Smith, G. R. (1997). An instrument for measurement of outcomes of care for schizophrenia. *Evaluation and the Health Professions, 20,* 96–108.

Dickey, B., Hermann R. C., & Eisen, S. V. (1998). Assessing the quality of psychiatric care: Research methods and application in clinical practice. *Harvard Review of Psychiatry, 6,* 88–96.

Doering, S., Muller, E., Kopcke, W., Pietzcker, A., Gaebel, W., Linden, M., et al. (1998). Predictors of relapse and rehospitalization in schizophrenia and schizoaffective disorder. *Schizophrenia Bulletin, 24,* 87–98.

Donabedian, A. (1980). *Explorations in quality assessment and monitoring. Vol. 1: The definition of quality and approaches to its assessment.* Ann Arbor, MI: Health Administration Press.

Eisen, S. V., Dill, D. L., & Grob, M. C. (1994). Reliability and validity of a brief patient-report instrument for psychiatric outcome evaluation. *Hospital and Community Psychiatry, 45,* 242–247.

Hendryx, M., Beigel, A., & Doucette, A. (2001). Introduction: Risk adjustment issues in mental health services. *Journal of Behavioral Health Services and Research, 28,* 225–234.

Hendryx, M., Dyck, D. G., & Srebnik, D. (1999). Risk-adjusted outcome models for public mental health outpatient programs. *Health Services Research, 34,* 171–195.

Hendryx, M., Moore, R., Leeper, T., Reynolds, M., & Davis, S. (2001). An examination of methods for risk-adjustment of rehospitalization rates. *Mental Health Services Research, 3,* 15–24.

Hendryx, M., Russo, J. E., Stegner, B., Dyck, D. G., Ries, R. K., & Roy-Byrne, P. (2003). Predicting rehospitalization and outpatient services from administration and clinical databases. *Journal of Behavioral Health Services and Research, 30*(3), 342–351.

Howard, K. I., Lueger, R. J., Maling, M. S., & Martinovich, Z. (1993). A phase model of psychotherapy outcome: Causal mediation of change. *Journal of Consulting and Clinical Psychology, 61,* 678–685.

Iezzoni, L. I. (Ed.). (1997a). *Risk adjustment for measuring health care outcomes* (2nd ed.). Ann Arbor, MI: Health Administration Press.

Iezzoni, L. I. (1997b). The risks of risk-adjustment. *Journal of the American Medical Association, 278,* 1600–1607.

Kramer, T. L., Daniels, A. S., Zieman, G. L., Williams, C., & Dewan, N. A. (2000). Psychiatric practice variations in the diagnosis and treatment of major depression. *Psychiatric Services, 51,* 336–340.

McClellan, M. B., & Newhouse, J. P. (2000). Overview of the special supplement issue. *Health Services Research 35*(5), 1061–1069.

Overall, J. E., & Gorham, D. R. (1962). The brief psychiatric rating scale. *Psychological Reports, 10,* 799–812.

Rubin, D. B. (1997). Estimating causal effects from large datasets using propensity scores. *Annals of Internal Medicine, 127,* 757–763.

Smith, G. R., Burnam, A., Burns, B., Clear, P. & Rost, K. M. (1998). *Major depression outcomes module: User's manual.* Little Rock: University of Arkansas for Medical Sciences.

Teague, G. B., Ganju, V., Hornik, J. A., Johnson, J. R. & McKinney, J. (1997). The MHSIP mental health report card: A consumer-oriented approach to monitoring the quality of mental health plans. *Evaluation Review, 21,* 330–341.

Young, A. S., Sullivan, G., Burnam, A., & Brook, R. H. (1998). Measuring the quality of outpatient treatment for schizophrenia. *Archives of General Psychiatry, 55,* 611–617.

Zani, B., McFarland, B., Wachal, M., Barker, S., & Barron, N. (1999). Statewide replication of predictive validation for the Multnomah Community Ability Scale. *Community Mental Health Journal, 35,* 223–229.

45 VALIDITY AND RELIABILITY IN FAMILY ASSESSMENT

Cynthia Franklin, Patricia A. Cody, & Catheleen Jordan

This chapter summarizes and discusses the reliability and validity of five measures of family assessment. Reliability is related to the consistency of a measure and is especially important when assessing measurement tools that will be used in clinical practice to guide the clinical decision-making process (Springer & Franklin, 2003). Reliability is established through four methods: test–retest, alternate form, split-half, and internal consistency. Validity addresses whether a tool measures what it is intended to measure. There are four types of validity: content validity, criterion validity, construct validity, and factorial analysis. Validity should be assessed in terms of the specific measurement tool and its intended use (Springer & Franklin, 2003). Managed behavioral health care and the subsequent demands for accountability in clinical practice require assessment tools and interventions that are known to be effective with clients and have well-established reliability and validity. Springer, Abell, and Hudson (2002) point out that despite an increase in accountability tools, the science of measurement and instrument development is very young. Much progress has been made on the psychometric development of valid and reliable assessment tools in the 25- to 30-year developmental period of marital and family therapy measures (Franklin & Jordan, 1999). The purpose of this chapter is to illustrate the importance of the development of psychometric measurement tools, which inform practice in marital and family therapy.

The measures reviewed in this chapter are empirically derived, based on systems theory, and were developed to assess families in marital and family therapy settings. Measures were derived from research on the classification and assessment of family functioning, as well as from clinical work with families, and are widely used in clinical settings (Jordan & Franklin, 2003). Five measures with good validity and reliability that are considered to be some of the best measures in clinical practice are reviewed in this chapter: the Beavers Systems Measures (Beavers, 1981, 1982; Beavers & Hampson, 1990); the McMaster Family Assessment Measures, also called the Family Assessment Device (FAD) (Epstein, Baldwin, & Bishop, 1982, 1983); the Moos Family Environment Scales (Moos & Moos, 1986); the Family Assessment Measure (Skinner, Steinhauer, & Sitarenios, 2000; Steinhauer, 1984), which is based on the Process Model of Family Functioning (Steinhauer, 1987); and the Olson Circumplex Family Model (Olson, 1986; Olson et al., 1985; Olson, Sprenkle, & Russel, 1979).

BEAVERS SYSTEMS MODEL

The Beavers Systems Model, originally called the Beavers Timberlawn Family Evaluation Scale, was developed over a 25-year period from clinical observations of both dysfunctional and healthy, competent families in treatment and research settings (Beavers, 1981, 1982; Beavers & Hampson, 1990; Beavers & Voeller, 1983). The first instruments were utilized in structural observation of family interaction in the here and now; they integrate family systems theory with developmental theory and are widely used in clinical practice. The model seeks to understand the health and competence of families in relationship to their ability to produce healthy and competent children and classifies families on the axes of family competence and family style. From this work, three assessment instruments have been developed: Beavers Interactional Scales, Family Competence and Style, and the

Self-Report Family Inventory (SFI). The first two scales are observational clinical rating scales, and the third is a self-report instrument completed by family members (Beavers & Hampson, 1990; Olson & Tiesel, 1993).

As they were tried and improved, the family competence and family style subscales were developed (Beavers, 2002). *Family competence* refers to a family's ability to negotiate, function, and deal effectively with stressful situations, whereas *style* addresses the manner and quality of family interaction (Beavers & Hampson, 2000). The competence axis classifies families into types that fall along a continuum according to their level of functioning: optimal, adequate, midrange, borderline, and severely disturbed. The style axis classifies families according to their quality of interaction: centripetal and centrifugal. Centripetal families turn outward and seek fulfillment in relationships outside the family. Centrifugal families turn inward and seek pleasure and gratification from within the family. Both family competence and style converge to produce levels of family functioning, which are believed to have implications for the types of difficulties children may have in relationship to psychiatric categories. Additionally, when the two dimensions of family competence and family style are combined, nine distinct family groups based on clinical observation and empirical research are diagrammatically defined. Three of these groups are considered functional, while six are problematic and require clinical intervention (Beavers & Hampson, 2000).

The validity and reliability of the Beavers Systems Model have been well documented since its initial inception in 1970 (Beavers & Hampson, 2000). The Interactional Competence Scale, designed to assess overall health and competence within 13 subscales (Beavers & Hampson, 1990), should be used by trained raters who observe the family discussing what they would like to see change in their family (Beavers & Hampson, 2000). Reliability is addressed by Beavers and Hampson (2000) in three areas: Interrater reliability Kappa coefficients ranged from .76 to .88, global competence Kappa coefficient was .86, and internal consistency across the 13 subscales had a Cronbach's alpha of .94. Beavers and Hampson (2000) cite Lewis, Beavers, Gossett, and Phillips (1976) and the original Timberlawn study as demonstrating the validity of the competence scale, which successfully discriminated clinical from nonclinical fam-

ilies. It has shown high construct validity and was shown by Epstein, Bishop, Ryan, Miller, and Keitner (1993) to correlate with the McMaster Family Assessment Device, which will be looked at later in this chapter ($r = .68$).

The Interactional Style Scale has eight subscales and is designed to measure the quality of family interaction. The interrater reliability Kappa coefficients ranged from .76 to .88 on the subscales, with a coefficient of .81 for the overall scale (Beavers & Hampson, 2000). They further noted a Cronbach's alpha of .88, indicating good internal consistency across the subscales. Beavers and Hampson (2000) acknowledge that validation work is still being done on this scale, but earlier studies by this team found that style may be an important predictor.

Development of the model is ongoing, as with all assessment models. The recent introduction of the self-report version of the family assessment instrument has added to the clinical utility of the model. The Self-Report Family Inventory (SFI) measures two dimensions of family functioning: (a) overall competence and (b) behavior and emotional style of functioning. The first dimension includes family happiness, optimism, problem solving, and parental coalitions; the second dimension includes conflict communication, cohesion, leadership, and emotional expressions (Pardeck, 2000). The SFI correlates well with observational scores, indicating that the self-report measure is roughly equivalent to observations (Beavers, 2002).

The SFI has five domains and may be completed by any family member over the age of 11. Cronbach alphas were found to range from .84 to .93 on internal consistency reliability and .85 or higher on test–retest reliability (Beavers & Hampson, 2000). Beavers and Hampson cite earlier work by Hampson, Beavers, and Hulgus done in 1989 that indicates canonical correlations of .62 or better with the Interactional Competence Scale, which shows good reliability between the self-report and the observer rating. Validity has also been shown to be strong in studies by discriminating between psychiatric diagnoses (Beavers & Hampson, 2000).

Drumm, Carr, and Fitzgerald (2000) conducted a study that compared the Beavers Model to the McMaster and Circumplex Models, which will be discussed later in this chapter. They found that the Beavers Model was the best at detecting clinical families in their study and had a particularly high level of sensitivity in determining clinical cases. Drumm et al. (2000) found significant differences between groups on the competence scale but not on the style scale. They found the competence scale to be an excellent unidimensional indicator of level of family functioning, with the style scale adding little in the way of descriptive or discriminative power (Drumm et al., 2000).

MCMASTER FAMILY MODEL

The McMaster Family Model (Epstein et al., 1982) is another widely used family assessment model that evolved out of clinical practice. The model was developed over a 15-year period with families at McMaster University in Canada, Brown University, and Butler Hospital Family Research Program. This model assesses whole systems functioning and evaluates family structure, organization, and transactional patterns that distinguish healthy from unhealthy families. Two assessment instruments have emerged from this work: the McMaster Clinical Rating Scale and a self-report family measure, the McMaster Family Assessment Device (FAD), version 3. These scales assess six dimensions of family functioning: (a) problem solving, (b) communication, (c) roles, (d) affective responses, (e) affective involvement, and (f) behavior control, as well as an overall family functioning assessment. Family problem solving describes how families solve both instrumental (e.g., financial) and affective (e.g., social support and nurturance) problems.

While there has been some debate over the past couple of years about whether the FAD scoring procedures should be reorganized to reflect higher-order factors from self-report measures (Ridenour, Daley, & Reich, 2000), Miller, Ryan, Keitner, Bishop, and Epstein (2000) argue that numerous studies indicate that the overall ecological validity of the scale suggests an absence in the utility for higher-order factors. Additionally, Miller et al. (2000) suggest that the most important issue regarding any scale is its clinical utility and validity, which the FAD has demonstrated repeatedly.

In regard to construct validity, the FAD has been correlated with theoretical constructs related to family functioning (Byles, Bryne, Boyle, & Offord, 1988; McFarlane, Bellissimo, & Norman, 1995). Drumm et al. (2000) found that the McMaster has a high level of sensitivity in detecting clinical cases (Epstein et al., 1983), which supports the Miller et al. (2000) assertion that the clinical utility is most important. In the Drumm et al. (2000) comparison study, the McMaster clinical rating scale showed the best ability to correctly detect families with children exhibiting both emotional and conduct disorders.

Bihun, Wamboldt, Gavin, and Wamboldt (2002) tested the FAD scale on children under the age of 12 years. They found that although reliabilities were lowest with young children (alpha = .48 to .79), there was good concurrent validity on measurements of family functioning on mothers' reports. They suggest that modifications to increase structure and simplicity would be needed if the scale were to be used with children under age 12. They note that improved reliability would strengthen the agreement with maternal report. The FAD scale has also been used in other cultures. Shek (2002) found good internal consistency, concurrent validity, and discriminant and construct validity across a range of samples in China. He found good psychometric properties but thought the factor structure might differ from the English version. Reliability of the Chinese FAD is suggested to be acceptable; however, the alpha values of the Chinese subscales were lower than the values based on the English version. Interestingly, Shek (2002) found that correlations between the Chinese FAD and a Chinese measure were high, indicating that the FAD does measure constructs that may be crosscultural.

MOOS FAMILY ENVIRONMENT SCALES

The Moos Family Environment Scales (FES) (Moos & Moos, 1986; Moos & Spinrad, 1984) evolved from research on the unique personality or attributes of social environments. The FES is a self-report measure that assesses whole-family functioning and is compatible with social and systems ecological theory. It has been widely used in both clinical research and practice and has been demonstrated to be an effective outcome measure. The FES evaluates families' perceptions of their social or interpersonal climate along three dimensions: interpersonal relationships, personal growth, and systems maintenance. Each of these dimensions is made up of subscales that evaluate diverse areas of family functioning.

Despite its popularity, the three-factor structure of the FES used across different groups of respondents has been shown to be problematic (Chipuer & Villegas, 2001). In particular, their study of wives' and husbands' responses to the perceptions of their family environment did not support the Moos and Moos (1986) three-factor model. Rather, they found evidence supporting a two-factor solution: cohesion versus conflict and an organization–control dimension. The discrepancy was found in how the subscales were grouped for different family members and was not a surprise to the researchers; they cite Chodorow (1978) and Gilligan's (1982) exemplary work showing that husbands and wives focus on different aspects of family functioning. They recommend using the two-factor second-order solution when comparing perceptions of spouses and to provide the best fit across data for wives and husbands (Boake & Salmon, 1983; Chipuer & Villegas, 2001; Fowler, 1981).

The psychometric properties of the FES are sufficient, however, to make this a useful instrument for group research if clinicians and researchers ensure that the subscales can be combined in the same way for different family members (Chipuer & Villegas, 2001). Despite the differences in factors, Chipuer and Villegas (2001) did find support for internal reliability. Internal consistency reliability estimates for the Form R subscales range from .61 to .78. Intercorrelations among the 10 subscales range from .53 to .45, indicating that the scales measure distinct characteristics with good consistency. Test–retest reliability ranges from .52 to .91 over 2-month, 3-month, and 12-month intervals, indicating that the scale is reliable over time (Moos & Moos, n.d.).

FAMILY ASSESSMENT MEASURE (FAM)

The Family Assessment Measure (Skinner, Steinhauer, & Sitarenios, 2000; Steinhauer, 1984), based on the process model of family functioning (Steinhauer, 1987), describes how to conduct family assessments based on seven dimensions: affective involvement, control, task accomplishment, role performance, communication, affective expression, and values and norms. Each of these dimensions is measured at three levels: whole-family systems, dyadic relationships, and individual functioning.

The FAM, following 20 years of work in developing the measure, has four self-report components, including the general scale, which is 50 items and nine subscales; dyadic relationship scales with 42 items and seven subscales; a self-rating scale with 42 items and seven subscales; and the brief FAM with 14 items. The FAM scales yield high alpha values: general scale = .94, dyadic relationship = .95, and self-rating = .89 (for adults), indicating good consistency reliability (the values for children were similar in these areas) (Skinner et al., 2000). Skinner et al. (2000) cite a study by Jacob (1995) that found test–retest reliability to be acceptable: mothers = .57, fathers = .56, and children = .66. The average length of time between testing was 12 days.

The literature consistently supports that FAM effectively and efficiently assesses family functioning; the validity has been supported by many studies (Skinner et al., 2000). Skinner et al. (2000) claim FAM to have good discriminant validity; if there is a strong a priori reason to believe that groups will differ, they state, FAM is capable of discerning the differences. They cite as support Jacob (1991); Skinner, Steinhauer, and Santa-Barbara (1995); and Forman (1988). Construct validity is cited in several studies. Bloomquist and Harris (1984) found a strong relationship between FAM and MMPI; Bloom (1985) reports that FAM correlates significantly with FACES, FES, and the Family Concept Q Sort (not discussed in this chapter); and Jacob (1995) found FAM to have high correlations with appropriate dimensions on FACES, FES, and FAD (Skinner et al., 2000).

OLSON CIRCUMPLEX FAMILY MODEL

The Circumplex Model is derived from systems theory and provides a classification schema for understanding marital and family functioning. The classification schema provides a typology of family functioning along three important dimensions: cohesion (emotional bonding), adaptability and flexibility (degree of change in family rites and structure), and communication (facilitative dimension). The communication dimension is considered important for establishing appropriate levels of the other two dimensions. Through research on more than 1,000 families over the last decade, Olson et al. (1985) have developed a number of empirically derived family inventories that measure these three dimensions of family life. Family assessment instruments, including the Family Satisfaction Inventory and the Family Crisis Oriented Personal Evaluation Scales (F-Copes), have been developed for the model.

One of the most famous of these self-report measures is the Family Adaptability and Cohesion Scale (FACES III), which measures the first two dimensions of the Circumplex Model: cohesion and adaptability and flexibility. The third dimension, communication, can be assessed with other inventories developed by the authors (e.g., Parent and Adolescent Communication Form). FACES III is a 20-item, normative-based, paper-and-pencil self-report inventory that operationalizes the Circumplex Model. The original Circumplex Model posits a curvilinear understanding of family functioning that emphasizes the need for balance in family relationships. Families falling along extreme dimensions of functioning in cohesion, adaptability and flexibility, or communication are believed to be at risk for dysfunction, while those falling into balanced or midrange dimensions are believed to be better adjusted. For example, in the cohesion dimension, families characterized at the two extremes of enmeshed or disengaged are both considered at risk for dysfunction, while those characterized as balanced between the these two extremes are considered to function well. The same idea applies to the adaptability and flexibility (change) dimension. Families characterized at the extremes of chaotic (too much flexibility and random change) or rigid (not enough flexibility and change) are at risk for dysfunction, and those characterized as balanced between these dimensions function well.

By categorizing families into 16 types, from lowest to highest on four categories each of the cohesion and adaptability dimensions, FACES III forms a helpful typology for understanding how various families function. It also provides a frame of reference for understanding what types of families may have dysfunctional characteristics; the ones falling into the extreme dimensions on the model (e.g., chaotically disengaged, chaotically enmeshed, etc.) tend to have greater dysfunction. The real key to family functioning, however, is not in the classification per se but in the amount of family life satisfaction experienced by the family members participating in the various family types. If individuals in the

family are satisfied with a chaotic or rigid family structure, then the type is considered to be functional for the individuals involved in that type of relational patterns. Fortunately, the FACES III instrument provides a way for family practitioners to calculate a family satisfaction score that makes it possible to determine the amount of family satisfaction derived by family members, thereby adding to the clinical utility of the model for a wider variety of families from different cultures.

Thomas and Olson (1993) found considerable research support for the curvilinear Circumplex Model using the Clinical Rating Scale (CRS) with 60 clinical families and 60 control families, but less support has been found for the self-report measure FACES III (Green, Harris, Forte, & Robinson, 1991). In response to criticisms concerning the validity of the FACES III measure, Olson and colleagues reconceptualized the Circumplex Model as a 3-D Circumplex model. The 3-D model is linear, and the FACES III, when used in conjunction with this model, is believed to provide a valid assessment of family functioning (Olson, 1991). Practitioners are instructed to use the 3-D model for their clinical assessments. The 3-D model, like the curvilinear model, measures only the cohesion and adaptability dimensions of the Circumplex Model. Each is measured on an 8-point continuum ranging from low cohesion (disengaged) to high cohesion (very connected) and from low adaptability (rigid) to high adaptability (very flexible). With the 3-D model, high scores on cohesion and adaptability are conceptualized as measuring balanced family types, while low scores on these two dimensions indicate extreme family types. Franklin and Streeter (1993) found support for the full 3-D Circumplex model but determined that the adaptability dimension lacked validity; they questioned whether the introduction of the 3-D model had been an improvement.

Another recent study, by Thomas and Zechowski (2000), challenged the validity of the FACES III as a means to operationalize the curvilinear dimension of the Circumplex Model constructs. The authors cite numerous studies to support their conclusions that two central concepts of the model—cohesion and adaptability—appear to be linear rather than curvilinear in relating to family functioning. Thomas and Zechowski note that the Clinical Rating Scale (CRS), rather than FACES, should be used to test the central hypotheses of the model, which include direct effects of cohesion and adaptability on family functioning, indirect effects of communication on family functioning through its facilitation of cohesion and adaptability, and an orthogonal relationship between cohesion and adaptability. They concluded that the direct relationships between cohesion and family functioning, communication and cohesion, and communication and adaptability were supported but not the direct relationship between adaptability and family functioning. Also, they found that instead of an orthogonal relationship (independent of one another) between cohesion and adaptability, these were significantly correlated. This recent test of the Circumplex Model using the CRS implies that therapists should help families raise levels of communication to promote healthy family cohesion, which is consistent with other popular models of marital and family therapy, such as emotionally focused marital therapy, integrative couple therapy, and functional family therapy.

To respond to the criticisms of the previous FACES measures, Olson and colleagues recently developed the FACES IV in hopes of contributing a reliable and valid self-report measure that will assess the Circumplex Model. (A copy of the items of the FACES IV measure may be obtained from Dr. Olson at the University of Minnesota, Department of Family Social Sciences.) Similar to its predecessors, FACES IV is a self-administered, pencil-and-paper, rapid assessment instrument. The current measure contains 24 items, measured on a 5-point Likert scale, to assess four dimensions (chaotic, disengaged, enmeshed, and rigid) representing the extremes of the Circumplex Model. The constructs cohesion (enmeshed, disengaged) and flexibility (chaotic, rigid) are inferred from the four subscales as being higher-order dimensions of those four subscales (Franklin, Streeter, & Springer, 2001).

Previous empirical research showed that attempts at changing the response format of the measure in order to enhance its ability to capture the extremes of the model failed to demonstrate an advantage. For this reason, the FACES IV follows the same rationale and response format as previous versions of the measure, with the exception that the items are worded in an extreme manner in an effort to assess dysfunction in the families who fell into the upper extremes of the model. Franklin et al. (2001), however, showed in a subsequent validity study that the FACES

IV continues to have difficulty with its validity and reliability. In a study of adolescents from pregnancy prevention programs in Texas, reliability was examined on each of four subscales, and confirmatory factor analysis and correlation analysis were used to examine the validity of the four subscales (Franklin et al., 2001). The McMaster Family Assessment Device, Multi-Problem Screening Inventory, and Social Support Behavior Scales were used to assess convergent and discriminant validity (Franklin et al., 2001).

Factor analysis showed that the items in the enmeshed and rigid domains loaded correctly, but the loadings were low; several items in the disengaged and chaotic domains split between the domains, indicating that there may be overlap between the two domains (Franklin et al., 2001). In addition, Franklin et al. (2001) found alpha levels for the four subscales of FACES IV to be at an acceptable level for research but not for clinical work: enmeshed (.75), disengaged (.79), rigid (.65), and chaotic (.76). Currently, Olson plans to release a revised FACES IV, which contains 20 additional items. The new revision, as well as reliability and validity data, will be available in the fall of 2003. Practitioners should currently use the FACES II or the linear version of the FACES III until it can be determined if the revision is able to resolve these difficulties. For updates on the FACES IV instrument, contact David Olson at Life Innovations or the University of Minnesota (dolson @lifeinnovations.com).

CONCLUSION

Much may be learned by carefully examining the validity and reliability of family measurement instruments. First, a careful examination informs practitioners about the best assessment and accountability tools currently available for use in practice. Second, an examination of the psychometric development of family measurement instruments helps practitioners comprehend the limitations of knowledge in their field, as well as the ongoing nature of the development of that knowledge. This is clearly illustrated by the rise and fall of the Circumplex Model and the subsequent validity and reliability problems found with the FACES instruments. At one time the Circumplex Model stood as one of the most popular and clinically appealing models for family practitioners to use, and the FACES instruments were considered to be great clinical helpers for measuring the family characteristics in that theoretical model. Subsequent psychometric work in the form of validity and reliability studies, however, raised many questions about the validity and reliability of the FACES measures. This is not to say that the model or the measure is totally discredited. To the contrary, such questions may yet spur the instrument and its curvilinear model to new leaps in knowledge and move forward the practice tools of marital and family therapy. All measurement instruments must open themselves to the same type of ongoing examination if they are to become effective accountability tools for marital and family practice. Ongoing validity and reliability analysis of family assessment and measurement tools must become a part of each practitioner's job as they learn to evaluate the assessment and accountability tools they use in their practices.

References

Beavers, W. R. (1981). A systems model of family for family therapists. *Journal of Marital and Family Therapy, 7,* 229–307.
Beavers, W. R. (1982). Healthy, midrange, and severely dysfunctional families. In F. Walsh (Ed.), *Normal family processes.* New York: Guilford.
Beavers, W. R. (2002, April 9). *The Beavers system model of family assessment.* Paper presented at the 2002 conference of the International Academy of Family Psychology. Abstract retrieved May 6, 2003, from http://www.iafpsy.org/
Beavers, W. R., & Hampson, R. B. (1990). *Successful families: Assessment and intervention* (pp. 73–102). New York: Norton.
Beavers, W. R., & Hampson, R. B. (2000). The Beavers systems model of family functioning. *Journal of Family Therapy, 22*(2), 128–133.
Beavers, W. R., & Voeller, M. N. (1983). Family models: Comparing the Olson circumplexmodel with the Beavers systems model. *Family Models, 22,* 85–98.
Bihun, J. T., Wamboldt, M. Z., Gavin, L. A., & Wamboldt, F. S. (2002). Can the Family Assessment Device be used with school-aged children? *Family Process, 41*(4), 723–732.
Bloom, B. L. (1985). A factor analysis of self-report measures of family functioning. *Family Process, 24,* 225–239.
Bloomquist, M. L., & Harris, W. G. (1984). Measuring family functioning with the MMPI: A reliability and concurrent validity of three MMPI scales. *Journal of Clinical Psychology, 40,* 1209–1214.

Boake, C., & Salmon, P. G. (1983). Demographic correlates and factor structure of the Family Environment Scale. *Journal of Clinical Psychology, 39,* 95–100.
Byles, J., Bryne, C., Boyle, M., & Offord, D. R. (1988). Ontario child health study: Reliability and validity of the General Functioning subscale of the McMaster Family Assessment Device. *Family Process, 27,* 97–104.
Chipuer, H. M., & Villegas, T. (2001). Comparing the second-order factor structure of the Family Environment Scale across husbands' and wives' perceptions of their family environment. *Family Process, 40*(2), 187–199.
Chodorow, N. (1978). *The reproduction of mothering: Psychoanalysis and the sociology ofmothering.* Berkeley: University of California Press.
Drumm, M., Carr, A., & Fitzgerald, M. (2000). The Beavers, McMaster and Circumplex clinical rating scales: A study of their sensitivity, specificity and discriminant validity. *Journal of Family Therapy, 22*(2), 225–239.
Epstein, N. B., Baldwin, L. M., & Bishop, D.S. (1982). *McMaster family assessment device(FAD) manual* (version 3). Providence, RI: Brown University/Butler Hospital Family Research Program.
Epstein, N. B., Baldwin, L. M., & Bishop, D. (1983). The McMaster family assessment device. *Journal of Marital and Family Therapy, 9*(2), 171–180.
Epstein, N. B., Bishop, D. S., Ryan, C., Miller, I., & Keitner, G. (1993). The McMaster model: View of healthy family functioning. In F. Walsh (Ed.), *Normal family processes* (2nd ed., pp. 138–160). New York: Guilford.
Forman, B. (1988). Assessing perceived patterns of behavior exchange in relationships. *Journal of Clinical Psychology, 44,* 972–981.
Fowler, P. C. (1981). Maximum likelihood factor structure of the Family Environment Scale. *Journal of Clinical Psychology, 37,* 160–164.
Franklin, C., & Jordan, C. (1999). *Family practice: Brief systems methods for social work.* Pacific Grove, CA: Brooks/Cole.
Franklin, C., & Streeter, C. L. (1993). Validity of the 3-D circumplex model for family assessment. *Research on Social Work Practice, 3*(3), 258–275.
Franklin, C., Streeter, C. L, & Springer, D. W. (2001). Validity of the Faces IV Family Assessment Measure. *Research on Social Work Practice, 11*(5), 576–596.
Gilligan. C. (1982). *In a different voice: Psychological theory and women's development.* Cambridge, MA: Harvard University Press.
Green, R. G., Harris, R. N., Forte, J. A., & Robinson, M. (1991). Evaluating FACES III and thecircumplex model: 2,440 families. *Family Process, 30,* 55–73.
Hampson, R. B., Beavers, W. R., & Hulgus, Y. F. (1989). Insiders' and outsiders' views of family:

The assessment of family competence and style. *Journal of Family Psychology, 3,* 118–136.

Jacob, T. (1991). *Comparison of athletic, depressed, and control families using the FAM-III.* Unpublished manuscript.

Jacob, T. (1995). The roles of the timeframe in the assessment of family functioning. *Journal of Marital and Family Therapy, 21,* 281–286.

Jordan, C., & Franklin, C. (2003). *Clinical assessment for social workers* (2nd ed.). Chicago: Lyceum.

Lewis, J. M., Beavers, W. R., Gossett, J. T., & Phillips, V. A. (1976). *No single thread: Psychological health in family systems.* New York: Brunner/Mazel.

McFarlane, A. H., Bellissimo, A., & Norman, G. R. (1995). Family structure, family functioning and adolescent well-being: The transcendent influence of parental style. *Journal of Child-Psychology and Psychiatry, 36,* 847–864.

Miller, I. W., Ryan, C. E., Keitner, G. I., Bishop, D. S., & Epstein, N. B. (2000). [Commentary—"Factor analyses of the family assessment device, by Ridenour, Daley, & Reich]. *Family Process, 39*(1), 141–145.

Moos, R. H., & Moos, B. S. (1986). *Family Environment Scale manual* (2nd ed.). Palo Alto, CA: Consulting Psychologists Press.

Moos, R. H., & Moos, B. S. (n.d.). *Family Environment Scale.* Retrieved May 5, 2003, from NOVA Southeastern University, Center for Psychological Studies Web site: http://www.cps.nova.edu/~cpphelp/FES.html

Moos, R. H., & Spinrad, S. (1984). *The social climate scales: An annotated bibliography.* PaloAlto, CA: Consulting Psychologists Press.

Olson, D. H. (1986). Circumplex model VII: Validation studies and FACES III. *Family Process, 26,* 337–351.

Olson, D. H. (1991). Commentary: Three-dimensional (3-D) circumplex model and revised scoring of FACES III. *Family Process, 30,* 74–79.

Olson, D. H., McCubbing, H. I., Barnes, H., Larsen, A., Muxen, M., & Wilson, M. (1985). *Family inventories: Inventories in a national survey of families across the family life cycle* (rev. ed.). St. Paul: University of Minnesota, Family Social Science.

Olson, D. H., Sprenkle, D. H., & Russel, C. S. (1979). Circumplex model of marital and familysystems: Cohesion and adaptability dimensions, family types and clinical applications. *Family Process, 18*(1), 3–28.

Olson, D. H., & Tiesel, J. (1993). *FACES III: Linear scoring and interpretation.* St. Paul: University of Minnesota, Family Social Science.

Pardeck, J. T. (2000). Clinical instruments for assessing and measuring family health. *Family Therapy, 27*(3), 178–187.

Ridenour, T. A., Daley, J. G., & Reich, W. (2000). Further evidence that the family assessment device should be reorganized: Response to Miller and colleagues. *Family Process, 39*(3), 375–381.

Shek, D.T.L. (2002). Assessment of family functioning in Chinese adolescents: The Chinese version of the Family Assessment Device. *Research on Social Work Practice, 12*(4), 502–524.

Skinner, H. A., Steinhauer, P. D., & Santa-Barbara, J. (1995). *Family Assessment Measure–III manual.* Toronto, Canada: Multi Health Systems.

Skinner, H. J., Steinhauer, P., & Sitarenios, G. (2000). Family assessment measure (FAM) and process model of family functioning. *Journal of Family Therapy, 22*(2), 190–210.

Springer, D. W., Abell, N., & Hudson, W. W. (2002). Creating and validating rapid assessment instruments for practice and research: Part 1. *Research on Social Work Practice, 12*(3), 408–439.

Springer, D. W., & Franklin, C. (2003). Standardized assessment measures and computer assisted assessment technologies. In C. Jordan & C. Franklin (Eds.), *Clinical assessment for social workers* (2nd ed.). Chicago: Lyceum.

Steinhauer, P. D. (1984). Clinical applications of the process model of family functioning.*Canadian Journal of Psychiatry, 29,* 98–111.

Steinhauer, P. D. (1987). The family as a small group: The process model of family functioning. In T. Jacob (Ed.), *Family interaction and psychotherapy* (pp. 67–115). New York: Plenum.

Thomas, V., & Olson, D. H. (1993). Problem families and the circumplex model: Observational assessment using the clinical rating scale (CRS). *Journal of Marital and Family Therapy, 19*(2), 159–175.

Thomas, V., & Zechowski, T. J. (2000). A test of the circumplex model of marital and familysystems using the clinical rating scale. *Journal of Marital and Family Therapy, 26*(4), 523–534.

46 STATISTICAL METHODS FOR ESTIMATES OF INTERRATER RELIABILITY

Charles Auerbach, Heidi Heft La Porte, & Richard K. Caputo

To assure interrater, or interobserver, reliability, much research in clinical fields relies on judges or raters who observe a common event. Bloom, Fisher, and Orme (1999) state that this type of reliability is used "to determine the extent to which two observers agree in their observations about whether, how often, or how long overt behaviors occur" (p. 48). Interrater reliability can be defined as the extent to which observations yield similar results from different judges. It is assumed that at least two judges independently rate a phenomenon. Orme and Gillespie (1986) suggest that a number of measures have been developed for the assessment of client problems. Often multiple observers of client problems use these measures. Ratings by consumers, providers, or other significant individuals are used to form consumer-specific sets of behavior. In these instances, there is a need to employ a method to rate the interobserver agreement. Interobservation is used widely in the research literature.

The use of percent agreement interrater reliability (IRR) does not provide for the likelihood that the degree of agreement differs from what would be expected by chance. As Waltz, Strickland, and Lena (1984) note, the simple calculation of a correlation like the Pearson's r measures only the consistency of how the raters assign scores. Thus, if two raters differ consistently on how they assign scores, the IRR will be high as measured by Pearson's r. Because of these issues, more appropriate statistics such as Cohen's kappa and interclass correlation coefficient (ICC) need to be considered (Laschinger, 1992). This chapter proceeds by showing inappropriate use of interrater reliability in the research literature. It then discusses how and under what conditions more accurate methods for quantification of interrater reliability can be employed.

EXAMPLE

Nasuti and Pecora (1993) assessed the interrater reliability of the Utah Risk Assessment Scales, a statewide system of risk assessment for child abuse and neglect used by intake and investigative workers in child protective services (CPS). The Utah Risk Assessment Scales are 32 scales that evaluate five areas of potential risk, including parent, child, and family functioning, type and nature of maltreatment, and intervention issues (Nasuti & Pecora, 1993). Each risk factor was rated using three to six anchored scales, ranging from adequate to severely inadequate, with operational definitions grounded in actual performance criteria attached to each anchor.

Two groups of CPS workers and supervisors were recruited from 22 local offices to serve as judges to assess the interrater reliability of the Utah Risk Assessment Scales. They were asked to assess risk levels in case material presented in three of eight randomly selected vignettes. The judges were asked to assess the degree of risk present in the vignettes in the behavioral, physical, emotional, and mental functioning of the parents and the children, as well as in the adequacy of the household in terms of sanitation, nutrition, and other factors. The degree of risk present in each vignette varied across the three major risk factors.

The 15 members of the first group of the CPS steering committee were considered to have the highest levels of experience and expertise. The second group of 56 workers and supervisors had varying levels of education and experience. The first group was used to establish expert rating levels of the presence of risk in the vignettes. All judges were trained in risk assessment (2 days of training) 2 to 6 months prior to participating in the study. Interrater reliability was assessed across raters for the same vignette using the Pearson's correlation coefficient. Nasuti and Pecora (1993) determined that the correlations, ranging from .56 to .85, were sufficient to suggest that interrater reliability was present and that these correlations "pose no threat to the interrater reliability because they represent the single best score for the vignette" (pp. 30–31).

A stepped-up estimated reliability composite was also derived using the Spearman-Brown prophecy formula, which markedly increased the correlations. For example, one vignette, with a Pearson's r of .568, had a stepped-up reliability estimate of .974.

Nasuti and Pecora (1993) cautioned that the stepped-up coefficients were based on summated scores representing the average rating for each vignette and therefore did not provide evidence that scores were consistent with what would have been predicted. To address this, they calculated means and standard deviations for both groups and used t tests to assess whether there were statistically significant differences in mean ratings between the two groups (CPS experts and CPS staff) to examine levels of agreement. In this example, the differences in scores between individual judges were completely dismissed as an area of assessment, a fact not mentioned in the discussion of study limitations. The ICC would have been a useful tool to examine the degree of homogeneity of ratings across judges as well as vignettes, which may have resulted in different conclusions about the amount of random error present in the ratings.

The case illustrates the need to decide on the most appropriate method to assess interrater reliability. We now proceed with a review of Cohen's kappa and a discussion of the interclass correlation coefficient.

COHEN'S KAPPA

Kappa is a widely used measure of the degree to which there is agreement between judges on how they rate the same object or persons. A judge can be a person or a diagnostic test that classifies a phenomenon on the basis of systematic predefined criteria. Kappa as developed by Cohen (1960) is expressed as

$$K = \frac{Po - Pe}{1 - Pe}$$

P_o represents the number of concordant items, and P_e represents the number of expected concordant items. Finally, $1 - P_e$ represents the number of expected nonconcordant items. To demonstrate, suppose nursing home residents and their respective spouses rate satisfaction with the facility as low, medium, and high. Table 46.1 displays the relationship between resident satisfaction and their corresponding spouses. The bolded diagonal scores display where there is agreement between them. Thus the number of concordant items is 66.

Table 46.2 displays what would be expected by chance. The degree of expected or chance concordance is 39.8. Kappa is simply a ratio between observed concordance (P_o) minus expected con-

TABLE 46.1 Observed Scores of Resident and Spouse Satisfaction

	Spouse satisfaction			
	Low	Medium	High	Total
Resident satisfaction				
Low	**42**	5	1	48
Medium	7	**19**	4	30
High	10	7	**5**	22
Total	59	31	10	100

TABLE 46.2 Expected Scores of Resident and Spouse Satisfaction

	Spouse satisfaction			
	Low	Medium	High	Total
Resident satisfaction				
Low	**28.3**	14.9	4.8	48.0
Medium	17.7	**9.3**	3.0	30.0
High	13.0	6.8	**2.2**	22.0
Total	59.0	31.0	10.0	100.0

cordance (P_e) and the expected divided by expected nonconcordant scores ($1 - P_e$).

The kappa would be $(.66 - .393) / (1 - .393)$ $= .44$. In other words, 44% of the scores are concordant if nothing more than chance concordance were in use.

Cohen's kappa ranges from -1 to 1. A value of 1 would indicate perfect agreement, and a value of -1 equals total disagreement. A value of 0 would indicate the rating between judges is no greater than what would be expected by chance.[1] Landis and Koch (1977) suggest the kappa interpretation scale shown in Table 46.3.

Kappa has its limits in that it is appropriate only with nominal or categorical data. Under certain conditions, it is also possible to obtain high-observed agreement but a low kappa (K) value (Feinstein & Cicchetti, 1990). Under the condition where the observed agreement (P_o) is high and the expected agreement (P_e) is large, the resulting kappa will be low. Using a constant value for P_o of .85 and P_e of .50, K would equal .70. If P_e was .78, k would equal .32. With a different value of P_e, K is reduced by half the amount (Feinstein & Cicchetti, 1990).

INTERCLASS CORRELATION COEFFICIENT

According to McGraw and Wong (1996), "The most fundamental interpretation of an ICC is that it is a measure of the proportion of a variance ... that is attributable to objects of measurement, often called targets" (p. 30). In the interclass correlation, the desired outcome is to have homogeneity of ratings between judges and variability attributed between subjects. If there is perfect agreement between judges, the ICC coefficient will be 1. On the other hand, if the rat-

ings between subjects do not vary but ratings between judges for each subject do, the ICC will be 0. The use of the ICC is preferable to kappa or Pearson's r when there is need to generalize the ratings of judges to similar judges in the future (Laschinger, 1992). Shrout and Fleiss (1979) present three basic forms of ICC. They are referred to as ICC(1,1), ICC(2,1), and ICC(3,1). They recommend that the researcher make clear which form of the ICC is being used so that the consumers can determine its appropriateness to the situation. For example, ICC(1,1) can be used in the situation where a set of judges rates some subjects but not necessarily all of them. Finally, if the researcher intends to generalize, ICC(2,1) and (3,1) would be the appropriate choice (Laschinger, 1992). Laschinger (1992) presents Shrout and Fleiss's (1979) formulas for estimating interrater reliability.

$$ICC(1,1) = \frac{MSP - MSE}{MSP + (k-1) MSE}$$

where k = number of raters, MSP = mean square persons / subjects, and MSE = mean square error from a one-way ANOVA.

$$ICC (2,1)$$
$$= \frac{MSP - MSE}{MSP + (k - 1) MSE + k(MSR - MSE) / n}$$

where n = number of persons, MSR = mean square raters, and MSE = total $MS - MSP - MSR$ from a two-way ANOVA.

$$ICC (3,1) = \frac{MSP - MSE}{MSP + (k - 1) MSE}$$

where variance components are obtained from a two-way ANOVA.

Shrout and Fleiss (1979) explain that if the effects of raters are not included in the index, the ICC is only a measure of interrater consistency, not concordance. Rater effects are included in formula ICC(2,1), which is therefore a measure of rater agreement. This is not the case for ICC(3,1), where the rater effect is not included and is a measure of consistency. The example presented earlier of nursing home satisfaction can be expanded to include a third judge, the resident's child. The coefficient for the ICC(1,1) would be .51, for the ICC(2,1) .51, and for the ICC(3,1) .53. Unlike the Pearson r or Cohen's kappa, a third judge can be easily included and, if model ICC(2,1) is used, a generalizable measure of rater agreement can be obtained.

TABLE 46.3 Kappa Interpretation Scale

Kappa value	Interpretation
Below 0.00	Poor
0.00–0.20	Slight
0.21–0.40	Fair
0.41–0.60	Moderate
0.61–0.80	Substantial
0.81–1.00	Almost perfect

COMPUTER APPLICATIONS

Five different forms of the ICC based upon the Shrout and Fleiss (1979) model can be obtained using SPSS 8.0 (1998) or higher. However, the terminology used by SPSS differs from that of Shrout and Fleiss (1979). The process of obtaining the necessary results is less complicated than with SAS (Choukalas, Melby, & Lorenz, 2000). As Table 46.4 displays, when data for ICC analysis is entered in SPSS, each rater becomes a variable while each target is a row. The data could represent each health care provider's rating of the cognitive level of six patients on a scale from 1 (lowest) to 10 (highest). The columns represent each provider while the rows represent their ratings of the cognitive level of six patients.

The ICC procedure can be found under Analysis / scale / reliability analysis / statistics. At this point the user needs to select

1. The type of model: one-way random, two-way random, or two-way mixed ANOVA
2. Type: consistency or absolute agreement

Each of the methods is appropriate under different conditions. According to Choukalas, Melby, and Lorenz (2000), the one-way model is most useful when the raters are not selected randomly from two different populations. The one-way model is more conservative and will produce smaller coefficients. The two-way model assumes that the observers have been selected randomly from two different populations. A fixed model would be used if the same two or more raters rated the same target. A mixed model would be appropriate if raters are randomly selected; as a result, agreement between any two observers would be of concern. Absolute agreement takes into account the magnitude of the rater's observation. On the other hand, like Pearson's r, consistency compares how each rater places a target. Because of these differences, absolute agreement is considered to be more accurate. The one-way model's only option is absolute agreement. If there is perfect agreement between raters, the one-way and two-way models will produce the same results. Another consideration is whether to use a single-item ICC or the average of the items. The single-item ICC is based upon the observations of single observers, while the averaged-item ICC is based upon the observations of multiple observers of the same target. If the analysis is based upon a rater's scale observations, the averaged ICC should be used (Choukalas, Melby, & Lorenz, 2000). SPSS automatically displays the single-item and averaged-item ICCs.

Using the data in Table 46.4, Table 46.5 displays the ICC coefficients derived for each of the models discussed.

The most conservative method, one-way random, which uses only absolute agreement, produces the smallest coefficient (.17). The two-way absolute model also yields smaller values.

CONCLUSION

When establishing interrater reliability, researchers need to carefully examine the nature of their data to select the most appropriate method of assessment. Some procedures may show consistency in raters noticing improvement or deterioration, but they show nothing in regard to the degree of agreement about the actual rating given. Similarly, some procedures that do attempt to identify percentage of agreement about the ratings do not consider the variation between raters when there are more than

TABLE 46.4 Data Entered for Interclass Correlation Coefficient

Target	Rater 1	Rater 2	Rater 3	Rater 4
1	1.00	9.00	2.00	5.00	8.00
2	2.00	6.00	1.00	3.00	2.00
3	3.00	8.00	4.00	6.00	8.00
4	4.00	7.00	1.00	2.00	6.00
5	5.00	10.00	5.00	6.00	9.00
6	6.00	6.00	2.00	4.00	7.00
7					

TABLE 46.5 Interclass Correlation Coefficients

	Two-way mixed	Two-way random	One-way random
Consistent agreement	.72	.72	
Absolute agreement	.29	.29	.17

two observers. The incorrect usage of procedures to determine the reliability of ratings is highly problematic, particularly in applied professions. If clinical practice is to be more appropriately informed by the results of empirical studies, such as testing the efficacy of social work or other human services interventions or evaluating the adequacy of standardized procedures, we must ensure that the process for making such determinations is accurate and thereby more appropriately useful. Only then can we be confident in applying what we learn to what we do in our practice.

Note

1. Expected values are calculated for each cell by multiplying the column total by the row total and dividing the product by the total number of scores. The expected nonconcordant scores are the number of nonagreeing scores occurring by chance.

References

Biggerstaff, M. A. (1994). Evaluating the reliability of oral examinations for licensure of clinical social workers in Virginia. *Research on Social Work Practice, 4*(4), 481–496.

Bloom, M., Fischer J., & Orme, J. G. (1999). *Evaluating practice: Guidelines for the accountable professional* (3rd ed.). Needham Heights, MA: Allyn & Bacon.

Choukalas, C. G., Melby, J. N., & Lorenz, F. O. (2000). *Technical report: Interclass correlation coefficients in SPSS.* Unpublished manuscript (Iowa State University Institute for Social and Behavioral Research).

Cohen, J. (1960). A coefficient of agreement for nominal scales. *Educational and Psychological Measurement, 20*, 37–46.

Feinstein, A. R., & Cicchetti, D. V. (1990). High agreement but low kappa: The problems of two paradoxes. *Journal of Clinical Epidemiology, 6*(43), 543–549.

Landis, J., & Koch, G. G. (1977). The measurement of observer agreement for categorical data. *Biometrics, 33*, 159–174.

Laschinger, H. K. (1992). Intraclass correlations as estimates of interrater reliability in nursing research. *Western Journal of Nursing Research, 14*, 246–251.

McGraw, K. O., & Wong, S. P. (1996). Forming inferences about some interclass correlation coefficients. *Psychological Methods, 1*, 30–46.

Nasuti, J. P., & Pecora, P. J. (1993). Risk assessment scales in child protection: A test of the internal consistency and interrater reliability of one statewide system. *Social Work Research and Abstracts, 29*(2), 28–33.

Orme, J. G., & Gillespie, D. F. (1986, March). Reliability and bias in categorizing individual client problems. *Social Service Review*, pp. 161–174.

Shrout, P. E., & Fleiss, J. L. (1979). Interclass correlations: Use in assessing interrater reliability. *Psychological Bulletin, 86*, 420–428.

Waltz, C., Strickland, O., & Lenz, E. (1984). *Measurement in nursing research.* Philadelphia: F. A. Davis.

ELEMENTS OF CONSUMER-BASED OUTCOME MEASUREMENT

Carol A. Snively

By informing the helper about how clients view their environment, subjective community quality measures can be useful tools for social work practitioners, especially mental health clinicians and community organizers. After defining relevant terms, this chapter provides a brief overview of community quality research. Research on the effect of community context on mental health outcomes is highlighted. Five measures of subjective community quality are then described. The chapter concludes with suggestions for instrument development and for using subjective community quality measures to improve clinical mental health and community practice outcomes.

DEFINING COMMUNITY CONCEPTS

The term *community* can be used to describe a variety of contexts (geographic, school, and workplace) but is limited to the discussion of geographic settings throughout this chapter. Boudon and Bourricaud (1989) list three elements of a community that are widely recognized as crucial: (a) a social network that is both resilient and flexible, (b) some symbolic ties to an object of identification, and (c) an identified group that is part of a larger society. These elements provide a foundation for my discussion of community quality.

According to Boudon and Bourricaud (1989), the symbolic tie of a community varies based on group members but could include ethnocultural identity, geographic location, residents' type of work, affiliation with a community institution (such as a school or a religious institution), the presence of a natural entity (such as a park or a lake), or the residents' socioeconomic status. A community defined by geographic location may comprise all of several different neighborhoods or parts thereof. While the level at which individual members use the community's name and subscribe to the symbolic ties varies, the included blocks or neighborhoods are generally perceived by most members of the larger setting (residents and nonresidents) to share one or more elements.

Community context refers to the state of organization or order within the community at any given time. Community organization is conceptualized as a continuum from extremely declined or disorganized to organized and vital (Ahlbrandt & Brophy, 1975; Birch, 1971; Connerly & Marans, 1988; Palen & London, 1984). Increases in physical disorder (e.g., litter, trash, and graffiti), combined with increases in social disorder (e.g., delinquent youth and increased social isolation among neighbors) and shifts in the economic base of the neighborhood, accelerate the rate of overall community decline (Skogan, 1990; Taylor & Covington, 1988). *Decline* has been described as a downward spiral of deviance and decay (Skogan, 1990). If the decline goes unchecked, the community will reach a state where the damage cannot be repaired (Ahlbrandt & Brophy, 1975).

Earlier research on community context sought to describe social and physical problems and explain variations in these problems within a given community and across neighborhoods that make up a given community. Contemporary community context research delineates the factors influencing a community's state of well-being, describes how communities change over time, and explores how community quality (the physical and social state) influences individual and familial well-being. The latter focus has great relevance to social work practitioners because it enhances our understanding of the "person-in-environment" by providing tools to quantify the individual's experience of his or her environment.

COMMUNITY QUALITY MEASURES

Objective indicators of community quality include both community- and individual-level measurement of demographics and resident characteristics. Aggregated statistics (community level) can be used to compare the problems of various neighborhoods within the community or to compare the problems of communities from different regions of the city, state, or country. Measures of economic status, residential mobility, cultural heterogeneity, crime and unemployment rates, family composition, and special housing policies are frequently used to estimate community decline because these factors have repeatedly been associated with neighborhood and community instability (Elliot et al., 1996). The same variables (e.g., economic status, residential mobility, racial or ethnocultural identity, employment status, and family composition) have frequently been used to predict the behavior (e.g., criminal activity) of individuals who live in declining neighborhoods.

Several subjective instruments of community quality have also been developed by sociologists and community psychologists to measure residents' knowledge of the number of specific physical and social problems present in their neighborhood (e.g., trash and litter, noise, and drug trafficking), the extent to which residents label the disorder as a community problem, and attitudes toward the neighborhood or community. The latter category includes a variety of instruments that measure general attitudes about the community (community, neighborhood, or residential satisfaction), feelings of connectedness to the physical characteristics or the social groups within the environment (community or neighborhood attachment, sense of community, or neighborhood cohesion), and the belief that the community will improve over time (community or collective efficacy).

COMMUNITY QUALITY RESEARCH

Comparisons of subjective community quality measures (e.g., resident responses to "How much of a problem are gangs in your neighborhood?") with aggregated objective measures of disorder (e.g., crime rates) provide some indication regarding the extent to which residents view their community in realistic terms. While this area of research needs further development, there is evidence that residents tend to be good reporters of their community quality. For example, Stiffman, Hadley-Ives, Elze, Johnson, and Dore (1999) found that the subjective measures of community disorder by youth residents matched objective measures of community quality. Since most research has focused on community problems, it is not known if residents are reliable informants regarding neighborhood strengths.

Research indicates that more positive community attitudes (e.g., high levels of attachment, satisfaction, sense of community, and community efficacy) are related to changes in objective community quality, both positive and negative. Increases in some types of disorder may increase residents' feelings of attachment to their neighborhood (Woldoff, 2002). Also, collective efficacy among residents has been associated with lower crime rates (Sampson & Raudenbush, 1999). Positive attitudes and improved social order may be related to residents' efforts to organize and defend their home environment through efforts such as an organized block watch.

Studies of the psychosocial effects of community quality demonstrate a relationship between collective resident attitudes about their community and the quality of individual resident life. For example, Theodori (2001) found that community satisfaction and community attachment are associated positively with individual well-being. Similarly, Ellaway, Macintyre, and Kearns (2001) found that perceived local problems and neighborhood cohesion were associated with self-assessed health, mental health, and recent symptoms.

The perception of community problems and disorder may be more important that the actual or objective level of disorder. For example, O'Brien and Ayidiya (1991) found that neighborhood attachment mediated the effect of objective and perceived neighborhood conditions on subjective quality of life. In the Stiffman et al. (1999) study, the perception of the neighborhood environment was found to have the only direct effect on adolescent mental health. Perception mediated the effects of the objective environment on adolescent mental health and was influenced by the presence of environmental support and exposure to violence. The following section further discusses research on community context and mental health.

COMMUNITY QUALITY RESEARCH AND MENTAL HEALTH

The relationship between community quality and resident mental health has received significant attention in recent years. Youth who reside in dangerous, violent, and stressful communities are now considered "at risk" because of their greater potential for poor developmental outcomes. These youth need not participate in violent activities for violence to have an impact on their lives. Watching others participate in or being victimized by community violence and simply being aware of violence that occurs within the community are experiences that affect the development of health and behavioral problems of adolescents who live in dangerous environments (Bowen & Chapman, 1996; Garbarino, 1999; Garbarino, Kostelny, & Dubrow, 1991; Richter & Martinez, 1993).

In addition, positive feelings about one's community appear to act as protective factors for at-risk youth. Despite the actual community level of order, teens who have a more positive view of their community tend to have better mental health outcomes (Stiffman et al., 1999). In addition, a strong psychological sense of community among teens is related to greater availability of social support (Pretty, Andrewes, & Collett, 1994).

More specifically, community quality has been linked with specific mental health concepts and diagnoses among persons of all ages. Community violence exposure has been linked to the diagnosis of posttraumatic stress disorder (Allen, 1996; Davies & Flannery, 1998; Foy & Goguen, 1998; Horowitz, Weine, & Jekel, 1995; Martinez & Richters, 1993). Stiffman et al. (1999) found that community perceptions had a strong influence on adolescent mental health, particularly externalized mental health problems (behavioral disorders).

But how can we apply this empirical relationship between community attitudes and mental health to practice? While this bridge has not yet been firmly built, the answer may be found in recent efforts to create more effective service provision models. The focus of clinical practice has been shifting in recent years from the provision of formal programs and services to integrative networks of formal and informal supportive services. Anecdotal reports and research have begun to document how the availability of informal supports positively influences mental health outcomes. For examples, see Burchard, Burns, and Burchard (2002) regarding the effectiveness of wraparound services for youth. As part of the effort to secure strong community-based intervention and support plans, the helping professional could benefit from understanding the extent to which each consumer feels part of the community. Then, efforts could be made to place consumers in geographic communities where they feel a greater connection. Also, service plans could include efforts to assist consumers in building a sense of community by establishing stronger informal support systems, including strategies to build relationships between consumers and their neighbors, instead of capitalizing only on those relationships that already exist and may be stressed to their capacity.

COMMUNITY QUALITY AND COMMUNITY PRACTICE

In addition to enhancing clinical practice, knowledge of community attitudes can improve community practice. According to Brodsky, O'Campo, and Aronson, (1999), strong community systems (healthy and viable communities) serve as a resource for residents, helping them resist social, psychological, and physiological problems. Healthy systems enable residents to grow individually and collectively, maintaining and improving their quality of life. Conversely, weak community systems (unhealthy communities) cannot provide resources for their residents; therefore, residents who live in such settings have higher risks for the development of social, psychological, and physiological problems. Very weak community systems can be life-threatening at times, causing residents to withdraw from community life and feel isolated and alienated. Residents with more favorable views of their community tend to be more actively involved in their community.

Research has documented the relationship between community attitudes and community organization activities. More favorable community attitudes are associated with greater involvement in formal community betterment efforts. A high level of community involvement (formal and informal) by residents strengthens community structure and enables residents to address problems as they develop; therefore, the community is able to resist the forces that produce social disorganization, as well as physical and economic decline. In regard to formal involvement, Carr, Dixon, and Ogles (1976) found that attitude toward the place of residence, perception of neighbors as active and potent yet stable, and a view of the future as promising and secure determined attitudes toward and participation in community organization activities. Also, Perkins, Florin, Richard, Wandersman, and Chavis (1990) found that residents' satisfaction with their block predicted participation in voluntary block associations.

Community attitudes also have an influence on informal community activities such as being a "good neighbor." Unger and Wandersman (1985) found that the perception of the physical and social environment affected neighboring activity. Silverman (1986) found the following factors influenced neighboring activities: attachment to the neighborhood, home ownership, housing density, perceptions of others as similar to oneself, and trust of neighbors.

Understanding how residents view their community can help social workers and other helpers assess the individual's potential for healthy outcomes. In addition, understanding the collective views of residents helps the social worker assess and evaluate community-level health status and organizational level. In the following section, instruments that measure subjective community quality, developed by sociologists and community psychologists, are described. While it is not possible to review all available community attitudinal instruments for this discussion, five scales with high reliability are presented to give the reader an idea of the kinds of instruments available for use in clinical and community practice.

COMMUNITY QUALITY INSTRUMENTS

Building on Sarason's (1974) seminal work, McMillan and Chavis (1986) defined *sense of community* as "a feeling that members have of belonging, a feeling that members matter to one another and to the group, and a shared faith that members' needs will be met through their commitment to be together" (p. 9). The Sense of Community Index (SCI), developed by Chavis, Hogge, McMillan, and Wandersman (1986), is widely used in community quality research for both youth and adult residents (see Hill, 1996). The SCI contains 12 items with four subscales: reinforcement of needs, membership, influence, and shared emotional connection (see Chavis, n.d.). Subjects respond with true (= 1) or false (= 0) in response to a directive that instructs them to think about their block. While different referents are acceptable (e.g., school, neighborhood, city, church), Chavis (n.d.) cautions against using "community" as the referent. The original research on the scale found that it explained only 25% of the variance in self-reported perceptions of sense of community. Pretty et al. (1994), the first to study the psychological sense of community among adolescents, found that there were some commonalities inherent in adult and adolescent responses to the SCI.

The Neighborhood Quality Scale (NQS) was created and used in Coulton et al. (1996), a study on the effects of neighborhood context on young children living in urban areas by adult caregivers (see Appendix in this chapter). The NQS consisted of 11 items. Subjects rate their response on a 10-item scale, 1 (mostly false) to 10 (mostly true). The NQS had high reliability in Coulton et al. (1996) (Cronbach alpha =.81, $N = 156$). As stated by the authors, the scale measures "judgments on the positive and negative aspects of their neighborhood and whether or not they would like to continue living in their neighborhood" (p. 16).

The Youth Community Opinion Scale (Snively, 2002) is an adapted version of the Coulton et al. (1996) Neighborhood Quality Scale (see Appendix to this chapter). It contains six items. Initial use of the scale with a purposive sample of 119 adolescents resulted in a Cronbach alpha of .8659. Subjects rate their response on a five-item scale: (a) not at all true, (b) a little true, (c) somewhat true, (d) very true, and (e) extremely true. A high score on the community opinion scale indicates overall satisfaction with their home community. Snively and Williamson (2001) found evidence that supports the notion that youths' perception of their community does not differ from adult residents' perceptions.

The indicators of disorder used in the Community Physical and Social Disorder Scales (Snively, 2002) were developed from Skogan's (1990) neighborhood crime studies (see Appendix). In Skogan's book, the results of five different studies are presented. These studies have a combined total sample size of slightly under 13,000 urban residents of 40 residential neighborhoods (mostly inner city but considered neither declining nor renewing). Residents were interviewed on a number of topics, including their victimization experiences, the extent of various forms of disorder in the neighborhood, neighborhood satisfaction, intent to move, fear of crime, and "other questions directly related to theories about neighborhood stability and change" (p. 19). From these studies, Skogan presents a list of community disorder problems (physical and social) that are most frequently mentioned across neighborhoods.

Skogan's indicators were rewritten for the study (Snively, 2002) to reflect people-first language and to separate the behavior of adolescents from that of children and adults. In addition, the definitions of certain terms (e.g., vandalism) were added to assist youth in responding to survey items, and other words were adapted to increase readability. Following these minor adaptations, six indicators of physical disorders and twelve indicators of social disorder, based on Skogan's work, were used in the scales.

The same Likert-type scale (1 to 5 response categories) is used for both the physical and social disorder instruments. In responding to items from the physical and social disorder scales, participants were asked to consider "How often do these things happen in your community?" and were given a choice of five Likert-type responses: (a) never, (b) a little of the time, (c) some of the time, (d) most of the time, and (e) all of the time. High scores on these scales indicate greater perceived disorder (physical or social) in the community. Cronbach alphas for these two scales were .8517 (physical disorder) and .9319 (social disorder) in the initial study (Snively, 2002).

SUMMARY AND CONCLUSION

Measures of the perceived community environment can be useful in establishing best practices for both clinical and community social work practitioners. Throughout the assessment process, community attitudinal measures can assist the clinical practitioner in assessing how the community influences the problems that cause the client/consumer to seek assistance and how the community influences the general well-being of the client/consumer. During discharge planning, community measures can inform the social worker's efforts to connect the consumer/client with community resources. While the development of additional measures is needed to assess informal resources for individual clients and to evaluate how receptive the client is to accessing informal community resources for support, these instruments provide a good start for helping professionals who are interested in incorporating community attitudes into assessment and discharge planning activities.

Knowledge of community problems is not enough to create change. Informing community residents about community problems and crime without more extensive efforts to organize residents may increase fear and pessimism about community change (Perkins et al., 1990). Organized community betterment efforts are needed to maintain a collective sense of hope that the community can improve over time (community efficacy). Community organizers can play an important role in assessing residents' knowledge of community problems and motivation for sustained involvement in community change activities. Measures are needed to assess community motivation for change, identify potential leaders for change efforts, and evaluate the success of community betterment strategies. Community attitudinal measures can assist in this process. While much work is needed in this area, attitudinal measures of community quality can begin to fill this void.

Appendix: Community Attitude Scale

My neighborhood is a good place to live.

My neighborhood is a good place to raise children.

The people moving into my neighborhood in the past year or so are good for the neighborhood.

I would like to move out of this neighborhood.*

There are some children in the neighborhood that I don't want my children to play with.*

The people moving into my neighborhood in the past year or so are bad for the neighborhood.*

For the most part, the police come within a

reasonable amount of time when they are called.

There is too much traffic in my neighborhood.*

There are enough bus stops in my neighborhood.

My neighborhood is conveniently located in the city.

If I had to move out of my neighborhood, I would be sorry to leave.

From Neighborhood Quality Scale (Coulton, Korbin, & Su, 1996).

* = Scores need to be reversed.

My community is a good place to live.
My community is a good place to grow up.
I would like to move out of my community.*
There is too much crime in my community.*
My community has become a better place to live in the past year.
I feel safe in my community.

From Youth Community Opinion Scale (Snively, 2002), adapted from Coulton, Korbin, & Su's (1996) Neighborhood Quality Scale.

*= Scores need to be reversed.

Community item	Problem
Physical	Litter or trash on the sidewalks and streets
	Graffiti on buildings and walls
	Abandoned cars
	Empty buildings where no one lives or works
	Vandalism (buildings, cars, or other property in the community that have been destroyed or damaged, except graffiti)
	Houses and yards that are not kept up
Social	Community people dealing drugs
	Community people using illegal drugs (like marijuana, weed or blunts, crank, crack, or any other nonprescription drugs)
	Community people drinking alcohol
	Gang activity
	Community adults without jobs hanging around the community
	Loud noises

Community people who seem mentally ill

Community people who seem homeless

Community people who seem to be selling sex (prostitution)

Groups of young children misbehaving (younger than teenagers)

Groups of teenagers misbehaving
Groups of adults misbehaving

Community physical and social disorder scales (Snively, 2002), developed from Skogan (1990).

References

Ahlbrandt, R. S., & Brophy, P. D. (1975). *Neighborhood revitalization.* Lexington, MA: D. C. Heath.

Allen, I. M. (1996). PTSD among African Americans. In A. J. Marsella, M. J. Friedman, E. T. Gerrity, & R. M. Scurfield (Eds.), *Ethnocultural aspects of post-traumatic stress disorder* (pp. 209–238). Washington, DC: American Psychological Association.

Birch, D. L. (1971, March). Toward a stage theory of urban growth. *AIP Journal,* pp. 78–87.

Boudon, R., & Bourricaud, F. (1989). (P. Hamilton, Trans.). *A critical dictionary of sociology.* Chicago: Routledge/University of Chicago Press. (Original work published 1982)

Bowen, G. L., & Chapman, M. V. (1996). Poverty, neighborhood danger, social support, and the individual adaptation among at-risk youth in urban areas. *Journal of Family Issues, 17*(5), 641–665.

Brodsky, A. E., O'Campo, P. J., & Aronson, R. E. (1999). PSOC in community context: Multi-level correlates of a measure of psychological sense of community in low-income, urban neighborhoods. *Journal of Community Psychology, 27*(6), 659–679.

Burchard, J. D., Burns, E. J., & Burchard, S. N. (2002). The wraparound approach. In B. J. Burns & K. Hoagwood (Eds.), *Community treatment for youth* (pp. 69–90). New York: Oxford University Press.

Carr, T. H., Dixon, M. C., & Ogles, R. M. (1976). Perceptions of community life which distinguish between participants and non-participants in a neighborhood self-help organization. *American Journal of Community Psychology, 4*(4), 357–366.

Chavis, D. M. (n.d.). *Sense of community index.* Retrieved January 15, 2002, from http://www.capablecommunity.com/pubs/SCIndex.PDF

Chavis, D. M., Hogge, J. H., McMillan, D. W., & Wandersman, A. (1986). Sense of community through Brunswik's lens: A first look. *Journal of Community Psychology, 14*(1), 24–40.

Connerly, C. E., & Marans, R. W. (1988). Neighborhood quality: A description and analysis of indicators. In E. Huttman & W. van Vliet (Eds.), *Handbook of housing and the built environment in the United States* (pp. 37–61). New York: Greenwood.

Coulton, C. J., Korbin, J. E., & Su, M. (1996). Measuring neighborhood context for young children in an urban area. *American Journal of Community Psychology, 24*(1), 5–32.

Davies, W. H., & Flannery, D. J. (1998). Post-traumatic stress disorder in children and adolescents exposed to violence. *Pediatric Clinics of North America, 45,* 341–353.

Ellaway, A., Macintyre, S., & Kearns, A. (2001). Perceptions of place and health in socially contrasting neighborhoods. *Urban Studies, 38*(12), 2299–2316.

Elliot, D. S., Wilson, W. J., Huizinga, D., Sampson, R. J., Elliot, A., & Rankin, B. (1996). The effects of neighborhood disadvantage on adolescent development. *Journal of Research in Crime and Delinquency, 33*(4), 389–426.

Foy, D. W., & Goguen, C. A. (1998). Community violence–related PTSD in children and adolescents. *PTSD Research Quarterly, 9*(4), 1–6.

Garbarino, J. (1999). *Raising children in a socially toxic environment.* San Francisco: Jossey-Bass.

Garbarino, J., Kostelny, K., & Dubrow, N. (1991). What children can tell us about living in danger. *American Psychologist, 46*(4), 376–383.

Hill, J. L. (1996). Psychological sense of community: Suggestions for future research. *Journal of Community Psychology, 24*(4), 431–438.

Horowitz, K., Weine, S., & Jekel, J. (1995). PTSD symptoms in urban adolescent girls: Compounded community trauma. *Journal of the American Academy of Child and Adolescent Psychiatry, 34,* 1353–1361.

Martinez, P., & Richters, J. (1993). The NIMH community violence project: II. Children's distress symptoms associated with violence exposure. *Psychiatry, 56,* 22–36.

McMillan, D. W., & Chavis, D. M. (1986). Sense of community: A definition and theory. *Journal of Community Psychology, 14*(1), 6–23.

O'Brien, D. J., & Ayidiya, S. (1991). Neighborhood community and life satisfaction. *Journal of the Community Development Society, 22*(1), 21–37.

Palen, J. J., & London, B. (1984). Through the glass darkly: Gentrification, revitalization, and the neighborhood. In J. J. Palen & B. London (Eds.), *Gentrification, displacement, and neighborhood revitalization* (pp. 256–266). Albany: State University of New York Press.

Perkins, D. D., Florin, P., Richard, R. C., Wandersman, A., & Chavis, D. M. (1990). Participation and the social and physical environment of residential blocks: Crime and community context. *American Journal of Community Psychology, 18*(1), 83–115.

Pretty, G.M.H., Andrewes, L., & Collett, C. (1994). Exploring adolescents' sense of community and its relationship to loneliness. *Journal of Community Psychology, 22*(4), 346–358.

Richter, J., & Martinez, P. (1993). Children as victims and witnesses to violence in a D.C. neighborhood. In L. A. Leavitt & N. A. Fox (Eds.), *The psychological effect of war and violence on children* (pp. 243–281). Mahwah, NJ: Lawrence Erlbaum.

Sampson, R. J., & Raudenbush, S. W. (1999). Systematic social observation of public spaces: A new look at disorder in urban neighborhoods. *American Journal of Sociology, 105*(3), 603–651.

Sarason, S. B. (1974). *The psychological sense of community: Prospects for a community psychology.* San Francisco: Jossey-Bass.

Silverman, C. J. (1986). Neighboring and urbanism: Commonality versus friendship. *Urban Affairs Quarterly, 22*(2), 312–328.

Skogan, W. G. (1990). *Disorder and decline: Crime and the spiral of decay in American neighborhoods.* New York: Free Press.

Snively, C. A. (2002). *Model analyses of factors affecting the neighboring activities of youth who reside in a revitalizing community.* Unpublished doctoral dissertation, Ohio State University.

Snively, C. A., & Williamson, L. B. (2001). Making murals: Creative strategies for youth and community development. In *Building on family strengths: Research and services in support of children and their families. 2001 conference proceedings.* Portland, OR: Portland State University, Research and Training Center on Family Support and Children's Mental Health [Electronic version]. Retrieved from http://www.rtc.pdx.edu/pgConf01more.shtml

Stiffman, A. R., Hadley-Ives, E., Elze, D., Johnson, S., & Dore, P. (1999). Impact of environment on adolescent mental health and behavior: Structural equation modeling. *American Journal of Orthopsychiatry, 69*(1), 73–86.

Taylor, R. B., & Covington, J. (1988). Neighborhood changes in ecology and violence. *Criminology, 26,* 553–590.

Theodori, G. L. (2001). Examining the effects of community satisfaction and attachment on individual well-being. *Rural Sociology, 66*(4), 618–628.

Unger, D. G., & Wandersman, A. (1985). The importance of neighbors: The social, cognitive, and affective components of neighboring. *American Journal of Community Psychology, 13*(2), 139–169.

Woldoff, R. A. (2002). The effects of local stressors on neighborhood attachment. *Social Forces, 81*(1), 87–116.

USING COMPUTER TECHNOLOGY IN THE MEASUREMENT AND PREVENTION OF COLLEGE DRINKING

48

Heather Harris & John S. Wodarski

Alcohol and drug abuse–related deaths, injuries, disease, and family disturbances are consequences that cannot be measured in monetary figures (Kenkel & Wang, 1999; Wodarski & Wodarski, 1993; Wolvar, 2002). The consequences of substance use and abuse include traffic accidents and fatalities, health problems later in life, suicide, school-related problems, temporary or terminal sickness, and absenteeism (Barr, Antes, Ottenberg, & Rosen, 1984; Perkins, 2002). Young adults are faced with daily decisions about the role that substance use will play in their lives.

There is a considerable problem with consumption of alcohol among college students. Young adults, in comparison with any other age group, have the highest prevalence of high-risk drinking (five or more drinks at any one sitting) (Hingson, Heeren, Zakos, Winter, & Weschler, 2003; Wechsler, Dowdall, Davenport, & Rimm, 1995). In comparing the prevalence of heavy drinking based on data from the national sample collected in the Monitoring the Future studies, Johnson, O'Malley, and Bachman (1994) report that college students (40.7%), unlike their noncollege peers (35.5%), more often engaged in heavy, high-risk drinking. Since college students consistently report a higher prevalence of heavy drinking than their noncollege peers, this discrepancy suggests that a proportion of high school seniors acquire heavy drinking behaviors upon entering or during their early college experience (Hingson et al., 2003; Johnson et al., 1994).

The goal of this pilot project is to determine whether feedback regarding drinking patterns will lessen future alcohol consumption as compared with those subjects who do not receive personalized informative feedback. Assessment and Feedback Information (AFI), which has two major components, will accomplish this.

The first component is primary prevention for freshmen arriving on campus with no alcohol use, and the second is for freshmen arriving with an alcohol use history. The long-term objective of this project is to change the behavioral and attitudinal norms of university students as they are entering freshmen. Another objective of the pilot project is to examine the variation in perceived drinking norms of college students and explore the relationship between perceived campus norms and personal alcohol abuse.

The college environment has a major impact on the development of a young adult. College provides young adults with a sense of independence through decreased influence of parents and increased self-determination and social norming. For many heavy-drinking students, the behavior of other students could become a standard for acceptable behavior. Individuals typically perceive their best friends' drinking as similar to their own (Agostinelli, Brown, & Miller, 1995; Wood, Read, Palfai, & Stevenson, 2001). One of the strongest variables correlated with college drinking is social influence (Hawkins, Catalano, & Miller, 1992).

Because of social norms, college students believe their amount of alcohol consumption is "normal" and within their peers' drinking habits. In fact, some studies suggest that students often overestimate both the acceptability and the actual drinking behavior of their peers (Wechsler, Molnar, Davenport, & Baer, 1999). Because most students maintain enough distance to conceal their drinking behavior from their parents, peers are usually the only ones who could approve or disapprove. Regardless of what consequences follow binge drinking, students feel accepted by their peers because the peers are normally approving of the drinking behavior (Wolburg, 2000).

Brief interventions have gained more momentum in the past decade. To date, there does not seem to be one intervention that works equally well for every subject. A need exists to establish programs that effectively reduce irresponsible use among the college population. This study will use computer technology and AFI to assist in decreasing the gap that currently exists between college drinking and what to do about the problem.

USING COMPUTERS IN THE PREVENTION AND EARLY INTERVENTION OF COLLEGE DRINKING

The agenda for this project centers on the collection of pilot data on the use of information technology in the prevention of irresponsible college drinking. The study involves the development of a comprehensive alcohol abuse prevention program to be delivered over the university computer network. Computer technology increasingly is being applied as an effective means for imparting knowledge and influencing college students' behavior (Rabasca, 2000). The proposed study will utilize this computer technology in the provision of feedback on drinking patterns in an attempt to reduce the incidence and magnitude of alcohol consumption among University of Tennessee students. Another goal of the intervention is to make students aware of their potential risk for developing a drinking problem. The Web site will give immediate feedback and individualized recommendations.

The following components of information technology will be applied on the prevention and early intervention Web site: computerized assessment of alcohol involvement, a brief computerized treatment intervention, referral sites, and a tracking system for the assessment and integration of service at the University of Tennessee.

The pilot project will target students entering as freshmen, the most vulnerable group for acquiring alcohol use or for increasing prior alcohol consumption patterns during the first year of their college experience. All entering freshmen will have the opportunity to participate in the study. After freshmen open their e-mail accounts, a link will appear on their screens. If they choose to participate in the study, students must agree upon and sign a confidentiality statement.

Similar to the BASICS treatment intervention for college students developed by Dimeff, Baer, Kivlahan, and Marlatt (1999), AFI focuses on empirically derived pragmatic strategies and approaches that have been shown to delay the acquisition of alcohol use or accelerate the "maturing out" of problematic patterns of alcohol consumption by enhancing students' motivation to avoid alcohol use entirely or reduce drinking risks by lowering consumption levels of beverage alcohol. Thus, AFI has a true primary prevention goal, preventing the acquisition of alcohol use during an at-risk period.

The AFI includes five components that are based on a common assessment protocol. Development of the computerized data collection screen and the feedback screens that will depend on them will occur during the initial 3½ month period after school begins in August 2003.

Component 1: General Information

A computerized self-report assessment obtains measures of a student's (a) typical drinking pattern and episodic drinking occasions, (b) expectations concerning alcohol use, (c) perceptions about the norms of college student drinking, (d) support for alcohol use in the student's peer group, (e) health risk behaviors, and (f) negative consequences stemming from alcohol use. Students' answers to these questions will help determine their level of alcohol consumption.

Component 2: The Nonuser

A distinguishing factor of the "using computers to prevent irresponsible college drinking" project is the explicit recognition that some students entering college have not begun alcohol use.

Screen I will present nondrinking students with an acknowledgment of their decision not to drink. It will present statistics on the negative consequences the student is missing by not drinking.

Screen II presents the distribution of weekly drinking activity in the college population. The percentage of nondrinkers will be highlighted.

Screen III will emphasize the factors that commonly influence alcohol use initiation: conformance to the behavior of friends (norms), expectations of the benefits of alcohol use, modeling by older students, and lack of "fun" activities.

Screen IV will present the student with information on how to recognize alcohol-related behaviors in other students and provide a listing of campus-based services that can be contacted to get help with the disturbances that can accompany alcohol use by students on campus (loud noise, aggressive behaviors, and alcohol overdose).

Screen V will again acknowledge the student's choice in not drinking as a legitimate, sound decision and part of the student's own choice for building a healthy lifestyle. It will then list campus organizations that are alcohol free.

Component 3: The Occasional User

Most students (54%) report having fewer than eight drinks per week (Johnson et al., 1994). This level of consumption places them in the low to moderate range for alcohol use. In preparing feedback to students in this category, a harm reduction approach will be followed. Students are encouraged to examine their use of alcohol and weigh the perceived benefits of use against the actual biological effects of alcohol and the risk of negative consequences such as hangovers, missed classes, and deterioration of school performance.

Screen I will present the student's weekly drinking habits recorded previously (General Information) with the weekly number of drinks in the college population.

Screen II will discuss alcohol, along with explanations of gender differences in metabolism of alcohol that affect blood alcohol levels (BAC).

Screen III reports the degree of peer support for alcohol use and discusses the influence that peer groups have on reinforcing potentially harmful behaviors.

Screen IV will discuss the effects alcohol has on mood and other mental states. Also, this screen will explain the basic effects of alcohol in general.

Screen V explores the negative consequences attributed to alcohol use. Feedback will be given on the level of negative consequences the student attributes to her or his alcohol use. This information will be obtained from the general information screen previously completed by the student.

Screen VI encourages the student to create a change plan with reduced consumption goals. During this screen, the student will complete an online version of the Alcohol Use Disorder Identification Test (AUDIT).

Screen VII will direct the student to campus activities that promote alcohol- and drug-free lifestyles.

Component 4: The Heavy Drinker

Analyses of data obtained in the 1995 National Survey of Adolescent Males indicate that approaches to collecting data on sensitive topics (such as substance use and sexual practices) that are based on computerized, self-administered data collection systems have been shown to be no less effective and for some types of information (drank alcohol weekly, ever smoked marijuana, drinking or drunk at the time of last sexual intercourse) more effective at obtaining responses than self-administered paper questionnaires (Turner et al., 1998).

Screen I will compare the student's weekly drinking habits recorded previously (General Information) with the weekly number of drinks in the college population.

Screen II will discuss alcohol, along with explanations of gender differences in metabolism of alcohol that affect blood alcohol levels (BAC).

Screen III reports the degree of peer support for alcohol use and discusses the influence that peer groups have on reinforcing potentially harmful behaviors.

Screen IV will discuss the effects alcohol has on mood and other mental states. Also, this screen will explain the basic effects of alcohol in general.

Screen V explores the negative consequences attributed to alcohol use. Feedback will be given on the level of negative consequences the student attributes to his or her alcohol use. This information will be obtained from the general information screen previously completed by the student.

Screen VI encourages the student to create a change plan with reduced consumption goals. During this screen, the student will complete an online version of the Alcohol Use Disorder Identification Test (AUDIT). Those scoring above 8 will be strongly encouraged to seek professional help.

Screen VII will allow students to identify settings in which they are likely to engage in drinking behavior, evaluate the risk of heavy drinking for that setting, and develop consumption targets as guides for controlling their alcohol consumption.

Screen VIII will direct the student to campus activities that promote alcohol- and drug-free lifestyles.

Component 5: Alcohol Dependence

Students whose information suggests they might be severely alcohol dependent or who have medical conditions for which the use of alcohol is contraindicated (e.g., possible pregnancy, ulcers, diabetes) will be strongly encouraged to abstain from alcohol use and to accept a referral to an abstinence-based treatment program. A listing of campus-based referral sources and contact numbers will be provided.

This project relies heavily on self-report measures. Farrell, Danish, & Howard (1992) suggest that in the proper circumstances (not in home or church) adolescents tend to be reasonably truthful in reporting drug use and other problem behaviors. The computer-based screen will be designed to induce participation and is expected to add a novelty dimension that generates a higher response rate than a mailed questionnaire.

Tracking System

Registration will be necessary to provide personalized feedback. The tracking system will require the individual's e-mail address, which is how feedback will be sent to them. Registration will also include a password, age, and gender of participant.

Current research points to a less invasive intervention being more acceptable than traditional group or individual counseling with college-age students. Because of this, there are several benefits of a computer-based intervention. First, the individual may be more likely to disclose personal and sensitive information if the information can be given via e-mail. Second, the individual who chooses to participate in the study is likely to already have an interest in the topic of alcohol consumption. Third, computer-based interventions offer low-cost, preliminary treatment options to serve a greater number of clients at one time (Squires & Hester, 2002).

If results of this project warrant it, the program can be applied across the student body with little or no adaptation and can be packaged and distributed as a low-cost intervention for colleges and universities nationally.

Limitations

The Web site contains a detailed disclaimer informing students that this program is not intended to provide therapy and is not a substitute for a therapist. The program should be implemented with early prevention and intervention in mind for entering freshmen students. The program allows the student to quit the program at any time, which could be problematic. It will be difficult to track students who do this or do not give accurate information. Another obstacle in the program is the use of self-reports. It would be ideal to have a number of self-report measures for each student to check for the reliability of the student's answers.

Case Illustration

The University of Tennessee will be the site of implementation for this pilot program. In light of the evidence of the severity of college drinking and particularly the problem at this university, it appears important to test the effectiveness of an alcohol prevention program that offers the reasonable probability of preventing alcohol use for entering students who do not drink and of preventing the transition to heavy drinking by students who currently use alcohol.

As previously mentioned, if results warrant, the program can be implemented across the student body with little or no adaptation, as well as packaged and distributed as a low-cost intervention for other colleges and universities.

CONCLUSION

Because of the stigma associated with alcohol problems, the computer program could alleviate some of the barriers to prevention and treatment. The information presented discusses a way in which college students can be targeted for alcohol prevention by utilizing computer technology. The technology allows students to feel a sense of anonymity while they are receiving help for their drinking problems. The anonymity available through a prevention program delivered on the Internet may also help reduce the barriers of stigmatization. The Web-based program should provide students a way of receiving help in the privacy of their own rooms or, at the very least, when and where they are ready to get some help.

The proposed study is intended to adapt brief intervention technology developed primarily in the alcohol treatment field to a computer-based delivery system. Brief interventions are among the least costly and the most efficacious interventions in the treatment armamentarium of alcohol abuse treatment providers. The Web site is a low-cost, low-maintenance program that can be promoted on a college campus as a voluntary alcohol information site.

References

Agostinelli, G., Brown, J., & Miller, W. (1995). Effects of normative feedback on consumption among heavy drinking college students. *Journal of Drug Education, 25*(1), 31–40.

Barr, H., Antes, D., Ottenberg, D., & Rosen, A. (1984). The mortality of treated alcoholics and drug addicts: The benefits of sobriety. *Journal of Studies on Alcohol, 45*(5), 440–452.

Dimeff, L., Baer, J., Kivlahan, D., & Martlatt, G. A. (1999). *Brief alcohol screening and intervention for college students (BASICS): A harm reduction approach.* New York: Guilford.

Farrell, A. D., Danish, S. J., & Howard, C. W. (1992). Relationship between drug use and other problem behaviors in urban adolescents. *Journal of Consulting and Clinical Psychology, 60,* 705–712.

Hawkins, J., Catalano, R., & Miller, J. (1992). Risk and protective factors for alcohol and other drug problems in adolescence and early adulthood: Implications for substance abuse prevention, *Psychological Bulletin, 112,* 64–105.

Hingson, R., Heeren, T., Zakos, R., Winter, M., & Wechsler, H. (2003). Age of first intoxication, heavy drinking, driving after drinking and risk of unintentional injury among U.S. college students, *Journal of Studies on Alcohol, 64*(1), 23–31.

Johnson, L., O'Malley, P., & Bachman, J. (1994). *National survey results of drug use from the Monitoring the Future Study, 1975–1993: Vol. 2. College students and young adults.* Rockville, MD: National Institute on Drug Abuse.

Kenkel, D., & Wang, P. (1999). Are alcoholics in bad jobs? In F. Chaloupka, M. Grossman, W. Bickel, & H. Saffer (Eds.), *Economic analysis of substance use and abuse.* Chicago: University of Chicago Press.

Perkins, W. (2002). Surveying the damage: A review of research on consequences of alcohol misuse in college populations, *Journal of Studies on Alcohol,* Suppl, 91–100.

Rabasca, L. (2000). Self-help sites: A blessing or a bane? *Monitor on Psychology, 31*(4), 28–30.

Squires, D., & Hester, R. (2002, March). Development of a computer-based, brief intervention for drinkers: The increasing role for computers in the assessment and treatment of addictive behaviors. *The Behavior Therapist,* pp. 59–65.

Wechsler, H., Dowdall, G., Davenport, A., & Rimm, E. (1995). A gender specific measure of binge drinking among college students, *American Journal of Public Health, 85*(7), 921–926.

Wechsler, H., Molnar, B., Davenport, A., & Baer, J. (1999). College alcohol use: A full or empty glass? *Journal of American College Health, 47,* 247–252.

Wodarski, J. S., & Wodarski, L. A. (1993). *Curriculums and practical aspects of implementation: Preventive health services for adolescents.* Lanham: University Press of America.

Wolburg, J. (2000). The "risky business" of binge drinking among college students: Using risk models PSA's and anti-drinking campaigns. *Journal of Advertising, 30*(4), 23–39.

Wolvar, A. (2002). Effects of heavy drinking in college on study effort, grade point average, and major choice, *Continuing Economic Policy, 20*(4), 415–428.

Wood, M., Read, J., Palfai, T., & Stevenson, J. (2001). Social influences processes and college student drinking: The mediation role of alcohol outcome expectancies, *Journal of Studies on Alcohol, 62*(1), 32–43.

SECTION VI
Assessment Tools and Measures

49 LOCATING MEASUREMENT TOOLS AND INSTRUMENTS FOR INDIVIDUALS AND COUPLES

Kevin Corcoran

One striking characteristic in the development of all sciences is how progress follows the lead first set by advances in measurement. Improvement in measures, it seems, is a predicate to other scientific development. In the behavioral sciences, measurement first allowed research to improve diagnoses and evidence the efficacy of theories for diagnostic-related groupings. Measurement has advanced to the current state where it is available for incorporation in the routines and procedures of everyday practice.

Currently, measures are available to ascertain just about any and every client problem, some which are seen frequently (e.g., measures of depression) and others that are seen rarely and usually by specialists (e.g., measures of Tourette's syndrome in children). In less than 30 years the availability of relevant and practical instruments has gone from a few (e.g., Beck, Ward, Mendelson, Mock, & Erbaugh, 1961; Locke & Wallace, 1959) to thousands. Many of the more frequently used instruments for clinical practice are centrally located in books, publishing houses, and Web sites. This chapter will consider one of the more practical types of measures for clinical practice, rapid assessment instruments, delineate recent sources for accessing a variety of tools, and describe a few of the most useful RAIs.

A RECENT TREND IN ASSESSMENT

A recent trend in assessment is how it has moved from broadband measurement tools for diagnostic purposes (e.g., the Minnesota Multiphosic Personality Inventory [MMPI]) to those that are narrowly tailored to a particular client problem. Previously, instruments such as the MMPI, the Rorschach, and various IQ tests were administered by a professional who submitted a diagnostic report in the form of a clinical evaluation or assessment. More often than not, this diagnostician was not the same person as the attending clinician. This role of measurement in clinical practice continues to have some value and will do so—to some degree—for years to come.

Along with the continued use of broadband instruments, clinical practice has witnessed the development of more practical measures that give more immediate feedback to the clinician, the client, or a managed care organization. These instruments are narrowband measures designed to ascertain a particular cognition, affect or emotion, and human performance. These instruments ascertain and quantify the observations of affect, behavior, or cognition in terms of the frequency, intensity, or duration. With such instruments, measurement is now something that most clinicians do frequently, and would do even more if the tools were more readily available.

This type of measurement tool is often called a *rapid assessment instrument* (RAI). A RAI is typically completed by the client as self-observation. With a little creativity, however, most RAIs can be adapted as a rating scale. As a rating scale, RAIs can be used by some relevant other to observe the client, such as a family member or the clinician. Further, sometimes a single item from a RAI is useful as an index or individualized rating scale. When used repeatedly over the course of the treatment, RAIs provide valuable feedback to monitor client change and evaluate practice because scores reflect changes in the clinical problem or attainment of a goal.

To be practical in ascertaining client change, RAIs must be relatively short, quickly and conveniently completed, and easily scored and interpreted. Anything short of these dimensions and measures in clinical practice will not be likely for busy providers. Additionally, if an RAI is to be useful and of probative value, it must have seven essential features: reliability, validity, utility, suitability, acceptability, sensitivity, and nonreactivity.

At a minimum, an RAI must be reliable and valid. A reliable and valid instrument is one that is consistent and accurate, respectively. Consistency takes three general forms: consistency between items that constitute the instrument (i.e., internal consistency); consistency between different forms of the same instrument (i.e., alternative or parallel forms reliability); and consistency when used over the course of time, such as a week or sessions of therapy (i.e., test-retest reliability). Reliability is typically expressed in a coefficient that has a maximum score of 1.0. Reliability coefficients greater than .80 are usually considered acceptable evidence that the instrument is consistent between its items, forms, or administration over time.

Whereas reliability is simply the consistency of an instrument, validity is nothing more than a way of estimating an instrument's accuracy. There are three general ways to estimate accuracy. One is to evaluate the content of the instrument to assess whether the items represent the domain of the variable (i.e., content validity). Another way to estimate the accuracy of an instrument is to evaluate its relationship to some established criterion; the criterion may itself be ascertained concomitant with the administration of the instrument (i.e., concurrent validity), or it may be an event that will occur in the future,

such as grades in graduate school as a criterion estimating the accuracy of the Graduate Record Examination (i.e., predictive validity). The third way to estimate the accuracy of an instrument is to determine how it is similar to some constructs while also being different from others (i.e., construct validity). (For a more thorough discussion, see Nunnally & Bernstein, 1994.)

In addition to using RAIs that have evidence of consistency and accuracy, clinicians need RAIs that have utility. *Utility* refers to some practical and added value for including measures in routine practice. RAIs have utility because they can help plan, monitor, and evaluate clinical services (Bloom, Fischer, & Orme, 2003). This is chiefly done by providing consistent and accurate feedback about changes in the client's problem or as an assessment of the attainment of a goal.

An instrument's utility is easily influenced by its length and ability to calculate and interpret the score. RAIs overcome these impediments in measurement by containing a limited number of items—often fewer than 50, unless the instrument is an adjective checklist, which can still be completed quickly even though it has more items.

RAIs are designed for easy scoring and are frequently expressed as total scale scores or as an average for the total number of items. Scores are easily interpreted by comparing them before, during, and after treatment, which is known as a *self-referenced comparison*. Self-referenced scores are conveniently interpreted to illustrate change by plotting them over time on graph paper. Client scores may also be interpreted by comparing them to a norm of similar persons from the general population and persons from a clinical sample. Such *norm-referenced comparison* is useful in managed care settings where treatment necessity must be demonstrated (see Corcoran & Vandiver, 1996). The comparison with the general population could be interpreted to illustrate how the client's problem is not typical and, therefore, is medically necessary; scores similar to a clinical sample would show how the client is just like those already warranting treatment.

A clinician will want to use RAIs that are also suitable and acceptable to his or her client. An RAI is *suitable* when its content is appropriate for the client's emotionality and comprehension, which is of course greatly influenced by his or her reading ability. Clients who may be experiencing psychotic symptoms are probably unlikely to complete an RAI with much accuracy, and a client who is unable to read the instrument clearly will not provide scores of much value. In essence, the practitioner must select an RAI that suits the client's circumstances, abilities, and social environment.

The RAIs must also be acceptable to the client. *Acceptability* refers to how the content of the instrument is seen by the client. If the content is offensive, it is unlikely that you will get any information at all, and such an instrument might even have an adverse consequence on the treatment process and the therapeutic relationship. Consider, for example, a couple who is in treatment for marital discord, including dissatisfaction with their sex life. Several instruments are available to measure sexual satisfaction, and it is easy to imagine how some content could offend a more reserved couple and yet seem trivial to others.

In addition to being suitable and acceptable, a useful RAI must be sensitive. *Sensitivity* refers to the instrument's ability to ascertain change in the behavior when change has in fact occurred. Clearly, this is a critical element when using an RAI over the course of treatment because change is therapy's very purpose. Any instrument that is not sensitive will not reflect what happened during the intervention. Many instruments, unfortunately, are not sensitive to observing real change. Sensitivity is particularly challenging in that it is contrary to the very idea of reliability, which is stability. How can an RAI be both sensitive and stable? The answer is that you want a measure that is stable when no change has occurred and, concomitantly, sensitive to observing difference in the client's behavior when it has occurred. When selecting RAIs for your routine use, you should avoid those that ascertain a trait of the client, as is found with personality disorders. These scores reflect a variable that is relatively enduring over time, settings, and persons, so change is less observable. RAIs are most sensitive when they ascertain a behavior state of a client, a behavior that is expected to change by the end of treatment.

The final critical criterion for selecting useful RAIs is to use those that are nonreactive. *Reactivity* refers to how the very process of measurement itself causes changes in the client's behavior. Continuing with the case of the couple whose sex life is not satisfying, the same instrument that might offend one couple might stimulate another. Although this may actually facil-

itate the treatment process, the challenge to the clinician is in determining if the change in scores is due to treatment or just filling out a questionnaire. If genuine and lasting change did result solely from completing instruments, there would be little need for clinicians; only psychometricians would be necessary.

If an instrument is reactive, it is very important to be judicial when interpreting the scores. With measures that are not nonreactive, you simply do not know why there are changes in the scores. This suggestion of caution, frankly, applies to all measures used in clinical practice, even those that are reliable, valid, suitable, acceptable, and sensitive. Scores on a measure may provide valuable observables of change in a client's problem, more material to aid clinical judgment.

LOCATING TOOLS

Locating tools for evaluating client change was once a formidable challenge. Clinicians who used measures had to either have known the research literature thoroughly or spend hours searching journals for any instrument even remotely relevant to the client's problem or treatment goal. This has all changed. In the past 15 years or so, many books have been published that describe instruments, and many even reprint the complete scale. An excellent Web site for 79 book sources of instruments is Tests and Measurement in Social Sciences (http://libraries.uta.edu/Helen/test&meas/tetmainframe.htm), and a number of recent volumes are listed in the bibliography.

Most measurement tools are first published in professional journals. As such, contemporary measures are also available in academic libraries. Many journals frequently include research reports on the development or revision of an instrument (e.g., *Journal of Consulting and Clinical Psychology* and *Research on Social Work Practice*), and others focus solely on measurement (e.g., *Psychological Assessment* and *Journal of Personality Assessment*). Although it is difficult to stay abreast of all the new instruments found in journals, it is useful to identify the major journals in one's specialty area and to review those frequently.

The last major source for locating instruments is the Internet, which includes not only all the major publishing houses that commercially market instruments and manuals but also networks of other Web sites where measures may be procured both commercially and from the public domain. The Internet usually includes books and journals on measurement. With this in mind, the Internet might seem like an easy place to find good RAIs. It is not. The Web, in fact, is probably the most difficult place to locate instruments because Web sites come and Web sites go away. Further, it seems that just about anyone can put materials on the Web, and the number of hits is unruly. For example, a search for *measures* yields over a million hits, and even *psychological instruments* gives nearly half a million. Unless you are willing to spend a few days and blurry eyes, the Web is not the easiest place for locating RAIs. Even with its power, the Web is still subject to human foibles. For example, the Albert Einstein College of Medicine references Joel Fischer's third edition of *Measures for Clinical Practice*, a rather striking error to this author.

The most useful Web sites are those that provide links to other relevant sites. One of the most valuable ones is Health and Psychosocial Instruments (HAPI; www.ovid.com), which includes measures of health, psychosocial sciences, organizational behavior, and library and information sciences. Also noteworthy is the ERIC/AE (http://erice.testcol.htm), a clearinghouse of major outlets of instruments. Finally, a wealth of information is available at the Web site Tests and Measures in the Social Sciences, cited earlier, which provides materials on nearly 9,000 instruments from 79 sources and is updated frequently.

EXEMPLARY INSTRUMENTS

As the preceding discussion suggests, if one is successful in locating instruments, the result will be too many instruments and not too few. Being overwhelmed with choices can be as difficult as being underwhelmed because there are too few instruments. For this reason, I would like to review just a few instruments that are particularly useful. Some are broadband in that they ascertain a range of attributes about a clinical condition; others are more focused to measure a particular clinical problem. Obtaining these measures for clinical use, though, is only a start, and soon the tools in one's toolbox of measures will expand.

Some broadband instruments that are partic-ularly useful are those that allow you to isolate the clinical problem in the event this is undetermined at intake. Along with the narrowband instruments discussed earlier, these instruments tend to capture the major clinical conditions seen in practice, including depression, anxiety, somatic complaints, psychotic conditions, and substance use. All these instruments have good to very good reliability and validity estimates.

The Symptom Questionnaire (SQ), by Robert Kellner (1987; in Corcoran & Fischer, 2000), is one of the most useful tools for the first phases of treatment. It consists of 92 adjectives to which the client endorses those that reflect his or her clinical condition, and it takes less than 5 minutes to complete. The SQ measures four major dimensions of clinical problems: depression, anxiety, somatization, and anger-hostility problems. It also measures four corresponding conditions of well-being: relaxation, contentment, somatic health, and friendliness. These subscales are particularly useful as an operationalization of a treatment goal, whereas the problem subscales nicely tap into the actual clinical problem to be decreased over the course of treatment. The internal consistency of each subscale is as high as .95, which is exceptional, and there is good evidence of test-retest reliability. Known-groups validity is evident by the distinction in score for psychiatric patients and the general population.

The Symptoms Checklist Revised (SCL-90-R), by Leonard Derogatis (1975; Derogatis, Lipman, & Covi, 1977), another useful broadband instrument, is one of the most recognized self-report measures of psychopathology. It has been translated into 20 languages. The SCL-90-R, which, as its title suggests, has 90 items, measures a broad spectrum of psychological conditions by means of the symptomatic distress. As a broadband measure it was intended to ascertain nine dimensions of psychiatric symptoms, although a number of studies question this assertion. For example, Clark and Watson's (1991) findings suggest the SCL-90-R measures general neurosis, as defined by feelings of inferiority and rejection, oversensitivity to criticism, self-consciousness, social distress, and perhaps depression and anxiety; in contrast, Steer, Clark, and Ranieri (1994) aver the SCL-90-R items measure chiefly distress of psychological symptoms, and then somatic anxiety, depression, irritability, and attention problems. Although the subscale structure of the SCL-90-R may not be consistent, the instrument is still a useful screening tool and outcome measure in clinical practice. Numerous studies have evidenced the reliability of the SCL-90-R, and its internal consistently tends to be above .90. The instrument has excellent validity, with scores that differ between psychiatric patients and the general population, as well as correlating with other similar measures of psychopathology.

The Oregon Mental Health Checklist (OMHRC), by Kevin Corcoran (in Corcoran & Fischer, 2000), is a 31-item checklist designed for adolescents, particularly those in the juvenile justice system. The instrument ascertains the presence of 31 symptoms arranged in descending order of clinical severity. As with other checklists, this one is very quick to complete, taking only about 2 minutes. The OMHRC has three parallel forms, one for completion by the youth, another for use by a parent, and a third for use by relevant others, such as a probation officer or clinician. Each of these three forms is accompanied by three separate instruments for use at a baseline and at 6- and 12-month intervals. The OMHRC is also available in Spanish. The forms have fairly good reliability (approximately .80), and there is significant interrater agreement between scores by parents and juvenile justice staff ($r = .48$). One appealing feature of the OMHRC is that it is not in the stream of commerce but has been put in the public domain and may be copied ad libitum.

SOME NARROWBAND INSTRUMENTS

In addition to the three broadband instruments discussed earlier, there are many others to learn about and integrate into routine practice. Often, though, a narrowband instrument will be more expedient and focused; it is for this reason that the subscales of a broadband measures will be more convenient to use. After a broadband measure is used at intake, it makes little sense to include the other subscales that are not relevant. In a sense, then, the subscales of broadband instrument may be used as a narrowband rapid assessment tool. Three areas to consider measuring are the three most common clinical conditions in the population: depression, anxiety, and substance abuse.

Depression

Depression is the most commonly seen mental health condition in practice, and not surprisingly, it has many exceptional instruments. As discussed by Nezu, Ronan, Meadows, and McClure (2000), there are literally hundred of instruments to ascertain depression; these authors review over 90 of them. Twenty-nine instruments are reprinted in Nezu et al. (2000), and 26 are reprinted in Corcoran and Fischer (2000).

One of the granddaddies of instruments for measuring depression is the Beck Depression Inventory (BDI), by Tim Beck (Beck, Ward, Mendelson, Mock, & Erbaugh, 1961), followed by the BDI-II (Beck, Steer, & Brown, 1996). Although it is one of the long-standing measures of depression in the field, unfortunately the BDI-II is available only from a commercial publishing house and is fairly expensive; at about $2 for each copy, its clinical utility for repeated use over the course of treatment is severely restricted. Thus, the BDI-II may not be the most recommended instrument simply because it is priced out of the market, especially when contrasted with those that are available for free or at a low cost.

The Generalized Contentment Scale (GCS), by Walter Hudson (1997; in Corcoran & Fischer, 2000), is a good example of a less expensive instrument; it is available for about 25 cents a copy. The GCS is a 25-item instrument with scores ranging from 0 to 100. The instrument has been developed with impeccable psychometric procedures and has exceptional reliability, with an internal consistency coefficient of up to .92. Validity is estimated with correlation between .76 and .85 with the BDI, and .92 with other measures of depression. The GCS has two cutting scores, one to indicate a clinically significant problem and the other to distinguish those with suicidal ideation. Because of the extensive research that has been done on the GCS, there are both general and clinical norms for comparison with the client's scores.

The Center for Epidemiologic Study Depressed (CES-D) Mood Scale, by Radloff, 1977; in Corcoran & Fischer, 2000), is a 20-item instrument designed to measure depression in the general population instead of a clinical population. It is also available as a 10-item short form. One unique feature of the CES-D is that instead of assessing the magnitude of depressive symptoms, as the other instruments do, it defines depressed mood from the view of its frequency. The internal consistency is .85 for a sample from the general population and .90 for a sample of psychiatric patients. It tends to be stable over time, with test-retest correlations between .51

and .67 for 2- and 8-week periods. Validity estimates are very good and include the ability to distinguish psychiatric patients from the general population. The CES-D is extremely valuable for illustrating how a client is more depressed than the general population, and therefore to assert that treatment is medically necessary.

Anxiety

Anxiety, like depression, is one of the most common mental health conditions in the country, although depression is seen most often for clinical services. Many instruments are available to measure anxiety. Anotony, Orsillo, and Roemer (2001) review 200 of them (of which about one third are brief reviews) and reprint 80. Twenty-six measure of anxiety are also available in Corcoran and Fischer (2000).

The Fear of Negative Evaluation (FNE), by David Watson and Ronald Friend (1969; in Corcoran & Fischer, 2000), is one of the most useful measures because it ascertains social anxiety, which is seen here as the result of perceived negative evaluations by others. The FNE is a 30-item instrument, but a 12-item short form may be used for even more rapid assessment. This measure is also available from the journal itself and from Corcoran and Fischer (2000) at no charge, or at least the authors say it may be copied. The internal consistency estimates range up to .94, and the instrument is stable over a 1-month period ($r = .78$). There is also exceptional known-groups validity.

The Social Avoidance and Distress (SAD) Scale, also by Watson and Friend (1969; in Corcoran & Fischer, 2000), is another useful measure of anxiety. This 28-item instrument ascertains anxiety from the perspective of the client's feelings of distress, discomfort, and fear, and the resultant avoidance of social situations. As a measure of avoidance, the SAD ascertains the opposite of the appropriate clinical intervention for anxiety, which is exposure; as such, the instrument has a close nexus between the client problem and the clinical intervention. Estimates of reliability are as high as .94, with test-retest reliability of .68 for a 1-month period. As with the FNE, the authors have granted assess to the instrument from the original journal article or by copying it from Corcoran and Fischer (2000).

Substance Abuse

Substance abuse—including abuse of drugs, alcohol, and tobacco—is another common client condition seen in practice, but it is more often seen in health promotion settings. One of the first steps in treating substance use is to determine the severity of use, which can be quite challenging; screening for drug and alcohol use is essential because denial is a common defense.

The Drug Abuse Screening Test (DAST), by Harvey Skinner (1983), and the Self-Administered Alcoholism Screening Test (SAAST), by Wendell Swenson and Robert Morse (1975), are two exceptional measurement tools; both are reprinted in Corcoran and Fischer (2000). The DAST is a 20-item instrument that measures problems associated with drug use, which helps get around a client's tendency to understate or deny a drug problem. The internal consistency coefficients range up to .92. Scores discriminate between persons with alcohol problems and those with drug problems and also correlate with drug use over the past month. The DAST is also available in a short 10-item form, and the author has made the instrument available at no pecuniary cost.

The SAAST is similar to the DAST but is directed to alcohol abuse. It is a 35-item self-administered instrument that is based on the Michigan Alcoholism Screening Test, which has an interview format. The SAAST has a parallel form, for use by a spouse; this form appears to have a 90% accuracy rate for identifying alcoholism, which is strong support for the instrument's validity. The original article does not report reliability, but scores do discriminate between an alcoholic patient and others. The instrument has a cutting score that allows the clinician to accurately diagnose alcoholism. The SAAST is available from the authors at no cost.

These instruments are useful at intake to identify problems with drugs or alcohol. They are not particularly useful, however, for measuring the magnitude of the substance use problem. One of the most convenient and useful measures of the magnitude of alcohol or drug use is to simply ask about the frequency of use in the past 30 days and the amount of use per day. This approach, which is used in federally funded research programs, would include the following questions to measure use of marijuana.

In the last month (30 days), on how many days did you use marijuana?
On those days you did use marijuana, how many times a day did you use it?

The items are then scored by multiplying the days of use by the amount of use to obtain a score on severity or magnitude. The instrument is available for use on a monthly basis and may be modified to fix any substance under consideration, such as alcohol, marijuana, cocaine, or zaldine. When it is used for alcohol assessment, the second item is also a measure of binge drinking, which is defined as having four or more drinks a day—a score that must be interpreted judiciously around major holidays such as New Year's Eve, a Passover seder, an Easter dinner, Thanksgiving, Christmas, Hanukkah, a 21st birthday, the Fourth of July, or other special events at which drinking is more likely. Clearly, it is possible to overdiagnose binge drinking without careful consideration of the client's circumstances.

CONCLUSIONS

The previous section reviewed but a few of the numerous tools for clinical practice. It is not even a single crystal on the tip of the proverbial iceberg, but hopefully it is a point of departure for assessing some of the more common clinical problems. The clinician will find, like most who start to use an instrument routinely in their practice, that he or she will want to accumulate a large number and variety of measures to assess a variety of problems and even the range of nuances presented by different clients with the same diagnostic condition. The need for measures in clinical practice is likely to be met with some RAI. The information presented in this chapter is intended to help the clinician identify and select rapid assessment tools for his or her toolbox. This information is valuable feedback for the client to work with as well.

References

*American Psychiatric Association. (2000). *Handbook of psychiatric measures*. Washington, DC, APA Press.

Anotony, M. M., Orsillo, S. M., & Roemer, L. (2001). *Practitioner's guide to empirically based measures of anxiety*. New York: Kluwer/Plenum.

Beck, A. T., Steer, R. A., & Brown, G. K. (1996). *Man-ual for the BDI-II*. San Antonio, TX: Psychological Corporation.

Beck, A. T., Ward, C. H., Mendelson, M., Mock, J., & Erbaugh, J. (1961). An inventory for measuring depression. *Archives of General Psychiatry, 4*, 561–571.

Bloom, M., Fischer, J., & Orme, J. G. (2003). *Evaluating practice: Guidelines for the accountable professional* (4th ed.). Needham Heights, MA: Allyn and Bacon.

Clark, L. A., & Watson, D. (1991). Tripartite model of anxiety and depression: Psychometric evidence and taxonomic implications. *Journal of Personality Assessment, 49*, 571–578.

*Corcoran, K., & Fischer, J. (2000). *Measures for clinical practice* (Vols. 1–2). New York: Free Press.

Corcoran, K., & Vandiver, V. L. (1996). *Maneuvering the maze of managed care: Skills of mental health practitioners*. New York: Free Press.

Derogatis, L. R. (1975). *The SCL-90-R*. Baltimore: Clinical Psychometrics Research.

Derogatis, L. R., Lipman, R. S., & Covi, L. (1977). SCL-90: An outpatient psychiatric rating scale, preliminary report. *Psychopharmacology Bulletin, 9*, 13–27.

Hudson, W. W. (1997). *The WALMYR assessment scales: Scoring manual*. Tallahassee, FL: WALMYR Publishing.

*Jones, R. L. (1996). *Handbook of tests and measurements for Black populations* (Vols. 1–2). Hampton, VA: Cobb and Henry.

Kellner, R. (1987). A symptom questionnaire. *Journal of Clinical Psychiatry, 48*, 268–274.

Locke, H. J., & Wallace, K. M. (1959). Short marital-adjustment and prediction tests: Their reliability and validity. *Marriage and Family Living, 21*, 251–255.

Nezu, A. M., Ronan, G. F., Meadows, E. A., & Mc-Clure, K. S. (2000). *Practitioner's guide to empirically based measures of depression*. New York: Kluwer/Plenum.

Nunnally, J., & Bernstein, I. (1994). *Psychometric theory*. New York: McGraw-Hill.

*Ponton, M. O., & Leon-Carrion, J. (2001). *Neuropsychology and the Hispanic patient: A clinical handbook*. Mahwah, NJ: Erlbaum.

Radloff, L. S. (1977). The CES-D scale: A self-report depression scale for research in general populations. *Applied Psychological Measurement, 1*, 385–401.

Skinner, H. A. (1983). The Drug Abuse Screening Test. *Journal of Addictive Behaviors, 7*, 363–371.

*Stanhope, M., & Knollmueller, R. (2000). *Handbook of community and home health nursing: Tools for assessment, intervention and education*. St. Louis, MO: Mosby.

Steer, R. A., Clark, D. A., & Ranieri, W. F. (1994). Symptom dimensions of the SCL-90-R: A test of the tripartite model of anxiety and depression. *Journal of Personality Assessment, 62,* 525–536.

Swenson, W. M., & Morse, R. M. (1975). The use of a self-administered alcoholism screening test (SAAST) in a medical center. *Mayo Clinic Proceedings, 50,* 204–208.

*Touliatos, J., Perlmutter, B. F., & Straus, M. A. (2001). *Handbook of family measurement techniques* (Vols. 1–3). Thousand Oaks, CA: Sage.

*Waltz, C. F., & Jenkins, L. S. (2002). *Measurement of nursing outcomes.* New York: Springer.

Watson, D., & Friend, R. (1969). Measurement of social-evaluative anxiety. *Journal of Consulting and Clinical Psychology, 33,* 448–457.

*Books reprinting instruments

50   OVERVIEW OF HEALTH SCALES AND MEASURES

David L. Streiner

Measurement is an essential component of most scientific research, whether it involves determining the temperature of stars, taking a patient's blood pressure, or assessing a person's attitudes and beliefs. In many of the "hard" sciences, such as physics or astronomy, there is little inherent difficulty, other than building the appropriate apparatus. The measurement itself is relatively objective, and subjective judgment plays a minor role. Although errors may still arise because of miscalibration or observer error (such as in noting the exact time a satellite transits its planet), greater accuracy and minimizing errors are usually achieved through technical solutions, that is, building a better instrument. In the "softer," human sciences, though, researchers are acutely aware of the fallibility of human judgment and the difficulties encountered in trying to measure subjective states. This is seen by sociologists attempting to measure belief systems, psychologists assessing traits or moods such as anxiety and depression, and health care researchers from a number of disciplines trying to measure patients' quality of life. The result has been the birth of a discipline called *psychometrics*, which

originally arose from psychology and education, with the aim of making the assessment of aptitudes and achievement more rigorous. Over the past few decades, psychometrics has grown to encompass the measurement of subjective states through the use of scales and questionnaires. This chapter outlines some of the basic principles involved in developing scales and ensuring that they indeed measure what they purport to. A more thorough description of the process can be found in Streiner and Norman's book (2004).

THE ITEMS

Although it may seem trivial to mention, all scales are composed of individual items. This is important to keep in mind, though, because if the items are poorly chosen or badly worded, nothing can rescue the test from deserved oblivion. The items must satisfy a number of criteria. The first relates to the two components of *content validity.* If we are measuring an attribute such as anxiety, the questions must cover all its aspects, such as physiological changes, behavioral manifestations, and the cognitive component; this is referred to as the *content coverage* of the scale. By the same token, the test should not include any items that are unrelated to the attribute, such as depression; this is called the *content relevance* of the test. The items can come from a number of sources: other scales (if done properly, this is called *adaptation* rather than *plagiarism*), theory, research, expert opinion, and, most important for clinical scales, patient interviews.

Once written, the items should be checked by people representative of the intended users to ensure that they are understandable, which usually means that they are worded at a sixth-grade reading level, and free from jargon terms (e.g., a "stool" to a physician does not have the same meaning as it does for the lay public, and confusing the two can lead to somewhat unusual responses).

The next step is to decide the format of the response options. The easiest to write are dichotomous ones, such as yes/no or agree/disagree. However, respondents often find these annoying to use because they want to say, "Yes, but . . ." One improvement over this format has a fancy name, a *visual analog scale*, to describe a simple concept: a line 10 cm (about 4 inches) long, along which a person can put a mark. For example, the stem of the question can ask, "How much pain are you currently experiencing?" One end of the line would be labeled "No pain at all" and the other "The worst pain imaginable." Where the person places a mark on the line then corresponds (at least theoretically) to the degree of pain. A third possible response option is an *adjectival scale*. As the name implies, this consists of a series of boxes, under each one of which is an adjective or phrase. Using the same stem, the adjectives may say "None/Slight/Moderate/Intense/Unbearable." Finally, a *Likert scale* is often used to measure attitudes and feelings. It is a bipolar scale, meaning that the person can express either positive or negative opinions for the same question, and usually has seven or nine alternative answers. One end is labeled, for example, "Strongly agree," the other "Strongly disagree," and there is a neutral point somewhere in the middle. Likert scales are perhaps the most widely encountered in daily life because they are used extensively by pollsters or companies assessing customers' reactions. This by no means exhausts the possible options of responding to test items; other response options, with their strengths and limitations, can be found in Streiner and Norman (2003).

RELIABILITY

Before one can say that an instrument is measuring what is intended, it is first necessary to establish that it is measuring *something* in a reproducible fashion. This property of the scale is known as *reliability*. There are a number of ways of assessing reliability, depending on the nature of the scale and what we want to know about it.

If the scale is self-administered, then the important property is *test-retest reliability;* that is, if a person fills out the scale today, his or her score should be nearly the same if it is completed again at some later time. How much later is a trade-off between competing demands. On the one hand, the interval between the initial test and the retest should be short enough that whatever is being measured has not changed. For extremely stable traits, such as intelligence or extroversion, this can be a number of years. For more labile states such as anxiety, depression, or how we feel about the current head of state, 1 or 2 weeks may be the upper limit. On the other hand, we want the interval to be long enough so that the person does not remember what he or she said the first time, and thus simply repeats the original answer in order to appear consistent, but responds to the items de novo. Needless to say, this is more of a problem with shorter scales than longer ones; it is easier to remember the responses to 5 items than to 500.

Some scales are completed by an observer evaluating the person, such as a nurse rating how psychotic a patient's behavior is, or a developmental psychologist assessing a child's reaction to being in a strange situation. The focus here is on the *interrater reliability* of the scale, or the degree to which the two observers, independently completing the form, agree with one another.

A third form of reliability is seemingly different from these two and looks at the *internal consistency* or *homogeneity* of the scale, which is the degree to which all the items are related to each other. This property is based on the assumption that a scale should be *unidimensional*, measuring only one attribute. This is desirable because homogeneity "speaks directly to the ability of the clinician or researcher to interpret the . . . score as a reflection of the test's items" (Henson, 2001, p. 177). That is, if the scale purports to measure risk-taking behavior, then all the items should tap some aspect of this—and therefore be correlated with one another—and not be measuring something else, such as suicidal ideation (although at times it may be difficult to differentiate between the two).

Not all scales, though, try to be homogeneous. Some, which more resemble checklists, consist of unrelated symptoms or events. For example, the Hassles and Uplifts Scale (Kanner, Coyne, Schaefer, & Lazarus, 1981) is a list of daily events that either annoy people or buoy them up. There is no reason to suspect that if one occurs, others must necessarily follow; in other words, the items need not be correlated with each other. Similarly, the General Health Questionnaire (Goldberg, 1979) consists of unrelated physical and psychological symptoms; the more a person endorses, the greater the probability of distress. Again, having one symptom does not increase the probability of having others. Naturally, estimates of internal consistency are not (or, at least, should not be) calculated for indices such as these.

All three types of reliability are expressed on a scale that ranges from 0 for a totally unreliable instrument to 1.0 for a perfectly reliable one (although one has yet to be developed). If the scale is to be used for research purposes, test-retest and interrater reliability should be at least .70; if it is to be used for clinical purposes, then the minimal value should be .85 to .90 (Nunnally, 1978; Streiner & Norman, 2004). For homogeneous scales, the most common index is Cronbach's alpha (Cronbach, 1951), which should be in the range of .80 to .90 (Streiner, 2003).

At a more formal level, reliability states that a person's score on a test (using the term *test* very broadly to cover everything from a paper-and-pencil questionnaire to a measurement of his or her weight) consists of two parts: the "true" score plus some error, or observed score = true score + error. We never actually see the true score; it would be the result we would get if the person were tested an infinite number of times and we took the average. In essence, the true score is always distorted to some degree by the error, which is caused by limitations of the scale itself, variation in the person from one occasion to the next, simply putting down the wrong answer, and a host of other sources. Reliability is the ratio of the variability among the observed scores for all the people in our sample divided by the variability of the sum of the observed scores plus the error scores. This simple equation has a number of implications. First, and most obviously, we can improve the reliability of a scale by reducing the error. Because we assume that the error is random, one way to reduce it is by increasing the number of measurements; that is, testing the person more often, or using more observers, or increasing the number of items on the scale. The rationale is that, as the number of measures increases, the random errors will cancel each other out.

The second implication is somewhat counterintuitive. It is that if everyone got the same score on a scale, the reliability would be zero. At first glance, you may think that if everybody always got the same score, reliability would be perfect, because all the raters would always agree on the number, and each retest would yield the same score. But if we go back to the definition of reliability, we can see that if the variability of the observed scores is zero, then the reliability must be zero. This leads to another way of thinking about reliability—it is the ability of the test to differentiate among people. If everyone scores the same on the test (a phenomenon we see all too often when graduate or medical students are all rated as "above average"), the scale is useless; we cannot differentiate among the people, and the test gives us no information that we did not have before.

The third implication is that we cannot talk about *the* reliability of a scale. Because reliability is a function of the variability of the scores, a test that may be reliable for one group of people may not be reliable for another. A measure that can differentiate degrees of physical impairment among people in the general population, where the impairment can range from none to very severe, for instance, may be useless for trying to discriminate among patients in an arthritis clinic, where the range of impairment is much narrower. Thus, we talk about the reliability of a scale *for a particular group of people*.

VALIDITY

Reliability is a property that a scale must have, but it is not sufficient. It tells us that we are measuring something in a reproducible manner, but it does not ensure that we are actually measuring what we think we are. For example, two phrenologists can agree completely that a person has a bump over the brain area they say corresponds to conscientiousness, but this does not guarantee that they are assessing this attribute. Thus, a scale must also be evaluated regarding its *validity*. We can think of validity in a number of ways. Perhaps the easiest is that validity tells us if the test is measuring what we think it is. A more accurate description, though, would be that "validating a scale is really a process whereby we determine the degree of confidence we can place on inferences we make about people based on their scores from that scale" (Streiner & Norman, 2004, p. 146). In other words, what can we safely conclude about a person who gets a score of 17 on a certain depression inventory or 105 on an intelligence test? What do we now know about these people that we did not know before we had access to these scores?

What this leads us to is similar to the caveat mentioned for reliability: Just as a scale is neither reliable nor unreliable in isolation, but only within the context of its use with specific groups, we do not "validate" a scale. Instead, "one validates not a measuring instrument but rather some use to which the instrument is put" (Nunnally, 1970, p. 133).

The ways in which we validate a scale are different in one important regard from the process of reliability testing. There are only a limited number of reliability indices—test-retest, interrater, and internal consistency. Validity testing, though, is a process of *hypothesis testing*, and as such, there are an unlimited number of studies, with an equally wide range of designs, that we can perform. For example, if we were developing a scale to measure anxiety, a few of the many hypotheses we can test are the following:

- If our scale is valid, then it should correlate highly with other, previously validated anxiety instruments.
- People who are attending an anxiety disorders clinic should score higher than people who are not.
- People at the clinic should score higher before therapy than after.
- Scores should be higher among students 1 week before their final exam than 1 week after it.
- Those who score high on the scale should do

worse on complicated cognitive tasks than those who score low.

Each of the studies that confirms a hypothesis further strengthens the validity of the scale. A negative study could indicate that (a) the hypothesis is right, but our scale is not valid, (b) the scale is valid, but our hypothesis is wrong, or (c) both the hypothesis is wrong and our scale is not valid. Only further studies can differentiate among these alternatives.

Although the types of studies we can perform are limitless, they generally fall within three broad classes: *content validity, criterion validity,* and *construct validity*. Content validity was already mentioned within the context of selecting and writing the items. Very briefly, it ensures that the entire domain is covered (*content coverage*) and that nothing but the domain is included (*content relevance*).

Criterion validity is used when there is another, validated way of measuring the outcome (what is often referred to as the *gold standard*); it comes in two flavors: *concurrent* criterion validity and *predictive* criterion validity. In the former, we administer our new scale and the other one at the same time and assess the degree to which they are correlated with each other. The issue is why, if another scale already exists, we are trying to develop a new one. Leaving aside the unworthy (if prevalent) reason that we want a scale with our name on it, there are still some legitimate aims: to develop one that is shorter, or easier to use, or less expensive, or that contains a somewhat different set of items. In fact, at times we are willing to accept a somewhat less valid new test because it is not as invasive as the current gold standard; this is the case with the skin test for tuberculosis, which is not as accurate as a chest X ray but does not subject the person to ionizing radiation.

With predictive validity, the aim is to estimate an outcome that will occur at some time after the new test is administered. For example, the gold standard for whether a person has Alzheimer's disease (AD) is a brain biopsy, which, naturally, can be done only after the person has died. Consequently, there is an ongoing search for tests (such as neuropsychological assessments or brain scans) that can predict which patients will have the pathognomonic signs of AD when a biopsy is performed 5 or 10 years later. Similarly, tests used for admission to college or graduate school were developed using predictive validity, where the outcome was successful grad-uation 4 or 5 years later. Needless to say, during the validation phase, the test itself could not be used as a basis for the decision to admit or not; otherwise, the test would be predicting itself, at least in part (a phenomenon known as *criterion contamination*).

The most common situation in test develop-ment, though, is that there is no gold standard, either because the existing scales are seriously deficient and more resemble lead than gold, or because we are entering into an area that is rel-atively new and uncharted. Under these circum-stances, we use *construct validity* to help us develop the instrument. A construct, in psycho-logical jargon, is a variable that cannot be ob-served directly but only inferred from its sup-posed effect on variables that we can observe. For example, although we talk about anxiety all the time, no one has ever seen it. What we do observe are various behaviors (such as avoidance of certain situations or poor performance under stress), physiological signs (e.g., rapid heart rate or sweatiness), and expressed thoughts ("I feel afraid" or "My stomach is in knots"). We hy-pothesize that these tend to occur together be-cause they are all the outward manifestations of the construct of anxiety. Similarly, a large vo-cabulary, knowledge about the world, and the ability to solve abstract puzzles are all reflections of the underlying construct of intelligence, which itself cannot be seen directly (according to some conservative politicians and professors, be-cause it exists in such small quantities). Under these circumstances, our only recourse in vali-dating a scale is to devise hypotheses based on our understanding of the construct, the same way we generated hypotheses about an anxiety scale earlier in this section. Thus, construct va-lidity includes criterion validity but goes beyond it, also forming hypotheses that do not involve already existing tests. Because there is no end to the hypotheses we can generate, or the different groups for whom we want our scale to be valid, scale validation is a never-ending task.

USEFUL SCALES AND WHERE TO FIND THEM

Literally thousands of scales are available. The vast majority were developed for one study and have never been used since; a far smaller num-ber have been accepted as the gold standards in

their areas, because of either their excellent psy-chometric properties or simply inertia. Before anyone undertakes the long and laborious task of trying to develop a new one, he or she should definitely see what already exists. The following list mentions some of the most widely used scales; it is followed by a number of resources that can help the searcher find others.

Minnesota Multiphasic Personality Inventory (MMPI). The revision of the MMPI, called the MMPI-2, is the most widely used objec-tive personality test. It consists of over 550 items, subdivided into many scales that tap personality traits and the presence of psy-chopathology. There are literally thousands of articles relating to its reliability and valid-ity with various populations.

The Beck Depression Inventory (BDI). A self-administered, 21-item scale used to measure the intensity of depression in a clinical pop-ulation.

Center for Epidemiological Studies–Depression (CES-D). Another short (20-item) depression inventory. However, the CES-D was vali-dated to be used in community surveys, so it is better than the BDI for nonclinical pop-ulations.

Medical Outcomes Study Short Form-36 (SF-36). This scale was designed as a generic in-dicator of health status in the general popu-lation. It is widely used as an index of quality of life, and taps physical functioning, role limitations, bodily pain, social function-ing, mental health, energy, and general health perceptions.

State-Trait Anxiety Inventory (STAI). There are two versions of the same 20 questions: the State form asks how the person feels right now; the Trait form has the person re-spond as he or she generally feels. This scale is used primarily in nonclinical groups.

McGill Pain Questionnaire (MPQ). Often re-ferred to as the "Melzak," after the author's name, the MPQ measures the sensory-discriminative, motivational-affective, and cognitive-evaluative aspects of pain. Al-though some find it long and difficult to complete, it is still regarded as the gold stan-dard in the area.

Katz Adjustment Scales. Originally developed to measure social adjustment in psychiatric patients, the scales are now more widely used, even in survey research. One set of scales is completed by the patient and another by a relative. Despite their widespread use, relatively little validity data exist.

General Health Questionnaire (GHQ). Also known as the "Goldberg," the GHQ is a self-completed 60-item questionnaire designed to detect those with a diagnosable psychiatric problem. The GHQ indicates that such a problem exists; it cannot be used to assign a diagnosis. Many short forms exist, used often as a screening test in community surveys.

Affect Balance Scale. The "Bradburn" is a 10-item scale used to measure people's psychological reactions, both positive and negative, to events in their daily lives. It is seen as an index of psychological well-being and has been used in large population-based surveys in Canada.

Locus of Control. Originally developed by Rotter, there are now a number of such scales designed for different groups (e.g., children) or concerning specific areas (primarily health). The scales tap the degree to which people believe that events in their lives are controlled by them, by fate or chance, or by other people.

1. Streiner, D. L., & Norman, G. R. (2004). *Health measurement scales: A practical guide to their development and use* (3rd ed.). Oxford: Oxford University Press.

   An appendix in this book lists many books and computer bases that either reproduce the tests and evaluate them or simply give a summary of their intended uses.

2. McDowell, I., & Newell, C. (1996). *Measuring health* (2nd ed.). Oxford: Oxford University Press.

   This book reviews 88 scales in the areas of physical disability, psychological well-being, social health, depression, pain, general health and quality of life, and mental status. Each scale is described in detail, often with example questions, and its reliability and validity are reviewed. An excellent guide.

3. Corcoran, K., & Fischer, J. (2000). *Measures for clinical practice* (3rd ed.). New York: Free Press.

   This is a two-volume set; volume 1 covers scales for couples, families, and children; volume 2 covers scales for adults. Each scale is reproduced in full, and there is a de-

scription of the norms, scoring, reliability, and validity. A very handy resource.

4. *The mental measurements yearbook.* Lincoln, NE: Buros Institute of Mental Measurements.

   The first eight editions of the *MMY* were edited by Oscar Buros, and the set is often referred to as "Buros." After his death, there have been various editors of this excellent series. The latest volume, the 12th in the series, is edited by Conoley and Impara. Only published tests are listed, and most are reviewed by two or more experts in the field.

5. Keyser, D. J., & Sweetland, R. C. *Test critiques.* Kansas City, MO: Test Corporation of America.

   As of 1994, there were 10 volumes in this series of critical evaluations of published tests; there do not appear to have been any additions since then. Unlike the *MMY*, there is only one review per test, and the reference list is representative rather than exhaustive. However, the reviews tend to be longer and more detailed than in the *MMY*.

6. *Directory of unpublished experimental measures.* Washington, DC: American Psychological Association.

   One of the few comprehensive sources of scales that have appeared in journals but have not been published commercially. As of this date, there are seven volumes in the series, listing over 7,000 scales, with a minimal description of each.

SUMMARY

In many areas of science, in order to understand something, we must be able to measure it accurately. Once we leave the realm of objectively observed phenomena and try to assess subjective, internal states such as attitudes, beliefs, opinions, or health states, we must devise scales that can be completed by the people themselves or by outside observers. Scale development consists of a number of steps, involving devising and evaluating the individual items on the instrument, deciding on an appropriate response format, establishing that the test yields reproducible answers when completed at different times or by different people, and finally assessing whether it is truly measuring what we think it is. This is a time-consuming process, but one that is necessary to ensure that what we say about a phenomenon is actually so.

References

Cronbach, L. J. (1951). Coefficient alpha and the internal structure of tests. *Psychometrika, 16,* 297–334.

Goldberg, D. P. (1979). *Manual of the General Health Questionnaire.* Windsor: NFER Publishing.

Henson, R. K. (2001). Understanding internal consistency reliability estimates: A conceptual primer on coefficient alpha. *Measurement and Evaluation in Counseling and Development, 34,* 177–189.

Kanner, A. D., Coyne, J. C., Schaefer, C., & Lazarus, R. S. (1981). Comparison of two modes of stress measurement: Daily hassles and uplifts versus major life events. *Journal of Behavioral Medicine, 4,* 1–37.

Nunnally, J. C. (1970). *Introduction of psychological measurement.* New York: McGraw-Hill.

Nunnally, J. C. (1978). *Psychometric theory* (2nd ed.). New York: McGraw-Hill.

Streiner, D. L. (2003). Starting at the beginning: An introduction to coefficient alpha and internal consistency. *Journal of Personality Assessment, 80,* 99–103.

Streiner, D. L., & Norman, G. R. (2004). *Health measurement scales: A practical guide to their development and use* (3rd ed.). Oxford: Oxford University Press.

51   CLINICIAN AND PATIENT SATISFACTION WITH COMPUTER-ASSISTED DIAGNOSTIC ASSESSMENT IN COMMUNITY OUTPATIENT CLINICS

Edward J. Mullen, Christopher Lucas, Prudence Fisher, & William Bacon

Community mental health clinics often have difficulty designing intake procedures that facilitate accurate and timely diagnostic assessments. A delay in accurate identification of patient clinical problems, symptoms, and diagnoses at intake impedes timely treatment for patients who, increasingly, are in need of immediate therapeutic services. Too often initial assessments are not accurate because of lack of information or expertise. Garfield (2001) has described many of the problems and issues pertaining to the clinical diagnosis of psychopathology, including varying interpretations of clinical diagnosis, reliability, and validity. Kutchins and Kirk (1997) present a comprehensive analysis of issues pertaining to arriving at meaningful diagnoses based on the *Diagnostic and Statistical Manual of Mental Disorders* (American Psychiatric Association,

1994). In validation studies comparing standardized diagnostic assessment instruments with clinician-based diagnoses, clinician assessments have been found less reliable (Piacentini et al., 1993; Schwab-Stone et al., 1996). To address these problems, computerized diagnostic assessment software programs, both lay-administered and self-administered, have been developed to serve as decision supports for busy practitioners (Mullen, 1989; Mullen & Schuerman, 1990; Schuerman, Mullen, Stagner, & Johnson, 1989). These programs can be designed to gather, analyze, and report information collected from patients and collaterals, for use by practitioners, thus facilitating rapid assessment. However, it is not known if such programs would be found useful by practitioners, patients, and collaterals in community mental health clinic settings.

In this chapter we report findings from a field experiment designed to examine how one such computerized diagnostic program is viewed by clinicians and patients (children, youths, and caretakers) when used to support intake diagnostic assessments in urban, community-based mental health clinics. We examine clinician assessment of the effects of a computerized, lay-administered diagnostic assessment protocol. We report findings about the extent to which clinicians found the protocol and information provided helpful; the extent to which it changed their clinical evaluations; and, whether they found it made the intake interviews more difficult or upsetting to patients. We report effects on clinician, patient, and caretaker satisfaction with the intake session, including patients' feelings of being understood and of being able to discuss their concerns.[1] These data were gathered in a randomized field experiment, conducted between October 1995 and June 1999, in which clinicians from four clinics were randomly assigned to two assessment conditions, namely, the computer-assisted condition or the routine intake assessment condition. We used a crossover design to assure that clinicians could be observed in each condition, as well as during a baseline phase. The subjects were 26 clinicians, 192 patients, and their caretakers (usually a parent). The clinicians were male and female social workers and psychologists. The patient sample included female and male African Americans, Hispanics, Whites, and Asians patients, ranging from 9 to 17 years old.

The diagnostic assessment instrument examined in this study is a lay-administered, computerized version of the National Institute of Mental Health (NIMH) Diagnostic Interview Schedule for Children (C-DISC-IV), based on the *DSM-IV* and *International Statistical Classification of Diseases and Related Health Problems* (ISD-10) (World Health Organization, 1992). The C-DISC was originally developed under NIMH auspices for use in epidemiological research, where it has been used extensively. However, little is known about its usefulness in clinical practice. This is the first published report of findings from a field experiment examining the C-DISC in community mental health clinic practice. The development of the NIMH DISC and its use in prior research have been described previously. For a fuller description of the C-DISC-IV, as well as its reliability, the reader is referred to Shaffer, Fisher, Lucas, Dulcan, and Schwab-Stone (2000). Data pertaining to its performance in epidemiological surveys is presented in Shaffer et al. (1996). Criterion validity has been examined using clinician-based diagnoses as the standard (Schwab-Stone et al., 1996). The C-DISC's reliability has been the subject of extensive research (Breton, Bergeron, Valla, Berthiaume, & St-Georges, 1998; Fisher et al., 1997; Shaffer et al., 2000; Shaffer et al., 1993). The C-DISC was developed specifically for use with children and youths aged 9 through 18.

All participants completed signed consent forms prior to participation in the research. The research protocol was approved by the Columbia University Morningside Campus Institutional Review Board (IRB) on December 16, 1994 (Protocol No. 94/95-196A). All subsequent protocol modifications received IRB approval. Annual IRB approvals were received through completion of data collection in 1999.

METHOD

Our data come from four New York City community mental health outpatient clinics.[2] We used a crossover experimental design such that in each clinic, data were gathered using a simple checklist during a prospective baseline phase detailing each clinician's normal assessment practice and satisfaction. Following prospective baseline, an experimental phase was implemented such that, in each clinic, half of the clinicians were randomly assigned to the C-DISC assessment condition, and the other half continued with baseline data gathering, using only the checklist to record assessment and satisfaction data. In the C-DISC condition the C-DISC was administered by lay interviewers to outpatients (i.e., children and youths) as well as their caretakers (usually a parent) immediately prior to their first intake meeting. The C-DISC output was printed at the interview's conclusion and given to the clinician prior to the intake interview.

Each clinic was assigned to the experimental phase as soon as an average of 3 baseline cases per clinician was completed in the respective clinic. Clinicians were to remain in the C-DISC assessment condition until the clinician had completed an additional 5 cases. At that point the baseline clinicians were to be switched over to the C-DISC assessment condition until they had completed 5 cases. Each clinician was to have completed an average of 13 cases, 5 in each of the two experimental phase conditions, and 3 in the baseline phase. However, as reported in the following, this goal of 5 cases in each of the experimental phase conditions was not realized.

Instruments

Following the initial intake meeting, clinicians were asked to complete a series of checklists that provided basic information regarding each child and youth, a clinician satisfaction checklist (four items pertaining to the intake interview for all assessment conditions and an additional six items for the C-DISC intervention-only condition). In addition to the clinician checklists, also immediately following the intake interview, children, youths, and caretakers were asked to complete separate checklists containing three satisfaction questions pertaining to the initial intake interview.[3] We present findings about the six items that record how the clinician assessed the effects of the C-DISC on the intake session; the four items from the clinician satisfaction checklist; and the child, youth, and caretaker satisfaction items (three items for each respondent).

Statistical Procedures

Clinician assessment of the effects of the C-DISC protocol on the intake session is examined in two ways. First, the frequency distribution for each of the six C-DISC variables is presented. Second, we then compute a mean for each clinician for each of the six variables to compensate for the fact that each clinician is rep-

resented in the distribution with more than one case, and therefore the assessments are not independent.[4] Accordingly, we present the mean of these clinician means together with 95% confidence intervals for these means.

Reports of feeling understood and of being able to discuss concerns are examined first by describing the responses of the total sample. We then report differences between the two assessment conditions. We report point estimates and confidence intervals for the combined C-DISC and checklist-only responses for each of the 10 items regarding clinician, caretaker, and patient assessment. The effects of condition (C-DISC and checklist-only conditions), clinician, and clinic were examined using the Statistical Package for the Social Sciences General Linear Model Univariate procedure (SPSS GLM) for a mixed-effects nested design model.[5] In this model clinician is nested within clinic. In each analysis the dependent variable is a specific "satisfaction" variable; assessment condition is treated as a fixed factor; clinic and clinician are treated as random factors. The design estimates the main effects of assessment condition as well as of clinic, the interaction effect of assessment condition by clinic, and the effect of clinician nested in clinic.[6]

Sample

Clinics

The four study clinics are operated by a large, urban, multiservice, nonprofit mental health social service agency serving clients with a wide range of religious, ethnic, and economic backgrounds. The clinics are state-licensed outpatient mental health clinics providing services for emotional and social problems. Services for adults and children include evaluation and assessment; crisis intervention; and, individual, couple, family, and group therapy.

Clinicians and Patients

The clinicians were either full-time or part-time professionals with master's or doctoral degrees in either social work or psychology. The psychologists were state licensed, and the social workers were state certified.

Four clinics participated in the study's experimental phase.[7] The analysis pertaining to how the clinicians assessed the effects of the C-DISC on the intake session includes those 21 clinicians who responded to any one of those six items. Those 21 clinicians provided responses pertaining to their intake sessions with 87 patients and caretakers. The analysis pertaining to the C-DISC and checklist-only condition contrasts includes the responses of 26 clinicians, 192 patients, and the patients' caretakers.[8]

Data were collected regarding patient gender, age, and ethnicity or race. The demographic characteristics of those 87 patients exposed to the C-DISC and, therefore responding to the C-DISC items, are shown in Table 51.1.

The demographic characteristics of the sample of 192 patients included in the analysis of the experimental phase contrasts are shown in Table 51.2.

The experimental condition groups do not differ in distribution of gender,[9] age,[10] or ethnicity and race.[11]

RESULTS

C-DISC Helpfulness

Clinicians were asked to what extent they agreed with the statement that the C-DISC had been helpful. As shown in Table 51.3 the modal view is "agree somewhat." However, most (57.5% or 50 respondents) disagreed with the statement or were neutral.

These responses were obtained from 21 clinicians assessing 87 cases. The clinicians' modal number of cases was five but ranged from one to five. Accordingly, some clinicians were overrepresented in the sample shown in Table 51.3, whereas others were underrepresented. To deal with this, we calculated each clinician's mean rating and averaged these means. This "mean of means" is a rating of "neutral."[12] The 95% confidence interval for these "clinician means" has a lower bound of 1.7 and an upper bound of 2.4, which is in the "neutral" range. Eighty-six percent (18) of the clinicians reported that the C-DISC had been "helpful" in at least one of their cases.

Changed Clinician Evaluation

Clinicians were asked to what extent they agreed with the statement that the C-DISC had changed their evaluation of the patients. As shown in Table 51.4, the modal response is "disagree strongly." In approximately 22% (19) of the cases the clinicians did agree that the C-DISC had changed the evaluation.

The mean of the clinician means is 1.41, midway between "neutral" and "disagree some-

TABLE 51.1. Demographics of Patients Exposed to C-DISC

Gender		Race/ethnicity				Age	
Female	Male	African American or Black	Latino/a	White	Other	Median and mode	Range
42 (48.3%)	45 (51.7%)	37 (42.5%)	26 (29.0%)	17 (19.5%)	7 (8%)	12 10	9–17

TABLE 51.2. Demographics of Patients in Experimental Phase

Gender[a]		Race/ethnicity[b]				Age	
Female	Male	African American or Black	Latino/a	White	Other	Median and mode	Range
89 (47.1%)	100 (52.9%)	62 (35.2%)	54 (30.7%)	44 (25%)	16 (9.1%)	13 10	9–17

a. Gender was available for 189 of the 192 patients.
b. Race/ethnicity was available for 176 of the 192 patients.

what." The 95% confidence interval for the mean has a lower bound of 1.0 and an upper bound of 1.7, in the "disagree somewhat" to "neutral" range. While the tendency was to disagree with this statement, approximately 57%

(12) of the clinicians report that the C-DISC had "changed" their evaluations in at least one of their cases.

Made Intake More Difficult

Clinicians were asked to what extent they agreed with the statement that the C-DISC had made their intake interviews with the patients more difficult. As shown in Table 51.5, the modal response is "disagree strongly."

The mean of the clinician means is 1.09, "disagree somewhat." The 95% confidence interval for the mean has a lower bound of 0.6 and an upper bound of 1.5, in the "disagree somewhat" range. Approximately 52% (11) of the clinicians report that the C-DISC had made their interviews "more difficult" in at least one of their cases.

Made Intake Interview with Caretaker More Difficult

Clinicians were asked to what extent they agreed with the statement that the C-DISC had made

TABLE 51.3 Agreement with Statement That C-DISC Was Helpful

	Frequency	Percent	Cumulative percent
Disagree strongly (0)	10	11.5	11.5
Disagree somewhat (1)	18	20.7	32.2
Neutral (2)	22	25.3	57.5
Agree somewhat (3)	33	37.9	95.4
Agree strongly (4)	4	4.6	100.0
Total	87	100.0	

TABLE 51.4 Agreement with Statement That CDISC Had Changed Intake Evaluation

	Frequency	Percent	Valid percent	Cumulative percent
Disagree strongly (0)	26	29.9	30.2	30.2
Disagree somewhat (1)	24	27.6	27.9	58.1
Neutral (2)	17	19.5	19.8	77.9
Agree somewhat (3)	15	17.2	17.4	95.3
Agree strongly (4)	4	4.6	4.7	100.0
Total	86	98.9	100.0	
Missing	1	1.1		
Total	87	100.0		

TABLE 51.5 Agreement with Statement that C-DISC Made Intake Interview with Children or Youths More Difficult

	Frequency	Percent	Valid percent	Cumulative percent
Disagree strongly (0)	40	46.0	50.0	50.0
Disagree somewhat (1)	12	13.8	15.0	65.0
Neutral (2)	7	8.0	8.8	73.8
Agree somewhat (3)	17	19.5	21.3	95.0
Agree strongly (4)	4	4.6	5.0	100.0
Total	80	92.0	100.0	
Missing	7	8.0		
Total	87	100.0		

their intake interview with the caretaker more difficult. As shown in Table 51.6, the modal response is "disagree strongly."

The mean of the clinician means is 1.0, "disagree somewhat." The 95% confidence interval for the mean has a lower bound of 0.5350 and an upper bound of 1.4107, in the "disagree somewhat" range. About 52% (11) of the clinicians report that the C-DISC had made their interviews "more difficult" in at least one of their cases.

Upset Patient

Clinicians were asked to what extent they agreed with the statement that the C-DISC interview had upset the patient. As shown in Table 51.7, the modal response is "disagree strongly" (50.6%).

The mean of the clinician means is 0.9, between "disagree strongly" and "disagree somewhat." The 95% confidence interval for the mean has a lower bound of 0.5 and an upper bound of 1.3, in the "disagree somewhat" range. One third (7) of the clinicians report that the

C-DISC had "upset" a patient in at least one of their cases.

Upset Caretaker

Clinicians were asked to what extent they agreed with the statement that the C-DISC interview had upset the caretaker. As shown in Table 51.8, the modal response is "disagree strongly" (59%).

The mean of the clinician means was 0.8, between "disagree strongly" and "disagree somewhat." The 95% confidence interval for the mean has a lower bound of 0.4 and an upper bound of 1.1, in the "disagree somewhat" range. Slightly over one fourth (28.6%) of the clinicians report that the C-DISC had "upset" a caretaker in at least one of their cases.

Assessment of Intake Experiences

Our research also examined questions about how clinicians, patients, and caretakers assessed their intake interview experiences. Tables 51.9 through 51.11 provide point estimates and con-

TABLE 51.6 Agreement with Statement that C-DISC Made Intake with Caretaker More Difficult

	Frequency	Percent	Valid percent	Cumulative percent
Disagree strongly (0)	45	51.7	56.3	56.3
Disagree somewhat (1)	11	12.6	13.8	70.0
Neutral (2)	8	9.2	10.0	80.0
Agree somewhat (3)	13	14.9	16.3	96.3
Agree strongly (4)	3	3.4	3.8	100.0
Total	80	92.0	100.0	
Missing	7	8.0		
Total	87	100.0		

TABLE 51.7 Agreement with Statement That C-DISC Upset Patient

	Frequency	Percent	Valid percent	Cumulative percent
Disagree strongly (0)	40	46.0	50.6	50.6
Disagree somewhat (1)	15	17.2	19.0	69.6
Neutral (2)	11	12.6	13.9	83.5
Agree somewhat (3)	10	11.5	12.7	96.2
Agree strongly (4)	3	3.4	3.8	100.0
Total	79	90.8	100.0	
Missing	8	9.2		
Total	87	100.0		

fidence intervals for responses to each of 10 questions designed to address those questions. The response choices with numerical equivalents are presented in table footnotes.[13] The clinicians' assessments of the intake experience are shown in Table 51.9.

As shown, all four mean assessments are near the "substantial" rating (a rating of 2 for "satisfaction" and 3 for the remaining variables), ranging from "not at all" to "fully" for the patient's ability to discuss concerns, and from "minimally ("partially or less") to "fully" for the other three assessments. The patients' assessments of the intake interview experience are shown in Table 51.10.

As shown, the patients rated their experiences with the intake interview very positively. Typically they were "very satisfied" (rating of 2), and they felt understood and able to discuss their concerns "fairly well" (rating of 2) to

"completely" (rating of 3). Nevertheless, the range for all three variables was from "not at all" to "completely." The caretakers' assessments are shown in Table 51.11.

Caretakers rated their experiences with the intake interview very positively. With little variation they were either "very satisfied" (rating of 2) or "completely satisfied" (rating of 3), and they felt understood and able to discuss their concerns "fairly well" (rating of 2) to "completely" (rating of 3). None were "not at all" satisfied; only one (.5%) did not feel understood at all; three (1.6%) reported they were not able to discuss their concerns at all.

In summary, these findings suggest a largely positive assessment of the intake interview by clinicians, patients, and caretakers, but with some small percentage more negative, especially among patients.

TABLE 51.8 Agreement with Statement That C-DISC Upset Caretaker

	Frequency	Percent	Valid percent	Cumulative percent
Disagree strongly (0)	46	52.9	59.0	59.0
Disagree somewhat (1)	12	13.8	15.4	74.4
Neutral (2)	11	12.6	14.1	88.5
Agree somewhat (3)	8	9.2	10.3	98.7
Agree strongly (4)	1	1.1	1.3	100.0
Total	78	89.7	100.0	
Missing	9	10.3		
Total	87	100.0		

TABLE 51.9 Clinician Assessment of Intake Interview Experience[a]

Assessment Variable	Mean (5% trimmed mean)	Standard deviation (range)	95% Confidence interval for mean
Satisfaction with intake session (recoded)[b]	1.98 (1.97)	.680 (1–3)	1.88–2.08
Understands patient's concerns[c]	2.87 (2.87)	.695 (1–4)	2.76–2.97
Patient's ability to discuss concerns[d]	2.60 (2.63)	.886 (0–4)	2.47–2.73
Caretaker's ability to discuss concerns[e]	2.97 (2.98)	.744 (1–4)	2.85–3.08

a. Clinician response choices were "not at all" (0); "minimally" (1); "partially" (2); "substantially" (3); and "fully" (4). Regarding the "satisfaction" variable, because so few "not at all" and "minimally" responses occurred (1.5%, $n = 3$), these were combined into "partially or less" (1), resulting in a scale of 1 to 3.

b. 174 of 192 (90.6%).

c. 175 of 192 (91.1%).

d. 174 of 192 (90.6%).

e. 174 of 192 (90.6%).

TABLE 51.10 Patient Experience of Intake Interview Experience[a]

Assessment Variable	Mean (5% trimmed mean)	Standard deviation (range)	95% Confidence interval for mean
Satisfaction after intake interview[b]	2.05 (2.06)	.796 (1–3)	1.94–2.17
Extent clinician understood concerns[c]	2.50 (2.56)	.645 (1–3)	2.41–2.60
Ability to discuss concerns	2.25 (2.28)	.743 (1–3)	2.14–2.36

a. Valid responses were available from 183 to 192 (95.3%) patients.

b. Patient response choices were "not at all satisfied," "slightly satisfied," "moderately satisfied," "very satisfied," and "completely satisfied." Because few "not at all satisfied" and "slightly satisfied" ratings were recorded, these two categories were combined with "moderately satisfied." The recoded categories are "less than very satisfied" (1); "very satisfied" (2); and "completely satisfied" (3).

c. For this variable as well as the next variable, "report of ability to discuss concerns," the ratings were "not at all," "slightly," "fairly well," and "completely." Because few "not at all" ratings were recorded, this category was combined with "slightly." The recorded categories are "slightly or less" (1); "fairly well" (2); and "completely" (3).

TABLE 51.11 Caretaker Assessment of Intake Interview Experience

Assessment Variable	Mean (5% trimmed mean)	Standard deviation (range)	95% Confidence interval for mean
Satisfaction after intake interview[a]	2.10 (2.11)	.729 (1–3)	1.99–2.20
Clinician understood concerns[b]	2.65 (2.71)	.562 (1–3)	2.56–2.73
Ability to discuss concerns	2.47 (2.52)	.616 (1–3)	2.38–2.56

a. 186 of 192 (96.9%) valid responses were included. Caretaker response choices were "not at all satisfied," "slightly satisfied," "moderately satisfied," "very satisfied," and "completely satisfied." Because few "not at all satisfied" and "slightly satisfied" ratings were recorded, these two categories were combined with "moderately satisfied." The recoded categories are "less than very satisfied" (1); "very satisfied" (2); and "completely satisfied" (3).

b. 187 of 192 (97.4%) valid responses were included in the analysis for this and the next variable. For this variable as well as the next variable, "caretaker's report of ability to discuss concerns," the ratings were "not at all," "slightly," "fairly well," and "completely." Because few "not at all" ratings were recorded, this category was combined with "slightly." The recoded categories are "slightly or less" (1); "fairly well" (2); and "completely" (3).

Experimental Condition Differences

We were interested in the extent to which clinician, patient, and caretaker assessments of their experiences with the intake interview differed between the C-DISC and checklist-only conditions. Accordingly, we used the GLM Univariate procedure as described previously to estimate the main effects of assessment condition as well as of clinic, the interaction effect of assessment condition by clinic, and the effect of clinician nested in clinic.[14]

In these analyses only one significant difference was found pertaining to the main effect of the assessment condition. Clinicians reported

that they thought caretakers were able to discuss their concerns to a greater extent in the C-DISC condition than in the checklist-only condition.[15]

However, contrary to this report from the clinicians, caretakers themselves reported a greater ability to discuss their concerns in the checklist-only condition than in the C-DISC condition in three of the four clinics.[16] A final significant finding was also an interaction effect between condition and clinic for a caretaker assessment, namely, the caretakers' assessment of the extent to which clinicians understood their concerns.[17] This significant difference was due to one clinic wherein clinicians were seen by caretakers as less understanding in the C-DISC condition than in the checklist-only condition. In other clinics, differences were not marked. These condition by clinic interaction effects were not predicted, and they are difficult to interpret. Similarly, it is difficult to explain the discrepancy between the clinicians' and caretakers' assessments on what would appear to be the similar factors. Nevertheless, inspection of the clinic mean ratings in the profile plots (not reproduced here) shows that one of the four clinics accounted for much of this variance. Accordingly, it may be that caretakers were reacting to some organizational factors, such as organizational climate, that may have been negatively affected by the presence of the C-DISC procedure (Schiff, 2000). It could also be that caretakers had experienced the C-DISC interview as opening up and identifying a number of patient symptoms and problem areas that were not explored or discussed in the subsequent intake interview with the clinicians. If this happened, it is understandable that the caretakers could experience these clinicians as providing less opportunity for discussion and being less understanding. However, since the C-DISC had opened up much for discussion it is possible the clinicians experienced the caretakers as better able to discuss their concerns after exposure to the C-DISC. This is an explanation that requires future research attention.

No other significant effects were found in the GLM Univariate analysis.

CONCLUSIONS

Generalizations from our findings are limited by two factors. First, our sample size was small. Fewer clinics, clinicians, and patients were secured for the study than originally planned, making the sample size smaller and more homogeneous. Second, the clinicians studied are highly skilled practitioners. They are experienced diagnosticians, with master's or doctoral training in social work or psychology, as well as extensive in-service training. They are routinely provided psychiatric consultation to assist initial diagnostic assessment. They practice in community mental health clinics operated by one of the nation's most reputable mental health organizations. Accordingly, the additional information provided by the C-DISC may not have had the effects it would have with less highly trained clinicians in less supportive clinics. With these sample limitations in mind, we draw a number of conclusions.

The finding that 86% of the clinicians say the C-DISC had been "helpful" in at least one of their cases is clinically important. Since clinicians in this study typically carried five cases, this indicates that for most clinicians, in at least one of five cases the C-DISC provided information that was deemed helpful. Indeed, for some clinicians the C-DISC was found to be helpful in even more of their cases because in the entire sample approximately two fifths of the cases reportedly benefited from the C-DISC information. The belief that a large number of well-trained clinicians would find the C-DISC overly intrusive or simply redundant is not supported by this finding.

Similarly, the value of the C-DISC information to the clinician is supported by the second major finding, namely, that the majority of clinicians (57%) reported that the C-DISC had "changed" their evaluations in at least one of their cases, and that in about one fifth of the cases (22.1%) the clinicians said that the C-DISC report had "changed" their evaluations. Again, these findings are especially noteworthy because the clinicians in this study were all well-trained, experienced practitioners. Although there is no clear guideline to determine how often the C-DISC information should be "helpful" or how often it should be influential in changing a clinical evaluation, arguably, the proportion of cases benefiting in this study is clinically significant.

Concerns regarding negative effects of the C-DISC are not supported by our findings, since approximately one half of the clinicians report that the C-DISC never made an interview with a child or youth or caretaker more difficult. Indeed, in approximately three quarters of the child and youth interviews and four fifths of the caretaker interviews, the C-DISC did not make the intake interviews "more difficult." Similarly, most clinicians reported that the C-DISC had never upset a child, youth, or caretaker whom they saw for intake interviews, and most children, youths, and caretakers in the study were not seen as upset by the C-DISC. These findings suggest that in most cases the benefits attributed by the clinicians to the C-DISC information are not offset by risks to patients or caretakers.

However, it is troubling to find that almost half of the clinicians reported that the C-DISC protocol made their intake interview "more difficult" for at least one of their patients and that this occurred in approximately one out of four cases. We did not ask about the reasons the C-DISC made the interviews more difficult. It is possible the increased difficulty was due to the amount of information provided from the computer reports, pressure felt from exposure to a new procedure being introduced into the intake process, or patients being tired out after completing the C-DISC interview. Similarly, the finding that one third of the clinicians reported that the C-DISC had "upset" a child or youth in at least one of their cases, and that approximately one of four clinicians report this for caretakers as well, is problematic. However, it should be noted that this perception may not have been a true reflection of how the patients and caretakers actually experienced the C-DISC. On balance, the benefits attributable to the C-DISC noted earlier (helpfulness and changing the evaluation) may well offset these negative perceptions. Nevertheless, if the C-DISC is to be introduced into routine clinical practice such as in populations similar to those in this study, this rate of perceived negative effects should be considered unacceptable. Additional research is needed to better understand why the C-DISC may be upsetting to some patients, as well as why it would make some intake interviews more difficult for clinicians. Especially useful in this regard would be qualitative studies, including focus group discussions with clinicians, patients, and caretakers. Also needed is further developmental work on the C-DISC, so as to minimize intrusiveness, possibly by shortening the protocol and experimenting with self-administration. Indeed, since completion of this study, the reports generated by the C-DISC have been modified significantly to make them more user (clinician) friendly. If the difficulty reported here was due to the clinician's need to wade through lengthy computer-generated reports, this might be lessened with the new versions. Also since completion of this study, the C-DISC interview has been modified so that it now takes less time to administer, which may make the protocol more palatable. Another possible way of increasing the acceptability and utility of the C-DISC procedure is to strengthen clinician control over its administration so that clinicians perceive it as a diagnostic aid that is under their control.

Our findings suggest a largely positive assessment of the intake interview by clinicians, patients, and caretakers. We have found no meaningful differences between the two assessment conditions other than those reported pertaining to the caretakers' experiences. We conclude that there is no evidence indicating that the introduction of a computerized assessment protocol such as the C-DISC would affect, one way or another, clinician or patient assessments of their experiences with the intake interview, when these are already largely positive. The reported effects on the caretakers' experiences deserve further study.

These findings are important, but those pertaining to other questions addressed in this study need to be examined before drawing firm conclusions. Questions remain regarding the C-DISC's effects on improving clinical assessment, increasing efficiency of the assessment, and improving treatment planning. As the data from this study are analyzed further, these questions will be addressed and reported in future publications.

ACKNOWLEDGMENTS The project described was supported by Grants Numbers 5 R01 MH53833, 5 P30 MH60570, and K20 MH01298 from the National Institute of Mental Health (NIMH). Its contents are solely the responsibility of the authors and do not necessarily represent the official views of the NIMH. This chapter is a revision of Mullen, E. J. (1999, October). *Using assessment instruments in social work practice.* Paper presented at the second annual meeting of the International Inter-centre Network for Evaluation of Social Work Practice: Researcher–Practitioner Partnerships and Research Implementation, Stockholm, Sweden.

Notes

This chapter is based on data and experiences from research conducted under subcontract to the Center for the Study of Social Work Practice (CSSWP) (New York State Research Foundation for Mental Hygiene Contract No. SDMHCU00642601). The multisite study was initially funded by the National Institute of Mental Health Grant No. 1R01MH052822-01 (02) (03). The principal investigator at the New York State Psychiatric Institute was David Shaffer, M.D., and the coinvestigators were Prudence Fisher, Ph.D., and Christopher Lucas, M.D. The investigators for the subcontract were principal investigator Edward J. Mullen, D.S.W.; coinvestigators Robert Abramovitz, M.D.; William Bacon, Ph.D.; and Bruce Grellong,

Ph.D. Prior investigators included Helene Jackson, Ph.D., and Jennifer Magnabosco, Ph.D. The CSSWP research coordinator is Gretchen Borges, M.S. The CSSWP research assistants were James A. Catalano, Ph.D.; Rachelle E. Kammer, M.S.; Steven P. Lohrer, Ph.D.; L. Donald McVinney, Ph.D.; Leslie M. Pereira, Ph.D.; Hilda P. Rivera, Ph.D.; Anne C. Singh Stephan, M.S.; Miriam Bellecca; and Danielle Barry, whose work contributed significantly to this chapter. The original plan included subcontracts for implementation in two locations, New Jersey and New York City. The CSSWP implemented the study in the New York City sites; this chapter is limited to those sites.

1. Data from this study have been used to address additional questions and issues. The association between organizational culture variables and satisfaction with intake sessions have been reported previously (Schiff, 2000). Issues pertaining to implementation of this study are examined in Mullen (1998). Congruence in problem identification is examined in Lynn et al. (in preparation). Effects on clinician diagnosis, symptom identification, and treatment planning will be examined in forthcoming publications.

2. The description of the design presented here refers only to those aspects pertinent to the data presented. Furthermore, as originally proposed, the design called for larger sample sizes (more clinics, clinicians, and patients), as well as lengthier phases. Because fewer clinics, clinicians, and patients were sampled than planned, design modifications were made. Power calculations described in the proposal were based on larger sample sizes than realized. Accordingly, those calculations are not pertinent here, and they are not presented because they would be misleading.

3. Also collected from the clinicians were data pertaining to number of visits taken to complete the initial assessment, diagnoses (36 items), current Global Assessment of Functioning score, a symptoms checklist (29 symptoms), a recommended treatment checklist (28 items), and a listing of clinical problems presented. In addition, patients and caretakers competed a problem list indicating what they had wanted to talk about in the interview. These data are not presented in this chapter but will be the subject of future publications.

4. We were curious about whether or not our assumption that there would be a "clinician effect" or "bias" would be supported by the data. Also, we were curious about whether or not there would be a "clinic effect." Accordingly, to examine the effects of clinicians and clinics on each of the C-DISC variable ratings, the SPSS's GLM Univariate procedure for a mixed-effects nested design model was used. In this model clinicians were nested within clinics. The dependent variable in each analysis was the specific C-DISC variable. In these six analyses, clinic was treated as a fixed factor with four levels, and clinician was treated as a random factor with varying levels in each clinic. In these analyses, "clinic" was treated as a fixed factor under the assumption that the four clinics constitute the entire set of clinics of concern. In each analysis, a custom model was specified, which included clinic as a factor and clinician nested within clinic. The Type III sum of squares method was used. When significant differences were found, to determine which clinics had clinicians that were significantly different, four sets of custom hypotheses were tested, one for each clinic. In only one of these analyses was the clinic effect significant, namely, pertaining to the variable "C-DISC helpfulness." The clinician (clinic) effect was significant in all six analyses ($p < =.10$ level, two-tailed).

5. SPSS for Windows, version 11.0.1 (Type III sum of squares method).

6. In these analyses, the omitted term, condition by clinician (clinic) becomes residual error. Throughout, alpha is set at .05, two-tailed.

7. The New York City site evaluation included data from 50 clinicians, eight clinics, and 352 patients. The 352 patients included 141 from the prospective baseline group; 97 from the C-DISC-administered assessment condition group (experimental phase); 95 from the checklist-only assessment condition group (experimental phase); and 19 cases in the retrospective baseline. Only data pertaining to the experimental phase are included in this analysis. Eighteen clinicians in four clinics completed the prospective baseline as well as both conditions during the experimental phase, providing data concerning 238 youths. Of these 18 clinicians, 12 had completed at least 3 cases in each of the 3 conditions. Nine clinicians completed at least 5 cases in both the experimental phase conditions (e.g., C-DISC and checklist-only conditions). Of these, 7 clinicians completed at least 3 cases in the prospective baseline as well.

8. Of these, four clinicians completed only C-DISC condition cases, and another four completed only checklist-only condition cases. In the analysis pertaining to clinician assessment of the effects of the C-DISC protocol on the intake session, one of the clinicians included in the C-DISC and checklist-only condition contrasts was excluded because that clinician provided no data regarding that clinician's two cases, although these were C-DISC condition cases. Also, in that analysis eight cases were excluded because no data were provided by the clinician for any of the C-DISC variables examined. Again, with only one exception, none of those clinicians provided data pertaining to the variables examined regarding the C-DISC and checklist-only condition contrasts. However, the data requested from their respective patients and caretakers were provided for all these cases, so the cases are included in those analyses. Variables measuring clinician assessments for those patients and caretakers are treated as missing data for all but one of these cases.

9. Pearson chi-square $= .149$, $df = 1$, $p = .70$.

10. $t = -.816$, $df = 174$, $p = .415$.

11. Pearson chi-square $= 6.906$, $df = 5$, $p = .228$.

12. The mean was 2.06 on a scale ranging from 0 ("strongly disagree") to 4 ("strongly disagree").

13. Missing values excluded cases pairwise.

14. As previously described, the design plan called for each clinician to complete five cases in each of the experimental conditions. However, only nine clinicians completed this many cases. Indeed, eight clinicians completed cases in only one of the experimental conditions. Nine others completed cases in both conditions, but fewer than five in each.

15. Estimated marginal means: C-DISC condition $= 3.129$ and checklist condition $= 2.818$; $F = 7.912$, $df = 1$, $p = .030$. The scale for this and all subsequently present clinician ratings ranged from 0 to 4, with 3 indicating "partially" satisfied.

16. For these condition by clinic estimated marginal means the statistics are $F = 2.609$, $df = 3$, $p = .054$; C-DISC condition $n = 96$, and checklist-only condition $n = 91$; clinic n's $= 32$, 18, 96, and 41, respectively.

17. For the condition by clinic estimated marginal means the statistics are $F = 3.109$, $df = 3$, $p = .028$; C-DISC condition $n = 96$, and checklist-only condition $n = 91$; clinic n's $= 32$, 18, 96, and 41, respectively.

References

American Psychiatric Association. (1994). *Diagnostic and statistical manual of mental disorders.* 4th ed. Washington, DC: American Psychiatric Association.

Breton, J., Bergeron, L., Valla, J., Berthiaume, C., & St-Georges, M. (1998). Diagnostic Interview Schedule for Children (DISC-2.25) in Quebec: Reliability findings in light of the MECA study. *Journal of the American Academy of Child and Adolescent Psychiatry, 37,* 1167–1174.

Fisher, P., Lucas, C., Shaffer, D., Schwab-Stone, M., Dulcan, M., Gaae, F., Lichtman, J., Willourghby, S., & Gerald, J. (1997, October). *Diagnostic Interview Schedule for Children, Version IV (DISC-IV): Test-retest reliability in a clinical sample.* Paper presented at the meeting of the American Academy of Child and Adolescent Psychiatry, Toronto, Canada.

Garfield., S. L. (2001). Methodological issues in clinical diagnosis. In P. B. Sutker & H. E. Adams (Eds.), *Comprehensive handbook of psychopathology* (3rd ed., pp. 29–51). New York: Kluwer Academic/Plenum.

Kutchins, H., & Kirk, S. A. (1997). *Making us crazy: DSM: The psychiatric bible and the creation of mental disorders.* New York: Free Press.

Lynn, C. J., Abramovitz, R., Bacon, W., Fisher, P. W., Grellong, B., Lucas, C. P., & Mullen, E. J. (in preparation). Urban child mental health need: Youth, parent, and clinician perspectives on presenting problems.

Mullen, E. J. (1989). The use of expert systems in research on community mental health services. In *Final Report-NH-90-NH-Workshop on Social Work Research and Community-Based Mental Health Services.* Bethesda, MD: National Technical Information Service, NIMH Division of Biometry and Applied Sciences.

Mullen, E. J. (1998). Linking the university and the social agency in collaborative evaluation research: Principles and examples. *Scandinavian Journal of Social Welfare, 7,* 152–158.

Mullen, E. J., & Schuerman, J. R. (1990). Expert systems and the development of knowledge in social welfare. In L. Videka-Sherman & W. J. Reid (Eds.), *Advances in clinical social work research* (pp. 67–83). Silver Spring, MD: National Association of Social Workers.

Piacentini, J., Shaffer, D., Fisher, P., Schwab-Stone, M., Davies, M., & Gioia, P. (1993). The Diagnostic Interview Schedule for Children–Revised Version (DISC-R): III. Concurrent criterion validity. *Journal of the American Academy of Child Adolescent Psychiatry, 32,* 658–665.

Schiff, J. (2000). *The measurement of organizational culture in mental health clinics and the correlation of cultural dimensions with satisfaction with service.* Unpublished doctoral dissertation, Columbia University.

Schuerman, J. R., Mullen, E. J., Stagner, M., & Johnson, P. (1989). First generation expert systems in social welfare. *Computers in Human Services, 4* (1–2), 111–122.

Schwab-Stone, M., Shaffer, D., Dulcan, M., Jenson, P., Fisher, P., Bird, H., Goodman, S., Lahey, B., Lichtman, J., Canino, G., Rubio-Stipec, M., & Rae, D. (1996). Criterion validity of the NIMH Diagnostic Interview Schedule for Children Version 2.3 (DISC-2.3). *Journal of the American Academy of Child and Adolescent Psychiatry, 35,* 878–888.

Shaffer, D., Fisher, P., Dulcan, M., Davies, M., Piacentini, J., Schwab-Stone, M., Lahey, B., Bourdon, K., Jensen, P., Bird, H., Canino, G., Regier, D. (1996). The NIMH Diagnostic Interview Schedule for Children Version 2.3 (DISC-2.3): Description, acceptability, prevalence rates, and performance in the MECA study. *Journal of the American Academy of Child and Adolescent Psychiatry, 35,* 865–877.

Shaffer, D., Fisher, P., Lucas, C., Dulcan, M., & Schwab-Stone, M. (2000). NIMH Diagnostic Interview Schedule for Children, Version IV (NIMH DISC-IV): Description, differences from previous versions, and reliability of some common diagnoses. *Journal of the American Academy of Child and Adolescent Psychiatry, 39,* 28–38.

Shaffer, D., Schwab-Stone, M., Fisher, P., Cohen, P., Piacentini, J., Davis, M., Edelbrock, C., & Regier, D. (1993). The Diagnostic Interview for Children–Revised Version (DISC-R): I. Preparation, field testing, interrater reliability, and acceptabil-

ity. *Journal of the American Academy of Child and Adolescent Psychiatry, 32,* 643–650.

World Health Organization. (1992). *International Statistical Classification of Diseases and Related Health Problems, 1989 revision.* Geneva: World Health Organization.

52 PSYCHOSOCIAL MEASURES FOR ASIAN PACIFIC AMERICANS

Marianne R. Yoshioka & Tazuko Shibusawa

Asian Pacific Americans (APAs) are one of the fastest growing minority groups in the United States. According to the 2000 census, there are approximately 12.5 million APAs, who constitute 4.5 percent of the U.S. population. In 2020 this number is expected to increase to 6% (Lai & Arguelles, 2003). APAs are a diverse population embracing approximately 50 ethnic groups (Chun, Enomoto, & Sue, 1996) and several religions, including Buddhism, Christianity, Hinduism, and Islam. These ethnic groups are often categorized within four large subgroups: East Asians (e.g., Chinese, Koreans, and Japanese); South Asians (e.g., Indians and Pakistanis); Southeast Asians (e.g., Vietnamese and Cambodians); and Pacific Islanders (e.g., native Hawaiian and Samoans). Currently, 15% of APAs identify as multiracial (Lai & Arguelles, 2003).

Past research suggests that APAs as a group present different psychosocial behavior patterns than do Caucasian Americans. Studies have found that, as a group, APAs present lower levels of self-disclosure in a therapeutic context (Steel,

1991); are less emotionally expressive in public interactions (Lai & Linden, 1993; Matsumoto, 1993); and are less assertive (Cheng, 1990). Okazaki (2000) reported that APAs, in comparison to White Americans, report more depressive symptoms (Chang, 1996; Okazaki, 1997); social anxiety symptoms (Okazaki, 1997; Zane, Sue, Hu, & Kwon, 1991); cognitive anxiety symptoms (Lai & Linden, 1993); and other signs of maladjustment (Abe & Zane, 1990). Although this evidence may seem very compelling, researchers and practitioners have questioned if these differences are a product of real difference in mental health behavior or a reflection of cultural bias in measurement. By using measures designed for non-APA populations with APA groups, an accurate appraisal of psychosocial phenomena may be masked by cross-cultural differences in language and behavior. The goal of this chapter is to examine the ways by which APA culture may influence the measurement of psychosocial phenomena and the types of measures that have been developed for use with this population.

IMPACT OF ASIAN CULTURE ON THE MEASUREMENT OF PSYCHOSOCIAL PHENOMENA

Despite the diversity across different APA ethnic communities, APAs share a number of traditional cultural traits that manifest in behavioral and cognitive preferences that distinguish them from White Americans. These cultural traits include collectivism, nonegocentric constructions of selfhood, emphasis on experience over verbal expression of emotions, and coping styles.

Collectivism

Traditional Asian cultures are collectivist in orientation and characterized by a respect for authority. In keeping with conceptions of selflessness, self-renunciation, or self in relation to others (Ho, 1995), Asian values emphasize harmonious interpersonal relationships and interdependence. The interests of the family take precedence over those of the individual (Kitao & Kikumura, 1976; Jung, 1969; Root, Ho, & Sue, 1986). For example, in the Filipino culture, value is placed on "smooth relationships," and conflicts between people are minimized (Agbayani-Siewert, 1994). People are discouraged from displaying anger or aggression and are expected to behave in a passive and cooperative manner (Agbayani-Siewert, 1994).

Within these traditions are powerful messages about the nature of personhood, health, and well-being that are the foundation on which experiences of wellness, illness, and proper behavior are understood and communicated. In traditional Asian cultures, individuals are identified in terms of family membership and are expected to sacrifice their desires for the sake of the family.

Sense of Self

European Americans are trained from a young age to be assertive (Yager & Rotheram-Borus, 2000). The importance of self-determination is emphasized, and children are taught that they can change their environment. Asians, on the other hand, are taught from a young age to be sensitive to their environment, to suppress one's wishes in the interest of the family and group, and to be able to mold oneself according to the demands of environment rather than individu-

alism (Stewart, Bond, Deeds, & Chung, 1999). These cultural values encourage behaviors that emphasize self-effacement rather than self-promotion.

Somatization

In Chinese philosophy, the mind and body are seen as integrated and related to the social context (Inouye, 1999; Ying, Lee, Tsai, Yeh, & Huang, 2000). As a result, psychological, physical, and social factors each contribute to the development of specific symptoms and illnesses (Ying et al., 2000). Physical illnesses are believed to be associated with illnesses of emotion or psyche. What is perceived as somatization in America is understood differently in Asia. It is not regarded as an inability or unwillingness to experience emotionally based disturbance but a reflection of the integration between mind and body (Kuo & Kavanagh, 1994).

Emotions

The ways in which emotions are experienced and articulated differ between Asian and Western cultures. Phenomena tend to be dichotomized in Western cultures, and experiences are judged as either good or bad, right or wrong, true or false. Asians, on the other hand, do not polarize their experiences but tend to see opposites flowing together (Bell, 1989). As such, it is more difficult for Asians to articulate emotions. In addition, in Asian cultures, emotions are experienced as interrelated entities. The origin of the word for feelings and emotions in East Asia is derived from China and is pronounced as *jyo* in Japanese, *chin* in Chinese, and *jeong* in Korean. Unlike in Western cultures, where emotions are thought to be located in the individual, *jyo* denotes an intersubjectivity where feelings are thought to be a shared experience. Therefore, emotions do not reside within oneself, as is conceptualized in the West. For example, in the Japanese language, when inquiring how someone is feeling, one asks, "How are things?" instead of "How are you feeling?" In therapy, a clinician will ask a client, "What kind of feeling do you become when this occurs?" rather than "How does it make you feel?" The subtle difference is that feelings are considered to be something that an individual takes on rather than something that inherently belongs to them.

Coping

Much evidence indicates that there are differences between APAs and other Americans in terms of appraisal of stress, common coping strategies, and the perception of optimism. The differences are not substantive as much as they are a matter of emphasis. The process of cognitive appraisal refers to the personal significance attributed to a given event by an individual (Park & Folkman, 1997) and is informed by the individual's beliefs, commitments, perceptions of available options, and level of optimism. Cognitive appraisal is also subject to both individual and cultural variation. The cultural context shapes the types of events that are perceived as stressors, their relative importance, and the kinds of coping strategies one employs (Phillips & Pearson, 1996). For example, forbearance of suffering is a valued behavior in Chinese culture because it demonstrates strength of character, an acceptance of fate, and repayment of debts inherited from one's ancestors (Phillips & Pearson, 1996). Hwang (1977) discusses the link between forbearance and the Taoist philosophy of non-action. This philosophy has its roots in the *I-Ching* (*Book of Changes*), in which a basic assumption is that the natural order of the world becomes apparent only if one does not try to control it. In more culturally syntonic terms, avoidant and withdrawal strategies are acts of fatalism, self-cultivation (i.e., striving to achieve self-moderation), and self-transcendence (i.e., striving to detach from one's troubles) (Yue, 2001). Pessimism is a component of Asian life orientations (Chang, 1996) and is tied to beliefs in fatalism. If one accepts that the mind and body are inseparable, then coping may be enhanced medicinally through the use of herbs (Char, Tseng, Lum, & Hsu, 1980). An emphasis on self-directed coping reflects a value on self-discipline.

ASSESSMENT MEASURES USED WITH ASIAN PACIFIC AMERICANS

These preferences for self-effacing behavior—an emphasis on forbearance and moderation, an acceptance of physical symptoms for what might be considered psychological phenomena—have implications for psychosocial measures. These range from normative responses unique to APAs, to the addition to or elimination of items

from established measures, to the creation of new instruments that specifically address aspects of APA culture. Table 52.1 depicts the four types of measures that have been used with APA populations: mainstream measures, adjusted mainstream measures, pan-Asian measures, and ethnic-specific measures. In this section we will review these four types of measures and present more detailed psychometric information about one measure within each category.

The first category of measures, mainstream measures, are those developed with non-APA populations that have been administered to APA samples to ascertain reliability and validity estimates. In some cases, the measure was translated prior to administration, and norms relevant to APAs may have been articulated. The content and number of items of these measures are the same whether the measure is administered to a non-APA or APA sample. Measures included in this group typically are focused on symptoms of illness. Table 52.1 presents some illustrations of such mainstream measures: the Geriatric Depression Scale (Brink et al., 1982); the Center for Epidemiological Studies–Depression (CES-D) scale (Radloff, 1977); the Rosenberg Self-Esteem Scale (Rosenberg, 1965); and the Impact of Events Scale (Horowitz, Wilner, & Alvarez, 1979). In each of these cases, there has been an empirical investigation of the reliability and validity of these measures for a general APA population or a specific ethnic population. In all cases, the researchers find evidence to support the unchanged use of these instruments for an Asian sample.

The second category, adjusted mainstream measures, is composed of instruments that were developed and validated with non-APA populations, but based on psychometric evaluation with an APA sample, they have undergone substantive change to enhance their suitability for APA populations. In each case, the original mainstream measure was adjusted by the deletion, addition, or rewording of items or by the reconfiguration of items within subscales. Illustrative measures include the GDS-SF for Asians (Mui, 1996), which suggests a different grouping of items within subscales for Chinese elders, and the CES-D-R for Koreans (Noh, Kaspar, & Chen, 1998). Although the CES-D has been tested and found to be reliable for APA populations (MacKinnon, McCallum, & Anderson, 1998), some researchers have gone further in examining whether it might be refined to fit better

TABLE 52.1 A Typology of Measures Used With APA Populations

Mainstream measures used with APA populations	Mainstream measures adjusted for use with APA populations	Pan-Asian measures designed specifically for APA populations	Ethnic-specific measures
Definition			
Instruments developed with and validated on non-APA populations that have been used with APA populations. They may or may not have been translated. Norms may be reported for pan-APA or ethnic-specific groups.	Instruments developed with and validated on non-APA populations. Based on psychometric analysis with APA populations, changes in item wording, the deletion or addition of items, and/or the development of new subscales have been recommended.	Instruments developed with and validated on APA populations. They are considered applicable and appropriate across APA subgroups.	Instruments developed with and validated on specific APA ethnic populations. They aim to measure some aspect of an ethnic-specific experience.
Examples			
Geriatric Depression Scale (Brink et al., 1982): A 30-item inventory designed to assess depression symptoms among geriatric populations. Has been used with multiple APA groups.	GDS-SF for Asians (Mui, 1996): A 16-item version of the GDS-SF with a unique distribution of items into subscales.	Asian Values Scale (Kim, Atkinson, & Yang, 1999): A 36-item scale assessing adherence to Asian cultural values.	Vietnamese Acculturation Scale (Nguyen, Messe, & Stollak, 1999): A 76-item measure that assesses level of involvement in both Vietnamese and U.S. culture
CES-D (Radloff, 1977): A 20-item scale that examines symptoms of depression in 4 areas: depressive affect, somatic symptoms, positive affect, and interpersonal relations. Has been used with multiple APA groups	CES-D-R Korean version (Noh, Kaspar, & Chen, 1998): A 20-item revision of CES-D scale; the 4 positively worded items have been reworded as negative items.	Loss of Face Scale (Zane & Yeh, 2002): A 45-item measure assessing the extent to which an individual engages in face-saving behaviors and/or avoids face-threatening situations.	Hawaiian Culture Scale: Adolescent version (Hishinuma et al., 2000): A 50-item measure that assesses involvement with 7 aspects of Hawaiian culture and lifestyle.
Rosenberg Self-Esteem (Rosenberg, 1965): A 10-item unidimensional scale designed to measure personal worth, self-confidence, self-satisfaction, self-respect, and self-deprecation.	Fear Survey Schedule for Hawaiians (Shore & Rapport, 1998): The FSSC-HI: A 84-item measure based on the 80-item FSSC–Revised (Ollendick, 1983).	Suinn-Lew Asian Self-Identity Acculturation Scale (Suinn, Rickard-Figueroa, Lew, & Vigil, 1987): A 21-item measure assessing level of Asian American identity (acculturation)	Cultural Values Conflict Scale for South Asian Women (Inman, Ladany, Constantine, & Morano, 2001): A 40-item measure assessing acculturative difficulties relevant to South Asian women.

(continued)

TABLE 52.1 A Typology of Measures Used With APA Populations (*continued*)

Mainstream measures used with APA populations	Mainstream measures adjusted for use with APA populations	Pan-Asian measures designed specifically for APA populations	Ethnic-specific measures
Impact of Events Scale (Horowitz, Wilner, & Alvarez, 1979): A 15-item measure of stress reactions following a traumatic event. It has been tested for use with Cambodians (Sack et al.,) and Chinese (Wu & Chan, 2003)	Beck Depression Inventory: Hmong Adaptation (Mouanoutoua, Brown, Cappelletty, & Levine, 1991): A 22-item version of the original 21-item BDI with changes to response options and item wordings.	Asian American Family Conflicts Scale (Lee, Choe, Kim, & Ngo, 2000): A 10-item scale that describes family conflicts found in Asian American families	Chinese Affect Scale (Hamid & Cheng, 1996): A 40-item measure that assesses negative and positive affect reflective of Chinese values of emotional expression.

the unique symptom patterns of APA populations in Asia and the United States. Currently, the CES-D in its original and adjusted forms is used in research with APAs. Both forms remain under examination, and no conclusions have been reached regarding which is more effective. Other examples of adjusted mainstream measures include the Fear Survey for Children: Hawaiian version (Shore & Rapport, 1998) and the Beck Depression Inventory: Hmong Adaptation (Mouanoutoua, Brown, Cappelletty, & Levine, 1991).

The third category of measures are pan-Asian instruments, which were developed with and validated on APA samples for use with APAs. They typically address behaviors and/or values common across multiple APA ethnic groups such as acculturation processes or aspects of conflict avoidance. Examples of pan-Asian instruments are the Asian Values Scale (Kim, Atkinson, & Yang, 1999); the Loss of Face Scale (Zane & Yeh, 2002); the Suinn-Lew Asian Self-Identity Acculturation Scale (Suinn, Lew, & Vigil, 1987); and the Asian American Family Conflicts Scale (Lee, Choe, Kim, & Ngo, 2000).

Finally, the fourth category consists of measures developed with and validated on a specific APA ethnic sample for use with that ethnic group. These instruments typically address some unique aspect of an ethnic community by including specific linguistic terms or references to specific cultural practices or experiences. Examples of ethnic-specific instruments include the

Vietnamese Acculturation Scale (Nguyen, Messe, & Stollak, 1999); Hawaiian Culture Scale: Adolescent version (Hishinuma, et al., 2000); the Cultural Values Conflict Scale for South Asian Women (Inman, Constantine, Ladany, & Morano, 2001); and the Chinese Affect Scale (Hamid & Cheng, 1996).

Impact of Events Scale: A Mainstream Measure Applicable to APA Populations

The Impact of Events Scale (IES; Horowitz et al., 1979) is a widely used 15-item measure that assesses the frequency with which experiences of "intrusions," "avoidance," and emotional numbing related to stressful events were experienced in the last week. A total distress score is calculated by summing responses across all items. A review of 40 studies (Sundin & Horowitz, 2002) of the psychometric properties of the IES finds that IES scores are sensitive to temporal differences in stress reactions and predictive of post–traumatic stress disorder (PTSD). Past research suggests that there may be a two- or three-factor structure (Yule, Bruggencate, & Joseph, 1994).

Sack et al. (1988) assessed the suitability of the IES for use with Khmer adolescents aged 13 to 25 years. A total of 209 youths participated in the research, 86% of whom had experienced a traumatic event. The sample was 48% female, 52% male. The participants had lived in the United States for an average of 7.9 years, (*SD*

= 3.5). Based on this sample, the Cronbach alpha was calculated to be .92.

The three-factor IES structure, identified by Yule et al. (1994), was replicated with the Khmer adolescents. Significant differences in IES item means were found between adolescents with a current PTSD diagnosis and those without a PTSD diagnosis.

The Center for Epidemiological Studies Depression Korean Version: A Mainstream Measure Adjusted for Use With APA Populations

The CES-D (Radoff, 1977) is a widely used and tested measure for assessing symptoms of depression. Its 20 items assess the number and duration of symptoms of depression over the preceding 2 weeks. The response for each symptom item is scored on a 4-point Likert scale: 0 = never or rarely (less then 1 day a week), 1 = sometimes or occasionally (1 or 2 days a week), 2 = frequently (3 or 4 days a week), and 3 = all the time or almost always (5 days or more a week).

Noh et al. (1988) have questioned the suitability of the 4 positive affect items of the CES-D for Asian populations. These items (e.g., "felt as good as other people," "enjoyed life") may be problematic due to cultural values regulating emotional expression. To address this, Noh and colleagues compared three versions of the CES-D: a Korean translation of the original 20-item scale (CESD-K-20); a Korean translation of a 16-item CES-D scale (4 positive items were deleted; CESD-K-16); and a Korean translation of a revised 20-item CES-D scale (4 positive items were reworded as negative items; CESD-K-R). Overall, the CESD-K-R was found to be the most valid and reliable measure of depression among Korean adults in comparison to the CESD-K-20 or the CESD-K-16.

A total of 1,039 Korean adults residing in the Toronto, Canada, area who immigrated at the age 17 or older were randomly selected to participate. Based on this sample, Noh et al. (1988) reported that the Cronbach alpha for the CESD-K-20 was .89, and for the CESD-K-R it was .90. The convergent validity of the revised items was found to be stronger than that for the positive items based on the strength of their correlation coefficients with scores on SCL-90 subscales and a measure of life events.

The Loss of Face Scale: A Pan-Asian Measure

The Loss of Face (LOF Scale; Zane & Yeh, 2002) is a 21-item unidimensional measure that assesses the extent to which one avoids situations and behaviors that are related to loss of face with regard to social status, ethical behavior, social propriety, or self-discipline (e.g., "I do not criticize others because this may embarrass them"). The measure uses a 7-point Likert scale ranging from 1 = strongly disagree to 7 = strongly agree. All items are scored in the direction of loss of face.

This measure has been tested with a diverse sample of undergraduate students including white and multiple Asian subgroups. The LOF measure has a Cronbach alpha of .83 and has demonstrated concurrent and discriminant validity. LOF scores correlate with other-directedness, self-consciousness, social anxiety, extraversion, and acculturation in predicted directions.

The Acculturation Scale for Vietnamese Adolescents: An Ethnic-Specific Measure

The purpose of the Acculturation Scale for Vietnamese Adolescents (ASVA; Nguyen et al., 1999) is to assess an adolescent's level of involvement in the Vietnamese and American cultures. It consists of 76 items nested within two subscales. The first subscale measures the level of involvement in Vietnamese culture (IVN), and the second measures the level of involvement in United States culture (IUS). Items reflect attitudes, behaviors, and values related to lifestyle, group interaction, family orientation, social behavior, and global involvement. The response set is a 5-item Likert-type, indicating the extent of agreement with each item. A shorter 50-item version is also available.

The ASVA was tested with a sample of Vietnamese junior high school students. The reliability of both subscales was excellent: IVN subscale = .92 and IUS subscale = .90. Subscales were developed based on a two-factor solution: involvement in Vietnamese (IVN) culture and involvement in United States culture (IUS). The IVN score was found to be significantly and positively correlated with Vietnamese-language fluency and items assessing involvement and relative importance of the Vietnamese culture ($r = .40–57$). The IUS score was found to be significantly and positively correlated with English-language fluency and overall ratings of level of involvement and importance of U.S. culture (.45–48).

DISCUSSION

When selecting measures for use with APA populations, the researcher or practitioner must address the issue of comparability, that is, the extent to which target construct is equivalent across cultural contexts or subject to cultural variation. Overall, although there may be some culturally unique qualities to symptom manifestation, the research indicates that there may be enough equivalence to allow most mainstream measures to be usable or at least adaptable to APA populations. Social phenomena, however, such as qualities of family relationship and acculturation experiences, appear to be much more culturally contingent. APA-specific measures may be more appropriate in these circumstances. Before using a measure with APA populations, one must also consider other issues of cross-cultural measurement that include quality of translation in terms of functional, conceptual, and metric equivalence.

References

Abe, J. S., & Zane, N. W. S. (1990). Psychological maladjustment among Asian and White American college students: Controlling for confounds. *Journal of Counseling Psychology, 37,* 437–444.

Agbayani-Siewert, P. (1994). Filipino American culture and family: Guidelines for practitioners. *Families in Society, 75,* 429–438.

Brink, T. L., Yesavage, J. A., Lum, B., Heersma, P., Adey, M., et al. (1982). Depressive symptoms and depressive diagnoses in a community population. *Archives of General Psychiatry, 45,* 1078–1084.

Chang, E. C. (1996a). Cultural differences in optimism, pessimism, and coping: Predictors of subsequent adjustment in Asian American and Caucasian American students. *Journal of Counseling Psychology, 43,* 113–123.

Chang, E. C. (1996b). Evidence for the cultural specificity of pessimism in Asians vs Caucasians: A test of a general negativity hypothesis. *Personality and Individual Differences, 21,* 819–822.

Char, W. F., Tseng, W. S., Lum, K. Y., & Hsu, J. (1980). The Chinese. In J. F. McDermott, W. S. Tseng, & T. W. Maretzki (Eds.), *People and cultures of Hawaii: A psychocultural profile* (pp. 53–72). Honolulu: University Press of Hawaii.

Cheng, S. K. (1990). Understanding the culture and behaviour of East Asians: A Confucian perspective. *Australian and New Zealand Journal of Psychiatry, 24,* 510–515.

Chun, C., Enomoto, K., & Sue, S. (1996). Health care issues among Asian Americans. In P. M. Kato & T. Mann (Eds.), *Handbook of diversity issues in health psychology* (pp. 347–365). New York: Plenum Press. *Gerontology, 53B,* 343–352.

Hamid, P. N., & Cheng, S. (1996). The development and validation of an index of emotional disposition and mood state: The Chinese Affect Scale. *Educational and Psychological Measurement, 56,* 995–1014.

Hishinuma, E. S., McArdle, J. J., Miyamoto, R. H., Nahulu, S. B., Makini, Jr., G. K., Yuen, Y. C., Nishimura, S. T., McDermott, J. F., Jr., Waldron, J. A., Luke, K. L., & Yates, A. (2000). Psychometric Properties of the Hawaiian Culture Scale–Adolescent Version. *Psychological Assessment, 12,* 140–157.

Ho, D. Y. F. (1995). Selfhood and identity in Confucianism, Taoism, Buddhism, and Hinduism: Contrasts with the West. *Journal for the Theory of Social Behaviour, 25,* 115–139.

Horowitz, M., Wilner, N. J., & Alvarez, W. (1979). Impact of events scale: A measure of subjective stress. *Psychosomatic Medicine, 41,* 209–218.

Hwang, K. (1977). The patterns of coping strategies in a Chinese society. *Acta Psychologica Taiwanica, 19,* 61–73.

Hwang, K. K. (1999). Filial piety and loyalty: Two types of social identification in Confucianism. *Asian Journal of Social Psychology, 2,* 163–183.

Inman, A. G., Ladany, N., Constantine, M. G., & Morano, C. K. (2001). Development and preliminary validation of the Cultural Values Conflict Scale for South Asian women. *Journal of Counseling Psychology, 48,* 17–27.

Inouye, J. (1999). Asian American health and disease: An overview of the issues. In R. M. Huff & M. V. Kline (Eds.), *Promoting health in multicultural populations* (pp. 337–356). Thousand Oaks, CA: Sage.

Jung, H. Y. (1969). Confucianism and existentialism: Intersubjectivity as the way of man. *Philosophy and Phenomenological Research, 30,* 186–202.

Kim, B. S. K., Atkinson, D. R., & Yang, P. H. (1999). The Asian Values Scale: Development, factor analysis, validation, and reliability. *Journal of Counseling Psychology, 46,* 342–352.

Kitao, H., & Kimura, A. (1980). The Japanese American family. In R. Endo, S. Sue, & W. Wagner (Eds.), *Asian Americans: Social and psychologi-*

cal perspective (Vol. 2, pp. 32–48). Palo Alto, CA: Science and Behavior Books.

Kuo, C., & Kavanagh, K. H. (1994). Chinese perspectives on culture and mental health. *Issues in Mental Health Nursing, 15*, 551–567.

Lai, J., & Linden, W. (1993). The smile of Asia: Acculturation effects on symptoms reporting. *Canadian Journal of Behavioral Science, 25*, 303–313.

Lee, R. M., Choe, J., Kim, G., & Ngo, V. (2000). Construction of the Asian American Family Conflicts Scale. *Journal of Counseling Psychology, 47*, 211–222.

Lin, N. (1989). Measuring depressive symptomatology in China. *Journal of Nervous and Mental Disease, 177*, 121–131.

Mackinnon, A., McCallum, J. A., & Anderson, I. (1998). The Center for Epidemiological Studies Depression Scale in older community samples in Indonesia, North Korea, Myanmar, Sri Lanka and Thailand. *Journals of Gerontology Series B—Psychological Sciences and Social Sciences, 53B*, P343–P352.

Matsumoto, D. (1993). Ethnic differences in affect intensity, emotion judgments, display rule attitudes, and self-reported emotional expression in an American sample. *Motivation and Emotion, 17*, 107–123.

Mouanoutoua, V. L., Brown, L. G., Cappelletty, G. G., & Levine, R. V. (1991). A Hmong adaptation of the Beck depression inventory. *Journal of Personality Assessment, 57*, 309–322.

Mui, A. (1996). Geriatric Depression Scale as a community screening instrument for elderly Chinese immigrants. *International Psychogeriatrics, 8*, 445–458.

Nguyen, H. H., Messe, L. A., & Stollak, G. E. (1999). Toward a more complex understanding of acculturation and adjustment: Cultural involvement and psychosocial functioning in Vietnamese youth. *Journal of Cross-Cultural Psychology, 30*, 5–31.

Noh, S., Kaspar, V., & Chen, X. (1998). Measuring depression in Korean immigrants: Assessing validity of the translated Korean version of CES-D scale. *Cross-Cultural Research, 32*, 358–377.

Okazaki, S. (1997). Sources of ethnic differences between Asian American and White American college students on measures of depression and social anxiety. *Journal of Abnormal Psychology, 106*, 52–60.

Okazaki, S. (2000). Asian American and White American differences on affective distress symptoms: Do symptom reports differ across reporting methods? *Journal of Cross-Cultural Psychology, 31*, 603–625.

Ollendick, T. H. (1983). Reliability and validity of the Revised Fear Survey Schedule for Children

(FSSC-R). *Behaviour Research and Therapy, 21*, 685–692.

Park, C. L., & Folkman, S. (1997). Meaning in the context of stress and coping. *Review of General Psychology, 1*, 115–144.

Phillips, M. R., & Pearson, V. (1996). Coping in Chinese communities: The need for a new research agenda. In M. H. Bond et al. (Eds.), *The handbook of Chinese psychology* (pp. 429–440). Hong Kong: Oxford University Press.

Radloff, L. (1977). The CES-D scale: A self-report depression scale for research in the general population. *Applied Psychological Measurement, 1*, 385–401.

Rezentes, W. C. III. (1993). Na Mea Hawaii: A Hawaiian acculturation scale. *Psychological Reports, 73*, 383–393.

Root, M., Ho, C., & Sue, S. (1986). Issues in the training of counselors for Asian Americans. In H. P. Lefley, P. B. Pedersen, et al. (Eds.), *Cross-cultural training for mental health professionals* (pp. 199–209). Springfield, IL: Thomas.

Rosenberg, M. (1965). *Society and the adolescent self-image.* Princeton, NJ: Princeton University Press.

Sack, W. H., Seeley, J. R., Him, C., & Clarke, G. N. (1998). Psychometric properties of the Impact of Events Scale in traumatized Cambodian refugee youth. *Personality and Individual Differences, 25*, 57–67.

Shore, G. N., & Rapport, M. D. (1998). The Fear Schedule for Children-Revised (FSSC-HI): Ethnocultural variations in children's fearfulness. *Journal of Anxiety Disorders, 12*, 437–461.

Steel, J. L. (1991). Interpersonal correlates of trust and self-disclosure. *Psychological Reports, 68*, 1319–1320.

Stewart, S. M., Bond, M. H., Deeds, O., & Chung, S. F. (1999) Intergenerational patterns of values and autonomy expectations in cultures of relatedness and separateness. *Journal of Cross-Cultural Psychology, 30*, 575–593.

Suinn, R., Rickard-Figueroa, K., Lew, S., & Vigil, P. (1987). The Suinn-Lew Asian Self-Identity Acculturation Scale: An initial report. *Educational & Psychological Measurement, 47*(2), 401–407.

Sundin, E. C., & Horowitz, M. J. (2002). Impact of Event Scale: Psychometric properties. *British Journal of Psychiatry, 180*, 205–209.

Sung, K. (2001). The kindness of mothers: Ideals and practice of Buddhist filial piety. *Journal of Aging and Identity, 6*, 137–146.

Wu, K. K., & Chan, K. S. (2003). The development of the Chinese version of the Impact of Event Scale-Revised (CIES-R). *Social Psychiatry and Psychiatric Epidemiology, 38*, 94–98.

Yager, T. J., & Rotheram-Borus, M. J. (2000). Social expectations among African American, Hispanic, and European American adolescents. *Cross-*

Cultural Research: The Journal of Comparative Social Science, 34, 283–305.

Ying, Y., Lee, P. A., Tsai, J. L., Yeh, Y., & Huang, J. S. (2000). The conception of depression in Chinese American college students. Cultural Diversity and Ethnic Minority Psychology, 6, 183–195.

Yue, X. (2001). Culturally constructed coping among university students in Beijing. Journal of Psychology in Chinese Societies, 2, 119–137.

Yule, W., Bruggencate, S. T. J., & Joseph, S. (1994). Principal components analysis of the Impact of Events Scales in adolescents who survived a ship-ping disaster. Personality and Individual Differences, 16, 685–691.

Zane, N. W., Sue, S., Hu, L., & Kwon, J. (1991). Asian-American assertion: A social learning analysis of cultural differences. Journal of Counseling Psychology, 38, 63–70.

Zane, N., & Yeh, M. (2002). The use of culturally-based variables in assessment: Studies on loss of face. In K. S. Kurasaki, S. Okazaki, et al. (Eds.), Asian American mental health: Assessment theories and methods (pp. 123–138). New York: Kluwer Academic/Plenum.

53 CRISIS ASSESSMENT MEASURES AND TOOLS

Albert R. Roberts

Throughout society, individuals, couples, and families are confronted with acute and situational crises. Millions of individuals and families encounter stressful life events and traumatic events. A growing number of these people are unable to cope with the traumatic event or accumulation of stressors and perceive themselves as being in a crisis state.

The most important first step in crisis intervention is a lethality and biopsychosocial assessment. Crisis intervention with persons in acute crisis must begin with a rapid and accurate assessment of lethality (i.e., level of suicide or homicide risk). This assessment should focus on affective reactions (i.e., anger, fear, sadness); cognitive perceptions (i.e., emotions and feelings, relationship losses); and behavioral actions (e.g., avoidance, immobility, drug abuse). Crisis assessment can provide necessary information to behavioral clinicians on the client's immediate needs. Accurate assessment requires the ability to gather information for rapid assessment in a manner that assures the individual that he or she has made the right decision and is in exactly the right place. Skilled clinicians working to complete an initial assessment are also establishing and building rapport while trying to bolster hope and confidence in the individual caller.

OVERVIEW OF THE BASICS OF CRISIS ASSESSMENT

The following presents an overview of crisis assessment. One should begin by planning and conducting a thorough biopsychosocial and crisis assessment. This involves a quick assessment of risk and dangerousness, including suicide and homicide/violence risk assessment, need for medical attention, positive and negative coping strategies, and current drug or alcohol use (Eaton & Ertl, 2000; Roberts, 2000). If possible, a

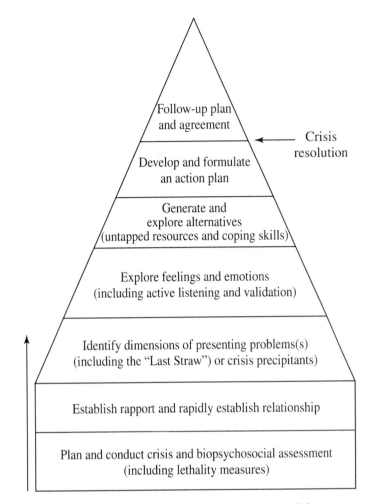

FIGURE 53.1 Roberts 7-Stage Crisis Intervention Model

medical assessment should include a brief summary of the presenting problem, any medical conditions, current medications (names, dosages, and time of last dose), and allergies. This medical information is essential to relay to emergency medical responders attempting to treat problems such as overdoses.

A drug or alcohol assessment should include information about drugs used, amount used, time of last use, and any withdrawal symptoms the client is experiencing. Any knowledge of angel dust, metamphetamine, or PCP ingestion should always precipitate a team crisis response with the police, due to the likelihood of violent and bizarre behavior.

The initial crisis assessment should examine resilience and protective factors, internal and ex-

ternal coping methods and resources, and the degree of extended family and/or informal support network. Many individuals in a precrisis or crisis situation isolate themselves socially and are unaware of and lack insight into which persons would be most supportive in their efforts at crisis resolution and recovery. The crisis clinician can facilitate and bolster clients' resilience by encouraging them to telephone or write a letter to persons who may well support their efforts at recovery. Seeking advice on how best to cope with a crisis related to self-destructive patterns such as polydrug abuse, binge drinking, self-injurious behavior, or depression can lead to overwhelming support, suggestions, advice, and encouragement from one's support network (Yeager & Gregoire, 2000).

A • Assessment/appraisal of immediate medical needs, threats to public safety and property damage
  • Triage assessment, crisis assessment, trauma assessment and the biopsychosocial and cultural assessment protocols

C • Connecting to support groups, the delivery of disaster relief and social services, and critical incident stress debriefing (Mitchell & Everly's CISD model) implemented
  • Crisis intervention (Robert's seven-stage model) implemented, through strengths perspective and coping attempts bolstered

T • Traumatic stress reactions, sequelae, and post-traumatic stress disorders (PTSDs)
  • Ten step acute trauma and stress management protocol (Lerner & Shelton), trauma treatment plans and recovery strategies implemented

FIGURE 53.2 ACT model

The ACT Intervention Model of Assessment, Crisis Intervention, and Trauma Treatment

Somatic stress, acute crisis, and psychological trauma frequently take place in the wake of unnatural, man-made disasters such as the terrorist mass murders of September 11, 2001. Most individuals have little or no preparation for such trauma-inducing events. The catastrophic nature of the World Trade Center and Pentagon disasters has impacted and threatened the safety of many American citizens. The important first step in determining the psychosocial needs of all survivors and their families and the grieving family members of the murder victims of a terrorist attack or other community disaster is assessment. The focus of this chapter is to examine the "A" (or assessment) component of the newly developed ACT Intervention Model for Acute Crisis and Trauma Treatment. I will briefly discuss psychiatric triage assessment and types of assessment protocols. I will then identify and discuss the components of a crisis assessment. Next I will enumerate and review the dimensions of the biopsychosocial and cultural assess-

ment. Finally, I will briefly list the types of rapid assessment instruments and scales used in mental health, crisis, and trauma assessments.

TRIAGE ASSESSMENT

Crisis counselors, crisis workers, first responders, or crisis response team members are often called upon to conduct an immediate debriefing under less than stable circumstances, and sometimes they have to delay the crisis assessment until right after immediate stabilization and support. With other disaster responses, an assessment can be completed simultaneously with the debriefing. According to many of the disaster mental health and crisis intervention specialists I have trained, ideally "A" (assessment) precedes "C" (crisis intervention), but in the rough-and-tumble of the disaster or acute crisis, the sequence is not always that linear (Roberts, 2002).

The first type of assessment by disaster mental health specialists and crisis workers in the immediate aftermath of a community disaster should be psychiatric triage. A triage or screening tool can be useful in gathering and recording information about the initial contact between the mental health specialist, and a person experiencing crisis or trauma reactions. The triage form should include the following:

1. Essential demographic information (name, address, phone number, e-mail address, etc.);
2. Perception of the magnitude of the traumatic event; and
3. Coping methods, any presenting problem(s), safety issues, previous traumatic experiences, social support network, drug and alcohol use, preexisting psychiatric conditions, suicide risk, and homicide risk (Eaton & Roberts, 2002).

Several hundred articles have examined emergency medical triage, but very few publications have discussed emergency psychiatric triage. Triage has been defined as the medical "process of assigning patients to appropriate treatments depending on their medical conditions and available medical resources" (Liese, 1995, p. 48). Medical triage was first used in the military to respond quickly to the medical needs of wounded soldiers. Triage involves assigning physically ill or injured patients to different levels of care, ranging from "emergent" (i.e., immediate treatment required) to "nonemergent" (i.e., no medical treatment required).

Psychiatric or psychological triage assessment refers to the immediate decision-making process in which the mental health worker determines lethality and referral to one of the following alternatives:

1. Emergency inpatient hospitalization;
2. Outpatient treatment facility or private therapist;
3. Support group or social service agency; or
4. No referral needed.

The "A" in my ACT Intervention Model refers to triage, crisis, and trauma assessments and referral to appropriate community resources. With regard to triage assessment, emergency psychiatric response should take place when the rapid assessment indicates that the individual presents a danger to himself or others and is exhibiting intense and acute psychiatric symptoms. These survivors generally require short-term hospitalization and psychopharmacotherapy to prevent them from harming themselves (e.g., suicide at-

tempts and self-injurious behavior) or other persons (e.g., murder and attempted murder). The small number of individuals needing emergency psychiatric treatment generally are diagnosed with moderate to high potential lethality (e.g., suicidal ideation and/or homicidal thoughts) and acute mental disorders (Roberts, 2002). In the small percentage of cases where emergency psychiatric treatment is indicated, these persons usually are suffering from a cumulation of several previous traumatic events (Burgess & Roberts, 2000).

Triage Assessment and Crisis Assessment

With regard to the other categories of psychiatric triage, many individuals may be in a pre-crisis stage as a result of ineffective coping skills, a weak support system, or ambivalence about seeking mental health assistance. These same individuals may have no psychiatric symptoms and no suicide risk. However, because of the catastrophic nature of the September 11 disaster, persons who have suddenly lost a loved one and have no previous experience coping with sudden death may be particularly vulnerable to acute crisis or traumatic stress. Therefore, in the weeks and months following September 11, it was imperative for all mental health professionals to become knowledgeable about timely crisis and trauma assessments.

Another type of triage assessment used almost exclusively by crisis intervention and suicide prevention programs is the Intervention Priority Scale. This scale, developed by the 24-hour mobile crisis intervention services of Community Integration, Inc., of Erie, Pennsylvania, should be used by other programs throughout North America. It allows a number from I to IV to be assigned at the time the triage information is collected, based on clinical criteria. Each number on the scale corresponds to an outside time limit considered to be safe for crisis response. Examples of a Priority I include requests for immediate assistance by police and emergency services personnel, suicide attempts in progress, suicidal or homicidal individuals with the means currently available, or individuals experiencing command hallucinations of a violent nature. Examples of a Priority II include individuals who are able to contract for safety or who have reliable supports present, individuals experiencing hallucinations or delusions, or individuals who are unable to meet basic human needs. Examples of a Priority III include individuals with fleeting suicidal ideation or major depression and no feasible suicide plan, or individuals suffering from mood disturbances. Priority IVs often include cases where there is no thought to harm self or others, no psychiatric symptoms are present, and no other situational crises exist (Eaton & Roberts, 2002).

CRISIS ASSESSMENT

The primary role of the crisis counselor and other clinical staff in conducting an assessment is to evaluate an individual in a crisis state in order to gather information that can help to resolve the crisis. Intake forms and rapid assessment instruments help the crisis clinician or mental health counselor to make better informed decisions on the type and duration of treatment recommended. Although crisis assessment is oriented to the individual, it must always include an assessment of the person's immediate environment and interpersonal relationships. As Gitterman (2002) eloquently points out in "The Life Model":

The purpose of social work is improving the level of fit between people and their environments, especially between people's needs and their environmental resources. . . . (The professional function of social work is as follows) . . . to help people mobilize and draw on personal and environmental resources for effective coping to alleviate life stressors and the associated stress. (p. 106)

Crisis assessment will facilitate treatment planning and decision making. Its ultimate goal is to provide a systematic method of organizing client information related to personal characteristics, parameters of the crisis episode, and the intensity and duration of the crisis, and utilizing these data to develop effective treatment plans (Roberts, 2002). In the words of Lewis and Roberts (2001):

Most intake workers have failed to distinguish between stressful life events, traumatic events, coping skills and other mediators of a crisis, and an active crisis state. Most crisis episodes are preceded by one or more stressful, hazardous, and/or traumatic events. However, not all stressed or traumatized individuals move into a crisis state. Every day thousands of individuals completely avert a crisis,

while many others thousands of individuals quickly escalate into a crisis states. (p. 208)

Therefore, it is extremely important to assess and measure whether or not a person is in a crisis state, so that individual treatment goals and an appropriate crisis intervention protocol can be implemented. For a detailed discussion of crisis-specific measurement tools and crisis-oriented rapid assessment instruments, see Lewis and Roberts (2001).

According to Eaton and Roberts (2002), the crisis worker should ask the client eight fundamental questions when conducting a suicide risk assessment. These include:

Are you/client having thoughts of self-harm?
Yes ( ) No ( ) Unknown ( );
Have you/client done anything to intentionally hurt yourself: Yes ( ) No ( ), If YES, describe _____
Do you feel there is hope that things can improve?
Yes ( ) No ( ), If YES, describe _____

Eaton and Roberts (2002) also delineate nine questions for measuring homicide or violence risk, such as

Have you/client made any preparations to hurt others? Yes ( ) No ( ), If YES, describe _____
(p. 92)

BIOPSYCHOSOCIAL AND CULTURAL ASSESSMENTS

Various methods of assessment have been designed to measure clients' situations, stress levels, presenting problems, and acute crisis episodes. These include monitoring and observations; a client log; semistructured interviews; individualized rating scales; goal attainment scales; behavioral observations; self-reports; cognitive measures; and diagnostic systems and codes (Pike, 2002; LeCroy & Okamoto, 2002).

Vandiver and Corcoran (2002) identify and discuss the biopsychosocial-cultural model of assessment as the first step in the clinical interview aimed at providing the necessary information to "establish treatment goals and an effective treatment plan." (p. 297). It is important for individual assessments to gather information on the following topics:

1. Current health status (e.g., hypertension) and past health status (e.g. diabetes), or in-

juries (e.g., brain injury); current medication use, and health and lifestyle behaviors (e.g., fitness exercises, nutrition, sleep patterns, substance abuse).

2. The psychological status of the client, including mental status, appearance and behavior, speech and language, thought process and content, mood and affect, cognitive functioning, concentration, memory, and insight and general intelligence. An additional critical area of assessment is the determination of suicidal or homicidal risk and possible need for an immediate referral.

3. The sociocultural experiences and cultural background of the client, including ethnicity, language, assimilation, acculturation, spiritual beliefs, environmental connections (e.g., community ties, neighborhood, economic conditions, availability of food and shelter), social networks and relationships (e.g., family, friends, coworkers). (Vandiver & Corcoran, 2002, p. 298)

The assessment process should provide a step-by-step method for exploring, identifying, describing, measuring, classifying, diagnosing, and coding health or mental health problems, environmental conditions, resilience and protective factors, positive lifestyle behaviors, and level of functioning. Austrian (2002) delineates the 10 basic components or elements of a biopsychosocial assessment:

1. Demographic data
2. Current and previous agency contacts
3. Medical, psychiatric, and substance abuse history
4. Brief history of client and significant others
5. Summary of client's current situation
6. Presenting request
7. Presenting problem as defined by client and counselor
8. Contract agreed on by client and counselor
9. Intervention plan
10. Intervention goals

Some of the most popular assessment tools include the following:

1. The *Diagnostic and Statistical Manual*-IV-TR (DSM-IV-TR) (APA, 2000; Williams, 2002; Munson, 2002);
2. Rapid assessment instruments (RAIs) such as the Brief Symptom Inventory, the Beck

Depression Inventory (BDI), the Derogatis Symptom Checklist–SCL-90, the Reasons for Living Scale, and the Impact of Events scale (see Corcoran & Fischer, 2000; Corcoran & Boyer-Quick, 2002).
3. Person-in-Environment (PIE) system (Karls, 2002); and
4. Goal attainment scales (Pike, 2002).

Clinician-Rated—Crisis-Specific Measurement Tools

Based on a literature search through four major databases (Psychlit, Sociofile, Infotrac, PubMed), three standardized, multidimensional instruments that are designed specifically for crisis assessment (not solely lethality) and on which the psychometrics are known are currently available for noninstitutionalized adults. All three instruments have a structured interview format. The first scale is the Crisis Triage Rating Scale (CTRS), which was developed by Bengelsdorf, Levey, Emerson, and Barile (1984). The interviewer using the instrument chooses one of five descriptive statements in each of the following three categories: dangerousness, support system, and ability to cooperate. Scores range from 3 to 25, and individuals with scores lower than 10 are recommended for inpatient treatment, and individuals with scores of 11 or more are recommended for outpatient treatment.

Myer, Williams, Ottens, and Smith (1994) developed the Triage Assessment Form: Crisis Intervention (TAF), which aids clinicians in assessing the type and severity of crisis experienced by college students. As with the CTRS, the clinician and not the client uses the instrument to quantify a crisis state. The TAF uses a three-dimensional model that includes affective responses to, cognitive perceptions of, and behavioral coping with the crisis situation.

The Suicide Assessment Checklist (Rogers, Alexander, & Mezydlo-Subich, 1993), otherwise known as the Crisis Line Suicide Risk Scale, is a two-part suicide risk assessment tool. The first part of the instrument is used to collect information on relevant demographic variables; the second part consists of counselor ratings of psychological, psychosocial, and clinical factors.

Crisis-Oriented Rapid Assessment Instruments (Self-Rated)

Several RAIs fall under this rubric. All are crisis-oriented, but only one of them is crisis-specific.

The Lewis-Roberts Crisis State Assessment Scale (CSAS) is the first short self-rated RAI that is designed to measure the magnitude of a crisis state. The CSAS, which was recently validated, measures two distinct constructs: perceived psychological trauma and problems in perceived coping efficacy (Lewis & Roberts, 2002). The global score is believed to indicate the magnitude of an individual's crisis state.

Corcoran and Fischer (2000) have compiled over 400 other RAIs in a wide range of problem areas; none, however, directly assesses the magnitude of a crisis state. There are five scales related to suicide in Corcoran and Fischer (2000), but the editors suggest also looking under depression and life satisfaction. A few of the scales not listed in Corcoran and Fischer (2000) that could possibly be appropriate for portions of a crisis assessment are the following:

1. Brief Psychiatric Rating Scale (Overall & Gorham, 1962);
2. Brief Symptom Inventory (Boulet & Boss, 1991);
3. Adult Suicidal Ideation Questionnaire (Reynolds, 1991);
4. Suicide Probability Scale (Cull & Gill, 1982);
5. Suicide Intervention Response Inventory (Cotton & Range, 1992); and
6. Hopelessness Scale (Beck, Weissman, Lesier, & Trexler, 1974).

CONCLUSION

Crisis workers and crisis counselors are usually available and on call 24 hours a day, 7 days a week. It is therefore critical for these professionals and paraprofessionals to be highly energetic, flexible, trained, and skilled in both lethality and biopsychosocial assessment. Each crisis worker should have at his or her fingertips a comprehensive list of community resources and referral sources, as well as Internet mental health resources. Finally, the crisis worker should be armed with the latest methods of documentation and evidence-based crisis intervention treatment protocols.

References

Austrian, S. (2002). Biopsychosocial assessment. In A. R. Roberts & G. J. Greene (Eds.), *Social workers' desk reference* (pp. 204–208). New York: Oxford University Press.

Beck, A. T., Weissman, A., Lester, D., & Trexler, L. (1974). The measurement of pessimism: The Hopelessness Scale. *Journal of Consulting and Clinical Psychology, 42,* 861–865.

Bengelsdorf, H., Levy, L. E., Emerson, R. L., & Barile, F. A. (1984). A crisis triage rating scale: Brief dispositional assessment of patients at risk for hospitalization. *Journal of Nervous and Mental Disease, 172,* 424–430.

Boulet, J., & Boss, M. W. (1991). Reliability and validity of the Brief Symptom Inventory. *Psychological Assessment, 3,* 433–437.

Burgess, A. W., & Roberts, A. R. (2000). Crisis intervention for persons diagnosed with clinical disorders based on the Stress-Crisis Continuum. In A. R. Roberts (Ed.), *Crisis intervention handbook: Assessment, treatment and research* (2nd ed., pp. 56–76). New York: Oxford University Press.

Corcoran, K., & Boyer-Quick, J. (2002). How clinicians can effectively use assessment tools to evidence medical necessity and throughout the treatment process. In A. R. Roberts & G. J. Greene (Eds.), *Social workers' desk reference* (pp. 198–204). New York: Oxford University Press.

Corcoran, K., & Fischer, J. (2000). *Measures for clinical practice: A sourcebook* (3rd ed., Vols. 1–2). New York: Free Press.

Cotton, C. R., & Range, L. M. (1992). Reliability and validity of the Suicide Intervention Response Inventory. *Death Studies, 17,* 185–191.

Cull, J. G., & Gill, W. S. (1982). *Suicide Probability Scale.* Los Angeles: Western Psychological Services.

Eaton, Y., & Ertl B. (2000). The Comprehensive Crisis Intervention Model of Community Integration, Inc. Crisis Services. In A. R. Roberts (Ed.), *Crisis intervention handbook: Assessment, treatment and research* (2nd ed., pp. 373–387). New York: Oxford University Press.

Eaton, Y., & Roberts, A. R. (2002). Frontline crisis intervention: Step-by-step practice guidelines with case applications. In A. R. Roberts & G. J. Greene (Eds.), *Social workers' desk reference* (pp. 89–96). New York: Oxford University Press.

Gitterman, A. (2002). The life model. In A. R. Roberts & G. J. Greene (Eds.), *Social workers' desk reference* (pp. 105–107). New York: Oxford University Press.

Karls, J. M. (2002). Person-in-Environment System: Its essence and applications. In A. R. Roberts & G. J. Greene (Eds.), *Social workers' desk reference* (pp. 194–198). New York: Oxford University Press.

LeCroy, C., & Okamoto, S. (2002). Guidelines for selecting and using assessment tools with children. In A. R. Roberts & G. J. Greene (Eds.), *Social workers' desk reference* (pp. 213–216). New York: Oxford University Press.

Leise, B. S. (1995). Integrating crisis intervention, cognitive therapy and triage. In A. R. Roberts (Ed.), *Crisis intervention and time-limited cognitive treatment* (pp. 28–51). Thousand Oaks, CA.: Sage.

Lev-wiesel, R. (2000). Posttraumatic stress disorder symptoms, psychological distress, personal resources, and quality of life. *Family Process, 39*, 445–460.

Lewis, S., & Roberts, A. R. (2001). Crisis assessment tools. In A. R. Roberts & G. J. Greene (Eds.), *Social workers' desk reference* (pp. 208–212). New York: Oxford University Press.

Myer, R. A., Williams, R. C., Ottens, A. J., & Schmidt, A. E. (1992). Crisis assessment: A three-dimensional model for triage. *Journal of Mental Health Counseling, 14,* 137–148.

Overall, J. E., & Gorham, D. R. (1962). The brief psychiatric rating scale. *Psychological Report, 10,* 799–812.

Pike, C. K. (2002). Developing client-focused measures. In A. R. Roberts & G. J. Greene (Eds.), *Social workers' desk reference* (pp. 189–193). New York: Oxford University Press.

Roberts, A. R. (2000). An overview of crisis theory and crisis intervention. In A. R. Roberts (Ed.), *Crisis intervention handbook: Assessment, treatment and research* (2nd ed., pp. 3–30). New York: Oxford University Press.

Roberts, A. R. (2002). The ACT Model of Assessment, Crisis Intervention, and Trauma Treatment. *Brief Treatment and Crisis Intervention, 2,* 1–17.

Roberts, A. R., & Roberts, B. S. (2000). A comprehensive model for crisis intervention with battered women and their children. In A. R. Roberts (Ed.), *Crisis intervention handbook: Assessment, treatment and research* (2nd ed., pp. 177–207). New York: Oxford University Press.

Vandiver, V. L., & Corcoran, K. (2002). Guidelines for establishing treatment goals and treatment plans with Axis I disorders: Sample treatment plan for generalized anxiety disorder. In A. R. Roberts & G. J. Greene (Eds.), *Social workers' desk reference* (pp. 297–304). New York: Oxford University Press.

Williams, J. B. W. (2002). Using the Diagnostic and Statistical Manual for Mental Disorders, fourth edition, text revision (DSM-IV-TR). In A. R. Roberts & G. J. Greene (Eds.), *Social workers' desk reference* (pp. 171–180). New York: Oxford University Press.

Yeager, K. R., & Gregoire, T. K. (2000). Crisis intervention application of brief solution-focused therapy in addictions. In A. R. Roberts (Ed.), *Crisis intervention handbook: Assessment, treatment and research* (2nd ed., pp. 275–306). New York: Oxford University Press.

54 OUTCOME MEASUREMENT SCALE WITH FAMILIES OF THE SERIOUSLY MENTALLY ILL

Phyllis Solomon & Jeffrey Draine

Frequently, practitioners and evaluators are in a position where they need to evaluate targeted brief group interventions that address specific diseases or conditions (Sands & Solomon, in press). These may be educational or support groups (Toseland & Rivas, 2001) or socioeducational groups that combine educational, socialization, and support functions. These groups usually meet for 1 or 2 sessions or possibly as many as 10 to 12 sessions for about an hour or two

(Brown, 1991). Given the highly targeted nature of these groups, frequently the objectives are to increase knowledge, a sense of self-efficacy in handling the problem or condition, and coping ability in cognitions and behaviors relevant to the particular condition. The intent of these programs is to improve the knowledge and ability of the participants in a defined area, such as children of alcoholics, various chronic medical conditions, or populations of family caregivers of an identified illness. Generally, there is little expectation that these brief interventions will improve participants' generalized self-efficacy or coping ability in all domains of living. Consequently, generalized measures of self-efficacy and coping cannot capture the expected effects of these interventions. Using these generalized measures would likely lead the evaluator to conclude that the groups are not effective in reaching their intended objectives. Such a global approach to measuring these concepts fails to recognize that families may have specialized coping capacities. For example, a woman who copes well in a high-profile job may feel at a loss when coping with the challenges of having an adult son with schizophrenia. She may draw on the some of the same strengths for both, but the specific coping behaviors necessary in the latter situation are what the intervention targets. Thus, a highly specified coping measure is necessary to capture these intended effects.

We generally employ measures that are easily accessible in the literature or in measurement books. We trust their reported sound psychometric properties. But when these measures are used to assess outcomes more broadly than that for which the intervention was intended, their validity is no longer retained. This situation frequently presents evaluators with the task of having to construct their own measures that have marginal or situational validity, at best.

This chapter will present an example of the construction of two measures to evaluate the outcomes of a family educational intervention for family members of adults with severe psychiatric illnesses. This intervention was delivered by a mental health professional and a peer consultant, who was a trained family member, and consisted of 10 weekly 2-hour sessions. The specific objectives of the educational program were to provide participants with an orientation to serious mental illness and its treatment; to help group participants to realize that they are not alone in their feelings and experiences, as there

are others in similar situations; and to offer guidelines for dealing more effectively with their ill relative, other family members, and the mental health service delivery system. Of the 2-hour weekly sessions, 30 minutes were allocated to new information about mental illness and its treatment, and the remaining time was used for developing group members' coping skills. Homework assignments were given at the end of the sessions to help participants apply the skills they learned in their own environmental situations with their interactions with their ill relative (Solomon, Draine, Mannion, & Meisel, 1996, 1997). The evaluators, in working with the providers, determined that the outcome objectives were to increase the knowledge of group participants about mental illness and its attendant treatments, to improve their sense of self-efficacy in managing the behaviors of their ill relative, and to improve their ability to cope with their relative's illness. The remainder of this chapter will focus on the development of the scales to measure the latter two outcome objectives.

DEVELOPMENT OF THE MEASURES

Self-Efficacy Measure

Self-efficacy theory asserts that behavioral change is contingent on an individual's personal sense of mastery expectations over the particular behavior—in other words, the degree to which an individual has beliefs or confidence in his or her ability to perform the necessary tasks involved in the behavior. According to this theory, two types of expectancies exert influence over an individual's behavioral performance. One is the belief that particular behaviors will achieve specific outcomes; the other is that the individual believes that he or she has the ability to successfully perform the particular behavior (Bandura, 1977, 1982). In reviewing the literature, we did not find any self-efficacy assessment instruments related to a family coping with a relative with mental illness. The self-efficacy measures seemed to be developed for changing specific behaviors such as dieting or smoking cessation. Consequently, we needed to construct our own measure.

Taking this theory into consideration, we constructed a measure based on a study by Hatfield (1983) in which she surveyed families of adults with mental illness who were members of

FIGURE 54.1 SMI Family Self-Efficacy Scale

How strongly do you agree or disagree that you are able to . . .

1 = strongly agree   **2** = agree   **3** = disagree   **4** = strongly disagree

1. Accept the fact that your disabled relative has a mental illness	**1**	**2**	**3**	**4**
2. Accept realistic goals for your disabled relative	**1**	**2**	**3**	**4**
3. Reduce nonproductive arguments with your disabled relative	**1**	**2**	**3**	**4**
4. Allow your disabled relative to do as much as he/she can for him/herself	**1**	**2**	**3**	**4**
5. Help your disabled relative to improve his/her hygiene	**1**	**2**	**3**	**4**
6. Understand psychiatric medications and their use	**1**	**2**	**3**	**4**
7. Understand side effects of psychiatric medication	**1**	**2**	**3**	**4**
8. Assist your disabled relative to comply with medication	**1**	**2**	**3**	**4**
9. Respond to psychiatric symptoms such as hearing voices, talking to self, or paranoid thinking of your disabled relative	**1**	**2**	**3**	**4**
10. Alleviate feelings of guilt and blame about your disabled relative	**1**	**2**	**3**	**4**
11. Reduce your feelings of anxiety concerning your disabled relative	**1**	**2**	**3**	**4**
12. Take time for your own personal life	**1**	**2**	**3**	**4**
13. Gain order and control over your household	**1**	**2**	**3**	**4**
14. Reduce friction over your disabled relative's behavior	**1**	**2**	**3**	**4**
15. Gain acceptance of your disabled relative by other family members	**1**	**2**	**3**	**4**
16. Get other family members to share responsibility for your disabled relative	**1**	**2**	**3**	**4**
17. Handle a crisis of your disabled relative	**1**	**2**	**3**	**4**
18. Locate needed resources for your disabled relative, e.g., housing, treatment, income maintenance	**1**	**2**	**3**	**4**

self-help organizations regarding the kinds of assistance that they as family members wanted from professionals. Hatfield's survey covered five domains: understanding mental illness and coping with behavior; coping with psychiatric symptoms and medications; getting supportive help for caregivers; improving family relationships; and linkage with community services. We then took the goals for therapy to which families responded on her survey and adapted these goal statements in such a way as to ask family participants to rate the extent to which they agree or disagree that they are able to do such things as accept realistic goals for their disabled relative; understand side effects of psychiatric medication; and get other family members to share responsibility for the disabled relative (see Figure 54.1).

The Families of Adults With Severe Mental Ill Sense of Efficacy or SMI Family Efficacy Measure, which we developed, contained 18 items using a Likert-type format of "strongly agree" to "strongly disagree" for rating each item. This met our needs in terms of being short and easy for respondents to complete. We had confidence in the measure's content validity, given that we exploited someone else's research on the topic of what skills and knowledge families felt they needed in coping with their relative with a mental illness. Because we did not have the time or resources to conduct our own validation assessment, which is often the case in evaluation studies, building on existing literature was one resourceful means for developing a measure.

Adaptive Coping Measure

Adaptation refers to efforts that individuals engage in their interactions with their environments and is best thought of as the fit between an individual's own environment and him or herself (Hatfield, 1987, p. 63). For individuals to be successfully adapted or to have good adaptive coping skills, they must have the motivation, capabilities, and skills to deal with social and environmental demands without being overwhelmed by discomfort and anxiety (Hatfield, 1987). Coping is a response to environmental stresses and "strains in order to prevent, avoid or control emotional distress" (Pearlin & Schooler, 1978, p. 3). Families of persons with severe mental illness engage in a variety of adaptive and maladaptive coping strategies in responding to the stresses they face. Adaptive coping involves applying behavioral strategies to the reduction of actual or potential stress. Carver and his colleagues (1989) delineated 13 categories of coping strategies to respond to stress. These include planning, seeking emotional support, use of denial, or disengagement.

Again, in seeking a scale to assess adaptive coping by families with a relative with a severe mental illness, we found general measures for coping, but nothing specifically geared to coping with this particular life stress. Our approach for constructing a targeted instrument to meet our needs was to adapt an existing measure, COPE, by Carver and his colleagues (1989), which had been evaluated and had good reported psychometric properties. It is important to consider whether a given tool is copyrighted and to operate within the parameters of copyright laws. The COPE instrument was composed of 15 subscales with a total of 60 items. Using 13 of these scales, we found that it was easy to minimally change the wording to meet our needs. For example, the original scale asked respondents what they do when they experience a stressful event; one item that stated "I try to grow as a person as a result of the experience" was changed to "I try to grow as a person as a result of my relative's mental illness." Another example from the original COPE scale was "I pray more than usual," which was changed for our purposes to "When I have a problem with my mentally ill relative, I pray." The same response choices, of 1 = I usually don't do this at all; 2 = I usually do this a little bit; 3 = I usually do this a medium amount; 4 = I usually do this a lot, as were used in the original COPE scale and were employed in the adaptation as well.

Minimal Assessment of the Psychometrics of These "Homegrown" Measures

At the time we were developing these measures, we happened to be conducting a research study

in which the sample consisted of persons with severe mental illness who were receiving case management services. Therefore, we were in a position in which we could ask a few of these participants if we could speak with their family member to test these measures. Although a practitioner may not be in a position of having an active research study on which to draw, he or she may have access to a similar service population that would be willing to test the measure. Another possibility is that the first time the intervention is offered, the evaluation may be used as a means to refine and assess the measures.

We were able to get 16 family members of the consumers in our study to participate in this pilot study. For such a small sample, the research assistant on the evaluation of the case management study was able to conduct the interviews with these family members. We recognized that this was a very small sample; therefore, what we were able to do was very limited. However, this sample would at least provide us with some preliminary assessment of these homegrown measures.

For reliability, we did test-retest and Cronbach's alpha on each of these measures. For use in guiding decision making and treatment planning with individual clients, Springer, Abell, and Nugent (2002) provide the following guidelines for acceptability of reliability coefficients:

$< .70$ = unacceptable
$.70-.79$ = undesirable
$.80-.84$ = minimally acceptable
$.85-.89$ = respectable
$.90-.95$ = very good
$> .95$ = excellent

The Family Self-Efficacy Measure produced excellent test-retest scores ($N = 10$, $r = .9805$, $p < .001$) and minimally acceptable internal consistency, with a Cronbach's alpha of .8419 ($N = 13$). For the validity assessment, we used Pearlin and Schooler's (1978) Mastery scale. Self-efficacy is usually viewed as situation-specific, whereas mastery is a sense of power in a generalized context. Therefore, the correlation between these two was hypothesized as possibly providing an assessment of the validity against a widely used brief measure, which contained only 7 items. However, the Mastery measure did not perform very well in this sample. It had poor test-retest reliability ($r = .1555$, N.S.) and barely acceptable internal consistency (alpha = .7329). Therefore, the fact that these two measures did not correlate at all did not surprise us. To further assess the Family Self-Efficacy scale, we correlated this measure with the adapted COPE measure ($r = .923$, $p < .001$). Based on the theories of self-efficacy and coping adaptation, we expected the two concepts to be related. In summary, we were thus able to determine that the measure seemed to have good reliability and some indication of validity.

The adapted coping measure for families of adults with severe mental illness was assessed in the same manner as the self-efficacy measure. The adapted coping measure had excellent test-retest reliability (.9107, $p < .001$, $N = 12$) and very good internal consistency, with a Cronbach's alpha of .8445 ($N = 16$). This measure also had good validity, being highly correlated with the COPE measure of Carver and associates (1989; $r = .9233$, $p < .001$, $N = 16$). Thus, this homegrown measure appeared to have good reliability and validity.

When we used these two homegrown measures in the full-scale study to evaluate the effectiveness of the psychoeducation, we found that they did well in terms of internal reliability. The Family Self-Efficacy measure had an alpha coefficient of .8074 ($N = 161$). The adaptive coping also had good internal consistency, with an alpha of .8226 ($N = 215$).

Because this adapted coping measure contained 51 items in the total measure, which includes both adaptive and maladaptive items, or 32 items in just the adaptive coping portion, we thought that shortening it would be beneficial for purposes of future evaluations of interventions with the same objectives. Both of these versions are relatively lengthy measures for use in evaluations. In the sample for the larger study, we conducted an analysis to assess whether we could shorten the measure. A stepwise multiple regression was performed to determine which smaller set of subscales might explain most of the variance in the total measure of adapted coping for families of adults with severe mental illness. We used the baseline measure of the evaluation study of the family education intervention for purposes of this analysis and found that three subscales containing 11 items explained 90% of the variance in the measure. The alpha reliability for this 11-item version had acceptable internal reliability (alpha coefficient = .76, $N = 222$; see Figure 54.2 for the

11-item version of the scale). This met our need for brevity while still retaining good psychometric properties.

CONCLUSION

One of the easiest means for developing specific outcome measures for particularized interventions for which there is not likely to be an existing instrument is to adapt available ones that measure the more generalized concept. A review of the literature may reveal a completed study whose survey questions can be adapted to form a scale. The other possibility, which requires more work, is to develop a measure totally from scratch. The literature review should help to develop some of the items and is indeed a key step used by scale developers. In addition, interviewing providers, researchers, and clients will provide information to formulate scale items. Further, conducting a focus group or two will help to refine, delete, or offer new items and will enhance the scale's content validity. The reality is that all too frequently we are not able to find brief measures that address the concepts we need for evaluation studies. There may be very lengthy measures that have been developed for research purposes but that do not work well for an evaluation study, or even for some research studies where numerous concepts are being assessed. These two measures worked well in the larger study. The self-efficacy measure was the one outcome measure for which the intervention had an effect (Solomon et al., 1996, 1997). Both of these measures need far more research to assess their reliability and validity. We have received a number of requests for this measure, indicating that the concept is well used in research on families of persons with severe mental illness.

References

Bandura, A. (1977). Self-efficacy: Toward a unifying theory of behavioral change. *Psychological Review, 84*, 191–215.

Bandura, A. (1982). Self-efficacy mechanism in human agency. *American Psychologist, 37*, 122–147.

Brown, L. N. (1991). *Groups for growth and change.* New York: Longman.

Carver, C., Scheier, M., & Weintraub, J. (1989). Assessing coping strategies: A theoretically based approach. *Journal of Personality and Social Psychology, 36*, 267–283.

FIGURE 54.2 Brief SMI Family Adaptive Coping Scale

We are interested in how family members respond when they confront a different or stressful situation with their mentally disabled relative. There are lots of ways to try to deal with these situations. These questions ask you to indicate what you generally do and feel, when *YOU* experience these situations. Obviously different situations bring out somewhat different responses, but think about what you usually do when you encounter these situations. Please try to respond to each item separately. There are no "right" or "wrong" answers, so choose the most accurate answer for *YOU*—not what you think "most people" would say or do. Indicate what *YOU* usually do when *YOU* experience each of these situations.

Use the following rating categories

    1 = I usually don't do this at all   **2** = I usually do this a little bit
    3 = I usually do this a medium amount   **4** = I usually do this a lot

1. I try to grow as a person as a result of my relative's mental illness.	1	2	3	4
2. I try to see my relative's mental illness in a different light, to see the strengths and positive characteristics of my relative.	1	2	3	4
3. I try to learn from the experience of having a mentally ill relative.	1	2	3	4
4. I try to get advice from someone about problems I have with my mentally ill relative.	1	2	3	4
5. I talk to someone to find out more about particular situations I encounter with my mentally ill relative.	1	2	3	4
6. I talk to someone who I think could do something concrete about problems I have with my mentally ill relative.	1	2	3	4
7. I ask people who have had similar experiences with their mentally ill relative what they did.	1	2	3	4
8. When I have a problem with my mentally ill relative, I put aside other activities in order to concentrate on this.	1	2	3	4
9. When I have a problem with my mentally ill relative, I focus on dealing with this problem and if necessary, let other things slide a little.	1	2	3	4
10. When I have a problem with my mentally ill relative, I try hard to prevent other things from interfering with my efforts at dealing with this.	1	2	3	4
11. When I have a problem with my mentally ill relative, I keep myself from getting distracted by other thoughts or activities.	1	2	3	4

Hatfield, A. (1983). What families want of family therapists. In W. R. McFarlane (Ed.), *Family therapy in schizophrenia*, (pp. 41–65). New York: Guilford.

Hatfield, A. (1987). Coping and adaptation: A conceptual framework for understanding families. In A. B. Hatfield & H. Lefley (Eds.), *Family interventions in mental illness*, (pp. 60–84). New York: Guilford.

Pearlin, L., & Schooler, C. (1978). The structure of coping. *Journal of Health and Social Behavior, 19*, 2–21.

Sands, R., & Solomon, P. (in press). Developing educational groups in social work practice. *Social Work with Groups.*

Solomon, P., Draine, J., Mannion, E., & Meisel, M. (1996). Impact of brief family psychoeducation on self-efficacy. *Schizophrenia Bulletin, 22*, 41–50.

Solomon, P., Draine, J., Mannion, E., & Meisel, M. (1997). Effectiveness of two models of brief family education: Retention of gains by family members of adults with serious mental illness. *American Journal of Orthopsychiatry, 67*, 177–186.

Springer, D. W., Abell, N., & Nugent, W. R. (2002). Creating and validating rapid assessment instruments for practice and research: Part 2. *Research on Social Work Practice, 12*, 805–832.

Toseland, R. W., & Rivas, R. F. (2001). *An introduction to group work practice* (4th ed.). Boston: Allyn and Bacon.

55

CONSTRUCTING AND VALIDATING ASSESSMENT TOOLS FOR SCHOOL-BASED PRACTITIONERS

The Elementary School Success Profile

Natasha K. Bowen, Gary L. Bowen, & Michael E. Woolley

Accurate and appropriate assessment is critical to the process of evidence-based practice. In Vandiver's "algorithm for using practice guidelines in a mental health setting" (2002, p. 735), for example, assessment is the starting point of intervention. And, according to Thyer (2002), the practitioner's use of a "systematic, hypothesis-testing approach" with every case starts with a "careful assessment" (p. 739). Without relevant, accurate, and complete assessment information, the practitioner is unlikely to design an appropriate and effective evidence-based intervention strategy. The quality of available assessment tools, therefore, potentially establishes the credibility of the entire subsequent evidence-based practice sequence. The quality of assessment tools, in turn, is related to the quality of the instrument development process. In this chapter we argue that involving end users and targeted populations in the process of developing assessment tools enhances their validity, reliability, and practical utility.

Using the development of the Elementary School Success Profile (ESSP) as an example, the chapter describes standard and innovative instrument development procedures. The ESSP is a comprehensive assessment tool for third- to fifth-grade children. The innovative procedures included, but were not limited to, qualitative methods to involve end users and the targeted population in the process of developing the instrument. Although we describe multiple strategies for involving site-level users of assessment tools in their development, we focus especially on how we involved children in the development process of the ESSP through the use of cognitive pretesting. Pretesting was conducted to ensure the *developmental validity* of self-report items for children—that is, to ensure that items were read, understood, and responded to by children in the manner expected by the instrument developers. Developmental validity is a critical, but often overlooked, criterion for high-quality assessments.

CONTEXT

The ESSP is a tool for school-based practitioners who require comprehensive understanding of students' social environments and current functioning in order to design appropriate individual and group interventions. Based on an ecological perspective, information about the neighborhood, school, friends, and family systems of children is collected, along with data on behavior, school performance, physical health, and psychological functioning. Children, parents, and teachers respond to items on the ESSP Child Form, Parent Form, and Teacher Form, respectively. The Child Form is a colorful, engaging computer program; the Parent and Teacher Forms are scannable paper-and-pencil questionnaires. Visual profiles that integrate the data from all three sources summarize findings at both the individual and group level. School staff use the profiles to guide intervention planning and monitor intervention results.

Our dedication to using a practice-based and rigorous development process for the ESSP stemmed from the experiences of senior members of the current research team with the development of the "parent" instrument of the ESSP, the School Success Profile (SSP; Bowen, Richman, & Bowen, 2002). The SSP is a comprehensive, self-report assessment tool for middle and high school students. It emerged from a collaboration between practitioners in the school-based, national dropout prevention program Communities in Schools (CIS) and members of the research team. Input was sought from stakeholders in the success of students—school staff, parents, community members, and students themselves. The SSP has been used for over 10 years by CIS staff and other practitioners in schools and has been completed by tens of thousands of students.

Practitioners familiar with the SSP requested a version of the instrument that could be used with younger children to help prevent the development of the problems that can lead to school failure and behavior problems in middle school and high school students. With funding from the National Institute on Drug Abuse and a partnership with a small computer technology firm, we launched a project to develop such an instrument. While acknowledging the need to collect some information from the original SSP from parents and teachers, we retained a child self-report component in the ESSP. Assuring the quality of data collected with the Child Form has been a major focus of the ESSP development process.

STUDY OVERVIEW

Consistent with the centrality of empirical findings to evidence-based practice in general, systematic research procedures play a central role in the development of assessment instruments. The goal of rigorous procedures is to ensure that instruments are valid and reliable. In the development of self-report instruments for children, developmental validity, as defined earlier in this chapter, is a special concern. One recommended set of scale development procedures includes determining what to measure through a review of relevant theory and existing measures, developing an item pool, choosing question and response formats, obtaining expert feedback on the item pool, collecting data from a test sample, and evaluating the items statistically (DeVellis, 1991). These standard procedures are primarily quantitative. It should be noted that some assessment tools comprise one scale, or set of items (i.e., questions) assessing one phenomenon (e.g., depression or life stressors). Others comprise a number of subscales (e.g., inattention, hyperactivity, impulsivity) that assess multiple dimensions of one general phenomenon (e.g., attention deficit/hyperactivity disorder). These instruments provide information about only one type of functioning or experience. Technically, scale development recommendations refer to the development of scales and/or subscales for assessing one phenomenon; however, the procedures can be extended to the development of instruments that include multiple scales, such as the ESSP.

Faced with the challenge of developing a comprehensive assessment instrument for school-based practitioners working with students in Grades 3 through 5, members of our research team designed a development process that included the standard instrument development steps listed earlier in this chapter, as well as a variety of additional procedures. Many of the additional procedures allowed us to incorporate feedback from parents, teachers, student services staff, and elementary school children themselves into the ESSP. Steps beyond the traditional scale development steps included reviewing literature on child development and instrument development methods (i.e., conducting a review that went well beyond the scope of the recommended literature review step), obtaining expert feedback at two stages of the development process instead of one, collecting feedback from teachers about aspects of the Child Form as it was being developed, cognitive pretesting of Child Form items, collecting feedback from parents and teachers about the length and content of the Parent and Teacher Forms, and collecting feedback from school staff about administration procedures and data summaries. In the following, we discuss the components of the ESSP development process, illustrating how we worked with individuals in elementary schools and others to enhance the validity, reliability, and practical utility of the instrument.

DEVELOPMENT OF THE ESSP: METHODS AND FINDINGS

Determining What to Measure Through a Literature Review

Like the SSP, the ESSP was designed from the start to be a multiple-scale instrument. The decision to assess multiple aspects of the social environment and child functioning stemmed both from ecological theory, which states that current performance is determined by characteristics of the major environments in which children function, and from our knowledge of the realities of the school practice setting. Because school-based practitioners encounter a wide range of referral issues, they require an assessment tool that provides (a) a comprehensive view of outcomes or functioning, (b) a comprehensive view of the potential individual and environmental contributors to problems, and (c) a view of individual and environmental strengths that can be harnessed in interventions. Our review of neighborhood, school, friend, and family factors relevant to elementary school students' current performance and future drug use helped us modify the list of risk and protective factors assessed with the middle and high version of the instrument to be developmentally appropriate for younger children. More important, however, our review of child development theory suggested that it was necessary to pay careful attention to both the wording of items on the Child Form and the overall format and length of the Child Form. At the same time, our review of methods for developing self-report instruments revealed a useful method for evaluating the appropriateness of the child self-report items—cognitive pretesting. Implications of these findings are discussed in more detail later.

Developing an Item Pool and Choosing Question and Response Formats

At the early stage of item pool development, our goal was to use our own expertise and existing literature and instruments to develop the best preliminary item pool possible. After identifying the factors that needed to be assessed with scales, our strategies for generating new items and modifying existing SSP items were informed by the cognitive developmental theory of Jean Piaget.

Piagetian developmental theory asserts that children go through a series of four developmental stages at approximately similar ages and in the same order: Stage 1, the sensory motor stage (birth to 2 years of age); Stage 2, the preoperational stage (2 to 6 years of age); Stage 3, the concrete operations stage (6 to 12 years of age); and Stage 4, the formal operations stage (ages 12 and older). As children advance through these stages, their understanding of the world, fund of knowledge, and ability to manipulate mental images expand (Miller, 1993). The development process is seen as a biologically guided trajectory that is influenced by the child's interaction with the environment (Wadsworth, 1996).

We focused our attention on the cognitive abilities of children in the concrete operations stage because the ESSP targets third to fifth graders. As the name implies, the concrete operations stage begins when children acquire the ability to perform operations, which are the cognitive processes of mentally representing environmental phenomena and mentally manipulating those representations to draw conclusions about the environment. The ability to perform operations is the minimal cognitive ability necessary to validly answer social information questions. However, the number of mental representations a child can manipulate at this stage is still limited. Also, as the name implies, children's operations are limited in this stage by the "concrete" nature of their thinking. Therefore, children's ability to perform operations is not only limited by the number of representations they can operate on, but also by the level of abstraction of the concepts they can represent.

Piagetian theory suggests that the ability of children to respond validly to any specific questionnaire item will be a function of the cognitive demands of that item. Items that demand abstract thinking, such as imagining hypothetical situations, interpreting the thoughts or feelings of others, or interpreting one's own thoughts, feelings, or behaviors, will likely fail. There is also likely to be a limit to the number of concepts in any one item that children in the concrete operations stage can successfully process. Finally, because response option sets must also be represented and operated upon, they, too, must be clear and concrete. Response options should add as little as possible to the cognitive demands of each item.

As part of the item pool development process, five experts reviewed the preliminary pool of items and provided feedback. All our experts had experience in developing instruments for children, and one is the author of a social science sourcebook on scale development. All were also experienced researchers. Two of the reviewers had expertise in education and child development, one specialized in early education and developmental disabilities, and one was a child and adolescent psychiatrist. Items in the pool were organized into scales within three categories: questions for children, questions for parents, and questions for teachers. The experts were asked to examine individual items for developmental appropriateness (for the child and adult respondents) and for regional, gender, or race/ethnic biases. They were also asked to assess the content validity of each of the proposed scales in the item pool. *Content validity* refers to the extent to which all aspects of a phenomenon, such as neighborhood safety, are covered in the pool of items for the scale designed to measure that phenomenon (Carmines & Zeller, 1979). Finally, they were asked to assess the content validity of the entire instrument, that is, to indicate if there were important environmental or individual factors related to child functioning that were missing from the proposed sets of scales.

The reviewers provided us with extensive feedback in each of the requested categories. Based on their feedback, we modified the response options for some items; reduced the overall number of response option sets; modified numerous items on the child, parent, and teacher forms; and added and deleted other items. At the conclusion of this item pool development substep, we believed the ESSP content for the Child, Parent, and Teacher Forms to be of high quality. At this point we created the scannable Parent and Teacher Form templates.

Choosing a Format for the Child Form

Theory and literature about the abilities of children in middle childhood led us to carefully consider formatting alternatives for the Child Form. Given the more limited vocabulary, comprehension, and attention skills of third to fifth graders (in relation to adolescents), it was clear that a half-hour, paper-and-pencil questionnaire would be unlikely to generate valid and reliable data from children. We decided to exploit computer technology to address these limitations. Under our supervision, programmers at a small computer technology firm designed a creative computerized format for the ESSP. Children's short attention spans are addressed through the use of a colorful, engaging interactive program. Children can select answers in two different ways (by clicking on a response or by typing the number of a response), can keep track of their progress through the program by watching characters make their way across the bottom of the screen, and are rewarded with short animations after each topical sequence of items. Large print and consistent formatting make each screen easy to negotiate. Lower reading abilities are accommodated through links to word definitions and a (future) toggle option to have items read aloud. These features, as well as graphics related to each topical domain (e.g., neighborhood, school, family, friends, health and well-being), promote reliable and valid responses by keeping children on task, providing cues about item content, and helping them understand questions and response options.

During the development of the prototype computerized Child Form, we again sought expert feedback. The five experts consulted previously focused their attention in this second review on the computer format and the presentation of items within that format. They also reviewed the revised content of the Child Form items. They provided useful feedback on the ease of the computer functions, the developmental appropriateness of the graphics, the format of the question pages, and item content. Examples of changes made based on their feedback included adding a "back" option for when children want to return to a question to change an answer, making it possible to skip animations (which might be necessary for children with seizure disorders), and changing the order and wording of some items.

In addition to seeking feedback from our academic and mental health experts, we also showed the prototype ESSP to 11 elementary school teachers and student services staff and asked for qualitative feedback about all aspects of the computerization. This step represented our first step into the actual practice setting to obtain the insights of potential users of the ESSP. Using their knowledge of third- to fifth-grade children's interests, life experiences, and exposure to other software, the school staff members were able to provide useful feedback about how children might respond to the ESSP. They reported, for example, that the ESSP's use of items in the form of statements instead of questions would be well received by children who dislike tests. They thought the animation leading up to the school items captured well the mood and environment of their school. They agreed that children would like the "status bar"—the group of figures walking across the bottom of the screen—telling them how far along in the ESSP they were. They also validated that the content of the ESSP reflected the issues of interest and concern among teachers and students services staff. The teachers offered suggestions about how to make ESSP animations reflect the experiences of more children—such as having some figures come to school by bicycle or walking and having some children greeted by one parent instead of two when they return home from school. Like the academic experts, the teachers made a number of helpful suggestions for improving the program and provided strong positive feedback about the quality, developmental appropriateness, and appeal of the program.

Cognitive Pretesting

Researchers creating assessment instruments typically rely on the "expertise" of adults, as described in the previous ESSP development steps. After the rigorous and high-quality development sequence the ESSP had undergone up to this point, it could have been considered ready for pilot testing and statistical evaluation. However, because the ESSP targets children between 7 and 11 years of age who are in a developmental stage in which their cognitive abilities are theoretically qualitatively different from those of adults, an additional development step was implemented: cognitive pretesting of the Child Form. Cognitive pretesting involves monitoring the thought processes of respondents while they complete a questionnaire to determine if they are comprehending questions and responding to them in the manner intended by the questionnaire developers.

Cognitive pretesting methods are derived from cognitive processing theories, such as information-processing theory. We collaborated with teachers and student services staff at two schools to pretest ESSP items with children. This development step proved invaluable for detecting items that contained vocabulary or sentence structures that proved difficult for some children, items that were interpreted differently

than intended by the adults who designed them, and response options that were inadequate.

Theoretical and Empirical Basis for Cognitive Pretesting

Children in the concrete operations stage of cognitive development think more concretely than adults, and their cognitive ability to represent and manipulate multiple concepts mentally is much more limited than that of adults. This combination effectively means children think differently than adults. The implication for scale developers is that adults cannot assume children will interpret items and answer options the way we intend, even when we attempt to take into account their developmental limitations while constructing items and answers. The best way to determine how children cognitively process instrument items is to consult them as the experts on how children read, interpret, and respond to instrument items through cognitive pretesting.

Cognitive pretesting is recognized as a qualitative technique for improving questionnaire design (e.g., Jobe & Mingay, 1989; Willis, Royston, & Bercini, 1991) by assessing how successfully respondents proceed through theoretical steps in processing information related to survey items. From an information-processing perspective there are four critical steps in responding validly to an instrument item: (a) comprehension (interpreting the question as the instrument developers intended); (b) orientation (understanding and adopting the appropriate perspective for the question); (c) judgment (comprehending the response options within the context of the question); and (d) response (providing an answer and a valid rationale for the answer) (DeMaio & Rothgeb, 1996; Hippler, Schwartz, & Sudman, 1987; Tourangeau, Rips, & Rasinski, 2000). Successful completion of these steps by children indicates that an item has developmental validity. If respondents have difficulties with any of the four information-processing steps, items can be modified, replaced, or deleted to increase the instrument's developmental validity.

Procedures for Cognitive Pretesting of the ESSP

Two rounds of cognitive pretesting were conducted with a total of 39 children. Modifications to items and to the testing procedures were made after each step. The primary cognitive pretesting technique used for testing the ESSP was "verbal probing" (Willis et al., 1991); testers asked children scripted questions about the ESSP items and about their responses to the items. First, teachers familiar with the child subjects were trained by the researchers in cognitive pretesting procedures and about federal human subjects research guidelines. Teachers were provided with all the materials necessary for testing a designated number of children. Children sat one at a time with a teacher and tested 15 predesignated questions from the prototype computerized Child Form. Upon advancing to a question to be tested, the teacher first asked the child to read the item aloud. If the child had trouble reading any word in the item, the teacher said the word aloud and asked if the child understood the word. Next the child was asked to put the question in his or her own words. (Because many items are very simply worded and were difficult to reword, this step has been modified. Children are now asked, "What does that question mean; what is it trying to find out from you?") Then the child was asked to choose an answer and to explain why he or she chose it. In the first round of cognitive pretesting, testers were trained to record in writing relevant observations about children's verbalizations. In the second round, the testing sessions were audiotaped, reducing the writing burden of teachers and providing the researchers with more complete data. The data were analyzed to determine if children could read questions fluently, if they understood the vocabulary used in questions, if they interpreted the questions as intended, and if their explanations for their responses were consistent with the intended meaning of the questions and the response options.

Findings from Cognitive Pretesting of the ESSP

Although the Child Form of the ESSP had undergone scrutiny by researchers, by experts in child development, education, and scale development, and by elementary school staff, cognitive pretesting of items with children revealed the need for further modifications to some items to improve their developmental validity. Not all items were read, understood, and responded to by children in the manner expected by adults who had contributed to the form's development. Although almost all of the items tested could be read with no difficulty by third graders with av-

erage or below-average reading ability, a few words proved problematic to some children. Examples of words that caused difficulty for one or two children were *bother, something, grownups, aches,* and *confused.* Some questions proved not to be concrete enough to be interpreted accurately by the children. For example, when asked if he had friends to play with outside of school, one child responded that he had friends to play with at recess (when he was *physically* outside of the school). A sequence of self-esteem items also proved to be too abstract. For example, in explaining his response to the item "I feel happy with myself," one child said, "Sometimes I feel happy and sometimes I don't." Another said, "I'm always happy." And a third said, "If you're not sad, you can be happy by yourself."

The identification of words that some children could not read, and phrases and items that some children misinterpreted indicated that cognitive pretesting was a valuable component of the ESSP development process. Results from the testing helped us make modifications to items and response options and helped us better understand the meaning of responses to Child Form items.

Collecting Data from a Test Sample

After making extensive revisions to the Child Form based on findings from the cognitive testing, we proceeded to a more standard instrument development step: conducting a pilot test. Data were collected from 102 students. Teacher data were collected on all 102 students, and parent data were obtained for 90 of the students. The principal goal of the collection of data from a test sample is usually to conduct statistical tests of items and scales. Our goal, in contrast, was much broader. In addition to obtaining data on enough cases to conduct preliminary statistical analyses, our purpose was to work closely with student services staff who administered the ESSP, and parents and teachers who completed the Parent and Teacher Forms to assess all aspects of the ESSP administration. Teachers and student services staff at an elementary school were trained using the detailed ESSP Administration Manual to collect parent, teacher, and child consent/assent and to administer the ESSP. A brief questionnaire was attached to the Parent and Teacher Forms, asking respondents for their feedback on the length and content of the forms. Questions with limited response possibilities (e.g., Which questions, if any, made you uncomfortable?), as well as open-ended questions (e.g., Do you have suggestions for improving the survey? Are there areas or issues *not* covered in the survey that you think are important for understanding the situation and needs of elementary school children?) were used. Finally, after the administration of the ESSP was complete, we sought qualitative feedback from school staff about how well the ESSP administration training and implementation procedures performed. We also provided them with the graphic individual and group summaries generated by the ESSP data, explained how to interpret the summaries, and asked for their feedback.

Seeking information from respondents and school personnel using the ESSP, like all previously described strategies to obtain and incorporate information from individuals at the intended ESSP practice sites, proved to be valuable. School staff provided us with both positive feedback about many aspects of the ESSP administration procedures and useful suggestions for improving the procedures. Based on their feedback, for example, we modified our administration procedures to better highlight the advantages of creating a team to share the responsibilities of administering the ESSP. We incorporated into the manual school staff suggestions about how teachers could be invited into the ESSP administration process to facilitate the collection of parent consent and distribution of Parent Forms.

A number of parents and teachers provided feedback on the Parent and Teacher Forms. Through the easy and inexpensive method of attaching a short questionnaire to the adult forms of the ESSP, we identified a number of response sets that were not adequate, as well as a construct ("neighborhood") that did not apply to some respondents in the rural setting in which the pilot test was conducted. Because a small number of parents questioned the need to ask about family income, we added language to a document in the parent consent package explaining that ESSP information about sensitive issues (such as family income and parent work and education status) are never seen by school personnel. The information is only reported in aggregate on the ESSP group summary profile.

The pilot test confirmed that collecting data from parents, even after they have consented to complete the ESSP and to allow their children to complete the ESSP, may be the biggest implementation challenge of the instrument. School staff responsible for the administration of the ESSP during the pilot test shared strategies they implemented and other suggestions for increasing the rate of return for the Parent Form. This information was incorporated into the ESSP Administration Manual.

Evaluating ESSP Items Statistically

The pilot test provided enough cases ($N = 102$) for preliminary statistical tests of ESSP items. We examined the distributions of items and reliabilities of scales. Preliminary tests indicated that Parent and Teacher Form scales performed very well—with almost all Cronbach's alpha reliabilities over .80. Not surprisingly, the lowest reliability coefficients were found among the Child Form scales. However, most Child Form reliabilities were in the .70 to .78 range. One inadequate scale, which asked children about adults at their school, was deleted from the Child Form. Item revisions and additions were made to other Child Form scales with marginal pilot test reliabilities. We expect the performance of the Child Form scales to exceed patterns of reliability commonly found in self-report instruments for children in the next round of statistical tests, which will follow the large-scale data collection of a pending study.

DISCUSSION AND CONCLUSION

The first step in the sequence constituting effective, evidence-based practice is the development of instruments that are valid, reliable, and appropriate for the intended practice setting and targeted population. Standard, quantitative instrument development procedures may not go far enough to ensure the validity and practice utility of instruments. Developmental validity, in particular, is a special concern in the development of self-report instruments for children. This chapter described the development of the ESSP as an example of how researchers developing instruments can augment the recommended basic steps in instrument development. We sought expert input twice instead of once, sought qualitative and quantitative feedback from adult respondents (parents and teachers) and end users of the instrument (teachers and student services staff), and sought extensive feedback from children in the age range targeted by the ESSP. In response to theory and empirical evidence about the cognitive abilities of third to fifth graders, we also developed an innovative format for the child component of the ESSP.

Involving end users and respondents in the development of assessment tools can increase the tools' validity, reliability, and practice utility. When developing self-report instruments for children, cognitive pretesting of items to promote developmental validity may be critical. The ESSP design strategy bridges quantitative and qualitative methods. Although the ESSP is a quantitative assessment tool, its development combined traditional scale development procedures, including statistical tests of reliability, with qualitative methods in a highly iterative process. Most notably, the qualitative procedure of cognitive pretesting was used to strengthen the developmental validity of the Child Form. In their recent handbook on mixed methods, Tashakkori and Teddlie (2003) describe such a combined use of quantitative and qualitative strategies in solving applied research problems as the "third methodological movement" (p. ix). A central tenet of this movement, which is anchored in pragmatism, is that quantitative and qualitative methods of inquiry are complementary rather than competing approaches.

We view the development of assessment tools like the ESSP as a process rather than a product. Our instrument development procedures have been designed to bolster the "validity argument" that it is possible to draw meaningful inferences from the self-reports of children and their parents and teachers (Kane, 1992). Both the reliability and the practical utility of assessment tools rest on the validity argument.

Although our instrument development procedures have increased our confidence in the ESSP as a valid assessment tool, work is already under way to further examine the cultural sensitivity and psychometric properties of the Child, Parent, and Teacher Forms with larger samples of respondents. We also plan to add an audio component to the Child Form that will help children with reading deficits complete the survey. Plans are also under way to develop a Spanish version of the Child and Parent Forms in the context of the increasing Hispanic/Latino population in the United States. Cognitive pretesting procedures will play an important role in these further tests and additions.

We have been approached by a number of schools and school systems that have an interest in using the ESSP. Few ecologically based and practice-focused assessment tools are available for practitioners who work with elementary school students. Although we have been reluctant to release the ESSP until we felt that it was ready for implementation, we learned a valuable lesson in developing the "parent" instrument of the ESSP, the SSP: The practice community can help refine the assessment tool. Consequently, we are working with several sites in testing the feasibility of the ESSP as an assessment tool that can be successfully implemented in elementary schools and used to guide intervention planning and monitor intervention results. Such collaboration is a distinctive and refreshing feature of evidence-based practice procedures.

ACKNOWLEDGMENT The ESSP was developed in collaboration with Flying Bridge Technologies with funding from the National Institutes of Health, National Institute on Drug Abuse (IRYZDA13865-01, 3RY1DA13865-0151, and 2RY2DA013865-02). Findings and opinions expressed in this chapter are those of the authors and not necessarily those of Flying Bridge Technologies, NIH, or NIDA.

References

Bowen, G. L., Richman, J. M., & Bowen, N. K. (2002). The School Success Profile: A results management approach to assessment and intervention planning. In A. L. Roberts & G. J. Greene (Eds.), *Social workers' desk reference* (pp. 787–793). New York: Oxford University Press.

Carmines, E. G., & Zeller, R. A. (1979). *Reliability and validity assessment* (Vol. 17). Beverly Hills, CA: Sage.

DeMaio, T. J., & Rothgeb, J. M. (1996). Cognitive interviewing techniques: In the lab and in the field. In N. Schwarz & S. Sudman (Eds.), *Answering questions: Methodology for cognitive and communicative processes in survey research* (pp. 739–742). San Francisco: Jossey-Bass.

DeVellis, R. F. (1991). *Scale development: Theory and applications.* Newbury Park, CA: Sage.

Hippler, H. J., Schwartz, N., & Sudman, S. (Eds.). (1987). *Social information processing and survey methodology.* New York: Springer-Verlag.

Jobe, J. B., & Mingay, D. J. (1989). Cognitive research improves questionnaires. *American Journal of Public Health, 79,* 1053–1055.

Kane, M. T. (1992). An argument-based approach to validity. *Psychological Bulletin, 112,* 527–535.

Miller, P. H. (1993). *Theories of developmental psychology.* New York: Freeman.

Tashakkori, A., & Teddlie, C. (Eds.). (2003). *Handbook of mixed methods in social and behavioral research.* Thousand Oaks, CA: Sage.

Thyer, B. A. (2002). Principles of evidence-based practice and treatment development. In A. R. Roberts & G. J. Greene (Eds.), *Social workers' desk reference* (pp. 739–742). New York: Oxford University Press.

Tourangeau, R., Rips, L. J., & Rasinski, K. (2000). *The psychology of survey response.* Cambridge: Cambridge University Press.

Vandiver, V. L. (2002). Step-by-step practice guidelines for using evidence-based practice and expert consensus in mental health settings. In A. R. Roberts & G. J. Greene (Eds.), *Social workers' desk reference* (pp. 731–738). New York: Oxford University Press.

Wadsworth, B. J. (1996). *Piaget's theory of cognitive and affective development* (5th ed.). White Plains, NY: Longman.

Willis, G. B., Royston, P., & Bercini, D. (1991). The use of verbal report methods in the development and testing of survey questionnaires. *Applied Cognitive Psychology, 5,* 251–267.

56 POST–TRAUMATIC STRESS DISORDER AND TRAUMA ASSESSMENT SCALES

Patrick Bordnick, Ken Graap, & M. Elizabeth Vonk

Mental health practitioners are often the first line of assessment for victims in crisis. Due to exposure to traumatic events, the initial screening and assessment can identify persons who warrant further evaluation for post–traumatic stress disorder (PTSD). Traumatic events are varied, but general categories include physical abuse, sexual assault, automobile accidents, workplace accidents, disasters (man-made and natural), and war. These events are ubiquitous; therefore, mental health practitioners need to develop a basic understanding of trauma and its associated symptoms in order to conduct valid clinical assessments. A key factor to consider is that early identification of traumatic stress and treatment can lead to the prevention of related physical and mental sequelae (Yarvis & Bordnick, 2003) (Figure 56.1). The type of traumatic event or time since exposure to the event may dictate different instruments and assessment techniques (e.g., difference between motor vehicle accident, rape, or war experience). In this chapter, general assessment strategies will be presented for mental health practitioners. The assessments described here assume that screening has indicated reasons to evaluate PTSD specifically and that adequate time for such an in-depth evaluation is available.

POST–TRAUMATIC STRESS DISORDER

PTSD can occur as a result of virtually any extreme (e.g., life-threatening) stressful situation in which one perceives a significant risk to his or her well-being (or to that of a loved one) and the experience results in intense fear, helplessness, or horror (American Psychiatric Associa-

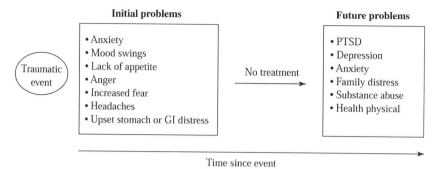

FIGURE 56.1 Progression of symptoms from exposure to the traumatic event

tion, 1994). Data from the National Comorbidity Survey indicated a lifetime prevalence of PTSD at approximately 7% in U.S. adults (Kessler, 1995). Further estimates indicate that over 5 million U.S. adults older than 18 years experience PTSD currently (American Psychiatric Association, 1994). The spectrum of symptoms can have an acute onset or be delayed until a later time. Symptoms manifesting in the first 3 months are specified as acute stage, and those that persist after 3 months may be specified as chronic. The progression of symptoms from exposure to the traumatic event is depicted in Figure 56.1. For example, a disaster responder who works on the scene of a collapsed building with mass causalities may first experience symptoms such as grief, anxiety, loss of appetite, and anger. These symptoms, if left unaddressed, may begin to interfere with psychosocial functioning and lead to both psychological disorders (PTSD, depression) and physical disorders (hypertension), or they may abate through the use of effective coping strategies. However, research on PTSD still has not identified the exact progression of symptoms from acute to chronic.

PREPARING FOR PTSD ASSESSMENT

A diagnosis of PTSD is made after a thorough evaluation of symptoms set forth in the fourth edition of the *Diagnostic and Statistical Manual of Mental Disorders* (American Psychiatric Association, 1994). Diagnosing PTSD differs from many other disorders in that the first criterion is the occurrence of a significant, often life-threatening, event to an individual or to a close relative. These events can occur in virtually any

aspect of one's life. Recent events in the United States and abroad have increased exposure to man-made disasters (terrorist events). Subsequently, professionals must be aware of this potential category of victims and events that may require assessment and treatment.

A thorough PTSD assessment may be complicated by the patient's difficulty in answering specific questions about the traumatic events, especially during the acute phase of the disorder. Assessors must be very sensitive to affective (mood state) changes that may ensue when difficult situations are described by patients. In some cases, the use of self-report instruments may provide an alternative method of gathering required information if patients become overly distressed during a clinical interview.

Unfortunately, it is not uncommon for a patient to present for evaluation and treatment after multiple traumas. Each trauma must typically be evaluated separately. It is critical to determine that the assessor is talking about a specific trauma for each symptom being evaluated. The temporal order of the traumas may also be informative in formulating a treatment strategy. A note of caution is warranted here. When attempting to evaluate trauma occurring in the past, retrospective recall of symptoms may present unique challenges to the evaluator (Hyman & Loftus, 1998). See also Banyard (2000) for a more complete review of the issues associated with traumatic memory. Many studies have suggested that retrospective recall can be contaminated with recent events and with events that never occurred. Additionally, specific time thresholds and sequences of events may be difficult to recall.

A final caution is included here that is not

specific to PTSD but is relevant to any diagnosis that is being offered in settings where patient motivations are not overtly understood. If there are issues of secondary gain associated with the diagnosis, additional rigor is often necessary to correctly categorize and quantify the trauma and its sequelae. After a formal diagnostic evaluation, an assessment of specific symptoms and related sequelae should be conducted, and validating information gathered from secondary sources may add credence to cases where there is doubt regarding the veracity of the self-report.

Preparing to assess PTSD includes attaining familiarity with the diagnostic criteria and an appreciation for the process one encounters after a trauma. In general, the type of trauma experienced is not critical, but one's perception of the risk involved appears to be central to the development of symptoms. Once an event has occurred, other symptoms organized loosely into categories of reexperiencing, increased arousal, and increased reactivity will often be present. If these symptoms continue for more than 30 days and lead to significant disruption in one's life, a diagnosis of PTSD may be appropriate. Importantly, many people who experience life-threatening events do not develop PTSD and find ways to cope with the events adequately. Whereas PTSD may be relatively well known among professionals, it is often unknown to those suffering with the symptoms and struggling to make sense of their world after a traumatic event. Thus a careful evaluation may be necessary to reveal the temporal relationship of symptom onset and the occurrence of a specific traumatic event.

BROADENING THE SCOPE WITH PTSD

PTSD affects many aspects of a patient's psychosocial functioning and can lead to a variety of self-destructive coping mechanisms. A comprehensive evaluation goes beyond simply assessing the formal symptoms and puts the disorder into the context of the patient's life so that treatment may be guided by the information provided.

Research suggests that depression co-occurs with PTSD (Davidson & Fairbank, 1993). In fact, lifetime prevalence rates of depression in veterans with PTSD are as high as 65% (Friedman, 1990). The presence of depression may also sug-

gest a need for medical or psychiatric referral. Substance abuse is commonly found in populations with PTSD (Bremner, Southwick, Darnell, & Charney, 1996; Chilcoat & Breslau, 1998; Dansky, Roitzsch, Brady, & Saladin, 1997; Epstein, Saunders, Kilpatrick, & Resnick, 1998). Substance abuse or dependence is usually addressed prior to beginning formal treatment for PTSD, because the presence of some substances will directly interfere with behavioral treatments. Also, after exposure to a traumatic event, stressors can occur in the family, leading to a deterioration of family function. The role of family functioning is critical to understand because behavioral treatment may initially lead to increased reexperiencing of symptoms, and the family may need to be more supportive during initial treatment.

CHOOSING ASSESSMENT INSTRUMENTS

In the preceding sections, we have suggested a broad approach to assessing PTSD. The information may be gathered in structured interviews or via self-report questionnaires.

More directed forms of interviews might be found in clinician-administered structured interviews designed specifically to evaluate symptoms of PTSD (Table 56.1). These scales focus on a specific event or events and one's reactions. They may be useful in evaluating the entire clinical picture as it relates to PTSD. Additionally, patient self-report instruments are used to determine the presence and severity of symptoms.

Slightly different evaluation measures have been developed for use with civilian and military populations. Additional care must be taken when dealing with child populations as well. Children's behavior after an event may be disrupted, and depending on their age and language development, children may not be able to verbally describe their experience.

In the following a number of techniques for evaluation are discussed. This is meant not to prepare the reader to conduct evaluations using the instruments discussed but to suggest possible instruments for use. Each instrument is accompanied by specific instructions and psychometric properties that must be understood prior to their use in the clinic. A list of suggested PTSD and traumatic stress assessment instruments is presented in Table 56.1

TABLE 56.1 Assessment Instruments

Name	Versions[1]	How to find or locate source
SCID-I	O H	http://cpmcnet.columbia. edu/dept/scid/
CAPS	H	National Center for PTSD Ncptsd@ncptsd.org www.ncptsd.org
PDS	O H	http://www.pearson assessments.com
BDI-II	O H	www.psychorpcenter.com
SCL90-R	O H	http://www.pearson assessments.com
IES	H	Corcoran K., & Fischer J. (2000). Measures for clinical practice: A sourcebook (3rd ed., Vol. 2, pp. 363–364). New York: Free Press. Horowitz, M. J., Wilner, N., & Alvarez, W. (1979). Impact of event scale: A measure of subjective distress. *Psychosomatic Medicine, 41,* 209–218.
ASI	O H	www.asimv.com www.deltametrics.com
IFR	O H	http://www.walmyr.com/ famscales.html

[1]O = Computer/online; H = Hard copy

DIAGNOSTIC ASSESSMENT

Three of the most widely used diagnostic instruments for PTSD will be reviewed. The information collected ranges from basic diagnostic criteria to in-depth comprehensive coverage of symptoms and impact on the patient's daily life. The instruments reviewed include Structured Clinical Diagnostic Interview for PTSD (SCID; First, Spitzer, Williams, & Gibbon, 2000), the Clinician-Administered PSTD Scale (CAPS; Blake et al., 1995), and the Posttraumatic Diag-

nostic Scale (PDS; Foa, Cashman, Jaycox, & Perry, 1997). In summary, this review includes instruments that suit a range of clinical settings and offer varying degrees of diagnostic and clinical information; it is not to be interpreted as a review of all instruments.

The SCID (PTSD module), a 21-item structured interview based on the *DSM-IV* criteria for PTSD, is is a subsection of the full SCID diagnostic evaluation for *DSM-IV* Axis I disorders (American Psychiatric Association, 1994; First, Spitzer, Gibbon, & Williams, 1994). The module interview includes specific questions designed to assess each criterion of PTSD and rate it on a 3-point Likert scale. The SCID (PTSD module) yields basic diagnostic information and takes approximately 15 to 45 minutes to complete. The SCID (PTSD) requires users to complete a training program. Its module can be administered alone or as a full SCID interview if other diagnostic categories are indicated.

The CAPS is a comprehensive assessment of both PTSD diagnostic criteria and clinical symptoms. The CAPS consists of 30 questions and takes approximately 1 hour to complete. Each of the *DSM-IV* criteria for PTSD is assessed, along with specific cognitive and behavioral symptoms (Blake et al., 1995). The CAPS has been shown to have acceptable reliability and validity (Mueser et al., 2001; Weathers, Keane, & Davidson, 2001). The CAPS interview yields specific information regarding impact on functioning, which can aid clinicians in setting up a treatment plan and therapeutic goals. The CAPS has been used in both clinical outcomes studies and research trials (Blanchard et al., 2003; Martenyi, Brown, Zhang, Prakash, & Koke, 2002). Based on the literature and this review, the CAPS would be useful as an outcome measure to empirically assess interventions or programs.

The PDS is a 49-item self-report instrument based on the *DSM-IV* criteria for PTSD and related symptoms. Patients can typically complete the questionnaire in 10 to 15 minutes (Foa et al., 1997). Though the PDS yields both diagnostic information for making a formal *DSM-IV* diagnosis and clinically relevant information regarding specific symptoms (e.g., nightmares, emotional reactions, physical problems) (Foa et al., 1997), caution must be used if one is going to depend on the PDS as the only source of information for a diagnosis. The PDS has adequate psychometric properties of reliability and validity and has been normed in several studies (e.g., Foa, Riggs, Dancu, & Rothbaum, 1993). In practice, the list of traumas in Section-A may reveal traumas other than the specific trauma that brought the patient into the current treatment. Descriptions of each event selected are requested in Section 2 and may be used to facilitate further inquiry and to facilitate treatment. Later sections correspond to the *DSM-IV* criteria for PTSD and to the specifiers for the diagnosis (e.g., acute or chronic) (Foa et al., 1997). The instrument is scored by first deciding if all six elements of the PDS are present and diagnostic criteria have been met. If diagnostic criteria are met, a severity score may be calculated by adding the response frequency scores for items 22 through 38. These scores may then be classified as mild (10 or less) to severe (greater than 35) (Foa et al., 1997). Qualified professionals may purchase the instrument from Pearson Assessment, Inc. (http://www.pearsonassessments.com/ assessments/tests/pds.htm).

Overall, these instruments provide assessment of the *DSM-IV* diagnostic criteria for PTSD (American Psychiatric Association, 1994). The SCID (PTSD module) (First et al., 2000; First et al., 1994) and the PDS (Foa et al., 1997) instruments are designed to provide diagnostic information for making a formal *DSM-IV* diagnosis of PTSD. The SCID (PTSD module) is suitable for clinicians who are limited by time due to clinical constraints or are in need of just a formal PTSD diagnosis. We recommend either the self-report PDS or the clinician-administered CAPS because these instruments offer the greatest utility for clinicians. The PDS and the CAPS provide both a diagnostic assessment of PTSD and a comprehensive assessment of relevant clinical symptoms (cognitive and behavioral), which is helpful in treatment planning, goal setting, and outcome evaluation.

CLINICAL CHARACTERISTICS AND SYMPTOMS

The Beck Depression Inventory-II (BDI-II; Beck, Steer, Ball, & Ranieri, 1996; Beck, Steer, & Brown, 1996) is a 21-item self-report instrument designed to assess depression according to the *DSM-IV* criteria. The BDI-II can be completed in approximately 5 minutes for persons aged 13 to 80 years (Beck et al., 1996). The BDI-II can

be completed confidentially on-line, and scoring reports can then be downloaded (Beck et al., 1996). The BDI-II is also available in hard-copy format for users without computers.

The Symptom Checklist 90-R (SCL-90-R; Derogatis, 1983) is a 90-item self-report measure that assesses psychological syndromes across the following nine scales: somatization, depression, obsessions-compulsions, hostility, psychoticism, paranoia, anxiety, phobic anxiety, and interpersonal sensitivity (Derogatis, 1983). In addition to the nine scales, the SCL-90-R consists of three global indices (global severity, positive symptom distress index, and positive symptom total). The SCL-90-R can be completed in approximately 10 to 15 minutes. Scoring and administration are available in hard-copy and on-line/computer formats.

The Impact of Event Scale (IES; Horowitz, 1979; Horowitz, Wilner, & Alvarez, 1979) is used to assess the impact of traumatic events on a patient's life. The IES is a 15-item self-report scale with which patients rate their difficulty over the previous 7 days. The IES consists of items to assess avoidance, intrusion, and stress related to the trauma. The scale has acceptable reliability and validity (see Corcoran & Fisher, 1994). Patients rate their level of difficulty on each item on a scale of 0 (not at all), 1 (rarely), 3 (sometimes), or 5 (often) (Horowitz, 1979; Horowitz et al., 1979). Scoring on the IES is straightforward and consists of summing the total scales for each item to arrive at an overall level of stress. Total scores range from 0 to 40, with higher scores indicating greater levels of stress. A clinical cutoff score of 26 has been established. Two subscales can be calculated to determine levels of avoidance and intrusion (Horowitz, 1979; Horowitz et al., 1979). The IES has been recommended as both an assessment tool and an outcome measure for monitoring clinical interventions (Corcoran & Fischer, 1994).

The Substance Abuse–Addiction Severity Index (ASI; McLellan et al., 1992; McLellan et al., 1986; McLellan, Luborsky, O'Brian, & Woody, 1980) provides an assessment of addiction severity across the following problem areas: employment, legal, psychiatric, drugs, alcohol, medical, and family/social. It consists of 147 items that focus on severity of problems in the previous 30 days and also over the patient's lifetime. The ASI yields both subject clinical indices and composite scores (McLellan et al., 1992;

McLellan et al., 1986; McLellan et al., 1980). It is available in several versions, including clinician administered and client administered (via computer). The latest version of the ASI is a multimedia version (ASI-MV). The ASI can be used as an outcome assessment tool for programs and individual clients.

The Index of Family Relations (IFR; Hudson, 1992, 1993) provides a rapid assessment for identification of family and relationship problems. The IFR is a self-report instrument that takes 5 to 10 minutes to complete. It consists of 25 items rated on a scale from 0 to 100. A clinical cutoff score of 30 is used to identify clinical problems in family relations (Hudson, 1992, 1993). The IFR is a general measure that provides an indicator of family problems and should be followed up with a full assessment battery if a more thorough evaluation is warranted.

SUMMARY

Due to the increasing need for mental health professionals to both diagnose and treat PTSD, mental health practitioners are playing a larger role in the identification and assessment of patients with this disorder. As is evident throughout this chapter, assessment of PTSD can be fairly straightforward or extremely complex depending on the type of trauma and the status of the patient presenting for treatment. Patients presenting for PTSD assessment are often experiencing difficulties across several areas of their lives. Mental health practitioners need to address the following areas in addition to PTSD diagnostic criteria: drug and alcohol use, depression, general psychopathology, impact of trauma, and family distress. The plethora of assessment tools for PTSD and related symptoms make it a challenge to select reliable and valid instruments. Our goal in this chapter has been to provide a review of the best instruments for social workers to utilize in research and practice. Mental health practitioners who are considering assessment strategies should keep in mind the utility of the instruments, the amount of time available, patient burden, costs, and uses of information obtained. All too often, mental health practitioners are left to weigh the costs versus the benefits when assessing patients. The instruments presented provide not only diagnostic information but also detailed assessment and identification of broader associated problems

associated with PTSD that are essential in formulating treatment plans and assessing outcomes.

References

American Psychiatric Association. (1994). *Diagnostic and statistical manual of mental disorders* (4th ed.). Washington, DC: Author.

Banyard, V. L. (2000, Fall). Trauma and memory. *PTSD Research Quarterly, 11*(4), 1–7.

Beck, A. T., Steer, R. A., Ball, R., & Ranieri, W. (1996). Comparison of Beck Depression Inventories-IA and-II in psychiatric outpatients. *Journal of Personality Assessment, 67,* 588–597.

Beck, A. T., Steer, R. A., & Brown, G. K. (1996). *Manual for the Beck Depression Inventory* (2nd ed.). San Antonio, TX: Psychological Corporation.

Blake, D. D., Weathers, F. W., Nagy, L. M., Kaloupek, D. G., Gusman, F. D., Charney, D. S., & Keane, T. M. (1995). The development of a clinician-administered PTSD scale. *Journal of Traumatic Stress, 8,* 75–90.

Blanchard, E. B., Hickling, E. J., Deviveni, T., Veazey, C. H., Galovski, T. E., Mundy, E., Malta, L. S., & Buckley, T. C. (2003). A controlled evaluation of cognitive behavioural therapy for posttraumatic stress in motor vehicle accident survivors. *Behaviour Research and Therapy, 41,* 79–96.

Bremner, J. D., Southwick, S. M., Darnell, A., & Charney, D. S. (1996). Chronic PTSD in Vietnam combat veterans: Course of illness and substance abuse. *American Journal of Psychiatry, 153,* 369–375.

Chilcoat, H. D., & Breslau, N. (1998). Posttraumatic stress disorder and drug disorders: Testing causal pathways. *Archives of General Psychiatry, 55,* 913–917.

Corcoran, K., & Fischer, J. (1994). *Measures for clinical practice: A sourcebook* (3rd ed.). New York: Free Press.

Corcoran, K., & Fischer, J. (1994). *Measures for clinical practice: A sourcebook* (3rd ed.). Vol. 2. *Adults.* New York: Free Press.

Dansky, B. S., Roitzsch, J. C., Brady, K. T., & Saladin, M. E. (1997). Posttraumatic stress disorder and substance abuse: Use of research in a clinical setting. *Journal of Traumatic Stress, 10,* 141–148.

Davidson, J. R., & Fairbank, J. A. (1993). The epidemiology of posttraumatic stress disorder. In E. B. Foa (Ed.), *Posttraumatic stress disorder: DSM-IV and beyond.* Washington, DC: American Psychiatric Press.

Derogatis, L. R. (1983). *SCL-90-R: Administration, scoring, and procedures manual-II.* Towson, MD: Clinical Psychometric Research.

Epstein, J. N., Saunders, B. E., Kilpatrick, D. G., & Resnick, H. S. (1998). PTSD as a mediator between childhood rape and alcohol use in adult women. *Child Abuse and Neglect, 22,* 223–234.

First, M., Spitzer, R., Williams, J., & Gibbon, M. (2000). Structured clinical interview for DSM-IV Axis I disorders (SCID-I). In American Psychiatric Association (Ed.), *Handbook of psychiatric measures* (pp. 49–53). Washington, DC: American Psychiatric Association.

First, M. B., Spitzer, R. L., Gibbon, M., & Williams, J.B.W. (1994). Structured Clinical Interview for DSM-IV Axis I Disorders—Patient Edition (SCID-I/P, Version 2.0). In B. R. Department (Ed.). New York.

Foa, E. B., Cashman, L., Jaycox, L., & Perry, K. (1997). The validation of a self-report measure of posttraumatic stress disorder: The posttraumatic diagnostic scale. *Psychological Assessment,* 445–451.

Foa, E. B., Riggs, D. S., Dancu, C. V., & Rothbaum, B. O. (1993). Reliability and validity of a brief instrument for assessing post-traumatic stress disorder. *Journal of Traumatic Stress, 6,* 459–473.

Friedman, M. J. (1990). Interrelationships between biological mechanisms and pharmacotherapy of posttraumatic stress disorder. In M. E. Wolf & A. D. Mosnaim (Ed.), *Post-traumatic stress disorder: Etiology, phenomenology, and treatment* (pp. 204–225). Washington, DC: American Psychiatric Press.

Horowitz, M. J. (1979). Impact of event scale. In J. Fisher (Ed.), *Measures for clinical practice: A sourcebook* (Vol. 2, pp. 275–276). New York: Free Press.

Horowitz, M. J., Wilner, N., & Alvarez, W. (1979). Impact of event scale: A measure of subjective distress. *Psychosomatic Medicine, 41,* 209–218.

Hudson, W. W. (1992). Index of family relations. In K. Corcoran (Ed.), *Measures for clinical practice: A sourcebook* (2nd ed., pp. 338–340). New York: Free Press.

Hudson, W. W. (1993). *Index of family relations.* Tempe, AZ: WALMYR Publishing.

Hyman, I. E., Jr., & Loftus, E. F. (1998). Errors in autobiographical memories. *Clinical Psychology Review, 18,* 933–947.

Kessler, R. C. (1995). Posttraumatic stress disorder in the national comorbidity survey. *Archives of General Psychiatry, 52,* 1048–1060.

Martenyi, F., Brown, E. B., Zhang, H., Prakash, A., & Koke, S. C. (2002). Fluoxetine versus placebo in posttraumatic stress disorder. *Journal of Clinical Psychiatry, 63,* 199–206.

McLellan, A. T., Kushner, H., Metzger, D., Peters, R., Smith, I., Grissom, G., Pettinati, H., & Argeriou, M. (1992). The fifth edition of the addiction severity index. *Journal of Substance Abuse Treatment, 9,* 199–213.

McLellan, A. T., Luborsky, L., Cacciola, J., Griffiths, J., Evans, F., Barr, H., & O'Brian, C. (1986). New data from the addiction severity index: Reliability and validity scores from three centers. *Journal of Nervous and Mental Disease, 173,* 412–423.

McLellan, A. T., Luborsky, L., O'Brian, C. P., & Woody, G. E. (1980). An improved diagnostic instrument for substance abuse patients. *Journal of Nervous and Mental Disease, 168*(1), 26–33.

Mueser, K. T., Salyers, M. P., Rosenberg, S. D., Ford, J. D., Fox, L., & Carty, P. (2001). Psychometric evaluation of trauma and posttraumatic stress disorder assessments in persons with severe mental illness. *Psychological Assessment, 13,* 110–117.

Weathers, F. W., Keane, T. M., & Davidson, J. R. (2001). Clinician-administered PTSD scale: A review of the first ten years of research. *Depression and Anxiety, 13,* 132–156.

Yarvis, J., & Bordnick, P. (2003). Psychological intervention for military mental health responders after 9/11. *U.S. Army Medical Department Journal.* Fort Sam, Houston, TX.

57

DIAGNOSIS AND ASSESSMENT OF COMORBID OPPOSITIONAL DEFIANT DISORDER AND OBSESSIVE-COMPULSIVE DISORDER

Gary Mitchell & Dawn Koontz

This chapter will focus on the diagnostic and assessment implications of comorbid oppositional defiant disorder (ODD) and obsessive-compulsive disorder (OCD) in children and adolescents. Treatment implications are discussed but are not explained in detail. For further information, the reader is referred to additional resources.

OVERVIEW OF ODD

Oppositional defiant disorder is defined by a pattern of negativity, noncompliant defiance to authority figures (e.g., parents, teachers, and other adults), and temperamental outbursts that impair a child's ability to function effectively in home, school, and peer environments. This maladaptive pattern of behavior must have endured for 6 months or longer for the diagnosis to be made accurately. Because of the pervasive behavioral disruptions caused by these disorders, ODD and conduct disorder (CD) continue to be the primary diagnoses of children and adolescents referred for mental health intervention (Frick, 1998; Kazdin, 1995). Research has shown that ODD can be validly diagnosed in children as young as those of preschool age (Keenan & Wakschlag, 2002).

More specifically, the fourth edition of the *Diagnostic and Statistical Manual of Mental Disorders* (American Psychiatric Association, 1994) lists the diagnostic criteria for ODD, including a pattern of negativistic, hostile, and de-

fiant behavior lasting at least 6 months during which the patient regularly engages in at least four qualifying behaviors, such as losing temper, arguing with adults, defying requests or rules, deliberately annoying people, blaming others rather than taking responsibility for behavior, becoming easily annoyed, angry, and resentful, and acting spiteful or vindictive. The *DSM-IV* is careful to note that these behaviors must occur more often than in peers of comparable age and developmental level. Criterion B in the *DSM-IV* states that the disturbance in behavior causes clinically significant impairment in social, academic, or occupational functioning. Because these patients often deny having problems, the clinician is most often in the position to determine if the impairment is clinically significant. Criterion C states that the behaviors do not occur exclusively during the course of a psychotic or mood disorder. Finally, Criterion D rules out conduct disorder or antisocial personality disorder. A related disorder, disruptive behavior disorder, not otherwise specified, is coded when the patient does not meet full criteria for ODD or conduct disorder but is significantly affected.

It is quite normal for most children to occasionally exhibit oppositional behavior. In fact, Vitiello and Jensen (1995) reported that in a nonclinical sample of children and adolescents in the community, the prevalence of oppositional symptoms was as high as 20% on the basis of *DSM-III-R* criteria (American Psychiatric Association, 1987). However, when the criterion of functional impairment was added, the rate dropped to 10%.

Unlike children and adolescents with conduct disorder, those with ODD have no history of breaking the law. Still, many experts believe that ODD is often a precursor to later development of conduct disorder. Moreover, aggressiveness, impulsivity, inattention, and general difficult temperament have been described as the main characteristics of children who are at greater long-term risk for developing a full-blown conduct disorder (Lehmann & Dangel, 1998).

One problem with research on ODD is that it is rarely researched in its pure form. Rather, research suggests that ODD is often comorbid with other psychiatric disorders. Most often, it is studied in relation to its comorbidity with other disruptive behavior disorders, such as attention deficit/hyperactivity disorder (ADHD) and conduct disorder. Less frequently, ODD is studied in relation to its comorbidity to other psychiatric disorders such as mood disorders (e.g., Capaldi, 1992) and anxiety disorders (e.g., Russo & Beidel, 1994). This makes it difficult, at best, to be clear about the true prevalence of ODD, but some suggest that the prevalence is somewhere between 2 and 16% (American Psychiatric Association, 1994), depending on how and where the research sample was obtained. Similarly, because of how researchers have historically grouped certain diagnostic conditions (e.g., anxiety disorders, disruptive behavior disorders, ODD, and CD), our review of the literature found no prevalence rates for the specific comorbidity of ODD and OCD in children and adolescents.

Diagnostic considerations are complicated by the presence of comorbid conditions. As previously noted, ODD would not be diagnosed if the behaviors occur only during an active mood disorder or a psychotic disorder. Children with ADHD often display oppositional behavior. If the clinician suspects ADHD, it should be ruled out. If the identified patient qualifies for a diagnosis of ADHD, the clinician must discern whether the behaviors are driven exclusively by the inattention and impulsivity related to this disorder or whether a comorbid diagnosis of ODD is appropriate. With ODD, the child is more likely than members of his or her peer group to interpret ambiguous social situations as hostile (Behan & Carr, 2000; Hogan, 1999). Thus, in these children the clinician can expect to find a low degree of perceived responsibility

for their own actions, with identified patients often focusing on other people's behavior as justification for their own.

Occasionally, behaviors associated with OCD in children and adolescents are mistaken for ODD. One study found that conduct disorder frequently was associated with subclinical OCD but not with OCD defined by *DSM-IV* clinical criteria (Valleni-Basile et al., 1994). Thus, in order to devise the best treatment intervention, it is important to determine whether the behaviors observed are driven by anxiety or by blatant noncompliance because the behaviors themselves can appear quite similar.

Anxiety-driven oppositional behavior can be triggered for various reasons that can be attributable to OCD rather than ODD. Parents and school professionals sometimes perceive OCD-related behaviors as "manipulative" and refer children for assessment based on this belief. Parents and caregivers may describe "tantrum" behavior, ranging from refusal to discontinue rituals to yelling and screaming, to crying, breaking items, verbally threatening, and even physically attacking. Additionally, these behaviors can last for extended periods—as long as 3 or more hours under certain conditions. Purposeful or accidental interference with rituals may initiate the oppositional behavior. Imagine a child who believes that interference with a particular ritual may result in the death of a parent; he or she is likely to be "oppositional" should somebody attempt to interfere. Forced separation from people or places that the child perceives to be "safe" in some way can have similar outcomes. A child who is forced to leave a bedroom perceived to be "uncontaminated" may become quite upset. Likewise, he or she might become upset if this "uncontaminated" area is unwittingly or purposefully "contaminated" by others. The child or adolescent may react oppositionally to a caregiver's attempts to discontinue engaging in rituals, such as discontinuing reassurance for harm obsessions or assistance in cleaning rituals. In all these situations, the oppositional behavior is driven by intense fear or anxiety.

Some children and adolescents with OCD are embarrassed about revealing their fears and would rather risk being perceived as oppositional than to admit the actual problem. Additionally, a child suffering from extreme anxiety may experience delays in social development and may interact with others in ways that are perceived to be deliberately annoying. Excessive focus on details and refusal to tolerate vague or ambiguous communications may be driven by OCD, but they are likely to frustrate others and may be perceived as oppositional.

ASSESSMENT OF ODD IN CHILDREN AND ADOLESCENTS

A thorough assessment is required to facilitate an accurate diagnosis of ODD versus OCD or comorbidity of the two. In general, an assessment should have clinical utility that allows the provider to make behaviorally specific treatment recommendations (Ollendick & King, 1998). Thus, the clinician should use assessment tools that are helpful in selecting the most appropriate treatment modality. This is particularly important in attempts to distinguish between ODD and OCD because treatments for anxiety differ significantly from those for oppositionality.

Most clinicians choose to use a multimethod and multi-informant assessment, which may include diagnostic interviews with the parent and child, direct behavioral observation of the child, parent and teacher rating scales, and some standardized and self-report measures for the youth. Additionally, school records can be a valuable source of information regarding academic, social, and behavioral problems in the classroom setting. In its recently published clinical practice guidelines for ADHD, the American Academy of Pediatrics (2000) also recommended using multimethod assessment tools with multiple informants. Moreover, it stated that other comorbid conditions such as ODD, CD, mood disorders, and anxiety should be ruled out. A multimethod assessment consisting of reliable and valid measures has the advantage of incorporating empirically based assessment with *DSM-IV* diagnostic criteria (Achenbach & McConaughy, 1996).

In addition to the information afforded the clinician from the diagnostic clinical interview and direct behavioral observation, parents and teachers are often asked to fill out behavioral rating scales that provide a broader and clearer picture of the child's behavior in multiple settings. Two of the most widely used behavior rating scales are the Child Behavior Checklist (CBCL; Achenbach & Rescorla, 2001) and the Behavior Assessment System for Children (BASC; Reynolds & Kamphaus, 1998). These behavioral ratings provide a current description of parents' and teachers' perceptions and direct observations of child and adolescent behaviors along a number of dimensions, including behaviors that are more suggestive of anxiety and/or oppositionality. Parent and teacher ratings are then compared in order to identify where the behaviors are occurring and to assess their intensity within the various settings. Youths who are older than 11 years of age can also fill out self-report versions of either the CBCL or the BASC.

After completion of a broad-based assessment of behavioral problems, most clinicians choose to gather more specific information about particular problem behaviors that were revealed. For instance, Barkley (1997) suggests having both parents and teachers complete the Disruptive Behavior Disorders Rating Scale to assist in the differential diagnoses of ODD, ADHD, and CD. Barkley (1997) also recommends having the parents complete the Home Situations Questionnaire (HSQ) to evaluate when problems with compliance occur and how severe the noncompliance is in each situation. Similarly, teachers can complete the School Situations Questionnaire (SSQ; Barkley, 1997) to evaluate the child's noncompliance in the classroom setting. For the assessment of defiant teenagers, the same type of instruments can be utilized (Barkley, Edwards, & Robin, 1999).

ASSESSMENT OF OCD IN CHILDREN AND ADOLESCENTS

As with the diagnostic assessment of ODD, evaluation of OCD in children and adolescents is determined through clinical interview, including one or more structured interviews or rating scales. March, Leonard, and Swedo (1995) indicate that the Yale-Brown Obsessive Compulsive Scale (Y-BOCS; Goodman et al., 1989) is the most widely used assessment instrument for OCD. For the evaluation of children and adolescents, the Children's Yale-Brown Obsessive Compulsive Scale (CY-BOCS) may be more developmentally appropriate (Scahill et al., 1997). March et al. (1995) also indicate that a structured interview such as the Anxiety Disorders Interview for Children (ADIS-C) can be helpful with assessment.

The process of assessment for OCD can be complicated for several reasons. Some patients may be embarrassed about symptoms and thus reluctant to discuss them. Parents are occasionally overly sensitive to possible symptoms due to family history of OCD, resulting in excessive focus on symptoms that might not meet diagnostic criteria. Some OCD-related behaviors might suggest the presence of a behavior disorder when none actually exists. Behaviors associated with some disorders may be mistaken for compulsions. For instance, children and adolescents with disorders along the autistic spectrum often display stereotypical behaviors that may be perceived as OCD rituals. As with the assessment of any disorder, comorbidity with other Axis I and Axis II conditions can cloud the diagnostic picture.

When the clinician suspects that the child or adolescent is embarrassed to discuss OCD symptoms, it can be helpful to normalize the condition. This can be accomplished through psychoeducation about OCD. Additionally, the clinician can attempt to address fears of embarrassment through discussion of similar presenting problems and positive treatment outcomes.

DSM-IV (American Psychiatric Association, 1994) diagnostic criteria for OCD include obsessions or compulsions (Criterion A) that are understood by the individual during some course of the disorder to be excessive or unreasonable (Criterion B). Additionally, the disorder results in marked distress, takes at least 1 hour per day, or causes significant interference with the person's performance or functioning (Criterion C). Criterion D differentiates OCD from eating disorders, trichotillomania-related hair pulling, body dysmorphic disorder, substance use disorders, hypochondriasis, paraphilia, and ruminations connected with major depressive disorders. Criterion E states that the disorder cannot be directly due to the use of a substance or to a general medical condition.

The *DSM-IV* accounts for developmental considerations by excluding children from Criterion B, thus allowing a child to be diagnosed despite his or her inability to question the validity of the obsessions or compulsions. The clinician must have an accurate understanding of the patient's ability to question the obsessions in order to develop an appropriate treatment plan.

TREATMENT OPTIONS FOR ODD

The use of pharmacotherapy with children and adolescents with ODD has shown limited effectiveness (Cantwell, 1989). Therefore, most research on the treatment of ODD focuses on intervention modalities that involve behavior management of the child, including parent training, token economies, and structural family therapy. Clinicians who value empirically supported treatment protocols can take advantage of manuals that guide the sessions in a methodical and sequenced manner (e.g., Barkley, 1997).

Forehand and Long (1996) provide detailed guidelines to assist parents in the behavior management of their noncompliant children. These guidelines include differential reinforcement and attention for positive versus negative behaviors, effective instruction giving, and use of time-outs. Other authors have also found these methods to be effective with children who display oppositional or undesirable behavior (e.g., Christophersen, 1994, 1998; Eyeberg & Robinson, 1982; Forehand & McMahon, 1981).

Token economies are frequently used with children who exhibit behavioral difficulties (Christophersen & Mortweet, 2001). Tokens (e.g., poker chips, pennies, marbles) are earned when the child engages in the target behaviors. The reader is referred to Barkley and Benton (1998) for more examples of specific token economies and their various uses.

Some studies have shown support for structural family therapy as a treatment for ODD. For example, Szapocznik et al. (1989) found that when structural family therapy was compared with psychodynamic therapy for boys exhibiting disruptive behavior, family functioning improved only with the structural family therapy intervention. Likewise, Barkley and colleagues (1992) found that structural family therapy was just as effective as behavior management training and problem-solving and communications training in reducing family conflicts, internalizing symptoms, externalizing symptoms, and improving the child's school adjustment.

The most widely used treatment manual for ODD is that developed by Russell A. Barkley. In the second edition of his comprehensive manual, *Defiant Children: A Clinician's Manual for Assessment and Parent Training* (1997), Barkley outlines a research-supported, 10-session behavioral training program for parents. The manualized treatment is designed to educate parents about the causes of noncompliance and then teach them how to use contingency management, time-out, application of structure through specific household and school rules, and preemptive planning for situations in which the child is more likely to be noncompliant. The 10 parent training sessions are scripted for the clinician, homework assignments are given, and the parents are provided handouts reiterating the key points of the session. Parents and teachers are encouraged to collaborate in order to identify, monitor, and reinforce positive behaviors and to impose consequences for the negative target behaviors.

TREATMENT OPTIONS FOR OCD

In a recent review of the literature on the pharmacological treatment of children with OCD, Grados and Riddle (2001) found that Selected Serotonin Reuptake Inhibitors (SSRIs) appear to be the "first-line pharmacological agents in the treatment of childhood OCD." Their review found that pharmacological treatment for children with OCD often included medications such as fluoxetine (Prozac), fluvoxamine (Luvox), paroxetine (Paxil), and sertraline (Zoloft). Further, they suggested that pharmacological intervention should be based on a thorough assessment of symptoms (e.g., CY-BOCS) based on the types of obsessions and compulsions and their intensity and severity. Frequent reevaluation at regular intervals can also be useful in determining how well the medication(s) and therapy are working. It should be noted, however, that the expert consensus treatment guidelines for OCD recommend that cognitive-behavior therapy (CBT) be used prior to medication with prepubescent children and prior to medication with adolescents with milder symptoms of OCD (March, Frances, Carpenter, & Kahn, 1997).

Cognitive-behavioral treatment plans for OCD in children can vary but generally have similar components. Kendall et al. (1991) suggest a template for treating anxiety disorders that includes relaxation training, specifically progressive muscle relaxation; "building a cognitive coping template," which includes challenging cognitive distortions and replacing them with more accurate beliefs; problem solving; contingent reinforcement of active participation in the therapeutic process; modeling of healthy behavior; and exposure therapy. Active involvement with the family occurs throughout treatment. March and Mulle (1998) describe a structured program for treating OCD that includes psychoeducation about the disorder and treatment, cognitive training, development of a hierarchy,

of anxiety-producing stimuli, graded exposure and response prevention with parent participation and use of positive reinforcement, and relapse prevention. Children are taught that OCD is a medical condition and are encouraged to externalize it as separate from their own identity. To do this, children are encouraged to "name the OCD" and commit to driving it out of their lives.

It is important for the clinician to understand the patient's level of insight into the validity of the obsessions and compulsions. Exposure and response-prevention treatment, by its nature, is anxiety provoking. Flooding exposure, which is simply a prolonged exposure to stimuli perceived to be extremely fearful, can elicit very high levels of distress. The effectiveness of flooding procedures is contingent on the child's understanding of the problem and the treatment rationale (Francis & Beidel, 1995).

When the clinician diagnoses OCD and the patient perceives no problem, the clinician may work with the patient to provide education and discern together whether a problem exists. In some cases, a child may be amenable to positive reinforcement strategies that provide incentives to engage in treatment protocols despite a lack of agreement regarding the problem. For reasons discussed in the preceding paragraph, these strategies may be limited in efficacy as the difficulty of exposure increases. Generally in these cases, the clinician will work with the parents to assist them in disengaging from accommodating behaviors that may serve to protect the patient from consequences of his or her compulsions and avoidance. This strategy sometimes increases the patient's discomfort enough to facilitate agreement with the clinician that a problem does indeed exist.

TREATMENT OF COMORBIDITY WITH OCD AND ODD

Though much can be said about the treatment of comorbid OCD and ODD, little has been written on the topic. It is clear that a pervasive pattern of inaccurate communication and refusal to follow protocols will undermine attempts to treat the OCD. Behavioral patterns related to ODD, including misrepresentation of the frequency and duration of compulsive behavior, as well as a pattern of refusal or unwillingness to follow through with behavioral assignments, contributes to a poor treatment outcome. It becomes clear that attempts to treat OCD without first attending to the oppositional behavior are unlikely to be effective. Additionally, premature attempts to treat the OCD are likely to frustrate the child and parents, resulting in exacerbation of feelings of hopelessness and undermining their trust in the efficacy of behavioral treatment. This may put the family at risk of avoiding the intervention necessary for recovery.

Mitchell and Koontz (in press) provide a discussion of treatment issues and strategies along with example cases. Mitchell and Pollard (1999) identify several considerations in the treatment of comorbid conditions, including issues of safety, patient preference, the impact of the disorders on the life of the patient and family, treatment history, and "the nature and relationship between existing disorders" (p. 111). Given the negative impact of a behavior disorder on efficacy of OCD treatment, sequencing considerations are simplified. The ODD should be sufficiently addressed before OCD treatment begins. Though conceptually there may be exceptions, the authors have not yet had a successful treatment outcome when this guideline was not followed.

References

Achenbach, T. M., & McConaughy, S. H. (1996). Relations between *DSM-IV* and empirically based assessment. *School Psychology Review, 25,* 329–341.

Achenbach, T. M., & Rescorla, L. A. (2001). *Manual for ASEBA school-age forms and profiles.* Burlington: University of Vermont, Research Center for Children, Youth, and Families.

American Academy of Pediatrics. (2000). Clinical practice guideline: Diagnosis and evaluation of the child with attention deficit/hyperactivity disorder. *Pediatrics, 105,* 1158–1170.

American Psychiatric Association. (1987). *Diagnostic and statistical manual of mental disorders* (3rd ed., Revised). Washington, DC: Author.

American Psychiatric Association. (1994). *Diagnostic and statistical manual of mental disorders* (4th ed.). Washington, DC: Author.

Barkley, R. A. (1997). *Defiant children: A clinician's manual for assessment and parent training* (2nd ed.). New York: Guilford.

Barkley, R. A., & Benton, C. M. (1998). *Your defiant child: 8 steps to better behavior.* New York: Guilford.

Barkley, R. A., Edwards, G. H., & Robin, A. L. (1999). *Defiant teens: A clinician's manual for assessment and family intervention.* New York: Guilford.

Barkley, R. A., Guevremont, A. D., Anastopoulos, A. D., & Fletcher, K. E. (1992). A comparison of three family therapy programs for treating family conflicts in adolescents with attention-deficit hyperactivity disorder. *Journal of Consulting and Clinical Psychology, 60,* 450–462.

Behan, J., & Carr, A. (2000). Oppositional defiant disorder. In Alan Carr (Ed.), *What works with children and adolescents: A critical review of psychological interventions with children, adolescents, and their families* (pp. 103–130). Philadelphia: Taylor and Francis.

Bernstein, G. A., Anderson, L. K., Hektner, J. M., & Realmuto, G. M. (2000). Imipramine compliance in adolescence. *Journal of the American Academy of Child and Adolescent Psychiatry, 39,* 284–291.

Brestan, E. V., & Eyeberg, S. M. (1998). Effective psychosocial treatments of conduct-disordered children and adolescents. *Journal of Clinical Child Psychology, 27,* 180–189.

Brown, R. A. (1999). Assessing attitudes and behaviors of high-risk adolescents: An evaluation of the self-report method. *Adolescence, 34,* 25–32.

Cantwell, D. P. (1989). Oppositional defiant disorder. In H. I. Kaplan & B. J. Sadock (Eds.), *Comprehensive textbook of psychiatry* (5th ed., pp. 1842–1845). Baltimore: Williams and Wilkins.

Capaldi, D. M. (1992). Co-occurrence of conduct problems and depressive symptoms in early adolescent boys: II. A 2-year follow-up at grade 8. *Developmental and Psychopathology, 4,* 125–144.

Christophersen, E. R. (1994). *Pediatric compliance: A guide for the primary care physician.* New York: Plenum.

Christophersen, E. R. (1998). *Little people: Guidelines for commonsense child rearing* (4th ed.). Shawnee Mission, KS: Overland Press.

Christophersen, E. R., & Mortweet, S. L. (2001). *Treatments that work with children: Empirically supported strategies for managing childhood problems.* Washington, DC: American Psychological Association.

Eyeberg, S. M., & Robinson, E. A. (1982). Parent-child interaction training: Effects on family functioning. *Journal of Clinical Child Psychology, 11,* 130–137.

Forehand, R. L., & Long, N. (1996). *Parenting the strong-willed child.* Chicago: Contemporary Books.

Forehand, R. L., & McMahon, R. J. (1981). *Helping the noncompliant child: A clinician's guide to parent training.* New York: Guilford.

Francis, G., & Beidel, D. (1995). Cognitive-behavioral psychotherapy. In John S. March (Ed.), *Anxiety disorders in children and adolescents* (pp. 321–340). New York: Guilford.

Frick, P. J. (1998). *Conduct disorders and severe antisocial behavior.* New York: Plenum.

Goodman, W. K., Price, L. H., Rasmussen, S. A., Mazure, C., Delgado, P., Heninger, G. R., & Charney, D. S. (1989). The Yale-Brown Obsessive Compulsive Scale: Vol. II. Validity. *Archives of General Psychiatry, 46,* 1012–1016.

Grados, M. A., & Riddle, M. A. (2001). Pharmacological treatment of childhood obsessive-compulsive disorder: From theory to practice. *Journal of Clinical Child Psychology, 30,* 67–79.

Hogan, A. E. (1999). Cognitive functioning in children with oppositional defiant disorder and conduct disorder. In Herbert C. Quay & Anne E. Hogan (Eds.), *Handbook of disruptive behavior disorders* (pp. 317–355). New York: Kluwer Academic/Plenum.

Kazdin, A. E. (Ed.). (1995). *Conduct disorders in childhood and adolescence* (2nd ed.). Thousand Oaks, CA: Sage.

Keenan, K., & Wakschlag, L. S. (2002). Can a valid diagnosis of disruptive behavior disorder be made in preschool children? *American Journal of Psychiatry, 159,* 351–358.

Kendall, P. C., Chansky, T. E., Freidman, M., Kim, R., Kortlander, E., Sessa, F. M., & Siqueland, L. (1991). Treating anxiety disorders in children and adolescents. In Philip C. Kendall (Ed.), *Child and adolescent therapy: Cognitive behavioral procedures* (pp. 131–164). New York: Guilford.

Lehmann, P., & Dangel, R. (1998). Oppositional defiant disorder. In B. A. Thyer & J. S. Wodanski (Eds.), *Handbook of empirical social work practice: Mental disorders* (Vol. 1, pp. 91–116). New York: Springer.

March, J., Frances, A., Carpenter, D., & Kahn, D. (1997). The expert consensus guideline series: Treatment of obsessive-compulsive disorder. *Journal of Clinical Psychiatry, 58*(Suppl. 4), 65–72.

March, J. S., Franklin, M., Nelson, A., & Foa, E. (2001). Cognitive-behavioral psychotherapy for pediatric obsessive-compulsive disorder. *Journal of Clinical Child Psychology, 30,* 8–18.

March, J., Leonard, H. L., & Swedo, S. E. (1995). Obsessive-compulsive disorder. In John S. March (Ed.), *Anxiety disorders in children and adolescents* (pp. 251–275). New York: Guilford.

March, J. S., & Mulle, K. (1998). *OCD in children and adolescents: A cognitive-behavioral treatment manual.* New York: Guilford.

Mitchell, G., & Koontz, D. (2004). Diagnosis and assessment of comorbid oppositional defiant disorder. In A. R. Roberts and K. Yeager (Ed.) *Evidence Based Research Manual.* New York: Oxford University Press.

Mitchell, G., & Pollard, C. A. (1999). Clinical management of co-morbidity in anxiety disorder patients. *Crisis Intervention, 5,* 109–118.

Ollendick, T. H., & King, N. J. (1998). Empirically supported treatments for children with phobic and anxiety disorders: Current status. *Journal of Clinical Child Psychology, 27,* 156–167.

Reynolds, C. R., & Kamphaus, R. W. (1998). BASC: Behavior Assessment System for Children. Circle Pines, MN: American Guidance Service.

Russo, M. F., & Beidel, D. C. (1994). Co-morbidity of childhood anxiety and externalizing disorders: Prevalence, associated characteristics, and validation issues. *Clinical Psychology Review, 14,* 199–221.

Scahill, L., Riddle, M. A., McSwiggin-Hardin, M., Ort, S. I., King, R. A., Goodman, W. K., Cicchetti, D., & Leckman, J. F. (1997). Children's Yale-Brown Obsessive Compulsive Scale: Reliability and validity. *Journal of the American Academy of Child and Adolescent Psychiatry, 36,* 844–852.

Szapocznik, J., Rio, A., Murray, E., Cohen, R., Scopetta, M., Rivas-Vazquez, A., Posada, V., & Kurtines, W. (1989). Structural family therapy versus psychodynamic child therapy for problematic Hispanic boys. *Journal of Consulting and Clinical Psychology, 57,* 571–578.

Valleni-Basile, L. A., Garrison, C. Z., Jackson, K. L., Waller, J. L., McKeown, R. E., Addy, C. L., & Cuffe, S. P. (1994). Frequency of obsessive-compulsive disorder in a community sample of young adolescents. *Journal of the American Academy of Child and Adolescent Psychiatry, 33,* 782–791.

Vitiello, B., & Jensen, P. (1995). Disruptive behavior disorders. In H. I. Kaplan & B. J. Sadock (Eds.), *Comprehensive textbook of psychiatry* (6th ed., pp. 2311–2319). Baltimore: Williams & Wilkins.

Waters, T. L., Barrett, P. M., & March, J. S. (2001). Cognitive-behavioral family therapy of childhood obsessive-compulsive disorder: Preliminary findings. *American Journal of Psychotherapy, 55,* 372–387.

58

ASSESSMENT MEASURES FOR SEXUAL PREDATORS

Step-by-Step Guidelines

Graham Glancy & Cheryl Regehr

As a result of recent legislative changes in both the United States and Canada regarding sexually violent predators (Glancy & Regehr, 2001; Zonona, 1999), mental health practitioners are increasingly being called upon to provide predictions regarding the future dangerousness of convicted sex offenders. Prediction of dangerousness based solely on clinical assessments for offenders of any kind and in particular sexual offenders, however, has proved to be remarkably inaccurate and to result in very low interrater reliability between professional assessors (Hilton & Simmons, 2001). Consequently, there has been considerable effort in the past decade to develop actuarial tools with the aim of improving predictive accuracy. Developers of the tools have reported favorable results in terms of predictive validity, but, nevertheless, considerable controversy exists about the place of actuarial testing in the assessment of sexual offenders (Zonona, 2000; Sreenivasan, Kirkish, Garrick, Wineberger & Phenixa, 2000). The original actuarial instruments focused exclusively on "static" or historical factors such as the age at first offence and the nature of violent offenses. The developers suggested that these tools for the prediction of dangerousness are accurate enough to be used in isolation and that adjunctive clinical assessments not only may fail to add to the predictive validity but in fact may be detrimental (Quinsey, Khanna, & Malcolm, 1998). Other authors stated that actuarial instruments should be used only in association with other clinical methods of evaluation. From this perspective, it has been argued that the use of risk appraisal instruments not only may fail to meet the standard for admissibility in court but also may be unethical according to some professional associations

(Sreenivasan et al., 2000). One judge, in reviewing the use of actuarial instruments in a case, stated, "None of these actuarial instruments seem to include whether the person has been or is being treated, whether he has been or is still incarcerated, is under house arrest or is comatose, although to the unsophisticated one or more of these would seem to bear heavily on future conduct" (In re *Valdez*, p. 6). Consequently, more recent actuarial instruments have included a clinical component.

This chapter will review the reliability and predictive validity of actuarial instruments for assessing the risk of recidivism for sexual offenders. We will then recommend adjunctive measures that we believe add to the accuracy of predictions. This is based on our contention that assessments of sexual predators must be thorough and completed by someone with expertise in the area for two main reasons. First, these assessments are hotly contested in courts, and second, the outcome of the assessment has profound implications for individual liberty and community safety.

ACTUARIAL RISK ASSESSMENT TOOLS

Actuarial scales are designed following retrospective research for factors associated with recidivism in offender populations. That is, typically the files of violent offenders are reviewed, and factors associated with violent behavior are determined. These factors are then combined and weighted, producing a score that is assumed to give an assessment of risk. Next, a particular violent offense is selected as the "index offense," and again, through the process of chart review research, the degree to which the weighted factors predicted subsequent offending is assessed. The model of analysis utilized to evaluate predictive validity typically utilizes a Receiver Operating Characteristic Analysis (ROC). In this analysis, the true positive rate (TRP = sensitivity) and the false positive rate (FPR = 1 − specificity) are plotted on a graph and result in a curve. The area under the curve (AUC) is the probability that the detection method will give a randomly selected violent person a higher score than a randomly selected nonviolent person. A perfect detection method would give an AUC score of 1.0, and a test that was no better than chance would give an AUC score of 1.5. The standard error scores are also reported to help the reader to assess the accuracy of the measure (for a straightforward and thorough discussion of this, refer to Mossman, 2000). In addition, the correlation (r) is frequently reported by researchers. This is the average correlation between test scores and sex offense recidivism. Studies addressing the predictive validity of tools have found variable results in part due to different populations studied, different definitions about what constitutes recidivism, and different lengths of time between the index offense and follow-up.

VRAG/SORAG

The history of actuarial scales for sex offenses starts with the Violence Risk Appraisal Guide (VRAG), which is an actuarial test designed to predict risk for general violence, followed by the development of the Sex Offense Risk Appraisal Guide (SORAG), which focuses more specifically on sexual crimes (Quinsey, Harris, Rice, & Cormier, 1998). These actuarial tests aim to estimate the long-term likelihood that an individual with a history of sexual offenses will commit any act of violence. The SORAG contains 15 items that address early childhood behavior problems, alcohol problems, sexual and nonsexual criminal history, age, marital status, and psychopathology. Several criticisms have been levied against early testing of these instruments, including broad definitions of violent offenses used by the developers, the use of static factors alone as predictors (e.g., age at first offense), and sampling strategies that were limited to high-risk offenders in a maximum security hospital who had limited opportunities for recid-

ivism in a natural setting. Predictive validity based on this sample resulted in a reported AUC of .80 (Harris, Rice, & Cormier, 2002), although an earlier study with the same sample yielded an AUC of .60 for sexual recidivism and .76 for violent recidivism (Rice & Harris, 1997). Subsequent studies, however, have also suggested reasonably good predictive validity. A study of 215 sexual offenders followed for an average of 4½ years reported an AUC of .77 for any reoffense, .69 for a serious reoffense, and .61 for a sexual reoffense (Barabaree, Seto, Langton, & Peacock, 2001). A Swedish study found an AUC of .68 with a cohort of personality-disordered individuals and an AUC of .60 for individuals with schizophrenia (Grann, Belfrage, & Tengstrom, 2000). In addition, a study of 106 Canadian federal inmates resulted in correlation of .32 with violent recidivism and .38 with recidivism in terms of any criminal activity (Glover, Nocholson, Hemmati, Bernfeld, & Quinsey, 2002).

MnSOST-R

The Minnesota Sex Offender Screening Tool–Revised (MnSOST-R) is a 16-item actuarial scale developed to assess long-term (6-year) risk of sexual recidivism among extrafamilial child molesters and rapists excluding incest offenders (Epperson, Kaul, & Hesselton, 1998). It includes both static and some dynamic factors related to the prediction of sexual recidivism. The scale was derived from a selected sample of 123 sexual reoffenders, a random sample of 120 nonsexual reoffenders, and a random sample of 144 non-reoffenders. The methodology used in developing the measure has been criticized on the basis of sample size and sample selection. A study by Barbaree et al. (2001) found an AUC of .65 for any reoffense, .58 for serious reoffense, and .65 for sexual reoffense. In that study, the MnSOST-R failed to meet conventional standards of significance in predicting recidivism.

RRASOR

The Rapid Risk Assessment for Sex Offense Recidivism (RRASOR) was based on the author's comprehensive meta-analysis of predictors of sexual offense recidivism in 61 studies (Hanson, 1997; Hanson & Bussiere, 1998). It was developed to assess the risk for sexual offense recidivism with a limited number of easily scored items that could be used by relatively untrained raters using commonly available information. Testing on the instrument is impressive in that highly varied samples from three countries were included. The scale is moderately accurate in predicting sexual recidivism (essentially equal to the VRAG and the MnSOST-R) but, according to the author, should not be used in isolation. The measure does not include phallometric testing, which is one of the strongest predictors in Hanson's meta-analysis. This was a deliberate move. The RRASOR was intended for use as a quick checklist, which includes only four items: prior sex offenses; being younger than 25; having any male victims; and having any extra-familial victims. A Swedish study reports an AUC of .72 for sexual recidivism of 1,384 offenders released from prison and an AUC of .63 for any type of violent recidivism (Sjostedt & Langstrom, 2001). The Barbaree et al. (2001) study reported an AUC of .60 for any reoffense, .65 for serious reoffense, and .77 for sexual reoffense.

Static-99

Hanson has to be given credit for not resting on his laurels but for instead moving forward to help design the Static-99. Collaborating with Thornton (1997), who produced the Structured Anchored Clinical Judgment-Minimum (SACJ-MIN) in 1998, the authors considered the possibility that a combination of the two scales would predict better than the original scale. The new scale was created by adding together items from RRASOR and the SACJ-MIN. The Static-99 was indeed more accurate than the RRASOR or the SACJ-MIN alone in predicting both sex offense recidivism and general violent recidivism, resulting in an AUC of .71 for sexual offenses and a correlation of .33 with sexual recidivism (Hanson & Thornton, 2000). A Swedish study of offenders released from prison similarly found an AUC of .76 for sexual recidivism and .74 for any violent crime (Sjostedt & Langstrom, 2001). Further, a Canadian study found AUCs of .71 and .70 (Barbaree et al., 2001). Hanson and Thornton present observed recidivism rates of 5, 10, and 15 years and divide scores on the Static-99 into low, medium low, medium high, and high. They conclude that the Static-99 showed a moderate predictive accuracy for both sexual recidivism and general recidivism and note that it is intended to be a measure of long-

term risk potential. They also point to the lack of dynamic factors, which could be useful in selecting treatment targets, measuring the change, and predicting when offenders are likely to recidivate; some caution is advised.

SONAR

In his early work, noted earlier, Hanson has always cautioned that actuarial scales should be used as part of an empirically guided clinical approach (Hanson, 2000). For the Sex Offender Need Assessment Rating (SONAR), Hanson and Harris (1998) organized the dynamic or changeable risk factors into a structured assessment procedure. They considered five so-called stable factors, which included intimacy deficits, negative social influences, attitudes tolerant of sex offending, sexual self-regulation, and general self-regulation, with four so-called acute factors, which are substance abuse, negative mood, anger, and victim access. They then tested the validity of the scale using data previously collected from 208 sex offenders who had recidivated sexually while on community supervision. They compared this group with a group of 201 sex offenders who had not recidivated and found that the scale showed a moderate ability to differentiate between recidivism and nonrecidivism ($r = .43$, AUC = .74) (Hanson & Harris, 2001). This is a new test that has not been independently validated, but again we must give credit to Hanson, who continues to improve upon his original instruments and analyses. This test begins to answer some of the criticisms that have been levied against actuarial testing.

PCL-R

Psychopathy appears to be a central construct relevant to sex offenders as well as other offender groups such as juvenile delinquents, adult offenders in general, and mentally disordered offenders. Research from a variety of sources has consistently demonstrated that high psychopathy scores are related to sexual offending (Seto & Lalumière, 2000). The Psychopathy Checklist (PCL) was developed by Hare (1991) to screen for psychopathy in criminal populations and to assess changes in psychopathic symptomatology over time. It is supported by a plethora of evidence describing its interrater reliability and validity. It is a historically based assessment procedure that requires at least a 2-

or 3-hour interview with the individual, where possible. In addition, corroborative information is generally needed. The PCL should be considered a psychometric test and is recognized by psychological associations as such. It is recommended that users take a training course; such courses are available from time to time in various jurisdictions. Nevertheless, the Psychotherapy Checklist-Revised (PCL-R) along with its manual, is a comparatively easy-to-use psychometric test with a very simple scoring system that does not require computer assistance. Results in a Canadian study of federal inmates have raised questions about the predictive validity because a correlation of only .14 was reported for violent recidivism and .22 for any recidivism (Glover et al., 2002). A second Canadian study with a similar population found AUCs of .71 for any reoffense, .65 for serious reoffense, and .61 for sexual reoffense (Barbaree et al., 2001).

HCR-20

The HCR-20 is a checklist of risk factors for violent behavior that includes 10 items that consider historical factors, 5 that consider current clinical variables, and 5 that address future risk management issues (Webster, Douglas, Eaves, & Hart, 1997). Clinical items include insight, negative attitudes, impulsivity, response to treatment, and active symptoms of a major mental illness. Risk management items address the feasibility of plans, exposure to destabilizers, social supports, treatment compliance, and stress. Studies by independent researchers evaluating the predictive validity of the HCR-20 have resulted in impressive findings (see Table 58.1). For instance, an AUC of .80 was found in a study of 40 severely disordered male forensic patients who were followed an average of 8 years after hospitalization. The researchers concluded that the clinical and risk management factors rather than the static factors contributed most to the predictive validity (Grann et al., 2000). A study of 101 subjects followed in the community in Sweden found an AUC prediction of .75 (Grann et al., 2000).

CLINICAL INTERVIEW

Although Quinsey, Khanna, and Malcolm (1998) have argued that the clinical interview is unnecessary and unhelpful when acutarial tests

are to be used, the prevailing standards in the field suggest that a clinical interview should be performed whenever possible (Zonana, 2000). The interview process should be extensive and ideally would include more than one interview, depending on the circumstances. It is certainly possible that the assessor may be denied access to the person being assessed, but efforts at gaining access should be clearly documented. Further, denied access to the patient should be explicitly mentioned in the conclusions as a caveat.

At the outset of the interview, the assessor should inform the client of the limits of the confidentiality inherent in the situation. First and foremost, it is imperative that the interviewer be clear in identifying the agency requesting the assessment and the intended nature and purpose of the assessment. It should also be made clear whether or not a report will be prepared, the form of this report (verbal or written), and to whom the report will be submitted. If the assessment is for legal purposes rather than clinical or inherently helpful purposes, this should be stated. Any other limits to confidentiality that may be relevant, such as the duty to warn and protect a third party or a child, should also be stated at the outset (Glancy, Regehr, & Bryant, 1998). It may be necessary to remind the client of these limits to confidentiality at various stages in the assessment process because some processes, such as a therapeutic alliance, may undermine his critical judgement (Regehr & Antle, 1997).

A full clinical interview should focus on a complete psychosocial history performed in the normal manner. However, there should also be a focus on the sexual offenses in order to define a pattern of offending, cognitive distortions, and the offense cycle. Other issues such as insight, judgment, and remorse are important. A history of the individual's participation in treatment and what he has learned in treatment can be particularly helpful. The individual should be asked about discharge plans, contingency plans, and future treatment options. Specific tests, some of which are easily administered, may help focus the interview and serve as memory aids, contributing to a more comprehensive interview.

CORROBORATING DATA

Corroborating data should be considered essential in the assessment of sexual predators. An

TABLE 58.1 Reliability and Predictive Validity of Violence Prediction Tests

	AUC	Correlation

VRAG	• Personality disorders .68
	  Schizophrenia .60[3]
	• 0.80[5]
	
	• Any reoffense .77
	  Serious reoffense .69
	  Sexual reoffense .61[6]
	• Sexual offense .60
	  Violent offense .76[7]
		• Violent recidivism .32
		  Any recidivism 0.38[4]
		• Sexual offense .17
		  Violent offense .44[7]

SORAG	• Any reoffense .76
	  Serious reoffense .73
	  Sexual reoffense .70[6]	

MnSOST-R	• Any reoffense .65
	  Serious reoffense 0.58
	  Sexual reoffense 0.65[6]	

RRASOR	• Sexual recidivism .68
	  Any violent rec. .64[1]
	• Sexual recidivism .72
	  Any violent recidivism .63[4]
	• Any reoffense .60
	  Serious reoffense .65
	  Sexual reoffense .77[6]
		• Sexual recidivism .28
		  Any violent recidivism .22[1]
		• Sexual recidivism .22
		  Any violent recidivism .17[4]

Static-99
1999
	• Sexual recidivism .71
	  Any violent recidivism .69[1]
	• Sexual recidivism .76
	  Any violent recidivism .74[4]
	• Any reoffense .71
	  Serious reoffense .70
	  Sexual reoffense .70[6]
		• Sexual recidivism .33
		  Any violent recidivism .32[1]
		• Sexual recidivism .22
		  Any violent recidivism .30[4]

SONAR 2000	• Multiple populations .74[2]	• Multiple populations 0.43[2]

PCL-R
1991
	• Any reoffense 0.71
	  Serious reoffense 0.65
	  Sexual reoffense 0.61[6]
		• Violent recidivism .01
		  Any recidivism .22[4]

HCR-20 1998	• .75[3] • .80[3]	

1. Hanson & Thornton, 2000
2. Hanson & Harris, 2001
3. Grann, Belfrage, & Tengstrom, 2000
4. Glover et al., 2002
5. Harris, Rice, & Cormier, 2002
6. Barbaree et al., 2001

TABLE 58.2 Strengths and Limitations of Violence Prediction Tests

	Strengths	Limitations
VRAG/SORAG 1998 VRAG—12 items plus the PCL-R SORAG—13 items plus the PCL-R	• Moderate ability to predict violence • Good for mentally disordered offenders	• Requires training for PCL-R • Includes any form of minor violence • Standardized on small number of high-risk offenders • No dynamic factors
MnSOST-R 1998 16 items	• Some dynamic factors • Easy to score	• Validation sample too small
RRASOR 1997 4 items	• Easy to score • Moderate ability to predict sexual violence • Well validated	• Simplistic • No dynamic factors
Static-99 1999 10 items	• Easy to score • Moderate ability to predict sexual violence • Well validated	• No dynamic factors
SONAR 2000 2 items	• Considers dynamic factors • May predict short-term and long-term risk of sexual violence	• Not yet well tested
PCL-R 1991 20 items	• Recognized psychological test • Well validated	• Requires training • No dynamic factors

interview with family members allows the assessor to compose a picture of the person within the context of his family and background. Specific family issues and dynamics may be helpful in understanding the person and would, therefore, be paramount in the design of a treatment plan. Also included in collateral information may be police synopses of the offenses, court transcripts, victim statements, and evidence. Previous records of treatment, counseling, or other contacts with mental health agencies are also helpful (see Table 58.2).

TESTING

Considering the magnitude of the issue under question when assessing sexual predators, testing should be as comprehensive as possible. Some of the methods of testing being addressed in this chapter require referral to other professionals with specialized training or credentials;

other methods are easily administered by social workers.

Psychometric Testing

Most psychometric testing must be conducted by a registered clinical psychologist. Some of the more general tests, such as the Minnesota Multiphasic Personality Inventory (MMPI) can be most helpful in determining the personality profile of the offender. In addition, a neuropsychological screen can assist in identifying neurological contributors (Langevin & Watson, 1996).

Biomedical Testing

A range of biomedical tests may also require referral but may be relevant and indicated in specific cases. This could include electroencephalograms, CT scans, and other imaging studies where it is felt that specific brain pathology may be relevant. Endocrine testing may also be helpful.

Sexual Preference Testing

Sexual preference testing should be considered a specialized field and should be attempted only by professionals with the requisite qualifications in the area. Three specific measures should be considered.

Penile Plethysmography

Initially described by Freund (1979), sexual preference testing, or phallometry, is the single best indicator of a paraphilia (Langevin & Watson, 1996). It involves the measurement of penile volume or circumference when the individual is confronted with a variety of standardized stimuli. The reported reliability coefficients are as high as .87 for the sensitivity of the test and as high as .95 for the specificity (Abel et al., 1994). The test can be invalidated by attempts to fake, although such attempts can often be detected. Penile plethsymography is primarily a clinical approach, and caution should be exercised when using this test in the legal context (Langevin, n.d.; Zonona, 1999). In many jurisdictions, especially Canada, it is routinely used in clinical and psycholegal assessments of sexual offenders referred to forensic services. In many other jurisdictions, it is used primarily as part of a comprehensive treatment approach (Scott, 1994). This test is particularly valuable in the clinical confrontation of nonadmitters who may subsequently admit to the offense, thereby facilitating treatment success.

We cannot emphasize strongly enough that phallometrics, like any other approach described in this chapter, should be considered as only one part of a complete assessment. It should be performed by a recognized lab using standardized test materials, an appropriate setting, and a procedure that respects the dignity of the client. Results should be scrutinized for faking, taking into account the client's mental state, his age, and any physical illnesses, such as diabetes, that may affect the results of testing.

Visual Reaction Time

A newer test that holds great promise has now been developed by Abel and colleagues (1998). This test has some advantages over phallometric testing in that it can be administered in an hour, requiring only a laptop computer, and it does not require the use of naked stimuli material. Although it is useful, at this stage it is debatable whether it has reached the accepted standard for admissibility in court (Krueger, Bradford, & Glancy, 1998). Impressive figures of the test's sensitivity and specificity have been reported but not adequately replicated at this time.

Polygraphy

Polygraphy (or the lie detector) is another test that has been used during the assessment and treatment of sex offenders. Again, it does not meet the standard for admissibility in court but can be used as an adjunctive test (Zonana, 1999).

Attitude and History Measures

Langevin and Watson (1996) and Zonana (1999) outline some specific tests that may be important in the assessment of sex offenders and people with paraphilia, which include the following: Clarke Sexual History Questionnaire (Langevin, Paitich, Handy, & Langevin, 1990); Abel and Becker Cognition Scale (Abel et al., 1984); Attitudes Towards Women Scale (Check, 1985); Burt Rape Myth Acceptance Scale (Burt, 1980); and Michigan Alcohol Screening Test (MAST; Selzer, 1971).

One problem with these tests is their transparency. Unlike the more sophisticated tests such as the MMPI, they do not have specific validity scales and are easily faked. In theory, they are very useful, and if the honesty of the client can be assured, they can play a vital role in the design of a treatment plan and also in the prediction of dangerousness. For instance, the Abel and Becker Cognition Scale identifies cognitive distortion in sex offenders, which can be modified in treatment (Abel et al., 1984). The MAST may identify alcoholism, which can be addressed in treatment, and is also an important variable in predictive instruments (Selzer, 1971). The Clarke Sexual History Questionnaire (Langevin et al., 1990) can give an indication of the number and severity of paraphilias present. It is obvious that caution needs to be used given the self-report nature of these instruments.

General Comments Regarding Actuarial Tests

Although we believe that it was Lord Kelvin who said, "Without measurement there can be no science," Esquirol countered with, "One should never be absolute in practice." Considerable controversy exists about the place of actuarial testing in the assessment of sexual offenders (Zonona, 2000; Sreenivasan et al., 2000). Most experts seem to agree that actuarial tests should be used only in association with other clinical methods of evaluation. It is argued that the use of risk appraisal instruments alone may not meet the standard for admissibility in court and may even be unethical according to some professional associations (Sreenivasan et al., 2000). In fact, in a Florida case, actuarial instruments were ruled inadmissable (In re *Valdez*, p. 6).

Although static factors may be easier to score and can often be gleaned from files, it would be unfortunate if these were the only criteria for a comprehensive assessment. Additionally, they do not assist the assessor in looking at unique relevant factors in an individual client, such as a client who may have a few past offenses and who presents with overwhelming urges to molest or is in a new situation where a child relative has moved into his house temporarily. It is true that the SONAR represents a development of previous tools in that it begins to address dynamic factors. We would agree with Sreenivasan and colleagues' (2000) conclusions that it is the responsibility of the clinician to understand how the individual risk factors are represented in a specific patient. They, like many commentators, have concluded that guided clinical judgment should be the norm.

CONCLUSIONS

We would conclude, therefore, that a comprehensive approach to the assessment of a sexual offender requires a combination of as many of the approaches described in this chapter as are feasible in the circumstances. Every effort should be made to complete a clinical examination and adjunctive testing as described here. Only in this way can the known risk factors be applied to an individual in the context of his current state and unique circumstances.

References

Abel, G., Becker, J., Cunningham-Rathner, J., Rouleau, J., Kaplan, M., & Reich, S. (1984). *Treatment of child molesters*. Atlanta, GA: Emory University School of Medicine.

Abel, G., Becker, J., Mittelman, S., Cunningham-Rathner, J., Rouleau, J., & Murphy, D. (1987). Self-reported sexual crimes of non-incarcerated paraphiliacs. *Journal of Interpersonal Violence, 2,* 3–25.

Abel, G., Huffman, J., Waberg, B., & Holland, C. L. (1998). Visual reaction time and plethysmography as measures of sexual interest in child molesters. *Sexual Abuse: A Journal of Research and Treatment, 10*(2), 81–95.

Abel, G., Lawry, S., Karlstrom, E. M., Osborne, C. A., & Gillespie, C. F. (1994). Screening test for pedophilia. *Criminal Justice and Behaviour, 21,* 115–131.

Badgely, R., Allard, H., McCormick, N., Proudhock, P., Fortin, D., Ogilvie, D., Rae-Grant, Q., Gelinas, P., Pepin, L., & Sutherland, S. (1984). *Sexual offenses against children* (Vol. 1). Ottawa, Canada: Canadian Government Publishers.

Barbaree, H., Seto, M., Langton, C., & Peacock, E. (2001). Evaluating the predictive accuracy of six risk assessment instruments for adult sex offenders. *Criminal Justice and Behaviour, 28,* 490–521.

Burt, M. (1980). Cultural myths and supports for rape. *Journal of Personality and Social Psychology, 38,* 217–230.

Check, J. (1988). Hostility toward women: Some theoretical considerations. In G. W. Russell (Ed.), *Violence in intimate relationships* (pp. 29–42). New York: PMA Publishing Corporation.

Epperson, D., Kaul, J., & Hesselton, D. (1998). *Final report of the development of the Minnesota Sex Offender Screening Tool–Revised*. Paper presented at the 17th Annual Research and Treatment Conference of the Association for the Treatment of Sexual Abusers, Vancouver, British Columbia, Canada.

Freund, K. (1979). Phallometric diagnosis with nonadmitters. *Behavioural Research and Therapy, 17,* 451–457.

Glancy, G., Regehr, C., & Bradford, J. (2001). Sexual predator laws in Canada. *Journal of the American Academy of Psychiatry and the Law, 29,* 232–237.

Glancy, G., Regehr, C., & Bryant, A. (1998) Confidentiality in crisis: Part I. The duty to inform. *Canadian Journal of Psychiatry 43,* 1001–1005.

Glover, A., Nocholson, D., Hemmati, T., Bernfeld, G., & Quinsey, V. (2002). A comparison of predictors of general and violent recidivism among high-risk federal offenders. *Criminal Justice and Behaviour, 29,* 235–249.

Grann, M., Belfrage, H., & Tengstrom, A. (2000). Actuarial assessment of risk for violence: Predictive validity of VRAG and the historical part of the HCR-20. *Criminal Justice and Behaviour, 27,* 97–114.

Grove, W., & Meehl, P. (1996). Comparative efficiency of informal (subjective impressionistic) and formal (mechanical, algorithmic) prediction procedures: The clinical statistical controversy. *Psychology, Public Policy and Law, 2,* 293–323.

Hanson, R. (1997). *The development of a brief actuarial risk scale for sexual offense recidivism* (user report). Ottawa, Canada: Department of the Solicitor General.

Hanson, R. (2000, October). *Using research to improve risk assessment for sex offenders.* Paper presented to the annual meeting of the American Academy of Psychiatry and the Law, Vancouver, British Columbia, Canada.

Hanson, R., & Bussiere, M. (1998). Predicting relapse: A meta-analysis of sexual offender recidivism studies. *Journal of Consulting and Clinical Psychology, 66,* 348–362.

Hanson, R., & Harris, A. (1998). *Dynamic predictors of sexual recidivism* (user report). Ottawa, Canada: Department of the Solicitor General.

Hanson, R., & Harris, A. (2001). A structured approach to evaluating change among sexual offenders. *Sexual Abuse: A Journal of Research and Treatment, 13,* 105–122.

Hanson, R., & Thornton, D. (2000). Improving risk assessments for sex offenders: A comparison of three actuarial scales. *Law and Human Behaviour, 24,* 119–136.

Hare, R. (1991). *Manual for the Revised Psychopathy Checklist.* Toronto, Canada: Multihealth Systems.

Harris, G., Rice, M., & Cormier, C. (2002). Prospective replication of the violence risk appraisal guide in predicting violent recidivism among forensic patients. *Law and Human Behaviour, 26,* 377–394.

Hilton, Z., & Simmons, J. (2001). The influence of actuarial risk assessment in clinical judgements and tribunal decisions about mentally disordered offenders in maximum security. *Law and Human Behaviour, 25,* 393–408.

In re: The Commitment of Robert Valdez. (2000). 6 Judicial Circuit Florida, Case no. 99-007373CI.

Krueger, R., Bradford, J., & Glancy, G. (1998). Report from the Committee on Sex Offenders: The Abel Assessment for Sexual Interest—a brief description. *Journal of the American Academy of Psychiatry and the Law, 26* 277–280.

Langevin, R., (n.d.). *Sexual preference testing: A brief guide.* Toronto: Juniper Press.

Langevin, R., Paitich, D., Handy, L., & Langevin, A. (1990). *The Clarke Sexual History Questionnaire Manual.* Etobicoke, Canada: Juniper Press.

Langevin, R., & Watson, R. (1996). Major factors in the assessment of paraphilias and sex offenders. *Journal of Offender Rehabilitation, 23,* 39–70.

Mossman, D. (2000). Commentary: Assessing the risk of violence—are "accurate" predictions useful? *Journal of the American Academy of Psychiatry Law, 28,* 272–281.

Quinsey, V., Harris, G., Rice, M., & Cormier, C. (1998). *Violent offenders: Appraising and managing risk.* Washington, DC: American Psychological Association.

Quinsey, A., V., Khanna, A., & Malcolm, P. (1998). A retrospective evaluation of the regional sex offender treatment program. *Journal of Interpersonal Violence, 13,* 621–624.

Regehr, C., & Antle, B. (1997). Coercive influences: Informed consent in court-mandated social work practice. *Social Work, 42,* 300–306.

Regehr, C., Edwardh, M., & Bradford, J. (2000) Research ethics with forensic patients. *Canadian Journal of Psychiatry, 45,* 892–898.

Rice, M., & Harris, G. (1997). Cross–validation and extension of the violent risk assessment guide for child molesters and rapists. *Law and Human Behaviour, 21,* 231–241.

Scott, L. (1994). Sex offenders. In A. Roberts (Ed.), *Critical issues in crime and justice* (pp. 61–76). Thousand Oaks, CA: Sage.

Selzer, M. (1971). The Michigan Alcohol Screening Test: The quest for a new diagnostic instrument. *American Journal of Psychiatry, 127,* 1653–1658.

Seto, M., & Lalumière, M. (2000). Psychopathy and sexual aggression. In C. Gatcono (Ed.), *The clinical and forensic assessment of psychopathy: A practitioner's guide* (pp. 333–350). Mahwah, NJ: Erlbaum.

Sjostedt, G., & Langstrom, N. (2001). Actuarial assessment of sex offender recidivism risk: A cross validation of the RRASOR and the Static-99. *Law and Human Behaviour, 25,* 629–645.

Sreenivasan, H., Kirkish, P., Garrick, T., Wineberger, L., & Phenixa, A. (2000). Actuarial risk assessment models: A review of critical issues related to violence and sex offender recidivism assessments. *Journal of the American Academy of Psychiatry and the Law, 28* 438–448.

State of Washington. (1991). Sexually Violent Predators Statute, Revised Code of Washington, Chapter 71.07.

Thornton, D. (1997). *A 16-year follow-up of 563 sexual offenders released from HM Prison Service in 1979.* Unpublished raw data.

Webster, C. D., Douglas, K. S., Eaves, D., & Hart, S. D. (1997). Predicting violence in mentally and personality disordered individuals. In C. D. Webster & M. A. Jackson, *Impulsivity: Theory, Assessment, and Treatment.* New York: Guildford.

Zonona, H. (1999). *Dangerous sex offenders: A task force report of the American Psychiatric Association.* Washington, DC: American Psychiatric Association.

Zonona, H. (2000). Sex offender testimony: Junk science of unethical testimony. *Journal of the American Academy Psychiatry and the Law, 28,* 386–388.

59

"OPTIMAL PRACTICE" CLINICAL NEUROPSYCHOLOGY

A Cautionary Tale and Revisionist Proto-Model

Nathaniel J. Pallone & James J. Hennessy

> There is a long-standing romance between the "true believer"
> and the too-easy answer.
>
> —John Tracy Ellis, 1949

In Lezak's (1995) definition, "Clinical neuropsychology is an applied science concerned with the behavioral expression of brain dysfunction" (p. 7). As if in amplification, Gilandas, Touyz, Beumont, and Greenberg (1984) state, "Clinical neuropsychology relates brain dysfunction to observable, empirically documented behavioral deficits" (p. 1). In optimal practice circumstances, the distinctive role of the clinical neuropsychologist is the specification and remediation of the cognitive, emotional, and behavioral consequences that follow and flow from medically verified neuropathology. Optimal practice circumstances are achieved, however, only when members of the several relevant medical and mental health professions—including (but perhaps not limited to) neurology, psychiatry, endocrinology, psychology, social work, and marriage and family counseling—function cooperatively and harmoniously in the interest of patients. In its turn, such cooperative and harmonious functioning requires both that each member of each profession experience a high level of security in his or her professional identity, understand the boundaries of his or her competence and those of his or her profession, and harbor no territorial urge to violate the scope of practice unique to other professions. Unfortunately, such optimal circumstances are not often encountered in the real world.

Were we to construct this paper in conventional fashion, we might proceed by

- reviewing data concerning the prevalence of neuropathology in the general population (estimated by the Federal Centers for Disease Control at 2%, as reported by Marino, 1999)
- acknowledging, if not attempting to catalog in detail, the enormous knowledge explosion in the neurosciences that has occurred since 1970 as a result of the introduction of technologically sophisticated brain-scanning devices (BEAM, CAT, fMRI, MRI, MRS, QEEG, rCBF, SPECT, SQUID, SQUIRM, and a seemingly ever-expanding array of related technologies) that make it possible to observe brain "events" (including the absorption and transfer of neurohormones) as they occur in real time so that functions and dysfunctions (pathologies) can be studied (and perhaps localized) with some precision[1]
- identifying the most frequent sources of neuropathology (including congenital defects; falls from cribs, sofas, ladders, bicycles; sports injuries; closed head injuries and traumatic brain injuries in motor vehicle or industrial accidents or victimization in criminal violence at any age)
- proceeding to an exposition of the areas of

the brain where pathology is most likely to yield those cognitive, emotional, or behavioral defects amenable to specification and modification by psychological (nonmedical) means (primarily, but not exclusively, the frontal lobe, held in the human species to be the seat of most "executive" functions, the temporal lobe, the hypothalamus, and the limbic system)[2]
- coming to rest with an encomium to the pioneers who fathered neuropsychology (Wechsler, Halstead, and Reitan in this country, Luria in what was then the Soviet Union, and their colleagues and coinvestigators).

Were we to proceed according to such an outline, we would surely parade before the reader a bewildering set of terms and facts more likely to obfuscate than to elucidate—and, in the process, leave an aftertaste of unflavored sawdust. Suppose, instead, that we begin this excursion with a cautionary tale intended to illustrate that, absent attention to neuropsychiatric and neuropsychological issues, mental health practitioners might readily misattribute the source of real-life problems faced by patients, in the process perhaps infringing, however unwittingly, the first canon in the oath of Hippocrates.

THE CAUTIONARY TALE: VERA AND MAX

We should emphasize that the setting in which our tale unfolds is a behavioral health clinic attached to the outpatient department of a university teaching hospital. In such a setting, owing to formal relations with the several academic departments represented by staff and interns and because interprofessional and interdisciplinary consultation can fairly readily be obtained, something approximating optimal clinical practice conditions is more probable than in stand-alone settings. As a matter of policy, all hospital staff are required to wear white lab coats, so that (save for green-clad surgeons entering operatories) there is no set of "vestments" peculiarly reserved to a priesthood; instead, neither patients nor staff members can differentiate on the basis of garb alone members of one profession from those of another. That circumstance by itself may, at the very least, trammel the more virulent expressions of that strain of one-

upmanship known euphemistically as interprofessional rivalry.

Alcohol: The Source of All Human Troubles?

Our focus is Max R, a man of 39 with a high school education followed by union-sponsored apprenticeship training in pipe fitting. He has long been employed as a journeyman pipe fitter in a factory that manufactures jams and jellies. His wife, Vera, 35, had until recently been a "soccer mom," but she now works on the 4-to-midnight shift as a packer in the shipping department in the same factory as her husband. The couple have a son, aged 11, and a daughter, aged 8, who attend a religious school. Prior to the instant situation, no member of the family had sought or received professional mental or behavioral health assistance.

Vera and Max were coerced into seeking the services of the clinic through direct court action. Ten days prior to the couple's first visit, police had been summoned because what appeared to be a turbulent argument had erupted between Vera and Max at about one o'clock in the morning. Alarmed neighbors had reported hearing loud voices and the sounds of smashing glass. Police had been called by an older, retired couple who had perhaps become overly sensitive to "distant early warning signals" of domestic violence; they told the 911 operator that they had not been awakened but were in fact watching an old movie when they were startled by the uncharacteristic noise emanating from next door. They had made similar calls in the past that involved other households in the neighborhood. Their sensitivity, however, had roots in the same mother lode of public sentiment that, subsequent to the trial of a well-known sports figure for the murder of his ex-wife (resulting in acquittal), prompted the township in which Vera and Max live to adopt a "zero-tolerance" policy toward domestic violence. The operative municipal statute, in effect, removes discretion from police in assessing whether an incident is of sufficient gravity as to require (or support) the lodging of formal charges and further requires that a "first incident report" shall result in a judicial order that the couple, or other disputants, involved seek mental health intervention. Following the pathway customary for pretrial diversion protocols, should the court judge such intervention effective and should no further complaints be lodged within the space of a year, the record of the initial complaint is to be expunged; otherwise, the initial complaint is to be advanced to arraignment and trial.

Responding officers noted in their report broken glass in the dining room, apparently the result of a vase having been hurled against a large mirror; the arm of a chair also had been broken. There was no evidence of physical injury to any member of the family, although they noted obvious anxiety in the children. There was a slight odor of beer on Max's breath, and a partially consumed six-pack (three cans down) was evident in the den. Max readily submitted to a saliva swab, but the result was negative for the presence of a toxic level of alcohol. Still, the officers noted in their report their view that alcohol had at least contributed in some way to the altercation. Both parents and children seemed to have returned to a state of relative calm, so the officers did not seek to remove anyone from the home. Instead, they issued a summons returnable in municipal court, with the distal result that Vera and Max had presented themselves to the clinic.

Especially if we have prejudged that alcohol is the source of all human troubles, how else can we construe the circumstances leading to the fracas but that Max had imbibed one too many and that the level of alcohol in his system, whatever the (perhaps falsely negative) results of the saliva screening test, was sufficient as to elicit a hostile response from Vera? It requires little in the way of empathetic imagination to construe Vera's reactions to the odor of alcohol when she returns from a long evening's work. If we encode the precipitating events in that fashion, we are likely to design a program of intervention that addresses Max's inability or unwillingness to monitor his alcohol consumption, as well as Vera's apparently exaggerated response to nontoxic alcohol use. Those interventions may do no major harm (and thus leave Hippocrates' canon unscathed). But unless we develop a comprehensive picture that accounts for all the variables that contributed to the fracas that brought Vera and Max to the clinic, those interventions may prove beneficial only at the periphery. To put the matter more succinctly, if alcohol is not the exclusive source of their distress, we might therapize Max's alcohol consumption and Vera's reactions thereto until the cows come home and still change very little.

Sexual Frustration: The Source of All Human Troubles?

During intake, Vera and Max provide a narrative of how the altercation had started. They agree on the basic outlines. Vera had returned to the home about 20 minutes past midnight; Max greeted her, telling her that, as planned, he had placed a frozen TV dinner in the oven for her at the appropriate time; Vera commenced her meal while Max continued his televiewing; there were verbal exchanges about trivial topics until Max heard Vera washing up in the kitchen. He then entered the kitchen and reminded Vera that they had previously agreed upon sexual congress when she got home from work. Vera declined, telling Max that she had had a hard day at the factory. Max retorted in some hostile fashion or another. Vera dismissed him, telling him to go back into the den and continue watching the Playboy channel or whatever other skin flick he had on.

At this point in the narrative, Max becomes visibly distressed, frowning and squirming in his seat. In response to an inquiry, he amplifies, "It was when she made that crack about 'being locked in the down position'—again. That's when I pounded on the arm of the chair and it broke and she threw the vase. And the next thing I know the cops are there."

We might inquire as to the meaning of the quaint phrase, even though its denotation seems clear enough. We used to have an old station wagon with an electric window that didn't work right, Vera says, because it sometimes got locked in the down position. That's the way it is with Bozo here (in clear reference to Max), especially when he's had a couple of beers.

Now the genesis of the altercation seems more richly textured, particularly if we have prejudged that sexual frustration is the source of all human troubles—even more so when lubricated by alcohol. We appear to have a problem of (at least partial) erectile dysfunction in a man entirely too young to be undergoing what is, still somewhat controversially, called "andropause." But, as the ads and commercials for Viagra ceaselessly remind us, a "quick fix" chemical remedy is now available and no longer (if the ads and commercials are to be believed) reserved primarily for those consumers whose hair has turned silvery gray. Still, that chemical remedy is not without some health risk; Viagra is essentially a vasoconstrictor (a substance that causes blood vessels to narrow), so that its use by patients with any sort of cardiac peculiarity is strongly discouraged. Absent a comprehensive urological examination, we cannot be certain that the chemical remedy is required; absent a comprehensive cardiological examination, we cannot be certain that the chemical remedy will, in fact, do no harm. (Happily, that judgment lies entirely within the scope of medical, not mental health, practice.) And "treating the symptom," as the psychoanalysts never tire of reminding us, is not to extirpate the source of that symptom.

Money: The Source of All Human Troubles?

We are, of course, curious about Vera's level of libido. So we inquire further: Max, when did this problem begin? Vera, Max is implying that your sexual interest has waned, evaporated, or perhaps even been directed elsewhere; is any of these the case? If so, when did that begin to happen?

The couple assert that there were few problems involving sex before Max stopped working. Max claims that it's all really Vera's fault, that her sex drive took a plunge when she went to work, that how can anyone expect him to maintain an erection when she's always in a hurry and, for her, it's got to be "Slam, bam, thank you ma'am" so she can get some sleep? Balderdash (or some word to similar effect), says Vera, I wouldn't have had to get a job except that your check is about half what it used to be. And, yes, I get home and you've been drinking beer, you've gained 20 pounds since you've been home I bet, doing nothing but sitting around all day watching that damn Playboy channel, and then you start grabbing practically as soon as I get in the door, sticky and dirty—real romantic, a real goddamned turnoff that is, when you want to do it on the couch in the den with those skinny naked babes running around and grunting on that screen, saying that's what makes you hot, and you can't keep it up anyway.

Other variables now seem to be peeping through. Let us explore Vera's decision to seek employment. No choice about it, Vera explains, he used to work 14, 16, sometimes 18 hours a week overtime at time and a half, sometimes double time. Now the disability check from the factory comes to half of straight time, so you do the arithmetic. (We observe, parenthetically, that if Max worked on average 16 hours per week at time and a half, he was being paid for 40 + 24 hours, or a total of 64 hours, while the disability check in effect pays him for 20 hours; Vera's arithmetic is unassailable.) And that's all there was for 6 months, our savings went down the tube, so I had to get a job. The people at the plant went out of their way to help us out, but that late shift was the only thing available. Besides, I'll quit as soon as he's medically cleared to go back to work; he knows that. Why, he had a checkup just a few days before that thing with the cops, hoping the docs would clear him to go back to work; but they didn't, said he still can't lift more than 20 pounds, kept him out for another 6 weeks at least, then another checkup.

Those who have prejudged that money is the source of all human troubles will not be surprised by these revelations. For the rest of us, a more nuanced picture of the dynamics that flowed, and that likely still flow, between Vera and Max begins to come into focus.

Neuropathology: The Source of Every Trouble Imaginable?

In order to understand the character of the injuries Max sustained on the job, we need to know something of his specific work activities. In daily life, one assumes that the pipes on which a pipe fitter works are those that deliver water or gas or remove waste, ranging in diameter perhaps from 1 to 12 inches. Not so within the industrial context; the pipes that Max fits together range in diameter from 18 to 42 inches and carry, in the form of heated viscous liquid, ingredients destined to find their way into jars as jam, jelly, or preserves—sugar, other sweetening agents, processed fruit, fruit juice reduced by boiling to spreadable consistency. Those pipes hang from structural steel beams at a height of 15 feet above the shop floor. When Max works on a pipe, he does so while standing in the carriage of an industrial-strength forklift. (If we consider the torque required to handle a wrench capable of opening a 36-inch pipe, we can understand why Max's capacity to lift 20 pounds or more repeatedly is relevant to his fitness to work; clearly, the factory cannot risk injury that might result in permanent disability.)

On the day of his accident, Max had been in the process of descending in the carriage when a malfunction caused it to plummet, rather than float slowly, to the shop floor. The impact sheared the safety harness Max is required to wear and hurled him, hard hat and all, out of the carriage. Witnesses could not recall whether his head struck the floor as he was thrown from the carriage, but he landed with a thud on his right side, lost consciousness, and remained unconscious for some minutes. EMT personnel from the industrial medical center under contract to the factory responded rapidly and took Max to the trauma unit in a nearby hospital specially designated to handle industrial accidents. Admitting diagnoses included dislocated shoulder, broken right elbow, cracked ribs, assorted cuts, abrasions, and contusions, and mild concussion; happily, the skull had not fractured. Max remained in the hospital for 9 days and was then placed on indefinite medical leave to recuperate at home until medically cleared to resume his normal work duties; he has reported on a regular basis to the industrial medical center for reevaluation, as required by his employer.

During the first weeks following hospital discharge, Max had been medicated on a fixed schedule by means of a powerful painkiller that, according to its manufacturer, has been associated with such undesirable side effects as "loss of coordination, confusion, irregular heartbeat, irregular breathing, extreme dizziness, anxiety or tremors," and he continues to take the medication as needed for shoulder pain. The medication is accompanied by a strong warning that the user is to abandon alcohol use; however, that admonition is frequently more honored in the breach than in the observance. (Under a specific, time-release formulation marketed under the name Oxycontin-80-TR, the active ingredients in this medication achieved considerable notoriety when it began to be distributed illegally on a wide scale as a street drug in the late 1990s.)

After the fractures healed, Max followed the program of physical therapy prescribed, and he has been examined to determine fitness to work every 4 to 6 weeks. Following each such examination, he had been pronounced not yet fit. Subjectively, in response to probing during intake, Max reported that he had experienced some blurring of vision for perhaps 10 days after discharge from the hospital, but beyond the obvious limitations on activity imposed as fractured bones knit thoroughly, he claimed no other residual effects, specifically denying (again in response to probing) difficulties in perception, cognition, memory, and so forth. For her part, Vera returned to the leitmotif involving sexual demands, alcohol, reduced income, and incessant televiewing of "girlie" shows—sometimes even in the presence of their children.

It is a matter of more than contextual interest that the malfunctioning forklift is leased to Max's employer by its manufacturer, a "household name" corporation, which also is under contract to provide regular inspection and maintenance so as to ensure worker safety. At the urging of his employer (and, probably, also thus to limit the employer's liability), Max has filed a claim with the lessor both for lost wages and for "pain and suffering." The couple has been given every reassurance by the human resources department at the factory that they will doubtless receive a handsome settlement, in time; but, as Vera says, the prospect of future windfall does not pay the mortgage or the tuition or the electric bill due the day after tomorrow.

Staff members at the clinic in our tale had been particularly sensitized (some might have said "brainwashed") to unlikely manifestations of lingering neuropathology. They have been constantly urged to probe for past history of head trauma (or other neurological damage) because, as the distinguished neuropsychiatrists Silver, Yudofsky, and Hales (1987, pp. 179–180) observe in the first edition of the American Psychiatric Association's semiofficial *Textbook of Neuropsychiatry*, "the patient, while providing a psychiatric history, may fail to associate current symptoms with head trauma. . . . The patient may present only the [obvious psychosocial or behavioral] symptoms for evaluation and treatment." According to these experts, the "prototypic examples of brain damage" that are not associated by the patient with current cognitive, emotional, or behavioral abnormalities include "the 10-year-old boy whose head was hit while falling from his bicycle, but who fails to inform his parents."

If such an apparently mild injury can result in psychological dysfunctions, how much more so in the case of Max, who suffered a medically verifiable concussion, especially since neuropsychiatrists Brown, Fann, and Grant (1994, pp. 15–16) declare flatly that "post-concussional disorders may represent one of the most common etiologies of neurobehavioral disorder"? For those who are even mildly disposed to so prejudge, it may seem that, with revelation of closed head injury resulting in concussion, the mother lode has been uncovered. But, if for no other reason than its implicit smugness, we should not be surprised if that conclusion proves only slightly less accurate than other premature judgments anchored in other pet prejudices.

ASKING BETTER QUESTIONS

Reductionism pivots on the belief that complex phenomena can be explained by single causes; the true believer searches constantly for *nothing but*. In contrast, the clinical scientist shuns explanations that reduce to a single pivot; he or she seeks *both/and* in efforts to understand the genesis of behavior. From that perspective, the principal role of the clinical neuropsychologist and clinical neuropsychiatrist in the assessment process may be to ask better and more comprehensive questions about both "causes" and "cures."

Under whatever specific nomenclature and in whatever work setting, mental health clinicians are called upon to integrate hard (e.g., from medical and/or psychological tests) and soft (e.g., from self-reports and reports of observers) data about patients so that appropriate questions can be asked and answered *both* about the genesis *and* the contextual dynamics that have contributed distally or proximally to "presenting problems" *and* about remedies likely to prove (at least) ameliorative, including the still-extant coping mechanisms of the afflicted parties. In that mix, the distinctive function of the clinical neuropsychologist is to search out the cognitive, emotional, and behavioral consequences (if any) to neuropathology (if any).

How will clinical neuropsychology contribute to better questions in the case of Max and Vera? What questions should be raised? What sources of information are to be accessed in response?

To be sure, closed head injury resulting in concussion might well account for many, or even most, of the problems presented by the couple at intake. If their report is accurate, either edema (swelling) or shearing of brain tissue, or both, ensued; and edema alone might well explain both impaired social judgment and perseveration on Max's part. As we noted elsewhere:

While the exterior of the skull at maturity is smooth and hard, the interior is relatively craggy, with many bony structures protruding. Even without skull fracture, a blow to the head sufficient to shift brain cells (themselves rather gelatinous in texture) within the skull may thus cause edema, with consequent "temporary" re-arrangement of spatial relationships among and between brain cells, or direct damage to cells, most of which do not regenerate, with consequent "loss" of function that may be associated with damaged cells. . . . The most worrisome consequence of such temporary spatial re-arrangement is that neurohormones may not be able to "find" the brain sites where they are typically metabolized and instead "spill over" onto unaccustomed sites, with effects that cannot readily be predicted. . . . Clinically, it has sometimes been reported edema is discernible for as long as 24 months following impact. But there is presently no medically reliable treatment that can hasten the process; what is left, then, is the task of helping the patient compensate for functions that are temporarily impaired or permanently lost. (Pallone & Hennessy, 1996, p. 48)[3]

In the couple's self-reports and the police incident report, we observe impaired social judgment in Max's singular devotion to (putatively) X-rated televiewing and in his apparent inability to understand that a demand, or even request, for sexual congress as soon as his wife returns from work is not likely to be welcomed. Frontal lobe dysfunction may account both for impaired social judgment and for what we take to be the essentially perseverative character of Max's demands in the absence of positive reinforcement and for what we can infer to be the compulsive use of alcohol, this time despite negative reinforcement from Vera. Even though these diagnostic categories are no longer available in the *Diagnostic and Statistical Manual of Mental Disorders* issued by the American Psychiatric Association, the World Health Organization's *International Classification of Diseases* still litanizes both Post-Concussion Syndrome (310.2) and Frontal Lobe Syndrome (310.0); should we not make those diagnoses, tell Max and Vera to wait until the swelling dies down, pat ourselves on the back, and call it a day?

ENTER THE ANTIREDUCTIONISTS

Reductionsists are at high risk for mistaking component parts for the whole. Wherefore: Let the revisionists and antireductionists have their say.

The first impediment we encounter is that neither diagnosis adequately accounts for Max's erectile dysfunction, intermittent or not. Indeed, were Max typically inebriated when he demands sexual congress with Vera and is then unable to perform, or able to perform only partially, there might be (as Shakespeare reminded us many a year ago) an explanation that accounts for both heightened interest and decreased ability; but there is no strong reason to believe that is the case here. Despite police impressions, swab results found Max's blood-alcohol level to be below toxic proportions. Alternately, it might be that the brain sites that govern erection (those at which the relevant neurohormones, including vasopressin and norepinephrine as well as testosterone, are metabolized and where they might interact with the metabolites of beverage alcohol) have been damaged; but there is no particular evidence of that. Rather than venturing deeply into neurochemistry, we might more simply inquire into whether Max heeds the warning on the prescription label for the painkiller he now uses intermittently. As worded by the manufacturer, the warning is unconditional: *Avoid alcoholic beverages, because they increase certain side effects of this drug.* Not unlike the majority of patients, Max may pretend to understand that the prohibition means only that he should not swig his pills down with a beer or a shot. If Max even occasionally uses the painkiller and alcohol in near juxtaposition, the former may potentiate the latter in such fashion that the *same* chemical cocktail *simultaneously* impedes sexual performance *and* produces an "impression" of inebriation even in the absence of a toxic concentration of alcohol in the blood. Unfortunately for our tidy root source explanation, that scenario seems to move in the direction of voluntary misbehavior. Still, can we not interpret Max's inability or unwillingness to comply with pharmacological safety precautions as an instance of impaired judgment, so that we are right back to the frontal lobe?

Next, there are contextual questions that only in the most tangential way impinge on whatever neuropathology Max sustained. Vera asserts that the family has fallen on hard times because Max's disability check comes to only about 30% of his usual weekly check, including both "straight" time and overtime. There seems no other way to interpret such data but to speculate that the family is accustomed to living well beyond its means, in a pattern that well preceded Max's injury. What dynamics account for that pattern of mercantile overconsumption? For that matter, is Max's typical overtime schedule itself a means of playing "keep-away" from Vera and

the children? (Indeed, there are enough such questions in the premorbid functioning of the family to warm the cockles of the heart of those who believe that family dysfunction is the source of all human troubles.) Any set of remedies we devise predicated solely on Max's neuropsychological and neuropsychiatric deficits will not address those preexisting dynamic patterns.

Finally, and most important, it is professionally irresponsible to conclude to *brain pathology on the basis of self-report*—or, indeed, on the basis of observations of mental health clinicians who are not physicians. Brain pathology is a medical diagnosis; it simply cannot be made by a nonphysician. Further, because one of the cognitive indicia discernible in patients who have sustained clinically significant head injury is confabulation, we should be especially wary of accepting without verification self-reports of any sort bearing upon any arena of behavior. Instead, we need to gather and to assess, whether from extant examinations (in Max's case, for example, at the point of admission to and discharge from the hospital, during subsequent outpatient examinations) *medical-neurological* data, including data from brain scans (if any). Indeed, it may *simultaneously* be the case that a patient sustains a head injury and afterward behaves uncharacteristically, but the two may not be related in any "causal" way. Borrowing from the lexicon of toxicology, Valciukas (1995) would term such a situation one in which the head injury, even though medically verified, has produced "no observable effect" cognitively, emotionally, or behaviorally. Thus, it is absolutely essential that there be *medical-neurological* confirmation of the *hypothesis* implicit in the "enriched" question(s) to which clinical neuropsychology has contributed.

AN "OPTIMAL PRACTICE" PROTO-MODEL ILLUSTRATING DIFFERENTIAL ROLES

In Figure 59.1, we offer a proto-model for optimal practice that illustrates differential professional roles and functions in neuropsychological assessment and rehabilitation. The model posits four distinct stages, from initial screening to provision of services responsive to patient requirements. We label it a proto-model because of the relative reversal of the roles played by the clinical neuropsychologist and the clinical neu-

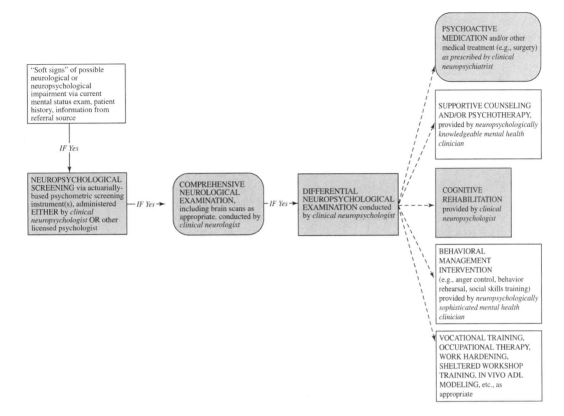

FIGURE 59.1 An optimal practice proto-model illustrating differential professional roles and functions in neuropsychological assessment and rehabilitation

ropsychiatrist when compared with what is purveyed in many texts dealing with clinical neuropsychology, the essential message in which seems to be *neuropsychology über alles*—or, less cryptically, that the findings, judgments, and/or opinions of the neuropsychologist based on results of psychometric examination should guide, not follow, those of the neurologist and neuropsychiatrist, even when the latter are grounded in advanced neuroimaging examination.

Neuropsychological Screening

In most versions of the mental status interview, and surely in that version that has become standard in clinical psychiatry (Hales & Yudofsky, 2002) and widely adopted by the other mental health professions, there are direct probes for recent or remote neurological injury, alongside to be sure probes for substance abuse of such severity as to raise the specter of neuropathology.

Whether observed directly in the intake interview or revealed as the patient provides his or her psychosocial history (or provided by the referral source), any of these *may* constitute "soft signs" of neuropathology: abnormalities in motor, memory, or receptive or expressive language functions; general disorientation; limited capacity to abstract; deficits in attention or concentration. Any such "soft sign" is sufficient to trigger a formal neuropsychological screening, precisely to initiate the process of differential diagnosis. (Is confabulation, for example, a function of neuropathology or of a psychosis that is categorizable as "functional" because it is relatively independent of neurophysiological dysunction?)

Such screening should be undertaken only by a licensed psychologist (i.e., one who is legally empowered under the laws of his or her state to administer and interpret standard psychological tests, not by other mental health clinicians who infringe upon that scope of practice, sometimes unaware that they are violating not merely the boundaries of the ethical code of their own profession but indeed the law of the state) *or* by a properly qualified clinical neuropsychologist. Corporations that publish tests are fond of offering for sale a wide variety of instruments they claim to be neuropsychological screening devices, which they are willing to sell to virtually any purchaser without regard to his or her background, training, or experience in psychometrics. Some such devices, in fact, turn out to have very little capacity to differentiate patients with medically verified neuropsychological dysfunction from examinees with no evidence of such dysfunction; nonetheless, their publishers purvey them to users who have no appropriate training or experience that qualifies them as competent administrators or interpreters.[4] In a current catalog, for example, one publisher hawks an instrument which it asserts can "quickly identify strengths and weaknesses in five cognitive domains . . . of adults with neurological impairments." The publisher is willing to sell the instrument to a purchaser who supplies his or her name, address, and telephone number and an "official purchase order number" and, ominously, who meets "no additional requirements." In contrast, other of this publisher's instruments are available for purchase only by those who hold a master's degree or a doctorate, sometimes with the additional requirement of membership in an appropriate professional organization. What conclusion can we draw but that, in the view of this publisher, identification of the "strengths and weaknesses in five cognitive domains" attributable to neuropathology is apparently a task of such trifling import that it can be undertaken by anyone with the price of the ticket, whatever his or her training and experience—or lack thereof?

Many tests sold as neuropsychological screening devices are, in fact, merely structured interview schedules relying on the self-reports of patients and, consequent to the high incidence of confabulation and memory impairment of patients with neuropathologic conditions, are scarcely to be relied upon. Two actuarially anchored (objective) instruments we have found most useful are the *Kaufman Short Neuropsychological Assessment Procedure* (Kaufman & Kaufman, 1994), with a pronounceable acronym (so well loved by publishers and some test purchasers), and the *Stroop Color and Word Test 2002* (Golden, 2002), recently revised by the lead developer of the Luria-Nebraska Neuropsychol-

ogical Battery. Each instrument provides norms that support an actuarial decision that further inquiry is necessary by citing "probabilities" that the patient examined, in fact, can be psychometrically "sorted" into one or more groups of patients with medically verified neuropathologies or into a group medically verified as free of neuropathology. (Technically, clinically relevant "reference range" values are provided, beyond which patients' scores can be taken as indicative of "probable" neuropathology, in the same way that body temperature of 103 degrees is interpreted not merely as an increment of one degree beyond 102 but as a signal of probable serious physical ailment sufficient to trigger more discerning medical examination.) Both instruments tend to "overpredict" (i.e., to yield a high ratio of "false positives"), but that is surely preferable to the obverse situation that yields a high ratio of false negatives.

In contrast to our insistence upon methods that are actuarially anchored, some clinicians continue to be enamored of projective techniques, whatever it is that is to be measured. Among them, and despite its lack of objective norms, the Bender Visual-Motor Gestalt Test is the instrument of choice (Lacks, 1984). Ironically, however, its publisher does not categorize it as either a neuropsychological screening test or neuropsychological test.

Comprehensive Neurological Examination

If, but only if, results of that screening are positive, in our proto-model the patient should be referred for comprehensive *neurological* examination conducted by a qualified (i.e., board-certified in this specialty) clinical neurologist. In an earlier era, as the writings of Ward Halstead and Ralph Reitan amply demonstrate, it was frequently the case that a comprehensive neuropsychological examination followed screening directly and often guided the examination subsequently conducted by the neurologist. But that way of doing things prevailed in a time long before the widespread availability of neuroimaging devices. Indeed, in many metropolitan areas today, the costs associated with a comprehensive neuropsychological examination are greater than those associated with a comprehensive neurological examination that includes neuroimaging.

Whether neuroimaging is undertaken is, of course, a decision to be made medically. For valid reasons, the neurologist may employ older, "office-bound" indices (tuning fork maintenance of attention, eye motion, heel-to-toe ambulation, etc.) either adjunctively or in lieu of neuroimaging and/or neuroendocrine and neurochemical analyses. Nonmedical mental health clinicians need to bear in mind that neuropathology is essentially a medical diagnosis and can be made or disconfirmed only be properly trained and licensed physicians. We would do well to realize that, whatever the venue (including the courts and the offices of third-party health care payers), it is the physician who will invariably have the last word. Interprofessional rivalry, or games of one-upmanship about who examines whom first, who is entitled to make what diagnosis, and the like—let alone the protocols that should be followed in a comprehensive neurological examination—are largely a colossal waste of time and do little to enhance the welfare of the patient. Even practicing neuropsychologists expend entirely too much effort in second-guessing neurologists; that energy could, and should, instead be directed to specifying the cognitive, emotional, and behavioral sequelae to medically verified neuropathology and to devising psychological methods and protocols to address those sequelae—functions they alone, as psychologists who have achieved expert knowledge in cognition and learning, are uniquely equipped to perform.

Differential Neuropsychological Examination

In our proto-model, if (but only if) results of the comprehensive neurological examination are positive, the next step is a *differential* neuropsychological examination to determine with some precision both the specific impairments in psychological functioning attributable to medically verified neuropathology *and* the intact resources within the patient upon which to anchor psychologically oriented methods of treatment. Although we label our position as revisionist, it is not entirely radical. Indeed, 20 years ago, during the adolescence, if not quite infancy, of neuroimaging and quite before imaging devices became as ubiquitous as they are today, Golden, Moses, Coffman, Miller, and Strider (1983) put it clearly: "In general, the neuropsychologist will rarely localize the effects of a [lesion] for a physician, since most [lesions] can be localized through neuroradiologic techniques. The neu-

ropsychologist is [instead] responsible for describing deficits due to [lesions]." Wonder of wonders, even one test publisher, in hawking new wares, has implicitly recognized the inevitability of the sequence we here describe. In advertising the Wilg-Nielsen Alzheimer's Quick Test, the Psychological Corporation (2003, p. 17) deposes that clinicians should "use the AQT in conjunction with brain imaging (e.g., CT scan, MRI, etc.) and other neuropsychiatric procedures in support of a differential diagnosis of Alzheimer's."

No single instrument is adequate to the purpose of differential neuropsychological examination. Instead, the "gold standards" are, respectively, the *Halstead-Reitan Neuropsychological Test Battery* (Reitan & Wolfson, 1992a) and the *Luria-Nebraska Neuropsychological Test Battery* (Golden, Purisch, & Hammeke, 1992). Neither protocol is a single "instrument" in the usual sense but instead a battery containing a variety of discrete measures that assess a spectrum of neurocognitive and neuromotor functions. Depending upon the severity of neuropathology, administration of the complete battery in either case may take many hours and require more than one sitting. Each protocol provides a number of discrete scores: Patterns of scores can be actuarially related (both via norm tables and through reference ranges) to specific types of brain dysfunction.

At its most ample, the Halstead-Reitan battery includes the Wechsler Adult Intelligence Scale and the Minnesota Multiphasic Personality Inventory, as well as the Wisconsin Card Sorting Test, the Category Test, and measures of aphasia, grip strength, bilateral sensory stimulation, and tactile form recognition. The Luria-Nebraska yields scores in arithmetic, handedness, intellectual processes, lateral dominance, memory, receptive language, rhythm, and visual perception. Administration and, in particular, interpretation of these protocols require high levels of knowledge and skill and should not be undertaken lightly; indeed, misinterpretation of results may readily lead to violation of the first canon in the Hippocratic oath.

Rehabilitation and Remediation

The final step in our proto-model is the provision of remedial or rehabilitative services of several sorts, predicated on carefully inventoried deficits as well as the patient's residual resources.

We have highlighted *cognitive rehabilitation*, the rehabilitative service most frequently associated with clinical neuropsychological intervention (Sohlberg & Mateer, 2001) and today often implemented with the assistance of desktop computers, with Reitan's REHABIT program (Reitan & Wolfson, 1988) and Bracy's (1997) OSS-COG the leading integrated protocols.

Other services may be required simultaneously or serially. Some can be provided only by a clinical neuropsychiatrist, ranging from neurosurgery in the most extreme cases to psychoactive medication in situations, for example, in which neuropathology has resulted in uncharacteristic irascibility or aggressivity. Other services can be adequately provided by properly licensed mental health clinicians with sensitivity to neurological and neuropsychological deficits. As we have seen in the case of Vera and Max, marriage counseling focused on financial issues will necessarily assume quite different dimensions when the source of insolvency is neurological dysfunction in one partner coupled with a certain intransigence in the other than when the source is lack of enterprise in either or the inability of one or the other to tolerate fellow workers.

TRAINING AND COMPETENCE IN CLINICAL NEUROPSYCHOLOGY

A little learning, the English poet Alexander Pope declaimed in 1711, is a dangerous thing; drink deep, he counseled, or taste not the Pierian spring, for "shallow draughts there intoxicate the brain, and drinking largely sobers us again."

Thoracic surgery is an advanced medical specialty; it is also what people who study vocational psychology call a "late-entry" career. To become a thoracic surgeon, one needs to (a) graduate from college, (b) graduate from medical school, (c) complete an internship of 1 year in a general medical-surgical hospital, (d) successfully undergo licensure examination by the state board of medical examiners, (e) complete a residency in general surgery spanning 2 to 3 years, (f) successfully undergo written and oral knowledge and competency examination leading to certification by the American Board of Surgery, (g) complete a further residency in thoracic surgery, and finally (h) successfully undergo written and oral knowledge and competency examination leading to certification by the American

Board of Thoracic Surgery. (The reader who wishes to trace this arduous pathway can begin a sojourn at the home page of the American Board of Medical Specialties, accessible through the Internet at www.abms.org.) After that final certification, and in order to maintain licensure as a physician as well as dual certification in general and thoracic surgery, one engages continuing education requirements of several sorts.

There is nothing quick or easy about that roadway, nor should there be; we should properly be quite cautious about to whom we entrust the opening of our chest cavities. We certainly trust the general medical practitioner to use a stethoscope appropriately to uncover irregular heart rhythms or lung contractions (analogous to neuropsychological screening in our revisionist proto-model), but we would not, on the evidence that he or she uses a stethoscope well, empower him or her to cut open our rib cage.

Why is it that mental health clinicians, physicians (some, but not all, neurologists, neurosurgeons, and neuropsychiatrists excepted), third-party health care payers, and the general public—none of whom has the slightest doubt that thoracic surgery is an advanced medical specialty—have not recognized that clinical neuropsychology is, in close analogy, also an advanced specialty, a late-entry career, that requires not merely licensure to practice psychology but also training and supervised experience that goes well beyond that required for licensure alone?

The American Board of Clinical Neuropsychology (accessible at www.theabcn.org), a constituent of the American Board of Professional Psychology, lists the following among the prerequisites for application for examination leading to its diplomate:

A doctorate in psychology;
State licensure;
Formal course work in basic neuroscience, functional neuroanatomy, neuropathology, clinical neurology, clinical neuropsychological assessment, *in addition to, and typically subsequent to, course work leading to the doctorate in professional psychology;*
Two years of post-doctoral experience in clinical neuropsychology; and/or
Completion of an accredited postdoctoral program in neuropsychology.

Contemplating that litany, one can readily understand that the board declaims, "ABCN board certification in clinical neuropsychology is strictly analogous to medical board specialty certification."

We invite the reader to contrast the requirements indicated as *prerequisites* for further examination of skill, understanding, and competence (both written and oral, and including case presentations) prior to laying legitimate claim to the title *clinical neuropsychologist* with the implicit promises from workshop organizers that instant expertise will follow a 3-day, or sometimes even 3-hour, training session. Or contrast ABCN's prerequisites with the implicit promises made by those test publishers who, mimicking the snake oil salesmen of an earlier era, seem to promise that, if you but buy our instrument(s) and administer it or them to a patient who should be better served, all will be revealed unto you.

Hippocrates, take cover. To be sure, the practice of clinical neuropsychology is not for the faint of heart—and much less for the untrained. A little learning is a dangerous thing.

TREATMENTS OF CHOICE, "BEST PRACTICES," OPTIMAL PRACTICE

As Wolman (1965) observed many moons ago, clinical medicine is the praxiological science par excellence. In contrast to those who decry the "medicalization" of the mental health professions, we retort that the mental health professions have only recently begun to emulate clinical medicine in earnest and, regrettably, are not yet sufficiently medicalized.

For many decades, clinical medicine has used the terms *disorder-specific treatment* and *treatment of choice*. The term disorder-specific treatment is employed to designate those modalities (whether pharmacological agents, surgical procedures, or other interventions or combination of interventions) that have been found *on an empirical basis* to be effective in relieving the symptoms of the disorder in question—at its empirical fundament, to be better than nothing. The empirical base may rest on experimental evidence in which a given treatment is contrasted with no treatment or even on accumulated clinical evidence that remains unchallenged. In contrast, the term *treatment of choice* denotes that *single* therapeutic modality that has been found, on an empirical basis, to be superior to other disorder-specific treatments.

If we use headache as an example, clinical medicine readily agrees that both (a) application of cold compresses to the affected areas of the skull and (b) the ingestion of such medications as aspirin, acetaminophen, and ibuprofen (perhaps enriched or, more technically, chemically potentiated, by the addition of codeine) constitute disorder-specific remedies, whereas manicure and pedicure do not. Were the physician called upon to identify the single treatment of choice, he or she would likely be hard-pressed to go beyond the elimination of ice pack application, yielding a situation in which disorder-specific medication is pronounced the treatment of choice—with, of course, manicure and pedicure as nonstarters. Whether a particular physician treats a particular patient (or even whether a particular patient self-medicates) through one or the other of the three competing pharmacological agents depends in some large measure on that patient's response to particular formularies. And, in the unlikely event that a particular patient proves intolerant (i.e., exhibits an allergic or otherwise paradoxical reaction) to each of the three agents, the physician is surely well justified in regarding the application of cold compresses as the treatment of choice *for that patient*.

Let us now move from the abstract to the real world—and, more particularly, to the real world of managed health care. Suppose the claims examiner for a third-party payer (typically, a recent graduate with a bachelor's degree in something called "risk management," which many interpret as a curriculum in learning how to say no before the question is asked) is called upon to authorize compensation for the provision of medication; a demurrer will be very difficult to justify. But if the same claims examiner is called upon to authorize compensation for the application of ice packs, doubtless the physician will be compelled to explain why a more cumbersome and therefore more costly treatment is deemed clinically necessary. And if the same claims examiner is called upon to authorize manicure, pedicure, or removal of the appendix to remediate a patient's headache, the demurrers are likely to fly with supersonic speed.

Note, please, that we have thus far inquired into neither frequency nor duration, nor, even more fundamentally, into whether headache is itself the disorder or but the outcropping or a more pervasive disorder. Clinical medicine can as readily successfully medicate the recurrent headache symptomatic of brain tumor as the transient headache attributable to interpersonal stress and excessive humidity. But to continue to medicate, or otherwise treat palliatively, the headache resultant from brain tumor without inquiry into its root source is to practice such shoddy clinical medicine as to invite Hippocrates to spin rapidly in the grave he has occupied for 2,400 years.

It has only been within the relatively recent past (and, one suspects, not without prodding from third-party payers in the managed health care industry; some future doctoral dissertation may provide the definitive history) that the mental health professions have begun to think in remotely analogous terms. Indeed, some 40 and more years ago, Robert Callis (1963) trenchantly compared the prototypical mental health professional to the "one-tool mechanic." If you bring your auto to the shop because the windshield wipers are not functioning properly, the one-tool mechanic takes his (back then, it was almost always "his," because equal opportunity for women to enter this noble field lay ahead) screwdriver and adjusts the mechanism that turns the wiper blades; and you drive away, happy as a clam. But if you bring your car to the shop because the left rear tire seems to be losing air, the same mechanic reaches for the same screwdriver—or, in a worst-case scenario, goes on to use that screwdriver to adjust the windshield wiper mechanism in the fixed belief that your left rear tire will thereby become rectified. To be sure, the one-tool mechanic has much in common with those true believers who hew to the conviction that the source of all human troubles is to be attributed to alcohol, money, sexual frustration, neuropathology, or any other pet ideological source. Forty years ago, as Callis intimated, the prototypical mental health professional was likely to describe himself or herself as a psychoanalyst, a nondirective counselor, an existential therapist, a behavior therapist—and not as a clinical scientist who applies the specific techniques of psychoanalysis, nondirective counseling, or existential or behavior therapy as and if appropriate both to the character of the problems (we had not yet come to prefer the euphemism "issues") presented by patients (analogue: headache) *and* in relation to patient characteristics (analogue: allergy to specific medication).

For reasons that are not entirely clear, variant terminology has emerged in the mental health

professions. Rather than adopt clinical medicine's hoary disorder-specific and treatment-of-choice (and, implicitly, irrelevant) distinctions, we have invented the terms *empirically supported treatment* and *empirically validated treatment*, with analogous but not identical meaning. Even more controversially, we have invented the rather ambiguous term *best practices*.

In at least a general sense, there has emerged reasonable empirical support about the effectiveness of specific treatments for specific mental and emotional disorders. The monumental undertaking by a task force of the American Psychiatric Association that resulted in publication of the massive four-volume *Treatments of Psychiatric Disorders* (Karasu, 1989) represented a landmark achievement in the codification of empirical knowledge about effective treatment modalities geared to disorders categorized according to the principal groups represented in the *Diagnostic and Statistical Manual of Mental Disorders*, with (admittedly as a secondary concern) some attention to patient characteristics (e.g., treatment of organic mental disorder in patients with liver disease versus lung disease). It is a fair assessment to say that the task force concentrated, in its pioneering effort, on identifying disorder-specific treatments, with but an occasional foray into assessment of treatments of choice. However, the third edition of that work (Gabbard, 2001), in two volumes that print to more than 3,100 pages, adopts as its focus no less than the identification and description of "optimal treatments" geared to the major *DSM-IV-TR* categories. Because these works are intended primarily for psychiatrists and other physicians, we are not surprised that there is relatively heavy emphasis on pharmacology and other medical interventions.

Although medical-pharmacological treatments are not ignored, psychosocial interventions predominate in Nathan and Gorman's *A Guide to Treatments That Work* (1998, 2002) and in Nathan, Gorman, and Salkind's (1999) companion volume, *Treating Mental Disorders: A Guide to What Works*. The latest edition of the "mother" work contains 26 chapters by leading figures in the treatment of a variety of disorders, ranging from substance abuse to compulsion to anorexia to sexual dysfunction. The companion volume is arranged in such fashion as to be optimally accessible to the mental health professional in the trenches—and in some reviews has been (wrongheadedly) faulted for its ease of use.

These works collectively have made important contributions to the knowledge base of empirically supported or empirically validated treatments, but there is far less unanimity about what constitutes "best practice," and not without good reason. To return to headache for a moment: In the real world, the patient is not limited to a single treatment modality—that is to say, he or she can readily opt to reach for *both* an aspirin *and* an ice bag and perhaps even switch the radio to mood music or whatever else he or she finds generally soothing. If it be the case that such a *combination* of disorder-specific treatments (and self-directed environmental manipulation) dependably (and thus empirically demonstrably, in a large cadre of patients) relieves the transient headache more rapidly than any single treatment acting alone, is not that combination definitive of "best practice"? Yet and still: Does it make a difference as to whether the patient applies the ice pack or takes the aspirin or tunes the radio first—that is to say, does the *sequence* in which disorder-specific treatments of choice are applied affect outcome? That is a ponderable question, and it is easy enough to construe the responsive research design.

We know, or think we know, some things about what works in the rehabilitation of people addicted to alcohol. In descending order (measured in proportion of cases showing sustained improvement over time), these "treatments" have proved effective: active participation in the programs of Alcoholics Anonymous (AA) for a period of at least 12 months; medication by means of antidepressants; and individual counseling or psychotherapy. This order provides the basis for proposing to a particular patient the *single* modality that is most likely to prove effective. But we do not live in an *either-or* world. If participation in AA and use of antidepressive medication is each likely to extirpate or reduce alcohol consumption, why not the two in tandem? And so on, as we add individual counseling to the mix, rather in close analogue to our headache sufferer who takes an aspirin, grabs an ice bag, and finds soothing music. Once again, we have ponderable questions. To answer those questions on an experimental basis, we need a rather large subject pool composed of "otherwise similar" alcoholics who resemble each other closely in age, socioeconomic status, level of education, onset of first use of alcohol, pattern of alcohol consumption in terms of typical dosage and frequency, and so forth; self-labeling by the patient ("I'm an alcoholic") simply will not do. From that pool, we need to extract eight subgroups, to which subjects are to be randomly assigned:

A control group, from whom we will withhold any treatment whatever—and who we will prevent from undertaking any sort of self-directed change in behavior (and good luck to us in that endeavor);

Group AA, who will participate in AA but not be placed on medication nor receive individual counseling;

Group MED, who will be placed on medication but will neither participate in AA nor receive individual counseling;

Group COUNS, who will receive individual counseling but will neither participate in AA nor be placed on medication;

Group AA+MED, who will both participate in AA and be placed on medication but will not receive individual counseling;

Group AA+COUNS, who will both participate in AA and receive individual counseling but not be placed on medication;

Group MED+COUNS, who will both be placed on medication and receive individual counseling; and

Group AA+MED+COUNS (a/k/a the "whole ball of wax" group), who will participate in AA, be placed on medication, and receive individual counseling.

Construction of those experimental groups masks all sorts of issues, ranging from real-world concerns to ethical conundrums. Among the real-world concerns is the resistance of many active AA participants to the use of psychoactive (or even potentially psychoactive) mood-altering substances of any sort—indeed, to the extent that aspirin enriched by codeine is avoided. Another is the sequence in which conjoint treatments are engaged; for example, it is not uncommon that participation in AA follows, and results from, individual counseling, but the obverse sequence is not altogether unknown. And our hypothetical investigation is fraught with all manner of ethical quandaries. If each of the three treatment modalities has been shown to be effective, what ethical justification can we offer for *withholding* effective treatment by assigning would-be patients to any experimental group save the last, or, more perversely, to that untreated control group that is an absolute necessity if we are to demonstrate that any one of the treatments considered by itself, let alone in various combinations, is superior to the mere passage of time? Is random matching of patient and treatment modality or modalities not precisely contrary to clinical goals? What salve do we use for our consciences should it come to pass that a member of that control group dies of a cirrhotic liver during the course of our investigation?

Even presuming that we can in one way or another overcome these issues, the characteristics of the subject pool from which we have drawn the members of each of our experimental (and control) groups constitute boundaries that severely limit the generalizability of our results. If our subject pool consists of blue-collar workers aged 30 to 35 who have been court-referred to treatment as a result of arrest for driving while intoxicated, on what basis do we generalize to white-collar workers aged over 65 who have been advised to seek treatment as a result of renal impairment? Still, if it turns out that, say, AA+MED produces superior results for subjects drawn randomly from a pool of blue-collar workers, we may have empirically identified what constitutes "best practice" in alcoholism rehabilitation *for this group*. That is surely better than nothing, but it represents an insufficient empirical basis on which to identify "best practice" or even a series of "best practice" permutations for alcoholics in general.

Of course, the bleakness of that overwrought account must be tempered by the sophisticated statistical tweaking involved in meta-analysis, whereby data from a number of studies across a spectrum of subjects (who really are not comparable to each other, but that limitation on generalizability is rarely recognized) are amalgamated so that "mean effect sizes" can be teased together. Since the technique was invented in an effort literally to demonstrate that psychotherapeutic treatment of some sort (any sort?) is better than nothing (Smith & Glass, 1977; Smith, Glass, & Miller, 1980), an extraordinarily large number of meta-analyses have appeared in the mental health professions—indeed, in the view of some commentators, with something like reckless abandon driven by the impulse to magnify small differences. That situation is in some contrast to clinical medicine, where one encounters meta-analyses with but sparing frequency

(Bailar, 1997; Kassirer, 1992). Perhaps clinical medicine has moved beyond the compulsion to tweak out mean effect sizes that demonstrate, say, that surgical removal represents the treatment of choice when confronted with a ruptured appendix.

Or perhaps it is the case that the mental health professions need *either* to admit that we have unfurled the banner that promises to identify best practices somewhat prematurely *or* to redefine the notion of best practices more modestly. In the main, the mental health professions have been able to demonstrate (a) that this or that treatment for this or that condition in this or that patient population is probably more efficacious than doing nothing (albeit most often measured in the crude pre- and posttreatment fashion for which we are so often excoriated by statistical purists) and (b) that this or that treatment for the same condition seems totally irrelevant. Those are no mean accomplishments, particularly when we understand that clinical medicine has had a head start of something like 2,300 years. But the present state of knowledge should compel us to admit that our notions of "best practice" are only in part empirically driven; in other parts, they are clinically driven, theory driven, and, if truth be told, aspirationally driven. Nor should we feel compelled to apologize for that state of affairs.

We have presented in this chapter what we have labeled an "optimal practice" proto-model for clinical neuropsychology. Its distinctive features are that it insists (indeed, consistent with customary standards for current mental status examination) that probing for "soft signs" of neuropsychological dysfunction should be a routine feature of any intake or psychosocial history interview in any mental health or social service installation; that if such probes are positive, a neuropsychological screening should be undertaken by a competent psychologist; that if results of such screening are positive, a comprehensive neurological examination should be conducted, including neuroimaging if indicated; that if results of such comprehensive neurological examination are positive, a comprehensive neuropsychological examination should be conducted to identify the cognitive, emotional, and behavioral consequences of medically verified neuropathology that are remediable through psychosocial treatment modalities. That proto-model is only in part empirically driven (some neuropsychological instruments are demonstrably more adept at identifying the consequences of one or another form of neuropathology than others), in part clinically driven, in part theory driven, in part driven by recognition of the real-world reality that advances in neuroimaging of the last three decades have so transformed clinical neurology—indeed, from an "approximate" to an "exact" clinical science—as to render interprofessional rivalry counterproductive and potentially harmful to patients; and in part driven by pious hope that tomorrow will be not only another, but a better, day.

SUMMARY

This chapter has presented a "revisionist," although not entirely revolutionary, view of clinical neuropsychology in optimal practice situations in the age of neuroimaging technologies, with particular focus on assessment of cognitive, emotional, and behavioral consequences of medically verified neuropathology. As a cautionary tale, we have sketched a case study replete with a sufficient panoply of interactively impinging variables to entice into misattritubution and misdiagnosis virtually any mental health clinician with an even mildly reductionist turn of mind. Indeed, in rendering that tale, we have had the temerity to suggest that it is all too easy for reductionists of one stripe to attribute to neuropathology real-life problems that have patently preexisted neurological injury. Not quite in passing, we have urged both clinical neuropsychologists and other mental health clinicians to abandon interprofessional rivalry with neurology and psychiatry and especially with clinical neurology and clinical neuropsychiatry. Further, we have described the training and experience required to lay claim to the title clinical neuropsychologist in optimal practice and have urged mental health clinicians (including doctoral-level psychologists without formal training and experience in neuropsychology) to belay misrepresenting their competence. Finally, we have limned whether the current state of knowledge in the mental health professions justifies the use of terms like *best practices*.

Notes

1. These topics are covered in detail in Daugherty and Rauch's (2001) volume on psychiatric neuroimaging and in Frackowiak's (2001) paper on the func-

tional architecture of the brain. Kosslyn's (1995) *Image and Brain* is also highly instructive, and works by Stuss and Knight (2002) and Miller and Cummings (1999) on frontal lobe functions are particularly useful. Several chapters in the American Psychiatric Association's 1,400-page semiofficial *Textbook of Neuropsychiatry and Clinical Neurosciences* (Yudofsky & Hales, 2002) are relevant and well illustrated. Those who prefer the computer screen to the printed page may wish to visit www.braininjury.com, a Web site organized by an attorney but containing links to a neurologist and a rehabilitation specialist, that nonetheless offers a glossary that defines and illustrates the more frequent neuroimaging modalities. Another useful Web site is maintained, at www.biausa.org, by the Brain Injury Association of America, an organization located in a Washington suburb that advocates and lobbies on behalf of the brain injured.

2. Beatty's (2001) masterful book *The Human Brain* is an up-to-date compendium of information about localization of function that also reviews remedial regimens and, not incidentally, contains handsome illustrations that portray routes followed through the brain by the more powerful neurohormones. *Neuropsychiatry and Behavioral Neuroscience* (Cummings & Mega, 2002) is highly informative, particularly for readers with some background in neurochemistry.

3. With the benefit of hindsight, we might add that some experts now believe that functions once performed by brain cells that have been permanently damaged can, through neuropsychological rehabilitation, be "relearned" by other, intact cells (Eslinger, 2002); "neuronal plasticity," considered a radical and unsupported notion as recently as 1990, has now entered the mainstream (Beatty, 2001). In addition, neurosurgeons have experimented with ways of relieving edema through microscopic surgery. Without question, the pioneers in neurocognitive rehabilitation have been Bracy (1983, 1997) and Reitan and Wolfson (1988, 1992b).

4. The *Mental Measurements Yearbook*, first organized by Oscar Buros at Rutgers University in 1933 and now published by the Buros Institute of Mental Measurement at the University of Nebraska at Lincoln (Plake & Impara, 2001), has become the encyclopedic resource for information on psychometric instruments, occupying in relation to psychological testing the same position the *Physician's Desk Reference* occupies in relation to pharmacotherapy. In cooperation with the federally supported Educational Resources Information Center Clearinghouse on Assessment and Evaluation at the University of Maryland, the Educational Testing Service (publisher of the SAT, GRE, etc.), Pro-Ed (which publishes educational tests), and George Washington University, the Buros Institute makes available to users information concerning 10,000 psychological tests at www.Ericae.net. In addition, the home page for the Association of Test Pub-

lishers can be accessed via the Internet at www.
testpublishers.org. From there, the user can further
gain access to information about virtually any psychometric instrument currently in print, albeit the
presentation will have something of a "sales pitch"
tinge. In forensic neuropsychology, the critical synopses of an array of widely used instruments provided
by Valciukas (1995) as Appendix A in his landmark
book is particularly useful, especially in the context of
recent U.S. Supreme Court rulings about the evidentiary value of "junk science."

References

Bailar, J. (1997). The promise and problems of meta-
analysis. *New England Journal of Medicine, 337,*
559–561.

Beatty, J. (2001). *The human brain: Essentials of behavioral neuroscience.* Thousand Oaks, CA:
Sage.

Bracy, O. (1983). Computer based cognitive rehabilitation. *Journal of Cognitive Rehabilitation, 1,* 1,
3–12.

Bracy, O. (1997). Teaching daily living skills to severely brain impaired individuals. *Journal of
Cognitive Rehabilitation, 15,* 5, 113–125.

Brown, S., Fann, J., & Grant, I. (1994). Post-
concussional disorder: Time to acknowledge a
common source of neurobehavioral morbidity.
*Journal of Neuropsychiatry and Clinical Neu-
rosciences, 6,* 1, 15–22.

Callis, R. (1963). Counseling. *Review of Educational
Research, 33,* 3, 179–187.

Cummings, J., & Mega, M. (2002). *Neuropsychiatry
and behavioral neuroscience.* New York: Oxford
University Press.

Daugherty, D., & Rauch, S. (2001). *Psychiatric neuroimaging research: Contemporary strategies.*
Washington, DC: American Psychiatric Press.

Eslinger, P. (2002). *Neuropsychological interventions:
Clinical research and practice.* New York: Guilford.

Frackowiak, R. (2001). The functional architecture of
the brain. In G. Edelman & J. Changeux (Eds.),
The brain (pp. 105–130). New Brunswick, NJ:
Transaction.

Gabbard, G. (2001). *Treatments of psychiatric disorders* (3rd ed., Vols. 1–2). Washington, DC:
American Psychiatric Press.

Gilandas, A., Touyz, S., Beumont, P., & Greenberg,
H. (1984). *Handbook of neuropsychological assessment.* New York: Grune and Stratton.

Golden, C. (Ed.). (2000). *LNNB handbook: Vol. 1. A
guide to clinical interpretation and use in special
settings.* Los Angeles: Western Psychological
Services.

Golden, C. (2002). *Stroop Color and Word Test 2002.*
Wood Dale, IL: Stoelting Scientific.

Golden, C., Moses, J., Coffman, J., Miller, W., &

Strider, F. (1983). *Clinical neuropsychology: Interface with neurologic and psychiatric disorders.*
New York: Grune and Stratton.

Golden, C., Purisch, A., & Hammeke, T. (1992). *The
Luria-Nebraska neuropsychological test battery.*
Los Angeles: Western Psychological Services.

Hales, R., & Yudofsky, S. (Eds.). (2002). *The American Psychiatric Press textbook of clinical psychiatry.* Washington, DC: American Psychiatric
Press.

Karasu, T. (Ed.). (1989). *Treatments of psychiatric disorders* (Vols. 1–4). Washington, DC: American
Psychiatric Press.

Kassirer, J. (1992). Clinical trials and meta-analysis:
What do they do for us? *New England Journal
of Medicine, 327,* 273–274.

Kaufman, A., & Kaufman, N. (1994). *Kaufman Short
Neuropsychological Assessment Procedure
(K-SNAP).* Circle Pines, MN: American Guid-
ance Service.

Kosslyn, S. (1995). *Image and brain.* Cambridge, MA:
Bradford Books/MIT Press.

Lacks, P. (1984). *Bender-Gestalt screening for brain
dysfunction.* New York: Wiley.

Lezak, M. (1995). *Neuropsychological assessment* (3rd
ed.). New York: Oxford University Press.

Marino, M. (1999). CDC report shows prevalence of
brain injury. *TBI Challenge, 3,* 3, 1, 13.

Miller, B., & Cummings, J. (1999). *The human frontal
lobes.* New York: Guilford.

Nathan, P., & Gorman, J. (Eds.). (1998). *A guide to
treatments that work.* New York: Oxford University Press.

Nathan, P., & Gorman, J. (Eds.). (2002). *A guide to
treatments that work,* 2nd ed.). New York: Oxford University Press.

Nathan, P., Gorman, J., & Salkind, N. (1999). *Treating
mental disorders: A guide to what works.* New
York: Oxford University Press.

Pallone, N., & Hennessy, J. (1996). *Tinder-box criminal aggression: Neuropsychology, demography,
phenomenology.* New Brunswick, NJ: Transaction.

Plake, B., & Impara, J. (Eds.). (2001). *Mental measurements yearbook.* Lincoln: University of Nebraska Press

Psychological Corporation. (2003). *Catalog for psychological assessment products.* San Antonio,
TX: Author.

Reitan, R., & Wolfson, D. (1988). The Halstead-Reitan
Neuropsychological Test Battery and REHABIT:
A model for integrating evaluation and treatment
of cognitive impairment. *Cognitive Rehabilitation, 6,* 10–17.

Reitan, R., & Wolfson, D. (1992a). *The Halstead-
Reitan neuropsychological test battery: Theory
and clinical interpretation.* Tucson, AZ: Neuropsychology Press.

Reitan, R., & Wolfson, D. (1992b). *Neuropsycholog-*

ical evaluation of older children. Tucson, AZ: Neuropsychology Press.

Silver, J., Yudofsky, S., & Hales, R. (1987). Neuropsychiatric aspects of traumatic brain injury. In R. Hales & S. Yudofsky (Eds.), *American Psychiatric Press textbook of neuropsychiatry* (p. 179–190). Washington, DC: American Psychiatric Press.

Silver, J., Yudofsky, S., & Hales, R. (2002). Neuropsychiatric aspects of traumatic brain injury. In S. Yudofsky & R. Hales (Eds.), *American Psychiatric Press textbook of neuropsychiatry* (4th ed., pp. 625–672). Washington, DC: American Psychiatric Press.

Smith, M., & Glass, G. (1977). Meta-analysis of psychotherapy outcome studies. *American Psychologist, 32* 752–760.

Smith, M., Glass, G., & Miller, T. (1980). *The benefits of psychotherapy.* Baltimore: Johns Hopkins University Press.

Sohlberg, M., & Mateer, C. (2001). *Cognitive rehabilitation: An integrative neuropsychological approach.* New York: Guilford.

Stuss, D., & Knight, (Eds.). (2002). *Principles of frontal lobe function.* New York: Oxford University Press.

Valciukas, J. (1995). *Forensic neuropsychology: Conceptual foundations and clinical practice.* New York: Haworth Press.

Wolman, B. (1965). *Handbook of clinical psychology.* New York: McGraw-Hill.

Yudofsky, S., & Hales, R. (Eds.). (2002). *American Psychiatric Press textbook of neuropsychiatry and clinical neurosciences* (4th ed.). Washington, DC: American Psychiatric Press.

60   DEVELOPMENT OF THE FATHERHOOD SCALE

Gary L. Dick

Fatherhood is evolving, and how a man is expected to act as a father has changed dramatically over time (Cabrera, Tamis-Lemonda, Bradley, Hofferth, & Lamb, 2000; Frank, 1998; Griswold, 1993; Lamb, 2000). Historically, in the broadest and most generalized conceptualization of fatherhood, the role of the father has evolved from the moral and stern patriarch of colonial days to the playful, nurturing, and involved father of today (Pleck & Pleck, 1997). However, these broad conceptualizations of fatherhood fail to take into consideration the various types of father involvement, which are influenced by ethnicity, race, geographic region, economics, and culture. Fathers play out different roles in different social contexts, and what constitutes the good father varies greatly between cultures (Lamb, 1997). In addition to refining ideal conceptualizations of the father role, it is also important to examine negative paternal involvement. Not all fathers today are good providers; some are cold, distant, abusive, and emotionally detached from their children. The paternal bond a father has with his child and the child's perception of the father's emotional availability, especially with adults, has long been overlooked as an aspect of fatherhood.

In recent years, there has been a growing interest in the patterns of fatherhood, which has led to an increase in the development of programs and services for fathers (Fagan, 2002). There is a proliferation of these new programs that emphasize responsible fatherhood, all influenced by a growing body of research that indicates a significant relationship between positive paternal involvement and children's cognitive, emotional, and social development (Lamb, 2000; Parke, 2000). Despite the increased interest in fatherhood, social work professionals up to this point have lacked a conceptual model that helps explain the importance of the father's emotional relationship to his children and an instrument to measure the paternal bond. This chapter presents the subscale Positive Paternal Emotional Responsiveness (PPER), from the Fatherhood Scale (see Dick, in press), to measure the paternal bond adults had with their fathers during their own formative years.

The early relationships adults had with their fathers often surface later as issues during the course of therapy with social workers. Social workers commonly encounter adult clients in direct clinical practice who have unresolved or ambiguous feelings about their relationships with their fathers. In using the PPER scale, social workers are able to help clients engage in discourse about these relationships and assist them in interpreting their experiences. Thus, meaning is given to the emotional relationship, which brings about an understanding of the extent of the paternal bond.

FATHERHOOD AND SOCIAL WORK PRACTICE

Despite the fact that adults' relationships with their fathers are often a central issue in therapy, fatherhood has long been an overlooked aspect of social work practice and research. There has been a paucity of literature in the social work journals on fatherhood, and until recently the field has lacked an instrument to measure adults' perceptions of their relationships with their fathers (Dick, in press). The keywords *father, fatherhood,* and/or *paternal* were used in an electronic search of the literature in social work abstracts from January 1998 through January 2003. Only 51 articles were found that mention one of these words in the abstract, and 47 articles included one of the words in the title. The two most frequent themes in the articles dealt with fathers and divorce (8 out of 47) and new fathers (6 out of 47).

Fathers enact multiple roles in carrying out their responsibilities to their children, and yet father identity often competes with other salient aspects of how men define themselves, such as self-definitions based upon the type of work a father performs ("I am a carpenter") or negative self-attributes based upon failings and shortcomings ("I am an unemployed, irresponsible alcoholic"). A father is cast in the good provider role, the gender role model, the moral father role, and the nurturer (Pleck & Pleck, 1997). Lamb (1997) conceptualized three main components of fatherhood: (a) the degree to which fathers engage in activities with their children; (b) how accessible they are to their children; and (c) and the level of responsibility a father displays to his children. More recently, in an attempt to broaden how scholars conceptualize father involvement, the Inventory of Father Involvement (IVF) was developed to include the father's support of the mother (Hawkins et al., 2002). While these frameworks provide social workers with conceptual models of paternal involvement, fatherhood is also unique in that it is socially constructed, culturally influenced, and individual in nature (Marsiglio, 1995; Park, 2000). One of the least understood aspects of fatherhood has been the degree to which adults felt an emotional bond with their fathers during their formative years.

IMPORTANCE OF THE PATERNAL EMOTIONAL RELATIONSHIP

It is important for social workers to understand the extent to which their clients' fathers were emotionally available to them. Fatherhood is multidimensional and dynamic. The childhood relationships adults had with their fathers may have shifted and changed as the father enacted various roles and responded to environmental circumstances. Fathers have been described as distant breadwinners (Pleck & Pleck, 1997), and in some cultures fathers have viewed their role as the good providers as more important than their emotional relationships with their children, often leaving that to the mother. The type of relationship a father had with his child and with the child's mother both directly and indirectly affects the child.

Rohner and Veneziano (2001), in their analysis of approximately 100 studies on parent-child relationships, found that children's perceptions of their father's acceptance or rejection and affection or indifference were as important as their mothers' love in predicting the social, emotional, and cognitive development of children and young adults. Others studies have found a relationship between father nurturance and self-esteem in adolescents (Buri, Kirchner, & Walsh, 1987; Buri, Murphy, Richtsmeier, & Komar, 1992). Fathers play a significant role in the emotional lives of their children. Men who grew up with fathers who were emotionally unavailable remember a lack of warmth in the relationship and, as such, now struggle with their own internal feelings of humiliation, vulnerability, and inadequacy (Dutton, 1998). In studying abusive men, Dutton (1998) found that the relationship with the father was a major contributing factor in the development of the abusive personality. Men who became abusive in intimate relationships had memories of their own fathers as cold, rejecting, and abusive. Rejection and emotional indifference by the father attack the core sense of self, leaving the adult child filled with feelings of shame, inferiority, and inadequacy.

The lack of paternal involvement in a child's life not only directly affects the child but also influences the mother's emotional state. Subsequently, this may reduce her emotional availability to her children (Jackson, 1999). The nonresident father's absence from the child's life, his infrequent contact with his child, and the mother's dissatisfaction with the amount of time, love, and money were found to be related to maternal depression in single African American mothers (Jackson, 1999). It is possible that for these women, a failed relationship with the child's father and his lack of empathic responses to support her emotionally reduce that sense of belonging to another. They may also exacerbate the sense of diminishing control she has over her own life and reactivate her own childhood experiences with paternal emotional failures.

SELF-PSYCHOLOGICAL THEORY

Children benefit from an emotionally responsive, empathic, and understanding father. Fathers provide important psychological functions that support the inner emotional life of their children. Self-psychology (Kohut, 1977) provides a theoretical framework for understanding the pathway for the development of a healthy bond between a father and his children. According to self-psychology, children require an empathic relationship with an emotionally responsive parent. The emotional attunement of the parent toward the child serves important psychological functions that contribute to the development of an internal self-structure in the child. Kohut (1977) believed that human beings need a certain kind of object relationship with a person whom they experience as an undifferentiated psychological part of the self. Kohut coined the term *selfobject* to represent the individual's subjective aspect of this important psychological relationship. Selfobjects are not the person, or the self of the other person, but they are the child's *subjective experience of the relationship* (italics added) (Bacal, 1995). When the father becomes a selfobject, he in essence becomes a critical component in the development of the child's sense of self.

Empathy is central to self-psychology, and parental empathic responses are what Kohut described as *selfobject functions*. The self is dependent upon the caretakers in the child's environment (and, in this case, the father) being able to continually provide certain psychological responses that support the emerging sense of self in the child. These selfobjects functions are (a) mirroring, (b) idealizing, and (c) twinship. *Mirroring* is the need to be admired, recognized, affirmed, accepted, and appreciated by a loving, emotionally responsive parent who responds to the child's innate sense of vigor, greatness, and perfection. *Idealizing* is the need to be part of, or linked to, an admired, calm, and respected other (Bacal, 1992), whereas *twinship* is the need to experience alikeness with a stable, wise, and calm idealized other. Psychologically speaking, the child needs to feel linked to a father he or she admires, who is stable, calm, wise, and emotionally present.

Self-psychology views empathy as a central process in the development of a healthy sense of self. The emotional responsiveness of the father and his ability to provide concern, warmth, compassion and understanding serve to support the development of a *cohesive sense of self* in his child. When a father is able to emotionally respond to his child by reducing his or her tension in a calm and soothing manner, these functions not only become an internalized part of the child's self-structure (Brandell, 2002) but also strengthen the paternal bond.

STEPS TAKEN IN DEVELOPMENT OF THE FATHERHOOD SCALE

The process of developing an instrument to measure fatherhood consisted of the following steps.

- Review of the research on fatherhood
- Review of theoretical perspectives on the role of the father
- Selecting self-psychological theory as a central framework for understanding the importance of the emotional relationship a father has with his children
- Review existing instruments measuring fatherhood
- Conceptualization of the ways fathers engage with their children and how they connect emotionally
- Constructing the scale (item development)
- Revision and refinement of subscales
- Analysis of the scale to test reliability and validity: expert review, factor analysis, and pilot testing the scale
- Revision (reducing the items in the scale)
- Second validation of the scale

THE FATHERHOOD SCALE

The Fatherhood Scale (FS; Dick, in press) measures perceptions of the types of relationships adults had with their fathers during their formative years. The FS was validated on 311 adult men whose mean age of the respondents was 34 years ($SD = 10.5$). The subjects used to validate the FS were mainly White (76%), with a mean income of $54,443 ($SD = $40,592). The majority (66%) reported that they had always lived with their fathers during childhood and adolescence. Forty percent of the participants had a college degree or higher, and 35% of their fathers had attained a college degree or a graduate degree.

A Cronbach's alpha coefficient of .98 was obtained for the FS. The FS has nine subscales that measure positive and negative paternal engagement, fatherhood roles, and paternal emotional responsiveness. Alpha levels on each subscale range from .80 to .96, and seven subscales had interitem correlatations above .85. Multiple items that measure the same construct are expected to be internally consistent, that is, to

measure the same phenomena (Pedhazur & Schmelkin, 1991). An instrument's reliability is represented through reliability coefficients that range from 0 to 1.0. In the development of an instrument, to measure or assess data on a client, it is important to make a decision about the acceptability of the magnitude of the reliability coefficient. Two important factors to consider are the decisions that will be made based on the scores, and the consequences of those decisions (Pedhazur & Schmelkin, 1991). In the early stages of construct validation it is acceptable for instruments to have modest reliabilities, such as .70 (Nunnally & Bernstein, 1994). When comparing groups, a reliability of .80 is adequate, whereas when important decisions regarding test scores (selection and placement) are made about individuals, a reliability of .95 is the desirable standard (Nunnally & Bernstein, 1994). The PPER scale attained an alpha level of .96, indicating that the items are highly interrelated and useful for assessing individual clients.

The FS measures four domains: (a) actual events that occurred with the father ("My father helped me with homework"); (b) subjects' perceptions of their fathers ("My father is mean"); (c) how subjects felt about their fathers ("I have warm feelings toward my father"); and (d) the emotional responsiveness of the father ("My father comforted me when I was feeling bad"), as perceived by the individual completing the instrument. The 13-item scale, PPER measures perceptions of emotional responsiveness, providing a measure of the paternal bond with the father, based upon the subjective experience of the adult child. Each item is ranked on a 5-point scale, ranging from 1 (never) to 5 (always). Higher numbers indicate positive paternal involvement.

POSITIVE PATERNAL EMOTIONAL RESPONSIVENESS SCALE

Positive Paternal Emotional Responsiveness measures the individual's perception of the emotional availability of his or her father and the degree to which the individual feels attached, emotionally close, and bonded to the father (see Table 60.1). This scale is for use with adults and measures the subjective experience of their relationships with their fathers. Theoretically, it is based upon the concepts of self-psychology.

TABLE 60.1 Positive Paternal Emotional Responsiveness Scale

Directions: Think about your emotional relationship with your father during your childhood and adolescence. Thinking about that person, answer each question by placing a number between 1 and 5 on the line before each question that most accurately reflects your perceptions of the emotional bond you had with your father or the person you identify as your father while you were growing up.

1 = Never
2 = Rarely
3 = Sometimes
4 = Often
5 = Always

1. ____ My father told me that I was a good boy/girl

2. ____ My father is a caring person

3. ____ During my childhood I felt close to my father

4. ____ I felt close to my father as a teenager

5. ____ I know my father cared about me

6. ____ My father comforted me when I was feeling bad

7. ____ My father made me feel special

8. ____ My father was loving toward me

9. ____ I have warm feelings for my father

10. ____ My father understood me

11. ____ I told my father I loved him

12. ____ My father praised me

13. ____ My father showed concern when I got hurt

ADMINSTRATION AND SCORING

Applicable Populations

The FS is usable with adult clients. The vocabulary and sentence structure are simple to make it applicable to a broad section of the population. The PPER scale is based on the loving, nurturing father role and represents a type of fatherhood more likely associated with a contemporary fatherhood ideal. In addition, the scale is useful for many ethnic groups, since it readily allows the client to elaborate on the cultural and ethnic similarities and differences in their experiences

in relation to the items on the scale. (For further information on fatherhood, refer to Fagan [2002].)

Referent Time Period

The scale has a retroflective design and measures an individual's subjective internal experience of his or her relationship with his or her father. Social workers should be less concerned with the number of times a client was praised by the father and more interested in the client's perceptions of the relationship, as well as the degree to which a client feels a bond with the father. The instructions on the scale ask about the emotional relationship during childhood and adolescence, which encompass a period of approximately 20 years. Adaptations may have to be made to take into consideration changes that affected the father's emotional availability, such as divorce, illness, death of the mother, and other stressors, including depression and/or drug and alcohol abuse. For example, a client at age 15 whose father goes though drug and alcohol treatment may experience very different emotional relationships with the father at different stages (or each stage) of the treatment. The client could be asked to complete the scale twice: the first time to evaluate the father-son relationship prior to treatment (or another significant event) and the other following treatment. The responses would then be discussed within follow-up therapy sessions.

Referent Event

There may be indications for using the scale based on a significant event in a client's life in addition to a global measure of the paternal bond. As a young individual goes through life, he or she may encounter multiple stressful situations and crisis events in which the emotional availability of the father is needed. The father's positive emotional responsiveness may be a major supportive factor leading to a new level of growth. If instead the father is distant and indifferent, this kind of response may leave the child feeling more vulnerable and alone, less cohesive, and detached from the father. Examples of crisis events in the life of an individual may include teenage pregnancy, trouble with the law, school failure, suicide, death of the mother, divorce of parents, sexual identity issues such as coming out, drug or alcohol abuse, or other situational stressful events.

Scoring

The rating responses are the same for both males and females. Each item is ranked on a 5-point scale, ranging from 1 (never) to 5 (always). The scores range from 13 to 65, with higher scores indicating a stronger bond and a more positive emotional relationship. Scores between 52 and 65 represent a strong paternal bond, where a consistently emotionally available father praised the child and was internalized as warm, loving, concerned, caring, and comforting. Lower scores represent a lack of a paternal bond or a form of paternal emotional deprivation. Scores between the range of 13 and 26 indicate an indifferent and emotionally distant father who provided minimal empathy and little, if any, attempt to understand and comfort his child. This represents a father who never or rarely praised his children, possibly leaving them feeling paternally emotionally abandoned. Scores within the middle range, between 27 and 51, represent a father who was occasionally experienced as caring, loving, and supportive. It may be useful for clients who report within the middle range to explore other environmental demands that may have been placed upon the father. For some clients, *father hunger* may be assessed, as they may report on what they desire emotionally from their fathers rather than on how they really feel.

Assessment

The scale measures the paternal bond adults had with their fathers in four domains: (a) specific emotionally responsive behaviors demonstrated by the father; (b) the adult's perception of his or her relationship with the father; (c) his or her feelings toward the father; and (d) his or her internalized relationship with the father. Although the relationship with the father is often discussed in the course of treatment, this scale provides a measure of the paternal bond and serves as a focus for deeper discussion. Other areas for assessment include the following:

- Level of paternal deprivation.
- Strengths in the paternal relationship.
- Father hunger, the longing for an emotional bond with the father.

- For men, the degree to which their relationships with their fathers served as a role model for their own fathering; for women, the degree to which their fathers served as a model for what they expect from the fathers of their children.

TREATMENT IMPLICATIONS

- Measure the paternal bond and question directly about the extent of the emotional relationship to bring the father issue into conscious awareness.
- Assist clients in verbalizing their relationship with their fathers (the intensity of the love and closeness, or the lack of any emotional connection).
- Assist clients in constructing their own perceptions of the paternal bond.
- Explore with clients how they think the relationship with their fathers affect (a) how they feel about themselves; (b) their relationships with significant others; and (c) what they learned from their fathers about work, love, family, education, friends, play, and other issues that may have surfaced in treatment.
- Use empathic approaches to understand clients' subjective experience of the relationship, remain nonjudgmental, and avoid labels. Thus, the social worker supports the social construction of a deeper meaning of a client's relationship with his or her father.
- Ask clients to think of specific meaningful experiences with their fathers and to share those experiences with you.
- Explore ways in which adults can rebuild, maintain, or enhance their relationships with their fathers.
- Amplify the strengths in the paternal relationship.
- For those clients who lack a strong supportive bond with their fathers, help them identify other males who can serve as father role models to provide important emotional relationships.

CONCLUSION

The PPER scale is an instrument that measures the adult client's paternal bond and serves as a stimulus for the social worker and client to engage in deeper dialogue about the paternal relationship. One of the most powerful aspects of the scale is the way in which it brings into the therapy session the client's thoughts and feelings about his or her father. It provides evidence of the client's perceptions of what occurred and the extent to which the father was emotionally responsive. The PPER scale can be used with other practice methods utilized in clinical social work practice. By also incorporating a genogram, social workers can map patterns of paternal emotionality in the family history and/or gather a social history from the client to determine contextual factors that may have been a source of work-family conflict for the father, thus limiting his emotional availability.

Additionally, by using the strengths perceptive, social workers can assist a client in articulating his or her own father bond, or the lack thereof, and identify the strengths in the paternal relationships or, possibly for the very first time, clearly identify the barriers, limitations, and reality of the lack of a positive paternal bond. The discourse that follows the administration of the scale can serve as a bridge from what clients report as the reality of the paternal bond to helping clients construct an emotional meaning of their relationships with their fathers. The use of this assessment instrument and the dialogue that follows can bring an evidence-based approach to treatment.

TEN OF THE MOST USEFUL WEB SITES ON FATHERHOOD

- National Center on Fathers and Families
  http://www.ncoff.gse.upenn.edu/
- National Fatherhood Initiative
  http://www.fatherhood.org/
- National Center for Fathering
  http://www.fathers.com/
- United States Department of Health and Human Services Fatherhood Initiative
  http://fatherhood.hhs.gov/index.shtml
- Center on Father, Family and Public Policy
  http://www.cffpp.org/index.html
- Child Trends
  http://www.childtrends.org/
- National Center for Children in Poverty
  http://www.nccp.org/index.html
- Office of Juvenile Justice and Delinquency Prevention: Report on Teenage Fatherhood and Delinquent Behavior

  http://www.ncjrs.org/html/ojjdp/jjbul2000_1/contents.html
- American Academy of Child and Adolescent Psychiatry
  http://www.fathersworld.com/resources/practice.html
- Children's Defense Fund
  http://www.childrensdefense.org/

References

Bacal, H. (1992). Contributions from self psychology. In R. Klein, H. S. Bernard, & D. L. Singer (Eds.), *Handbook of contemporary group psychotherapy* (pp. 55–85). Madison, CT: International Universities Press.

Bacal, H. A. (1995). The essence of Kohut's work and the progress of self psychology. *Psychoanalytic Dialogues, 5,* 353–366.

Brandell, J. R. (2002). Using self psychology in clinical social work. In A. R. Roberts & G. J. Greene (Eds.), *Social workers' desk reference* (pp. 158–162). New York: Oxford University Press.

Buri, J. R., Kirchner, P. A., & Walsh, J. M. (1987). Familial correlates of self-esteem in young American adults. *Journal of Social Psychology, 127,* 583–588.

Buri, J. R., Murphy, P., Richtsmeier, L. M., & Komar, K. K. (1992). Stability of parental nurturance as a salient predictor of self-esteem. *Psychological Reports, 71,* 535–543.

Cabrera, N. J., Tamis-Lemonda, C. S., Bradley, R. H., Hofferth, S., & Lamb, M. E. (2000). Fatherhood in the twenty-first century. *Child Development, 71,* 127–136.

Dick, G. L. (in press). The fatherhood scale. *Research on Social Work Practice.*

Dutton, D. G. (1998). *The abusive personality: Violence and control in intimate relationships.* New York: Guilford.

Fagan, J. (2002). Fathering programs and community services. In A. R. Roberts & G. J. Greene (Eds.), *Social workers' desk reference* (pp. 563–567). New York: Oxford University Press.

Frank, S. M. (1998). *Life with father: Parenthood and masculinity in the nineteenth-century American North.* Baltimore: John Hopkins University Press.

Griswold, M. (1993). *Fatherhood in America: A history.* New York: Basic Books.

Hawkins, A. J., Bradford, K. P., Palkovitz, R., Christiansen, S. L., Day, R. D., & Call, V. R. (2002). The inventory of father involvement: A pilot study of a new measure of father involvement. *Journal of Men's Studies, 10,* 183–196.

Jackson, A. P. (1999). The effects of nonresident father involvement on single Black mothers and their young children. *Social Work, 44,* 156–166.

Kohut, H. (1977). *The restoration of the self*. New York: International Universities Press.

Lamb, M. E. (Ed.). (1997). *The role of the father in child development* (3rd ed.). New York: Wiley.

Lamb, M. E. (2000). The history of research on father involvement: An overview. *Marriage and Family Review, 29*, 23–42.

Marsiglio, W. (1995). Fatherhood scholarship: An overview and agenda for the future. In W. Marsiglio (Ed.), *Fatherhood: Contemporary theory, research, and social policy* (pp. 1–20). Thousand Oaks, CA: Sage.

Nunnally, J. C., & Bernstein, I. H. (1994). *Psychometric theory* (3rd ed.). New York: McGraw-Hill.

Parke, R. D. (2000). Father involvement: A developmental psychological perspective. *Marriage and Family Review, 29*, 43–58.

Pedhazur, E. J., & Schmelkin, L. P. (1991). *Measurement, design, and analysis: An integrated approach*. Hillsdale, NJ: Erlbaum.

Pleck, E. H., & Pleck, J. H. (1997). Fatherhood ideals in the United States: Historical dimensions. In M. E. Lamb (Ed.), *The role of the father in child development* (pp. 33–48). New York: Wiley.

Rohner, R. P., & Veneziano, R. A. (2001). The importance of father love: History and contemporary evidence. *Review of General Psychology 5*, 382–405.

61

CONSTRUCTING AND VALIDATING A SPECIFIC MULTI-ITEM ASSESSMENT OR EVALUATION TOOL

Anna C. Faul & Michiel A. van Zyl

In the wake of the accountability era, evidence-based practice has been adopted in the social welfare field. Evidence-based practice aims to develop best-practice methods for social workers that will increase their accountability. The approach requires social workers to put their practice behavior under the control of data, either data that they themselves collect or data that they obtain from the professional literature, and to be skeptical of methods with weak or non-existent empirical support (Dangell, 1994; Bloom & Fischer, 1982).

An integral part of the philosophy of evidence-based practice is the use of methodology to construct and validate multi-item assessment or evaluation tools. Practitioners need to have

adequate tools to accurately assess and monitor change in client functioning. According to Springer, Abell, and Hudson (2002), the fields of measurement and instrument development are still in their adolescence.

In developing an assessment or evaluation tool consisting of multiple items, one or a combination of four different measurement theories can be used. *Classical measurement theory* is often used in the development and initial validation of instruments. *Generalizability theory* helps us to assess the dependability of clinical cutting scores of measurement tools, and *item response theory* provides information on the interplay between samples and measurement error. Sometimes a multiple-choice measure is the preferred option for evaluating an intervention such as a training program, and *theory related to multiple-choice question design* is appropriate. Selecting the appropriate theory to use and understanding the basic assumptions and intent of each theory may be very confusing to the social work practitioner or even researcher.

In the first section of this overview, each of these theories will be discussed and the implications on choice of theory for study design, sampling, methods of analysis, and expected results outlined. The second section contains a more detailed discussion and step-by-step procedures for the validation of a rapid assessment instrument, using classical measurement theory. Classical measurement theory provides a sound foundation for thinking about scale validation. Once methods associated with this theory have been mastered, one can more easily understand other approaches and methodologies.

MEASUREMENT THEORIES AND THEIR APPLICATION

Classical Measurement Theory

Classical measurement theory was developed during the 1920s and is currently the most frequently used theory for instrument development and validation purposes in social work. This theory is based on the true-score model developed by Spearman in 1904, which consists of two theoretical concepts, namely, true scores and error scores (Nurius & Hudson, 1993; Nunnally & Bernstein, 1994). These concepts are theoretical because it is impossible to obtain the absolute true score or the absolute error score for any client. However, it is possible to say that a true score is that which reflects what the client is actually experiencing, and that an error score is the gap between actual experience and what is perceived as that experience. Any observed score (O) is therefore equal to the true score (T) plus the error score (E) and can be presented in the form of the following equation: $O = T + E$ (Nunnally & Bernstein, 1994; Nurius & Hudson, 1993, p. 213).

According to classical theory, reliability is based on the amount of error in an observed score for an individual or a population of individuals. If the amount of error is quite small, the scale developer can claim that he or she has developed a highly reliable measurement tool. If,

however, the amount of error is quite large, the scale developer has developed an unreliable measurement tool (Nurius & Hudson, 1993).

Part of classical measurement theory is the domain-sampling model. According to this model, any particular measure can be composed of responses to a random sample of items from a hypothetical domain of items. The purpose of any particular measurement will be to estimate the measurement that would be obtained if one could employ all the items in the domain. The score a subject would obtain if it were possible to test the whole domain is referred to as the *true score*. A sample of items is reliable to the extent that the score it produces correlates highly with these true scores (Nunnally & Bernstein, 1994). Classical measurement theory is discussed in a more detailed later section that focuses on the construction of a rapid assessment instrument.

Generalizability Theory

Generalizability theory (G-theory) was originally introduced by Cronbach and colleagues (Cronbach, Gleser, Nananda, & Rajaratman, 1972; Cronbach, Nageswari, & Gleser, 1963) in response to limitations of the popular true-score model of classical reliability theory. With G-theory, classical reliability theory is reinterpreted as a theory regarding the adequacy with which one can generalize from a sample of observations to a universe of observations from which it was randomly sampled. G-theory acknowledges that the reliability of an observation depends on the universe about which the investigator wants to draw inferences. Because an assessment instrument may be generalized to many different universes, it may vary in how reliably it permits inferences about these universes. One instrument can therefore be associated with different reliability coefficients. G-theory requires investigators to specify a universe of conditions over which they wish to generalize. When new assessment and evaluation tools are designed, the extent to which different conditions can be associated with different observations needs to be taken into account (Matt, 2001).

In G-theory the set of all possible admissible conditions of measurement is called the *universe of admissible observations*. An infinite set of items constitutes a universe of items that is called a *facet* of measurement. In G-theory any condition of a measurement procedure is a facet. An observed score is used in a single-facet design as an estimate of a universe score to generalize over a universe of measurements called the *universe of generalization*. The theory of measurement error, known in G-theory as the variance of the error δ, focuses upon the errors involved in using an observed score as an estimate of a universe score (Brennan, 1983; Cronbach et al., 1972). Whenever one wants to make relative comparisons of scores, δ is the error variance of concern (Brennan, 1983). The *absolute error variance* $\sigma^2(\Delta)$ is used to make absolute decisions regarding a person, such as how his or her universe score compares with a set standard (Brennan, 1983).

A *decision study* (D-study) is another core concept in G-theory. It refers to a single-facet measurement of a random sample of items from the universe of items being administered to a random sample of persons from a population. Conducting two D-studies offers the advantage of generalizing (a) over all items in the universe of items and over all occasions in the universe of occasions (i.e., over both facets), and (b) over the actual number of items in a measure and over all occasions in the universe of occasions.

The error terms σ(δ) and σ(Δ) and the generalizability coefficients vary depending on the generalizations one wishes to make for different universes of generalization and the universe of generalization desired for a given measurement application. The effect of fixing a facet as a means of standardizing a measurement procedure is that error variances are smaller, and the generalizability coefficients larger, for the restricted universe of generalization (Cronbach et al., 1972). Consequently, the scope of generalization is limited, and there may be a decrease in validity (Kane, 1982). The variance components can be used to determine ways of minimizing the contribution of measurement error brought about by specific conditions of measurement.

G-theory is useful in the development of clinical cutting scores, by considering the 95% confidence intervals for a person's universe, or true, score for different facets and generalizations. G-theory can also be used in "adaptive testing," a concept that will be discussed in a later section, when item responses are nested under persons (Brennan, 1983). Another use for G-theory is when different observers use rating scales to evaluate a series of individuals with re-

spect to multiple attributes. Two observers may disagree with each other because their judgments contain random measurement error or because they respond to different attributes. The more observers differ in what they consider an attribute to be, the less they will be able to generalize their rating to other possible observers (Nunnally & Bernstein, 1994).

Item Response Theory

Item response theory (IRT) is a powerful extension of classical measurement theory. Although IRT developed from classical measurement theory, it is conceptually somewhat different and more complex than classical measurement theory. In fact, classical theory can be seen as a special case of IRT. Classical measurement theory estimates the level of an attribute as the sum of responses to individual items, whereas IRT generally uses the response pattern. IRT is normally used in research where abilities are evaluated (Nunnally & Bernstein, 1994).

When we use classical measurement theory only to develop instruments, we do not know how the instrument performs at different levels of the construct measured. IRT provides the methodology to evaluate important additional characteristics of a measurement tool that classical measurement theory does not provide. IRT provides more detail in describing measurement error, and these descriptions are sample invariant, making wider application of measurement procedures possible and enhancing their use in practice.

A great advantage of IRT for evidence-based practice is that it makes possible "adaptive testing," a procedure that allows items to be administered one at a time to a respondent. Items presented subsequent to the first are dependent on previous responses, thereby decreasing response burden and increasing relevance (Spineti & Hambleton, 1977). IRT also opens the possibility of developing instruments for specific purposes with the advantage of preknowledge of how they will perform (Nugent & Hankins, 1989, p. 469). This can be achieved by selecting items whose parameters are known with confidence to build an instrument with a desired test-information curve.

Unidimensionality—which requires that a scale measure a single construct—is one of the basic assumptions of most current IRT models.

In IRT models, unidimensionality is a sufficient condition for local independence which is the assumption that the probability of an individual responding to an item in a given manner is unaffected by his or her response to other items (this does not mean that items are uncorrelated). A primary assumption of IRT models has to do with a monotonic increasing function of an individual's response to a given item. The probability of an individual responding to a given item in a particular manner is a monotonic increasing function (called the item-response function or item-characteristic curve) only of the individual's level of the trait being measured. It is further assumed that the metric for this trait can be chosen such that the item-characteristics curve for each item is the normal ogive, usually operationalized as the logistic ogive. Finally IRT models assume that items are scored dichotomously by using 1 or 0. The 1 indicates the "presence" of some construct or trait, whereas 0 indicates its "absence."

The item-response function is investigated by means of the logistic-shape of the item-characteristic curves for all items on a scale. If an iterative routine is used, convergence to a solution will indicate that all items on a scale can be represented by logistic curves, and this assumption will appear to be plausible. Local independence and unidimensionality can be investigated by means of procedures used in classical measurement theory such as the factor loading test and factor analysis. The last assumption concerns the scoring of items as either 1 or 0. If all requisite assumptions are met, IRT analysis can proceed.

IRT two-parameter normal and two-parameter logistics models describe the following parameters of item performance: the item-discrimination parameter, referred to as the a value, and the b parameter, which gives the level of trait being measured on a "theta" scale at which the item maximally discriminates among individuals who manifest different traits. These parameters are sample invariant and can be applied to any sample of the same population, but they may or may not be invariant across samples drawn from different populations. The a parameter describes the maximum amount of discrimination between levels of the trait measured that an item can provide, or the maximum slope of the item-characteristic curve. The theta (θ) scale is the metric scaling of the trait measured by the

instrument, usually in terms of standard deviations (SDs) from the mean (i.e., the mean is scaled at 0, with an SD of 1.0). An individual's trait level is estimated from the pattern of responses to the set (an n-element response vector) of items that constitutes the measurement instrument. Maximum-likelihood or Bayesian estimation procedures are used to estimate a person's trait level. The individual's response vector is scaled in the θ metric. The two-parameter logistic model allows use of an optimally weighted scale score to estimate the level of the construct measured.

The item-characteristic curve is obtained by plotting the probability of a person responding to an item with 1 against θ, the different levels of trait being measured. The vertical axis represents the probability of the presence of the trait of responding with a 1, and the horizontal axis represents the θ metric. The probability of θ, or $p(\theta)$, is the person's *true score* on the item; the sum of these scores is the *true test score*. The mathematical form of the two-parameter logistic model illustrates that $p(\theta)$ is a function of θ and an item's a and b values:

$$p(\theta) = \frac{1}{1 + e^{-1.7a(\theta - b)}}$$

The test-characteristic curve is the sum of items' $p(\theta)$ values at each θ level across the items of a measurement instrument. This curve relates the true score on the instrument to the θ metric. The regression of total test score on θ is intimately related to the test-characteristic curve. The test-characteristic curve in IRT is linked to the standard error of measurement in classical measurement theory, but the test information curve provides us with the best or greatest amount of "information" of measurement error.

The concept of "information" supplants reliability in IRT. Information concerns the precision of measurement at different levels. The higher the level of the test information curve, the more precise the measurement and the less error of measurement (and vice versa). Ideally the test information curve should be a relatively straight line across the range of measured levels, indicating equally precise measurement all along the θ continuum. It is possible that an instrument has a high classical reliability without giving sufficient information at critical levels of θ. The test-information curve illustrates the value of IRT models.

Theory Related to Multiple-Choice Question Design

Theory related to multiple-choice (MC) design emanated from both classical measurement theory and IRT. Which theory is preferable is a matter of continued debate, although most would agree that IRT offers distinct advantages over classical measurement theory. Irrespective of the theory used, specific knowledge of validation methods peculiar to MC is essential.

When we want to develop a test to evaluate student or client learning in the context of training or education, MC questions are often used because they offer obvious advantages associated with objectivity and cost-effectiveness considerations. The focus of these tests is usually on a certain domain of knowledge to be learned, and a test is a sample of that domain. Responses to items in MC tests usually form a pattern, which is investigated to evaluate the suitability of items and the validity of the measure. Both classical measurement theory and IRT can be used to evaluate item responses. There are several ways to study item response patterns; we will discuss approaches to item difficulty, item discrimination, the role of guessing, and distracter evaluation.

Items have different levels of difficulty. The natural scale for item difficulty is the percentage of respondents who answer the item correctly. The probability of a correct response depends on the floor of the item, that is, the outcome of examinees with no knowledge who are guessing randomly. With a three-option item the floor is 33%, and with a four-option item it is 25%. The natural difficulty of an item is based on the performance of all persons for whom the test has been developed. This value, also known as the p-*value*, is difficult to estimate in classical measurement theory unless the item has been tested on a very representative group of test takers. IRT allows us to estimate item difficulty without being too concerned about the composition of the sample. Most IRT models require large testing programs involving 500 or more test takers.

The ability of an item to sensitively measure the differences between test takers is an important characteristic. Therefore, we are interested in establishing whether test takers with more knowledge do better on an item than those with less knowledge. Item discrimination can be estimated in several ways. The product-moment

(point-biserial) relationship is used in classical measurement theory. The weakness of this estimate is that discrimination is underestimated if the range of scores is restricted, for example, when the instruction is good and all the students work hard. One of the IRT models often used in practice, the one-parameter item response model (known as the *Rasch model*), ignores item discrimination and surprisingly often provides satisfactory results. With other IRT models, for example, the two-parameter and three-parameter models, item discrimination is proportional to the slope of the option characteristic curve at the point of inflexion (Lord, 1980). In other words, an item is most discriminating in a particular range of scores. The *eta coefficient*, derived from the one-way analysis of variance, is another method to estimate item discrimination. It provides unique information about item discrimination when polychotomous, as opposed to dichotomous, scoring methods are used. The size of the eta coefficient depends on the differential nature of item options.

With classical measurement theory, contrary to general belief, guessing is not a serious problem, despite the fact that an element of guessing exists in MC. The probability of getting a higher than deserved score decreases with the length of the test. With a 10-item test, with each item having four options, the probability of 10 correct random guesses is only .0000009. The third parameter of the 3-item response model is guessing, which makes it possible to study the influence of guessing on items. Even so, the influence of guessing is small in relation to that of the discriminator parameter. Polychotomous scoring models often incorporate information about guessing into scoring procedures.

The quality of distracters influences the performance of a test. A distracter should appeal to low scorers who do not know the knowledge domain of the test. High scorers, those who have mastered the knowledge area being tested, should avoid distracters. Distracters that are unrelated to test performance should be replaced. Frequency tables of option choices according to score groups, trace lines, and statistical indexes are used to study responses to distracters. A nonmonotonic pattern in the frequency table is viewed as undesirable. Most statistical indexes to study distracter performance that are not based on trace lines have serious shortcomings and probably should not be used. The characteristics of trace lines in the evaluation of item performance make them attractive for distracter analysis. Trace lines are graphical depictions of option performance as a function of total performance. The correct answer should have a monotonically increasing trace line and a distracter should have a monotonically decreasing trace line. Trace lines make item analysis meaningful and easily interpretable.

Except for classical measurement theory, the other theories discussed are often difficult to master for the novice scale developer. Most of these theories require complicated statistical analysis techniques that usually are not available in frequently used statistical packages like the Statistical Package for the Social Sciences (SPSS). It is, however, important that these other theories are recognized in the field of scale development. When practitioners and researchers enter the field of scale development and scale validation, it is wise to start with the design and validation of instruments based on the classical measurement theory. With this theory, scales can easily be validated with basic methods in SPSS. Once this theory is mastered, the more advanced scale developers can start investigating the possibilities offered by the other theories.

The rest of this chapter describes the construction of an assessment tool, along with the underlying assumptions of classical measurement theory. Rapid assessment instruments (RAIs)—which usually consist of one or more unidimensional scales—will be used in this discussion. The development of unidimensional as opposed to multidimensional measures is especially relevant to this discussion, given their widespread use in social work. Following this discussion, the process of validating the newly developed tool will be outlined. The underlying assumptions of classical measurement theory will be illustrated throughout the discussion.

THE CONSTRUCTION OF A RAPID ASSESSMENT INSTRUMENT

It is very important to develop a scale within a specific theoretical framework. Identifying the theoretical framework before the scale is developed forces researchers to think about their data ahead of time and allows them to incorporate the reasons they select certain items for their scale (cf. Nunnally & Bernstein, 1994; see Box 61.1, Operational Definitions of Constructs).

After a detailed analysis of the theoretical

BOX 61.1 Operational Definitions of Constructs

After a careful analysis of the literature on social functioning, the following operational definition of social functioning has been defined in a study where a scale was designed to measure social functioning:

Social functioning relates to the behavioural patterns of the individual in the different roles and systems that the individual forms part of in his environment. The individual reacts with congruence among the four dimensions of his inner world to situations in his environment. The individual experiences himself and his world on two distinct levels that relate to achievement, satisfaction and expectation on the one hand and to frustration, stress and helplessness on the other hand. Optimal social functioning assumes that the positive forces will be stronger than the regressive forces. The social functioning of the individual always takes place in a specific time frame that is integrated with the developmental phase in which the individual is functioning. (Faul, 1995, p. 158)

framework, the specific assessment areas that are going to be measured must be identified and operationally defined. It is important to operationalize only one construct for a unidimensional scale and to write down the definition in clear terms. Everyone must understand the construct as it is defined. Specificity in operationalizing attributes is essential, particularly when they involve subjective phenomena like feelings and thoughts. This definition will then guide the scale developer in the design of the specific items that will measure the construct (Nurius & Hudson, 1993; Hudson, 1994; see Box 61.2, Constructs, Their Definitions and Related Attributes).

After the construct has been defined, the scale developer moves to the phase in which the actual scale development will take place. The step consists of writing the items that will make up the completed assessment scale. The domain sampling model of measurement—that there is an infinite pool of possible items that can measure a construct—is used here as a guideline. The skill lies in choosing the specific items that will lead to high content validity, that is, doing a good job of representing the domain that the re-

BOX 61.2 Constructs, Their Definitions and Related Attributes

When a scale is developed that measures social functioning, it must be clearly specified what assessment areas will be used. In the study on social functioning, six constructs were defined that were used to measure social functioning, namely, *achievement, satisfaction,* and *expectation* as positive indicators of social functioning, and *frustration, stress,* and *helplessness* as negative indicators of social functioning to relate to the three-dimensionality of the polarity of social functioning. After identification of these six constructs, each construct was operationally defined and attributes were identified that relate to each construct. For the sake of this chapter, only the satisfaction subscale will be used as an example.

The following definition for satisfaction was offered as it relates to optimal social functioning:

Satisfaction is the unique expression of an individual as to the feelings of well-being he attaches to his life. These feelings have no specific "objective" roots, but are characterized by the unique interaction of the individual with his environment. It represents an overall judgment of a person's life satisfaction that has to do with a person's cognitions and a person's affect. (Faul, 1995, p. 189)

After a careful analysis of different theoretical approaches to satisfaction, the following attributes have been identified to describe satisfied people:

- Work leads to intrinsic satisfaction.
- Experience their lives as full of meaning and direction.
- Feel content with life.
- Have a healthy circle of friends.
- Experience overall quality of life.
- Warm and friendly.
- Feel in control of their own fate.
- Experience sense of security.
- Want to keep things as they are.
- Spend time on hobbies, visits, and entertainment.
- Have good relationships with others.
- Social skills are well developed.
- Strong self-esteem and self-respect.
- Behave in an extrovert manner because of previously successful interaction with people.

searcher is trying to measure (Hudson, 1994; Nunnally & Bernstein, 1994).

Questions or statements can be used when the items are designed. Some researchers consider questions better than statements because questions avoid the problem of compliance tendency. Others think statements are preferable, especially when the researcher is interested in determining the extent to which respondents maintain a particular attitude or perspective. This attitude is then summarized in a fairly brief statement, and the respondents are asked whether they agree or disagree with it. In the end, personal preference will determine which method to use.

Hudson (1994) recommends either the two-step method or the list method in the creation of the initial item pool. The *three-step method*

consists of the following prominent steps: (a) Define the construct to be measured in clear, unambiguous terms; (b) ask one question that will measure the defined construct; and (c) write the number of items the scale developer wants to include that ask the same question in a different way. The *list method* consists of the following steps: (a) write down one attribute of the defined construct: an affect, behavior or judgment; (b) write an item based on that attribute; and (c) repeat these two steps until the required number of items have been generated (see Box 61.3, Design Items for a Scale).

One of the most frequently asked questions with respect to scale construction is how long the scale should be. According to Hudson (1982, 1994) and Nunnally and Bernstein (1994), the reliability of a scale increases with length; scales

BOX 61.3 Design Items for Scale

For the satisfaction subscale, the list method was used to develop the following items (Faul, 1995, pp. 271–272):

1. I feel cheerful.
2. I have the ability to retain my sense of humour under difficult circumstances.
3. I feel good about the course my life is taking at present.
4. I am satisfied with my relationships.
5. I experience peace of mind in my circumstances.
6. I am usually sincere in my relationships.
7. I feel joyful.
8. I feel happy.
9. I am at ease in my relationships with others.
10. I like things the way they are.
11. I am friendly.
12. I feel satisfied with my present accomplishments.
13. I feel satisfied with the standard of my life.
14. I enjoy my relationships.
15. I accept my circumstances.

with many items are usually more reliable than those with only a few. The law of diminishing returns is applicable here: The gain in reliability is smaller when one moves from 11 to 20 questions than when one moves from 1 to 10 questions, and even smaller when one moves from 21 to 30 questions. Hudson (1982) gives the following guidelines: "If a reliability of .60 or greater cannot be obtained by using 20 to 30 items for a single unidimensional scale, then the scale should be discarded, and the entire measurement task should be reconsidered (p. 149).

After a number of items have been designed, the next step is to scale them. Scaling items has to do with the development of a specific rule for assigning values to them to obtain an indication of the level or magnitude of the variable for a specific person. When values are assigned, a small value must indicate that the person has a low level or magnitude of the variable that is being measured, and a large number must indicate that the person has a high level or magnitude of the variable (Hudson, 1982).

When it is important for the researcher to measure the intensity of a specific variable, or the psychological meaning an individual attaches to a specific variable, a very useful approach is to make use of *category partition scaling*, or Likert scaling, named after Rensis Likert, who in 1932 wrote a classic article discussing the properties and uses of a category partition scale. This kind of scaling consists of breaking up a continuum into a collection of equal intervals or categories. With this kind of scaling, a problem that is common in the social sciences, namely, assigning values for a single item in such a way that the resulting item scale is a truly continuous variable, is overcome by partitioning the score continuum into a small number of categories (Hudson, 1982; Nurius & Hudson, 1993; Spector, 1992).

Different strategies can be used to name the categories on a category partition scale. One option is to define only the end points of the continuum. Another is to name all the categories. Another option is called the semantic differential format, in which respondents are asked to choose between two opposite positions, for example, ugly versus attractive (Spector, 1992).

If the scale developer decides to use category partition scaling, the next step is to decide on the number of response categories to be used for each item. At a minimum, every scale must be scored with two response categories. There is no theoretical upper limit to the number of response categories. The reliability of a scale increases when the categories on the scale increase. However, the law of diminishing returns again plays a role: The gain in reliability is greater when one moves from 2 to 9 categories than when one moves from 9 to 16 categories. In the end it is better to have too many rather than too few categories. But, because of the law of diminishing returns, a really large number of categories may be of little benefit and may influence the measurement sensitivity of the person who is completing the scale in a negative manner (Hudson, 1982; Nunnally & Bernstein, 1994; Spector, 1992). The magic number of categories is 7 ± 2. When a scale is developed, it would be best to use 7 categories, but it is possible to go as low as 5 or as high as 9 (Faul, 1995, p. 53).

If desired, a formula can be developed for use in scoring the new assessment tool. Hudson (1982, 1992) suggests a formula where the final score will always range from 0 to 100 and provision is made for respondents who did not complete all the questions. In this formula, missing items are replaced with the mean item score. However, Hudson (1992) warns that total scores should not be computed unless 80% or more of the items have been completed. The formula is as follows (Hudson, 1992, p. 18):

$$S = \frac{(\text{sum } X - N)(100)}{N(K - 1)}$$

where S = final score
X = item responses
N = number of correctly completed items
K = the largest item response permitted

The final step in the development of an assessment tool is to write instructions for the respondents. If the respondents do not understand how to answer the items, serious errors can be introduced. To avoid such errors, every measurement tool should contain clear instructions and introductory comments where appropriate (Rubin & Babbie, 1989; Spector, 1992; see Box 61.4, Instructions for Respondents).

SCALE VALIDATION WITH CLASSICAL MEASUREMENT THEORY

Study Design

In a validation study, the central research questions are: Is the newly designed instrument reliable? Is the newly designed instrument valid?

A background information sheet should always be used as part of instrument validation research. The background information is used to describe the characteristics of the sample and is also useful in investigating construct validity because it is normally hypothesized that the total scores on a scale would correlate poorly with these background variables. The background information normally consists of questions regarding the age, gender, education, marital status, income, length of marriage, number of children, and number of persons in the household (Hudson, 1982).

If only a unidimensional scale is to be validated, it is important to include two to four more scales in the research package to be able to investigate the different kinds of validity. If a multidimensional scale that consists of a collection of unidimensional scales is to be validated,

---

BOX 61.4 Instructions for Respondents

In the design of a scale to measure social functioning, the following instructions were written (Faul, 1995, p. 278):

With this questionnaire we would like to get an impression of your experiences in daily life in order to get an overall picture of your social functioning. In the list that follows, grade yourself on how often during the past week you have experienced the described feeling. Grade yourself as quickly and as honestly possible. Do not speculate too long before you answer. The first answer that comes to mind is usually the correct one. Place the relevant number next to each statement, using the following scale:

1 = *Never*	5 = *Often*
2 = *Rarely*	6 = *Mostly*
3 = *Sometimes*	7 = *Always*
4 = *Half the time*	

---

it is not necessary to include more scales (Hudson, 1994).

Sampling

When the aim of a research study is to generalize statements to populations on the basis of the sample that has been studied, the sample must be representative of that particular population. In validation studies the aim is not to represent any well-defined population. What is important is to obtain enough diversity and variability to permit examination of the reliability and validity of the newly developed measurement tool. Cronbach's coefficient alpha, which is used to test for reliability, is based on interitem correlations, and its value can be affected by homogeneity of subject responses to scale items. Therefore, heterogeneity in the sample in terms of experiences in the construct being measured is very important so that estimates of reliability and validity will not be artificially attenuated by small standard deviations and interitem correlations within the scale (Hudson & Pike, 1995).

In the light of the preceding explanation, it is clear that a representative probability sample is not necessary for validation studies. A nonprobability sampling technique that is much less expensive can be used, as long as heterogeneity can be guaranteed. Hudson prefers a convenience sampling technique through which heterogeneity can be ensured (see Hudson & Decker, 1994; Hudson, Nurius, Daley, & Newsome, R. D., 1990; Hudson, 1994). In convenience sampling, the researcher merely chooses the closest living persons as respondents. This is a very cost-effective sampling method that saves a lot of time (Bailey, 1982).

Orme and Hudson (1995) conducted a study in which confidence intervals were used to select sample sizes that ensure precise, efficient, and powerful estimates of the effects of variables. Their method suggests using a sample size of between 450 and 550 cases, which will comfortably satisfy the requirements of the hypothesis tester, power analyst, and parameter fitter. This suggestion leads to much more cost-effective and time-effective studies when validity studies of newly developed measurement tools are undertaken. It is relatively easy and efficient to gather a convenient sample of between 450 and 550 cases rather than a random sample of between 2,000 and 3,000 cases. This helps the researcher who does not have enough funds available to validate a newly developed measurement tool. Hudson (1994) also reasons that if high reliability and validity can be established with a sample size as small as 450 to 550 cases, it can definitely be said to be a good measurement tool. A small sample that produces high reliability and validity is better than a large sample that produces moderate reliability and validity. When large samples are used, errors of measurement are averaged out when average scores are computed. This is important when scale developers try to validate a scale for use with single clients because in this situation one cannot count on large numbers to reduce the effects of measurement error. In working with individual clients, one must be able to trust the basic accuracy of the measure (Hudson, 1994; Nurius & Hudson, 1993). As a general guideline Hudson (1994) suggests a sample of 300 or more cases.

Data Analysis

Investigating Reliability

According to Neuman and Kreuger (2003), reliability means dependability or consistency. It implies that the same thing is repeated or recurs under identical or very similar conditions. It addresses the question: To what degree does the measurement of a variable produce consistent results under similar circumstances (Weinbach & Grinnell, 2001)?

As already discussed, classical measurement theory, with its notion of true and error scores, forms the basis of reliability analysis. Reliability is based on the amount of error in an observed score for an individual or a population of individuals. If the amount of error is quite small, the scale developer can claim that he has developed a highly reliable measurement tool (Nurius & Hudson, 1993, p. 213; cf. Carmines & Zeller, 1979; Nunnally & Bernstein, 1994).

Reliability estimates range from .0 to 1.0. It is important to know how high this estimate must be for the scale developer to claim that he has developed a reliable measurement tool. A satisfactory level of reliability depends on how a measure is used. Nunnally and Bernstein (1994) and Nurius and Hudson (1993) distinguish between reliability standards for use in scientific applications (e.g., to compare different groups) and reliability standards for use in clinical applications. For large-sample scientific work, a reliability coefficient of .60 or greater is acceptable. According to Nunnally and Bernstein (1994), "Increasing reliabilities much beyond .80 in basic research is often wasteful of time and energy" (p. 265). On the other hand, a reliability of .80 may not be nearly high enough in making decisions about individuals. Group research is often concerned with the size of correlations and with mean differences among experimental treatments, but in clinical work, exact scores are important to make decisions about individuals (Nunnally & Bernstein, 1994). Therefore, measurement tools that will be used to make decisions about a single individual should have a minimum reliability of .80 (Carmines & Zeller, 1979; Nurius & Hudson, 1993). The latest version of Nunnally and Bernstein (1994) even suggests that a reliability of .90 is more appropriate when working with individuals.

Internal consistency measures are often used to assess reliability. Cronbach (1951) developed a simple equation to average all the different possibilities of split-half reliability. His coefficient, called the *alpha coefficient,* has become the most widely used measurement of reliability (Carmines & Zeller, 1979; Hudson, 1992; Nunnally & Bernstein, 1994). It is safe to conclude that when reliability is estimated for multiple-item scales in social work, the best way to do so is to compute the alpha coefficient (cf. Carmines & Zeller, 1979; Nunnally & Bernstein, 1994). Hudson (1982, 1992) did not compute any other kind of reliability when he established reliability for the numerous measurement devices he developed. The simplicity of the alpha coefficient can be seen from its equation (Cronbach, 1951; Hudson, 1994; Nunnally & Bernstein, 1994):

$$\alpha = (k/k - 1)(1 - \sum \frac{s^2}{s_0^2})$$

where k = number of items
s^2 = variance of items
s_0^2 = variance of total scores

Reliability coefficients based on correlations can be influenced by differences in the variance and SD of a measurement scale that may occur between samples. Therefore, homogeneous samples can affect the reliability coefficients by giving lower estimates of reliability, which is one of the important shortcomings of these coefficients. A specific feature of the alpha coefficient is that it is based on interitem correlations through its derivation from the generalized Spearman-Brown or GSB formula that can be seen in the following equation:

GSB = $k\bar{r}/(1+(k-1)\bar{r})$
where $\bar{r}$ = the correlation between any pair of items on a scale
$\bar{r}$ = the mean of all possible pairwise item correlations (the number of such correlations is N= $(k^2-k)/2$ where k is the number of items on the scale)

Its value can therefore be affected by homogeneity of subject responses to scale items (Hudson, 1992; Carmines & Zeller, 1979; Hudson & Pike, 1995).

To compensate for this mentioned problem with reliability coefficients, it is recommended that the standard error of measurement (SEM) also be computed before final conclusions are made with regard to the reliability of a measurement tool. The SEM, which is an estimate of the SD of the errors of measurement, is computed with the following formula (Hudson, 1992; see Nunnally & Bernstein, 1994, for a technical discussion of the SEM):

$$SEM = S_0{}^* \left(\sqrt{1-r_{tt}}\right)$$

where S_0 = standard deviation of the observed scores
r_{tt} = coefficient alpha

A great advantage of the SEM is that its value is not influenced by differences in the variance and SD of a measurement tool from one sample or population to the next.

If a measurement tool has a very small SEM, it can be said that the scale developer has produced a reliable measurement tool in terms of its measurement error characteristics. If it has a large SEM, it can be said that the developer has produced an unreliable measurement tool in terms of its measurement error characteristics. The primary disadvantage of the SEM is that there are no clear criteria for judging what is a small or large SEM. Hudson (1992) adopted a rule of thumb stating that the SEM should be approximately 5% (or less) of the range of possible scores when scored over a range from 0 to 100. Generally speaking, a good measurement tool, from a measurement error point of view, is one that has a large coefficient of reliability and a small SEM in relation to the overall range of possible scores (Hudson, 1982, 1992; see Box 61.5, How to Do a Reliability Analysis with SPSS).

Investigating Validity

According to Neuman and Kreuger (2003, p. 177) validity suggests truthfulness and refers to the match between the way a researcher conceptualizes a construct in a conceptual definition and a measure. Furthermore, validity also means that the construct is measured accurately. It is possible that an instrument measures the concept in question, but that the concept is not measured accurately. However, it is not possible to have an accurate measure, if the concept in question is not measured (Williams, Unrau, & Grinnell, 1998).

This distinction is vital to validation because it is quite possible for a measuring instrument to be relatively valid for measuring one kind of phenomenon but entirely invalid for measuring other phenomena. Thus, one validates not the measuring instrument itself but the measuring instrument in relation to the purpose for which it is being used (Carmines & Zeller, 1979).

A measurement tool is not either valid or invalid. Like reliability, validity is seen as a matter

BOX 61.5 How to Do a Reliability Analysis with SPSS

```
RELIABILITY
/VARIABLES = {varlist}
/FORMAT = NOLABELS
/SCALE(ALPHA) = ALL/MODEL = ALPHA
/SUMMARY = TOTAL.
```

RELIABILITY ANALYSIS—SCALE (ALPHA)
Item-total Statistics

	Scale mean if item deleted	Scale variance if item deleted	Corrected item-total correlation	Squared multiple correlation	Alpha if item deleted
Item1	59.3168	119.4351	.7723	.6921	.9610
Item2	59.6139	115.2613	.8189	.7473	.9600
Item3	59.4931	117.6790	.7959	.7128	.9605
Item4	59.4851	117.6352	.7496	.6310	.9613
Item5	59.3545	116.7451	.8244	.7349	.9599
Item6	59.5129	116.6710	.8254	.7256	.9599
Item7	59.5723	116.4159	.7601	.6275	.9611
Item8	59.5762	116.4471	.7957	.6795	.9604
Item9	59.5287	115.4798	.8448	.7536	.9595
Item10	59.4713	118.3806	.7172	.5893	.9619
Item11	59.4970	116.6791	.7886	.7149	.9605
Item12	59.6475	114.0382	.8458	.7791	.9594
Item13	59.5267	116.8569	.7377	.7419	.9616
Item14	59.5446	115.8914	.7916	.7877	.9605
Item15	59.7267	119.0522	.6746	.4772	.9627

Reliability Coefficients   15 items
Alpha = .9632   Standardized item alpha = .9635

What is important here is to see how the reliability coefficient can be improved if items are deleted. In this example, there were no items that would improve the already excellent alpha score if they were deleted.

of degree. Two measurement tools can both be valid in terms of the construct that is being measured, but one can be seen as a more valid tool than the other because it does a better job than the other in measuring the construct in question. In the establishment of validity, a measurement tool is judged in relation to one or more well-defined criteria. The validity of a scale can be described by computing a validity coefficient. Such coefficients are nearly always obtained as a proportion estimate or as a correlation coefficient and therefore have a theoretical range of values from 0 to 1.0. Sometimes validity coef-

ficients are not computed, and validity is judged only in relation to a specific criterion (Hudson, 1982, 1992).

Validity coefficients tend to be much smaller than reliability coefficients, and according to Downie and Heath (1967, in Hudson 1982), they tend to range between .40 and .60, with a median of about .50. Any measurement tool with a validity coefficient higher than .50 can therefore be seen as among the best 50% of all scales in terms of its validity (Hudson, 1982). Although the median of .50 can be used as a criterion for validity standards, Nurius and Hudson (1993) recommend that one can regard any measurement tool with a validity coefficient in excess of .60 as valid.

It is important to ensure content validity (adequacy of sampling the items on which people are measured) in terms of a well-formulated plan and procedure of scale construction *before* the actual scale is developed rather than evaluate this *after* construction. Careful selection and design in the initial stages will help to ease the task of validation later (Carmines & Zeller, 1979; Franzen, 1989; Nunnally & Bernstein, 1994).

Construct validity refers to "the ability of a measurement tool to measure the specific theoretical construct it was designed to measure" (Hudson, 1992, p. 45). With construct validity, the relation between the scale and its underlying theory is constantly at issue. Any particular measure can be thought of as having construct validity to the extent that results obtained from it would remain the same if other measures in the domain were used (Nunnally & Bernstein, 1994). Construct validity is related to content validity. However, content validity "refers largely to the sampling of the construct domain and the *construction* of a measurement tool while construct validity refers to the *performance* of the device with respect to theoretical expectations" (Hudson, 1982, p. 101).

Both content and construct validity can be investigated with the use of confirmatory factor analysis, which essentially consists of methods for finding clusters of related variables. Each such cluster or factor consists of a group of variables whose members correlate more highly among themselves than they do with variables outside the cluster. Such correlations can be seen as the factorial composition of measures and play a part in content and construct validity. Factor analysis is important to content validity in suggesting how to revise instruments. It also provides some of the tools necessary to define internal structures and cross-structures for sets of variables in construct validity (Nunnally & Bernstein, 1994).

Hudson (1982, 1992) recommends the use of confirmatory factor analysis and, more specifically, a kind of a priori, hypothesis-testing factor analysis, namely, the multiple-group method to investigate content and construct validity. The multiple-group method is designed "to show whether some well-specified hypothesis matrix will do a good job of accounting for the pattern of correlations among a specific set of variables that are supposed to represent a specific set of well-defined factors" (Hudson, 1992, p. 46; see Nunnally and Bernstein, 1994, for a full discussion of multiple-group confirmatory factor analysis).

If a measurement tool is constructed as a multi-item instrument, two hypotheses can be made: Each item measures the construct in question and not another construct, and each item will have a higher correlation with another measurement tool that measures the same construct, and it will have a lower correlation with other construct measures.

When multiple-group confirmatory factor analysis is used to investigate content and construct validity, it provides a method to test the hypothesis that items correlate well with the variables (constructs, factors) they are supposed to correlate with and that they correlate poorly with the variables (constructs, factors) they are not supposed to correlate with. According to Hudson (1982), this method is mathematically identical to a special form of item analysis, which makes it possible to avoid the complicated mathematics of factor analysis (cf. McAdams, 1990).

He explains this special form of item analysis as follows:

If R denotes the matrix of correlations among all the items for two or more scales (with units on the main diagonal) and H denotes a hypothesis matrix that specifies all the explicit hypothesis concerning which items load on which factors, then the factor loadings that are needed to confirm or deny those hypotheses can be obtained as:

$$S = RHD^{-\frac{1}{2}}$$

where D is the diagonal of $H'RH$ and

$$P = D^{-\frac{1}{2}}H'RHD^{-\frac{1}{2}}$$

contains the correlations among the factors. (Hudson, 1982, p. 109)

According to Hudson (1982, 1992), the great advantage of this method is that such results can be obtained by computing only Pearson product moment correlations:

In order to compute the factor loading matrix S, all that is needed is to compute a total score for each scale involved in the analysis and to then correlate every scale item with each of those total scores (an indication of content validity and construct validity at the item-level of analysis. The matrix, P, is obtained by correlating all of the total scores with each other (an indication of construct validity at the scale-level of analysis). This procedure is direct; it is powerful as an hypothesis-testing procedure; it requires no rotation; it produces an oblique solution; and it is simple to use. (Hudson, 1982, p. 109; cf. McAdams, 1990)

To summarize, the following steps must be followed to investigate content validity and construct validity on the item level of analysis:

1. Prepare a correlation matrix with all items included and investigate the item correlations. As a general rule of thumb, these item correlations need to be >.30 consistently.
2. Remove all unwanted item self-correlations. This step is important because the correlation of any scale item with its own total score is a part-whole correlation (it is a correlation between an item with itself and the sum of $K - 1$ items). The presence of this item-self correlation can produce an inflated picture of the content validity of a scale (Hudson, 1992).
3. Investigate the corrected item-total correlations. As a general rule of thumb, these correlations need to be >.45. Items that do not correlate highly with their own total score should be removed to ensure unidimensionality. The mean of these corrected item-total correlations can be treated as a coefficient of *content validity*. This coefficient should be >.50.
4. The previously mentioned coefficient of content validity, unlike the other scale-total correlations, can also be seen as an indication of *convergent and discriminant construct validity at the item level of analysis*. (See Box 61.6.)

Many times, scale developers validate their original investigation of reliability, content validity, and construct validity on the item level of analysis with confirmatory factor analysis. Factor analysis is used to confirm the dimensionality of the scale in terms of the predicted structures. In the case of RAIs, unidimensionality is desired for each scale. Factorial validity informs us about the number of domains we are dealing with, but not what the interpretation of each domain is or what is measured by that domain.

Other types of validity must be determined to capture these psychometric properties. Factor analysis involves statistical techniques that are used in an iterative manner to detect coherent subsets in a single set of variables that are relatively independent of one another. Sometimes a *principal component analysis* (PCA) solution may include more than one factor, without multidimensionality being confirmed, an aspect often ignored by researchers. In these situations it is necessary to use both PCA and *principal factor analysis* (PFA). If one factor is not extracted after the first PCA, results can be used to identify which items load on specific factors, and/or to eliminate items with relatively low factor loadings on the main factors. Given the number of factors identified by the PCA procedure and the specific items that make up each factor, a PFA will confirm or reject unidimensionality.

To test for *convergent and discriminant construct validity at the scale level of analysis*, the following steps should be followed:

1. Develop three a priori hypotheses concerning their relationship with one another and with a number of other variables. These hypotheses are: (a) The newly developed scale will correlate the lowest with a set of basic social background variables such as age, sex, ethnicity, marital status, family size, et cetera. It is believed that the kinds of personal and interpersonal relationship problems that are measured by social workers have little to do with "who we are" as represented by background social characteristics. Members of all social status groups are vulnerable to problems that can be encountered in the individual's effort to fit within his environment (Class I criterion variables). Class I criterion variables will usually give an indication of *discriminant construct validity at the scale level of analysis*. (b) There will be a number of variables that are expected to have only moderate correlations with the particular scale to be evaluated. This list of variables will vary from one scale to the next (Class II criterion variables). Class II criterion variables will usually give an indication of beginning evidence of *convergent construct validity at the scale level of analysis*. (c) There will be a group of variables that will have the highest correlations with the scale to be evaluated. Theory will guide

BOX 61.6 How to Do a Content and Construct Validity Analysis with SPSS on the Item Level of Analysis.

RELIABILITY
/VARIABLES={varlist}
/FORMAT = NOLABELS
/SCALE(ALPHA) =ALL/MODEL=ALPHA
/STATISTICS=CORR
/SUMMARY=TOTAL.

RELIABILITY ANALYSIS—SCALE (ALPHA)

Correlation matrix

	Item1	Item2	Item3	Item4	Item5
Item1	1.0000				
Item2	.7127	1.0000			
Item3	.7567	.7424	1.0000		
Item4	.6085	.6385	.6800	1.0000	
Item5	.7346	.6858	.7123	.6830	1.0000
Item6	.6618	.7598	.6478	.6188	.7547
Item7	.6514	.6867	.6519	.5591	.6415
Item8	.6106	.7091	.6630	.6534	.6509
Item9	.6889	.7458	.7023	.7033	.7272
Item10	.5262	.5537	.5462	.5020	.5950
Item11	.5976	.6262	.6236	.5823	.6205
Item12	.6062	.7268	.6613	.6482	.6679
Item13	.5369	.5433	.5182	.5446	.6549
Item14	.5507	.5961	.5883	.6561	.6830
Item15	.5893	.6010	.5945	.4983	.5762

	Item6	Item7	Item8	Item9	Item10
Item6	1.0000				
Item7	.6531	1.0000			
Item8	.6874	.7036	1.0000		
Item9	.6948	.7070	.7563	1.0000	
Item10	.6102	.5585	.5887	.6050	1.0000
Item11	.6786	.5755	.6259	.6780	.7171
Item12	.7083	.6322	.6805	.7575	.6908
Item13	.6352	.5461	.5627	.6139	.6051
Item14	.6797	.5595	.6205	.6456	.6236
Item15	.5857	.5684	.5450	.5571	.4812

	Item11	Item12	Item13	Item14	Item15
Item11	1.0000				
Item12	.7970	1.0000			
Item13	.6266	.6915	1.0000		
Item14	.6802	.7274	.8409	1.0000	
Item15	.5437	.5812	.5023	.5449	1.0000

These correlations should consistently be >.30. It is clear from this example that all the items adhere to this rule.

RELIABILITY ANALYSIS—SCALE (ALPHA)

N of Cases = 505.0

Item-total Statistics

	Scale mean if item deleted	Scale variance if item deleted	Corrected item-total correlation	Squared multiple correlation	Alpha if item deleted
Item1	59.3168	119.4351	.7723	.6921	.9610
Item2	59.6139	115.2613	.8189	.7473	.9600
Item3	59.4931	117.6790	.7959	.7128	.9605
Item4	59.4851	117.6352	.7496	.6310	.9613
Item5	59.3545	116.7451	.8244	.7349	.9599
Item6	59.5129	116.6710	.8254	.7256	.9599
Item7	59.5723	116.4159	.7601	.6275	.9611
Item8	59.5762	116.4471	.7957	.6795	.9604
Item9	59.5287	115.4798	.8448	.7536	.9595
Item10	59.4713	118.3806	.7172	.5893	.9619
Item11	59.4970	116.6791	.7886	.7149	.9605
Item12	59.6475	114.0382	.8458	.7791	.9594
Item13	59.5267	116.8569	.7377	.7419	.9616
Item14	59.5446	115.8914	.7916	.7877	.9605
Item15	59.7267	119.0522	.6746	.4772	.9627

The important column here is the "corrected item-total correlation" column. SPSS removes the unwanted self-correlations. All the individual item-total correlations should be above >.45. In this example, the items adhere to this rule. The mean of this column provides a content validity coefficient.

the scale developer to decide what variables these will be (Class III criterion variables). Class III criterion variables will give an indication of *convergent construct validity at the scale level of analysis.*

2. Summarize the construct validity findings by averaging all the correlations between the newly developed scale and each of the Class I, Class II, and Class III criterion variables.

3. Compare the summarized correlations for the three class criterion variables to see whether the hypotheses that were made are confirmed. (See Box 61.7.)

SUMMARY AND CONCLUSIONS

This chapter has discussed measurement theories that can be used by practitioners and researchers to develop assessment or evaluation tools for use in evidenced-based practice. Classical measurement theory is the easiest to understand and the one that is recommended for the novice scale developer. SPSS can easily be used with this theory to test the reliability and validity of newly designed measurement tools. If this is a field that interests the practitioner–researcher, the other theories can be investigated and used to further improve newly designed assessment or evaluation tools.

The field of scale development and scale validation still has a long path to follow. However, it has become an important part of evidenced-based social work practice and will be utilized more and more by practitioners and researchers alike. The mystery that was typically associated with the scale development process and the "exclusive" rights that were given to researchers to utilize these processes are all practices of the past. Practitioners need to become knowledgeable in this area and use their skills to develop relevant and valid assessment and evaluation tools for use in their practice settings. If they do

BOX 61.7 How to Do a Construct Validity Analysis on the Scale Level of Analysis

CORRELATIONS
/VARIABLES={VARLIST}
/PRINT = TWOTAIL NOSIG
/MISSING=PAIRWISE.

Correlations

		SATISF	GENDER	YMARRIED	ACHIEVE	EXPECT
SATISF	Pearson Correlation	1	−.118	−.111	.768	.745
	Sig. (2-tailed)	.	.008	.016	.000	.000
	N	505	505	472	420	490
GENDER	Pearson Correlation	−.118	1	.227	−.102	−.087
	Sig. (2-tailed)	.008	.	.000	.035	.051
	N	505	521	486	431	503
YMARRIED	Pearson Correlation	−.111	.227	1	−.170	−.023
	Sig. (2-tailed)	.016	.000	.	.001	.614
	N	472	486	486	406	469
ACHIEVE	Pearson Correlation	.768	−.102	−.170	1	.700
	Sig. (2-tailed)	.000	.035	.001	.	.000
	N	420	431	406	431	416
EXPECT	Pearson Correlation	.745	−.087	−.023	−.700	1
	Sig. (2-tailed)	.000	.051	.614	.000	.
	N	490	503	469	416	503

**Correlation is significant at the .01 level (2-tailed).
*Correlation is significant at the .05 level (2-tailed).

The correlations between SATISF (total score for the satisfaction subscale), GENDER and YMARRIED (years married) are an indication of discriminant construct validity, because the Level I hypothesis stated that there should not be a relationship between satisfaction and these background variables.

The correlations between SATISF, ACHIEVE (total score for the achievement subscale), and EXPECT (total score for the expectation subscale) are an indication of convergent validity because the Level III hypothesis stated that there should be a high correlation between these three subscales, due to the theory on social functioning that stated that these concepts are correlated. In this example, no Level II hypothesis was defined.

not make this part of their practice, the evidence-based movement of this century has the danger of not living up to its promises.

References

Bailey, K. D. (1982). *Methods of social research* (2nd ed.). New York: Free Press.
Bloom, M., & Fischer, J. (1982). *Evaluating practice: Guidelines for the accountable professional.* Englewood Cliffs, NJ: Prentice-Hall.
Brennan, R. (1983). *Elements of generalizability theory.* Iowa City, IA: ACT Publications.
Carmines, E. G., & Zeller, R. A. (1979). *Reliability and validity assessment.* London: Sage.

Cronbach, L. J. (1951). Coefficient alpha and the internal structure of tests. *Psychometrika, 16*, 297–334.
Cronbach, L. J., Gleser, G. C., Nanada, H., & Rajaratman, N. (1972). *The dependability of behavioral measurements: Theory of generalizability for scores and profiles.* New York: Wiley.
Cronbach, L. J., Nageswari, R., & Gleser, G. C. (1963). Theory of generalizability: A liberation of reliability theory. *British Journal of Statistical Psychology, 16*, 137–163.
Dangell, R. F. (1994). Is a scientist-practitioner model appropriate for direct social work practice? In W. W. Hudson & P. S. Nurius (Eds.), *Contro-*

versial issues in social work research. Boston: Allyn and Bacon.

Faul, A. C. (1995). *Scale development in social work.* Unpublished doctoral dissertation, Rand Afrikaans University, Johannesburg, South Africa.

Franzen, M. D. (1989). *Reliability and validity in neuropsychological assessment.* New York: Plenum.

Hudson, W. W. (1982). *The clinical measurement package: A field manual.* Homewood, IL.: Dorsey Press.

Hudson, W. W. (1992). *WALMYR assessment scales scoring manual.* Tempe, AZ: WALMYR Publishing.

Hudson, W. W. (1994, March). *Developing short-form assessment scales.* Paper presented at the annual meeting of the Council on Social Work Education, Atlanta, Georgia.

Hudson, W. W., Nurius, P. S., Daley, J. G., & Newsome, R. D. (1990). A short-form scale to measure peer relations dysfunction. *Journal of Social Service Research, 13,* 57–69.

Hudson, W. W., & Pike, C. K. (1995, March). *Reliability and measurement error in the presence of homogeneity.* Paper presented at the annual meeting of the Council on Social Work Education, San Diego, California.

Kane, M. (1982). A sampling model for validity. *Applied Psychological Measurement, 6,* 125–160.

Lord, F. M. (1980). *Applications of item response theory to practical testing problems.* Hillside, NJ: Erlbaum.

Matt, G. E. (n.d.). Generalizability theory [On-line]. Available: http://www.sciencedirect.com/science/article/B6WVS-46RRTJ6-10/2/42d5d1264df49c6f195c0acfd2f2aadc

McAdams, D. P. (1990). *The person: An introduction to personality psychology.* San Diego, CA: Harcourt Brace Jovanovich.

Neuman, W. L., & Kreuger, L. W. (2003). *Social work research methods: Qualitative and quantitative applications.* Boston: Allyn and Bacon.

Nugent, W. R., & Hankins, J. A. (1989). The use of item-response theory in social work measurement and research. *Social Service Review, 63,* 447–473.

Nunnally, J. C., & Bernstein, I. H. (1994). *Psychometric theory* (3rd ed.). New York: McGraw-Hill.

Nurius, P. S., & Hudson, W. W. (1993). *Human services practice, evaluation, and computers: A practical guide for today and beyond.* Pacific Grove, CA: Brooks/Cole.

Orme, J. G., & Hudson, W. W. (1995). The problem of sample size estimation: Confidence intervals. *Social Work Research, 19,* 121–127.

Rubin, A., & Babbie, E. (1989). *Research methods for social work.* Belmont, CA: Wadsworth.

Spector, P. E. (1992). *Summated rating scale construction: An introduction.* London: Sage.

Spineti, J, & Hambleton, R. (1977). A computer simulation study of tailored testing strategies for objective-based instructional programs. *Educational and Psychological Measurement, 37,* 139–158.

Springer, D. W., Abell, N., & Hudson, W. W. (2002). Creating and validating rapid assessment instruments for practice and research: Part 1. *Research on Social Work Practice, 12,* 408–439.

Weinbach, R. W., & Grinnell, R. M. (2001). *Statistics for social workers.* Boston: Allyn and Bacon.

Williams, M., Unray, Y. A., & Grinnell, R. M. (1998). *Introduction to social work research.* Itaschah, IL: Peacock Publishers.

SECTION VII
Program Evaluation Strategies

62 EMPOWERMENT EVALUATION

David Fetterman

Empowerment evaluation is the use of evaluation concepts, techniques, and findings to foster improvement and self-determination (Fetterman, 2001; Fetterman, Kaftarian, & Wandersman, 1996). It is guided by a commitment to truth and honesty (Fetterman, 1998). It is designed to help people help themselves and improve their programs using a form of self-evaluation and reflection. Program participants—including clients, consumers, and staff members—conduct their own evaluations; an outside evaluator often serves as a coach or additional facilitator, depending on internal program capabilities. By internalizing and institutionalizing self-evaluation processes and practices, a dynamic and responsive approach to evaluation can be developed.

There are three steps involved in helping others learn to evaluate their own programs: (a) developing a mission, vision, or unifying purpose; (b) taking stock or determining where the program stands, including strengths and weaknesses; and (c) planning for the future by establishing goals and helping participants determine their own strategies to accomplish program goals and objectives. In addition, empowerment evaluators help program staff members and participants determine the type of evidence required to document and monitor progress credibly toward their goals. These steps combined help to create a "communicative space" (Vanderplaat, 1995) to facilitate emancipatory and "communicative action" (Habermas, 1984).

MISSION

The first step in an empowerment evaluation is to ask program staff members and participants to define their mission. This step can be accomplished in a few hours. An empowerment evaluator facilitates an open session with as many staff members and participants as possible.

Participants are asked to generate key phrases that capture the mission of the program or project. This is done even when an existing mission statement exists, because there are typically many new participants and the initial document may or may not have been generated in a democratic open forum. Proceeding in this fashion allows fresh new ideas to become a part of the mission, and it also allows participants an opportunity to voice their vision of the program. It is common for groups to learn how divergent their participants' views are about the program, even when they have been working together for years. The evaluator records these phrases, typically on a poster sheet.

Then a workshop participant is asked to volunteer to write these telescopic phrases into a paragraph or two. This document is shared with the group, revisions and corrections are made in the process, and then the group is asked to accept the document on a consensus basis: That is, they do not have to be in favor of 100% of the document; they just have to be willing to live with it. The mission statement represents the values of the group and, as such, represents the foundation for the next step, taking stock.

TAKING STOCK

The second step in an empowerment evaluation is taking stock. This step can also be conducted in a few hours. It has two sections. The first involves generating a list of key activities that are crucial to the functioning of the program. Once again, the empowerment evaluator serves as a facilitator, asking program staff members and participants to list the most significant features and activities associated with the program. A list of 20 to 25 activities is sufficient. After generating this list, it is time to prioritize and determine which are the most important activities meriting evaluation at this time.

One tool used to minimize the time associated with prioritizing activities involves voting with dots. The empowerment evaluator gives each participant five dot stickers and asks the participants to place them by activities that the participant wants to evaluate as a group. The participant can distribute them across five different activities or place all five on one activity. Counting the dots easily identifies the top 10 activities. The 10 activities with the most dots become the prioritized list of activities meriting evaluation at that time. (This process avoids long arguments about why one activity is valued more than another is, when both activities are included in the list of the top 10 program activities anyway.)

The second phase of taking stock involves rating the activities. Program staff members and participants are asked to rate how well they are doing concerning each activity on a 1 to 10 scale, with 10 as the highest level and 1 as the lowest. The staff members and participants only have minimal definitions about the components or activities at this point. Additional clarification can be pursued as needed; however, detailed definition and clarification become a significant part of the later dialogue process. (The group will never reach the rating stage if each activity is perfectly defined at this point. The rating process then sets the stage for dialogue, clarification, and communication.)

Typically, participants rate each of the activities, while in their seats, on their own pieces of paper. Then each is asked to come up to the front of the room and record his or her ratings on a poster sheet of paper. This allows for some degree of independence in rating. In addition, it minimizes a long stream of second-guessing and checking to see what others are rating the same activities.

At the same time, there is nothing confidential about the process. Program staff members and participants place their initials at the top of the matrix and then record their ratings for each activity. Contrary to most research designs, this system is designed to ensure that everyone knows and is influenced by each other's ratings (*after* recording them on the poster sheet). This is part of the socialization process that takes place in an empowerment evaluation, opening up the discussion and stepping toward more open disclosure—speaking one's truth.

The taking-stock phase of an empowerment evaluation is conducted in an open setting for three reasons. The open setting (a) creates a democratic flow of information and exchange of information; (b) makes it more difficult for managers to retaliate, because they are in an open forum; and (c) increases the probability that the disclosures will be diplomatic, because program staff members and participants must remain in that environment. Open discussions in a vacuum, without regard for workplace norms, are not productive. They are often unrealistic and can be counterproductive.

Staff members and participants are more likely to give their program a higher rating if they are only asked to give an overall or gestalt rating about the program. Consequently, it is important that program staff members and participants be asked to begin by assessing individual program activities. They are more likely to give some activities low ratings if they are given an equal opportunity to speak positively about, or rate, other activities highly. The ratings can be totaled and averaged by person and by activity. This provides some insight into routinely optimistic and pessimistic participants. It allows participants to see where they stand in relation to their peers, which helps them calibrate their own assessments in the future. The more important rating, of course, is across the matrix or spreadsheet by activity. Each activity receives a total and average. Combining the individual activity averages generates a total program rating, often lower than an external assessment rating. This represents the first baseline data concerning that specific program activity. This can be used to compare change over time.

All of this work sets the tone for one of the most important parts of the empowerment evaluation process: dialogue. The empowerment evaluator facilitates a discussion about the ratings. A survey would have accomplished the same task up to this point. However, the facilitator probes and asks why one person rated communication as a 6, whereas two others rated it as a 3 on the matrix.[1] Participants are asked to explain their ratings and to provide evidence or documentation to support them. This plants the seeds for the next stage of empowerment evaluation (planning for the future), in which participants will need to specify the evidence they plan to use to document that their activities are helping them accomplish their goals. The empowerment evaluator serves as a critical friend during this stage, facilitating discussion and making sure everyone is heard, but at the same time being critical and asking, "What do you mean by that?" or requesting additional clarification and substantiation about a particular rating or viewpoint.

Participants are asked for both the positive and negative basis for their ratings. For example, if they give communication a 3, they are asked why a 3. The typical response is because there is poor communication, and they proceed to list reasons for this problem. The empowerment evaluator listens and helps record the information, then asks the question again, focusing on why it was a 3 instead of a 1. In other words, there must be something positive to report as well. An important part of empowerment evaluation involves building on strengths; even in weak areas, there is typically something positive that can be used to strengthen that activity or other activities. If the effort becomes exclusively problem focused, all participants see are difficulties, instead of strengths and opportunities to build and improve on practice.

Some participants give their programs or specific activities unrealistically high ratings. The absence of appropriate documentation, peer ratings, and a reminder about the realities of their environment—such as a high dropout rate, guns being brought on campus by students, and racial violence, in a high school—help participants recalibrate their ratings. Participants are reminded that they can change their ratings throughout the dialogue and exchange stage of the workshop, based on what they hear and learn from their peers. The ratings are not carved in stone. However, in some cases, ratings stay higher than peers consider appropriate. But the significance of this process is not the actual rating so much as it is the creation of a baseline, as noted earlier, from which future progress can be measured. In addition, it sensitizes program participants to the necessity of collecting data to support assessments or appraisals.

After examining four or five examples, beginning with divergent ones and ending with similar ratings (to determine if there are totally different reasons for the same or similar ratings), this phase of the workshop is generally complete. The group or a designated subcommittee continues to discuss the ratings, and the group is asked to return to the next workshop for planning for the future with the final ratings and a brief description or explanation of what the ratings meant. (This is normally shared with the group for review, at a time in which ratings can still be changed, and then a consensus is sought concerning the document.) This process is superior to surveys because it generally has a higher response rate—close to 100%, depending on how many staff members and participants are present—and it allows participants to discuss what they meant by their ratings, to recalibrate and revise their ratings based on what they learn, thus minimizing talking past each other about certain issues or other miscommunications such as defining terms differently and using radically different rating systems. Participants learn what a 3 and an 8 mean to individuals in the group in the process of discussing and arguing about these ratings. This is a form of norming, helping to create shared meanings and interpretations within a group.

PLANNING FOR THE FUTURE

After rating their program's performance and providing documentation to support that rating, program participants are asked, "Where do you want to go from here?" They are asked how they would like to improve on what they do well and not so well. The empowerment evaluator asks the group to use the taking-stock list of activities as the basis for their plans for the future—so that their mission guides their taking-stock phase, and the results of their taking stock shapes their planning for the future. This creates a thread of coherence and an audit trail for each step of their evaluation and action plans.

Goals

Program staff members and participants are asked to list their goals based on the results of their taking-stock exercise. They set specific goals associated with each activity. Then the empowerment evaluator asks members of the group for strategies to accomplish each goal. They are also asked to generate forms of evidence to monitor progress toward specified goals. Program staff members and participants supply all of this information.

Empowerment evaluators are not superior or inferior in the process. They are equals. They add ideas as deemed appropriate without dominating discussion. The evaluator's primary role is to serve as a coach, facilitator, and critical evaluative friend. Empowerment evaluators must be able to serve as facilitators, helping program members and participants process and be heard. Evaluators must also be analytical and critical, asking or prompting participants to clarify, document, and evaluate what they are doing, to ensure that specific goals are achieved. If the evaluator is only critical and analytical, the group will walk away from the endeavor. The empowerment evaluator must maintain a balance of these talents or team up with other coaches from within the group or outside the group who can help them maintain this balance.

The selected goals should be established in conjunction with supervisors and clients to ensure relevance from both perspectives. In addition, goals should be realistic, taking into consideration such factors as initial conditions, motivation, resources, and program dynamics. They should also take into consideration external standards, such as accreditation agency standards, superintendent's 5-year plan, board of trustees dictates, and board standards.

In addition, it is important that goals be related to the program's activities, talents, resources, and scope of capability. One problem with traditional external evaluation is that programs have been given grandiose goals or long-term goals that participants could only contribute to in some indirect manner. There is no link between an individual's daily activities and ultimate long-term program outcomes in terms of these goals. In empowerment evaluation, program participants are encouraged to select intermediate goals that are directly linked to their daily activities. These activities can then be linked to larger, more diffuse goals, creating a clear chain of reasoning and outcomes.

Program participants are encouraged to be creative in establishing their goals. A brainstorming approach is often used to generate a new set of goals. In such a process, individuals are asked to state what they think the program should be doing. The list generated from this activity is refined, reduced, and made realistic

after the brainstorming phase, through a critical review and consensual agreement process.

There are also a bewildering number of goals to strive for at any given time. As a group begins to establish goals based on this initial review of their program, they realize quickly that a consensus is required to determine the most significant issues to focus on. These are chosen according to (a) significance to the operation of the program, such as teaching in an educational setting; (b) timing or urgency, such as recruitment or budget issues; and (c) vision, including community building and learning processes.

Goal setting can be a slow process when program participants have a heavy work schedule. Sensitivity to the pacing of this effort is essential. Additional tasks of any kind and for any purpose may be perceived as simply another burden when everyone is fighting to keep their heads above water. However, any individual interested in a specific goal should be asked to volunteer to be responsible for it, as a team leader, to ensure follow-through and internal accountability.

Developing Strategies

Program participants are also responsible for selecting and developing strategies to accomplish program objectives. The same process of brainstorming, critical review, and consensual agreement is used to establish a set of strategies, which are routinely reviewed to determine their effectiveness and appropriateness. Determining appropriate strategies, in consultation with sponsors and clients, is an essential part of the empowering process. Program participants are typically the most knowledgeable about their own jobs, and this approach acknowledges and uses that expertise—and in the process, puts them back in the driver's seat.

Documenting Progress

Program staff members and participants are asked what type of documentation or evidence is required to monitor progress toward their goals.[2] This is a critical step. Each form of documentation is scrutinized for relevance, to avoid devoting time to collecting information that will not be useful or pertinent. Program participants are asked to explain how a given form of documentation is related to specific program goals. This review process is difficult and time-consuming but prevents wasted time and disillusionment at the end of the process. In addition, documentation must be credible and rigorous if it is to withstand the criticism that this evaluation is self-serving. (For additional discussion on this topic, see Fetterman, 1994.)

The entire process of establishing a mission, taking stock, and planning for the future creates an implicit logic model[3] or program theory, demonstrating that there is nothing as practical as a good theory of action, especially one grounded in participants' own experiences. (For additional discussion about program theory, see Bickman, 1987; Chen, 1990; Connell, Kubisch, Schorr, & Weiss, 1995; Cook & Shadish, 1994; McClintock, 1990; Patton, 1989; Weiss, 1998, pp. 55–71; Wholey, 1987.)

BASELINE COMPARISON AND A CULTURE OF EVIDENCE

The taking-stock step creates a baseline self-assessment of the program. The plans-for-the-future step represents the intervention or treatment. Conventional evaluation tools, such as interviews, surveys, focus groups, and observations, are used to determine if the strategies are working or accomplishing the group goals. These minitests represent an ongoing feedback mechanism, providing corrective feedback for decision making. Program staff members and participants can make midcourse corrections before it is too late. If the evaluative feedback indicates that the strategies are not working, then it is time to change the strategies. Approximately 3 to 6 months later, another formal taking-stock session is conducted. The first taking-stock findings are compared with the follow-up or second taking-stock findings to document change over time. Once again this is used for corrective feedback, confirming the effectiveness of certain strategies that should be maintained or enhanced and the ineffectiveness of other strategies that need to be revisited and changed. The cyclical process helps to internalize the logic of evaluation and builds an evaluative folk culture as well as a culture of evidence.

COLLABORATION

Empowerment evaluation is a collaborative group activity, not an individual pursuit. An evaluator does not and cannot empower anyone; people empower themselves, often with assistance and coaching. Empowerment evaluation can create an environment that is conducive to empowerment and self-determination. This process is fundamentally democratic, in the sense that it invites (if not demands) participation, examining issues of concern to the entire community in an open forum. As a result, the context changes: The assessment of a program's value and worth is not the end point of the evaluation—as it often is in traditional evaluation—but is part of an ongoing process of program improvement. This new context acknowledges a simple but often overlooked truth: Merit and worth are not static values. Populations shift, goals shift, knowledge about program practices and their value changes, and external forces are highly unstable. By internalizing and institutionalizing self-evaluation processes and practices, a dynamic and responsive approach to evaluation can be developed to accommodate these shifts. As Usher (1995) explains, "By developing the capacity to monitor and assess their own performance, program managers and staff can risk the mistakes that often occur with innovation. This is because they can detect problems and make midcourse corrections before the results of errors due to planning or execution become widely apparent and costly. Having the capacity and responsibility to obtain such information about program operations and impact thus empowers managers and staff to explore new ways to enhance their performance" (pp. 62–63).

Both value assessments and corresponding plans for program improvement—developed by the group with the assistance of a trained evaluator—are subject to a cyclical process of reflection and self-evaluation. Program participants learn continually to assess their progress toward self-determined goals and to reshape their plans and strategies according to this assessment. In the process, self-determination is fostered, illumination generated, and liberation actualized. Value assessments are also highly sensitive to the life cycle of the program or organization. Goals and outcomes are geared toward the appropriate developmental level of implementation. Extraordinary improvements are not expected of a project that will not be fully implemented until the following year. Similarly, seemingly small gains or improvements in programs at an embryonic stage are recognized and appreciated in relation to their stage of development. In a fully operational and mature program, moderate improvements or declining outcomes are viewed more critically.

PROCESS USE

Empowerment evaluation ensures that each voice is heard in the chorus, but when the performance begins it is the chorus that is heard. Empowerment evaluation is about building capacity, building community, and building a future. Teaching evaluation logic and skills is a way of building capacity for ongoing self-assessment—enhancing the capacity for self-determination. According to Patton (1997), "Participation and collaboration can lead to a long-term commitment to use evaluation logic and techniques thereby building a culture of learning among those involved" (p. 156).

Moreover, "learning to see the world as an evaluator sees it, often has a lasting impact on those who participate in an evaluation—an impact that can be greater and last longer than the findings that result from that same evaluation, especially where those involved can apply that learning to future planning and evaluation situations" (Patton, 1997). This is process use. This is ownership.

CONCLUSION

Empowerment evaluation is similar to many other forms of evaluation. Many of the same tools are used, including interviews, surveys, focus group, and observations. The only difference is that empowerment evaluation overturns conventional evaluation and wisdom.[4] The group is in charge of their own evaluation, instead of the evaluator. The evaluation is a collaboration, instead of an individual or external enterprise. The evaluator is a coach or critical friend, rather than an external expert. The focus is on self-determination, capacity building, internal accountability, and program improvement. At every step, the evaluation process becomes more responsive to the context and culture of the group. Diversity is a valued contribution, adding to instead of subtracting from the effort.

Empowerment evaluation adheres to evaluation standards (Fetterman, 2001). It does not operate in a vacuum. It is conducted in the context of existing external standards and requirements. In addition, internal or empowerment evaluation and external evaluation are not mutually exclusive. They work together very well. They strengthen each other. The difference between empowerment and many forms of conventional evaluation, however, is that program staff members and participants take charge of their own lives. They act as self-motivated and actualized individuals with intermediate objectives associated with larger group or organizational goals. They internalize and institutionalize evaluation. They create a dynamic and creative learning organization[5] that can be sustained in one format or another for a lifetime.

Notes

1. See Fetterman (1998) for additional information about this example. Briefly, we learned that the participants were talking past each other, or at least they were speaking on different levels of analysis. The individuals who rated communication a 3 stated that communication was poor in the school. However, the dean rated communication a 6 because he was assessing communication in the school from a larger perspective. He thought we communicated much better than other departments in the Institute.

2. See Linney and Wandersman (1991, 1996) for self-help documents to facilitate the process of documenting processes, outcomes, and impacts.

3. See Dugan (1996) for an illustration of how logic models are used in empowerment evaluations.

4. This chapter is based on a plenary presentation about empowerment evaluation at the Stauffer Symposium on Applied Psychology at the Claremont Colleges. The program was titled Evaluating Social Programs and Problems: Visions for the New Millennium. For additional updated information, refer to the empowerment evaluation Web site at: http://www.stanford.edu/~davidf/empowermentevaluation.html

5. See Preskill and Torres (1999) for an excellent dialogue about evaluation and organizational learning.

References

Bickman, L. (1987). Using program theory in evaluation. In L. Bickman (Ed.), *New directions for program evaluation: No. 33* (pp. 5–18). San Francisco: Jossey-Bass.

Chen, H. (1990). Issues in constructing program theory. In L. Bickman (Ed.), *New directions for program evaluation: No. 47. Advances in program theory* (pp. 7–18). San Francisco: Jossey-Bass.

Connell, J. P., Kubisch, A. C., Schorr, L. B., & Weiss, C. H. (Eds.). (1995). *New approaches to evalu-*

ating community initiatives: Concepts, methods, and contexts. Washington, DC: Aspen Institute.

Cook, T., & Shadish, W. (1994). Social experiments: Some developments over the past fifteen years. *Annual Review of Psychology, 45,* 545–580.

Dugan, M. (1996). Participatory and empowerment evaluation: Lessons learned in training and technical assistance. In D. M. Fetterman, S. Kaftarian, & A. Wandersman (Eds.), *Empowerment evaluation: Knowledge and tools for self-assessment and accountability.* Thousand Oaks, CA: Sage.

Fetterman, D. M. (1993). *Speaking the language of power: Communication, collaboration, and advocacy (translating ethnography into action).* London, England: Falmer.

Fetterman, D. M. (1994). Steps of empowerment evaluation: From California to Cape Town. *Evaluation and Program Planning, 17*(3), 305–313.

Fetterman, D. M. (1996). Empowerment evaluation: An introduction. In D. M. Fetterman, S. Kaftarian, & A. Wandersman (Eds.), *Empowerment evaluation: Knowledge and tools for self-assessment and accountability* (pp. 13–14). Thousand Oaks, CA: Sage.

Fetterman, D. M. (1998). Empowerment evaluation and accreditation in higher education. In E. Chelimsky & W. Shadish (Eds.), *Evaluation for the 21st century: A handbook.* Thousand Oaks, CA: Sage.

Fetterman, D. M. (2001). *Foundations of empowerment evaluation.* Thousand Oaks, CA: Sage.

Fetterman, D. M., Kaftarian, S., & Wandersman, A. (Eds.). (1996). *Empowerment evaluation: Knowledge and tools for self-assessment and accountability.* Thousand Oaks, CA: Sage.

Habermas, J. (1984). *The theory of communicative action: Vol. I.* Boston: Beacon Press.

Linney, J. A., & Wandersman, A. (1991). *Prevention Plus III: Assessing alcohol and other drug prevention programs at the school and community level: A four-step guide to useful program assessment.* Rockville, MD: U.S. Department of Health and Human Services, Office of Substance Abuse Prevention.

Linney, J. A., & Wandersman, A. (1996). Empowering community groups with evaluation skills: The Prevention Plus III Model. In D. M. Fetterman, S. Kaftarian, & A. Wandersman (Eds.), *Empowerment evaluation: Knowledge and tools for self-assessment and accountability.* Thousand Oaks, CA: Sage.

McClintock, C. (1990). Administrators as applied theorists. In L. Bickman (Ed.), *New directions for program evaluation: No. 47. Advances in program theory* (pp. 19–33).. San Francisco: Jossey-Bass.

Patton, M. (1989). A context and boundaries for theory-driven approach to validity. *Evaluation and Program Planning, 12,* 375–377.

Patton, M. (1997). Toward distinguishing empowerment evaluation and placing it in a larger context. *Evaluation Practice, 18*(2), 147–163. Retrieved June 23, 2003, from http://www.stanford.edu/ ~davidf/patton.html

Preskill, H., & Torres, R. (1999). *Evaluative inquiry for learning in organizations.* Thousand Oaks, CA: Sage.

Vanderplaat, M. (1995). Beyond technique: Issues in evaluating for empowerment. *Evaluation, 1*(1), 81–96.

Weiss, C. H. (1995). Nothing as practical as good theory: Exploring theory-based evaluation for comprehensive community initiatives for children and families. In J. P. Connell, A. C. Kubisch, L. B. Schorr, & W. H. Weiss (Eds.), *New approaches to evaluating community initiatives: Concepts, methods, and contexts.* Washington, DC: Aspen Institute.

Weiss, C. H. (1998). *Evaluation* (2nd ed.). Upper Saddle River: NJ: Prentice Hall.

Wholey, J. (Ed.). (1987). *Organizational excellence: Stimulating quality and communicating value.* Lexington, MA: Lexington Books.

63

THE SEVEN SECRETS OF A SUCCESSFUL VETERAN EVALUATOR

C. Aaron McNeece

How do we know whether or not a program works, under certain conditions? Planning and implementing systematic program evaluations is the answer. According to one leading text (Royse, Thyer, Padgett, & Logan, 2001), program evaluation is "applied research used as a part of the managerial process" (p. 11). It is a formalized step-by-step strategy to assess an agency's effort, measure a program's effectiveness in reaching its goals, or compare the relative efficiency of two or more programs in the use of resources (Tripodi, 1983). Practitioners and administrators use program evaluations to assess client progress, to make decisions about agency operations and program changes, and to measure costs and outcomes of a program. That is the technical side of program evaluation.

The information presented below is intended to be of practical value. It was inspired by the kind of highly useful information provided by Carol H. Weiss (1972) in her classic book on program evaluation, the most helpful evaluation book I have ever read. It is not the kind of technical information that is ordinarily found in modern textbooks. The case studies are composites of evaluations that I or my colleagues have conducted during the last three decades. All of these events did occur, except not in the same sequence or the same programs that are described below. All of the names have been changed, of course, to protect those individuals who may still be untenured.

CASE 1: THE COUNTY DELINQUENCY PREVENTION PROGRAM

John Jones was a young assistant professor who was being pressured by his dean, and constantly reminded by the chair of his school's promotion and tenure committee, that he should be doing funded research as early as possible in his career. He knew that getting a sizable federal grant to conduct basic research was very difficult and that the time lag between application and funding could be a year or more. So he put the machinery in motion to write an R01 proposal, but he also began to make contact with state and local agencies to see what kind of "easy" evaluation money was available.

Just by chance he was having lunch with an acquaintance from another department whose wife happened to be an executive assistant to the secretary of the local school board. John's colleague informed him that the County School District (CSD) had just received a grant from a private foundation to launch a delinquency prevention program, and that the school board was looking for someone to conduct an evaluation of the program. Even though Dr. Jones had no experience in delinquency or delinquency prevention, he decided to submit a proposal. He read the description of the delinquency prevention project in the grant award, but he could find nothing specific about the project's objectives. Dr. Jones's evaluation proposal was equally vague, promising only to conduct both process and outcome evaluations and to make recommendations to the school board regarding the program at the end of the next academic year.

The school board invited Dr. Jones to come to their next meeting. Much to his surprise, they voted unanimously to award him a contract for $20,000 to evaluate the program. After the meeting, the assistant superintendent walked him to his car. He put his hand on Dr. Jones's shoulder and said, "We've heard many good things about you, Dr. Jones. I know you will be able to conduct an evaluation that shows just how *great* a program this really is, since we are going to ask the XXX Foundation for twice as much money next year." Dr. Jones almost fainted.

Dr. Jones had been promised (verbally) that he would be able to randomly assign at-risk students to the prevention program and to a control group, and his research design was predicated on random assignment. In his first meeting with the assistant principal and guidance counselors at the school where the project would take place, he discovered that random assignment was not going to happen. The teachers had already submitted to the assistant principal a list of names of students that "we know will benefit from the program," and the principal and assistant principal both agreed.

Participation in the delinquency prevention program was voluntary, and the school scheduled students in the program to meet during the one free period each day, a time that was ordinarily reserved for field trips and extracurricular activities. Most of the eligible students declined to participate. The assistant principal decided to assign students to the program as a punishment for minor violations of the rules, such as tardiness and truancy.

Dr. Jones had intended to use actual delinquent behavior as an indicator of the program's outcome, but he didn't realize how difficult it was to get access to juvenile records. In fact, his university's Human Subjects Review Committee refused to give him permission to even request those records. In the end, he settled on a number of indicators such as tardiness, absences, behavioral reports, and grades.

At the end of the year Dr. Jones submitted his report to the school board, indicating that on each one of these indicators, the students in the delinquency prevention program were either no different from other students in this school, or they fared worse. He also pointed out that the way the program was implemented was not, in his opinion, consistent with the description of the program he had been given a year earlier. He was unable to make any recommendations about modifying the program, because he didn't know exactly why the program wasn't working. But because it wasn't working, he recommended that the program be discontinued. When the school board didn't respond to his report, Dr. Jones released a copy to the local newspaper.

The school superintendent issued a terse statement to the press, saying that "the evaluation conducted by Dr. Jones is deficient in the sense that he didn't really measure any outcomes related to delinquent behavior. We made a mistake employing an evaluator who was not an expert in this area." He also stated that "I have spoken with the teachers, and they all agree that this is a good program." Not only did they continue the program in this particular school, but the next year they implemented it in a second junior high school. Dr. Jones is still on the school board's blacklist.

CASE 2: DRUG COURTS

Charles Brown contracted with the state Department of Law Enforcement (DLE) to evaluate all of the state's drug courts. Before becoming a professor with a major university, Dr. Brown had extensive experience as a probation officer, where he worked with substance-abusing clients who were mandated to receive treatment by the courts. DLE wanted to make sure that its funding for the drug court program was being spent in the most effective manner, and the contract with DLE specified exactly how drug courts were to be evaluated. It just happened that the Drug Courts Program Office (1997) had issued a definitive statement about the key components of drug courts. Dr. Brown and DLE also agreed that, in addition to those components, drug court outcomes should be measured. (Dr. Brown and DLE officials had actually begun discussing how to evaluate drug court programs about 18 months earlier, just after the federal legislation was passed that provided the funding for this research.) The outcome measures included (a) treatment completion rates, (b) posttreatment drug use, and (c) posttreatment rearrest rates. The first measure was obtained from court records, the latter two from client interviews and statewide arrest records. In addition, Dr. Brown was charged with making an assessment of the appropriateness of treatment provided through the drug courts. It was left up to him to define appropriateness. Before the evaluation began, a meeting was held with drug court judges and other personnel. Dr. Brown solicited their input regarding the evaluation, and their cooperation was promised. It was decided that a similar meeting would be held each quarter.

The evaluation report found that two of the

state's drug courts did not meet the definition of a drug court, according to the standards of the Drug Courts Program Office (1997). A preliminary draft of the report had been shared with the two presiding judges. A meeting was held with the DLE administrator, personnel from both courts, and Dr. Brown. Both courts agreed to work toward meeting the standards, and DLE agreed to fund them for an additional year.

All of the drug courts were found to have higher treatment completion rates and lower rates of posttreatment drug use and rearrest than similar clients who went through the regular criminal courts. The two courts with the highest success rates also provided intensive probation supervision for clients, with probation caseloads about half the size of those in the other courts. Dr. Brown noted in his report that some of the differences were probably due to the fact that drug court clients were different, because many of them agreed to go to drug court in order to have their criminal records expunged at the completion of their treatment. This was very important for some clients, because a felony drug record would result in termination of employment.

Dr. Brown also noted that, although about half of the drug courts required acupuncture as a component of treatment, it had no appreciable effect on outcomes. In fact, Dr. Brown had heard several of the drug court clients complain about being required to "get stuck every week." His final report also recommended that acupuncture be voluntary, rather than mandatory, and that probation caseloads be reduced. DLE agreed and required all of the drug courts to implement those recommendations within 2 years as a condition of continued funding. (Before the year was over, however, a client sued one court because of the obligatory acupuncture. The client won, and the state supreme court administrator notified all drug courts to immediately make acupuncture voluntary.)

CASE 3: COMPREHENSIVE SERVICES FOR COCAINE-ADDICTED PROSTITUTES

Lucy Anderson, director of a private consulting firm, submitted a bid and won a contract with the county administrator to evaluate a state-funded program for cocaine-addicted prostitutes or Comprehensive Services for Cocaine-Addicted Prostitutes (CSCAP). The program provided employment counseling, job-readiness training, temporary shelter, and referral to substance abuse and mental health counseling to a group of about 40 streetwalking prostitutes. The agreement called for an assessment of the efficacy of each type of service provided, as well as outcome measures for each client (treatment completion, employment, recidivism, etc.). Information was obtained through agency records, police records, and client interviews. Six months into the evaluation, it appeared that the program was working very well. Most clients were in treatment and working at legitimate jobs.

Seven months into the evaluation, a sudden budget crisis befell the state, and funding for county social service programs was cut drastically. The county chose to eliminate the CSCAP program in order to continue funding a health care program for high-risk children. The women were given two weeks' notice that they would have to find other housing and that all of their services would be discontinued. Dr. Anderson's evaluation contract was also terminated, but she was given 90 days from the termination date to complete a report. She had made a preliminary assessment of the efficacy of the services, but the services no longer existed for these clients. She decided to continue tracking them, however, for the 90 days left in her contract. Because of their criminal justice system involvement, most were relatively easy to find. What her final report indicated was that, at the point that program funding was terminated, CSCAP seemed to be working. However, 3 months later, 43% of the clients were back on the street, engaged in prostitution, and using cocaine, and 37% were in jail or prison. Only 5% had managed to continue in legal employment. The rest had disappeared. Law enforcement and correctional services for these clients cost almost three times as much as the services that had been provided by CSCAP.

The report was well received by the county commission, but as they explained, they had to make a choice between funding a program for sick children or crack-using prostitutes. "It's a no-brainer," one of the commissioners stated in an interview with the local newspaper. The report was shared with the county's senior legislator in the state senate, but she was a member of the minority political party and had little influence with the committee that handled this particular budget. The program was never revived.

SEVEN SECRETS

1. Have the right *motivation*. In Case 1, both Dr. Jones and the school board had questionable motives for evaluating the delinquency prevention program. Dr. Jones was being pressured to get funding, and he was ready to jump at the first opportunity, whether it was right or wrong for him. The school board's motive was apparently to do a whitewash (Weiss, 1972). They told him at the beginning that he was expected to show that the program was successful. Given that caveat, he shouldn't have been surprised when the school board ignored his recommendations. In an ideal situation (such as Case 2), the motives of the evaluator and the funder are congruent and consistent with commonly accepted reasons for evaluating programs, such as determining a program's effort, effectiveness, or efficiency (Tripodi, 1983). Be aware that there are frequently reasons for doing an evaluation that don't meet these criteria. In addition to the whitewash, evaluations are sometimes undertaken as a way of torpedoing a program. In other instances someone may propose an evaluation simply as a way of delaying any changes in the program (Weiss, 1972).

2. Have *knowledge* of the program and the client population. Dr. Jones's lack of knowledge about delinquency gave the school board a perfect opportunity to undermine his recommendations regarding the delinquency prevention program. On the other hand, Dr. Brown's expertise (Case 2) in substance abuse and probation strengthened the funder's confidence in his recommendations. His familiarity with the justice system also led him to identify some possible sources of differences between drug court clients and other clients that could account for much of the variation in outcomes. In this particular state, anyone who held a professional license or certificate relating to employment would have had it revoked if convicted of a felony or a misdemeanor drug offense. Lawyers, doctors, nurses, realtors, teachers, and child care workers all had a strong incentive to choose and complete the drug court program in order to have their criminal records expunged. Dr. Anderson also had considerable experience working with justice system clients and with local law enforcement agencies. She located almost all of the women who had gone back into prostitution just by asking police officers.

3. *Plan* the evaluation as carefully as possible. This does not mean that there won't be changes during the course of the evaluation. Dr. Brown began the planning process as soon as he knew that federal funding was going to be available to evaluate drug courts. In fact, he was the person who alerted DLE to the possibility that funding was going to be available for this research. He actually lent DLE one of his graduate research assistants for a semester to help them write the federal grant proposal. When DLE was funded, they immediately thought of him as their first choice as an evaluator. When he began his study of the drug courts, he had prepared a very comprehensive Gantt chart that connected all activities with both resource allocations and time lines. This presents a stark contrast with Case 1, in which Dr. Jones began planning the evaluation only a week before the school board's decision. Because he knew very little about delinquency prevention, most of the week was spent hastily skimming the literature for ideas. If Dr. Jones had taken the time to have planned the evaluation thoughtfully, he might never have sought (and won) the contract.

4. Be *flexible*. In Case 3, Dr. Anderson had carefully planned and designed the CSCAP evaluation, but she abruptly changed the nature of the evaluation. It seemed to be the logical course of action. The evaluation question changed from "How effective is the program?" to "What happens to these clients without the program?" The sudden termination of the program was a sort of natural experiment that offered an opportunity to ask questions that were not possible to ask at the beginning of the study. Dr. Brown kept his methodology flexible enough to consider adjunctive therapies, such as acupuncture, and to eventually make recommendations about their use. Overhearing some clients' remarks about acupuncture led him to focus on some of the unanticipated consequences of the treatment. Dr. Jones missed an opportunity to modify his evaluation to look into possible reasons for the program's failure. Instead of using a black-box model, he could have

taken a limited number of external factors into consideration—such as the fact that students avoided the delinquency prevention program because it interfered with field trips. He also avoided dealing with the problem of stigmatization. Only a month or two into the school year, both students and teachers openly talked about the students in the delinquency prevention program as "juvenile delinquents" and "hoods." By the end of the year, the clients themselves were calling each other "JD." (Dr. Jones considered himself a quantitative researcher, and he was not particularly interested in questions that were perhaps best answered through qualitative research.) The issue of stigmatization was not mentioned in his final report.

5. Develop appropriate *relationships* with other actors in the task environment. Dr. Brown had worked with DLE administrators for several months prior to beginning the evaluation, and there was a strong element of trust in the relationship. DLE trusted Dr. Brown to carry out an objective, informative evaluation, and Dr. Brown trusted that DLE would take his recommendations seriously. Dr. Brown also began the evaluation by establishing a close working relationship with drug court staff. Dr. Jones's relationships with school personnel were practically nonexistent. He didn't know any of the school administrators prior to beginning the evaluation. Dr. Anderson had only the most formal and superficial relationship with county administrators. A closer relationship might have allowed her to avoid the surprise of an early termination of the program and its evaluation. Good relationships between the evaluator and program personnel may convince them to buy into the evaluation. The key is in convincing the staff that the evaluation will yield information that will in some way help them manage or improve the program. All evaluations are intrusive to some extent. They take staff time away from important functions, such as providing services to clients. A good initial relationship with the evaluators may minimize the staff's perception that the evaluation disrupts their routine. It may also socialize them to being receptive of feedback from the evaluators.

6. Know the *politics*. Dr. Anderson was un-

aware of the politics of county social services. Even the casual observer might have been aware of the strong possibility of budget cuts and of the relative priority of programs and services. In the local political environment, the choice of using limited funds for a program for sick kids rather than continuing a program for crack-addicted prostitutes really was a no-brainer. Dr. Jones also could have easily discovered that the delinquency prevention program he was selected to evaluate was the result of a political battle (school versus sheriff's department) over control of prevention resources. And he should have known from the beginning that the reputations of several school board members and administrators were riding on the success of this program. Dr. Brown was aware of the politics of the drug court program. (It was strongly opposed by state attorneys in two large metropolitan areas, because they believed it was "coddling criminals.") Dr. Brown refused to be drawn into the debate when a newspaper reporter ask to interview him regarding a drug court client who had suddenly stopped treatment, assaulted his probation officer, and robbed a liquor store. His only comment was, "It is too early in the evaluation to reach any conclusions." Some evaluations seem to be more fraught with political considerations. For instance, any evaluation of the DARE[2] program must be conducted in the context of a highly politicized social issue. The evaluator should recognize from the outset that most, if not all, of the participants already have made up their minds about the effectiveness of DARE, and the facts from an evaluation are not likely to change many of those opinions. In many cases, DARE has become an ideology and, therefore, not subject to scientific questioning.

7. Know how to appropriately *disseminate* the evaluation report. Much good advice has been given elsewhere about writing an evaluation report (Royse, Thyer, Padgett, & Logan, 2001) and about the dissemination of research (Harrison & McNeece, 2001). The most effective way to disseminate the results of a program evaluation depends on the target audience and what that audience hopes to achieve. Dr. Brown released his report to an agency that was eager to ensure that the drug court programs achieved max-

imum effectiveness. They had encouraged him to make recommendations about improving the program, and they acted on those recommendations. Dr. Jones, on the other hand, made a terrible mistake by releasing a copy of his report to the newspaper. There were other organizations in the community (the sheriff's department) that might have been able to use the report in a more effective way to lobby for appropriate changes in the program. Dr. Anderson's sharing of her report (indirectly) with a state legislator was an exercise in futility. (There actually was a sympathetic member of the majority party on that same committee who would have used the information to try to convince the governor that eliminating such programs across the state was penny-wise and pound-foolish.) The format of the report can also make a tremendous difference. In my experience, one should not present a report replete with numbers and Greek letters to a legislative committee (or city council, county commission, etc.), unless it is accompanied by color-coded pie charts or bar graphs that lend themselves to easy interpretation.

SUMMARY

Evaluation is as much an artistic as a technological process. Even the best evaluation, based on its scientific and technological merits, may be a complete waste of effort if the political context is not taken into account, the motives of the relevant parties are not understood, and the evaluator has not carefully planned the evaluation and taken care to establish good working relationships with all concerned parties. The answer to the question "Does it work?" is much more complex than one might think, even when objectives have been clearly identified. The DARE program works, in the sense that parents feel good about doing something to prevent drug abuse, school officials feel safer having a police presence in the schools, and police like having a more positive relationship with schools. The question of whether DARE reduces substance abuse may not be the central concern of "Does it work?"

Notes

1. Gantt charts are bar graphs that help plan and monitor project development or resource allocation on a horizontal time scale.
2. Drug Abuse Resistance Education.

References

Drug Courts Program Office. (1997). *Defining drug courts: The key components.* Washington DC: U.S. Department of Justice, Office of Justice Programs.

Harrison, D. F., & McNeece, C. A. (2001). Disseminating research findings. In B. A. Thyer (Ed.), *The handbook of social work research methods.* Thousand Oaks, CA: Sage.

Royse, D., Thyer, B. A., Padgett, D. K., & Logan, T. K. (2001). *Program evaluation: An introduction* (3rd ed.). Belmont, CA: Brooks/Cole–Wadsworth Thompson Learning.

Tripodi, T. (1983). *Evaluative research for social workers.* Englewood Cliffs, NJ: Prentice Hall.

Weiss, C. H. (1972). *Evaluation research: Methods of assessing program effectiveness.* Englewood Cliffs, NJ: Prentice Hall.

64

INTEGRATING PROGRAM EVALUATION AND ORGANIZATION DEVELOPMENT

Charles McClintock

The fields of program evaluation and organization development (OD) have existed on parallel paths for the past 50 years or so, with relatively little contact. OD evolved mainly in the corporate sector as a means of improving organizations through humanizing systems of work. Program evaluation emerged largely from the public sector, with an emphasis on accountability and performance (Campbell & McClintock, 2002). Each profession faces a comparable challenge of integrating key skills, practices, and values from the other. Program evaluation has empirical methods as its core competency. Although the field's commitment is to provide data about program performance, it has evolved to include the utilization of evaluation results for program improvement. The OD field rests on skills for group, organization, and system change. Humanistic and inquiry values lie at the core of these efforts, but they are increasingly expected to empirically document the outcomes of change interventions.

This chapter identifies ways in which each profession can incorporate the core competencies of the other to support organizational learning. For program evaluators, this change means using empirical methods in ways that involve organizational and community stakeholders in opportunities for shared understanding and achieving desired change. For OD professionals, the challenge is to incorporate empirical methods such as surveys, case studies, and experiments as a means of learning and strengthening accountability for results. Integrating the skills and goals of the two professions yields a model of organizational learning based on evaluative in-

quiry (Preskill & Torres, 1999; Rowe, 2002; Waclawski & Church, 2002). The term *OD evaluation* summarizes this ideal and is meant to identify professional practice that integrates empirical activities into change interventions from the outset to the finish.

When linking evaluation and OD, it is important to avoid idealized rational models of organizational learning that are unlikely to be found in practice. The notion of the continuously changing and learning organization is often a fiction that is not feasible, given the limits of human dynamics, resources, or political constraints. In fact, Weick and Westley (2001) argue that organizational learning can be thought of as an oxymoron, in that the process of organizing requires order, stability, and formalization, whereas learning requires forms of disorder such as questioning existing arrangements, experimentation, and ongoing dialogue.

However, organizing need not require rigid systems, and learning need not be associated with continuous or fundamental change. March (1991) notes a distinction between learning as exploring and exploiting. Evaluating interventions in an organizational context that favors exploration would focus on reflecting on assumptions, values, goals, and structures. This is a broad-based type of inquiry often associated with organizations engaged in strategic planning or a search for significant innovations. When the organizational context is more bureaucratic, with well-defined rules, structures, and roles, it is possible to exploit these existing routines by evaluating small variations aimed at making them more cost-effective. Part of the task for the

OD evaluator is to find various locations on this continuum of exploration of new alternatives to exploitation of existing programs, from which to encourage data-based learning.

STRATEGIES AND SKILLS FOR OD EVALUATION

Historically in the field of program evaluation, there has been a distinction between summative and formative evaluation, in which the former approach is concerned with determining the program's impact on specified outcomes and costs, and the latter emphasizes program improvement (McClintock, 1986). Summative evaluation seeks to make causal inferences that link program activities to outcomes. Formative evaluation is more concerned with improving the program's capacity to achieve outcomes than with proving that it was the program that produced them. Similar research methods might be used for either approach, but formative evaluation would include methods for individual, team, and organizational learning based on evaluation findings.

OD professionals seeking to employ evaluative inquiry in the spirit of formative evaluation can rely on several comprehensive treatments of the field that include step-by-step methods and practices (e.g., Patton, 1997; Preskill & Torres, 1999). In contrast, the following strategies and skills represent four key challenges for the practice and long-term success of OD evaluation—assessing the context, developing a model for data collection, integrating OD evaluation with organizational and program learning needs, and developing skills needed by the OD evaluator.

Assessing the Context of OD Evaluation

Assessing the context for an OD evaluation provides a framework that will guide all subsequent activities. Significant aspects of context include the history of the program or organization, change in executive leadership or other issues of power and coalition, what is known from theory and practice about how to accomplish the intended improvement, and specific information needs for program improvement from the intended users of evaluative inquiry. It is important to assess the context based on considerable

professional experience in the area of change as well as knowledge of theory and research that pertain to the issue, to ensure accurate appraisal. OD evaluation is likely to be more expensive than traditional stand-alone OD or program evaluation efforts, hence the need for the careful consideration of context.

An example from the nonprofit sector illustrates one approach to assessing context (McClintock, 2003). In this hypothetical case, an evaluation has been requested for a sex education program to reduce teen pregnancy and sexually transmitted disease. The context issue in this case is whether to focus the evaluation on the sex education program or on a broader collaboration among a group of community agencies that can help improve youth health and development—for example, schools, parents, community agencies, business, and the local media might address education, employment, and recreation opportunities for youth, as well as their needs for information and services related to sexuality.

A dilemma facing single human service programs is that, by themselves, they account for a small portion of the variance in outcomes, yet they draw a disproportionate share of the attention. There is a 40-year history of efforts to address this stark reality of social policy and human service programs, variously referred to as service integration, coordination, and collaboration (Marquart & Konrad, 1996). In this case, adolescent sexuality is complex and not readily or substantially influenced by any single initiative. Undesirable outcomes are driven by a broad array of forces: socioeconomic structure, culture, media, geography, and family and community resources, not to mention the "gentle" dynamics of adolescent human development.

OD evaluation that focuses on this kind of community collaboration is not simple, but it is more likely to honestly address what is required to achieve desired goals. Basing this analysis of context on research and practice knowledge strengthens its chances of producing desired change. Figure 64.1 depicts a diagram showing the factors involved in collaboration in the human services based on knowledge from research and practice (McClintock, 1998).

The diagram in Figure 64.1 helps the evaluator orient to those general aspects of collaboration that need attention in this particular situation (e.g., internal alignment factors among collaborators that might be considered in imple-

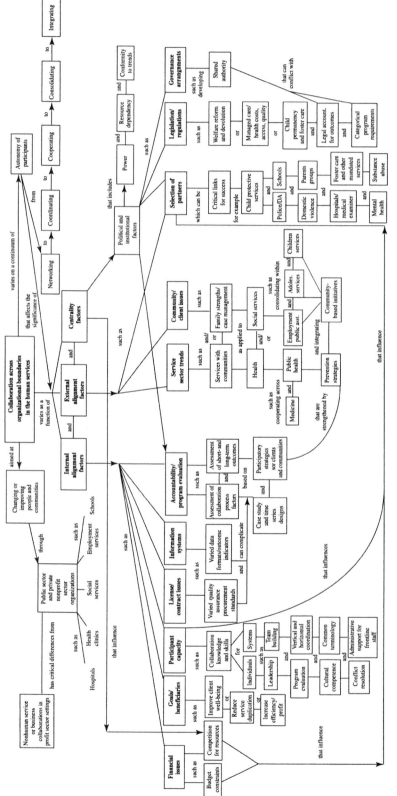

FIGURE 64.1 Example of context for organization development evaluation: research and practitioner knowledge about collaboration.

menting collaboration, centrality of the collaboration in the community context to gain support, external alignment issues such as building on a family strengths model). Each of the factors deemed to be critical in this context might be a focus of evaluation and OD activity.

Developing a Model for OD Evaluation Data Collection

We use models to help us conceptualize and visualize the otherwise unseen dimensions of organizations and programs, and to identify the key means and ends that will be the focus of OD evaluation. One approach to creating a program model is to diagram its values, inputs, processes, and outputs/outcomes and their interconnections through concept maps and diagrams. Figure 64.2 shows a concept map that was used to guide data collection for a hospice seeking to improve its services and outcomes (McClintock, 1990b). The map was developed from research literature, input from hospice professionals, and interviews with agency staff, volunteers, and client caregivers. The resulting diagram organizes hospice care into hierarchically related concepts, including the guiding assumptions (top row of concepts), service components or care activities (middle three rows of concepts), and the causal processes by which hospice is expected to affect client outcomes (bottom row of concepts). Questionnaire and interview guides were developed keyed to each of the concepts in Figure 64.2. The concept map also served as a means of dialogue about the data and a basis for planned change to improve hospice services. The time involved at the outset of the study in developing this model was rewarded by gathering data of greatest value to those who would use the information as a basis for program improvement.

Integrating OD Evaluation With Organizational and Program Learning Needs

Organization and program learning can be thought of as optimal combinations of disorder and disorder such that systematic inquiry is sustained while new alternatives are explored. (Weick & Westley, 2001). This view is similar to a conception of formative evaluation that combines uncertainty reduction about program performance through evaluative inquiry with

uncertainty enhancement through questioning assumptions, values, and structures (McClintock, 1986). Both views recognize that organizing requires stability and question answering, whereas learning requires variability and question raising. How might these notions of organizational and program learning be linked to OD evaluation?

Based on my previous research (McClintock, 1990a), I developed a framework to categorize a wide range of organizing and evaluation activities found in corporate and nonprofit settings. The framework combines three forms of OD with three ways in which evaluation results are used and serves as a basis for integrating OD evaluation with organizational and program learning.

Organization Development Activities

OD has many definitions and theoretical as well as practitioner underpinnings. It is a concept and practice that intersects with related fields such as industrial/organizational psychology, human resource development, and organizational theory and behavior. From its conceptual founding in the work of Kurt Lewin to more recent treatments, OD has stressed group process, systemic intervention, humanistic values, and action-based research (Waclawski & Church, 2002). Three main activity foci that relate to organizational learning are proposed, on the basis of this long history and wide range of concepts and practices.

- *Exchanging and coordinating:* Organizations are faced with fragmentation, redundancy, information overload, and unpredictable streams of attention and energy from employees (Cohen, March, & Olsen, 1972). Groups and individuals seek cost-effective ways of exchanging information and coordinating with others that will inform, stimulate, and convince them to pay attention to a particular issue. Exchange and coordination may be formalized through coalitions and ongoing processes for exploring and affirming basic values and purposes, with the ultimate purpose of identifying underlying concepts and commitments that will guide individual and collective action.
- *Deciding and acting:* Notwithstanding rational models of decision making in which many alternatives are carefully evaluated

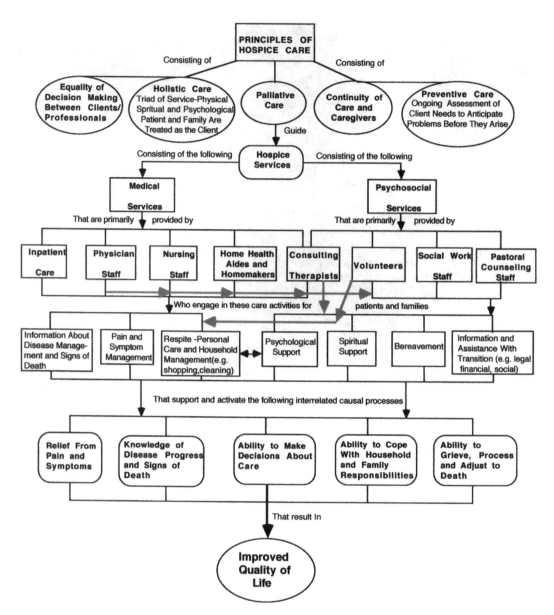

FIGURE 64.2 A Model for OD Evaluation Data Collection in Hospice Care.

prior to calculated choice, the social psychological basis of action and decision often requires that options be narrowed or simplified and attention directed to a single alternative (Brunnson, 1982). Organizations make use of standard operating procedures, formalized goals, constraints, and regular reminders as ways of narrowing alternatives and stimulating decision and action. The dynamic of deciding and acting is to prioritize, align, focus attention, and reduce resistance to change,

but ideally to do so in a spirit of experimentation where action is viewed as the operational definition of a hypothesis that can be revised.

• *Monitoring and evaluating:* Organizations are expected to account for the resources they use—to boards, auditors, stockholders, and stakeholders—and to identify the resulting outcomes and benefits (Wholey, 2001). This can be a very difficult task, especially in nonprofit organizations, because resources are usually not allocated in terms of program objectives, implementation easily diverges from plans, and there is often disagreement about what outcomes to measure or how to operationally define them. The tasks associated with monitoring and evaluating consist of scanning the environment for external influences, using participatory and multiple methods of inquiry to design studies and to gather and interpret findings, and clarifying accountability for program change and improvement.

Uses of Evaluation Findings

Leviton and Hughes (1981) describe three strategic uses for evaluation findings: (a) conceptual use that educates about new ways of defining problems and solutions, (b) instrumental use that focuses on improving programs and can function to motivate change, and (c) symbolic use in which information helps persuade people. Leadership in organizations can be thought of in a similar way as a process for managing cultures of learning that will educate, motivate, and symbolize meaning (Barrett, 1995; Bennis, 1989).

- *Educating:* This function can include processes for reviewing program history and context, assessing stakeholders' information needs, and clarifying implicit models of change and implementation that will lead to action experiments. The data-driven approaches to OD would include a wide range of empirical methods to scan the environment, make comparisons across programs as well as within programs over time, and make use of data from information systems, archives, surveys, and interviews. The overall aim of this kind of evaluation use is enlightenment and learning.
- *Motivating:* A second main use of evaluation findings is sometimes referred to as instrumental, wherein data are directly applied to program change and improvement. Motivation is a linking concept that focuses on engaging individual energy and collective action to produce change. Creating coalitions, clarifying priorities, making action plans, and engaging individuals in data collection, monitoring, and feedback are important means–ends activities in this area.
- *Persuading:* Evaluation findings are often used to persuade others through the symbolic activities of assessing vision and mission. Af-

firming values, creating a culture of learning through dialogue, aligning actions with espoused beliefs, dealing with resistance to change and fear of negative evaluation findings, and assigning accountability for change are all important aspects of the persuasive form of evaluation use. It is also important to provide the resources necessary to support program success if people are going to be persuaded that change will be meaningful.

Table 64.1 shows the nine-cell conceptual framework that combines evaluation use with OD. The OD evaluation activities are shown in each cell. This framework integrates OD and evaluation in support of organizational learning.

Developing Skills for OD Evaluation

There is considerable overlap between the principles of good practice in evaluation and OD (Rowe, 2002), yet there are few education and training programs that attempt to develop both skill sets in the same individual. The OD evaluator would possess core skills from each profession, as shown in Table 64.2. For program evaluation, these would be empirical methods skills such as using research designs and methods of sampling to make comparisons and render judgments of causality; employing empirical methods for gathering data and making representations of reality; and using statistical, simulation, and qualitative methods for analyzing data and substantiating interpretations or conclusions. OD core skills would consist of establishing trusting and respectful relationships, effective communications, diagnostics, and facility with motivation and change dynamics, whether aimed at individuals, groups, organizations, or communities.

CONCLUSION

This brief overview of ways to integrate program evaluation and OD rests on a broader vision of professional development and aspiration. Each profession has a technical core of expertise that defines its competence and societal privilege. Yet, making a difference in the world and not just in one's technical role as a practitioner requires the capacity to act in ways that have a broader systemic view. For example, access to quality health care is part of the context of every

TABLE 64.1. A Framework for Integrating Organization Development and Evaluation Activities

Use of Evaluation Findings

	Educate/ Explore	Motivate/ Apply	Persuade/ Symbolize
Organization Development Activities Exchange/ Coordinate	Review the history of the program or reasons for the intervention. Identify information needs of different stakeholders. Clarify implicit models that underlie change and program implementation. 1	Create coalitions among people with related interests. Link individual and program goals. Write plans for achieving cross-unit or collaborative goals. 2	Affirm values, people, and futures through appreciative inquiry. Create a culture that supports learning. Assess areas most ready for evaluation and change. 3
Decide/ Act	Identify change goals and decisions that are needed. Synthesize and contrast ideas across groups. Explore process variations as action experiments. 4	Clarify priorities and incentives for change. Convene decision and action plan groups. Identify types of data most likely to be valued by program members. 5	Align actions with espoused beliefs. Clarify resources necessary for program success. Work on resistance to change related to negative evaluation findings. 6
Monitor/ Evaluate	Scan for external influences and trends. Design comparisons across programs and/or within them over time. Use information systems archives and survey/interview data. 7	Engage program members in inquiry tasks. Monitor critical success factors in implementation. Provide feedback on program improvement activities. 8	Use multiple methods to portray inquiry findings. Convene dialogue about evaluation implications. Assign accountability for program change and improvement. 9

physician's daily work. CEO business decisions play a critical role in the stability of employee and retiree families and communities. In addition, doctors, lawyers, teachers, and social workers all function simultaneously as change agents and evaluators of their interventions.

The OD evaluator envisioned here represents this combination of technical and social orientations and is captured by the phrase *scholar–practitioner* (McClintock, in press). This term expresses an ideal of professional excellence grounded in theory and research, informed by experiential knowledge, and motivated by personal values, political commitments, and ethical conduct. Scholar–practitioners are committed to the well-being of clients and colleagues, to learning new ways of being effective, and to conceptualizing their work in relation to broader organizational, community, political, and cultural contexts. Scholar–practitioners explicitly reflect upon and assess the impact of their work. Their professional activities and the knowledge they

TABLE 64.2 Skills for OD Evaluation

Empirical Methods Skills

Applying research designs and methods of sampling to make comparisons and cause–effect claims	Employing empirical methods for gathering data, measuring, and making representations of reality	Using statistical, simulation, and qualitative methods for analyzing data and drawing conclusions

Organization Development Skills
(for individuals, groups, organizations, or communities)

Establishing trusting and respectful relationships	Engaging in effective communications	Applying diagnostic models and methods	Using motivation and change dynamics

develop are based on collaborative and relational learning through active exchange in communities of practice and scholarship.

The fields of program evaluation and OD have developed along separate paths for the past 50 years. It can be hoped that integrating these fields around the ideal of the scholar–practitioner will not take as long a period of time.

References

Barrett, F. J. (1995). Creating appreciative learning cultures. *Organizational Dynamics, 24*(2), 36–48.

Bennis, W. (1989). *Why leaders can't lead.* San Francisco: Jossey-Bass.

Brunnson, N. (1982). The irrationality of action and action rationality: Decisions, ideologies and organizational actions. *Journal of Management Studies, 19,* 29–44.

Cohen, M. D., March, J. G., & Olsen, J. P. (1972). A garbage can model of organizational choice. *Administrative Science Quarterly, 17,* 1–25.

Leviton, L. D., & Hughes, E. F. (1981). Research on the utilization of evaluation: A review and synthesis. *Evaluation Review, 5,* 525–548.

March, J. G. (1991). Exploration and exploitation in organizational learning. *Organization Science, 2,* 71–87.

Marquart, J. M., & Konrad, E. L. (Eds.). (1996). *New directions for program evaluation: No. 69. Evaluating initiatives to integrate human services.* San Francisco: Jossey-Bass.

McClintock, C. (1986). Toward a theory of formative evaluation. In D. S. Cordray & M. W. Lipsey (Eds.), *Evaluation studies review annual, Vol. 11* (pp. 205–223). Beverly Hills, CA: Sage. (Reprinted from *New Directions for Continuing Education, 24,* 77–95,)

McClintock, C. (1990a). Administrators as applied theorists. In L. Bickman (Ed.), *New directions for program evaluation: No. 47. Advances in program theory* (pp. 19–33). San Francisco: Jossey-Bass.

McClintock, C. (1990b). Evaluators as applied theorists. *Evaluation Practice, 11,* 1–14.

McClintock, C. (1998, Spring). Cross-agency collaboration: Research findings and practitioner experience. In C. McClintock (Ed.), *Healthy communities: Concepts and collaboration tools.* New York State College of Human Ecology Policy Perspectives Seminar.

McClintock, C. (2003). The evaluator as scholar practitioner change agent. *American Journal of Evaluation, 24*(1), 91–96.

McClintock, C. (2003). The scholar-practitioner. In A. DiStefano, K. Rudestam, & R. Silverman (Eds.), *Encyclopedia of distributed learning.* Thousand Oaks, CA: Sage.

Patton, M. Q. (1997). *Utilization-focused evaluation: The new century text* (3rd ed.). Thousand Oaks, CA: Sage.

Preskill, H., & Torres, R. (1999). *Evaluative inquiry for learning in organizations.* Thousand Oaks, CA: Sage.

Rowe, W. (2002, November 7). *Integrating evaluation and organizational development: New standards and competencies for evaluation professionals.*

Paper presented at meeting of the American Evaluation Association, Washington, DC. Available from Fielding Graduate Institute, Santa Barbara, CA.

Waclawski, J., & Church, A. H. (Eds.). (2002). *Organization development: A data-driven approach to organizational change*. San Francisco: Jossey-Bass.

Weick, K. D., & Westley, F. (2001). Organizational learning: Affirming an oxymoron. In S. T. Clegg, C. Hardy, & W. R. Nord (Eds.), *Handbook of organization studies*. Thousand Oaks, CA: Sage.

Wholey, J. S. (2001). Managing for results: Roles for evaluators in a new management era. *American Journal of Evaluation, 22*(2), 343–347.

65 PROCESS VERSUS OUTCOME EVALUATION

Michael J. Smith

The field of program evaluation consists of broad concepts that are descriptive and overlapping, but nonetheless useful. The distinction between process and outcome evaluation is a case in point. So is the distinction between process evaluation and program monitoring, and outcome evaluation and impact assessment. The inconsistencies and overlap between these terms can be a source of confusion and annoyance for both the beginning student and the expert evaluator. Nevertheless, they provide a rich context and a way to organize your approach to evaluation.

PROCESS EVALUATIONS

In program evaluation, process evaluation activities are related to identifying targets, determining if the program conforms to its design, examining issues of program implementation in the initial design, and testing programs. As such, process evaluations are essential to a quality program-planning process. Because evaluation is not always tied to the early stages of program development, one might assume that many program planning and development processes are flawed because a process evaluation has not been conducted.

Process evaluations are characterized by more informal types of research design and data collection. This could include collecting qualitative data on the program while it is in progress, use of agency reports, small surveys, and other informal types of data collection, such as some direct observation of the program. All or some of these data collection strategies could be used to examine what goes on inside the program. Process evaluations are more *descriptive* about the program rather than being *predictive* about the program's achievement of its goals and outcomes. The descriptive areas of the program can be how many people are attending or participating, the interventions or activities of the program, issues in the planning and implementation of the program, staff activities and practices, and client response to the initial program efforts.

Process evaluations are closely related to another evaluation activity, *program monitoring*. In fact, experts in the field of program evaluation say that process evaluations and program monitoring may be indistinguishable. One possible distinction is that process evaluation is a one-time activity, whereas program monitoring is ongoing (Rossi, Freeman & Lipsey, 1998, p. 67).

Program monitoring focuses on what is happening in the program and assesses program operations. Was the projected need for the program substantiated by people who showed up to use the service? Is there a need for the program? Is there a program design? What is the design? Is it a good one? Is the design appropriate for those served? The purposes of monitoring include determining whether the program is being implemented as planned, which outreach methods are being used to get people into the program, how many clients are being seen, whether people are connecting to the program, and whether they are getting services.

Program monitoring is achieved through a number of informal methods that might include, for example, making use of agency data about the program and determining if the program reached its intended audience or target population. Did the program serve those it was supposed to serve? What are the patterns of program use and utilization? What changes have taken place since the program was implemented? Monitoring studies often look at data from the organization's management information system to help determine how many in the target population the program is reaching, what treatment is being given, and so on.

One way to distinguish process evaluation from program monitoring might be related to the depth of data collected. Process evaluations can produce more in-depth, qualitative descriptions that give a flavor of how the program or intervention is being delivered, whereas program monitoring utilizes more structured data about the program.

EXAMPLE OF A PROCESS EVALUATION STUDY

The overlap between the methodologies and purposes of process evaluations and program monitoring studies can be seen in this example. Program administrators for a comprehensive, on-site program of social, health, and senior services to the elderly requested a program evaluation. The goal of the program was to help seniors live independently and prevent nursing home placement for residents residing in a naturally occurring retirement community (NORC), a co-op housing program with a high

concentration of seniors. The program evaluators had to decide what type of program evaluation to conduct.

A process evaluation rather than an outcome evaluation was chosen because the purpose was descriptive rather than predictive. Because not enough information was available about what the program did and how it worked, the purpose of the study was to develop thorough descriptions of the program model and its components, to assess program planning and implementation, and to identify program and outcome variables that could be used in later outcome-oriented evaluations. Process evaluations are more formative studies that are usually a first step along the road to the development of goal or outcome evaluations.

A process evaluation was planned because the primary data sources were descriptive and qualitative. Program evaluators conducted in-person interviews with staff, using primarily open-ended questions. This allowed staff to provide thorough descriptions of program processes and how the program worked. Qualitative interviews were also conducted with selected seniors who had used a full range of services from the program to get the client's perspective on program services. Because the primary type of data was qualitative, the study more clearly fit the definition of a process evaluation. If the data collected and analyzed were more structured and quantitative, the study might be more appropriately classified as a program monitoring study.

In fact, these qualitative data sources were supplemented with additional, more structured data, such as data from the agency's client and management information system. These were data on the characteristics of the seniors served and the types of services received. If the primary source of data was structured or closed-ended interviews of staff and clients with rating scales and yes/no checklists, supplemented with data from the agency information system, the study would more correctly be labeled a program monitoring evaluation.

VALUE OF A PROCESS EVALUATION

Process evaluations are especially useful in documenting the subtle factors that might make the program a success. For example, in the evaluation of services to seniors in the cooperative housing program, researchers asked program staff about the program philosophy and goals. Analysis of the qualitative data and direct quotes from program staff reflected their perceptions of program purposes and goals, revealing their strong commitment and dedication to the goals of the program and their enthusiasm and commitment in working together to prevent nursing home placement:

Working together to keep the clients at home, safe, in a livable manner. We're not big on nursing homes. . . . We pool our heads to keep them at home.

To keep clients at home is our main goal and we are all committed to that. To keep them safe and at home.

People stay in their own homes as long as possible. Homebound people can stay here and not be placed in nursing homes. It's great, especially for people whose families live far away.

In addition to goals and philosophy, one social worker gave a good description of comprehensive, community-based services:

[Our goal is] to help the elderly function in the community and give them community supports. We educate the elderly about services. We give them a lot of service. We are involved with nurses, lawyers, their relatives. We help assist the hospital social workers whose caseloads are high. We quiet down our clients. We make phone calls to reassure them.

We offer case management, case assistance, advocacy; we'll get people Pampers, assist them with will writing. . . . We've got nurses here. We can get people physical or occupational therapists. We can get them home care or assistance with daily living. We make sure they have enough food. If they can't go out, we make sure the housekeeper gets food or we get volunteers to get food. On two or three occasions, I've gone out and bought food myself.

Documentation of a community of workers and a community spirit between workers and seniors was something that could be described well through a process evaluation. "We have great communication between the staff and the seniors. Accessible services. A genuine concern. We have a tight community here. Everyone watches out for each other. There's an openness and innovation. Let's try this or that. Seniors are actively involved in doing things, planning and help setting up programs."

When asked what makes this NORC program distinctive from other programs, staff also provided data on program features and components of the program model. For instance, concerning on-site services, staff said, "We have doctors' offices in the housing complex and the hospitals have outpatient departments within a few blocks. Our services are all in one spot. As a tenant, you have lived here all your life. You are used to one geographic area and you don't have to move."

Likewise, workers provided excellent descriptions of each of the services provided, including case management services, security services at the co-op, home care, financial management, discharge planning, day treatment, medical services, nursing care, psychiatric services, casework counseling, bill paying, and legal services. The qualitative interviews with program staff and the seniors served provided thorough descriptions of the services and how they were used. This added greatly to the documentation of the program model and its components in this process evaluation.

OUTCOME EVALUATIONS

If the program has had some time to mature and achieve its goals, and we have already conducted process evaluations or program monitoring studies, we might move to conducting goal-oriented or *outcome evaluation* studies. Outcome evaluations focus on what happens to clients or patients after their participation in the program (Weiss, 1997, p. 32). These studies focus on assessing program goals or outcomes, the program's level of success, its usefulness, and its failures. What are the goals and outcomes the program is trying to achieve? What other outcomes might have also happened (unanticipated or serendipitous goals or outcomes)? The data for these studies could include the ratings by clients of whether or not they thought certain goals or outcomes were achieved. Because the goals of many programs include increasing knowledge, improving attitudes and behavior, increasing skills, or changing a condition in a person, outcome evaluations often make use of pre-post data.

Just as process evaluations are closely aligned with program monitoring studies, outcome evaluations are closely related to *impact assessment* studies. Impact assessments are more formal research designs to show that it was the intervention and not some other factors that caused the effect or outcome. Impact assessments "usually compare information for participants and non-participants to tease out the effects of the program or they can use repeat measures over time with program participants to determine if the program is achieving its goals" (Rossi, Freeman, & Lipsey, 1992, p. 236). Impact assessments usually employ experimental and quasi-experimental designs to help fulfill these criteria. Experimental designs are those in which participants are randomly assigned to a treatment group, a control group, or to different types of treatment groups. Quasi-experimental designs study the group in the program and then try to find a sample of similar clients who are not in the program. Impact assessments are the most rigorous types of designs and the most summative types of studies, in which researchers hope to uncover the true or net effects of the program.

EXAMPLE OF AN OUTCOME EVALUATION STUDY

In the study of the NORC program of comprehensive services to seniors living in a co-op housing program, there are a number of possibilities in terms of outcome studies. If the goal of services is provision of services that are pleasing to the clients served, then client satisfaction surveys (in which seniors rate the types of services they have received) could be used as an initial measure of outcome. Consumer satisfaction surveys are probably somewhere between program monitoring and outcome evaluation. Given the large variety of senior services that were provided in the NORC program, seniors could be involved in rating their overall satisfaction with services and with rating individual services that were provided. They could rate the quality of home care services provided, the degree to which they were engaged with their case managers, their use of co-op security staff, their use of financial management services, access to medical services, use of nursing services, and so on. The data produced could examine average ratings for each service and overall ratings of the program. Analysis could then separate the seniors in this group into types (in terms of functional ability, seriousness of medical diagnosis, involvement of family, etc.) to determine which types of seniors rated services higher or lower.

For example, if seniors with greater deficits in their ability to perform activities of daily living were receiving more services that they rated highly than seniors who needed less assistance in such activities, we could make some educated guesses that services were at least directed toward cases in which nursing home placements may have been prevented. This would be a first step on the road to outcome assessment.

Another form of outcome evaluation would be to have clients rate whether or not the program achieved certain goals. Questions asked might include, for example, "Did the program help you get medical care?" "Did the program prevent isolation by providing contact or telephone reassurance?" "Did the program help you pay bills and keep your finances straight?" "Were emergency services available?" Essentially, clients would be rating the degree to which program goals were achieved.

A later and somewhat less subjective approach to outcome evaluation would be a pre- and pre-post services study in which clients were surveyed before services were received and then at a later date, when substantial services were in place. Pre- and post-measures can be taken on a variety of standardized scales and indices. For example, evaluators could study feelings of isolation, anxiety over the increased frailties of old age, feeling safe and secure at home, depression, and worries about the future to see if there were reductions in isolation, anxiety, depression, and worries about the future, and increases in safety and security. So, for example, results could show that, on a 20-point scale, feelings of isolation had an average score of 15.5 before services were received but decreased to 9.5 after the senior received a year of comprehensive services.

If the researchers planned an impact assessment study, they would employ an experimental or quasi-experimental design. For example, in a quasi-experimental design, we could conduct a post services or a pre-post study on the group in the comprehensive services program. We could also select a housing site with similar clients who do not have a NORC comprehensive service program. We could study both groups over time to determine if, for example, the nursing home placement rate was lower for those in the NORC program. Although we could not assume that the two groups of clients are similar, we could also study their functional abilities on an Activities of Daily Living Scale, dementia rates, number of family members involved, level of depression, and so on. If we found no differences in the characteristics of the seniors on these variables, we could assert with more confidence that it was the program services that created a reduction in nursing home placement.

Whether it is process evaluation or program monitoring, outcome evaluation or impact assessment, the type of program evaluation selected may be less important then getting into the evaluation game. Feedback and data from staff and clients can only result in more productive program planning processes and improved, more creative programming and interventions.

References

Rossi, P., Freeman, H., & Lipsey, M. (1998). *Evaluation: A systematic approach.* Thousand Oaks, CA: Sage.

Weiss, C. (1997). *Evaluation: Methods for studying programs and policies.* Upper Saddle River, NJ: Prentice Hall.

66 DATA QUALITY FOR INTERNATIONAL SERVICE EVALUATION

Natalia E. Pane

SUMMARY

As the call for greater accountability spreads, so does the need for high-quality data. But how do you ensure good data if you are not the one collecting it? This chapter and the one that follows offer some contextual information and give some practical tips on how to improve data quality based on practices within the U.S. federal government agencies and national organizations.

Data Quality for International Service Evaluation begins by presenting some contextual information and the role of evaluation. We then turn to examine the fundamental change agents, humans, and the factors that drive change within us.

The next chapter offers practice-based examples of data-quality improvement procedures, including a discussion of suggestions for displaying data, a critical aspect of data use. Finally, this chapter closes with some lessons learned.

Many of the examples in both chapters are drawn from the author's work assisting clients undergoing significant organizational change, particularly the U.S. Department of Education (the Department). The views expressed throughout this chapter do not represent the Department or any other group, but reflect the author's individual thoughts and experiences.

WHAT IS ALL THIS ACCOUNTABILITY STUFF?

Accountability is the word of the day. Leaders in the public and private sectors want to see proof that their funds are having an effect. The way to assess whether there has been an effect is to collect data about it. Accountability, by definition, means that data are being collected. The data are then assessed, and that assessment yields a decision about further funding.

Yet, today's accountability is not—and does not have to be—simply another wave of post hoc evaluations that come too late, draw inaccurate conclusions, and leave programs misunderstood and ultimately cut from funding due to poor decision making. When accountability comes only at the end and from outside a program, it serves only as a deterrent to others and is about as effective as the death penalty in deterring behavior (i.e., arguably ineffective).

WHAT ARE ALL THESE DATA FOR?

Accountability can be a system in which funding agents hold their funded programs accountable for collecting and using information to manage their programs better. Because both groups have agreed that the goals of the program were important, the area that can be changed is how the program is implemented, and data can be incredibly useful there.

Data managers today are talking about performance management: Data are collected and immediately used to inform local decisions and improve local management without any overall evaluative judgment on the program. Data are collected and used as a regular part of program management, monthly, weekly, daily. If results show that an aspect of the program is not working, it gets changed. If another aspect appears to be working, it gets replicated.

ACCOUNTABILITY IS ABOUT KNOWING WHAT IS OCCURRING AND IMPROVING MANAGEMENT ON THE BASIS OF THAT KNOWLEDGE, NOT ABOUT MAKING QUICK EVALUATIVE (GOOD/BAD) CONCLUSIONS

A simple example of performance management would be monitoring and adjusting your progress on a cross-country U.S. trip. Your goal is to go from New Jersey to California, roughly 3,000 miles, in 6 days. Each day, you track the miles you have gone, which is your one key performance measure. You expect to go 500 miles a day, but the first 2 days, due to bad weather, you travel only 500 miles total, one sixth of your trip. But you have used two days, one third of your travel time. So, you adjust by increasing your mile-per-day goal to 700, so you can still achieve your goal.

If you did not track your mileage, you might not be aware of the delay and be able to readjust your daily goals accordingly. Performance management necessitates a stream of data, and that data had better be reliable and valid or you might be making the wrong management decisions.

WHAT ARE HIGH-QUALITY DATA?

There used to be an advertisement for a high-resolution printer that showed a picture of a tree. The caption read something like "With *their* printer, you see a tree. With *our* printer, you see a bonsai." If you then looked at the picture again, you would notice that there were ladybugs on the tree. You then realized that the proportion of ladybugs to the tree suggested that, indeed, this tree was not a full-sized tree in a forest, but rather a bonsai or dwarf tree. The advertisement was suggesting that the resolution on their printers was so good that you could distinguish small insects, and thus *you could see more clearly the underlying reality of the picture.* The same is true with data quality: The higher the data quality, the greater your ability to see what is really happening. In the case, for example, of program management, higher data quality allows you to understand more clearly what effects your program is having, and because you have a clearer picture of reality, you are able to make better decisions about program management.

The level of data needed to see at the level of resolution necessary to manage programs is far greater than the resolution needed to make broad policy or evaluative decisions about whether or not the program should be funded. New, detailed, and high-quality data are clearly needed.

WHERE IS THE PUSH FOR ACCOUNTABILITY COMING FROM?

The current movement toward accountability, at least as driven in the United States by the federal government, specifically by Congress,[1] is more a redirection of evaluations. Evaluations still must examine long-term impacts,[2] but there is an increasing focus on the process evaluation components. These process components, it is argued, may be used much more for management than we have used them in the past. In evaluators' language, this is a shift in focus from the all-or-none impact evaluation to process evaluation.

Many decentralized government bodies, including federal and state agencies in the United States, face major challenges in obtaining high-quality data on the performance of their programs. For example, the U.S. Department of Education accounts for only about 7% (about $32 billion) of the nation's investment (about $450 billion) in kindergarten through 12th-grade education. In addition, the system is highly decentralized, which means that the Department of Education must collect data through a series of intermediaries, including states, districts, and schools, each with different histories, contexts, and goals.

"Most agencies lack the reliable data sources and systems needed to develop, validate, and verify performance information" was Congress's response to the first performance reports submitted to them in 1999. The Department of Education's report was among them. With the best data presented together in one document, the Department's need for high-quality data could not have been more apparent. Data quality improvement became a Department priority.

Although some increase in accountability (top-down) would drive changes, improvements in program data had to come from the local offices and data providers themselves (bottom up). The Department of Education had to have a multipronged approach, and that approach became the Data Quality Initiative. This initiative was later recognized as exemplary by the Senate Governmental Affairs Committee, the U.S. General Accounting Office (GAO, 1999), and nationwide associations. The Department undertook four basic steps to drive a systemic change in data quality:

Step 1: Set data quality goals.
Step 2: Assess current data quality.
Step 3: Develop, implement, and support improved data-collection systems.
Step 4: Provide feedback and increase accountability.

The more prominent components (both successful and unsuccessful) of this initiative are pre-sented as examples in this chapter. For a more detailed description of the process, please see Ginsburg & Pane (in press).

If you are not the person collecting data on the program you are evaluating, then you have a problem similar to that faced by the Department of Education. You must rely on those people to collect accurate data, which may not be their first priority. For example, Michael may represent a foundation that gave a grant to support a homeless shelter. He may reasonably want to know if the foundation's money had any effect. From the shelter director's (Jane's) perspective, each minute spent on data collection is a minute that she is not providing services. How can you convince Jane to make data collection a priority? The first answer is by making the data useful to her, by showing her things about her shelter that help her provide services, but there are also other ways.

This chapter and the next are meant to be practical guides to making your way out of this predicament. They present strategies for both using your data and simultaneously increasing their quality.

CRITICAL ELEMENT 1: DATA USE

Federal agencies in the United States are notorious for collecting data that are not used. It is not uncommon to see a room stacked with hundreds of thick reports sent in from grantees and states that are simply collecting dust. Managers say that they want to use the data but do not know how. The grantees who send in the reports catch on quickly that their data are not used and change their approach, giving the report as little time and effort as possible. Several grantees each year do not even bother to submit a report and have yet to suffer any consequences.

- *No matter what else you do, use the data that you collect.* To leave the data unused is a clear signal to your data providers that you do not care about the data or, by extension, the quality of the data, so why should they? There are no consequences for providing poor-quality data. If you do not use the data (or examine it very carefully, which would follow from using the data), you will not be able to provide feedback about the acceptability or lack thereof of data quality. Absent that information, the providers will naturally assume that the data are at an acceptable level of quality, or worse, some may continue to drop the level of quality and wait to see when you notice.

- *Remember that everyone wants to provide good data.* Since data may be used to represent or summarize people's work—their programs or projects—it seems logical that no one would want to submit poor-quality data that inaccurately represent their work.[3] However, data providers, just like the rest of us, have limited time, so they are forced to prioritize. If there are no consequences for submitting poor data, then there are no reasons for them to make data quality a priority.
- *If you already collect data that you do not use, stop and start over.* Rather than collecting data that are not used, collect none at all. Take a year to determine what are the core (at most, 10) pieces of information that will further your goals and *how will you use this information once it is collected.* Then collect only that core information, no matter how tempting it may be to get more. If you do not use that information within a year, do not collect it again. Revise your plans and start over.
- *Begin to use the data as soon as you get it.* Inherent in the discussion so far is the assumption that if you use the data, your data providers will know that you are using it. This is not always the case. So, the first thing that you should do is to show the providers that you are using the data that they submitted. One of the easiest yet most effective strategies is simply to show people how they compare to others. For example, when the electric company sends your bill, it could also show you how your electricity usage compares to all of your neighbors' usage. If you used twice the electricity than the next highest neighbor, you might look into why you use so much more power than your neighbors. Maybe you would even change your electricity habits. Comparisons can be powerful motivators if the right comparison groups are selected. The best motivators will be ones tailored to the data collection audiences. Some media in which to present the data immediately include a postcard of achievements, newsletter, annual report, Web site ranking, comparison chart, and top 10 list.

The remainder of the chapter discusses how to motivate change through examples of change levers. The next chapter provides examples of these strategies.

CRITICAL ELEMENT 2: CULTURAL COMPETENCY

If you ever wondered why people are talking about cultural competency, read *The Spirit Catches You and You Fall Down* by Anne Fadiman (1997). She tells the story of Lia, a Hmong child born in California in 1981, who by 1988 was brain dead because of a series of cultural misunderstandings and resulting overmedications. The medical community did not understand the Hmong animist approach to healing, and the family could not understand the strange medications of Western medicine. The two groups did not understand each other and did not take any point to stop and communicate what was important to each.

A culturally competent evaluator starts with that communication: what is important to him or her and what is important to his or her data providers. Then, working with the data providers, the evaluator finds common ground that serves both goals and is achievable within the norms of the cultures or subcultures. If you do not ask what is important, you will likely end up with poor-quality data, because your data collection serves no clear purpose.

Culture is an issue in every evaluation. Even in one office building, the subcultures in different offices may have huge impacts on your data collection. If the head of one division, for example, puts priority on other things, you will not get the attention to data quality that you need.

THE CHANGE LEVERS MODEL

Changing data quality, like most changes, is all about people. To improve data quality, all you really need to do is get people to focus on data, to make data collection a priority. But how do you get people to make that change? The same way you would any other type of change: by appealing to what is important to them.

Six such psychological motivations are presented around the hexagram in Figure 66.1: get rewards, gain control, avoid punishment, learn, compete, and belong. These are *change levers*,

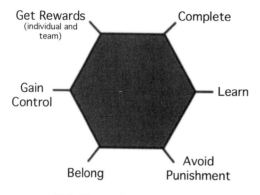

FIGURE 66.1 Change Levers.

the potential underlying motivating factors of change. They are not meant to be comprehensive; you are the best judge of what motivates your teams. However, we can use these levers as examples.

These factors work for teams as well as individuals, in fact, some even appear to be more beneficial for an organization to use with teams.[4] For example, gaining control over their environment can be a powerful motivator for some people. These people might be your entrepreneurs and might respond best, for example, to being given a new assignment with few constraints but accountability for results.

The next chapter provides detailed examples of the levers and how each has been applied in various settings.

Notes

1. For example, the Government Performance and Results Act (1993) and corresponding guidance Circular A-11 from the Office of Management and Budget require agencies to adopt a strategic planning and performance measurement–based approach to program management and budgeting.

2. In fact, some would argue that evaluation by definition has an evaluative (good or bad) component, but the term is used broadly here.

3. Regular data collections that remove the judgment and focus on management improvement tend to alleviate the tendency for data providers to exaggerate successes or hide failures.

4. Rewarding teams is better for an organization because it encourages teamwork instead of individual focus, which can lead the individual to also seek career advancement outside the team.

References

Fadiman, A. (1997). *The spirit catches you and you fall down: A Hmong child, her American doctors, and the collision of two cultures.* New York: Farrar, Straus, & Giroux.

General Accounting Office. (1999, February). *Agency performance plans: Examples of practices that can improve usefulness to decision-makers.* GAO/GGD/AIMD-99-69.

Ginsburg, A. & Pane, N. (in press). Decentralization does not mean poor data quality: A case study from the U.S. Department of Education. In R. Schwartz, J. Mayne, & J. Toulemonde (Eds.), *Assessing evaluative information: Prospects and pitfalls.* Somerset, NJ: Transaction Publishers.

THE DATA WHISPERER

67 *Strategies for Motivating Raw-Data Providers*

Natalia E. Pane

SUMMARY

This chapter offers practice-based examples of data-quality improvement procedures, including a discussion of suggestions for displaying data, a critical aspect of data use. The examples are organized around the change-lever model presented in the preceding chapter. Finally, the chapter closes with some lessons learned.

As in the preceding chapter, many of the examples are drawn from the author's work assisting clients undergoing significant organizational change, particularly the U.S. Department of Education (the Department). The views expressed throughout this chapter do not represent the Department or any other group, but reflect the author's thoughts and experiences only.

EXAMPLES OF IMPROVEMENT STRATEGIES

Change levers are simply the things that motivate us. In this case, the change levers refer to what motivates change in a social or organizational setting. For example, if you are a competitive person, you will respond best (produce more) in a competitive environment.

When thinking about how to motivate people to focus on data quality, the same drivers, or change levers, might apply. What would motivate that competitive person to pay attention to his or her data? Publish comparisons. Show how one group stacks up against another on key dimensions that are important to you. In doing so, you will be spurring and defining the parameters of the conversation. Look at what happened

when *U.S. News & World Report* began publishing rankings of colleges and universities; very quickly, they shaped the way in which people evaluate schools, and the dimensions that they selected have a significant impact. (The universities probably pay very close attention to exactly how each dimension is measured and rated.)

Examples of motivation strategies that you might employ (a sample of change levers) are presented around the hexagram in Figure 67.1. The left side of the diagram relates more to groups over whom you have direct control, while the right side focuses more on strategies in which you have less or indirect control. The majority of the remainder of the chapter describes some examples of these strategies in greater detail. Note that the process is the same: Determine what is important to your data providers and try to develop a strategy that addresses that need.

The examples below show that, by drawing people's attention to data, you will also improve the data. It is perhaps not a direct route, but a spiral of continuous improvement. As more attention is focused on the data, more errors are noted. As those errors are improved, new ones are found. And so the process moves forward.

Direct Control: Examples to Use in Your Organization

Focus on Leadership's Vision

How many organizations claim that their vision is clear, but when employees are asked what the vision is they each produce different answers? How clear are the vision and goals of your or-

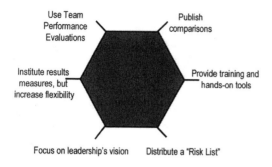

FIGURE 67.1 Examples of Change Levers.

ganization or team? Would your staff prioritize a list of mission-related tasks the same way that you would? If they would not, you are not alone. You need both an internal communication plan and rewards for people who work toward your vision.

For example, at the U.S. Department of Education, Secretary Paige continuously finds new ways to put his vision before each staff member in the department. Posters of the new strategic objectives have been placed all over the building. Pocket-sized minibooks of the objectives were given to all staff. Each of the four elevators now has a full-door-sized poster of one of the four principles of the department (accountability, flexibility, options for parents, and research). In addition, performance agreements are linked to the strategic plan, and all training done out of the training center must be directly related to the plan. The secretary also developed a multi-year plan for keeping the new values of the organization in the forefront of people's minds. The secretary has made it clear to everyone in the department what is important to him, and that influences decisions made up and down the organization.

Institute Results Measures, but Increase Flexibility

If you deal with many different data providers and no one solution would work for all, then you may want to hold each accountable for results while not specifying how each must get there. For example, a principal might tell teachers that they can choose the teaching methods for their classrooms, with only a few constraints (e.g., no corporal punishment), but that

they will be held accountable for raising test scores. This same idea may be applied to the improvement of data quality. You set the standard of quality at which data providers need to be, but the providers determine how they will get there.

For example, the Department of Education developed a "data attestation" process. Data managers were told that they would be held accountable to the department's newly drafted data quality standards. If a manager's data did not meet the standards, that manager was required to submit a plan for how he or she would meet the standard. The real emphasis was on the plan for improvement. There was a general amnesty regarding current level of data quality. That is, it did not matter how bad the data were at the beginning: The central question concerned what could be done now to collect better data next year. Thus, the purpose of the exercise was to get managers talking about data quality, to put data quality on their priority lists. The managers turned over their data quality assessments and recommendations to their bosses and then on up the chain to the senior department leaders. The leadership then reviewed the assessments and recommendations and attested (signed their names) to the soundness of their data or their plans for improvement.

Two things went wrong with the attestation process. First, there was too much detail at the top level to make the information meaningful. Programs assessed their data quality based on each program performance indicator. Although this was the most logical and complete method, it meant that each program would fill out multiple assessments. With over 100 programs, managers were quickly overwhelmed with paper. Condensing the attestations, for example, by database system, may be a better way to proceed. Second, there was not enough follow-through. The process was successful in getting managers at every level to think about and plan to improve data quality. However, because the managers never got through all the papers, there were no consequences for not doing the improvements that managers said they would do. A more successful approach might have been to publish the plans for improvement in the department's annual report, leaving the public and Congress to hold the office accountable.

Link Team or Individual Performance Evaluations to the Improvement of Data Quality

If you use performance evaluations in your organization, consider adding data quality and data use as dimensions on which teams and people are rated. For example, the team may be responsible for sharing comparison or trend data with data providers or for using data to determine where or in what area to provide technical assistance.

Alternatively, rewarding individuals or teams for improvements to data quality on a regular basis might also be effective. Manufacturing plants have been known to give weekly paychecks of different colors that include different levels of bonuses for teams who perform well. Applied to improving data quality, you might give out a ruler or tape measure each month to the office that makes the most improvements or develop similar rewards. Although these rewards may be small, you will be keeping the improvement of data quality on people's minds.

Indirect Control: Examples to Use Outside Your Organization

This area is one of the hardest for people to embrace but is particularly important as the data chains grow longer and more spread out. Even when you do not have direct control over the data providers, there are still ways to increase the quality of the data that they provide.

Distribute a Risk List

Comparisons are made more powerful when attention is drawn to the extremes. For example, many organizations produce best and worst lists. Cities in the United States are rated for an array of qualities including their traffic, pollution, growth, and even proportions of unmarried individuals.[1] Human Rights Watch (2000), for example, publishes a list of the "Top Ten Worst Offenders" in their report *Punishment and Prejudice: Racial Disparities in the War on Drugs.*

This type of list can be an effective means to draw attention, both positive and negative, to issues that are important to your organization. By increasing the attention to the issues, you likely will also increase the attention to the data underlying those rankings. For example, as achievement testing takes hold in U.S. schools, the attention paid to the construction of the tests has increased commensurately. Many people oppose the use of testing under the No Child Left Behind Act, but as people get more involved in the process, the construction of the tests improves.

Government agencies can also publish this type of information. In 1999, the U.S. Environmental Protection Agency (EPA) began publishing a ranking of states in their Toxic Release Inventory (TRI) report. EPA launched the TRI in part to help communities hold industry accountable for pollution. In Pennsylvania, the report's numbers seem to be causing a stir: "With the addition of the TRI reports, the heretofore low-key give and take about power plant emissions has become a pitched debate with no middle ground." People began talking about the data. "Until the TRI reports began to detail the emissions, 'No one even realized the chemicals that were in the air,' [a resident near a major plant] said" (Gazarik, 2002).

On a smaller scale, within the U.S. Department of Education, one program office decided to rank its states on key indicators—aspects of program outcomes that they thought were most important—and sharing those rankings with the states. The Office of Special Education Programs began distributing pages that simply ranked each state on each indicator (for example, the percentage of disabled students integrated into regular classrooms). When they first released these data they received all kinds of calls, nearly all complaints, but the states began paying more attention to these factors. Program staff in one state even went to their state legislature to change the way they collected data (their state data definitions) so that they could then comply with the collection and be included in the ranking.

Provide Training and Hands-on Tools

For some people, the best motivator is an opportunity to learn. Many people do not devote attention to data collection because they do not understand how it could serve their purposes or they do not understand what purposes it does serve. Teaching people about data, data use, evaluation, and even basic statistical issues may result in their providing better data—and those who provide it may even use the data themselves.

The Department of Education's inspector general found that two of the three most frequently identified barriers to successful collection of program performance data were related to staff training: Staff lacked an understanding of (a) information processing, evaluation, and reporting and (b) analyzing and interpreting performance measurement data. The department reacted to this finding by developing and providing a series of hands-on tools and training around them.

The first tool to be developed by the Department of Education's Planning and Evaluation Service (PES) and the American Institutes for Research (AIR) was a book of plain-language data quality standards. To develop these standards, staff reviewed and adapted standards used elsewhere, such as the department's own National Center for Education Statistics and those found in performance measurement literature (e.g., Hatry, 1999; Olve, Roy, & Wetter, 1999; Wholey, Hatry, & Newcomer, 1994). Many data quality concepts, such as validity of measures, accuracy of definitions, and reporting for use are integral across all types of data collections.

The data quality standards were eight standards for judging program data and related operations (see below). An important decision was made to write the standards in clear, nontechnical language; the standards were designed for the average person, not a statistician.

1. **Validity:** Data adequately represent performance. Have the objective, performance indicator and data been scrutinized to be sure that they all describe the phenomena of interest?
2. **Accurate Definitions:** Definitions are correct. Have clear, writrten definitions of key terms (including inclusions/exclusions) been communicated to data providers?
3. **Accurate Counts:** Counts are correct. Are counts accurate; e.g., is double counting avoided?
4. **Editing:** Data are clean. Have you discussed large changes or unusual findings with the primary data providers to see if they might be due to editing errors?
5. **Calculation:** The math is right. Have the + or − confidence intervals been reported for sample data?

6. **Timeless:** Data are recent. Do data meet decision-making needs?
7. **Reporting:** Full disclosure is made. Are data-quality problems at each level reported to the next level?
8. **Burden Reduction:** Data collected are used. Are all data that are collected actually used?[2]

To facilitate the use of the standards, a data quality checklist[3] was created. This checklist listed 3 to 10 questions for each standard to assist program staff unfamiliar with data issues to evaluate the extent to which their data met the standards. For example, under the calculation standard, there is the question: "Are missing data procedures applied correctly?" For those who might not understand the question and the importance of accounting for missing data, the checklist has a section that explains each question and offers examples of meeting and not meeting the criterion. Developing the standards was only the first and perhaps the easiest step, but implementing them has been challenging.

Programs and outside organizations adopted and adapted the standards and checklist to meet their needs. Internally, the Office of the Inspector General (OIG) began using the standards to evaluate program offices (OIG, 1998).

The data quality training classes are 3-hour classes in which the participants learn about the basic issues underlying data quality, are walked through the standards, use the checklist in a hands-on exercise, and discuss strategies and plans for improving the data quality in their offices. Data quality classes are open to all department staff and almost always have a waiting list. The popularity of the classes suggests that employees understand the importance of data quality to accountability as well as to the improvement of their programs and ultimately their success.

For several years, as a part of this initiative to improve data quality, the department teamed with AIR to offers guidebooks, prepared presentations, and specialized training sessions that offices may use to educate their grantees and data providers on the importance of data quality.[4] Because the department's data-quality problems begin long before the data come to the Department, emphasizing the importance of data quality throughout the data-provision chain (for

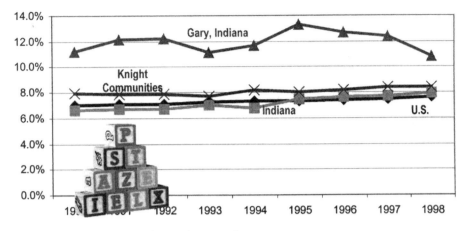

FIGURE 67.2 Knight Foundation data graph.

example, at state and local education agencies) is a key objective of department training.

Publish Comparisons

When rankings are too extreme, simple comparisons may be more effective. For example, the Knight Foundation used comparison data to assist their grantees in setting community priorities. Knight provided each of their 26 supported regions with data on 70 indicators describing their region (usually a metropolitan area). For example, they provided data on the number of low-birth-weight babies, the availability of housing, and the achievement test scores of students. See Figure 67.2, which shows the Knight Foundation's graph of data on low-birth-weight babies for Gary, Indiana. Notice how Gary stands out from the other comparison groups; Gary has a noticeably higher rate of low-birth-weight babies. The power of this kind of visual display often comes from the fact that people have not seen such comparisons made before. Showing community leaders in Gary this kind of graphic allows them to identify needs in their community that they otherwise might not have seen.

Forcing comparisons such as those in the Knight Foundation graph can be powerful displays. Choices of ways to display data are a natural outgrowth of using the data. During the 1980s, the Department of Education published a state-by-state wall chart, a controversial document that for the first time compared states on student outcomes. Every year, this publication

produced the department's largest press conference. The department is now planning to publish program outcomes results on a state-by-state basis in a wall-chart format that should have similar effects on reinforcing improvements in data timeliness and accuracy for program data.

DISPLAY OF DATA

Using your data is the most important step you can take to improving your data, and how you then present your data is a part of that process. Here is a list of the top 10 things to remember when designing graphs and other data displays:

1. Every graph or chart should be a comparison; do not must present one group or one element. Make comparisons? They enrich context and understanding.
2. Don't exaggerate; you lose the trust of your audience (e.g., although the data reports a 20% increase in text scores, the accompanying picture shows a picture increasing in size by 40%).
3. Only use pictures and design elements that directly relate to your point; especially avoid using purely decorative elements (e.g., does the 3-D component really make your point better?).
4. Add details if they are important (e.g., exceptions to the data) but exclude unnecessary details (such as underlining or placing text in boxes).
5. Don't be afraid to make many compari-

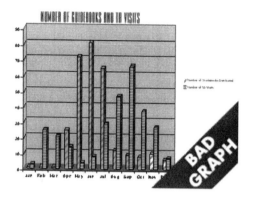

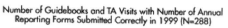

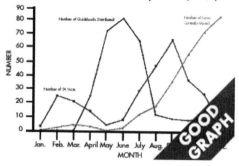

FIGURE 67.3 Bad graph, good graph comparison.

sons, so long as you keep the comparisons simple.

6. Avoid legends whenever possible; label data directly (e.g., put the label directly on the pie slice of the pie graph). Don't make the reader work to read your chart.

7. Find a publication that creates effective graphs and charts (e.g., the *New York Times*). Use these examples to design templates that fit your needs that you can use over and over.

8. Use color and similar elements (e.g., cross-hatching) to highlight. Don't use all colors in the spectrum on one graph; for example, use shades of blue for one group and shades of green for another.

9. Make sure all labels are complete and as close to their data as possible. The title should give all necessary information (e.g., population(s) reported, dates, and sample sizes) and be able to stand alone and make sense. Begin the vertical scale at zero, unless there is a clear scale break (//) and label each axis.

10. All graphs should have source notes; from where did the data come? If multiple sources, list all.[5]

The most useful tip from the list is Item 7, "Find charts in your field or generally that are done well." Hiring someone to make the templates mentioned in Item 7 might even be worthwhile if, for example, these are charts that you will use every year in an annual report.

An example of the application of some of these recommendations appears in the two charts that follow. In the first example (left), a program manager, Fiona, is showing her manager the team's efforts over the last year to increase the number of annual reporting forms submitted correctly. Since the program has repeatedly had sites send the forms in filled out incorrectly, Fiona decided to write a guidebook on how to fill out the forms and to send her staff on site visits to give technical assistance (TA) on filling out the forms. In the first graph, labeled the "Bad Graph," Fiona shows only the number of guidebooks distributed and the number of TA visits. The graph shows that the number of guidebooks peaked earlier than the number of site visits, but that's all it shows. In the "Good Graph," Lisa forces you to see how the number of forms submitted goes up a little with the guidebook, but increases the most with the addition of the TA visits.

Additional ways that the second graph is better include the following: (a) The line graph (good graph) is clearer and doesn't use needless graphics such as the different and distracting lines in the bars of the bad graph, (b) the good graph's title gives the time frame and number of data points contained in the graph, (c) the good graph labels the axes, (d) the good graph labels the lines directly instead of abstracting to a legend, and (e) the good graph avoids other extraneous decorations by avoiding a 3-D look and not using tick-marks or a gray background that might distract the reader.

CONCLUSIONS

The lessons I have learned from working with various federal agencies and organizations undergoing significant changes in the ways that they think about, approach, and collect data include the following:

- Always use every data element or cease collecting them immediately.
- Accept whatever level of data quality currently exists while demanding plans for improvement, and hold offices and people accountable for implementing those improvements.
- Obtain better data on fewer, more important items rather than collecting poor data across a broad set of categories.
- Build accountability into existing systems and avoid creating new, separate, paperwork-based systems.
- Hate mail can be a good thing; it means people are paying attention.
- Introduce incentives to give reporting units a reason for using the data themselves (e.g., send all comparison data and lessons learned information back to the reporting units in a reader-friendly format).
- Think creatively about data quality improvement. Remember that even if your organization is not in direct control of the data collection, there are still ways to impact the quality of data.
- Change systems of numbers, but even more, change systems of people. The initiative is best carried out as a partnership among leadership, managers, staff, states, and grantees.

Data quality is a continuum, and the goal is to move continuously in the direction of improved data quality. To improve data quality, the first step is to draw attention to the data. Get people to look at the numbers. If they are not yet high-quality data, present them anyway, but with all appropriate disclaimers.

Notes

1. For example, see the Road Information Program for car-related rankings and Forbes.com for a list of the best U.S. cities to be single.

2. The standards, full checklist, and presentations on each are available, free of charge, in electronic format by e-mailing the author *npane@air.org* or at *http://www.air.org/eqed/defaultnew.htm.*

3. The long and short versions of the checklist are available free from AIR at the Establishing Quality Education Data Web site (http://www.air.org/eqed/defaultnew.htm).

4. Some of these presentations, including data quality training materials and guidebooks, are available from AIR from their Web site (http://www.air.org/eqed/defaultnew.htm).

5. This list is based in part on the National Center for Education Statistics Standards for Tabular and Graphical Presentations and the work of Edward Tuft as well as the author's own experiences.

References

Gazarik, R. (2002). PA ranks among worst states for toxic emissions. *Tribute-Review*, November 18, 2002.

General Accounting Office. (1999, February). *Agency performance plans: Examples of practices that can improve usefulness to decision-makers.* GAO/GGD/AIMD-99-69.

Ginsburg, A., Noell, J., & Plisko, V. (1988, Spring). Lessons from the wall chart. *Educational Evaluation and Policy Analysis, 10*(1), 1–12.

Ginsburg, A., & Pane, N. (in press). Decentralization does not mean poor data quality: A case study from the U.S. Department of Education. In R. Schwartz, J. Mayne, & J. Toulemonde (Eds.), *Assessing evaluative information: Prospects and pitfalls.* Somerset, NJ: Transaction.

Government Accounting Office. (1999). *Agency performance plans: Examples of practices that can improve usefulness to decision-makers.* GAO/GGD/AIMD-99-69, February 1999.

Hatry, H. (1999). *Performance measurement: Getting results.* Washington, DC: Urban Institute.

Human Rights Watch. (2000, May). Top ten worst offenders. *Punishment and prejudice: Racial disparities in the war on drugs, 12* (2G). Retrieved June 23, 2003, from http://www.hrw.org/reports/2000/usa/

Keel, J., Hawkins, A., & Alwin, L. (1999, December). *Guide to performance measure management 2000.* SAO No. 00-318. Austin, TX: Texas State Auditor's Office.

Office of the Inspector General, U.S. Department of Education. (1998, September). *Moving toward a results-oriented organization: A report on the status of ED's implementation of the results act.* Document #ACN 17-70007.

Olve, N., Roy, J., & Wetter, M. (1999). *Performance drivers: A practical guide to using the balanced scorecard.* West Sussex, England: Wiley.

Road Information Program. (2002, September 30). Study ranks top 50 high accident corridors in Washington State [Press release]. Retrieved June 23, 2003, from http://www.tripnet.org/state/WashingtonRelease093002.pdf

Wholey, J., Hatry, H., & Newcomer, K. (1994). *Handbook of practical program evaluation.* San Francisco, CA: Jossey-Bass.

68 NEEDS ASSESSMENTS: A STEP-BY-STEP APPROACH

Douglas Leigh

Public and private sector organizations alike are increasingly aware of the usefulness of collecting data regarding their effectiveness, not only after program implementation through evaluation but also as part of organizational planning initiatives. Needs assessment provides a means for providing clear direction in selecting the right solutions to the challenges and opportunities at hand, while building shared commitment to an organization's future direction. It is a formal process that identifies needs as gaps in results between what is and what should be, prioritizes those needs on the basis of the costs and benefits of closing versus ignoring those gaps in results, and selects the needs to be reduced and eliminated (Kaufman, Oakley-Browne, Watkins, & Leigh, 2003). Needs assessment is not a technique that identifies only the current situation of an organization without also identifying what should be (Kaufman & Watkins, 1999). Doing so tends to justify preferred solutions and initiatives simply because they are popular or have been the methods of choice in the past. In addition, needs assessment is not a wishes, wants, demand, or market analysis (Watkins & Leigh, 2001). Although customers, vendors, and associates *are* critical planning partners in a needs assessment, such audiences commonly press for short-term cost savings at the expense of ensuring that real problems are resolved in the long run, in the absence of an agreed-on structure for identifying problems before choosing solutions. Needs assessment, then, is a valuable approach for not only solving problems but also for accurately identifying them and their causes.

Needs assessments identify gaps between current and desired results that occur both within and outside an organization in order to provide useful information for decision making. One approach to conceptualizing the stages of a needs assessment project is represented by the performance accomplishment model (Kaufman, Watkins, & Leigh, 2001). This framework (see Figure 68.1) provides a high-level depiction of the relationship between needs assessment and the allied processes of planning, causal analysis, objective setting, and solution consideration.

STEP 1: PREASSESSMENT

The first step of conducting a needs assessment is largely a logistical one. First, as important as bottom-up organizational involvement is to implementing change, systemic undertakings such as needs assessments typically require the initiating and sustaining sponsorship of top leadership (Bolman & Deal, 1997; Conner, 1993). Those in charge of overseeing the day-to-day conduct of needs assessments accomplish this by clarifying the problem of the status quo to organizational leadership (Bridges, 1991; Kanter, 1983).

Once sponsorship for the assessment is secured, assessment team members should be identified. Because all organizations impact both internal and external planning partners, care should be taken to draw participation from three distinct groups: (a) executives, leaders, and managers; (b) internal clients (employees and associates); and (c) external clients (such as vendors and customers, as well as members of the surrounding community). These partners provide perspectives and perceptions about reality as they experience and sense it, and also lend credibility to the process because they are seen as legitimate representatives (Kaufman et al., 2003).

Needs assessment team members should be selected according to their levels of power and

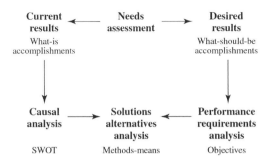

FIGURE 68.1 Performance accomplishment model.

authority, long-term commitment to the organization, technical expertise, and authentic leadership skills and competencies. The composition of the project team should make clear the unique contribution to be made by each member. On the basis of these characteristics, smaller teams should be formed to carry out the major functions outlined in the performance accomplishment model depicted in Figure 68.1. Last, project plans should be developed—typically using Gantt or PERT charting techniques—that clarify the project time line, individual and team roles and responsibilities, and major en-route milestones in the needs assessment.

STEP 2: SCOPING

Reaching agreement on the scope and use of needs assessments is a necessary precursor to undertaking such projects. First, project members and senior leadership should come to consensus regarding the purpose of the assessment: identifying, prioritizing, and selecting gaps in results for closure. These three aspects of needs assessment require that *needs* be defined solely as discrepancies between current and desired results, rather than deficiencies in processes or resources. Needs are gaps in individual, small-group, organizational, or societal results, not perceived shortages of personnel, resources, finances, training, or service provision. This approach to needs and needs assessment allows better informed decisions to be made regarding the prioritization of problems for resolution, the identification of redundancies in services or products, and the detection of previously unforeseen opportunities for providing services and meeting currently unmet needs.[1]

The second task of scoping involves identifying the primary clients and stakeholders to whom organizational results are delivered and from whom results data are to be collected. There are three levels of needs—and three corresponding levels of results—as defined by Kaufman (1992, 1998, 2000): (a) Mega level needs in which external stakeholders and society are the clients, (b) Macro level needs in which the organization itself is the client, and (c) Micro level needs in which individuals and teams within the organization are the clients. Needs assessments at the Mega level serve to identify discrepancies in societal outcomes—for example, self-sufficiency, disabilities, and environmental sustainability. At the Macro level, needs assessments identify gaps in organizational outputs, such as measures of return on investment, customer satisfaction, and merchandise defect rates. Micro level needs assessments provide decision makers with information about gaps in the products produced by individuals and teams—for instance, deliverables, staff satisfaction, absenteeism, and accident rates. Because each level of results may be best understood only in relation to the level immediately above it (Gilbert, 1996), it is preferable to address all three levels of results in a needs assessment project. Such a systemic examination of connections inside and outside the organization better ensures that individual and team products are aligned with organizational outputs so that external clients and the community are not harmed by an organization's efforts and instead receive products and services that enhance their quality of life.

Having agreed on the purpose, use, and approach for the needs assessment, project members should specify the questions to be answered by the assessment. At this point, it may be clear what some of those questions are. However, assessors should remain open to the inclusion of new questions as the project progresses. These questions will emerge as clients and stakeholders gain deeper understandings of the organization's challenges and opportunities, and as the project team learns more about the assessment process. Although assessment questions can span a variety of topics and will differ widely depending on the organizational context, they should relate to all three levels of results. As initially developed, these questions will be general, such as the following: Is the organization having any unintended effects on the environment and surrounding community? Did restructuring efforts have a positive impact on production? How well are employees performing on skill tests after training? After questions have been developed (and approved by sponsors), the next task is to identify gaps in results.

STEP 3A: IDENTIFYING WHAT IS

Needs assessments typically involve a substantial amount of new data collection, especially when no prior needs assessment has been conducted or evaluation data collected. However, because many organizations regularly collect results data, the first aspect of this step is to review the data currently available. Results data related to the questions developed in Step 2 may be gleaned from annual reports, documentation from previous projects and program evaluations, audits, and internal correspondences, among other sources. On the basis of what-is data not available from extant sources, requirements should be developed for new or supplemental data to be collected. From these requirements, data collection methods should then be identified. These may include direct observation, individual interviews, group interviews (focus groups), document searches, questionnaires or surveys, criterion tests, assessment centers, critical incidents, artifacts or work products, review of public data, and accessing research and statistical databases.[2] In most cases, hard (independently verifiable performance) and soft (opinions and perceptions) data should both be collected. This allows soft data regarding stakeholders' feelings about a situation to be corroborated with (or disconfirmed by) the hard data. After these data sources have been identified, a data collection plan should be prepared that specifies the time frame for collection, stakeholders from whom data will be collected, documents to be reviewed, individuals and teams responsible for each data source, specific questions to be answered, and procedures for gaining approval of the findings.

STEP 3B: IDENTIFYING WHAT SHOULD BE

Concurrent with the collection of what-is data, project members should also identify required or what-should-be results. As with the previous step, extant data should first be explored to determine what information already exists about Micro, Macro, and Mega level objectives. Such information may come from a variety of sources, including prior organizational visioning efforts, mission statements, organizational plans, needs assessments, and evaluations. Based on relevant data not available from these materials, two distinct methods for specifying what-should-be are used. First, leadership in the organization should undertake planning efforts to derive objectives at the Mega level (defined as an Ideal Vision, a measurable statement of the kind of world the organization hopes to contribute toward for the future), the Macro level (as a Mission Objective, which provides a performance-based statement of an organization's overall intended results to be delivered), and the Micro level (in the form of a Function Analysis that specifies the building-block results necessary for accomplishment of the Mission Objective and Ideal Vision).[3]

A second useful method for specifying what-should-be results comes from the collection of various stakeholders' perspectives on the objectives that the organization should be pursuing at the Micro, Macro, and Mega levels. The methods for collecting this soft data are identical to those discussed in Step 3a, though the nature of the questioning should focus on perceptions of results to be accomplished. A practical technique for economizing on stakeholders' time is to use opportunities for collecting what-is results data to also collect what-should-be data. To this end, the plan for the collection of what-should-be data should be developed at the same time that the data collection plan described in Step 3a is prepared.

STEP 4: ANALYZING CAUSES OF WHAT IS

With results data having been collected, needs assessments turn to the identification of the underlying causes for the results currently being achieved by the organization. This information can inform what practices should be continued or expanded in the future, as well as those to be discontinued or complemented by other methods and tools. SWOT (strengths, weaknesses, opportunities, threats) analysis is a technique that provides an indication of the factors to be considered in determining such operational requirements and tactics. As organizational brainstorming activities, most SWOT-analysis models ask two binary questions of the factors influencing an organization: Is this factor a benefit or cost? and Is a factor occurring inside or outside this organization? Beneficial factors internal to the organization are termed *strengths*, external factors are considered *opportunities*, internal costs are referred to as *weaknesses*, and external costs are designated as *threats*.

SWOT analysis can be made more useful for making decisions concerning resource allocation by considering independently verifiable data such as fiscal resources, market share, external impact on the surrounding communities, and measures of legislative support (Leigh, 2000). This requires that two additional questions be asked of each potential SWOT factor: How much is each factor currently and potentially costing the organization? and How much control does the organization have over each factor? Based on the answers to these questions, better informed decisions can be made regarding what existing assets to amplify or sustain, what liabilities to improve or fix, and what factors to simply monitor over time.[4]

STEP 5: ANALYZING PERFORMANCE REQUIREMENTS

Needs assessment does not end with the identification and prioritization of needs (gaps in results at the Mega, Macro, and Micro levels). The efforts described in Step 3b, "Identifying What Should Be," are useful for specifying the overarching results to be accomplished by an organization. Step 5 of the needs assessment process further clarifies those results as measurable objectives, or performance requirements, at the Mega, Macro, and Micro levels.

Performance requirements detail the measurable evidence necessary to demonstrate that an intervention has achieved desired results. They also help provide personnel performance appraisal standards and supply criteria for the evaluation and continuous improvement of human resources. In addition, they can be of assistance in identifying valid interventions and defining new organizational purposes.

A simple mnemonic device for developing performance requirements is represented by the acronym PQRS. First, objective statements should specify the *p*erformer who is expected to achieve the desired result. Next, relevant *q*ualifying criteria should be delineated, typically by

indicating the time frame over which a result is to be accomplished. Last, the *r*esults (ends) to be accomplished should be clearly and unambiguously stated, along with the *s*tandards or conditions under which the result or performance will be demonstrated. Performance objectives never include how a result will be achieved. A hypothetical example from a manufacturing organization (with PQRS attributes in parentheses) might be "Production line workers (P) will reduce the amount of scrap (R) produced this year by 10% less than the previous year (Q), as certified by the Waste Reduction Committee's yearly status report (S)."

STEP 6: ANALYZING SOLUTIONS REQUIREMENTS

Although the steps previously described serve to identify needs as gaps in results between what-is and what-should-be, those needs cannot be selected for reduction and elimination until they have been prioritized on the basis of the costs and benefits of closing versus ignoring those needs. Project team members are likely to have unearthed many possible solutions up to this point. Working with other partners and stakeholders, the assessment team should consider current solutions (identified in Step 4) and should explore new alternatives for resolving existing problems and capitalizing on new opportunities. Two approaches are used for deciding between competing solutions. The first of these involves determining the advantages and disadvantages of possible solutions in terms of the ability of each to meet the performance requirements (specified in Step 5). Depending on the nature of the organization and the solution, such advantages and disadvantages may include availability, reliability, quality, perceived adequacy, costs of solutions, duration of results, required time, personnel requirements, and applicable policies and regulations.

A second filter for choosing between alternative solutions involves examining the costs and benefits of closing versus ignoring gaps in results (Leigh, 2003). This approach, called cost-consequences analysis (CCA), develops coarse-grained, prospective return-on-investment estimates for potential solutions. It ensures that the costs and benefits of both problems and potential solutions are considered before committing to any solution. Specifically, CCA compares the costs and benefits of potential interventions against the often unconsidered cost to ignore a need. In the process, it may be discovered that the cost to close a gap in results exceeds the benefits of doing so.

For each gap identified in Steps 3a and 3b, the project team should generate a CCA ratio of the costs and benefits of closing the gap versus the cost to ignore it. Financial estimates in this step will assist in making pragmatic decisions regarding the prioritization of gaps as well as verifying value added once solutions have been implemented.[5]

STEP 7: PRIORITIZING AND SELECTING NEEDS

Once gaps in results are determined, causal analysis is conducted, performance requirements specified, and alternative solutions considered, the project team may move forward with prioritizing and selecting needs for closure, monitoring, or abandonment. This is done on the basis of CCA data that provided estimates of the costs and benefits of closing versus ignoring gaps in results.

First, needs should be listed in order of magnitude from the greatest to least discrepancy between what-is and what-should-be. Next to each of these needs, CCA data should be provided, indicating the cost of status quo (the cost of ignoring gaps in results), the cost of alternative solutions (the cost of closing gaps in results), and the anticipated benefits of closing gaps in results (the benefits of solutions). Project members will find it useful to caucus with project sponsors to decide which needs to seek to resolve, which to monitor over time for change, and which to abandon due to solutions being more costly than the problem identified.

For example, a productivity problem caused in part by a communication blockage might cost an organization $150,000 per year in rework and lost clientele. A new communications infrastructure might cost $15,000 and yield $125,000 per year. Thus, for a $15,000 investment, the productivity problem would be reduced from $150,000 to $25,000 per year ($150,000 minus $125,000). By implementing additional solutions, supplementary benefits might be realized.

In prioritizing and selecting needs, the project team should above all consider the ability to meet performance requirements. Although it would be preferable for organizations to select only those solutions that will accomplish all of the desired results at the Mega, Macro, and Micro levels, limited budgets, personnel, and time may make the closure of some gaps in results untenable . . . for the time being. On the other hand, selecting too few needs for resolution is likely to bring the usefulness of the organization into question.

STEP 8: POSTASSESSMENT

The final task involved in conducting a needs assessment is the writing of a comprehensive report of the project and its findings, preparing evaluation and performance improvement plans, and determining next steps. The project team should communicate the findings of the project through a variety of outlets. It is recommended that, in addition to the written report, a briefing be made to project sponsors to help minimize miscommunication of the project and clarify its findings and recommendations. This information will be of assistance to senior leadership as they complete their planning efforts (described in Step 3b). The project report itself should consist of several sections, including an introduction, a description of the technical approach, a detailed presentation of findings (supplemented by graphics when appropriate), discussion, conclusions, recommendations regarding solutions to be implemented, and relevant appendices.

As what-should-be data tend to be relatively stable over time, successive needs assessments are likely to be much simpler to conduct. This is because the more time-consuming step of strategic planning has only to be modified on the basis of current organizational realities. This allows for subsequent needs assessments to focus more fully on the collection of what-is data. To prepare for the next round of needs assessment, plans for evaluation and continuous improvement of solutions to be implemented as well as the project itself should be developed as a final stage of postassessment.

SUMMARY

Needs assessments serve to distinguish performance gaps and opportunities in measurable, results-focused terms (Leigh, Watkins, Platt, & Kaufman, 2000). The technique identifies gaps between current and desired results and places them in priority order for resolution based on the cost to meet the need as compared with the cost of ignoring it. A useful needs assessment provides decision makers the necessary data for selecting solutions, tools, and interventions that have the greatest probability of accomplishing results that are beneficial to internal and external partners alike.

Notes

1. In addition, this approach is compatible with both the intent and the requirements of the U.S. Government Performance and Results Act (GPRA). See Kaufman et al. (2001).

2. For a complete discussion of advantages and disadvantages of each of these methods, see Chapter 5 of Kaufman et al. (2003).

3. Details of these strategic, tactical, and operational planning efforts are beyond the scope of this chapter; more information can be found in Kaufman et al. (2003).

4. See Leigh (2000) for a step-by-step description of conducting this form of analysis.

5. See Muir, Watkins, Kaufman, and Leigh (1998), Kaufman and Watkins (1996), and Chapter 7 of Kaufman et al. (2001) for more information regarding CCA.

References

Bolman, L. G., & Deal, T. E. (1997). *Reframing organizations: Artistry, choice, and leadership*. San Francisco: Jossey-Bass.

Bridges, W. (1991). *Managing transitions: Making the most of change*. Reading, MA: Addison Wesley.

Conner, D. (1993). *Managing at the speed of change: How resilient managers succeed and prosper where others fail*. New York: Villard Books.

Gilbert, T. (1996). *Human competence: Engineering worthy performance* (Tribute ed.). Washington, DC: International Society for Performance Improvement.

Kanter, R. M. (1983). *The change masters: Innova-tions for productivity in the American corporation*. New York: Simon & Schuster.

Kaufman, R. (1992). *Strategic planning plus: An organizational guide* (Rev. ed.). Newbury Park, CA: Sage.

Kaufman, R. (1998). *Strategic thinking: A guide to identifying and solving problems* (Rev. ed.). Arlington, VA: American Society for Training & Development and International Society for Performance Improvement.

Kaufman, R. (2000). *Mega planning: Practical tools for organizational success*. Thousand Oaks, CA: Sage.

Kaufman, R., Oakley-Browne, H., Watkins, R., & Leigh, D. (2003). *Strategic planning for success: Aligning people, performance, and payoffs*. San Francisco: Jossey-Bass/Pfeiffer.

Kaufman, R., & Watkins, R. (1996). Cost-consequences analysis. *Human Resources Development Quarterly, 7*(1), 87–100.

Kaufman, R., & Watkins, R. (1999). Needs assessment. In D. Langdon (Ed.), *The resource guide to performance interventions*. San Diego, CA: Jossey-Bass.

Kaufman, R., Watkins, R., & Leigh, D. (2001). *Useful educational results: Defining, prioritizing, and accomplishing*. New Jersey: Proactive.

Leigh, D. (2000). Causal-utility decision analysis (CUDA): Quantifying SWOTs. In E. Biech (Ed.), *The 2000 Annual, Volume 2, Consulting* (pp. 251–265). Jossey-Bass/Pfeiffer.

Leigh, D. (2003). Worthy performance, redux. *PerformanceXpress*. International Society for Performance Improvement newsletter. (Available online: http://www.performancexpress.org/0306)

Leigh, D., Watkins, R., Platt, W., & Kaufman, R. (2000). Alternate models of needs assessment: Selecting the right one for your organization? *Human Resource Development Quarterly, 11*(1), 87–93.

Muir, M., Watkins, R., Kaufman, R., & Leigh, D. (1998). Cost-consequences analysis: A primer. *Performance Improvement, 37*(4), 8–17.

Watkins, R., & Leigh, D. (2001). Performance improvement: More than just bettering the here-and-now. *Performance Improvement, 41*(8), 10–15.

69

BUDGETING AND FISCAL MANAGEMENT IN PROGRAM EVALUATIONS

Leon Ginsberg

There is an old concept, which applies to many fields, that suggests that understanding anything usually involves understanding the money involved. Some criminal investigators, reporters, and evaluators say that one should "follow the money." And it is true that gaining a detailed understanding of almost any human endeavor is best achieved by looking at the financing of that endeavor. Where does the money come from, how is it spent, how is it accounted for?

Of all the means for evaluating social programs, none is quite so pervasive and important in the total scheme of management and planning as examining the agency's finances—how they are secured, budgeted, accounted for, and audited. This chapter describes the ways in which fiscal data are used in the evaluation of agencies.

For most social agencies, nothing is quite as dramatic as the annual budget process, the day-to-day accounting for the funds that are expended, and the periodic audits of agencies. It is likely that more agencies are changed in major ways or even forced to close because of fiscal evaluations than for any other reasons. Evaluations that are based on experimental research designs, monitoring, and other kinds of studies of the content of agency functioning are often significant factors in an agency's operations. However, they are not as commonly important to the agency's well-being and the well-being of agency staff as the fiscal evaluations.

AUDITING AND ACCOUNTING

Funding organizations, whether they are governmental or voluntary, are always interested in and concerned about the organization's finances. They want to know that the funds they have provided to the agency are well spent. Voluntary organizations' boards of directors expect careful accounting and satisfactory audits from their chief executive officers. They are legally responsible for the appropriate and responsible fiscal maintenance of the organizations.

Therefore, the information in this chapter is of special importance to agency managers. However, professional staff throughout the organization are also responsible for the proper fiscal operations of the organization. Therefore, because almost all social workers are employed by organizations, this information is important to most professional social workers and to students who are studying to become professional social workers. Even private practitioners are obligated by partners, tax authorities, and the social welfare community to operate in fiscally responsible ways, and therefore correct accounting, auditing, and budgeting are crucial for them, as well.

WORKING WITH ACCOUNTANTS AND AUDITORS

There are times in social welfare agencies when top officers such as executive directors do not exercise supervisory authority over fiscal staff members and do not establish viable relationships with auditors and others who fiscally evaluate the agency. It is, some may think, a fact about the functioning of social workers that they are either intimidated by or lack knowledge of fiscal matters. Some may suggest that there is a relationship between an interest in the human services professions and a lack of interest in and a perception of lack of skill in mathematical activity. Social work educators encounter that kind of phenomenon with some frequency when they teach research and statistics or other subjects that are quantitative in nature.

However, it is of vital importance for social workers and other human services personnel to maintain their authority over accounting activities. It is not unusual to find social service agencies in which the fiscal staff exercise the top authority and therefore, in effect, run the organizations. A failure to take into account these kinds of activities leads to the situation that one often sees in human services organizations—a situation in which the manager of the program checks every decision with the fiscal officer because the manager has little understanding of the financial situation or processes. That, in effect, makes the fiscal officer the primary manager of the program or service.

A manager of a social welfare organization or a unit in such an organization need not be an expert on fiscal issues or in accounting to exercise the proper authority over that series of functions. One need only understand the fiscal system, be able to tell when moneys are and are not being properly expended, and be able to determine the extent to which a program is operating within its budget to effectively function as a supervisor of fiscal matters. Turning all fiscal matters over to a fiscal specialist, with little or no supervision, is an abdication of the management role.

It is usual in social agencies that the functions and the authority are decentralized. That is, the top staff member or chief executive officer has authority over all units, but each individual unit head is responsible for the activities of his or her unit. Therefore, each unit head must be concerned about and should carefully monitor fiscal activities in his or her purview. For example, an agency that has programs for children, families, and the elderly is likely to have someone in charge of each of those age-group programs. The person in charge of each age-group program should know about and watch the budget of the program and should watch the ways in which expenditures are made, recorded, and accounted for. In essence, it is impossible to be in charge of all or part of a program unless one has fiscal knowledge about it and exercises control over it.

FISCAL OPERATION KNOWLEDGE

Learning about accounting processes and the like is achievable by taking a single course, perhaps, or by reading and understanding a textbook on basic accounting principles. But even without that kind of special preparation, most managers can learn what they need to know by talking to the financial staff of the organization, who usually are and certainly should be quite anxious to share information with program supervisors.

So effective social workers who manage programs or parts of programs work toward good relationships with fiscal staff members, and each should have a good understanding of what the other wants to achieve. The priorities of the program manager are programmatic—serving more people, serving people more effectively, meeting standards for effective service, and perhaps expanding the program. The fiscal staff has a greater interest in making sure that the finances are correctly handled and that funds are properly accounted for.

One of the interesting elements about these processes is that they are fundamentally universal in the human services. Every social agency of any size has a budget for which it is responsible and that displays the planning of its fiscal activities and serves as a device for monitoring the organization's functions. Every human services organization also has an accounting system of some kind. That is, in some way it collects information and keeps records on the receipt and expenditure of its funds. Almost all are also audited periodically. Those that receive grants and those that are part of government are, most often, annually, audited.

AUDITING AND AUDITORS

Relationships with auditors pose a special picture for social workers, especially managers. Auditors are, ideally, independent of the management of the organization. Their purpose is to determine the extent to which the organization complies with the regulations under which it operates, which may be the organization's own or those imposed by some external force such as a higher level government body, a large organization of which the social welfare program is a part, or a funding source.

The purpose of auditors is to inspect the financial and other aspects of the organization and to provide an opinion about the fiscal functioning of the organization. They may find the organization is properly functioning and properly accounting for all of its activities. Or, as an alternative, it may say that the organization is functioning adequately except in certain areas, and those areas are listed as *findings*.

Auditing and the roles of auditors have been subjects of major controversy in the United States in recent years. Some corporations were found to have employed accounting and auditing firms to consult with them on their management and fiscal procedures as well as auditing them for compliance with legal regulations. Of course, that sort of dual relationship creates a potential conflict of interest in which the auditors are reluctant to criticize the organization's fiscal procedures for fear of losing the consulting business. In several celebrated cases, accounting and auditing firms (for instance, Arthur Andersen, LLP) were found guilty of improperly or incorrectly auditing the firms they both consulted for and evaluated.

A federal body was established in 2002 by the federal government to supervise and regulate the accounting industry. The Public Company Accounting Oversight Board was established through the Sarbanes-Oxley Public Company Accounting Reform and Investor Protection Act of 2002 ("Accounting Reform," 2003.) Until then, accountants were primarily bound by their professional ethics, especially Certified Public Accountants, who are certified by the states. Auditing firms that once both kept accounts for organizations and audited them began separating those functions and turning over one or the other of them to a different firm, to make sure audits are independent. The Federal Accounting Standards Advisory Board (http://www.fasab.gov) promulgates standards for federal government accounting entities, such as those that receive federal grants.

Some states have established laws to regulate public accountants. California's licensed accountants have to meet higher standards. The state requires a cooling-off period of 1 year before an auditor who has examined a public company can take a job in the same company as a financial officer. California auditors must also keep records that an outsider can follow, and they must keep those records for 7 years. And the state also requires that a majority of the members of the Board of Accountancy, which certifies accountants, be public members rather than accountants ("Accounting Reform," 2003). The Governmental Accounting Standards Board (http://www.gasb.org) sets standards for state and local government accounting and financial reporting. A private organization, the American Institute of Certified Public Accountants Financial Accounting Standards Board, sets standards for the profession's accounting and auditing practices.

Audits are conducted by a variety of professionals and specially educated people. The top persons in accounting and auditing firms and in agency fiscal positions are Certified Public Accountants. Many others have degrees or experience in financial management. They may have studied accounting in high school, technical school, or in higher education, or they may have learned much of their skill on the job.

Managers who are in the process of being audited often find it important to meet with auditors prior to the beginning of the audit and to be quite open and complete in their provision of information to the auditors. Auditors are usually entitled to see all information pertaining to the organization. Seeming to withhold information from the auditors may send a signal that there is something wrong.

It is also important for social work management and those who direct programs in social agencies to stay in close touch with the auditors during the audit process (which may take several weeks or even months in a large organization) and to be certain that they understand and follow up when any possible errors or findings arise.

It is also important to understand what the audit may have found after the process is completed. If possible, the organization should correct any errors that may be identified so that the final audit report can indicate that errors were found but corrected.

TYPES OF AUDITS

The financial audit is the most common evaluation device that one encounters in social welfare and other human services organizations. However, there are other kinds of audits. Performance audits are also part of the evaluation of human services organizations. These examine the actual activities of the organization's employees to determine the extent to which they are carrying out the activities for which they are paid. There are also audits of organizational results or outcomes. That is, audits are conducted to determine the extent to which an organization is meeting its goals. The organization may also be audited on the efficiency with which it operates, such as determining the cost for each unit of service such as a single day of child day care, the conduct of a mental health treatment session, the investigation of a child abuse report, the provision of each meal to participants in a Meals on Wheels program, and the real costs of health screening for participants in a program.

It is not uncommon for social agency executives and other staff members to lose their jobs because of audits. It is perhaps the most common reason for changes in executive leadership of social agencies. That does not mean that agency executives are dishonest or that audits tend to uncover sensational, dramatic examples of managerial malfeasance. In fact, many audit results are rather minor and technical. An expenditure or even a series of expenditures might have been coded improperly, charging one account rather than another. Or an allocation of funds may be improper. A worker may be paid from one account for activities that should have been charged to another account.

Matters such as these are important, particularly when the funds come from grants or contracts with government that specify the ways in which the moneys are to be expended. Even though it may look to the board or other governing bodies with authority over the organization as if some malfeasance is responsible for misuse of funds, sometimes the problem is due to errors in the accounting process, instead.

In one organization with which the author is familiar, there was a significant audit exception to a unit's using generic (or, as the auditors referred to them, "dime store") receipts. That is, instead of using official, numbered receipts that were in the control of the organization, the financial staff used receipts that could be purchased anywhere. These could be misused in a variety of ways that might involve fraud and theft. That was not the case, and there was never any evidence of fraud or theft. However, the organization was instructed to begin using official receipts that could reliably be tracked and accounted for.

There are other similar examples to which auditors may take exception but which are not criminal in nature or not particularly improper. For example, on one travel voucher in an organization, a worker who lived 75 miles from the site of a 2-day meeting submitted a request for reimbursement for 300 miles of travel. On further investigation, the auditors determined that the worker had commuted back and forth from his home to the meeting twice rather than staying in the hotel room that would have been provided. Had the accountant who approved the expenditure noted on the expense voucher what the worker had done, there would have been no problem for the auditors to find. However, without an explanation, it appeared that the traveler was billing twice the required number of miles to attend the meeting.

On too many occasions, however, there are real cases of fraud. In one organization, the manager and staff members took travel expenses for trips that they did not take. The organization paid for automobile mileage when the employees used their personal cars to visit distant sites, which was part of their job. But the employees would create false trips of 200 miles (or 400 miles round-trip), often on several occasions during a week. Because there was no hotel bill to document their presence in the remote site, it would have been difficult to prove that they had not actually taken the trips. However, the auditors interviewed people who were supposed to have been visited to verify that the workers had actually made the trips, which was one way of detecting the fraud. And in one case, the auditors discovered that an employee had submitted a request for compensation for a round-trip during specific hours, although it was documented that the worker was in a distant city, on another trip, during those same hours.

BUDGETS AND BUDGETING

One of the more important ways in which social programs are audited or evaluated is by looking at their budgets. Setting up a budget is a major activity in agency planning. The budget is simply the organization's plan of activity translated into numbers. Evaluators can determine with a high degree of accuracy the organization's real priorities and interests by examining the budget. An organization that says its primary focus is on, for example, preventing child abuse, but that has little or no budget for prevention personnel, may be doing something entirely different, such as expending most of its money on fund-raising or other activities.

Classic items in a budget, particularly those in a governmental or nonprofit organization budget (Carmichael, Dropkin, & Reed, 1998), include salaries; employee benefits; payroll taxes; professional and other contract services fees; supplies; telephone; postage and shipping; occupancy or rent; interest expense (for a nonprofit rather than a governmental organization); rental, purchase, or maintenance of equipment; printing; and publications.

One of the usual functions of accountants in an organization is to keep careful track of how the organization's funds are being expended. Ideally, an organization's budget is followed in every aspect of the organization's functioning. If there are to be variations from the budget, permission is typically required, in governmental organizations, from a controlling organization higher than the operational group that spends the budget or, in a nonprofit organization, if the deviation is large, from the board of trustees or directors. Of course, accountants also determine that the proper authorization has been provided by personnel with the power to allow the expenditure.

An organization that is spending at a rate much larger than the budget had projected is in danger of expending all of its funds before the fiscal year ends. However, similarly, an organization that has spent little of its budget is not necessarily an organization that is frugal, although some might think that would be the case, but rather an organization that is probably not doing its job. Spending money is one of the things organizations do in pursuing their objectives, and not spending means that they are not carrying out their purposes.

So the agency's budget is one of the many ways in which accounting processes in human services organizations are typically quite different from those in profit-making companies. It is also quite different from a personal or family budget.

LINE-ITEM AND PROGRAM BUDGETING

There are many different kinds of budgets and budgeting processes. The line-item budget is the most traditional. It includes the categories described above—items of expenditure. However, the program budget is one of the more commonly used alternative forms of budgeting. It divides the expenditures into purposes or programs, and the specific items of expenditure, such as personnel, travel, and rent, are subsumed under the programs. The theory is that it is impossible to know what an organization is actually doing just by examining its expenditures on

a budget category. However, studying how much of the budget is spent on specific programs yields much more useful information. Audits may include an examination of both kinds of budgets, and many organizations maintain both kinds.

ACCOUNTING PROCESSES

Effective organizations have well-trained accountants on their staffs or contract for the services of well-trained accountants from professional accounting firms. These people know about the various kinds of accounting, keep careful records (documenting all of the organization's transactions), and maintain appropriate fiscal records for the agency. Organizations make sure that the funds available are sufficient to carry out the expenditure. They make certain that the budget allows for the particular expenditure, and they make certain that the organization's bylaws or other operating rules allow for the kind of expenditure that is being made.

MULTIPLE FUNDING SOURCES

In most human services agencies, there are many sources of funds. The organization may have income from fees, income from grants or contracts from private foundations or governmental bodies, donations from those who support the organization's activities, and, in some cases, endowments that provide interest and dividends to the organization, which can be used for some operating expenses. The complexity of multiple sources of funds is such that agency accounting personnel and frequently agency administrators are required to expend extensive periods of time making certain that the expenditures are legal and proper and within the rules of the funding sources.

For example, a $50,000 grant or contract from a governmental agency will usually come with a specific budget, often a budget that has been proposed by the organization staff members who wrote the proposal for the receipt of the funds. Every grant and contract operates under a variety of specific rules and regulations. For example, some funding organizations will not allow the expenditure of funds for the purchase of equipment. They approve of the expenditure of funds for the rental of equipment (equipment includes items such as computers, printers, copy machines, and dictating equipment), whereas others may allow for the purchase of equipment under the terms of the grant or contract but will not allow for payment of rental costs.

Similarly, the personnel line item in a grant or contract budget may not allow for the employment of nonprofessional personnel. In other words, the personnel funds may have to be spent exclusively for social workers, in some cases. In others, personnel costs are not as limited. Obviously, accountants and managers must be constantly familiar with what the external fund may provide or may not provide. These are important issues, because many grants and contracts, as indicated, require the organization to provide an audit at the end of the grant or contract period. That may sometimes be a condition for receiving additional funds from the organization, or it may lead to a requirement that the organization replace all or part of the funds that were provided, if the audit does not show proper expenditures of the moneys within the terms of the grant or contract.

VARIETIES OF RULES AND REGULATIONS

Auditors and accountants who work with human services organizations recognize that organizations are held fiscally responsible in various ways. For example, there are different accounting rules approved by the professional accounting organizations for nonprofit agencies (Carmichael et al., 1998). There are different rules and regulations used in governmental organizations. Governmental organization rules and procedures are promulgated under generally accepted accounting principles (GAAP). These are applied to state and local governments (Bailey, 1998). There are also specific guides for voluntary health and welfare organizations (American Institute of Certified Public Accountants, 1994a, 1994b). Once these rules and procedures are established for nonprofits, governmental bodies, and voluntary health and welfare organizations, accountants and auditors throughout the nation generally accept and begin to apply them by advising their organizations of their accounting and auditing obligations. The Web sites for these organizations are given in the reference list for this chapter. These can guide interested persons to the latest versions of the auditing and accounting rules, based on federal and state legislation. The Practitioners Publishing Company converts these rules and procedures into guide books (such as Carmichael et al., 1998) that auditors and accountants may use in carrying out their duties. Organizations for accountants and auditors also sponsor workshops and seminars that further assist in learning about and applying financial accounting and auditing rules.

DONATIONS

A special issue in human services organizations is the receipt and handling of donations. It is a matter of evaluation to determine the extent to which an organization uses contributions in the ways specified in its publicity and planning. It is important for some organizations to be quite clear about their policies for the receipt of funds and for the acknowledgment of those funds to contributors. That is because voluntary contributions are tied very closely to the tax laws. When individuals, families, foundations, and corporations make gifts to human services organizations, they often do so as part of their overall tax strategy. That is, they are entitled to deductions from their income taxes for contributions they make to appropriate organizations.

The first step in the whole process of receiving such contributions is to ensure that the organization has received appropriate status from the U.S. government as an organization that is able to receive funds that are tax deductible. The most familiar term is the 501(c)(3) organization, which is a religious, scientific, literary, educational, or charitable organization. Such an organization must apply for 501(c)(3) status, and when it is granted, the organization may receive voluntary contributions that are tax deductible. However, this is not the only kind of organization that can receive tax-exempt funds. There are 25 other designations for organizations that can receive funds and contributions that will constitute tax deductions for the contributors. The 25 other kinds of categories of tax-exempt organizations include associations, professional organizations, employee associations, social clubs, and recreation clubs. These organizations may receive funds, such as dues, that may be allowable as business expense tax deductions but not as charitable organizations. For example, the National Association of Social Workers is not a charitable organization under 501(c)(3) but is an association that can receive tax-exempt payments and contributions as a nonprofit, professional association. The National Association of Social Workers also has a 501(c)(3) or a charitable organization associated with it for which it can solicit and receive contributions (many other such groups have similar organizations associated with them). Churches and some similar religious organizations are exempt from the requirement of obtaining tax-exempt status from the government. Instead, they are assumed to be appropriate organizations for the receipt of contributions for their operating expenses, construction of buildings, and other fiscal activities.

There are many other complicated rules about receiving funds, as opposed to simply spending them. Individuals, families, and organizations may give an organization *in-kind* contributions. For example, contributions may be in the form of paintings, furniture, stocks and bonds, or other noncash items. Precisely how those are valued is often up to the individual who provided them, who must document the value of the products and the basis for determination of that value for tax deduction purposes.

Furthermore, the organization, in order to give credit to the contributor for a noncash or cash contribution of a certain amount or more ($250.00 when this chapter was written), must provide a formal, written receipt. A canceled check, which once was documentation acceptable to tax authorities, no longer qualifies as sufficient documentation of the contribution. Now there must be a written receipt from the recipient organization.

All of this becomes quite complicated with certain kinds of fund-raising activities. For example, when an organization has a dinner as a fund-raiser, the organization must specify how much of the cost of the ticket for the dinner is a tax-deductible contribution and how much is the fair market value of the dinner itself. Similarly, when people purchase items at agency auctions, the organization must specify the fair market value of the items purchased, and only the difference between that value and the actual payment is considered a contribution to the organization.

All of these matters are also factors in the evaluation of the organization's efficacy. That is, the organization may have fund-raising activities that cost almost as much as the funds raised by the activities. There are organizations that evaluate charities and other fund-raising organizations to determine the actual costs of their fund-raising efforts (Alexander & Rogonese, 1995; Council of Better Business Bureaus, Inc., 2003). Some organizations spend more than half of the proceeds from their functions on their fund-raising. A good rule of thumb is for an organization to spend no more than 10% of its proceeds on the actual cost of the event or program. The Council of Better Business Bureaus suggests that at least half of fund-raising efforts be spent on programs and that no more than 35% of proceeds be spent on fund-raising. No more than half of the proceeds of fund-raising should be spent on the combination of fund-raising costs and administration of the organization.

These matters are, in some states, regulated by state government. In many states it is the office of the secretary of state that regulates and evaluates charities for their fund-raising costs. Some state secretaries place a more positive face on this activity. In South Carolina (with which the author is most familiar), the secretary of state announces Angel Awards for organizations that hold their fund-raising costs down to 10%, or well below the costs of the functions they sponsor. Organizations are then able use their designation as "Angels" in their fund-raising appeals to the public. One of the reasons that United Way organizations are popular with contributors is that they generally raise funds for a cost of only a small percentage of the proceeds of their campaigns. They do so by using large numbers of volunteers, by running large and intense public campaigns, and by representing multiple agencies in their communities.

PROFIT-MAKING ORGANIZATIONS

It should be clear that not all human services organizations are either governmental or nonprofit. There are many proprietary or profit-making organizations in the human services. Many of these are in the medical field. Nursing homes, private clinics, child day care centers, and some mental health programs are profit-making organizations. Therefore, they operate under different rules than do the nonprofit and governmental organizations. However, many operate on grants and on contracts as well as through reimbursements from government agencies. Many nursing homes, for example, receive substantial portions of their income from Medicaid and, in a few cases, from Medicare. (Medicaid is a federal–state program for low-income people that can provide long-term care for people who need it. Medicare, the program for older adults, limits its expenditures for long-term care to relatively short periods of time in connection with discharges from hospital stays.) Governmental organizations that provide funds to proprietary or profit-making organizations have a right to audit the organizations and frequently to determine the actual and reasonable costs of the services they provide. A very specific formula is used by Medicaid and Medicare for determining cost. By law, Medicaid agencies and Medicare, when dealing with hospitals and long-term care facilities such as nursing homes, pay fees related to the audited costs of those services.

After health care organizations such as those described have been audited by governmental bodies, the government may owe the health care facility more for its services than it had provided initially, or it may be entitled to a refund from the facility. The costs in the case of proprietary organizations include profits for the owners of the company. However, in many ways there are few differences between nonprofit and profit-making companies. The only real difference is that the funds received that exceed the cost of the services provided are, in the case of nonprofit organizations, used to improve the services of the organization, to improve salaries for the employees, or to start new services. However, profits are never distributed to a board of directors or other owners who may be stockholders because they are not allowed to make or distribute a profit. In the case of profit-making organizations, they can distribute funds to the owners or stockholders of the company. However, in the nonprofit organization, the profits may sometimes be used to bolster the salaries of the top executives.

CONCLUSION

The financial aspects of agency operations are regularly subjected to evaluation. Few other elements of the agency's functions are likely to be so consistently reviewed for compliance with policies and for the purposes of evaluating the functioning of the organization. The whole issue of fiscal accounting and accountability is complex and is the subject of many statutes, policies, and guides in the field of accounting.

This chapter has outlined some of the basic issues of which social workers should be aware in their work in organizations. Accounting, budgeting, and auditing, as well as the specifics of managing donations and reporting fiscal operations, are covered in the chapter. All of these subjects are of special importance to agency managers as well as all other managerial staff in human services agencies.

References

Accounting reform: Watching the watchdogs. (2003, March). *Consumer Reports*, p. 6.

Alexander, I. A., & Rogonese, C. D. (1995). *Annual charity index*. New York: Council of Better Business Bureaus, Inc.

American Institute of Certified Public Accountants. (1994a). *Audit and accounting guide: Audits of certain nonprofit organizations*. New York: Author.

American Institute of Certified Public Accountants. (1994b). *Industry audit guide: Audits of voluntary health and welfare organizations*. New York: Author.

Carmichael, D. R., Dropkin, M., & Reed, M. L. (with Militio, V. R., Eason, S. B., Fransen, K. W., & Holland, S. E.). (1998). *Guide to audits of nonprofit organizations* (11th ed., Vols. 1–3). Fort Worth, TX: Practitioners.

Council of Better Business Bueaus, Inc. (2003). BBB wise giving alliance standard for charity accountability. Retrieved July 22, 2003, from http://www.give.org/standards/newcbbbstds.asp

70

CONSTRUCTING AND USING LOGIC MODELS IN PROGRAM EVALUATION

Thomas Chapel

Program evaluation presents us with a paradox. Although far fewer evaluations are conducted than is desirable, the *desire* to evaluate seems to come naturally and almost instinctively. That is, most of us want to know what makes a difference and, given the chance, will choose that course of action likely to produce the greatest impact. Many obstacles block the exhibiting of this instinctive evaluation behavior.[1] Chief among these are misunderstanding the components of good evaluation—ironically, usually an *overestimation* of the required level of scrutiny, rigor, and time and resources—missteps in determining a useful and feasible evaluation focus, and inattention to integrating evaluation results into planning and program improvement. Fortunately, these obstacles can be overcome if evaluation design is based on an accurate and comprehensive program description. Although many approaches can produce good program descriptions, at the Centers for Disease Control and Prevention (CDC), we promote logic models as the most effective way. This chapter introduces the concept of logic modeling and, using a few crosscutting examples inspired by CDC and other public health programs,[2] will demonstrate how a logic model can improve both program evaluation and the likelihood that evaluation results will be used to make a difference. Cases on which we will draw include the following:

- *Childhood lead poisoning prevention.* Lead poisoning is the most widespread environmental hazard facing young children, especially in older inner-city areas, which even at low levels has been associated with reduced intelligence, medical problems, and developmental problems. The main sources of lead poisoning in children are paint and dust in older homes with lead-based paint. Public health programs address the problem through outreach and screening of high-risk children, identifying those with elevated blood lead levels, assessing their environments for sources of lead, and case managing both their medical treatment and the correction of their environment. Programs usually must rely on partnerships with others to accomplish the actual medical treatment and the reduction of lead in the home environment.

- *Affordable home ownership program.* The program aims to provide affordable home ownership to low-income families by identifying and linking funders/sponsors, construction volunteers, and eligible families, who together build a house over an 8-week period. At the end of the period, the home is sold to the family using a no-interest loan.

- *Division of violence prevention.* CDC's mission in violence prevention is to prevent violence-related injuries and deaths through surveillance, research and development, capacity building, and leadership (National Center for Injury Prevention and Control, 2002).

- *Comprehensive cancer control.* CDC defines comprehensive cancer control as an integrated and coordinated approach to reducing cancer incidence, morbidity, and mortality through prevention, early detection, treatment, rehabilitation, and palliation. Important components of comprehensive cancer control planning include enhancing infrastructure, mobilizing support through education, using data and research, and building partnerships (National Center for Chronic Disease Prevention and Health Promotion, 2002).

BACKGROUND

Program evaluation is one of 10 essential public health services (Public Health Functions Steering Committee, 1994) and a critical organizational practice in public health (Dyal, 1995). Until recently, however, there has been little agreement among public health officials on the principles and procedures for conducting such studies. In 1999, CDC published *Framework for Program Evaluation in Public Health*. The framework defined effective program evaluation as "a systematic way to improve and account for public health actions by involving procedures that are useful, feasible, ethical, and accurate" and specified six steps in conducting good evaluations of public health programs (see Figure 70.1).

Although there is little radical or new about the CDC framework steps, they have helped broaden and improve evaluation at CDC in two ways. First, the framework elevates the definition of *good evaluation* to evaluation that is used, that is, evaluation that successfully accomplishes the last step, *ensure use and share lessons*. Second, by depicting the steps in a circle, the framework emphasizes that the steps build on each other. By doing a good job of engaging stakeholders and describing the program, we ensure the best choice of focus, the most credible evidence gathering, and the strongest justification of our conclusions.

LOGIC MODELS

Logic models are the main tool employed in the CDC Framework's second step, *describing the program*. Logic models are graphic depictions of the relationship between a program's activities and its intended effects. Two words in this definition bear emphasizing. The term *relationship* is used in the following sense: Logic models convey not only the steps or components of the program's activities, but also the link or *relationship* between those components and effects or outcomes. *Intended* is used in this sense: Logic models depict expected, or *intended*, effects or outcomes of a program's activities, rather than reality, at any point in time. As the starting point for evaluation and planning, the model serves as an outcomes road map that depicts the logic behind the program; that is, of all activities that could have been undertaken to address this

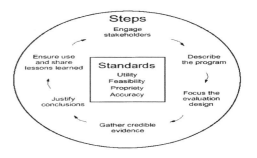

FIGURE 70.1 CDC's framework for program evaluation.

problem, we chose these activities because, if implemented *as intended*, they should lead to the effects depicted. Over time, evaluation, research, and day-to-day experience will deepen the program's understanding of what works and doesn't work, and the model will change accordingly.

The insights gained from developing the logic model are used in other framework steps. In particular, the model process organizes the discussion with stakeholders in the prior step and helps identify disagreements among them. And once the big picture of a program has been depicted in the logic model, it sets the stage for choosing the best evaluation focus in the next step.

Experts disagree on the best way to construct logic models and even on the terms used to label their components.[3] In developing the CDC Framework, we restricted ourselves to two terms, *activities* and *effects*, but, in practice, we find that the following four components are usually displayed in a comprehensive logic model.[4]

- *Inputs* are the resources on which the program is dependent to effectively mount its activities.
- *Activities* are the actual work that takes place as part of the program and that is performed by the program and its staff.
- *Outputs* are the direct products of a program's activities; often they are tangible services or products that can be counted.
- *Effects*, often called outcomes or impacts, are the intended changes that we hope will result from program activities and outputs. These may occur in a sequence from short term to long term.

Although these distinctions work well in theory, in practice the classifications are usually fuzzier. In particular, distinguishing outputs from effects or outcomes is often problematic. As a general rule, we restrict the term *effect* to changes in someone or something other than the program and its staff.[5]

Constructing Simple Logic Models

Although we may have a good understanding of our activities and effects, the act of composing a picture helps clarify implicit assumptions about the relationship of activities and intended effects, and the sequence in which effects will occur. Fortunately, logic models need not be complicated to yield these insights. In fact, a useful logic model can be constructed in four simple steps:

1. *Develop a list of activities and intended effects.* To stimulate thinking about activities and effects, some or all of the following three approaches may help develop a comprehensive list. The list should be displayed as two-column table, one of activities and one of effects.
   (a) *Review information on the program,* extracting from it anything that meets the definitions of activity or of effect.
   (b) *Work backward from effects.* When a program is given responsibility for a new or large problem, there may be clarity about the big change (most distal effect) the program is to produce, but about little else. Here, working backward from the distal effect by asking "how to" will help identify the factors, variables, and actors that will be involved in producing change.
   (c) *Work forward from activities.* Sometimes there is clarity about activities but not about why they are part of the program. Moving forward from activities to intended effects by asking "So what? Then what happens?" is often helpful in elaborating downstream effects of the activities.
2. *Subdivide the lists to display any time sequence.* Expand the two-column table to four to six columns. Place the activities and effects in the columns, depending on the order in which they are expected to occur. That is, do some occur first, or must some occur to serve as a platform for others?
3. (Optional) *Add any inputs and outputs.* Add a column to the left of the activities and insert any inputs, using the definition given earlier. Add a column to the right of the activities and insert any outputs.
4. *Draw arrows to depict causal relationships.* The multicolumn table of inputs, activities, outputs, and effects that has been developed so far may be enough detail, depending on the purposes for which the model will be used. For conveying in a global way the components of a program, it almost certainly will suffice. However, when the model is being used to set the stage for planning and evaluation discussions, the model should include arrows that show the causal relationships among activities and effects. Arrows can go in a variety of directions. Activities may feed into other activities or lead to selected effects. Early effects may lead to later effects or back to inputs, and later effects may cycle back to change how the program does its activities.
5. *Clean up the logic model.* Early versions are likely to be sloppy, and a nice, clean one that is intelligible to others often takes several tries.

Figures 70.2 through 70.5 show this process for CDC's childhood lead poisoning prevention (CLPP) program. Figure 70.2 shows the list of activities and effects extracted from information about the program. This is subdivided into early and late activities and effects in Figure 70.3, and then inputs and outputs are added in Figure 70.4. A final logic model that includes the implied causal relationships is presented in Figure 70.5.

Elaborating the Simple Model

Often the simple models that result are sufficient to begin planning or evaluation discus-

- Activities
  - Outreach
  - Screening
  - Case management
  - Referral to medical tx
  - Identification of elevated kids
  - Environmental assessment
  - Environmental referral
  - Family training
- Effects/Outcomes
  - Lead source identified
  - Families adopt in-home techniques
  - EBLL kids get medical treatment
  - Lead source gets eliminated
  - EBLL reduced
  - Developmental "slide" stopped
  - Q of L improved

FIGURE 70.2 CLPP Program: activities and effects.

Early Activities	Later Activities	Early Effects	Later Effects
If we do...	*And we do...*	*Then....*	*And then...*
Outreach	Case mgmt of EBLL kids		
Screening	Refer EBLL kids for medical treatment	EBLL kids get medical treatment	EBLL reduced
ID of elevated kids	Train family in in-home techniques	Family performs in-home techniques	Develop'l slide stopped
	Assess environment of EBLL child	Lead source identified	Quality of life improves
	Refer environment for clean-up	Lead source removed	

FIGURE 70.3 CLPP Program: sequencing of activities and effects.

Inputs	Early Activities	Later Activities	Outputs	Early Outcomes—	Later Outcomes
Funds	Outreach	Do case mgmt	*Pool (#) of eligible kids*	EBLL kids get medical treatment	EBLL reduced
Trained staff for screening and clean up	Screening	Refer for medical treatment	*Pool (#) of screened kids*	Family performs in-home techniques	Develop'l slide stopped
R'ships with orgs	ID of elevated kids	Train family in in-home techniques	*Referrals (#) to medical treatment*	Lead source identified	Quality of life improves
Legal authority		Assess environ't	*Pool (#) of "leaded" homes*	Lead source removed	
		Refer house for clean-up	*Referrals (#) for clean-up*		

FIGURE 70.4 CLPP Program: activities, effects, inputs, and outputs.

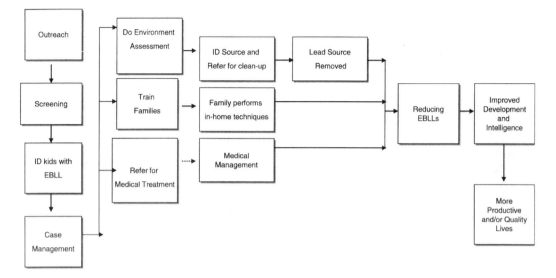

FIGURE 70.5 CLPP Program: "causal" roadmap.

sions. But typically, models will benefit from some elaboration, especially of the effects side of the model. Either or both of the following elaborations may make the model more useful.

Elaborating Distal Effects

Sometimes the simple model will end with the short-term effects or even outputs. Although this may reflect a program's mission, usually the program has been created to contribute to some larger purpose, and depicting this in the model leads to more productive strategic planning discussions later. This elaboration is accomplished by asking "So what? Then what happens?" of the last effect depicted in the simple model, and by continuing to ask that of all subsequent effects until more distal ones are included.

Figures 70.6 and 70.7 illustrate the process of elaboration for the affordable home ownership program. Figure 70.6 displays the very simple logic model that might result from a review of the narrative about this program. Figure 70.7 shows the model for this same program after elaborating the effects by asking "So what? Then what happens?" of key stakeholders. Note that the original five-box model survives as the core of the elaborated model, but the intended effects now include a stream of more distal effects for both the new home-owning families and also for the communities in which houses are built. As discussed later, developing and re-

viewing the elaborated model should motivate the organization to examine whether enough activities are in place to produce this expanded set of effects.

Elaborating Intermediate Effects

Sometimes the initial model presents the program's activities and its most distal effect in detail, but with a gap in between. In this case, the goal of elaboration is to better depict the program logic that links activities to the distal effects. Depicting this step-by-step road map to a difficult distal destination helps the model persuade skeptics that progress is being made in the right direction, even when the destination has not been achieved, and aids the program in examining how far progress is being made and what can be done to accelerate it.

The CDC division responsible for violence prevention offers a good illustration. The mission can be displayed as a simple logic model in Figure 70.8. However, the process of elaboration leads to the more thorough model in Figure 70.9 in which the same activities disclosed in the initial model produce the major distal effect.

The final step in developing logic models is determining the appropriate level of detail. This depends on the use to which the model is being put and the main audience for the model. A very global model will work best for stakeholders such as funders and authorizers, but program

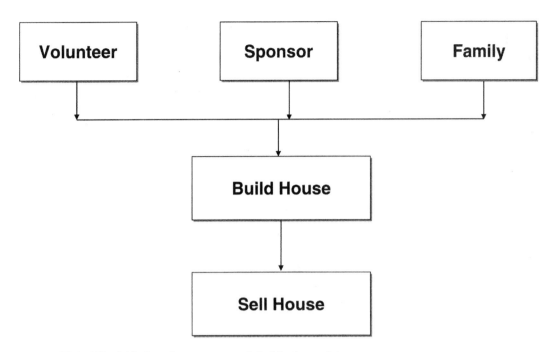

FIGURE 70.6 Affordable housing program: global logic model.

staff may need a more detailed model that reflects day-to-day activities and causal relationships. Sometimes, more than one model is necessary to meet these various needs. In these cases, it is most helpful to develop a global model first. Then all others are viewed not as different models, but as a single model at different levels of resolution or magnification. For example, when using Mapquest or a similar locator program, the user can zoom in or zoom out on the road map, depending on the detail needed, but understands intuitively that these are based on the same underlying map. The family of related models ensures that all players are operating from a common frame of reference. Even when some staff are dealing with a discrete part of the program, they are cognizant of where that part fits into the larger picture.

CDC's comprehensive cancer control program includes a family of related models. Figure 70.10 shows the global model for this program, whereas Figure 70.11 zooms in on this global model to provide more detail for those involved in day-to-day planning and implementation. All elements of the global model are displayed in the more detailed version, but the latter model indicates that the partnership component of the global model comprises a detailed list of inter-

mediaries and that embedded between program activities and effects is a set of change agents who are the levers for the system and individual behavior changes specified in global model. Engaging and working with these intermediaries and change agents is likely to be a priority focus for day-to-day efforts of program staff, even those these intermediaries and agents are not displayed in the global model.

USING LOGIC MODELS

At this point, the program using the CDC Framework approach has a logic model that depicts inputs, activities, outputs, and effects and may even have a family of related models of greater or lesser resolution. The logic model produces clarity for the program and its staff, and sometimes that is all it is intended to do. But, more often, the logic model sets the stage for discussions of strategy and evaluation. At CDC, logic models have been helpful in a variety of ways. In setting research agendas, logic models can help because they display the *implied* causation in the program logic. Using the model, program and research staff can examine where implied causation is supported by evidence,

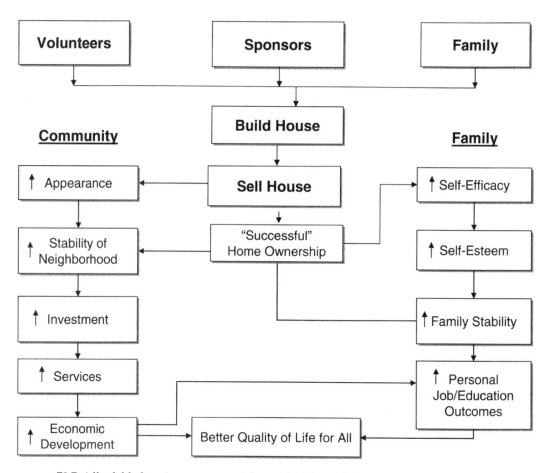

FIGURE 70.7 Affordable housing program: elaborated logic model.

where major evidence gaps exist, and which of those gaps are highest priority because they are on the critical path by which the program's activities produce its intended effects. In strategic planning, the logic model can graphically depict the program's mission and vision, thus setting the stage for examining progress on key effects, and which activities can be added or strengthened to accelerate it.

But the use of logic models at CDC grew mainly from an evaluation need. As mentioned, the logic models developed in the describing-the-program step prove useful at two other steps in the framework. First, the logic model process makes engagement of stakeholders more effective. Whether engaging stakeholders happens before or after the program description, these two steps are iterative. And the creation of the logic model aids in early identification and resolution of disagreements among key stakehold-

ers. As we have learned the hard way, stakeholders may disagree with some or all of the following:

• The activities that constitute the program
• The intended effects of the program
• The order in which effects are expected to occur
• The activities which are expected to produce the effects
• Which intended effects constitute success for the program

The resulting convergence of opinion is essential to good evaluation. Some stakeholders provide the credibility and access required to implement the evaluation successfully. And ensuring a consensus evaluation focus creates a market for the evaluation results, thus enhancing the chances that the results will be used to make a change.

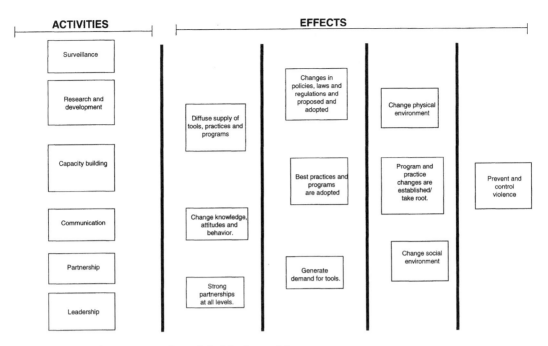

FIGURE 70.8 Violence prevention: global logic model.

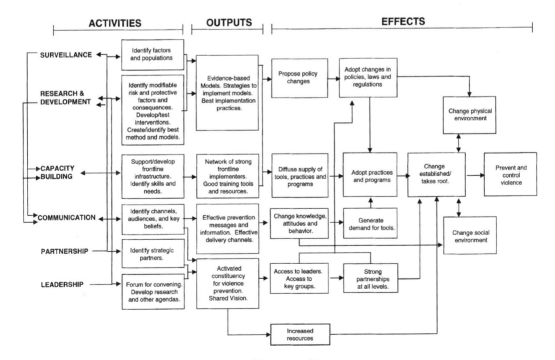

FIGURE 70.9 Violence prevention: elaborated logic model.

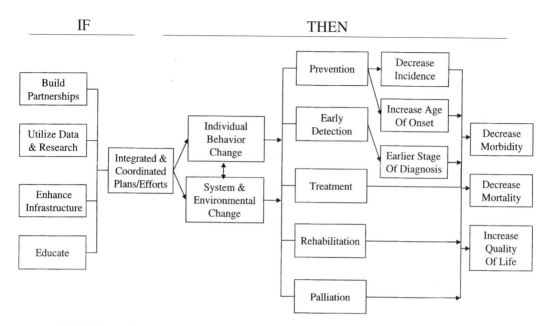

FIGURE 70.10 Comprehensive cancer control: global model.

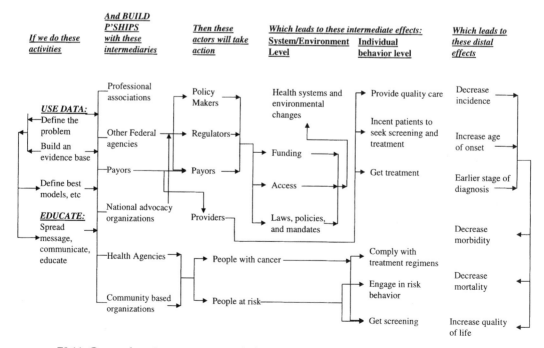

FIGURE 70.11 Comprehensive cancer control: detailed local model.

In designing an evaluation of a tuberculosis intervention in homeless shelters, stakeholders agreed on the list of intended effects of the program, including *improve quality of life for people with TB, increase access to medical care,* and *complete the TB drug regimen.* However, logic models developed by small groups revealed important differences in the sequencing of effects. Some saw the sequence as *complete drug regimen* leads to *access to medical care,* which leads to *improve quality of life,* whereas others displayed it as *improve quality of life* leads to *access to medical care* leads to *complete drug regimen.* Clearly, there were differences in the underlying program logic. These needed to be resolved because the resources, partnerships, and activities implied by each road map were significantly different.

Second, logic models frame the decisions on evaluation focus that must be made in the framework's third step, *focusing the evaluation design.* In the past, program evaluation tended to be overidentified with summative evaluation, conducted when the program had run its course and intended to answer the question, Did the program work? Consequently, a key question was, Is the program ready for evaluation? By contrast, the CDC Framework views evaluation as an ongoing activity over the life of a program that asks, Is it working? Consequently, a program is always ready for some evaluation, although the relevant evaluation questions are going to differ over the life of the program. The logic model, because it presents the big picture of the program, sets the stage for these focus discussions. Because the model displays the sequence of effects from short-term to most distal, a discussion of what we can expect to achieve at this point in the life of our project is not seen as an excuse for not reaching distal effects, but as a logical milestone on the journey to those effects. Likewise, an evaluation that includes only process evaluation can be justified using the model as an integral first step to producing even the early effects depicted there.

Determining the correct evaluation focus is a case-by-case decision. But several guidelines can help. Information gathered during earlier stakeholder discussions is a key resource in this step, including answers to questions such as Which stakeholders will use the evaluation results and for what purpose? Which effects need to be measured to meet that use? Beyond the users of the evaluation, are there other key stakeholders who are committed to specific effects, that is, who see those effects as markers of program success? By depicting all activities and effects and their relationships, the logic model makes these discussions smoother and more efficient.

In deciding on an evaluation focus on the effects side of the model, the needs of stakeholders must be balanced against other considerations, including the following:

- How long has the program been in place? It is unrealistic to expect a new program to achieve distal effects, even if these effects are among those that are most important to stakeholders.
- How intensive an effort is the program? Even at maturity, a small, unambitious effort cannot realistically be expected to make significant contributions to distal effects.

Because the logic model shows the sequence of effects and the relation of activities to effects, it can help frame the decisions about focus on the effects side of the model, especially when applying these guidelines produces choices that are contrary to preferences of stakeholders.

Finally, resources and logistics may influence the decision about evaluation focus. Some effects are quicker, easier, and cheaper to measure. Other effects may not be measurable at all. In the short run, at least, these facts may skew the decision about evaluation focus toward some effects as opposed to others.

The elaborated logic model for the affordable housing program was important because it clarified that, whereas program staff were focused on production of new houses, important stakeholders such as community-based organizations and faith-based donors were committed to more distal effects (e.g., changes in life outcomes of families or effects on outside investment in the community). The model led to a discussion of reasonableness of expectations and, in the end, to an expansion of evaluation indicators to include some of these more distal effects.

The CLPP program presented earlier is an example of an ambitious and complicated effort that can be expected to achieve its distal effects, but over time. In the early stages of implementing a CLPP program in a new city, evaluation might be expected to focus on outputs and short-term effects, such as number of children screened and number of children with elevated blood lead levels identified and referred. When the program had matured, it would be reasonable to expect program efforts to lead to sustained reductions in the elevated blood lead levels and to make a significant change in the overall prevalence of elevated blood lead levels in the community.

Process Evaluation Focus

When the rules for setting the effects focus are applied, we may conclude that no effects should be part of the current focus. Even when the focus includes some effects, a strong evaluation focus usually includes some process evaluation—unless there is absolute certainty that effects will be achieved. Evaluation serves not only to justify the program to outside stakeholders but also to produce insights for program improvement. Limiting evaluation to measurement of effects runs the risk of demonstrating that the program was a failure, but with little insight into why the program didn't work. Process evaluation helps unravel the mystery of program failure by examining issues of implementation fidelity: Were the program's activities actually implemented as intended? As with the effects focus, when evaluation resources are limited, only the most important issues of implementation fidelity can be included. Here are some usual suspects that (a) compromise implementation fidelity, (b) should be considered for inclusion in the process evaluation focus, and (c) can be readily identified in the logic model.

- *Transfers of accountability:* When a program's activities cannot produce the intended effects unless some other person or organization takes appropriate action, there is a transfer of accountability.
- *Dosage:* The intended effects of program activities such as training, case management, and counseling may presume a threshold level of participation.
- *Access:* When intended effects require not only an increase in consumer demand but also an increase in supply of services to meet it, then the process evaluation might include measures of access.
- *Staff competency:* The intended effects may presume well-designed program activities that are delivered by staff who are not only technically competent but are also matched appropriately with the target audience. Measures of the match of staff and target audi-

ence might be included in the process evaluation.

Our childhood lead poisoning logic model illustrates many of these process issues. As the model makes clear, reducing elevated blood lead levels presumes that the house will be cleaned, medical care referrals will be fulfilled, and specialty medical care will be provided. All of these are transfers of accountability beyond the program—to the housing authority, the parent, and the provider, respectively. For provider training to achieve its effects, it may presume completion of a three-session curriculum—a dosage issue. Case management results in medical referrals but presumes adequate access to specialty medical providers. And because lead poisoning tends to disproportionately affect children in low-income urban neighborhoods, many program activities presume cultural competency of the caregiving staff. Each of these components might be included in a process evaluation of a CLPP program.

PUTTING IT ALL TOGETHER

Thanks to effective use of logic modeling, a program is now well on the road to effective program evaluation. The model has produced clarity on program activities and effects and has ensured consensus among stakeholders on activities and effects. The existence of the model has helped the discussion of evaluation focus occur productively and swiftly and has ensured that all stakeholders are in agreement on which effects and activities should be part of the current evaluation focus. This up-front investment of time in developing a road map pays off by creating a market for the evaluation results from the start, thus ensuring that evaluation results will be used to make a difference.

Notes

1. For a thorough discussion of evaluation capacity building and obstacles to building it, see Milstein, Chapel, Wetterhall, et al. (2002).
2. These cases are composites of multiple CDC efforts, which have been simplified and modified to better illustrate teaching points. While inspired by real CDC and community programs, they may or may not reflect the current operation of these programs.
3. Some good sources of information on construction and use of logic models in evaluation include

Harvard Family Research Project: http://www.gse
.harvard.edu/hfrp/; Kellogg Foundation Logic Model
Development Guide: www.wkkf.org; University of
Wisconsin-Extension: http://www1.uwex.edu/ces/
lmcourse. In addition, the Community Tool Box
(http://ctb.ku.edu) is a helpful resource for most issues related to planning and evaluation of community
programs, including construction of logic models.

4. These definitions of terms have been adapted
from Office on Smoking and Health (2001).

5. Although the CDC Framework uses *effects* as
the label for results of program activities and outputs,
others use *outcomes* or *impacts*. And to distinguish
early from later effects, some will modify their term
of choice with *short-term, mid-term,* or *long-term,*
whereas others use terms such as *proximal* (close to
the intervention) and *distal* (far from the intervention) or *upstream* and *downstream*. One source of
confusion is the variable use of the terms *outcomes*
and *impacts*. Some use one or the other of these labels
in place of *effects*, whereas others use *outcomes* for
early effects and *impacts* for more distal ones; still
others reverse this usage.

References

Centers for Disease Control and Prevention. (1999).
    Framework for program evaluation in public
    health. *Morbidity and Mortality Weekly Report,*
    48(RR-11), 1–40.

Dyal, W. W. (1995). Ten organizational practices of
    public health: A historical perspective. *American
    Journal of Preventive Medicine, 11*(6, Suppl. 2),
    6–8.

Milstein, B., Chapel, T. J., Wetterhall, S. F., et al.
    (2002, Spring). Building capacity for program
    evaluation at the Centers for Disease Control and
    Prevention. In D. W. Compton, M. Baizerman,
    and S. H. Stockdill, The art, craft, and science of
    evaluation capacity building. *New Directions for
    Evaluation, 93.*

National Center for Chronic Disease Prevention and
    Health Promotion. (2002, March 25). *Guidance
    for comprehensive cancer control planning*. At-
    lanta, GA: Centers for Disease Control and Pre-
    vention.

National Center for Injury Prevention and Control.
    (2002). *Preventing violence: A public health
    framework*. Atlanta, GA: Centers for Disease
    Control and Prevention.

Office on Smoking and Health. (2001, November). *In-
    troduction to program evaluation for compre-
    hensive tobacco control programs*. Atlanta, GA:
    Centers for Disease Control and Prevention.

Public Health Functions Steering Committee. (1994,
    Fall). *Public health in America*. Retrieved June
    24, 2003, from http://www.health.gov/
    phfunctions/public.htm

PROGRAM EVALUATION
This Is Rocket Science

71

Kenneth R. Yeager

How could the space shuttle *Challenger* catas-
trophe and the deaths of all crew members
have been prevented?
How safe is health care?
Can medical errors be prevented?

Can process measurement and effective quality
programming prevent unnecessary fatalities?

This chapter examines processes associated with
estimation of safety in arenas where minimal

tolerance exists for error. Process measurement and evaluation is recommended as a tool to contribute to reduction of critical errors.

The space shuttle program was begun in the early 1970s with the concept of creating reusable craft for transporting people and cargo into space. When the first shuttle, *Columbia*, was launched in 1981, it represented the realization of a new era of reusable spacecraft. One year following the introduction of *Columbia*, the space shuttle *Challenger* rolled off the assembly line as the second of the new U.S. fleet of reusable spacecraft. Two others were to follow: *Discovery* in 1983 and *Atlantis* in 1985.

The space shuttle *Challenger* flew nine successful missions. The final mission was much like any other. *Challenger* was scheduled to conduct scientific experiments and to deliver cargo into space, specifically a tracking satellite to observe the tail of Halley's Comet. The most notable and unique function of this mission was the Teacher in Space Program. Sharon Christa McAuliffe, the first teacher to travel into space, was selected from more than 11,000 applicants from the education profession for entrance into the astronaut ranks.

Challenger's crew consisted of Mission Commander Francis R. Scobee; Pilot Michael J. Smith; Mission Specialists Ronald E. McNair, Ellison S. Onizuka, and Judith Resnik; and Payload Specialist Gregory B. Jarvis. The flight was short. Seventy-three seconds into the flight, *Challenger* exploded, killing the entire crew, while millions watched in dismay as a ball of fire consumed the crew.

Investigations were launched and surprising revelations came to light as a result. By now, most are familiar with the failure of the solid booster rockets' O-ring system, leading to catastrophic failure. Less understood by the general public but equally significant were investigations conducted by Nobel Prize recipient Richard P. Feynman as part of the Presidential Commission on the Space Shuttle *Challenger* Accident. This report brought to light enormous differences of opinion as to the probability of vehicle failure with loss of human life. Estimates of risk ranged from roughly 1 in 100 to 1 in 100,000, with higher figures coming from working engineers and the very low figures coming from NASA management. Estimates on the part of NASA management indicating 1 chance in 100,000 would imply that one could put up the shuttle each day for 300 years, expecting to lose only

one ship during that time period. Such estimates led Feynman to ask, What could be the cause of management's fantastic faith in the machinery? It appears that, for whatever purpose (whether for internal or external consumption), the management of NASA exaggerated the reliability of this product to the point of fantasy (Presidential Commission on the Space Shuttle *Challenger* Accident, 1986).

In Feynman's conclusions there are remarkable indications of a movement away from critical measurements in quality control programming and increasing reliance on assumptions of a lack of risk based upon previous absence of failures (essentially, the perspective is that quality is the absence of tragedy). A notable quote can be found in Feynman's review that applies to any discipline where technology and human life intersect. Feynman states, "For a successful technology, reality must take precedence over public relations, for nature cannot be fooled" (Presidential Commission on the Space Shuttle *Challenger* Accident Report, 1986, p. 69).

This remarkably powerful statement has its place in both the health care and human services fields. Donald Berwick, MD (1999), in his report to the National Academy of Sciences Institute of Medicine, indicated that more people die each year in the United States from medical errors than from highway accidents, breast cancer, or AIDS. Berwick's publication "To Err Is Human" presents studies showing between 44,000 and 98,000 people die each year as a result of mistakes by medical professionals (Berwick, 2000).

Much like the space shuttle scenario, an opposing view is presented by the American Medical Association, which reports that while any error that harms a patient is one error too many, "overwhelmingly the system of medicine in the United States is safe. . . . When you consider the millions of doctor/patient interactions each day" (Hayward & Hofer, 2001). The question remains: how safe is health care? The answer: There are startling levels of risk and harm to patients.

Bates et al. (1995) studied two of the most highly regarded hospitals in the world to determine degree of risk. This study indicated serious or potentially serious medication errors in the care of 6.7 out of every 100 patients. The Harvard Medical Practice Study, which reviewed over 30,000 hospital records in New York State, found that injuries from care itself occurred in

3.7% of hospital admissions. This study concluded that over half of the injuries were preventable, and that 13.6% of the errors resulted in death (Brennan et al., 1991). If these figures can be extrapolated to U.S. health care in general, then over 12,000 Americans die each year as a result of preventable errors in the health care system they turn to for healing.

More recent estimates indicate that progress has been made in reducing medical errors, and that in 2002 fewer than 3% of patients experienced severe medical errors. However, recent research indicates that mistakes are more common in complex cases. For example, Jessica Santillan died February 22, 2003, after receiving a heart–lung transplant from a donor with the wrong blood type. Slonim, LaFleur, Ahmed, and Joseph (2003) indicated in the March 2003 edition of *Pediatrics* that errors occur in approximately 11% of cases involving children with complex medical conditions.

What then is the method of reducing medical errors? What mechanism or combination of mechanisms will cut equally between fantasy and harsh reality for health care and human services? What becomes the process to measure efforts on the part of health care practitioners and human service workers toward and through processes of implementing best practices and evidence-based care? One answer is process measurement, designed to accurately capture problematic areas and to track initiatives designed to enhance the care delivered. Without accurate measurement, practitioners are left to believe that the practices in place are the most effective available. Accurate measurement is the key to scientifically based outcomes aligned with the application of best practices and evidence-based practice.

ASSUMPTIONS FOR MEASUREMENT

Assumptions for measurement are key to the utilization of process measurement. They will be mentioned but not elaborated on in this chapter, because they are thoroughly covered in other chapters. However, a brief discussion is required. Measurements must be valid, reliable, and designed to facilitate understanding and improved performance. But although measurements must be accurate, it is not true that they have to be overly complex or involve hours of statistical analysis to be effective. In fact, the most suc-

cessful measurements are those that are easily understood and easily linked to program goals and objectives. As a result, these measurements (a) can be utilized to drive organizational safety goals, (b) can be tied to current best practice applications, (c) can provide the opportunity for feedback from all staff persons, (d) can provide critical understanding to complex processes and emerging trends among populations served, (e) can provide critical clues into process improvement, and (e) can be utilized as a clear and accurate communication mechanism both internally and externally (Yeager, 2002).

USING STATISTICAL CONTROL CHARTS

Control charts (see Figure 71.1) are easy-to-use charts that make it easy to see both special and common cause variation in a process. They are called control charts, or sometimes Shewhart charts, after their inventor, Walter Shewhart, of Bell Labs. There are many different subspecies of control charts that can be applied to the different types of process data that are typically available (Austin, Gibb, Milos, Scott, & Raborn, 2002; Murray & Frenk, 2000; Wheeler & Chambers, 1992). All control charts have three basic components:

- A center line (AVG), usually the mathematical average of all the samples plotted
- Upper (UCL) and lower statistical control limits (LCL) that define the constraints of common cause variation
- Performance data plotted over time

Statistical control charts (shown in Figure 71.2) look at variation, seeking special causes and tracking common causes. Special causes can be spotted using several tests:

- 1 data point falling outside the control limits
- 6 or more points in a row steadily increasing or decreasing
- 7 or more points in a row on one side of the centerline
- 14 or more points alternating up and down

TYPES OF ERRORS

Control limits (shown in Figure 71.2) on a control chart are commonly drawn at 3's from the

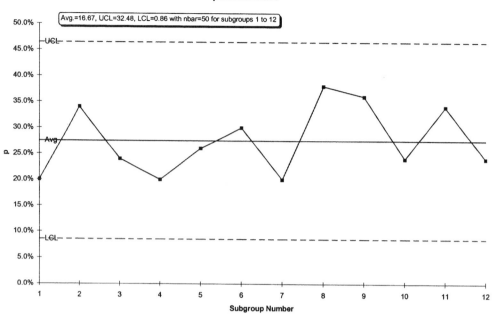

FIGURE 71.1 Control chart.

centerline because 3-sigma limits are a good balance point between two types of errors:

- Type I or alpha errors occur when a point falls outside the control limits, even though no special cause is operating. In this case, observation of process is required; however, hastily taken actions may only serve to disrupt a stable process.
- Type II or beta errors occur when a special cause is missed because the chart isn't sensitive enough to detect it. In this case, the problem exists beyond awareness and contin-

ues undetected until a time when critical mass accumulates and a problem is identified.

All process control is vulnerable to these two types of errors. This is because 3-sigma control limits balance the risk of error. Normally distributed data, data points will fall inside 3-sigma limits 99.7% of the time when a process is in control. This limits unnecessary evaluation while providing assurance that unusual causes of variation will be detected (Gunther & Hawkins, 1999; Murray & Frenk, 2000)

RESPONDING TO VARIATION: SPECIAL CAUSES

As processes are affected by special cause variation, they are considered to be unstable, or out of control. Removing special causes when they are harmful or integrating them into practice when they are beneficial is an important part of quality process improvement. Prompt response to special cause variation occurs when variation is identified early and the data used to identify them is timely (Murray & Frenk, 2000).

The following steps are required when special cause variation is identified:

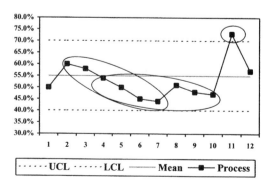

FIGURE 71.2 Statistical control chart.

1. Control any damage or problems with an immediate, short-term fix.
2. Search for the cause: Conduct a root-cause analysis by asking what was out of the ordinary. Examples include unexpected volume, a change in staff, or new materials. Data collection is critical, because it provides the basis for a complete analysis, noting details and tractability factors about the identified or recorded event.

Once you have discovered the special cause, you can develop a longer term remedy. Most special causes have a negative impact on the output of the process and need to be removed.

Occasionally, a special cause can have a positive impact, depending on the nature of the process. If this is the case, find ways to capture and integrate it into the system (Carey & Lloyd, 1995; Gunther & Hawkins, 1999; Murray & Frenk, 2000).

Avoid these mistakes:

• Changing the process to accommodate a special cause.
• Blaming individuals; chances are that the problem would have occurred regardless. This is a process of learning, and working with staff will improve processes.
• Identify differences between individual and system problems. Utilize education and system change to address problems as they arise.
• It's important not to stop when you've eliminated special causes of variation. Remember that identification of a common cause variation is only a part of a process of systematic quality improvement (Gunther & Hawkins, 1999; Murray & Frenk, 2000).

RESPONDING TO VARIATION: COMMON CAUSES

It is possible to improve a process despite the presence of statistical control. In stable processes, enabling a gradual tightening of specification limits and an overall attention to detail can improve quality, reduce staffing, and lower cost. Improving a stable process is somewhat more difficult than improving an unstable process. By definition, a stable process has no special causes of variation to indicate the need for change.

Therefore, process at this level requires looking at all data about the process, not simply what made one point different from the others.

Common causes of variation are hidden in the system; however, this does not mean that they are unavoidable. It is very possible to improve processes and enhance patient and client safety while reducing common cause variation. Experience has shown that integration of direct care staff familiar with a process yields numerous ideas for improvements that can make a significant impact, even on a sound process.

There are many different ways to search for and remove common causes. Probably the most well-known is experimentation, but you can also use stratification. Either of these methods may be helped by disaggregation of data.

Experimentation

In quality improvement in health care and human services, the process for experimentation with a process is the plan-do-check-act (PDCA) cycle described by Walter Shewhart and W. Edwards Deming, essentially an iteration of the scientific method (Deming, 1986; Yeager, 2002). The PDCA cycle stresses experimentation and observation as the means of discovering truth.

• In the planning stage, the problem is recognized and analyzed, and possible solutions formulated.
• In the doing stage, the most likely or effective solution is implemented in a test site.
• The checking stage is used to compare results of the test solution and the original method.
• The acting stage involves replacing the old method with the successful solution.

The search for common causes is just one of the many arenas in which the PDCA cycle can be used. This process is frequently implemented as a guide to overall process improvement, of which searching for common cause is only a small part.

The PDCA cycle calls for creative thinking and analytic thinking; it (PDCA cycle) is essential to process improvement. Analytic thinking encourages an exchange of ideas and processes to contribute to overall improvements in safety and care. Honest examination on a consistent basis is an important factor. Consistent feedback from all levels of care frequently leads to breakthrough paradigm shifts leading to processes beyond current and accepted ways of thinking about a process. However, creativity must not outweigh common sense. Process improvement must be monitored and regulated by analysis of data combined with convergent thinking that leads to a clean and coherent process (Yeager, 2002).

Stratification

Sometimes experimentation is not necessary, and common causes can be found using stratification of data. Stratifying data is essentially the separation of data into categories. Stratification often occurs iteratively as part of the data collection process—data are stratified at one level, then in one of the categories created by this stratification it is stratified again, and so on. If questions are posed at the most general level of data collected, then the information may lead to a superficial answer; however, if the data are stratified at different levels, links may begin to appear. The process of sorting data into multiple levels of groups with shared characteristics offers an opportunity to pinpoint the root cause of a problem. For example, if violent patients on a psychiatric unit are examined by primary diagnosis only, one may miss the presence of secondary or lesser ranks of substance abuse and potential substance withdrawal leading to increased levels of agitation and thus acting out on an inpatient level. Such processes can lead to increases in restraint or seclusion episodes.

Stratification can be accomplished by using Pareto charts, bar charts, or pie charts, all charts that can display counts of things in different categories. Even a cause-and-effect diagram could be used to build a tree of branching characteristics, each one being stratified further and further until root causes are reached (Carey & Lloyd, 1995; Gunther & Hawkins, 1999; Murray & Frenk, 2000).

Two common mistakes are made when stratifying data. First, it is easy to conclude too much from the stratification. Don't take small differences between category totals too seriously. Look for major differences instead; try stratifying the data using different stratification variables. Second, and more important, avoid the temptation to jump to a conclusion that an irregularly patterned category is the cause of the problem. The category may only provide a clue as to where to look for the cause, rather than being the cause (Gregiore, Rapp, & Portner, 1995).

Disaggregation

The process of disaggregating data or viewing its components individually can at times enhance experimentation or stratification. Frequently, in process improvement, it is difficult to view processes separately, because overlaps sometimes occur. Actively studying the components separately may assist in identifying a problem that exists in one process but that is hidden in another process. In the process of disaggregation, parts of the processes are viewed separately, yet it is important that they are still viewed as parallel processes working toward the same shared goal (Gregiore et al., 1995).

Disaggregation is the process of bringing pieces into view rather than actually separating them, permitting persons searching for improvement the opportunity to see both the forest and the trees. As with other quality improvement processes, searching for common causes through disaggregation relies heavily on regular meetings between managers and direct line staff, with both working together to examine distinct parts of the process so that all of the pieces can be discussed in the context of the entire system (Gregiore et al., 1995).

CONCLUSION

Clearly a link exists between program evaluation in health and human services. That link is the value of human life. As discovered from the examination of the *Challenger* disaster, the application of successful technology requires that reality take precedence over public relations. Clear and accurate assessment of data is required if health care and human services are to move forward in the development of technology. Measurement and open, honest communication of data are a must for health care and human service providers and administrators. If current standards of health care and provisions for human services are to be maintained, practitioners and administrators must not fall victim to subtle and apparently logical arguments that lead to critical alterations in safety criteria to facilitate increases in volume, throughput, and time savings. If practitioners accept false arguments that appear logical without implementing quality improvement and systematic program evaluation, they are at risk of providing care in an environment that is believed to be safer than it truly is. We must always remember that nature cannot be fooled.

References

Austin, M., Gibb, K. H., Milos, N., Scott, D. A., & Raborn, W. (2002, December). Understanding variation in revenue and expenses: Control charts can point the way to appropriate action to manage undesirable performance variation. *Healthcare Financial Management Magazine*, pp. 70–74.

Bates, D. W., Cullen, D., Laird, N., Petersen, L., Small, S., Servi, D., et al. (1995, July 5). Incidence of adverse drug events and potential adverse drug events: Implications for prevention. *Journal of the American Medical Association, 274*(1), 29–34.

Berwick, D. (2000). To err is human. In L. T. Kohn, J. M. Corrigan & M. S. Donaldson (Eds.), *To err is human: Building a safer health system* (p. 26). Washington, DC: National Academic Press.

Brennan, T. A., Leape, L. L., Laird, N. M., Herbert, L., Localio, A. R., Lawthers, A. G., et al. (1991). Incidence of adverse events and negligence in hospitalized patients: Results of the Harvard Medical Practice Study. *New England Journal of Medicine, 324*(6), 370–376.

Carey, R. G., & Lloyd, R. C. (1995). *Measuring quality improvement in healthcare: A guide to statistical process control applications*. Milwaukee, WI: ASQ Quality Press.

Deming, W. E. (1986). *Out of crisis*. Cambridge: Massachusetts Institute of Technology.

Gregiore, T., Rapp, C., & Portner, J. (1995). The new management: Assessing the fit of total quality management and social agencies. In B. Gummer & P. McCallion (Eds.), *Total quality management in social services: Theory and practice*. Albany, NY: Professional Development Program of Rockefeller College.

Gunther, J., & Hawkins, F. (1999). Making TQM work: Quality tools for human service organizations. New York: Springer.

Hayward, R. A., & Hofer, T. P. (2001). Estimating hospital deaths due to medical errors: Preventability is in the eye of the reviewer. *Journal of the American Medical Association, 286*, p. 219.

Murray, C. J. L., & Frenk, J. (2000). A framework for assessing the performance of health systems. *Bulletin of the World Health Organization, 78*(6), 717.

Presidential Commission on the Space Shuttle *Challenger* Accident. (1986, June 6). *Report (in compliance with Executive Order 12546 of February 3, 1986)*: Vol. 1. Retrieved June 25, 2003, from http://science.ksc.nasa.gov/shuttle/missions/51-l/docs/rogers-commission/table-of-contents.html

Slonim, A. D., LaFleur, B. J., Ahmed, W., & Joseph, J. G. (2003). Hospital-reported medical errors in children. *Pediatrics 111*, 617–621.

Wheeler, D. J., & Chambers, D. S. (1992). *Understanding statistical process control* (2nd ed., pp. 37–39). Knoxville, TN: SPC Press.

Yeager, K. R. (2002). Concepts of continuous quality improvement. In A. R. Roberts & G. J. Greene (Eds.), *Social workers' desk reference* (pp. 766–771). New York: Oxford University Press.

72

THE EVALUATION OF TRAINING FOR LEADERS OF FOSTER AND ADOPTIVE PARENT SUPPORT GROUPS

Elizabeth King Keenan

Numerous support groups for foster and adoptive parents currently exist in a New England state. Attendance tends to be uneven and inconsistent, and group member interaction in many support groups centers around airing problems without moving to a problem-solving or supportive stance. Support group leaders are employees of either a private nonprofit agency (the Connecticut Association of Foster and Adoptive Parents) or a public agency that provide services for foster and adoptive families. Administrators from both agencies report that many current leaders lack knowledge of group leadership skills to respond to these difficulties. Administrators thus decided that a once-monthly 9-month training for current group leaders would facilitate the development of their skills to increase attendance and improve the quality of the interaction at the foster and adoptive parent support group meetings.

This author conducted both the training and evaluation. The training intervention was created in consultation with the two agency administrators who identified the need for increased leader skills, specifically in the areas of recruitment and group facilitation. In reviewing the literature, this author found several training curriculums for leaders of foster or adoptive parent support groups (Brown & Wiedemeier, 1995; McNitt & Wasson, 1996; North American Council on Adoptable Children, 2002), but I noted that most are not presented in an ongoing format. In addition, this author found no research studies that examined the relationship between training and leader skills for leaders of foster or adoptive parent support groups. The

training was therefore designed to include an evaluation component that would generate empirical data regarding the relationship between the training intervention and the identified outcomes, which were as follows:

1. Group leader participation in training will result in increased leader skills as measured by the pre/post training group leader self-confidence questionnaire (see Appendix A).
2. Group leader participation in training will result in an increase in the number of parents attending the leader's support group, as measured by the final group monitoring form (see Appendix B).
3. Group leader participation in training will result in the leader's ability to report the presence of mutual aid dynamics and obstacles to mutual aid processes during support group meetings, as measured by the final group monitoring form.

These are all intermediate outcomes contributing to the ultimate outcome of foster and adoptive parents interacting with each other to obtain information and support (Shulman, 1999). The outcomes were based on the needs identified by the agency administrators and were supported by group work research that states that leader skills are a necessary but insufficient condition for successful group outcomes (Burlingame, Fuhriman, & Johnson, 2001; Corey & Corey, 1997; Yalom, 1995).

The training curriculum drew on several group models (Corey & Corey, 1997; Toseland & Rivas, 2001) but was largely based on Shulman's mutual aid model (1999) because of the match between the theoretical conceptualization and the support group purpose. Schwartz conceptualized mutual aid as an "alliance of individuals who need each other, in varying degrees, to work on certain common problems" (Schwartz, 1961, p. 18). Shulman (1999) has identified 10 processes of mutual aid: sharing data, all-in-the-same-boat phenomenon, developing a universal perspective, mutual support, mutual demand, individual problem solving, rehearsal, strength-in-numbers phenomena, discussing a taboo area, and emergence of new perspectives. He has also specified obstacles that interfere with the development of mutual aid in a group: trouble finding common ground or interests among members; difficulty negotiating rules, norms, procedures, or roles; and communication difficulties due to social taboos and norms, differences in cultural norms, or individual communication styles. The leader's role, according to Shulman, is to "help the group members create the conditions in which mutual aid can take place" (p. 303). Leader skills, then, emerge from this role. For this training, the following skills were identified: (a) ability to engage with prospective group members, (b) ability to create a shared purpose with group members, (c) ability to model expectations for group interaction, (d) ability to monitor the presence of mutual aid dynamics and obstacles to mutual aid, (e) ability to respond to conflicts and other obstacles to mutual aid, and (f) ability to elicit feedback from group members.

The training curriculum focused on the mutual aid processes and corresponding leader skills. The first training session was 6 hours long. Each subsequent monthly training session was 3 hours in duration and was structured in the following manner: The session began with a didactic component during which a specific aspect of mutual aid or leader skills was presented and discussed, drawing on leader experiences for illustrations; the group leaders then privately targeted goals for their specific groups, reviewing progress at the next training meeting; finally, the leaders gathered in small groups to provide mutual aid to each other as they discussed specific concerns in their own groups. The didactic content was only partially constructed prior to the training. After the first two trainings, content was selected in consultation with leaders, responding to the needs they identified.

Contextual information is also useful for understanding the challenges in measuring outcomes. Although the public and private agencies share similar goals when providing services for foster and adoptive families, there is also tension between the two systems that emerges both programmatically as well as between particular employees of each agency. In addition, there is some variation in how programs are implemented based on the region of the state in which the services are delivered. Agency staff from both agencies are also required to attend various trainings throughout the year, including this training. Public agency staff have not always found trainings to be helpful, stating that it places a demand on their time because they are expected to still attend to their caseloads. Program politics thus played a role in how the training was received by the group leaders (Gabor, Unrau, & Grinnell, 1998).

CHALLENGES IN MEASURING OUTCOMES

The evaluation component used the same materials that were used for the training itself. Knowing that group leaders have many other responsibilities in addition to the support group, training materials were designed to be completed primarily during the training sessions. Training materials included a pre/post training leader self-efficacy instrument, a monthly support group monitoring form of mutual aid dynamics and leader skills, monthly reviews of leader goals, a leader demographic form, and a training evaluation form. The evaluation analyzed data from the pre/post training leader self-efficacy instrument, the final monthly support group monitoring form, and the training evaluation form (see Appendixes A, B, and C). Research participation had no direct bearing on the participants' employment in either agency. Both agencies consented to the evaluation component of the training, participants provided their consent, and institutional review board approval was obtained.

Challenges in measuring outcomes centered around the following areas: (a) interactions between multiple stakeholders and this author's insider/outsider roles, (b) group leader distrust and lack of interest in research participation, (c) the evolution of the intervention over the course of the training, (d) confounding factors affecting outcomes, and (e) lack of access to the support group members.

Multiple Stakeholders and Insider/Outsider Role

As noted above, the agency administrators created the training intervention, requiring their staff (the group leaders) to attend. Seidman (1998) notes that participants have a heightened awareness of the hierarchical nature of relationships between evaluators and participants when evaluations have agency sponsorship, because the evaluator is often perceived as aligned with the administrators. This author had met with the administrators but not with any participants prior to the first day of training, so many participants responded to me as an outsider in a position of authority, and they wanted to know what my contact had been with the agency administrators. This hierarchical alignment was reinforced by my position at a state university, because many viewed me as disconnected from them. They did not view a university professor as having useful knowledge for their work, because universities do not always focus on applied research or the relationship between research and practice (Greenwood & Levin, 2000). This author attempted to alter this perception by emphasizing my insider role as someone who has worked for many years in agencies, has group work experience, and would be the trainer, but this was only somewhat successful. The sponsorship of the training evaluation by the administrators coupled with my university position thus resulted in some initial distrust between the participants and this trainer/evaluator (Royse, Thyer, Padgett, & Logan, 2001).

This distrust from participants can be attributed to the differing interests and positions of the multiple stakeholders in the evaluation. The administrators were interested in obtaining empirical data regarding the outcomes of the training for their own program monitoring, whereas the participants were wary because they were the focus of the evaluation and thus did not completely trust that the evaluation would not be used to evaluate their employee performance. Rossi, Freeman, and Lipsey (1999) state that difficulties in communicating with the multiple stakeholders can result in misunderstandings regarding the purpose and use of the evaluation, which then affects participation in the evaluation. They note that evaluation is inherently about providing empirical data to support judgments, so stakeholders who are being evaluated will have concerns about the how evaluation results will be used. The meaning and importance of the evaluator's findings will thus vary depending on the stakeholder's position.

This distrust was addressed on the first day of the training. This trainer/evaluator was forthcoming about the contact I had had with the administrators. This trainer/evaluator also informed participants about my agency and group leader experience and elicited their perspectives regarding their training needs and how the support groups had been functioning. The majority of the participants agreed with the administrators regarding the current state of support groups, but they disagreed on the intervention to achieve change. Most of the participants thought change would occur when they had an opportunity to talk with each other, to find solutions to their problems. The problems they identified dealt with systemic issues of communication and collaboration in and between the agencies, plus differing expectations of support groups by administrators, leaders, and group members. Thus, a consensus regarding the current functioning of the support groups was achieved in the first hour, but there were differing ideas regarding how to create improvements. This tentative consensus quickly unraveled, however, when the evaluation component of the training was presented.

Distrust and Lack of Interest in Research Participation

After introductions and mutual contracting regarding support group needs and training focus were completed, I then presented the evaluation component as a way to evaluate how well the training helped the group leaders respond to the needs of the foster and adoptive parent support groups. Adler and Adler (2002) state that persons are often reluctant to participate in research because of the history of ethical violations in research, and because research is often viewed as intruding into people's private lives or fostering social control. Many group leaders questioned how their confidentiality would be maintained. Identification numbers were used, with the code sheet kept locked in this author's office, but this did not seem satisfactory to some. In addition, others were not at all interested in supporting research because they did not think it would generate any important knowledge for them. This speaks to the continued disconnect between research and practice in the social work field, because many practitioners are unaware of the research applicable to their work, and researchers struggle with methodologies that capture the multiple factors influencing results in naturalistic studies (Gambrill, 2003).

The distrust was most clearly evident when this trainer/evaluator presented the informed consent form for their review and signature. Although the consent form's intent is to ensure the protection of participants, the amount of information now required turns it into a formidable document that reinforces this author's position of authority and dominance (Seidman, 1998). I attempted to describe the purpose and content of the informed consent form in informal language, but many participants once again viewed me as an outsider who was more aligned with administration and the university than with them. Fine, Weis, Weseen, and Wong (2000) have also found great difficulties in obtaining informed consent in their qualitative research. They state that preliminary rapport frequently unravels when discussing the informed consent form, highlighting the differing needs of researchers and participants. Institutional review board requirements for informed consent strive to provide safeguards for participants but also appear to have the unintended consequences of creating potential barriers between researcher and participant. Thus, although there were 45 participants at the first training session, only 25 elected to participate in the evaluation component.

Evolving Intervention and Confounding Factors

Although this trainer/evaluator used a specified curriculum, I selected monthly components in collaboration with group leaders on a month-by-month basis. This kept the content attuned to the specific group leader needs and increased my credibility with the participants. A flexible curriculum presents no problem when conducting a preliminary evaluation of this particular training, but does present a problem if this training is being scientifically tested, because that requires specific protocols of the intervention to determine if it is being reliably implemented (Rosen & Proctor, 2002). This is a continuing dilemma for me, because I am modeling the training in the manner that I am recommending

that the leaders use in conducting their support groups, that is, by flexibly selecting content in collaboration with the participants (Shulman, 1999). Articulating the specific details of a flexible curriculum thus appears challenging.

Additional confounding factors also presented challenges to measuring outcomes. As noted above, there were variations in agency service delivery depending on the region in which services are offered. Some group leaders therefore had more support from their administrators in the form of time and attention from the administrator. Other group leaders had more resources in the form of space, child care, refreshments, and office supplies. These factors most likely affected the ability of group leaders to effectively recruit and facilitate support groups. In addition, some groups tended to have a more educational focus, whereas others had a combination of mutual aid and education. Thus, the support groups are a heterogeneous variation of education, mutual aid, or a combination of the two.

Lack of Access to Group Members

Measurement of ultimate outcomes was hindered by the inability to access the group members themselves, who could have provided data regarding their experience of the support groups and leader skills. In response to the challenges of measuring outcomes, I decided to use a one-group pretest–posttest design (Royse et al., 2001), given the length of time involved in the training. The confounding factors identified above were included in the evaluation materials. Intermediate outcomes were selected, given the lack of access to support group members. If the evaluation data provided support for the training's effect on intermediate outcomes, a subsequent study could then measure ultimate outcomes with support group members.

SELECTING ITEMS FOR MEASURES OF OUTCOME AND EVALUATION INSTRUMENTS

As discussed in earlier sections, the foster and adoptive parent support group meetings had been characterized by infrequent or inconsistent attendance and a tendency to remain focused on problems rather than progressing into a supportive, problem-solving stance. The training curriculum thus focused on issues of group formation and the facilitation of mutual aid, drawing largely on Shulman's (1999) group model. Training handouts were developed to reinforce the didactic information, emphasizing monitoring of mutual aid dynamics, obstacles, and leader skills.

The training handouts were also designed as the evaluation measures so that no visible distinction would be made between those who were or were not participating in the evaluation component of the training. Evaluation measures targeted the three outcomes identified in the introduction: leader self-efficacy, support group attendance, and leader reporting of mutual aid dynamics and leader skills in support group meetings. These are intermediate outcomes that have been shown to be necessary conditions for ultimate outcomes of group member provision of mutual aid (Burlingame et al., 2001; Corey & Corey, 1997; Yalom, 1995). This author searched for but did not find standardized measures of monitoring mutual aid processes and leader skills, and thus I developed my own. I first created a pre/post training self-confidence questionnaire (see Appendix A). This was selected because counselor self-efficacy had been moderately positively related with various outcomes, including skills training (Larson & Daniels, 1998). The items in the questionnaire were taken from the training curriculum, and the standardized format of self-efficacy questions was used. Since the training was 9 months in duration, there would be sufficient time between the pre- and posttraining administration of this instrument to allow for change to occur.

The monthly support group monitoring form (see Appendix B) was developed so that participants could track the monthly attendance of their support groups, the presence of mutual aid dynamics and obstacles to mutual aid, and the leader skills they used during each meeting. The specific items were taken from Shulman's (1999) group model of mutual aid. In addition, this trainer/evaluator added two additional items to address confounding factors: I asked for a specification of the type(s) of group (e.g., education, mutual aid, social action, combination) in order to determine the degree to which mutual aid was being fostered, and I also added an additional obstacle to Shulman's list to determine if there were obstacles in obtaining necessary resources for the group. (These instruments have face validity with Shulman's theoretical concepts. Reliability has not yet been established for either of these instruments.)

Finally, an evaluation of the training was devised for participants to report the degree to which the training components facilitated the development of their skills (see Appendix C). The first four items addressed the primary components of the training: didactic presentation of mutual aid dynamics and leader skills, small group experience, individual group leader goal setting and review, and monitoring of interactions and leader skills during support group meetings. The next four items addressed the global aspects of the training: presentation of material, usefulness of material, and overall ratings of the trainer and the training. Space was also provided to add comments regarding the most and least useful components and suggestions for future training. The format was modeled after other training evaluation forms.

DISCUSSION

Two primary areas of concern emerged during this training evaluation: (a) My activities as trainer and evaluator conflicted on the first day of training, and (b) the training and evaluation of training placed differing demands on the structure of the training curriculum as intervention.

Evaluators and trainers both need to establish rapport with participants. Tensions arise, however, when evaluation is conducted as formal research, because it introduces additional requirements and interests. So, although social workers are encouraged to evaluate their practice, the findings can only be disseminated beyond the immediate place of practice if informed consent and institutional review board approval are obtained. When this is presented to potential participants, additional interests enter the relationship, including the researcher's self-interests, because the results will no longer remain just within the agency.

Stakeholder interests are frequently discussed in evaluation literature (Gabor et al., 1998; Royse et al., 2001), but the interests of the evaluator and outside interests are not always explicitly discussed, particularly in relation to the impact on sample participation. Thus, adding the formal evaluation component to this training increased the number of stakeholders involved, and the stakeholders hold varying social positions: the administrators as sponsors of the training/evaluation, the group leaders as participants in the training and thus part of the object of evaluation, my own position as both insider to the training and outsider to the agencies, the institutional review board's position as provider of oversight to the project (because it provided approval), and those other professionals as interested parties who will read about the evaluation results. Although evaluation can be viewed as inquiry for learning (Rallis & Rossman, 2000), evaluation is more likely to be viewed as judgment, particularly by less powerful stakeholders, unless those stakeholders are incorporated in the preparatory process. This would also include a clear explication of the self-interests of all stakeholders so that potential research participants are informed about the nature of the relationships as well as the research protocols.

How could this have been implemented in the training evaluation? This trainer/evaluator could have been more forthcoming about my self-interests in conducting the evaluation. When I described the details of the evaluation, I emphasized the importance of learning how well the training worked, for the group leaders' benefit and for other group leaders from their agencies who might participate in the future. I could have also stated that in my university position, I am interested in collecting data to support and inform practice guidelines for the social work field in general, and that the mechanism for doing so is through presentations and publications. That information was in the informed consent form, but I did not speak about my self-interests so directly. Although coming clean with my self-interests would have highlighted my university status more than my prior agency experience, it would have provided an explanation for why I was interested in the formal evaluation. Thus, I could have emphasized both my insider experience with agencies and groups and my outsider interests in generating social work knowledge.

I could have also met with a number of group leaders prior to the training to elicit their perspectives about the curriculum and evaluation. This would have required administrative support, because the trainings occurred during work hours, but I could have explained that the meeting would enhance the overall success of the training and evaluation. This could have been resolved by structuring a training planning meeting on the day of the first training, delaying the formal start of the training until the following month. The planning meeting would have focused on the group leaders' experience with support groups, ideas for training needs, and ideas for evaluation. By eliciting their participation prior to the training, the position of the least powerful stakeholders would have been incorporated in the overall design of the training and evaluation, thus increasing the likelihood of their investment in the project (Royse et al., 2001). The planning meeting would have then created relationships between me and the administrative sponsors as well as the training participants prior to the beginning of the training. My error was forgetting that the social position of the group leader stakeholders would impact their perception of the usefulness of evaluation as a dimension of practice.

Another option would have been to present the evaluation component in the second training session, at which point the participants would have had more time to interact with me as the trainer/evaluator. The above strategy for talking about my self-interests could have been discussed at that time. The delay, however, would have caused problems with the one-group pretest–posttest research design. Obtaining pretest data in the second training session would have introduced the confounding factor of the training they had already received. The planning meeting would also introduce a confounding factor, unless it was structured into the training curriculum.

This leads to the second primary area of concern: Training and evaluation of training placed differing demands on the structure of the training curriculum as intervention. As noted above, administrators and group leaders shared consensus in the assessment of current support group functioning but differed slightly in their perspectives for intervention: Administrators stated that group leaders needed skills training, and group leaders stated the need to problem-solve systemic problems regarding support, resources, and expectations with each other. In the trainer role, I drew upon group theory that recommends the mutual creation of a contract for work (Shulman, 1999). The training curriculum thus contained content on mutual aid dynamics and leader skills but also incorporated Shulman's content on negotiating systems and social action, to respond to the group leaders' requests. This has resulted in greater rapport between this trainer and the group leaders, because their needs are being responded to and respected.

What was gained through mutual contracting, however, became a methodological concern for outcome assessment, because the intervention shifted slightly throughout the training, from an emphasis on training group leaders to serving as a resource for information regarding mutual aid and leader skills that addressed their self-identified concerns. Credible outcome evaluation requires that the key components of the intervention be articulated in order to evaluate the relationship between the intervention and outcomes (DePoy & Gilson, 2003; Rosen & Proctor, 2002). If this training calls for mutually contracted curricular decisions, then perhaps the mutual contracting becomes the intervention, rather than the curriculum itself, or perhaps the intervention is specified as having process (mutual contracting) and content (mutual aid curriculum) components so that both are measured. This dilemma is similar to the challenges in psychotherapy research, in which the relationship (both the bond and the agreement on goals) has been found to play a necessary role in addition to the specific technique or intervention protocol (Lambert & Barley, 2001; Tryon & Winograd, 2001). Differentiating process and content elements of the training curriculum appears to be a useful response to this dilemma. Future evaluations of this training will therefore emphasize both process and content when replicating the intervention.

CONCLUSION

This evaluation of training for leaders of foster and adoptive parent support groups highlighted the construction of outcome measures that were also used as training materials, so that no visible distinction would be made between those group leaders who did or did not choose to participate in the formal evaluation. Tensions between the training and evaluation were discussed, emphasizing the need to meet with all stakeholders prior to the training, as well as the option of disclosing my own self-interests, as the trainer/evaluator, in order to establish relationships with the least powerful stakeholders, the group leaders. Finally, the intervention was redefined as comprised of both process and content components to provide the necessary specification for outcome assessment.

APPENDIX A: GROUP LEADERSHIP SELF-CONFIDENCE QUESTIONNAIRE

Circle the number that says how confident you are today that you can:

1. *Describe the key purposes of a foster/adoptive parent support group.*

1	2	3	4	5
not at all confident	slightly confident	somewhat confident	very confident	completely confident

2. *Outline the tasks involved in forming a foster/adoptive parent support group.*

1	2	3	4	5
not at all confident	slightly confident	somewhat confident	very confident	completely confident

3. *Clearly explain the group purpose and leader/member roles at the beginning of a meeting.*

1	2	3	4	5
not at all confident	slightly confident	somewhat confident	very confident	completely confident

4. *Facilitate the creation of a shared agenda/focus among parents at a meeting.*

1	2	3	4	5
not at all confident	slightly confident	somewhat confident	very confident	completely confident

5. *Ask for and respond to differing ideas for meeting focus.*

1	2	3	4	5
not at all confident	slightly confident	somewhat confident	very confident	completely confident

6. *Monitor the match between group agenda/focus and a meeting's discussion.*

1	2	3	4	5
not at all confident	slightly confident	somewhat confident	very confident	completely confident

7. *Explain how a discussion has strayed, and select a skill that fits with the reason to guide the discussion back to its focus.*

1	2	3	4	5
not at all confident	slightly confident	somewhat confident	very confident	completely confident

8. *Monitor the levels of participation among all members.*

1	2	3	4	5
not at all confident	slightly confident	somewhat confident	very confident	completely confident

9. *Select skills to encourage shifts in participation among members.*

1	2	3	4	5
not at all confident	slightly confident	somewhat confident	very confident	completely confident

10. *Review group focus and style for new group members or members who come sporadically.*

1	2	3	4	5
not at all confident	slightly confident	somewhat confident	very confident	completely confident

11. *Respond to conflicts between members.*

1	2	3	4	5
not at all confident	slightly confident	somewhat confident	very confident	completely confident

12. *Ask for and respond to feedback regarding the usefulness of the group for the members.*

1	2	3	4	5
not at all confident	slightly confident	somewhat confident	very confident	completely confident

APPENDIX B: SUPPORT GROUP MONITORING FORM

1. Approximate number of persons in attendance: Sept._____ April/May_____
2. Have any new members joined the group between September and April/May?
   _____ yes _____ no   If yes, approximately how many?_____
3. Describe the group format by selecting from the following, and list as many as apply:
   1. education/speaker   2. support group/mutual aid   3. social action   4. social gathering
   Group format in September:_____
   Group format in April/May:_____
4. Presence of mutual aid dynamics   (Provide 2 numbers—the first for September and the second
   for April/May—example: 2/3)
   Rank from 1–5: 1 = not at all present; 2 = slightly; 3 = somewhat; 4 = very much; 5 =
   present throughout

____ Sharing data	____ Discussing a taboo area
____ All-in-the-same-boat phenomena	____ Developing a universal perspective
____ Mutual support	____ Mutual demand
____ Individual problem solving	____ Rehearsal
____ Strength-in-numbers phenomena	____ Emergence of new perspectives

5. Presence of obstacles to mutual aid (Provide 2 numbers—the first for September and the second
   for April/May—example: ⅔)
   Rank from 1–5: 1 = not at all present; 2 = slightly; 3 = somewhat; 4 = very much; 5 =
   present throughout
   _____ Trouble finding common ground/interests among members.
   _____ Difficulty negotiating rules, norms, procedures, or roles.
   _____ Communication difficulties due to social taboos and norms, differences in cultural
   norms, or individual communication styles.
   _____ Difficulty obtaining necessary resources (money, space, child care, etc.)
6. Leadership skills you used to foster mutual aid (Provide 2 numbers—the first for September
   and the second for April/May—example: 2/3)
   Rank from 1–5: 1 = did not use; 2 = used briefly; 3 = somewhat; 4 = frequently; 5 = used
   throughout meeting
   _____ Modeled expectations for group interaction with your behavior and comments
   _____ Checked in with parents and reviewed group focus at beginning of group
   _____ Monitored who was participating in group discussion
   _____ Monitored and responded to conflicts or stalls in group discussion
   _____ Asked members for verbal feedback of group and focus for next meeting

APPENDIX C: SUPPORT GROUP LEADER TRAINING EVALUATION FORM

1. *The information on group dynamics and leader skills was useful for my work.*

1	2	3	4	5
strongly disagree	disagree	neither agree nor disagree	agree	strongly agree

2. *The group experience helped me understand how groups function.*

1	2	3	4	5

3. *The action planning and review helped me focus on specific areas for growth.*

1   2   3   4   5

4. *The support group monitoring form helped me notice group interactions and my leader skills during the group meetings.*

1   2   3   4   5

5. *The trainer presented the material in an understandable and engaging manner.*

1   2   3   4   5

6. *Overall, the group training has provided me with knowledge and skills that I can use when leading parent support groups.*

1   2   3   4   5

7. *Overall, I rank the instructor as . . .*

1	2	3	4	5
poor	fair	good	very good	excellent

8. *Overall, I rank the training as . . .*

1   2   3   4   5

Please describe the most useful aspects of the training.

Please describe the least helpful aspects of the training.

Please list any suggestions for further trainings.

References

Adler, P.A., & Adler, P. (2002). The reluctant respondent. In J. F. Gubrium & J. A. Holstein (Eds.), *Handbook of interview research: Context and method* (pp. 515–535). Thousand Oaks, CA: Sage.

Brown, J. H., & Wiedemeier, J. K. (1995). *Parent group manual: Part I.* St. Paul, MN: North American Council on Adoptable Children.

Burlingame, G. M., Fuhriman, A., & Johnson, J. E. (2001). Cohesion in group psychotherapy. *Psychotherapy, 38*(4), 373–379.

Corey, M. S., & Corey, G. (1997). *Groups: Process and practice* (5th ed.). Pacific Grove, CA: Brooks/Cole.

DePoy, E., & Gilson, S. F. (2003). *Evaluation practice: Thinking and action principles for social work practice.* Pacific Grove, CA: Brooks/Cole.

Fine, M., Weis, L., Weseen, S., & Wong, L. (2000). For whom? Qualitative research, representations, and social responsibilities. In N. K. Denzin & Y. S. Lincoln (Eds.), *Handbook of qualitative research* (2nd ed., pp. 107–131). Thousand Oaks, CA: Sage.

Gabor, P. A., Unrau, Y. A., & Grinnell, R. M., Jr. (1998). *Evaluation for social workers: A quality improvement approach for the social services* (2nd ed.). Boston: Allyn & Bacon.

Gambrill, E. D. (2003). From the editor: Evidence-based practice: Sea change or the emperor's new clothes? *Journal of Social Work Education, 39*(1), 3–23.

Greenwood, D. J., & Levin, M. (2000). Reconstructing the relationships between universities and society through action research. In N. K. Denzin & Y. S. Lincoln (Eds.), *Handbook of qualitative research* (2nd ed., pp. 85–106). Thousand Oaks, CA: Sage.

Lambert, M. J., & Barley, D. E. (2001). Research summary on the therapeutic relationship and psychotherapy outcome. *Psychotherapy, 38*(4), 357–364.

Larson, L. M., & Daniels, J. A. (1998). Review of the counseling self-efficacy literature. *Counseling Psychologist, 26,* 179–218.

McNitt, M. L., & Wasson, S. (1996). *Adoptive parent support group manual: A user guide to developing and maintaining an active support group to help adoptive families and children.* Lansing, MI: Michigan Foster and Adoptive Parent Association.

North American Council on Adoptable Children (2002). *Training and assistance available for parent groups.* Retrieved August 5, 2002, from http://www.nacac.org/pg_training.html.

Rallis, S. F., & Rossman, G. B. (2000). Dialogue for learning: Evaluator as critical friend. In R. K. Hopson (Ed.), *How and why language matters in evaluation* (pp. 81–92). San Francisco: Jossey-Bass.

Rosen, A., & Proctor, E. K. (2002). Standards for evidence-based social work practice: The role of replicable and appropriate interventions, outcomes, and practice guidelines. In A. R. Roberts & G. J. Greene (Eds.), *Social workers' desk reference* (pp. 743–747). New York: Oxford University Press.

Rossi, P. H., Freeman, H. E., & Lipsey, M. W. (1999). *Evaluation: A systematic approach* (6th ed.). Thousand Oaks, CA: Sage.

Royse, D., Thyer, B. A., Padgett, D. K., & Logan, T. K. (2001). *Program evaluation: An introduction* (3rd ed.). Belmont, CA: Brooks/Cole.

Schwartz, W. (1961). The social worker in the group. In *New perspectives on services to groups: Theory, organization, practice* (pp. 7–34). New York: National Association of Social Workers.

Seidman, I. (1998). *Interviewing as qualitative research: A guide for researchers in education and the social sciences* (2nd ed.). New York: Teachers College Press.

Shulman, L. (1999). *The skills of helping individuals, families, groups, and communities* (4th ed.). Itasca, IL: F. E. Peacock.

Toseland, R. W., & Rivas, R. F. (2001). *An introduction to group work practice* (4th ed.). Boston: Allyn & Bacon.

Tryon, G. S., & Winograd, G. (2001). Goal consensus and collaboration. *Psychotherapy, 38*(4), 385–389.

Yalom, I. D. (1995). *The theory and practice of group psychotherapy* (4th ed.). New York: Basic Books.

DOCUMENTING CHANGE IN ADDICTION TREATMENT SYSTEMS

A Model for Evaluation and Examples of Its Use

Dianna L. Newman, Jennifer A. Smith, Margaret M. Geehan, & Gail Viamonte

The original concept of professional development emphasized the training of specific knowledge and skills need to practice (Filby, 1995). In the 1980s, professional development began to focus on the improvement of professionals' thinking and decision making in unfamiliar practice situations. In fact, an overview of the various models of professional development (Telelearning, Inc., 1999) indicates that most of the current models emphasize the importance of a link between theory and practice, incorporating collaborative reflection, and the development of skills and dispositions that will shape ongoing learning from experience (Elmore & Burney, 1997). Of major importance are professional development activities that incorporate the development of a clear sense of purpose, a shared vision, and the building of collaborative culture (Elmore & Burney, 1997). Thus, the elements of a holistic approach to professional development are thought to lead to the improvement of professional practice on a deeper and more lasting level than the more traditional skills-only approaches that focus on changing discrete parts of an organizational system rather than the system as a whole. Proponents of this approach believe that change in any complex organization or social system will be ineffective and short-lived, if the fact that systems have many interrelated parts and change in one of these demands attention to other parts is not taken into account (Schalock, Fredericks, Dalke, & Alberto, 1994).

The interest in holistic systemic change has been particularly evident in the educational arena in response to federal legislation that mandates the reform of classroom instruction to accommodate students with special needs (Heggelund et al., 1985) and the increased use of instructional technology (Valdez et al., 1999). This call for documentation of organizational improvement is an outgrowth of federal initiatives such as the Child and Adolescent Service System Program (CASSP) and the Robert Wood Johnson Mental Health Services Program for Youth (Heggelund et al., 1985). These private and federal mandates require that change be assessed throughout the entire system to ensure the incorporation and assimilation of more holistic organizational practices.

More recently, this need for documentation has expanded to include all aspects of education and mental health (Heggelund et al., 1985). Specifically, the addiction field is one domain in the mental health arena that is in need of systemic change. Although there have been significant advances in substance abuse treatment research, which have resulted in treatment providers' and researchers' increased understanding of the effectiveness and key elements of various treatment alternatives (Fuller & Hiller-Sturmhoefel, 1999), a substantial body of research illustrates the equivocal nature of treatment outcomes with individuals addicted to drugs or alcohol (Joanning, Quinn, Thomas, & Mullen, 1992; Telch,

Hannon, & Telch, 1984). There appears to be differential effectiveness in this clinical population, with alcoholism showing greater responsiveness to treatment than addictions to other substances (Fuller & Hiller-Sturmhoefel, 1999).

The equivocal nature of these results may be indicative of a need for more holistic professional development in substance abuse counselors. Fuller and Hiller-Sturmhoefel (1999) propose that treatment providers may be unaware of the collaborative, collateral use of various treatment approaches; they also propose that these professionals could benefit from continued education or professional development in addictions treatment. Empirical investigation supports this suggestion concerning the importance of ongoing education of professionals working in the addictions field. Wilcoxon and Puleo (1992) and Hall, Amodeo, Shaffer, and Bilt (2000) found that most professionals reported considerable need for and interest in expanding their knowledge in substance abuse treatment issues. In addition, empirical investigation reveals that practitioners who have participated in professional development activities report continued use of newly acquired knowledge (Sobell, Sdao-Jarvie, Frecker, Brown, & Cleland, 1997) and more optimistic attitudes toward treatment outcomes for substance-abusing clients (Amodeo, 2000).

Based on the aforementioned findings (Amodeo, 2000; Hall et al., 2000; Sobell et al., 1997; Wilcoxon & Puleo, 1992), the need for more holistic professional development for professionals working in the substance abuse field becomes clear. Specifically, professionals have voiced the need for continuing education in substance abuse assessment, advanced clinical techniques, and dual diagnosis issues (Hall et al., 2000). To ensure the continued use of acquired knowledge in practice, professionals prefer that material be presented in a holistic manner rather than in the traditional skills-only method (Schalock et al., 1994). As a result, more programs of professional development in the addictions field are now being developed. Along with this change is a need to provide more evidence of the impact of these programs on the system.

This chapter uses a systems change model that takes into account the holistic nature of systems, documents change at various levels in the system, and shows how it can be used in the addictions field (Newman, Smith, & Geehan, 2000). The model collects information from various stakeholder groups to assess the change process within and across these groups, as well as the facilitators and barriers to change. According to this model, the change process is cyclical and encompasses three main stages, each with its own subphases. The first stage, initiation, involves three subphases: (a) the development of a shared vision, (b) development of objectives, and (c) development of plans and strategies for implementation. This stage addresses the conflicts between various stakeholders that may serve as barriers to change (Bridges, 1986; Schalock, 1994) and focuses on the development of a shared purpose and plans for change.

The second stage, implementation, consists of four subphases: (a) activities, which apply the previously developed strategies; (b) intermediate outcomes; (c) formative evaluation; and (d) subsequent modification of the intermediate outcomes. Without the achievement of a shared vision across stakeholders, the implementation of changes could not successfully occur (Bridges, 1986; Schalock, 1994). The third and final stage (impact) includes (a) any observable changes that occur as a result of the previous stages, (b) summative evaluation of these changes, and (c) a revisioning process that involves a reassessment of the original vision. This stage is the ultimate goal of systems change initiatives but cannot be successfully attained without the development of a shared vision, plans for change, and implementation of those plans (Bridges, 1986; Schalock, 1994).

This chapter documents the systems change process for case studies in the addictions field. Each case study was analyzed according to the three stages of change and their corresponding subphases. To facilitate the documentation of the change process, the projects were viewed in terms of the activities, learning, use, and outcomes that occurred at each subphase in the model. Also, barriers and facilitators to change were documented at each level. The systems change findings also will be discussed in relation to key components of professional development models.

METHODOLOGY

A mixed methodology was used for the evaluation of the change process in each case study. Interviews were conducted with program developers, administrative staff, clinical staff, faculty, and students to gather perceptions regarding the process and outcomes of change. Observations of staff presentations and community meetings at the organizations also were used to document change processes and outcomes. Finally, post-surveys were mailed to participants in the implemented curriculum to evaluate its effectiveness and occupational relevance.

RESULTS

Case Study 1

Case Study 1 documents efforts to design and implement a treatment model of addiction that would incorporate the larger context and would result in improved client outcomes. Presented in Table 73.1 is the documentation of the initiation phase of the systems change process for the first case study. The implementation phase of change is presented in Table 73.2, and the impact phase is presented in Table 73.3.

The initiation phase of systems change incorporated the development of a vision shared by clinical staff at a local hospital as well as administrative and teaching staff at a collaborating educational institution. Meetings were the vehicle used to increase the understanding and acceptance of the model in staff at both institutions. The discussions began as informal philosophical debates of the model and progressed into formal discussions of how to implement the model with clients.

This progression was facilitated by allowing clinical staff time to experiment with the model individually. These "trial runs" served as starting points for discussion, facilitated the psycho-

TABLE 73.1 Process Analysis of Systems Change for Case Study 1: Initiation Phase

	Activities	Learning	Use	Outcome
Vision	• Staff meetings to discuss the new model • Discussions between program developer and faculty	• Increased understanding of the new approach • Increased faculty understanding of the model	• Informal conceptualization of clients' use of the model • Informal discussions of model with current students	• Increased belief in the utility and validity of the model • Decision to design a course implementing the new model
Objectives	• Further discussion of model with clinical team regarding how to implement the model • Scheduling of meetings with administration	• Increased understanding of how to use the model • Administrative awareness of and increased faculty dedication to the model	• Formal conceptualization of model with current caseload • Written draft of prospective course content	• Increased understanding of and comfort with applying the model • Written request for addition of new course
Plans and strategies	• Formal team discussions of the use of model • Submission of written request to administration	• Clarification of the pros and cons of using the model with clients • Increased administrative understanding of the model	• Refined use of model with clients • Administration approves the addition of the new course	• Planned procedural changes based on pros and cons • Design of course syllabus

TABLE 73.2 Process Analysis of Systems Change for Case Study 1: Implementation Phase

	Activity	Learning	Use	Outcome
Activities	• Discuss which intake procedures should be changed and how treatment decisions will be made • Advertise new course in university course offerings booklet and through flyers	• All staff understand how to implement the new procedures and how to make treatment decisions • Continue to edit and revise syllabus, lectures, and assignments	• Implement new procedures and meeting formats • Obtain student enrollment in course	• Adopt new procedures on trial basis • Design course geared toward currently enrolled students
Intermediate outcomes	• Discuss barriers to implementation • Implement the new course	• Increase understanding of barriers and shared solutions • Increase student understanding of the model	• Try new solutions • Assign homework, administer tests, and arrange for field trips to apply student knowledge	• Maintain revised procedures • Increase student learning of a new treatment approach
Formative evaluation	• Formulate recommendations for change based on trial use • Ask students to complete course evaluation forms	• Understand others' concerns and how to change • Evaluate and understand where change is needed	• Generate concerns regarding the model • Modify the course based on student feedback	• Discuss concerns at next meeting • Design revised syllabus, lectures, tests
Modification	• Brainstorm ways to circumvent client resistance and staff turf losses and provide informal training on this topic • Implement new course	• Understand boundaries of current role and client concerns • Increase student understanding	• Intervene with clients to reduce resistance, and respect boundaries of other staff • Provide assignments for students to apply knowledge	• Accept new intake procedures and treatment planning processes • Refine course from previous year, resulting in increased student learning

logical transition process, and ultimately resulted in the unified acceptance of the model. Once the model was accepted and refined in light of clinical staff feedback, formal procedural changes could be planned. Common barriers at this phase of change included the anticipation of

loss and increased workload for clinical staff. The main facilitators of change were the open discussion forums and the potential positive outcomes for clients.

The implementation phase of change in Case Study 1 incorporated the procedural changes at

TABLE 73.3 Process Analysis of Systems Change for Case Study 1: Impact Phase

	Activity	Learning	Use	Outcome
Change	• Continued implementation of procedures • Continued offering of course	• Increased awareness of the client, significant others, and therapist in the addiction problem • Increased student knowledge and competency	• Increased client self-reflection, active work on relationships with significant others; therapist reformulation of treatment strategies • Broadening of addictions knowledge or application of knowledge to clients	• Increased client resistance to treatment and temporary psychological discomfort associated with change and insight • More effective clinical strategies, increased knowledge, more positive attitudes toward clients
Summative evaluation	• Discussion of client issues and barriers to implementation • Discussion of student feedback and concerns	• Awareness of new solutions from team discussions • Awareness of what needs to be changed for students	• Implementation of new solutions • Implementation of course changes	• Client acceptance of treatment, increased honesty, and increased motivation • Course more applicable to student needs
Revision	• Discussion of the initial goals • Discussion of the initial course objectives	• Comparison of goals and outcome • Comparison of objectives and outcome	• Provision of what was lacking (e.g., training) • Reassessment of objectives and purpose	• Modification or expansion of the vision to lead to more satisfied and competent staff and improved client outcomes • Modification or expansion of objectives to lead to more satisfied and competent pre-professionals

the hospital and the offering and redesign of a course at the college. Overall, the initial activities of the implementation phase at both institutions progressively evolved through shared feedback and training. At the hospital, the implementation phase began with staff discussions regarding specifically how the intake procedures and treatment planning meetings should change to accommodate the new treatment model.

These changes were tentatively implemented and discussed in terms of issues and barriers at future meetings. Regular staff meetings were scheduled to allow for the continued discussion of issues and concerns. Procedures were refined according to shared concerns and implemented on a more permanent basis.

Procedural changes at the hospital included new intake interviews and informed consent procedures with clients, such that significant others, family members, and probation officers became an active part of treatment. Also, treatment-planning methodologies were changed to a team approach, whereby interventions and treatment decisions were made on a team basis rather than solely by the primary therapist.

The course at the collaborating educational institution included both lecture and hands-on learning approaches. The lectures were designed by the instructor based on meetings with hospital staff, and hands-on field trips were arranged with the hospital to allow students to observe staff presentations of the model. The course was refined based on student feedback from university course evaluations. Interviews with students indicated that the course was highly informative and directly applicable to clients. Although most students did not have current caseloads to which they could apply these treatment concepts, they anticipated that this information would be useful for them as future clinicians.

Commonly identified barriers at the hospital included a lack of formal training in the model, clients' resistance to the involvement of others in their treatment, the increased volume of necessary paperwork, and the territoriality and defensiveness of clinical staff regarding their conceptualizations and interventions. This territoriality continues to be a delicate issue, as therapists and social workers must redefine their roles to accommodate the team approach to treatment. The open discussion format of staff meetings and the regularity of these meetings, however, were identified as significant facilitators of the change process. Barriers identified by students at the college included lack of time to complete the course assignments and lack of caseloads in which to apply the knowledge. Facilitators included the field trips and lecture style of the instructor.

The impact phase of the change process was the final phase in Case Study 1, whereby the new procedures or activities continued to be implemented and revised until the initial goals or objectives were met. If the initial goals were not met, the original vision, strategies, or activities were revised to address the needs of the stakeholders. If the initial goals were met, the vision was expanded to incorporate future needs.

At the hospital, the original vision included the utilization of a more comprehensive treatment approach to better serve client needs and improve client outcome. To accomplish this vision, considerable procedural changes were necessary, which resulted in short-term resistance by both staff and clients. Ultimately, however, clinicians became more competent and were better able to meet client needs. Also, clients became more self-reflective, motivated, and honest in treatment. Given that this original vision was accomplished, the revisioning process incorporated a provision of more formal training to staff and greater allocation of resources to this treatment approach.

At the college, the initial vision was to provide students with the necessary knowledge to treat addictions clients. To accomplish this vision, the course needed to provide students with lectures, field trips, homework assignments, and examinations. Students reported that their knowledge base increased considerably and their attitudes toward addictions clients became more positive, which indicates that the original objectives were accomplished. The revisioning process, therefore, included a modification of the original vision, such that students were able to achieve these same positive outcomes with a workload that was more feasible.

Case Study 2

The second case study presents a curriculum model for addictions at various educational levels that is rooted in competencies developed and published as a technical assistance publication (TAP 21, 1998) under the auspices of joint national professional associations and governmental agencies. Presented in Table 73.4 is the documentation of the initiation phase of the systems change process for the second case study.

This project cycled through the initiation phase of change in its development of an idea and a tentative plan for multilevel curricula for substance abuse. The initiation phase of change for this project was challenged by the possible impediment to the professional status of addictions counselors who have not acquired college degrees. Discussions among project directors served as the main vehicle of change, whereby philosophical underpinnings of the curriculum and the barriers to its implementation were discussed. The main barrier to implementation is the possible detrimental occupational effects of this curriculum for addictions counselors who do not possess college degrees. The recognition of this problem and the continued discussion of its

TABLE 73.4 Process Analysis of Systems Change for Case Study 2: Initiation Phase

	Activity	Learning	Use	Outcome
Vision	• Discussions between program developers regarding the need for a chemical dependency degree rooted in the counselor competencies	• Increased understanding of the competencies and how they relate to clinical practice	• Continued discussions of the competencies and how they relate to various levels of educational training	• Decision to design a degree ladder that will delineate which counselor competencies should be taught at various educational levels (associate's, bachelor's, master's, and doctoral levels)
Objectives	• Discussions of which competencies pertain to each educational level	• Mapping of a concrete plan of which competencies match with each degree level	• Discussion of how curricula could be developed and modified to incorporate the respective competencies	• Creation of sketch of curricula for each level rooted in their respective competencies
Plans and strategies	• Discussions of implications of this curriculum for recovering addicts without a degree	• Increased awareness of the possible negative implications for recovering addicts, who constitute a large sample of addictions professionals	• Further discussions of how the development of this degree ladder would not impede the occupational status of recovering addicts who have no degrees	• Tentative plans of how to implement curriculum at various educational levels without impinging on the professional status of addictions professionals who have no degrees

resolution eventually led to a modified vision that moved to the implementation level of change.

Case Study 3

Case Study 3 investigated the implementation of a new degree program with only minor revisions to existing courses and the development of one new course. Presented in Table 73.5 is the documentation of the initiation phase of the systems change process for the third case study, and its implementation phase is Table 73.6. The initiation phase of change incorporated the development of an empirically validated curriculum that would allow for institutional change in structured methods. Initially, there was an attempt to gain administrative support for the vision of a graduate degree specifically in substance use.

The initiation phase of change has progressed over the course of the past two and one half years from the proposal of an idea to conducting a research program and development of an empirically validated curriculum for a new degree in substance abuse. The vision (a substance abuse curriculum based on counselor competencies) has been slowly implemented through the

TABLE 73.5 Process Analysis of Systems Change for Case Study 3: Initiation Phase

	Activity	Learning	Use	Outcome
Vision	• Program developer/faculty member recognizes the need for a master's degree specifically for substance abuse	• Becomes aware of the need for this degree to be grounded in counselor competencies	• Proposes the idea of a new degree program to administrative staff during a meeting	• Administration encourages empirical support for this curriculum
Objectives	• Applies for and obtains funding for the research and develops a research program to test the efficacy of the counselor competencies	• Obtains empirical results regarding the necessity for Technical Assistance Publication (TAP) 21 competencies in substance abuse curricula	• Schedules another meeting with administration and presents the empirical results	• Administration grants approval to develop a tentative degree program
Plans and Strategies	• Modifies existing courses from BSW program to reflect necessary master's requirements and develops one new course that will complete the sequence	• Presents the curriculum to administration and is denied permission to implement the new program due to a lack of teaching staff and financial resources	• Obtains approval to implement the new course as a summer offering to pilot its efficacy and begin the change process • Begins informal discussions with the dean of a related department, so that the change can be considered a new track in lieu of a major change	• Schedules future meetings with administration regarding the new plan that will require fewer resources (only one adjunct and no application process to the state)

modification of existing courses and the offering of a new course as a summer elective.

Activities for the implementation phase of change included the modifications of current courses based on empirical findings and the design of a new summer course, such that these courses reflect state-of-the-art knowledge regarding counselor competencies and substance abuse treatment. Intermediate outcomes include the continued offering of courses that had been modified, as well as the official administrative

approval to offer a new summer course that eventually would be integrated into the proposed master's degree program. The implementation of the courses resulted in increased student learning and increased administrative support for the incorporation of a new graduate degree program for counseling in chemical dependency. Additionally, formative evaluation feedback from students based on course evaluations was used to modify and refine the courses for future implementation.

TABLE 73.6 Process Analysis of Systems Change for Case Study 3: Implementation Phase

	Activity	Learning	Use	Outcome
Activities	• Design curriculum for new course and revise curricula for existing courses; advertise new course in university course offerings booklet and through flyers	• Continue to edit and revise curricula based on research findings; devise syllabi, lectures, and assignments	• Obtain prospective student enrollment in course	• Design course geared toward currently enrolled students
Intermediate outcomes	• Obtain administrative approval for new course; implement new and revised courses	• Obtain increased administrative support for courses and proposed master's degree program	• Assign homework, administer tests	• Increase student learning and administrative support
Formative evaluation	• Ask students to complete course evaluation forms	• Evaluate and understand where change is needed	• Modify the course based on student feedback	• Design revised syllabi, lectures, tests
Modification	• Implement new course	• Increase student understanding	• Create assignments for students to apply knowledge	• Refine course from previous year, with increased student learning

A major concern or barrier to the continued implementation of the revised and new courses was the lack of resources to allow for the hiring of qualified instructors to teach the newly developed courses. Facilitators of the change process included frequent meetings and increased communication between the program developer and administrative staff, which enhanced administrative support for the proposed graduate degree program.

Case Study 4

Presented in Table 73.7 is the documentation of the initiation phase of the systems change process for the fourth case study, assistance to and improvement of managed care, and the subsequent implementation phase of change (presented in Table 73.8). The initiation phase of change was characterized by the formation of focus groups and committees consisting of stakeholder groups integral to the establishment of a common purpose and formulating an effective plan of action. The shared vision was to provide improved integration of services and better service delivery in reaction to managed care. The agreed-on plan of action focused on the creation of a curriculum and trainer manual that reflect jointly developed state competencies for working with clients with co-occurring disorders, or mentally ill substance abusers (MISA), and establishing contacts and collaboration with key specialists and agencies. To accomplish this goal, committee members assumed various roles and decided how to best distribute existing resources.

The implementation phase of change consisted of a concentrated search for relevant literature and references related to MISA consortium guidelines and the communication with curriculum specialists and MISA experts. The formulation of a team consisting of these specialists and experts to design and develop the

TABLE 73.7 Process Analysis of Systems Change for Case Study 4: Initiation Phase

	Activity	Learning	Use	Outcome
Vision	• Formation of focus groups and committees of relevant stakeholder groups	• Increased communication and collaboration among stakeholder groups	• Continued communication and meetings with committee members to identify a common purpose for the change	• Agreement among stakeholder groups regarding the importance of better integration and delivery of services
Objectives	• Meeting to identify how improved integration and delivery of services could be translated into practice	• Identification of training curriculum as a key means of transferring knowledge into practice	• Meetings regarding the resources needed to develop a curriculum	• Preliminary decisions regarding the effective distribution of financial and staffing resources
Plans and Strategies	• Meetings to discuss effective distribution of resources and roles of individual committee members	• Increased awareness of needs and their respective resource demands	• Decisions regarding the distribution of financial and staffing resources	• Decision to design a train-the-trainer manual reflecting state mentally ill substance abusers (MISA) standards

manual was established, and the first draft of the manual was completed. This training manual was then used in a pilot study, and formative evaluation feedback was obtained regarding the validity of the content and the training process.

DISCUSSION

Findings from the case studies reflect a holistic approach to change, given the focus on the development of a shared vision or purpose for change as well as the emphasis on the need for a collaborative culture. To accomplish the agreed-on vision, each systems change project rejected a piecemeal approach to change and instead drew in the various interrelated parts of its respective systems to establish a collaborative, participatory change effort. This collaborative effort often entailed the establishment of networks and regular communication lines in and across agencies as well as across various organizational

levels. As a result of this shared vision and agreement between various stakeholders, implementation plans were better accomplished, and change more readily occurred.

Key elements of professional development that were illustrated throughout the case studies were the link between theory and practice and the emphasis on collaborative reflection. In order to create and develop effective educational resources such as the MISA curriculum and the new degree program in chemical dependency, it was imperative that the knowledge gained through recent research in substance abuse treatment be reflected in the curriculum in such a way that it can be effectively manifested in practice settings. The incorporation of collaborative reflection also was demonstrated across the case studies through the emphasis on a shared vision, the regular communication among stakeholder groups, and the use of formative evaluation feedback.

The importance of effective treatment ap-

TABLE 73.8 Process Analysis of Systems Change for Case Study 4: Implementation Phase

	Activity	Learning	Use	Outcome
Activities	• Literature review on mentally ill substance abusers (MISA) consortium guidelines	• Increased awareness of need to establish contacts with MISA and curriculum specialists	• Establishment of contacts with MISA expert and curriculum design specialists	• Formation of a team composed of stakeholder groups and specialists, to devise a training manual
Intermediate outcomes	• Team meetings to discuss curriculum design issues	• Establishment of a concrete outline or plan regarding the content of the manual	• Review of the plan by specialists and experts and continued collaboration and communication between these individuals	• Development of first draft of training curriculum
Formative evaluation	• Pilot training of first draft of training curriculum and administration of evaluation surveys	• Increased understanding of the barriers to the training process	• Continued discussion regarding effective approaches and shared solutions to identified barriers	• Obtaining formative evaluation data regarding the training process
Modification	• Meetings among stakeholders to discuss evaluation results for the pilot training and how to refine the manual	• Increased understanding regarding the need for evaluation data	• Continued communication with evaluation staff and consideration of how evaluation data can enhance the existing manual	• Use of evaluation feedback to refine training manual

proaches cannot be overemphasized, and these are contingent upon the continued use of knowledge acquired through professional development activities. The holistic nature of the change process exhibited throughout the four case studies enhanced the knowledge base and clinical skills of project directors and all others who participated in the professional development activities. Because all individuals involved in the systemic change efforts were professionals in the addictions field (including educators, clinicians, and students in training), a greater potential for true transfer of knowledge into practice and a correspondingly greater subsequent impact on addictions clients were realized.

References

Amodeo, M. (2000). The therapeutic attitudes and behavior of social work clinicians with and without substance abuse training. *Substance Use and Misuse, 35*(11), 1507–1536.

Bridges, W. (1986). Managing organizational transitions. *Organizational Dynamics, 15*(1), 24–33.

Elmore, R. F., & Burney, D. (1997). *Investing in teacher learning: Staff development and instructional improvement in Community School District #2, New York City.* New York: National Commission on Teaching and America's Future. (Eric Document Reproduction Service No. ED 416 203)

Filby, N. N. (1995). *Analysis of reflective professional*

development models. San Francisco: Far West Laboratory for Educational Research and Development. (Eric Document Reproduction Service No. ED 393857)

Fuller, R. K., & Hiller-Sturmhoefel, S. (1999). Alcoholism treatment in the United States: An overview. *Alcohol Research and Health, 23*(2), 69–77.

Hall, M. N., Amodeo, M., Shaffer, H. J., & Bilt, J. V. (2000). Social workers employed in substance abuse treatment agencies: A training needs assessment. *Social Work, 45*(2), 141–156.

Heggelund, M., Haring, N. G., Lynch, V., Pruess, J., Soltman, S., & Zodrow, N. (1985). Systems change: A case study. *Remedial and Special Education, 6*(3), 44–51.

Joanning, H., Quinn, W., Thomas, F., & Mullen, R. (1992). Treating adolescent drug abuse: A comparison of family systems therapy, group therapy, and family drug education. *Journal of Marital and Family Therapy, 18,* 345–356.

Newman, D. L., Smith, J., & Geehan, M. M. (2000). Systems change in the human service domain: A model for documenting and evaluating change. A paper presented to the American Evaluation Association, Honolulu, Hawaii.

Schalock, M. D., Fredericks, B., Dalke, B. A., & Alberto, P. A. (1994). The house that traces built: A conceptual model of service delivery systems and implications for change. *The Journal of Special Education, 28*(2), 203-223.

Sobell, L. C., Sdao-Jarvie, K., Frecker, R. C., Brown, J. C., & Cleland, P. A. (1997). Long-term impact of addictions training for medical residents. *Substance Abuse, 18*(2), 51-56.

TAP 21. (1998). *Addiction counseling competencies: The knowledge, skills, and attitudes of professional practice.* Technical Assistance Publication Series 21. Rockville, MD: Addiction Technologies Transfer Centers National Curriculum Committee, U.S. Department of Health and Human Services.

Telch, M. J., Hannon, R., & Telch, C. R. (1984). A comparison of cessation strategies for the outpatient alcoholic. *Addictive Behavior, 9,* 103–109.

Telelearning, Inc. (with Laferriere, T., Breuleux, A., Baker, P., & Fitzsimons, R.). (1999). *Working group on professional development: In-service teachers professional development models in the use of information and communication technologies. A report to the SchoolNet National Advisory Board.* Author. Retrieved June 25, 2003, from http://www.tact.fse.ulaval.ca/ang/html/pdmodels.html

Valdez, G., McNabb, M., Foertsch, M., Anderson, M., Hawkes, M., & Raack, L. (1999). *Computer-based technology and learning: Evolving uses and expectations.* Chicago: North Central Regional Educational Laboratory.

Wilcoxon, S. A., & Puleo, S. G. (1992). Professional development needs of mental health counselors: Results of a national survey. *Journal of Mental Health Counseling, 14*(2), 187–195.

74

INNOVATIVE APPROACHES TO RISK ASSESSMENT WITHIN ALCOHOL PREVENTION PROGRAMMING

Lori K. Holleran, Young-mi Kim, & Kathy Dixon

Alcohol use by underage children is widespread. In 2001, about 10 million youth aged 12 to 20 (28.5% of this age group) reported drinking alcohol in the month prior to the survey interview (National Household Survey on Drug Abuse [NHSDA], 2001). Furthermore, there is a trend toward younger and younger ages of initiation, with 11% of teens reporting that they had their first drink before age 11 (American Academy of Pediatrics, 1998). The percentage of children reporting alcohol use in the past 30 days increased with age from youth to young adulthood, from 2% at age 12 to 65% at age 21 (NHSDA, 2001). The combination of youth and alcohol results in other risky and dangerous behaviors including cigarette use, violence, vandalism, high-risk sexual behavior, and drunk driving (Bonomo et al., 2001; McClelland & Teplin, 2001; NHSDA, 2001; Staton et al., 1999).

PREVENTION PROGRAM DESIGNS

Historically, prevention programs focused on information only, that is, teaching about alcohol without a social or experiential component. A number of studies, however, found that information provision alone fails to produce reduction in drug use (Botvin, Baker, & Dusenbury, 1995; Bukoski, 1985; Tobler & Stratton, 1997), and that some programs led to an increase in use of substances (Falck & Craig, 1988).

In lieu of information provision, recent research supports the efficacy of life skills (skills related to successful functioning regarding achievements and interpersonal relationships)

and resistance training interventions (skills related to effectively refraining from risky behaviors). A wealth of empirical evidence supports the efficacy of social skills–based prevention messages (Botvin et al., 1990; Botvin et al., 1995; Scheier & Botvin, 1997; Schinke, Tepavac, & Cole, 2000). Alcohol prevention programs designed for youth are more effective when they provide the opportunity to learn and practice life skills and resistance strategies when faced with a drug-use dilemma (Botvin et al., 1995).

The primary impetus for this shift in intervention techniques is the increasing emphasis on risk with relation to alcohol. Risk assessment is key in every aspect of alcohol prevention, from assessment through program design and program evaluation. The context for examining risk is the resilience model.

RISK AND RESILIENCE

For over a decade, primary prevention scientists have recognized that risk factors and protective factors influence child outcomes (Cowen & Work, 1988). By focusing on risk and protective factors that are believed to be mutable (including social skills), prevention efforts aim to eliminate, reduce, or mitigate negative outcomes by interrupting the pathogenic process and enhancing resiliency (Hawkins, Catalano, & Associates, 1992; Lorion, Price, & Eaton, 1989). The risk and resilience model represents a shift in focus from concentrating on psychopathology to trying to understand the process of healthy human development despite adverse environmental con-

TABLE 74.1 Research-Based Risk Factors

Community:

- High availability of drugs
- Community laws and norms favorable toward drug use
- Low community safety; high violence
- Instability: Transitions and mobility
- Low neighborhood attachment and community disorganization
- Extreme economic deprivation and poverty
- Negative community attitudes toward youth
- Lack of youth recreation opportunities
- Lack of cultural resources

Family:

- Family history of problem or high-risk behavior
- Family management problems (e.g., lack of structure and limits)
- Family conflict
- Favorable or rigid parental attitudes and involvement in problem behavior
- Incidence of child abuse, neglect, and trauma
- Tension around cultural identity, acculturative stress, or both

School:

- Early and persistent antisocial behavior
- Academic failure in school
- Absenteeism and dropout
- Lack of commitment in school
- Lack of cultural grounding and resources, language difficulties, or both

Individual and peers:

- Alienation and rebelliousness
- Lack of social bonding
- Friends who engage in a problem behavior
- Favorable attitudes toward the problem behavior
- Early initiation of problem behavior
- Constitutional factors (e.g., genetic predisposition to chemical dependency)
- High incidence of drug and alcohol use
- Stressful events, multiple stressors, or both
- Problematic health status (physical and mental)
- Tension concerning cultural identity, acculturative stress, or both

ditions (Masten, 1994). This model is a strengths-based conceptualization with a focus on client strengths, adaptation, healing, wellness, coping skills, positive self-concept, self-efficacy, and competence (Greene & Conrad, 2001; Saleeby, 1996). The model uses epidemiological methods and builds an ecological-developmental theory to identify factors at multiple systems levels (e.g., individual, family, neighborhood, or community) that are associated with the occurrence of certain outcomes (Nash & Bowen, 1999). It conceptualizes the range of possible outcomes as a dynamic, transactional balance between risk factors, stressful life events, and protective mechanisms on multiple layers of environmental, interpersonal, and individual interaction (Fraser, 1997).

The knowledge of what places an individual or group at risk for a certain negative outcome, coupled with awareness of the factors that buffer some individuals from that outcome, allows more effective programs to be developed. This perspective is important to the creation of prevention programs that enhance resilience and minimize risk. It is especially crucial to consider resilience when examining minority youth, in order to consider contextual stressors and structural barriers (Holleran & Waller, in press).

KEY CONCEPTS AND DEFINITIONS

Risk is defined as a psychosocial adversity or event that would be considered a stressor to most people and that may hinder normal functioning (Masten, 1994). The concept of risk is understood as a dynamic process rather than a causal mechanistic model (Greene & Conrad, 2001).

Resilience is defined as the capability of individuals to cope successfully in the face of significant change, adversity, or risk. This capability changes over time and is enhanced by protective factors in the individual and environment (Stewart, Reid, & Mangham, 1997, p. 22). Resilience is influenced by diversity, including ethnicity, race, gender, age, sexual orientation, economic status, religious affiliation, and physical and mental ability. It is expressed and affected by multilevel attachments, both distal and proximal, including family, school, peers, neighborhood, community, and society. In addition, it is affected by the availability of environmental resources (Greene & Conrad, 2001, p. 41).

Protective factors are defined as circumstances that moderate or mediate the effects of risks and enhance adaptation (Masten, 1994). Risk factors and protective processes exist and interact on a variety of levels with individual, familial, societal, or cultural manifestations. Resilience intercedes by reducing risk's effects, reducing negative chain reactions, establishing and maintaining self-esteem and self-efficacy, or opening opportunities (Smokowski, 1998).

RESILIENCE-BASED PREVENTION

Reducing vulnerability and risk is an approach for primary prevention: "Risk factors should guide intervention efforts, and the goal of intervention should be to reduce the effect of specifically targeted risk factors significantly" (Fraser & Galinsky, 1997, p. 268). This approach to promoting positive outcomes lies in increasing practical and skill-based resources and mobilizing protective processes (modifiable mediators) and key protective factors that buffer the individual and family and potentially the community against stress and risk.

INTERSECTING THEORETICAL FRAMEWORKS

Ecological Model

Ecological models are comprehensive health promotion models that are based on the reciprocal relationship between an individual and his or her environment (Bronfenbrenner, 1979, 1995). The defining feature of an ecological model is that it takes into account interpersonal factors, social and cultural environments, and physical environments that influence health behaviors and how these factors relate to people at individual, interpersonal, organizational, and community levels. Ecological programming for alcohol prevention considers the complexity of interacting factors in individual, interpersonal, organizational, and community realms (Marsiglia, Miles, Dustman, & Sills, in press; Perry et al., 1996). One of the models that hones in on the specific ecological factors contributing to alcohol use and abuse behaviors by youth is the social development model.

Social Development Model

Hawkins et al. (1992) developed the social development model (SDM) that incorporates social learning theory (Bandura, 1977), social control theory (Hirschi, 1969), and differential association theory (Sutherland, 1973). The SDM identifies etiological and developmental mechanisms affecting prosocial and problem behavior outcomes. The SDM is an appropriate theoretical model to examine various sources of risk and protection for alcohol misuse because it incorporates relationships among predictors including family, peers, school, and community systems (Lonczak et al., 2001).

A significant emphasis of the SDM is the concept of social bonding, which is described as attachment, commitment, involvement, and belief. The concept of social bonding is significant for understanding and preventing adolescent alcohol misuse, given the fact that when adolescents feel bonded to individuals or systems whose norms disapprove of problem behaviors as adolescent alcohol misuse, they tend to adopt similar norms. Four elements of social bonding have been shown as inversely related to alcohol misuse. Specifically, Hawkins et al. (1992) noted strong attachment to parents; commitment to schooling; regular involvement in church activities; and belief in the generalized expectations, norms, and values of society as inversely related to alcohol misuse. The SDM also targets adolescents' skills, opportunities, involvement, and reinforcement, thus affecting the socialization process (social bonding) with parents, schools, and community (Petratis, Flay, & Miller, 1995). A related theory that focuses on the development of deviant behaviors in youth is problem behavior theory.

Problem Behavior Theory

Problem behavior theory (PBT; Jessor, Donavan, & Costa, 1991) is a social-psychological framework that integrates cognitive-affective characteristics, interpersonal factors, and learning and ecological factors (Donavan, 1996; Petratis et al., 1995). This theory posits that adolescents' problem behaviors are consequences of interaction between the person and the environment. Problem behavior is defined as "socially disapproved behaviors that depart from the conventional norms of the larger society" (Donovan, 1996, p. 380). The primary focus of PBT is on the relationships among four systems of psychosocial influences: the personality system, the perceived environment system, the social environment system, and the behavior system. Thus, the PBT framework hypothesizes that the personality system and the perceived environment system affect each other and that they directly affect the behavior systems.

The personality system refers to an individual's values and expectations for achievement and independence, internal-external control, alienation, self-esteem, and personal control (which is organized into three structures: motivational-instigation structure, personal belief structure, and personal control structure; Jessor et al., 1991). The perceived environment system focuses on attachments to family and peers as environmental risks toward involvement in problem behaviors such as substance abuse. The perceived environmental risks to problem behavior consist of lower parental support and controls, lower levels of pressure from friends, lower parent–friend compatibility, greater peer influences than parental influence, lower parental disapproval of problem behavior, and greater peer approval for and models of problem behavior (Jessor, 1987, 1998).

The social environment system, as distinct from the perceived environment, is constituted of "variables that locate individuals in the larger social structure and that characterize the more objective aspects of the context of social interaction and experience in daily life" (Jessor et al., 1991, p. 32). The explanatory variables of the system include such factors as income, educational level, occupational status, and family composition. Risk assessment is a complicated task due to the complexity of interacting factors, as illustrated in the theoretical frameworks presented and the following exemplars.

INNOVATIVE APPROACHES TO RISK ASSESSMENT: EXEMPLARS

To illustrate innovative risk assessment techniques, this chapter presents two complementary models. The first is primarily quantitatively based and the second is qualitatively based. The models are described, and strengths and limitations are noted. Finally, a project is presented that incorporates aspects of risk assessment and demonstrates the operationalization of risk and resilience frameworks.

The Prevention Risk Indicator Services Monitoring System (PRISMS)

Risk profiles entitled PRISMS were developed by the New York State Office of Alcoholism and Substance Abuse Services (OASAS) to facilitate research-based prevention planning for adolescents in New York. Originally funded through a Center for Substance Abuse Prevention (CSAP) grant, the profiles are produced annually by OASAS for New York City and upstate New York counties. The PRISMS employ a research-based risk framework to predict youth alcohol and other drug consequences using community indicators. The framework is based on the concept of risk and protection; certain risk factors increase the likelihood of alcohol and substance abuse problems, whereas protective factors safeguard against or reduce the effects of alcohol and other drug abuse risks.

The PRISMS ecological framework further hypothesizes that risk factors operate in different levels or different domains, and that the relationship between certain risk factors and increased risk for alcohol and drug abuse holds true at both the individual and the community levels. Based on this research-driven ecological risk framework, the PRISMS profiles group 64 risk indicators into 15 risk constructs through factor analysis. The risk constructs are then placed into either the Community or Youth Risk Index. Five alcohol and five drug consequence indicators are factor analyzed into the Youth Alcohol Consequences Index and the Youth Drug Consequences Index, respectively. Thus, the PRISMS risk profiles consist of four indexes: the Community Risk Index (CRI), Youth Risk Index (YRI), the Youth Alcohol Consequences Index, and the Youth Drug Consequences Index. Data related to the PRISMS and statistical Geographic Information Systems (GIS) mapping information can be viewed at the NYS OASAS Web site(http://www.oasas.state.ny.us/hps/datamart/DataMart.htm).

Environmental risk factors that potentially impact all individuals in a community are placed in the CRI. Risk constructs measuring community disorganization (urban residence, poverty, violence, and crime) and alcohol and drug exposure form an index of risk affecting the entire community's population. The CRI represents risk that can be addressed through universal, communitywide environmental prevention strategies such as media campaigns, public educational programs, multiagency coordination and collaboration, and modifying alcohol advertising practices. The YRI is computed from risk factors reflecting youth whose family environments, behavior, or psychosocial development place them at greater risk for alcohol and substance abuse. Selected and indicated prevention strategies such as prevention counseling, resistance skills training, parent skills education, and self-help groups for children of substance abusers targeted to schools, peer groups, families, and individual youth can reduce youth alcohol and substance abuse risk. The Youth Alcohol and Youth Drug Consequences Indexes are computed from indicators that represent consequences for youth (e.g., arrests for driving while intoxicated, drug arrests, treatment admissions) resulting from their abuse of alcohol or other substances. The Youth Consequences Indexes may help estimate need for indicated prevention strategies, early intervention, and adolescent treatment.

One of the major strengths of the PRISMS profiles is the predictive ability of the risk indexes. The CSAP-funded study found that the Community and Youth Risk Indexes accounted for 62% of the variance in later youth alcohol consequences and 65% of the variance in later youth drug consequences. When current youth consequences were entered into the model, the risk indexes accounted for 84% of the variance in later youth alcohol consequences and 72% of the variance in later youth drug consequences, significantly enhancing the predictive ability of the model. Given the predictive ability of the indexes, the profiles are a useful tool to guide the development of community prevention services. Community prevention programs can hopefully mitigate the effects future negative youth alcohol and drug consequences by addressing and reducing the risk factors outlined in the Community and Youth Risk Indexes. The county-level risk information provided in the PRISMS profiles can also alert local governments, planners, and service providers to those domains where risks and negative consequences are greatest. In addition, the profiles' broad-based risk framework and selected prevention strategies can be effective in identifying and reducing violence, teen pregnancy, crime, school absenteeism, and other social problems, as well as youth alcohol and drug use.

On the other hand, the PRISMS have some limitations. The profiles principally measure social problems or risk factors; indicators that measure protective factors are, for the most part, unavailable. The PRISMS profiles cannot identify high-risk neighborhoods within counties, because county-level indicators cannot capture subcounty statistical variations. In addition, relationships among risk indicators and constructs found at the county level may not imply a similar relationship at the individual level. To ascertain protective and risk factors at the individual level and identify high-risk neighborhoods in the community, the PRISMS profiles need to be used in conjunction with local need assessment efforts, such as ethnographic studies; student, household, and special population surveys; and treatment need estimates. Another limitation of the profiles is that cultural and institutional factors such as the tourism industry, colleges, or alcohol and drug treatment facilities in the county are not adequately captured by the risk indicators in the profiles. Refined need assessments may be combined to investigate local and cultural effects on youth alcohol and drug abuse, as illustrated in the next exemplar.

Ethnography and Risk Assessment: The DRS Project's Innovations

In light of the information presented in this chapter, strategies are needed that accurately assess the alcohol problems and needs of individuals in communities and that combine the strengths of researchers and community to create effective prevention curricula for youth (Gosin, Dustman, Drapeau, & Harthun, 2003). The Drug Resistance Strategies (DRS, 2002) project models the use of what the DRS research team terms Participatory Action Research (PAR) methodology in order to create the keepin' it REAL drug and alcohol resistance strategies curriculum. The project is built on the premise that effective prevention efforts must involve ownership by the agency, interventionists, and the participants (Marsiglia, Holleran, & Jackson, 2000; Mrazek & Haggerty, 1997). The researchers note that if an outside agency is used, that agency's investment and sense of ownership of the program should be assessed. In the DRS project, school and community participants took ownership and were responsible for multiple stages of creation and implementation of the program including videos, which are an integral part of the curriculum. Teachers and students contributed lesson modifications and evaluations, suggestions for supplemental activities, and the actual production of instructional videos that are an integral part of the curriculum.

The project began as an ethnographic study of youth peer relationships in the area that would ultimately be a primary site for the prevention project. Ethnography refers to a social scientific description of a people and the cultural basis of their identities (Vidich & Lyman, 1994). This is especially critical when studying underserved populations and unique cultures (Marsiglia & Holleran, 1999). The ethnographic research is naturalistic and based on participant observational fieldwork and interpretations of observed data. The research methodology consists of (a) conceptualization and preparation for the study; (b) intensive participant observation in the field setting; (c) data collection through informal contacts, semistructured interviews, and focus groups; and (d) analytic reflection on the data. The process was not linear; information-gathering processes and directions were reevaluated throughout the research via weekly interdisciplinary team meetings and e-mailed notes and memos.

This was followed by a pilot study in which university researchers, in conjunction with the school staff and involved youth, began to identify adolescents' primary areas of risk. This program focused particularly on perceptions of drug resistance strategies, with the objective of learning the situations under which strategies were effective or ineffective. The researchers learned the following: (1) there are differences in resistance to alcohol and other drugs (both styles of resistance and susceptibility), (2) resistance is important beyond the initial refusal, (3) the critical role of peer pressure in resistance training, and (4) the significance of communication skill levels in resistance training. Having discovered that drug risk and involvement begin before high school, the project researchers targeted middle school students in their next phase of prevention testing and research. In this phase, supported by an externally funded grant, researchers developed the keepin' it REAL prevention curricula using research from the pilot that identified drug resistance strategies used by adolescents. The students then created 5 video-based performance lessons, which were incorporated into 10 lessons to be implemented by teachers in the classroom.

The curriculum was taught in 35 middle schools in Phoenix. Using data collected from the previous studies, an interdisciplinary team of researchers began testing the effectiveness of the program. Results showed the program to be effective in reducing drug use and pro-drug-use attitudes up to 12 months after the program was taught, with culturally grounded versions of the program being the most effective. Part of the reason for the effectiveness of the project was

the sense of trust and ownership that came from the community in which the program was eventually implemented. In addition, the youth who helped create the project were essentially the experts in the particulars of alcohol risk in their communities and lives (Holleran, Reeves, Dustman, & Marsiglia, 2002).

Developmental Assets Model: The Georgetown Project's Innovative Response to Risk

In light of the important role of risk and protective factors in augmenting the health and welfare of youth, the developmental assets framework provides concrete strategies for initiating, developing, and strengthening protective factors for children, families, and communities (Scales, 1999; Scales, Benson, Leffert, & Blyth, 2000).

In the late 1980s, while many community groups were augmenting their economic development, the Georgetown Project was busy focusing on human development, by recognizing and minimizing gaps in services for youth and families. By 1995, in a community whose population had grown 60% in 5 years, there were increasing concerns regarding drugs and alcohol. A task force was appointed to explore and find solutions. The team included representatives from the following entities and agencies: the City of Georgetown, the surrounding county, the local independent school district, Southwestern University, University of Texas School of Social Work, law enforcement, Ministerial Alliance, Georgetown Hospital, private health care providers, and local businesses. After 18 months of planning, in 1997, the Georgetown Project emerged (2001). This communitywide coalition immediately set out to promote asset-building (i.e., actions or activities that contribute to the positive development of children and adolescents) opportunities for the community youth.

The model is comprehensive and is applied at all levels of community. All of the Georgetown schools embrace the 40 assets model, a strengths-based, research grounded prevention model. The local departments of corrections work in a proactive mode, returning to walking a beat (as opposed to prior mode of reacting only to emergency calls) and being responsible for specific youth and families instead of responding to emergencies. Youth sit on advisory councils and planning boards. In fact, the Georgetown

Youth Advisory Board, appointed by the city council, provides a vehicle for youth voices and hosts a teen court and a youth summit to build youth leadership. The model pervades the community, in parenting programs, health agencies, recreational agencies, and public programs such as the library. The Georgetown Project's Board of Advisors brings more than 40 agencies and organizations together regularly to identify needs and close the gaps in services. This process has resulted in a variety of grants implementing many youth and family initiatives and shifting norms with regard to risk behaviors. Similar multimodal interventions based on models of risk and resilience are critical for prevention of alcohol use and abuse among youth.

References

American Academy of Pediatrics (1998). *Caring for your adolescent: Ages 12 to 21* (pamphlet).

Bandura, A. (1977). *Social learning theory.* New York: General Learning Press.

Bonomo, Y., Coffey, C., Wolfe, R., Lynskey, M., Bowles, G., & Patton, G. (2001). Adverse outcomes of alcohol use in adolescence. *Addiction, 96,* 1485–1496.

Botvin, G. J., Baker, E., & Dusenbury, L. (1995). Long-term follow up results of a randomized drug abuse prevention trial in a white middle class population. *Journal of the American Medical Association, 273*(14), 1106–1112.

Botvin, G. J., Baker, E., Dusenbury, L., Tortu, S., & Botvin, E. M. (1990). Preventing adolescent drug abuse through a multimodal cognitive-behavioral approach: Results of a 3-year study. *Journal of Consulting and Clinical Psychology, 58*(4), 437–446.

Bronfenbrenner, U. (1979). *The ecology of human development: Experiments by nature and design.* Cambridge: Harvard University Press.

Bronfenbrenner, U. (1995). Developmental ecology through space and time: A future perspective. In P. Moen, G. H. Elder, & K. Luscher (Eds.), *Examining lives in context: Perspectives on the ecology of human development.* Washington, DC: American Psychological Association.

Bukoski, W. J. (1985). School-based substance abuse prevention: A review of program research. In S. Ezekoye, K. H. Kumpfer, & W. J. Bukoski (Eds.), *Childhood and chemical abuse: Prevention and intervention.* New York: Hayworth Press.

Cowen, E. L. & Work, W. (1988). Resilient children, psychological wellness, and primary preventions. *American Journal of Community Psychology, 16,* 591–607.

Donovan, J. E. (1996). Problem-behavior theory and the explanation of adolescent marijuana use. *Journal of Drug Issues, 26*(2), 379–404.

Drug Resistance Strategies Project. (2002). *Keepin' it REAL.* Funded by the National Institutes of Health through the National Institute on Drug Abuse (NIDA/NIH R01 DA05629). Retrieved June 25, 2003, from http://keepinitreal.asu.edu/index.htm

Falck, R., & Craig, R. (1988). Classroom-oriented, primary prevention programming for drug abuse. *Journal of Psychoactive Drugs, 20*(4), 403–408.

Fraser, M. W. (1997). *Risk and resilience in childhood: An ecological perspective.* Washington, DC: NASW Press.

Fraser, M. W., & Galinsky, M. I. (1997). Toward a resiliency based model of practice. In M. W. Fraser (Ed.), *Risk and resilience* (pp. 265–275). Washington, DC: NASW Press.

Georgetown Project. (2001). *The Georgetown Project: Building a healthy community for children and youth.* Georgetown, TX: Author. Retrieved June 25, 2003, from http://www.georgetownproject.com/

Gosin, M. N., Dustman, P. A., Drapeau, A. E., & Harthun, M. L. (2003). Participatory action research: Creating an effective prevention curriculum for adolescents in the Southwestern U.S.. *Health Education Research: Theory and Practice, 18,* 363–379.

Greene, R. R., & Conrad, A. P. (2001). Basic assumptions and terms. In R. R. Greene (Ed.), *Resiliency: An integrated approach to practice, policy, and research* (pp. 29–62). Washington, DC: NASW Press.

Hawkins, J. D., Catalano, R. F., & Associates. (1992). *Communities that care: Action for drug abuse prevention.* San Francisco: Jossey-Bass.

Hirschi, T. (1969). *Causes of delinquency.* Berkeley: University of California Press.

Holleran, L. (2003). Chicano/a youth of the Southwest borderlands: Perceptions of ethnicity, acculturation, and race. *Hispanic Journal of Behavioral Sciences, 25*(3).

Holleran, L., Reeves, L., Dustman, P., & Marsiglia, F. F. (2002) Creating culturally grounded videos for substance abuse prevention: A dual perspective on process. *Journal of Social Work Practice in the Addictions, 2*(1), 55–78.

Holleran, L., & Waller, M. A. (2003). Sources of resilience of Chicano/a youth: Forging identities in the borderlands. *Child and Adolescent Social Work, 20*(5).

Jessor, R. (1987). Problem-behavior theory, psychological development, and adolescent problem drinking. *British Journal of Addiction, 82,* 331–342.

Jessor, R. (Ed.). (1998). *New perspectives on adoles-*

cent risk behavior. New York: Cambridge University Press.

Jessor, R., Donavan, J. E., & Costa, F. M. (1991). *Beyond adolescence: Problem behavior and young adult development.* New York: Cambridge University Press.

Lonczak, H. S., Huang, B., Catalano, R. F., Hawkins, J. D., Hill, K. G., Abbott, R. D., Ryan, J. A., et al. (2001). The social predictors of adolescent alcohol misuse: A test of the social development model. *Journal of Studies on Alcohol, 62*(2), 179–189.

Lorion, R. P., Price, R. H. & Eaton, W. W. (1989). The prevention of child and adolescent disorders: From theory to research. In D. Shaffer, I. Philips, & N. B. Enzer (Eds.), *Prevention of mental disorders, alcohol and other drug use in children and adolescents* (pp. 55–95). Rockville, MD: Office of Substance Abuse Prevention and American Academy of Child and Adolescent Psychiatry, Prevention Monograph #2 (DHHS Publication No. ADM 89-1646).

Marsiglia, F. F., & Holleran, L. (1999). I've learned so much from my mother: An ethnography of a group of Chicana high school students. *Social Work in Education, 21*(3), 220–237.

Marsiglia, F. F., Holleran, L., & Jackson, K. M. (2000). Assessing the impact of internal and external resources on school-based substance abuse prevention. *Social Work in Education, 22*(3), 145–161.

Marsiglia, F. F., Miles, B. W., Dustman, P. A., & Sills, S. K. (2003). Ties that protect: An ecological view of protective factors influencing urban adolescent substance use. *Journal of Ethnic and Cultural Diversity in Social Work, 11.*

Masten, A. S. (1994). Resilience in individual development: Successful adaptation despite risk and adversity. In M. C. Wang & E. W. Gorden (Eds.), *Educational resilience in inner-city America: Challenge and prospects, 1994.* Hillsdale, NJ: Erlbaum.

Masten, A. S. (1999). Commentary: The promise and perils of resilience research as a guide to prevention intervention. In M. D. Glantz & J. L. Johnson (Eds.), *Resilience and development: Positive life adaptation* (pp. 251–258). New York: Kluwer Academic/Plenum.

McClelland, G. M., & Teplin, L.A. (2001). Alcohol intoxication and violent crime: Implications for public health policy. *American Journal on Addictions, 10*(Suppl.), 10–85.

Mrazek, P. J. & Haggerty, R. J. (1994). *Reducing the risks for mental disorders: Frontiers for preventive intervention research.* Washington, DC: National Academy Press.

Nash, J. K., & Bowen, G. L. (1999). Perceived crime and informal social control in the neighborhood as a context for adolescent behavior: A risk and resilience perspective. *Social Work Research, 23,* 171–186.

National Household Survey on Drug Abuse. (2001). *The NHSDA Report* [Online]. Retrieved June 25, 2003, from http://www.samhsa.gov/oas/Dependence/toc.htm.

Perry, C. L., Williams, C. L., Mortenson, S. V., Toomey, T. L., Komro, K. A., Anstime, P. S., et al. (1996). Project Northland: Outcomes of a community wide alcohol use prevention program during early adolescence. *American Journal of Public Health, 86,* 956–965.

Petratis, J., Flay, B. R., & Miller, T. Q. (1995). Reviewing theories of adolescent substance use: Organizing pieces in the puzzle. *Psychological Bulletin, 117*(1), 67–86.

Saleebey, D. (1996). The strengths perspective in social work practice: Extensions and cautions. *Social Work, 41*(3), 296–305.

Scales, P. C. (1999). Reducing risks and building developmental assets: Essential actions for promoting adolescent health. *Journal of School Health, 69*(3), 113–119.

Scales, P. C., Benson, P. L., Leffert, N., & Blyth, D. A. (2000). The contribution of developmental assets to the prediction of thriving outcomes among adolescents. *Applied Developmental Science, 4*(1), 27–46.

Scheier, L. M. & Botvin, G. J. (1997). Expectancies as the mediators of the effects of social influences and alcohol knowledge on adolescent alcohol abuse: A prospective analysis. *Psychology of Addictive Behaviors, 11,* 48–64.

Schinke, S. P., Tepavac, L., & Cole, K. C. (2000). Preventing substance use among Native American youth. Three-year results, *Addictive Behaviors, 25*(3), 387–397.

Smokowski, R. P. (1998). Prevention and intervention strategies for promoting resilience in disadvantaged children. *Social Service Review, 72*(3), 336–364.

Staton, M., Leukfield, C., Logan, T. K., Zimmerman, R., Lynam, D., Milich, R., et al. (1999). Risky sex behavior and substance abuse among young adults. *Health & Social Work, 24*(2), 147–155.

Stewart, M., Reid, G., & Mangham, C. (1997). Fostering children's resilience. *Journal of Pediatric Nursing, 12,* 21–31.

Sutherland, E. H. (1973). *On analyzing crime.* Ed. Karl Schuessler. Chicago: University of Chicago Press.

Tobler, N. S., & Stratton, H. H. (1997). Effectiveness of school-based drug prevention programs: A meta-analysis of the research, *Journal of Primary Prevention, 18*(1), 71–128.

Vidich, A. J., & Lyman, S. M. (1994). Qualitative methods: Their history in sociology and anthropology. In N. K. Denzin & Y. S. Lincoln (Eds.), *Handbook of qualitative research* (p. 23–59). Thousand Oaks, CA: Sage.

SECTION VIII
Practice-Based Qualitative Research Exemplars

75

QUALITATIVE EVALUATION APPLICATION OF REFLECTIVE PRACTICE IN DIRECT CARE SETTINGS

Ian Shaw

I am no longer sure that it is worth expending too much effort on trying to agree on what we mean by qualitative evaluation. The diversity and lack of realistic shared expectations about evaluation frustrated the late Lee Cronbach and his colleagues quite some time ago. They were only slightly exaggerating when they remarked that

If any single intellectual sin is responsible for the present chaos, it is the readiness to make general assertions that supposedly apply to all evaluations. (Cronbach et al., 1980, p. 51)

I suspect they were right when they argued that "a theory of evaluation must be as much a theory of political interaction as it is a theory of how knowledge is constructed." Within this climate, evaluation's "role is not to produce authoritative truths but to clarify, to document, to raise new questions, to create new perceptions" (pp. 52–53). In carrying this out, the boundaries between research and evaluation are none too clear. Cronbach had himself previously espoused a distinction between conclusion-oriented and decision-oriented research, with evaluation falling in the latter category, but came to reject that as overly simple in that evaluation rarely enables a direct decision.

We do not have to accept the view that evaluation methods will be molded in a deterministic way by the paradigm position of the evaluator to recognize that evaluation questions are nonetheless shaped by our paradigm-like starting points. Greene identifies four main positions in program evaluation. She names these as postpositivism, pragmatism, interpretivism, and critical or normative evaluation (Greene, 1994).

The typical evaluation questions addressed by *postpositivist* evaluation are

- Are the desired outcomes attained and attributable to the program?
- Is this program the most efficient alternative?

Pragmatic evaluations focus on questions such as

- Which parts of the program worked well and which need improvement?
- How effective is the program with respect to the organization's goals and to the beneficiaries' needs?

Interpretivist evaluation typically starts by asking how the stakeholders experience the program, either individually or coconstructively.

Critical, normative evaluation addresses questions such as

- In what ways are the premises, goals, or activities of the program serving to maintain power and resource inequities in society?

• How might the evaluation process challenge these structured inequities?

Two naturally occurring but highly contrasting examples will help illustrate the practical significance of this argument. Wholey and Whitmore were both interested in evaluating prenatal programs. Note how their paradigm-like starting points shape the very different kinds of questions they ask. Wholey describes the preliminary assessment of the evaluability of the Tennessee Pre-Natal Program. Whitmore also describes the evaluation of an education program for single expectant mothers in a low-income area of Halifax, Nova Scotia (Whitmore, 1990, 1994; Wholey, 1994). Wholey's position is basically postpositivist, whereas Whitmore embraces critical evaluation.

The Tennessee Department of Public Health ran a 5-year project "Toward Improving the Outcome of Pregnancy" (TIOP) from 1977 to 1982. An evaluation of the program was funded for the final year. Wholey led an assessment aimed to plan the evaluation activities that would be most useful. He involved budget staff, senior management and executive staff, a deputy commissioner of health, senior project staff, and others in work and policy groups. Following this exercise, various design options were put forward.

• Success in meeting statewide standards
• Intraprogram comparisons among TIOP projects and counties
• Before and after comparisons and interrupted time-series analyses using birth data
• Before and after and time-series data comparing TIOP counties with others not served by TIOP
• Before and after and time-series analyses comparing TIOP projects offering different services at different costs

Agreement was reached in the light of this to focus on success in reducing numbers of low birth weight infants, as a surrogate indicator of risk of infant morbidity and mortality and of learning disability. Program representatives thought this was both a realistic goal and one for which they could be held accountable. Infant mortality targets were also kept on the advice of the deputy health commissioner, who believed questions would later be asked on this indicator.

The key guiding principles in this project were reliance on expert definitions, measurement and operationalization, control features of the design, accountability, and achievability. The program in which Whitmore was involved had run for 3 years when the evaluation was invited and reflects a very different set of steering principles. Whitmore offered to facilitate a participatory inquiry. As many as possible of the women who had previously used the service were contacted and invited to apply to join the evaluation team. Four women were appointed, with the brief to formulate the design, collect and analyze data, and present the results. Whitmore describes participatory research and evaluation as combining

investigation, education and action in an effort to improve the social and economic conditions under which people live. Its main goals involve broad social change, justice and equality, achieved by seeking to empower less powerful constituents. (Whitmore, 1990, p. 216)

Data collection was based on unstructured interviews and questionnaires. There were understandable difficulties. The women found it difficult to separate the data from their own opinions. There were group tensions, which led to one member leaving. Contact with the media proved "extremely destructive to our collective process and ultimately to group cohesiveness" (1990, p. 221). There were also communication and trust difficulties.

Yet the net results were positive. They had successful contacts with the advisory group, addressed a conference, and took a university class. In addition, Whitmore and the group concluded that there had been gains at individual, group, and wider social environment levels (see Table 75.1).

If what counts as *evaluation* is best left partly an open question, so, likewise, what we mean by *qualitative* evaluation is none too obvious. (See, for example, Hammersley, 1992, for a challenge to conventional positions on qualitative research.) Williams wisely avoids stirring up debate about the hallmarks of qualitative inquiry and collates a helpful list of criteria by which we may decide if a qualitative or naturalistic evaluation is appropriate (Williams, 1986). It will be appropriate, he suggests, in circumstances when

1. Evaluation issues are not clear in advance.
2. Official definitions of the evaluand are not

TABLE 75.1 Outcomes of Prenatal Program Evaluation

Level of practice	Component of empowerment
Individual	Self-confidence
	Knowledge and skills
	Enthusiasm and enjoyment
Group	Overcoming isolation
	Developing trust
Environment	Educational opportunities
	Speaking to outside groups
	Challenging the social service system
	Employment opportunities

sufficient, and insider perspectives are needed.

3. "Thick description" (Geertz's phrase) is required.

4. It is desirable to convey the potential for vicarious experience of the evaluand on the part of the reader.

5. Formative evaluation, aimed at improving the program, policy, or practice, is appropriate.

6. The outcome includes complex actions in natural settings.

7. Evaluation recipients want to know how the evaluand is operating in its natural state.

8. There is time to study the evaluand through its natural cycle. The true power of naturalistic evaluation is dissipated if there is not time to observe the natural functions of the evaluand in their various forms.

9. The situation permits intensive inquiry, without posing serious ethical obstacles.

10. The evaluand can be studied unobtrusively, as it operates, and in an ethical way.

11. Diverse data sources are available.

12. There are resources and consent to search for negative instances and counterevidence.

13. There is sufficient customer and end user agreement on methodological strategy.

Williams's list is helpful because it manages to be practical, thought provoking, and relatively specific without losing value as a set of working rules. It is not a complete or final list. For example, qualitative data have some strengths on which evaluators do not always capitalize. Later I refer briefly to ways in which qualitative evaluations can assess aspects of causality.

Part of the title of this chapter is "Reflective Practice in Direct Care Settings." I am not too finicky about definitions of reflective practice. Whatever the focus, the reflective research method can be characterized as following four stages in a cyclical process, a cycle closely akin to an experiential learning cycle that may be iterated until no more understanding can be elicited: immersion in experience, reflection-on-action, conceptualization, and action (Gould, 1999). The first stage is of concrete experience, the immersion of the researcher in the situation as it presents itself, be it an agency or the world of the service user. A shared definition is sought with workers or service users of what the problem is, how it has emerged, the context, contributory factors, and their effects. This is likely to proceed through a mixture of data collection methods such as participant observation, dialogue, and documentary sources. From this engagement develops an initial perspective on the situation, its boundaries, and significance. The second stage of inquiry becomes reflection on the emergent picture. This may be in a range of contexts such as groups of participants, supervisory relationships, or internal mental reflection. Third, a provisional conceptualization of the issues develops, perhaps as a written document, but it may be also represented in more unusual or creative media such as video, oral reports, metaphors, or visual images (Gould, 1996; Gould & Taylor, 1996). In the fourth stage, the analysis set out in the third stage is translated into prescriptions for action, which are then tested and evaluated in practice. This may then lead into further cycles of experience, reflection, conceptualization, and action.

DIRECTIONS IN QUALITATIVE EVALUATION

Developments in qualitative evaluation are marked by a creative fluidity. For example, there is a growing recognition that while qualitative evaluation cannot resolve the problems of causal conclusions any more than quantitative evaluation can, it can nonetheless assess *causality* "as it actually plays out in a particular setting"

(Miles & Huberman, 1994, p. 10; cf. Shaw, 2003). Qualitative evaluation methodology not only is well equipped to address the local outworking of cause and effect but also enriches the *choice of methods* in ways that are relevant to evaluative purposes.

Qualitative methodology also provides a strong purchase on the evaluation of *direct service delivery*—a main emphasis of this chapter. Thinking and practice in the evaluation field have been too much influenced by ideas of evaluation as being equivalent to *program* evaluation and have given insufficient attention to evaluation of direct practice and service delivery.

Qualitative evaluation has also made a distinctive contribution to the question of how evaluation might be *useful* for policies, programs, projects, and professional practice. At the broadest level, evaluation would be judged useful if it demonstrably contributed to one or more of the following.

- Added better policies, services, and practice
- Strengthened the moral purpose of professional practice
- Promoted methodological rigor, scope, depth, and innovation
- Strengthened the sense of a profession's intellectual nature and location

Careful specification is always needed of what we mean when we speak of evaluation being "useful." For instance, everyday discussions of evidence-based practice frequently proceed on a misconception at this point. Practice is not and cannot be "based" on evidence in the straightforward and unproblematic way envisaged by some of its advocates. Qualitative evaluation gets us beyond this likely impasse by its capacity to do the things Cronbach said are the core of evaluation: to clarify, document, raise new questions, and create new perceptions. The following series of examples illustrates the potential of practical evaluation choices to open out these larger issues.

ASSESSING EVALUABILITY

The example we gave from the work of Wholey was about assessing the feasibility of carrying out an evaluation. Wholey has developed relatively precise criteria for making these sorts of decisions, and I have discussed these elsewhere (Shaw, 1999, pp. 124–125). Assessing evaluabil-

ity is an important starting point, but his approach lends itself more readily to a quantitative, accountability model of evaluation. Example 1 illustrates a different approach to evaluability assessment.

Example 1: Evaluability Assessment

Pulice describes a stakeholder-focused evaluability assessment in his discussion of qualitative evaluation methods in the public sector with seriously mentally ill adults (Pulice, 1994). He recommends identifying relevant constituency groups at all levels and completing preliminary interviews with key informants on the reason for the evaluation request, the likely time frames, and their views regarding intended uses of the evaluation. He also advises a literature search of legislation, agency documents, and committee reports "to determine the nature and content of documentation relative to the evaluation question" (p. 307).

He then suggests that the evaluators develop a preliminary taxonomy of the identified constituency groups in terms of their likely role as advocates, planners, facilitators, monitors, or managers. Finally, he recommends conducting semistructured interviews that focus on the broad evaluation questions. It would be possible to use focus groups for this stage.

Evaluability assessments will reflect the underlying perspectives of the evaluators. For example, critical evaluators may wish to explore—with a view to mitigating—the potential for imposing their own worldviews on those participating in the evaluation. Where such imposition seems unavoidable, it may be decided that evaluation is not feasible. Evaluators who commence from a constructivist and relativist standpoint will wish to explore the feasibility of an authentic evaluation that takes local context into account and empowers stakeholders. Rodwell and Woody believe that

Constructivist methods to determine evaluability are very appropriate when the goal is to have all possible stakeholding groups involved in the process, while having problems emerge from observation, from experiences, and from the data. (Rodwell & Woody, 1994, p. 319)

They describe a proposal for an evaluation of a clinic setting, which went astray. "We ignored the context of our deeds" (p. 324). When, following the evaluability assessment, the proposal was made, it was turned down, on the grounds that it did not follow the research policy of the agency, that it threatened the homeostasis of the organization through having too broad a focus and too short a time frame to accomplish it, and that such detailed study was not needed but that the agency wanted comparison studies with similar services and using quantitative methods. The authors believe their failure stemmed in part from not taking criteria of authenticity into account. Such assessments can "create a referent in a not so rational program evaluation environment" (p. 326).

CHOOSING METHODS

I said a moment ago that qualitative evaluation methodology enriches the choice of methods in ways that are relevant to evaluative purposes. My own view is that qualitative evaluators do not need to identify a set of evaluation-specific methods. Evaluation inquiry is evaluative when it is marked by one or more evaluative purposes, and the forms taken by evaluation fieldwork are contingent on purpose. Evaluation methods will neither be entirely the same as, nor completely different from, those of qualitative research in general. For this reason I am reluctant to rule any methods of inquiry out of court. But I am equally unwilling to recommend the routine adoption of even the most apparently relevant methodological devices. Methodological automatism will produce awkward, clumsy evaluations, lacking both rigor and relevance.

An example may help. Suppose a qualitative evaluator wishes to explore professional decision making in a direct care setting, and she is uncertain of whether to use interviews or observation methods. One route to deciding the relative benefits and limitations of using interviewing or observation methods within qualitative evaluation is to directly compare the gains and limitations of each and to distinguish the knowledge claims made by each. Example 2 illustrates how this worked out in one such study.

Example 2: Choosing Methods for Exploring Professional Decision Making

McKeganey, MacPherson, and Hunter (1988) report a comparison between interviewing and observation undertaken as part of a study of professional decision making when people were to be offered a place in a home for the elderly. Their interests were in aspects of the microprocesses of decision making and to understand discretion and variations in such decisions. Table 75.2 summarizes the points of comparison and the weight that the research team attached to each of these in the context of their study.

The researchers concluded that it was difficult to use observation to focus on individual decisions because decisions occur across several contexts. Interviews, by contrast, can cover every decision point. They decided in the light of this to target the contexts for their observation in the light of prior interview outcomes. Interviewing was also judged stronger as a means of triangulating accounts by different professionals. They furthermore recognized that "There may be a tendency for interviewers and interviewees to concentrate on only the formal components of the decision making process," whereas "one of the benefits of observational work is precisely the capacity to focus attention upon the informal aspects of professionals' decision making"

TABLE 75.2 Interviewing or Observation for Evaluating Professional Decision Making

Aspects of professional decisions	Interviews	Observation
Data level	Individuals	Processes
Decision points	Multiple	Few
Triangulation of accounts	Strong	Less strong
Components of decisions	Formal	Informal
Routine decisions	Less strong	Strong
Nondecisions	Weak	Weak
Rationality or nonrationality of decisions	Overstate rationality	Strong on nonrationality
Disclosure of private accounts	Less strong	Adequate

Developed from McKeganey, MacPherson, and Hunter, 1988.

(McKeganey et al., 1988, p. 16). This formal-informal aspect was also reflected in their judgment that taken-for-granted dimensions of decisions may be harder for people to articulate in interviews and better accessed via observation.

Interviews may tend to re-create past decisions as if they were more rational than in fact they were. McKeganey et al. conclude that observational work can tap the more chaotic character of present decisions. Finally, they believe that professionals may use private decision categories that include moral or pejorative aspects—perhaps especially when the demand for a service outstrips the supply and they are obliged to ration. They concluded that interviews would be less likely to disclose these elements and that observation would at least problematize the grounds of decision making.

An important caveat is in order. Method choices made as a consequence of any such comparison must not be treated as absolute but contextualized within the specific study. We cannot transfer the pros and cons of Table 75.2 lock, stock, and barrel to all evaluations where a method choice of this kind is being made. There is no absolute reason, for example, why either interviews or observation methods cannot elicit nondecisions. These researchers have clearly contextualized their assessment of the two methods, and other evaluators must do likewise.

POLICIES AND CASE STUDY EVALUATION

Qualitative evaluation can also enrich the understanding of how social policies work in direct care settings. The application of case study designs to evaluation illustrates this point. "The case for case studies in qualitative evaluations rests on a confluence of their responsive political-value stance and their underlying interpretivist assumptions" (Greene, 1994, p. 538).

Evaluators are sometimes guilty of talking too loosely about "cases." Atkinson and Delamont are correct to chide us that "What counts as a 'case' is . . . much more problematic than 'case-study' researchers seem to allow for" (Atkinson & Delamont, 1993, p. 207). But, despite a slight hedging of his bets, Stake helpfully says,

The case is a special something to be studied, a student, a classroom, a committee, a program, perhaps, but not a problem, a relationship, or a theme. The

case to be studied probably has problems and relationships, and the report of the case is likely to have a theme, but the case is an entity. The case, in some ways, has a unique life. (Stake, 1995, p. 133)

Case studies may address either single or multiple cases. There are various rationales for focusing on a single case. Yin (1994) distinguishes critical cases (which allow the testing of a well-formulated theory), extreme or rare cases, and revelatory cases (a phenomenon hitherto inaccessible to scientific investigation). For example, voluntary welfare agencies may set up projects that reflect a novel model of intervention they wish to develop, local educational authorities may set up small numbers of innovative but relatively costly curriculum innovations, and government departments routinely introduce innovative or imported forms of dealing with offenders. Studies of critical or rare cases are possible in these cases. Changing public attitudes to the benefits or risks of a hitherto unimpeachable project may open up the possibility of revelatory case study evaluations in a previously no-go area of practice.

Innovations are frequently introduced in several locations simultaneously and therefore allow the possibility of multiple rather than single case studies. Multiple case studies can be achieved by setting up "projects which are specifically designed as a series of ethnographic studies in different settings, selected on criteria developed from existing theory to provide the most significant dimensions for comparison" (Finch, 1986, p. 185). Finch suggests the advantage of a central team that guides the analytic themes and categories at the design stage but does not dictate the research methods. Alternatively, multiple case studies could be done sequentially by planning cumulative comparative studies. While we should not expect this to yield an easy linear development of knowledge, it does provide opportunity for interdisciplinary evaluation and would be a significant advance on most current case study evaluation. Example 3 illustrates a multisite case study in a school setting.

Example 3: Multisite Case Study

Burgess and others (1994) report a multisite case study of the introduction of records of achievement into high schools in an English Midlands county. A researcher and two seconded teachers each spent a term in one of the schools, working with teachers and pupils and, where possible, participating in activities relating to the record of achievement process.

The four schools were "illustrative of the range of schools which existed in the authority" (Burgess et al., 1994, p. 131) and enabled comparisons between urban and rural schools, selective and nonselective schools, schools serving predominantly working-class and middle-class populations, and all-white and multiethnic schools. The schools also varied in the extent to which they had introduced the scheme.

Individual reports were written on each school, plus a thematic report. Thematic issues such as the significance of time and school-specific issues were both addressed. They stressed the interconnectedness of resources, selection of sites, and analysis and also implied some dangers in placing too much weight on local context. For example, they argued that the possibility of cross-case analysis stemmed from posing similar themes to the schools at the commencement of the evaluation.

The authors claim, "Overall the strength of the study rested in its comparative nature. The research design facilitated the examination of a wide range of substantive educational issues in different contexts" (p. 136). It is clear from this example that the authors were interested in the cases at more than one level. Part of their argument deals with holistic analyses of each school, but they are also apparently interested in differences of class, school admission policies, and rural or urban location. We can readily envisage direct care settings in which analogous considerations would be relevant. Yin (1994) uses the term *embedded* to describe case studies of this kind, where there is more than one unit of analysis.

The emergence of case studies has also reflected a concern about power relationships in organizations and in the relationship between evaluators and member–stakeholders. In response to this, case studies can serve at least moderate emancipatory purposes. Example 4 is an interesting and unusual illustration of this approach.

Example 4: Case Study for Practitioners and Researchers

Bogdan and Taylor report a multisite case study evaluation of 40 programs that aimed to promote the integration of people with learning disabilities and multiple disabilities into the community (Bogdan & Taylor, 1994). They aimed to develop a model of evaluation that partially resolves the conflicting orientations of practitioners and researchers by combining appropriately skeptical rigor with research that will "help conscientious practitioners—people who are leading the reforms in the direction of integration" (p. 295).

They studied each of the 40 projects through a rolling program of eight brief case studies a year over 5 years. "We consciously tried to find places that can teach us about how people with severe disabilities can be integrated into the community" (p. 298).

Consistent with their theoretical orientation, they started with a deliberately vague definition of integration. "We treat the concept of integration as problematic, something to be investigated rather than assumed. We want to learn about how agencies . . . define and accomplish integration" (Bogdan & Taylor, 1994, p. 297).

Their approach resulted in much easier access, and ironically people were more candid about dilemmas of practice than they may otherwise have been. Short reports were produced in the professional press on each project, and when the reports focused on negative aspects of less than exemplary agencies, the agencies were allowed the choice of whether or not their names were mentioned.

The sites were selected through purposive sampling methods, which combined asking key informants to nominate good programs and then undertaking telephone interviews. They wished to identify innovative and exemplary programs rather than build a probability sample. They were interested in generalizing "patterns that transcend individual cases" (p. 300). They were also interested in theorizing and "developing sensitizing concepts and grounded theory that transcend the commonsense ideas of the people we study" (p. 300), although they do not discuss how they think generalizing works or offer any reflection of the relationship between lay and scientific concepts.

EVALUATING PROGRAMS

We have already given an example of how qualitative evaluation in direct care settings may be focused on program issues, in the case of Wholey and Whitmore's two different projects on prenatal programs. Though there is no single good practice model for qualitative program evaluation, there are a number of questions whose answers set the broad parameters of a qualitative stance on evaluation. Qualitative program evaluators

- Will consider the *process* of program activities and delivery prior to considering program outcomes
- Will be mistrustful of program delivery and evaluation that depend heavily on assumptions of *rational decision making*
- Should not ignore the significance of *theorizing* about programs
- Will be less enthusiastic about the value of *accountability* models of evaluation
- Include a range of positions on the place of program evaluation in contributing to *social change*

The last 15 years have seen a partial revival of faith in outcome-focused effectiveness evaluation, under the rubric of evidence-based policy and practice. This has been stimulated by the political commitment of several Western governments to management-by-effectiveness approaches, public sector accountability, and the adoption of performance indicators for schools, hospitals, direct care agencies, and the whole gamut of public sector services.

I am not convinced that the problems this raises have been adequately resolved by the present generation of evidence-based evaluators. Rationalist ideas of efficiency do not sit comfortably with ideas of democratic participation. Cronbach goes as far as to say that "Rationalism is dangerously close to totalitarianism" (Cronbach et al., 1980, p. 95). In response to arguments that quasi-experimental designs are convincing and plausible, he and his colleagues say tartly that

The demand that an argument be "convincing" is nothing more than a rationalist attempt to define a category of conclusions that in no way rest on belief and values; in evaluation it is an attempt to place decisions outside politics by establishing an inescapable conclusion. (p. 292)

There is a further problem too little appreciated. The question "Does it work?" is a skeptical question and "functions as an exclusionary gatekeeper" (Bogdan & Taylor, 1994, p. 296). Even

assuming that design problems could be solved, the question still would not be helpful to practitioners. "Conscientious practitioners do not approach their work as skeptics; they believe in what they do" (p. 297). Bogdan and Taylor have worked to develop what they call "optimistic research." "We have evolved an approach to research that has helped us bridge the gap between the activists, on the one hand, and empirically grounded skeptical researchers, on the other" (p. 295). We noted in Example 4 how the main focus of their research has been on questions of how people with severe disabilities can be integrated into the community. Rather than ask whether services are effective, they ask, "What does integration mean?" and "How can integration be accomplished?"

I would not want to leave the impression that qualitative evaluation replaces an outcomes focus with a process one. The development of case study designs and the use of simulation methodology provide two contrasting illustrations of the development of qualitative design solutions analogous to designs, which entail a degree of control and can thus approach outcome questions. For example, Donald Campbell's early position was that "one-shot" case study designs are uninterpretable with regard to causal attribution. However, through exchanges with Becker and Erikson, he came to the position that the analogy of degrees of freedom provides a major source of discipline for interpreting intensive, cross-cultural case studies. The logic entails testing a theory against the predictions or expectations it stimulates, through a general process he describes as pattern matching, based on the premise that "experimental design can be separated from quantification" (Campbell, 1978, p. 197). He developed a perspective that entailed a mutual commitment to both ethnography and comparative studies.

Campbell's approach was developed in Yin's account of case study research (Yin, 1994). Patton has also illustrated how "well-crafted case studies can tell the stories behind the numbers, capture unintended impacts and ripple effects, and illuminate dimensions of desired outcomes that are difficult to quantify" (Patton, 2002, p. 152; cf. Shaw, 2003).

Simulations offer a rather different design solution for qualitative inquiry and have the potential to provide "a unique and innovative tool that has not yet been widely applied" (Turner & Zimmerman, 1994, p. 335). They have two main applications: first, as an evaluative test for service discrimination and, second, as a qualitative proxy for control within a natural setting. The first application is essentially an export from the social psychology laboratory, which offers some control over stimuli but also suffers from some of the laboratory risk of, for example, artificiality and demand characteristics. But it is the second application that is more relevant for our purposes. One particular example of simulation—the simulated client—represents an advance on the use of vignettes in policy evaluation. Those who evaluate the process of professional practice come face to face with the invisibility of practice. How may we learn the ways in which lawyers, teachers, general medical practitioners, or social workers practice? How would different professionals deal with the same case? Wasoff and Dobash used a promising innovatory method in their study of how a specific piece of law reform was incorporated into the practice of solicitors (Wasoff & Dobash, 1992, 1996). The use of simulated clients in "natural" settings allowed them to identify practice variations that could be ascribed with some confidence to differences between lawyers rather than the artifacts of differences between cases. Example 5 gives a hypothetical but feasible extension of this method to evaluation in direct care settings.

Example 5: Simulations

Suppose that you wish to carry out a qualitative evaluation of decisions made by housing managers, medical staff, and social workers regarding the allocation of care management packages. Evaluators using simulated clients might prepare a small number of detailed case histories designed to test the practice decisions under consideration. A researcher or evaluator takes on the role of the client in the case history. The housing manager, relevant medical staff, and social workers each interview the "client" within the "natural" setting of their work. Assuming a constant script, the differences in professional response can be attributed with moderate confidence to actual professional differences.

There are limitations to the application of simulation methods. The method needs additional resources to prepare the case material, perhaps to act the role of clients, and to reflect on the quite detailed material that results from transcriptions of the interviews. The cost is therefore likely to be relatively high, and it requires reasonably high levels of research skills. However, the use of simulated clients has several things going for it. First, some researchers, especially insider researchers who have completed professional training programs, are likely to be familiar with the "family" of role-playing methods from which it is drawn. Second, other methods are not always feasible for practical or ethical reasons. Simulated clients overcome the ethical problems of seeking the cooperation of genuine clients. Above all, third, it makes practice visible. It will be clear from the brief description that the method could not be a tool for evaluating particular cases but would focus on specific *kinds* of practice.

EVALUATING DIRECT PRACTICE

Reflective practice raises a particular agenda and a wide range of topics available to qualitative social work researchers to explore through reflective methods, including (adapted from Jarvis, 1999)

- The changing nature of practice
- The relationship between professional education and practice
- How practitioners develop practical knowledge
- The development of expertise
- The development and characteristics of tacit knowledge
- The development of professional identity
- The relationship between practice and continuing professional development

To keep the discussion concrete, I want to illustrate aspects of this through the use of life histories in qualitative evaluation. The study of the life story is an area where ethnography and clinical methods have at times been close. As Cohler puts it,

Understood as . . . a presently recounted past, experienced present, and anticipated future, the concept of narrative is central both to the systematic study of lives over time and to the effort to intervene in order to reduce the experience of personal distress. (Cohler, 1994, p. 167)

The proximity is well illustrated by Bowen's account of "the delights of learning to apply the life history method to school non-attenders"

(Bowen, 1993). He had about 12 meetings with each of four people who had currently or recently experienced serious education problems, ending up with 8 or 9 hours of audiotaped conversations. Three of these people wrote autobiographies of between 5,000 and 12,000 words.

A related approach is that represented by the growth of interest in "life course sociology." It should be emphasized that such methods are not intrinsically "evaluation" and have usually been developed by researchers who would not regard their work as evaluation. Hence we need to cultivate and graft these methods onto evaluative purpose. Life course analysis "places change and development at the heart of the analysis and seeks to explore the inevitable temporal dimension of our lives and experiences" (Morgan, 1985, p. 177). Example 6 illustrates how life course interviews can help evaluatively minded researchers or practitioners understand and respond to housing issues.

Example 6: Housing Biographies

Clapham, Means, and Munro point out that housing research has tended to rely on snapshot pictures, with little idea of how people reach their present housing position. They advocate seeing old age, and housing in old age, as "stages in the life course which can only be understood by reference to previous experience and the attitudes and choices of people and the opportunities open to them during the whole life course" (Clapham et al., 1993, p. 133).

Researchers proceed by constructing a personal biography through in-depth qualitative interviews, to understand how they reached their present housing situation. The interview focus is on why certain options were chosen and others rejected. It incorporates a recognition that class, gender, and ethnic differences do not disappear with old age. Unlike a purely biographical approach, distinctions are made between the different types of time in which housing pathways are structured. These include individual time (age, state of health, etc.), family time (the stage of the family life cycle at which certain decisions were made or imposed), and historical time (the prevailing economic, social, and political conditions).

ACTION RESEARCH AND QUALITATIVE EVALUATION

We have given space at several points to developing ways in which empowerment and action research commitments are part of qualitative evaluation. Participatory researchers give greater or lesser emphasis to five commitments:

- Participation by the people being studied
- Respect for popular knowledge in agreeing, conducting, and reporting research
- A liberatory focus on issues of empowerment
- An educative dimension through consciousness raising
- Political action and social transformation

"We ourselves are reluctant to separate epistemology from ideology, findings from yearnings" (Stake, 1997, p. 471). Thus Stake poses the central challenge of evaluation approaches where personal and political changes are seen as the main and perhaps sole measure of validity. Whitmore's account of an evaluation of a prenatal program for single, pregnant mothers illustrates how positive outcomes may on balance be achieved. The evaluation was carried out over several months by four women who had themselves been through the program, with Whitmore as consultant to the project. There were tensions in the group, and communication failures. One member left and another protested to Whitmore that

> Our world is different from yours. The fear is that people always want to humiliate you, put you down (for being on welfare). . . . We have a different lifestyle from you. We just don't trust people the way you do. (Whitmore, 1994, p. 92)

Whitmore concluded that she could never entirely share the worlds of the women with whom she worked. "My small words were often their big words. What I assumed was 'normal talk,' they saw as 'professor words'" (p. 95). Martin arrived at similar conclusions from her own feminist participative research, concluding that such research "places unrealistic expectations on the extent to which the researched can become involved in the research process" and that "even when problems are a major concern to people (the researched) they have work and private lives which usually take priority, whereas research IS work for the researcher"

(Martin, 1994, p. 142). But the strength of their final achievements is evidence that participatory evaluation with oppressed groups is not only political rhetoric.

CONCLUSION

We commenced this chapter on reflective practice in direct care settings with a recognition of ways in which evaluation questions are shaped by our paradigm-like starting points. Two naturally occurring but highly contrasting examples from the work of Wholey and Whitmore illustrated the practical significance of this argument.

Thinking and practice in the evaluation field have been too much influenced by ideas of evaluation as being equivalent to *program* evaluation and have given insufficient attention to evaluation of direct practice and service delivery. We have developed this argument in a deliberately practical way through a series of examples:

- Evaluability assessment
- Purpose-led choice of qualitative methods
- Understanding how social policies work in direct care settings, through the application of case study designs
- Qualitative methods for evaluating programs in ways that widen conventional assumptions regarding outcome program evaluation
- Qualitative evaluation of direct practice
- Action research

References

Atkinson, P. & Delamont, S. (1993). Bread and dreams or bread and circuses? A critique of case study research in evaluation. In M. Hammersley (Ed.), *Controversies in the classroom*. Buckingham: Open University Press.

Bogdan, R., & Taylor, S. (1994). A positive approach to qualitative evaluation and policy research in social work. In E. Sherman & W. Reid (Eds.), *Qualitative research in social work*. New York: Columbia University Press.

Bowen, D. (1993). The delights of learning to apply the life history method to school non-attenders. In B. Broad & C. Fletcher (Eds.), *Practitioner social work research in action*. London: Whiting and Birch.

Burgess, R., Pole, C., Evans, K., & Priestley, C. (1994). Four studies from one or one study from four? Multi-site case study research. In A. Bryman & R. Burgess (Eds.), *Analysing qualitative data*. London: Routledge.

Campbell, D. (1978). Qualitative knowing in action research. In M. Brenner & P. Marsh (Eds.), *The social context of methods*. London: Croom Helm.

Campbell, D. (1979). Degrees of freedom and the case study. In T. Cook & C. Reichardt (Eds.), *Qualitative and quantitative methods in evaluation research*. Beverly Hills, CA: Sage.

Clapham, D., Means, R., & Munro, M. (1993). Housing, the life course and older people. In S. Arber & M. Evandrou (Eds.), *Ageing, independence and the life course*. London: Jessica Kingsley.

Cohler, B. (1994). The human services, the life story, and clinical research. In E. Sherman & W. Reid (Eds.), *Qualitative research in social work*. New York: Columbia University Press.

Cronbach, L., Ambron, S., Dornbusch, S., Hess, R., Hornik, R., Phillips, D., et al. (1980). *Toward reform of program evaluation*. San Francisco: Jossey-Bass.

Finch, J. (1985). Social policy and education: Problems and possibilities of using qualitative research. In R. Burgess (Ed.), *Issues in educational research: Qualitative methods*. London: Falmer.

Finch, J. (1986). *Research and policy: The uses of qualitative methods in social and educational research*. London: Falmer.

Fook, J. (2000). Reflexivity as method. In J. Daly & A. Kellehear (Eds.), *Annual review of health social sciences*. Bundoora, Australia: Palliative Care Unit, La Trobe University.

Greene, J. (1994). Qualitative program evaluation: Practice and promise. In N. Denzin & Y. Lincoln (Eds.), *Handbook of qualitative research*. Thousand Oaks, CA: Sage.

Gould, N. (1996). Introduction: Social work and the crisis of the professions. In N. Gould. & I. Taylor (Eds.), *Reflective learning for social work*. Aldershot, England: Arena.

Gould, N. (1999). Qualitative practice evaluation. In I. Shaw & J. Lishman (Eds.), *Evaluation and social work practice*. London: Sage.

Gould, N., & Taylor, I. (Eds.). (1996). *Reflective learning for social work*. Aldershot, England: Arena.

Hammersley, M. (1992). *What's wrong with ethnography?* London: Routledge.

Jarvis, P. (1999). *The practitioner–researcher*. San Francisco: Jossey-Bass.

Martin, M. (1994). Developing a feminist participative research framework. In B. Humphries & C. Truman (Eds.), *Rethinking social research: Antidiscriminatory approaches in research methodology*. Aldershot, England: Avebury.

McKeganey, N., MacPherson, I., & Hunter, D. (1988). How "they" decide: Exploring professional decision making. *Research, Policy and Planning*, 6(1), 15–19.

Miles, M., & Huberman, A. (1994). *Qualitative data analysis: An expanded sourcebook*. Thousand Oaks, CA: Sage.

Morgan, D. (1985). *The family: Politics and social theory.* London: Routledge.

Patton, M. Q. (2002). *Qualitative research and evaluation methods.* Thousand Oaks, CA: Sage.

Pulice, R. (1994). Qualitative evaluation methods in the public sector: Understanding and working with constituency groups in the evaluation process. In E. Sherman & W. Reid (Eds.), *Qualitative research in social work.* New York: Columbia University Press.

Rodwell, M., & Woody, D. (1994). Constructivist evaluation: The policy/practice context. In E. Sherman & W. Reid (Eds.), *Qualitative research in social work.* New York: Columbia University Press.

Schon, D. (1983). *The reflective practitioner: How professionals think in action.* New York: Basic Books.

Shaw, I. (1999). *Qualitative evaluation.* London: Sage.

Shaw, I. (2003). Qualitative research and outcomes in health, social work and education. *Qualitative Research, 3*(1), 25–44.

Stake, R. (1995). *The art of case study research.* Thousand Oaks, CA: Sage.

Stake, R. (1997). Advocacy in evaluation: A necessary evil? In E. Chelimsky & W. Shadish (Eds.), *Evaluation for the 21st century.* Thousand Oaks, CA: Sage.

Turner, M., & Zimmerman, W. (1994). Acting for the sake of research. In J. Wholey, H. Hatry, & K. Newcomer (Eds.), *Handbook of practical program evaluation.* San Francisco: Jossey-Bass.

Wasoff, F., & Dobash, R. (1992). Simulated clients in "natural" settings: Constructing a client to study professional practice. *Sociology, 26*(2), 333–349.

Wasoff, F., & Dobash, R. (1996). *The simulated client: A method for studying professionals working with clients.* Aldershot, England: Avebury.

Whitmore, E. (1990). Empowerment in program evaluation: A case example. *Canadian Social Work Review, 7*(2), 215–229.

Whitmore, E. (1994). To tell the truth: Working with oppressed groups in participatory approaches to inquiry. In P. Reason (Ed.), *Participation in human inquiry.* London: Sage.

Wholey, J. (1994). Assessing the feasibility and likely usefulness of evaluation. In J. Wholey, H. Hatry, & K. Newcomer (Eds.), *Handbook of practical program evaluation.* San Francisco: Jossey-Bass.

Williams, D. D. (1986). When is naturalistic evaluation appropriate? In D. D. Williams (Ed.), *Naturalistic evaluation.* New Directions in Program Evaluation, No. 30, San Francisco: Jossey-Bass.

Yin, R. K. (1994). *Case study research.* Thousand Oaks, CA: Sage.

76

QUALITATIVE RESEARCH WITH BATTERED WOMEN

A Continuum Based on 501 Cases

Albert R. Roberts

This study developed a new classificatory schemata for chronicity in battered women. It was developed from the narratives of 501 battered women. The goal was to describe different types of battering relationships, psychosocial characteristics of the victim and abuser, and the duration of abuse in order to enhance our understanding of the ways in which battering relationships occur and endure.

SCOPE OF THE PROBLEM

Violence among current and former intimate partners is pervasive in American society. Every year an estimated 8.7 million women are abused by their partners (Roberts, 1998; Roberts, 2002). Two national studies have provided methodologically rigorous estimates of the prevalence of woman-battering. Tjaden and Thoennes (2000) said that 25% of their female respondents reported some form of violence. Straus and Gelles (1991) estimated that approximately 16 percent of American couples had encountered family violence incidents. Each year, for the past 20 years approximately 1.5 to 2 million women have needed emergency medical attention as a result of domestic violence (Roberts, 1998; Straus, 1986). Annual estimates indicate that approximately, 2,000 battered women are killed by their abusive partners, and the majority of these homicides take place after the victim has tried to leave, separate from, or divorce their batterer. In addition, 750 chronically battered women have killed their mates each year as a result of explicit terroristic or death threats, post-traumatic stress disorder (PTSD), and/or recurring nightmares or intrusive thoughts of their own death at the hands of the batterer (Roberts, 1998).

The aftermath of domestic violence assaults has a destructive impact upon the battered woman and her children (Stark and Flitcraft, 1988; Carlson, 1996). There are high rates of medical problems, mental disorders, miscarriages, abortions, alcohol and drug abuse, increased risks of rape, and suicide attempts. Each year more than 10 million children witness woman battering in the privacy of their own homes. The impact of growing up in a violent home often results in an intergenerational cycle of violence.

Typologies

Typologies and continua can provide a useful tool for identifying and assessing violence risk among battered women. The major advantage of continua and other assessment tools is that they provide clinicians with diagnostic indicators so that they can intervene before violence escalates

and hopefully prevent permanent injuries and death.

The continuum of the duration of woman battering ranges from short-term (e.g., one to three incidents over a 6-month period) to chronic (e.g., 20 years); severity ranges from less severe violence such as a push, slap, or punch to the very severe acts such as choking, blows to the head, specific death threats, and attempted murder. This chapter documents the duration, severity, and lethality of woman battering within each of five levels, in the words and experiences of the interviewees. Some of the victims had observed their mother being battered on and off for many years. In general, these women blamed themselves and accepted the violence by their partner as part of marriage or a cohabiting relationship. In other cases, the women refused to stay with a partner who was assaulting them, and they ended the relationship shortly after the violence began.

METHODOLOGY

The study sample came from four sources: There were 501 battered women in the sample.

1. Battered women who have killed their partners were found at a large state women's prison in the northeastern part of the United States ($N = 105$).
2. Three suburban New Jersey police departments ($N = 105$).
3. Three battered women's shelters in New Jersey ($N = 105$).
4. A convenience subsample of 186 formerly abused women was drawn by inviting 30 graduate students in two sections of my MSW Family Violence course, and 15 criminal justice honor students to locate and interview 1 to 3 friends, neighbors, or relatives who have been battered during the past 4 years.

The final sample included women from different income levels and educational and racial backgrounds.

All of the interviewers were college seniors or graduate students. Each interviewer received 30 hours of training on interviewing skills and qualitative research on woman battering. The training included role playing and practice interviews. The woman battering questionnaire was prepared, pretested, and modified. It consisted of a 39-page standardized interview schedule to guide the interviews.

The first 210 interviews were conducted by the author and seven student interviewers. In general, the depth and patterns of information collected in these interviews seemed to be of high quality. The second phase consisting of approximately 300 additional interviews were based on a police department sample, a shelter sample, and a modified snowball sample of formerly abused women conducted by my graduate students. These interviews also included detailed information and in-depth responses.

FINDINGS

In this study, the 501 battered women had three experiences in common: they had experienced one or more incidents of physical battering by their partners; they had experienced jealous rages, insults and emotional abuse; and over one-fifth of the victims received terroristic and/ or death threats from their abusive partner. Some of the women were hit a few times and left the batterer permanently. Others were assaulted intermittently over a period of several months to 2 years before leaving the batterer and filing for divorce. The majority of the women endured chronic abuse for many years before permanently ending the relationship (Roberts, 2002). The extent and degree of chronicity of battering is plotted on a continuum of woman battering among the 501 cases.

Table 76.1 describes a woman battering continuum based on five levels. The definition of each level is selective and limited to the data obtained from this New Jersey statewide sample of battered women in prison, shelters, police departments, and the community.

Continuum

Level 1+, Short-Term Victims

The nature and level of physical abuse experienced by short-term abused women was determined from interviews with 94 battered women who reported experiencing one to three misdemeanor abusive incidents by their boyfriend or partner. Most of the victims were high school or college students in a steady dating relationship. The overwhelming majority of the women were not living with the abuser. The abusive acts could usually be classified in the mild to moderate range of severity, e.g., pushing, slapping, and punching with no broken bones or permanent injuries. Most of these women were between 16 and 25 years of age and ended the relationship with the help of a parent or older brother. Short-term victims generally call the police or their parents and ask for help. Most of the women in this level were middle class.

Level 2+, Intermediate

The level and duration of battering of women in this category ranged from 3 to 15 incidents over a period of several months to 2 years. The 104 battered women in this category were usually living with the abuser in either a cohabiting or marital relationship. None of the women in this level had children. The women ended the relationship with the help of the police, a family member, or a friend after a severe battering incident. Many of the women had sustained severe injuries such as a broken jaw, stitches, broken ribs, and/or a concussion. These women often obtained a restraining order and moved out to a safer residence. Most of the women in this level were middle class.

Level 3+, Intermittent/Long-Term

The intensity of each incident is usually severe, and the duration of battering is 5 to 40 years. Most women in this category are economically and socially dependent upon their husbands. In addition, they are often religious and would not divorce for that reason. They are nurturing and caring mothers and want to keep the family together for the sake of the children. There may be no physical violence for several months, and then because of pressures (e.g., at his job) the husband vents his anger and frustration at his wife by beating her. Most of these 38 women are middle or upper class and rarely go to the hospital. When they go to their family physician for treatment, they have an excuse for the causation of the injury (e.g., accident-prone).

Level 4+, Chronic and Severe with a Regular Pattern

The duration of battering was 5 to 35 years, with the intensity of the violence increasing over the

TABLE 76.1 Duration and Severity Level of Woman-Battering Continuum

1+	2+	3+	4+	5+
Short-term (N = 94)	Intermediate (N = 104)	Intermittent long-term (N = 38)	Chronic and predictable (N = 160)	Homicidal (N = 105)
Less than 1 year (dating relationship); mild to moderate intensity	Several months to 2 years (cohabiting or married); moderate to severe injuries	Severe and intense violent episode without warning; long periods without violence, then another violent episode; married with children	Severe repetitive incidents; frequent, predictable pattern; violence often precipitated by alcohol or polydrug abuse; married with children	Violence escalates to homicide, murder precipitated by explicit death threats and life-threatening injuries (cohabiting or married)
1–3 incidents	3–15 incidents	4–30 incidents	Usually several hundred violent acts per woman	Numerous violent and severe acts per woman
Usually middle-class and steady dating relationship (severity, e.g., push, shove, and sometimes severe beating; woman leaves after first or second physically abusive act; caring support system, e.g., parents or police)	Usually middle-class and recently married or living together (severity, e.g., punch, kick, chokehold, or severe beating; woman leaves due to bruises or injury; caring support system, e.g., new boyfriend or parents)	Usually upper-middle or upper social class, staying together for children or status/prestige of wealthy husband (woman stays until children grow up and leave home; no alternative support system)	Usually lower socioeconomic or middle-class, often devout Catholic with school-age children at home (abuse continues until husband is arrested, is hospitalized, or dies; husband is blue-collar, skilled, or semiskilled)	Usually lower socioeconomic class, high long-term unemployment, limited education (majority of battered women; suffers from PTSD and BWS)

Copyright (2001): Albert R. Roberts, reprinted by permission.

years. The 160 battered women who comprised this category all reported a discernable pattern of abuse during the recent past (e.g., every weekend, every other weekend, every Friday night, etc.). Many of the batterers (68%) had serious drinking problems including binge drinking, drunkenness, and blackouts. However, about three-fourths battered their partners when they were sober. After many years, especially when the children are grown and out of the house, the battering becomes more extreme, more predictable, and includes the use of weapons, forced sex, and generalized death threats. The injuries for these victims are extensive and include sprains, fractures, broken bones, stitches, head injuries, etc., that require treatment in the hospital emergency room.

Level 4.5, Subset of Chronic with a Discernable Pattern—Mutual Combat

Twenty-four of the 160 *level 4* cases fit the mutual combat category. This mutual combat and chronic category sometimes led to dual arrests, and at other times the police arrested the partner who appeared to have the lesser injuries. The level of violence was usually severe, and the duration of woman battering in this category lasted from 1 to 25 years. The study identified two types of mutual combat. In the first type, the man initiated a violent act such as punching the woman and she retaliated (e.g., slapping or punching him back). He then retaliated more violently by beating her severely. In the second type of mutual combat, the woman retaliates for physical or emotional abuse and uses a weapon (typically a knife) to get back at him. The ten battered women in this category either had a chronic alcohol or drug problem or a history of violent aggressive acts in adolescence (e.g., cutting another girl, boy, or adult with a knife). In 14 of the 24 cases, both the abusive male and the female had a drug problem. Generally, there were severe injuries to one or both parties. Most of the women in this level were lower class. Many of these couples separated after a few years.

Level 5+, Homicidal

The duration of the battering relationship in this category is generally 8 years or longer, although the range is two years to 35 years. The majority of these women are usually in a common law relationship (cohabiting for seven years or longer), in a marital relationship, or recently divorced. The overwhelming majority (59.2%) of these women lacked a high school education and the skills to earn a decent income on their own (Roberts, 1996). Almost half (47.6%) of the homicidal battered women had been on public assistance for many years during the battering episodes.

The 105 women in this category began at Level 2 and usually escalated to either Level 4 or Level 5 for several years, after which the death threats became more explicit and lethal. Also, in a number of cases, the victim had finally left the abuser and obtained a restraining order, which he violated. Most of the women in this category suffered from post-traumatic stress disorder (PTSD) and some had attempted suicide. The most significant finding related to the homicidal battered women is that the overwhelming majority (65.7%) of the women received specific lethal death threats in which the batterer specified the method, time, and/or location of their demise (Roberts, 1996, p. 41).

SHORT-TERM ABUSE EXAMPLES

Most of the victims who were abused for several months were in a steady dating relationship as illustrated with Angela, victim of a relatively short-term abusive relationship. She was an 18-year-old high school senior, from a middle-class family, when her boyfriend started abusing her. Her career goal was to go to college and graduate

school and become a psychologist. The abuse started after going steady for 3 months. Her boyfriend was very controlling; he did not want her to have any self-confidence. During the 6 months of abuse before Angela broke up with her boyfriend, most of the abuse consisted of his pushing, shoving, slapping her, and forcing her to have sexual intercourse. She got pregnant and when she told her boyfriend about the pregnancy, he punched her in the stomach so hard that she lost the baby. The next week he was very apologetic and he tried to force her to have oral sex. She was upset about the miscarriage: "I tried to leave and started screaming at him. He hit me in the back with a golf club until my spine went into a spasm and I passed out." She was taken to the hospital, and her parents refused to let her see him again (Roberts, 2002).

INTERMEDIATE ABUSE

Most of the 104 battered women at the intermediate level were battered for less than 2 years. There were no warning signs prior to each abusive incident. There was no pattern with regard to the intervals between each incident. The overwhelming majority of the women in this category were college educated and deeply in love with their partners. Most of these victims left the batterer right after the abuse escalated to one final violent attack, as illustrated in the case example of Josephine. When her husband broke her jaw she realized that her life was in danger and he did not love her anymore.

Josephine came from a family that enjoyed spending a lot of time together and found it important to remain close. She attended college and then later graduate school, where she received her masters in counseling. While she was in graduate school she got engaged. The night of her engagement was the first night her fiancé abused her, but she ignored the abuse and blamed it on her own provocation and figured it would not occur again. However, after they married, the abuse escalated. Not only did she frequently receive bruises all over her body, but she was verbally abused. Although at the time Josephine was learning about woman battering in graduate school, she chose to ignore the abuse and deny it was actually happening to her. It wasn't until 1 year later, when her husband broke her jaw, that she decided to leave and get help. She never received emergency treatment for her jaw, but she called Women's Space and went to a private counselor. She went to Women's Space for approximately 3 months and her sessions with the private counselor finished in December of 1994. Josephine admits she denied the abuse because she wanted her marriage to work. She often wonders and cannot believe how naive she was, considering she had taken several courses in school of woman battering. Today, she still has problems with her jaw because of the lack of emergency care. Nevertheless, she feels her life has gotten back together and is in a new relationship and was married in January 1996. In her new relationship they went for premarital counseling. She feels it was very important to find out if they were good for each other. She believes that many problems could have been avoided if she would have done it the first time.

INTERMITTENT/LONG-TERM

The battered women in this category are usually married with several children. Most neighbors and the community rarely know about the violent abuse these women endure over the years. The violent assaults come without warning and can rarely be prevented. Since most of the batterers are successful wage earners, charming from time-to-time, and kind to their children, the battered women become traumatically bonded to them. These women are highly dependent, very materialistic and status seeking, and/or totally focused on caring for their children and keeping the family together despite the costs to their self-esteem and mental health.

Arlene is a 39-year-old woman with three children. She was a debutante who earned her bachelor's degree from Radcliffe. She came from a very wealthy New York family. Her mother was a socialite and her father was a chief executive officer of a Fortune 100 company. She married immediately after graduating from college without having had a job. She was aware that for 27 years her father had intermittently abused her mother. Her mother was never hospitalized, but was occasionally treated by the family physician. She thought her mother deserved to be abused because she had done something wrong. The first incident occurred on Arlene's honeymoon, and she felt that she deserved it. She has been intermittently abused for the past 17 years. In describing the violent

episodes, she describes periods of traumatic violence and periods of calm. Sometimes 6 to 9 months would go by between incidents. During those periods she wanted to believe that it would never happen again. She doesn't feel her husband will kill her because he only put her in the hospital twice. She plans to remain in the relationship for the sake of her children and because she enjoys her social prominence, which she feels would be compromised with a divorce because there would be such a bitter legal battle (Roberts, 2002).

CHRONIC AND SEVERE ABUSE WITH A REGULAR PATTERN

The women that are grouped in this category have been abused for years. The abuse escalates until it occurs either weekly or several days a week. These women are highly dependent, both emotionally and economically on the batterer. They have low self-esteem and often have an alcohol or drug problem. In many cases, the abuse ends only after the victim receives some type of "jolt" that causes her to leave the relationship, such as severe medical injuries to herself or the children, or the husband is hospitalized for alcoholism or polydrug abuse, or hearing about other battered women who were killed.

Naomi is a 34-year-old single parent who was chronically abused by her husband for 7 years. She is a high school graduate and has worked for the same company for the past 14 years as a customer service representative. Her father was an abuser. She described her injuries as follows:

Broken nose, he's tried to choke me so many times I feel that when I get older I will have cancer of the throat. I have bruises all over my body. I have a bad back and on three different occasions my eye has been swollen from his punches. He likes to punch me in the mouth. He does it without warning. The last time he strangled me in the kitchen I faked passing out, and he left. He might have killed me if I didn't fake passing out.

Naomi finally left her husband after attending a support group for battered women. In her own words: "I sat there and listened to their stories. It made me feel helpless because some women were battered for 25 years. I felt I was taking on their problems instead of helping myself. I decided I had to leave him. I went to the court and got a restraining order."

MUTUAL COMBAT SUBCATEGORY OF CHRONIC BATTERING

Most of the women involved in mutual combat exhibited violent behavior during adolescence. These women often grew up in low income single-parent families with a parent or siblings who had criminal histories. Their proneness to violence was influenced by the heavy stress of being a teen mom, unemployed and on welfare, and growing up in a drug subculture. Almost half of these 24 violent women had a criminal record for drug dealing and prostitution. The women reported that they often got involved in drugs to help their abusive partners. The case illustration of Lynn reveals the negative influence of a violent environment and neighborhood.

Lynn grew up fast and learned about violence and death at age 13. The critical incident during early adolescence that had a major impact on her life was the death of her father for whom she cared deeply. Lynn described this major loss, long delayed grief, repressed anger and rage, teen pregnancy at 16 and violence. "My father was stabbed. . . . I would have let everyone down."

Many of the women in the mutual combat category exhibited violence and acting-out behavior in early adolescence. In the words of Lynn:

My father was stabbed when I was 13. He was being robbed. My pop was my pride and joy. I come from a family of 10 and I'm the second oldest. I had a lot of responsibility. I'm my father's only child so I grieved alone—he did everything for me and when he was gone I really missed him. I had to grow up real fast and alone because I was so close to him. But no one should have helped me then. I had to deal with it myself. After all the pain's inside so no one can make it feel better. When I lost my dad I became cold to the world, and never cried about it. All the anger built up inside me, and once I heard these girls coming into my ex-boyfriend's apartment, and the first one that came inside I stabbed the shit out of her. I stabbed her 14 times. But no one found out it was me. I kept it to myself like I do everything else in life. People on the streets, they all know me as a bad ass. I couldn't cry when my dad died. I would have let everyone down.

For the past 10 years, Lynn and her husband were involved in mutual combat. She described her recollection of the violent incidents and the events which seemed to precipitate the violence:

He'd bring drugs in the house and tell me that he was the King, and I better suck his big black dick, swallow him. I'd say no way, he'd say my clothes will be off in 10 seconds. He'd drop his pants, and I'd pull my knife, then he would start punching me. . . . he knows I would then cut him.

Lynn described the last battering incident as the worst: "I think he had the same injuries. I filled out the papers and got a restraining order."

Lynn's future goals related to woman battering are as follows:

I don't think I am even gonna get away from him. Three years from now I'll still be fighting for my life. In 10 years I will still be fighting, if I'm not dead by then. I mean he'll never let me alone. He'll haunt me for the rest of my life.

HOMICIDAL BATTERED WOMEN

The battered women who kill their violent partner in self-defense usually have a low level of education and have witnessed their mother being battered throughout their childhood. The intergenerational cycle of violence continues since these women often cohabit or marry young to escape from a dysfunctional and abusive home. They often are teen moms with alcohol and substance abuse problems.

Maribell grew up in a home where her parents were always fighting. She got married at 18 and left home. Her husband had an alcohol and drug problem. The abuse got worse after she got pregnant.

Critical incidents during childhood:

My mother and father fighting. Always big fights and the police or ambulance would come. A few times a month over just normal things. Usually the neighbors called the police. It was usually physical and verbal. I tried to forget most of it so I can't remember one particular incident. We never talked about it.

Reasons for abuse:

The dinner burnt, or I talked to a guy. I couldn't look at a man while I was talking. It would happen over anything. I don't remember the exact details of the incident. A guy came over visit my brother, and Ron called me to the door and said someone is here to see you and the guy said he was looking for my brother. The guy left and we started arguing and fighting over it. He was drinking that day. Verbal argument to begin with. I can't remember if it got physical. I guess it did. I told him to get out and he wouldn't. Somehow or another I picked up a knife and he kept coming towards me and I hit him with the knife. I remember doing it once but the police report said 3 times. I thought it was his shoulder but it was further down. A kitchen knife. He fell to the floor and there was blood all over. I tried to stop the bleeding and he was talking to me. So then I grabbed the phone and I couldn't dial. I ran to a neighbor to get help and they called the police. The police came and we waited for an ambulance. Then they arrested me. He went to the hospital and I went to the police station and gave a statement and tried to protect him. I don't know why. I knew when he got out I'd be in worse trouble than I was at the police station. Can't remember what I told them. Throw out the plea bargain, that's what they kept telling me. My statement for 2 years, I tried to remember it and I can't.

Charged me with murder one and weapons charge (knife).

Dropped all of it and charged me with aggravated manslaughter. I took a plea bargain for 20 years flat sentence. They offered me 30 with 10 stip while I was on bail. My lawyer told me to take the 20 flat. Served 2 years already. June 1994. First parole hearing.

He died that day.

The police came immediately. The one police officer was nice 'cause they knew us, my mother. The person I gave the statement to wasn't very nice.

CONCLUSION

The prediction of both the duration and severity of woman battering are among the most complex issues in forensic risk assessment and the social sciences. Nevertheless, the courts, mental health centers, family counseling centers, intensive outpatient clinics, day treatment and residential programs, public mental hospitals, and private psychiatric facilities rely on clinicians to advise judges in civil commitment and criminal court cases. This chapter provides a new framework or continuum for evaluating battered women and improving risk assessments of dangerousness. The author's study of the duration and chronicity of battering can be used to facilitate court decisions on whether or not battered

women are at low, moderate, or high risk of continued battering and/or homicide.

All assessment continua or typologies should start with an evaluation of the harm and injury of the victim, duration and chronicity of violent events, and the likelihood of the victim escaping and ending the battering cycle. The continuum conceptualized in this chapter provides a classificatory schema by which forensic specialists and clinicians can make reasonably clear predictions of lethality and a likely repeat of the violence. The short-term and intermediate types seem to be amenable to crisis intervention, brief psychotherapy, support groups, restraining orders, and a relatively brief period of recovery. The prognosis for the chronic/long-term category, whether it be intermittent or a weekly pattern of battering, is much more negative. The chronic recidivist cases are frequently put into a life-threatening situation. However, when there are specific death threats and a loaded handgun in the house, the short-term and intermediate battering cases can also escalate to a code blue—life and death situation. In chronic cases, the human suffering, degradation, and emotional and physical pain sometimes ends in permanent injuries to the victim, or the death of the batterer or the battered woman. At other times, the chronically battered woman temporarily escapes to a shelter, a relative's home, or the police precinct. In many of the latter cases, the victim returns to the batterer or is dragged back to the violent home. Finally, a small but growing number of chronically battered women leave the batterer and stay free of violence because they are empowered through a support group and counseling or other forms of therapeutic intervention.

It is important for health care and mental health professionals and criminal justice practitioners to document the duration and intensity of battering histories among clients in order to provide the best possible care and effective intervention strategies.

References

Astin, M. C., Lawrence, K. J., & Foy, D. W. (1993). Risk and resiliency factors among battered women. *Violence and Victims, 8,* 17–28.

Browne, A. (1987). *When battered women kill.* New York: Free Press.

Carlson, B. E. (1996). Children of battered women: Research, programs and services. In A. R. Roberts (Ed.), *Helping battered women: New per-*

spectives and remedies (pp. 172–187). New York: Oxford University Press.

Cascardi, M., O'Leary, D., Schlee, A., & Lawrence, E. (1993). *Prevalence and correlates of PTSD in abused women.* Paper presented at the twenty-seventh annual conference of the Association for the Advancement of Behavior Therapy, Atlanta.

Federal Bureau of Investigation. (1992). *Crime in the U.S.: 1991.* Washington, DC: U.S. Government Printing Office.

Roberts, A. R. (1996). *Helping battered women: New perspectives and remedies.* New York: Oxford University Press.

Roberts, A. R. (1998). *Battered women and their families: Intervention strategies and treatment approaches* (2nd ed.). New York: Springer.

Roberts, A. R. (Ed.). (2002). *Handbook of domestic violence intervention strategies.* New York: Oxford University Press.

Stark, E., & Flitcraft, A. (1988). Violence among intimates: An epidemiological review. In V. B.

Van Hasselt, R. L. Morrison, A. S. Bellack, & M. Hersen (Eds.), *Handbook of Family Violence* (pp. 293–317). New York: Plenum.

Straus, M. A. (1986). Medical care costs of intrafamily assault and homicide. *Bulletin of New York Academy of Medicine, 6*(5), 556–561.

Straus, M. A., & Gelles, R. J. (1991). How violent are American families: Estimates from the National Family Violence Resurvey and other studies. In M. Straus & R. Gelles (Eds.), *Physical violence in American families: Risk factors and adaptations in 8,145 families* (pp. 95–112). New Brunswick, NJ: Transaction Publishers.

Tjaden, P., & Thoennes, N. (2000). *Extent, nature, and consequences of intimate partner violence: Findings from the national violence against women survey.* Washington, DC: National Institute of Justice, U.S. Department of Justice.

Walker, L. A. (1984). *Battered women syndrome.* New York: Springer.

USING QUALITATIVE RESEARCH TO ENHANCE PRACTICE

77

The Example of Breast Cancer in African American Women

Julianne S. Oktay & Eunice Y. Park-Lee

There has been a recurrent emphasis on the importance of utilizing research results to improve practice in social work and other health professions (Rosen, 1994; Rosen, 1996; Rosen, Proctor, & Staudt, 1999). However, advocates for a closer connection between research and practice tend to equate *research* with *quantitative research*, and the potential of qualitative research to improve practice has received little attention. This chapter discusses several ways that qualitative research can contribute to improved practice, using the example of breast cancer in African American women as an illustration. Specifically, qualitative studies are especially valuable in helping practitioners gain an in-depth understanding of new populations and new problems, design new interventions, and evaluate what is going on in existing programs.

The latest trend in practice research, evidence-based practice (EBP), grows out of a concern that professionals rely too heavily on practice wisdom, anecdotal experience, or authority in making clinical decisions (Rosen, 1994). As a result, clients or patients do not always get the most effective treatment available. Developed in the field of medicine, EBP encourages practitioners to define a specific population (subpopulation) with a specific problem and to identify a specific intervention (Sackett, Richardson, Rosenberg, & Haynes, 1997). Then they are expected to review well-designed research studies on this intervention with this subpopulation (Cochrane Library, 2003) and to consider this evidence as practice decisions are made (Gibbs & Gambrill, 2002). EBP is being rapidly accepted as the standard of practice in social work (Cournoyer & Powers, 2002), and educators are beginning to incorporate it into graduate programs in social work (Howard, McMillen, & Pollio, 2003)

The EBP model of practice may inadvertently overlook qualitative studies relevant to practice, because EBP is based on the assumption that certain research designs produce more trustworthy results than others, experimental design being the gold standard. In a health or mental health setting, this generally means that an intervention (e.g., a particular treatment) is given to a randomly chosen population with specified characteristics. Outcomes are defined in advance (e.g., decrease in symptoms of disease, or increase in desirable behavior), and quantifiable measures are identified for each of the desired outcomes. The results of these studies can be summarized, compared, and interpreted by practitioners. As a result, experimental studies are ideal for practitioners who use the EBP model. However, to enhance practice, it is important that practitioners seek qualitative as well as quantitative research.

To understand how qualitative research can contribute to clinical practice, some description of qualitative research is needed. Qualitative research is done in natural settings, using the words and behaviors of people as data (Erlandson, Harris, Skipper, & Allen, 1993). Research questions are broad and often descriptive rather than specific and causal (Maxwell, 1996). In qualitative research, the goal is to provide an insider perspective (Fetterman, 1998). Because the focus is on the perspective of the patient or client, hypotheses and research variables are not defined in advance by the researcher. Qualitative researchers use open, unstructured interviews and participant observation instead of the structured instruments and fixed choices employed in quantitative research. The results of qualitative research may be very detailed descriptions of settings, programs, or populations (for examples, see Faidman, 1997; Liebow, 1993; Meyerhoff, 1978). Because the insider (emic) perspective is studied, the exact nature of the research question or the population may change as the study progresses (Maxwell, 1996). It is difficult to use qualitative research findings in the EBP model, because the results of qualitative research cannot be easily summarized or compared with those of other studies. Why, then, is there a need for qualitative studies in practice research?

First, the classic theories that underlie most clinical practice, such as those of Freud, Erikson, and Piaget, were based on qualitative data (Reissman, 1994). Also, there is a strong similarity between the methods of qualitative research and those of clinical practice (Gilgun, 1994). Qualitative research is especially valuable when practice involves new problems, new populations, new interventions, or all of these. One characteristic of health and mental health fields such as social work is that these fields change rapidly. New populations with new problems constantly develop as society changes. Today's clinicians work with populations that were unknown to earlier generations. Some examples would be immigrant populations from Asia (e.g., Hmong, Korean), Central America, and Eastern Europe; individuals with diagnoses that are new (e.g., dual diagnosis, post-traumatic stress disorder); the very old (85 or older) and their families; clients suffering from the effects of terrorism; and adults who survived cancer as children. Social work, for example, is a very fluid field that is justifiably proud of its historical ability to react to new problems as they arise, designing new services as they are needed.

In rapidly changing fields, practitioners need to learn about new populations, new problems and new services, long before evidence on the effectiveness of specific interventions (as required by the EBP model) becomes available.

However, qualitative research is well suited to areas about which little is known. Good qualitative studies tend to ask questions that can be answered by providing description (asking what happened in terms of observable events), interpretation (asking about the meaning of these things for the people involved), or theory (asking how these effects can be explained) (Maxwell, 1996). In addition, qualitative research can provide intricate details about phenomena such as feelings, thought processes, and emotions that are difficult to learn about through more conventional, quantitative research (Strauss & Corbin, 1998). This research has the potential to improve social work practice by increasing practitioners' understanding of clients and families in new areas of practice (Oktay, 2003; Oktay & Walter, 1991). It can increase sensitivity to the cultural context the client brings to the clinical encounter. It also has the potential to provide in-depth understanding of complex settings, such as the organizational context of the clinical encounter.

A second situation in which traditional, quantitative, outcome-based research is of little help to practitioners occurs when the literature review shows that a commonly used intervention does not in fact achieve the expected results. This, too, is an area in which qualitative research can be of value. Qualitative research is good at describing an intervention in detail, from the perspective of the insiders—clients or workers. It can also be used to help practitioners understand what is actually going on when an intervention is applied—which is not always what the developers of the intervention or the policy intended. Padgett (1998), for example, suggests that "qualitative methods excel when used to explore the inner workings of the black box—the process dimension of program evaluation. They complement the quantitative findings by providing more in-depth understanding of how the experimental intervention succeeded (or failed)" (p. 9).

This chapter illustrates several ways that qualitative research can contribute to improved practice, using the example of breast cancer in African American women as an illustration. Qualitative research studies in this field illustrate how practitioners can use qualitative studies to (a) understand the beliefs and knowledge of minority populations, (b) design culturally sensitive interventions, and (c) evaluate the implementation of these interventions.

BACKGROUND

In spite of many advances in early detection and treatment, large numbers of American women (212,000) are diagnosed with breast cancer each year, and about 38,000 die of the disease (American Cancer Society, 2003). One factor that determines whether or not a woman survives is the stage of the cancer at the time it is diagnosed. Women whose disease is detected in an early stage (in situ, Stage 1, or Stage 2) have a much better survival rate than do women whose cancer is detected in the later stages. One disturbing finding related to breast cancer statistics is that although African American women are less likely than white women to develop breast cancer, they are more likely to die from the disease (American Cancer Society, 2003). The most important reason for this difference is that African American women are more likely to be in advanced stages of breast cancer at diagnosis (Douglas, Bartolucci, Waterbor, & Sirles, 1995; Eley et al., 1994).

Because of this, practitioners have been encouraged to develop interventions that will increase breast cancer screening among African American women. Of the three primary methods of detection of breast cancer (mammography, clinical breast exam, and breast self-exam), mammography is the most highly recommended because it can detect a cancer when the tumor is much too small to be felt in a breast exam. Therefore, much effort has been focused on increasing mammography use by African American women.

Factors known to influence participation in mammography programs, including mammogram cost, insurance coverage, and physician's recommendations for breast cancer screening (Blustein, 1995; O'Malley, Earp, & Harris, 1997; Urban, Anderson, & Peacock, 1994), were targeted in early programs aimed at African American women. For example, the New Hanover Breast Cancer Screening Program (funded by the National Cancer Institute) attempted to reduce barriers to breast cancer screening (Fletcher et al., 1993) by coordinating media campaigns and social events and by providing low-cost mammography and free clinical breast exams. Unfortunately, evaluation of these programs showed that mammography use increased only in the white women, so that after the interventions, the racial gap in mammography use actually widened (from 11% to 17%).

These early failures suggested that a better understanding of the cultural beliefs and knowledge about breast cancer in African American women was needed (Lannin, Mathews, Mitchell, & Swanson, 2002; Lannin et al., 1998; Tessaro, Eng, & Smith, 1994). Qualitative research was ideal for this situation because of its emphasis on the insider perspective and its strength in describing culture. The following section illustrates how qualitative research methods helped practitioners gain a better understanding of the way African American women perceive and respond to the threat of breast cancer.

AFRICAN AMERICAN BELIEFS AND KNOWLEDGE ABOUT BREAST CANCER

Three studies illustrate how qualitative research contributed to effective practice in reducing breast cancer mortality in African American women. Tessaro and colleagues (1994) began their study by recruiting community residents to help the researchers develop a conceptual framework. Next, they conducted focus group interviews with 132 members from 14 social networks of older African American women. The focus group participants included female members of churches, participants at senior citizens centers, health care providers, and sons and husbands of older African American women in the community. Another example is a study by Mathews, Lannin, and Mitchell (1994), who examined cultural conceptions of breast lumps and breast cancer using in-depth interviews with 26 African American women who were diagnosed at an advanced stage of breast cancer. A third example is the work of Phillips and colleagues (1999), who conducted three focus group interviews with 26 African American women of varied socioeconomic status (from teachers to service workers and the unemployed).

These studies found that the African American women who participated were not very worried about getting breast cancer and often thought of it as primarily a white woman's disease. A second important finding was that they attributed breast cancer to factors such as stress, heartbreak, violence, injury, or sex, and some thought that breast lumps were dangerous only when impure blood in the body moves up as a result of a blow or bruise to the breast. These qualitative studies also found that breast cancer

was a hush-hush subject among these African American women. They preferred to consult other women about "female problems," rather than to involve professional health providers. Also, there was a tendency to consult health providers only for serious problems, not for prevention.

Another barrier to breast cancer screening and treatment was that some African American women felt that the treatments (including mammograms) were worse than the disease, actually causing the cancer to spread, in addition to causing loss of the breast and hair. Some women felt that cancer is always a fatal disease, and thus all treatments are futile. Regarding mammography specifically, the researchers learned that most African American women who participated were not aware that mammograms could detect cancers long before they could be felt. Furthermore, these views on breast cancer screening and treatment contributed to reliance on alternative treatments. The most often cited alternative treatment included prayer and a reliance on the healing power of God.

In sum, these qualitative studies showed that the African American women studied held a set of beliefs about the cause, detection, and treatment of breast cancer that made early detection unlikely. This knowledge was critical for practitioners to begin to design and implement effective interventions acceptable to African American women.

DESIGNING CULTURALLY SENSITIVE INTERVENTIONS

Once practitioners have a good understanding of the cultural beliefs and concepts of the target population, they can develop culturally sensitive interventions. Several communitywide interventions were developed on the basis of the qualitative research findings just discussed. Two examples of these interventions are the Witness Project and the Save Our Sisters (SOS) Project.

The Witness Project developed a role model intervention based on focus group interview data in combination with a theoretical educational model (Bailey, Erwin, & Belin, 2000). The intervention used female African American breast cancer survivors as role models and (a) incorporated a spiritual component, (b) emphasized each individual's responsibility for her own health, (c) challenged the fatalistic view that cancer is a death sentence, and (d) reduced the stigmatization of the disease by having role models share their breast cancer experiences in public. The intervention incorporated the concept of witnessing that is familiar to many Southern African American women. African American breast cancer survivors, referred to as witness role models (WRMs), shared their breast cancer experiences in churches. The WRMs focused on their own discoveries of breast lumps, the treatment process, personal philosophy concerning survival, and the benefits of early detection through breast self-exam and mammography (Erwin, Spatz, & Turturro, 1992). Following the witnessing, participants in the intervention program discussed their concerns with the WRMs. This intervention has been shown to be effective in empowering African American women to take responsibility for their health and practice early detection behaviors (Erwin, Spatz, Stotts, & Hollenberg, 1999).

The SOS Project was developed from the findings of Tessaro and colleagues' (1994) qualitative study. Because older African American women seek other women in their social networks for female-specific concerns, "natural helpers" who were active members of church-based women's groups were used to increase mammography screenings in a North Carolina county (Eng, 1993; Eng & Smith, 1995). These lay health advisors reached out to older women in their social networks to break the silence about breast cancer. After education on various topics such as breast cancer, breast cancer screening, women's attitudes toward mammography, talking one on one, and giving presentations, the lay health advisors talked to women about breast cancer screening, supported them through the process of getting mammograms, and raised community awareness through presentations at community events and places such as beauty parlors, nutrition sites, and churches. The SOS network was linked to formal health care agencies, eventually forming the North Carolina Breast Cancer Screening Program (Earp, Altpeter, Mayne, Viadro, & O'Malley, 1995).

The Witness Project in Arkansas and the SOS Project in North Carolina illustrate how solid qualitative research can be used to design effective interventions for populations that have previously been outside the traditional health care system. By building on existing cultural structures (e.g., churches, natural social networks) and knowledge and beliefs that interfered with early detection (e.g., that cancer was a white

woman's disease, and that cancer was fatal), these projects were able to reduce the rate of breast cancer mortality in African American women.

EVALUATING THE IMPLEMENTATION OF INTERVENTIONS

It is not always enough to design interventions based on a solid understanding of the target community. Because interventions take place in the real world of practice (not in pure, laboratory settings), practitioners also need to know how their interventions are actually working. This type of exploration is especially important when interventions do not have the expected results. Qualitative research can shed light on the black box of interventions by describing what occurs from the perspective of the staff and the participants. Once again, the case of breast cancer detection in African American women is used to provide an example.

The North Carolina Breast Cancer Screening Program (NC-BCSP) combined qualitative studies and quantitative outcome studies to evaluate their interventions (Altpeter, Earp, & Schopler, 1998; Bishop, Earp, Eng, & Lynch, 2002; Earp et al., 1995; Earp et al., 2002; Earp et al., 1997; Flax & Earp, 1999). The NC-BCSP, a community-based intervention program, targeted changes at several levels, ranging from individuals and their social networks to institutions and policymakers (Altpeter et al., 1998). To increase mammography use among older African American women in eastern North Carolina, the NC-BCSP intervention created an extensive network of lay health advisors (LHAs) in the community and community outreach specialists who linked the LHAs to local health care system (e.g., local health departments, health centers; Bishop et al., 2002; Earp et al., 1998). Both LHAs and community outreach specialists were African American women who lived in the local community.

Quantitative outcome studies found the intervention model to be effective in increasing mammography use among women in intervention counties (Earp et al., 2002). However, quantitative research often creates a black box, leaving what actually happens that brings about the changes unclear. Documenting the process of interventions can help others replicate these interventions through providing insights on critical elements that have contributed to program successes or failures (Patton, 1990). Moreover, "findings on unintended deviations from the original plan can offer insights to policymakers and funding agencies on why programs may or may not be achieving their expected effects" (Bishop et al., 2002, p. 234). With these goals, a qualitative study was conducted by the NC-BCSP to evaluate how the program had been translated into actual practice. The researchers conducted document review and in-depth interviews with 24 LHAs with varying activity levels (e.g., high, moderate, low) and with four community outreach specialists. The study revealed that, although the natural helper model was followed in large part, the program implementation departed from the plan in several unanticipated ways. The findings found that recruitment of natural helpers was sometimes problematic. Because a limited time was allowed to identify and recruit LHAs, some women were included even though they did not have the recommended natural helper characteristics. Another problem was that since the LHAs were already natural helpers in their communities who had been advising individuals on a variety of topics, they were reluctant to limit their activities to breast cancer screening. The qualitative interviews gave voice to the perspectives of the LHAs, who suggested that the program goals be expanded to include other health issues. Eventually, the program was expanded in response, accepted outreach to a broader range of women, and incorporated education on other health problems of concern to African American women.

By evaluating the implementation process of the intervention, unexpected deviations from the original plan were found that offered insights on the black box of the intervention. These showed that an LHA needed a broader intervention than the one originally defined. The NC-BCSP illustrates how a program can be strengthened by undertaking and applying qualitative research.

CONCLUSION

This chapter has illustrated several ways that qualitative research can be used to improve practice. The case of breast cancer screening was used to show how practitioners have used qualitative research to help them gain an in-depth understanding of a population that needed services, to build a culturally sensitive intervention based on that understanding, and to evaluate their interventions. Although much of the current focus in practice research is on EBP, which emphasizes quantitative research methods, qualitative research will always be needed in fields like social work, where new problems and new populations constantly arise. Qualitative methods should also be used to understand what actually happens in real-world interventions and to improve programs based on this understanding. In fields where rapid change is common, practitioners need to be able to use both qualitative and quantitative research findings, if they are to be effective.

References

Altpeter, M., Earp, J. A., & Schopler, J. H. (1998). Promoting breast cancer screening in rural, African American communities: The "science and art" of community health promotion. *Health & Social Work, 23*(2), 104–115.

American Cancer Society. (2003). *Breast cancer facts & figures 2001–2002.* Atlanta, GA: American Cancer Society.

Bailey, E. J., Erwin, D. O., & Belin, P. (2000). Using cultural beliefs and patterns to improve mammography utilization among African-American women: The Witness Project. *Journal of the National Medical Association, 92,* 136–142.

Bishop, C., Earp, J. L., Eng, E., & Lynch, K. S. (2002). Implementing a natural helper lay health advisor program: Lessons learned from unplanned events. *Health Promotion Practice, 3*(2), 233–244.

Blustein, J. (1995). Medicare coverage, supplemental insurance, and the use of mammography by older women. *New England Journal of Medicine, 332,* 1138–1143.

Cochrane Library. (2003). *Index to abstracts to Cochrane reviews.* Retrieved July 11, 2003 from http://www.cochrane.org/cochrane/revabstr/main index.htm

Cournoyer, B. R., & Powers, G. T. (2002). Evidence-based social work: The quiet revolution continues. In A. R. Roberts & G. J. Greene (Eds.), *Social workers' desk reference* (pp. 798–806). New York: Oxford University Press.

Douglas, M., Bartolucci, A., Waterbor, J., & Sirles, A. (1995). Breast cancer early detection: Differences between African American and white women's health beliefs and detection practices. *Oncology Nursing Forum, 22*(5), 835–837.

Earp, J. L., Altpeter, M., Mayne, L., Viadro, C. I., & O'Malley, M. S. (1995). The North Carolina Breast Cancer Screening Program: Foundations and design of a model for reaching older, African American, rural women. *Journal of Breast Cancer Research and Treatment, 35*(1), 7–22.

Earp, J. L., Eng, E., O'Malley, M. S., Altpeter, M., Rauscher, G., Mayne, L., et al. (2002). Increasing use of mammography among older, rural African-American women: Results from a community trial. *American Journal of Public Health, 92,* 646–654.

Earp, J. L., Viadro, C. I., Vincus, A. A., Altpeter, M., Flax, V., Mayne, L., et al. (1997). Lay health advisors: A strategy for getting the word out about breast cancer. *Health Education and Behavior, 24,* 432–451.

Eley, J. W., Hill, H. A., Chen, V. W., Austin, D. F., Wesley, M. N., Muss, H. B., et al. (1994). Racial differences in survival from breast cancer: Results of the National Cancer Institute Black/White Cancer Survival Study. *Journal of the American Medical Association, 272*(12), 947–954.

Eng, E. (1993). The Save Our Sisters Project: A social network strategy for reaching rural black women. *Cancer, 72*(Suppl.), 1071–1077.

Eng, E., & Smith, J. (1995). Natural helping functions of lay health advisors in breast cancer education. *Journal of Breast Cancer Research and Treatment, 35*(1), 23–29.

Erlandson, D. A., Harris, E. L., Skipper, B. L., & Allen, S. D. (1993). *Doing naturalistic inquiry: A guide to methods.* Newbury Park, CA: Sage.

Erwin, D. O., Spatz, T. S., Stotts, R. C., & Hollenberg, J. A. (1999). Increasing mammography practice by African American women. *Cancer Practice, 7*(2), 78–85.

Erwin, D. O., Spatz, T. S., & Turturro, C. L. (1992). Development of an African-American role model intervention to increase breast self-examination and mammography. *Journal of Cancer Education, 7*(4), 311–319.

Faidman, A. (1997). The spirit catches you and you fall down: A Hmong child, her American doctors, and the collision of two cultures. New York: Farrar, Strauss & Giroux.

Fetterman, D. M. (1998). *Ethnography.* Newbury Park, CA: Sage.

Flax, V. L., & Earp, J. L. (1999). Counseled women's perspectives on their interactions with lay health advisors: A feasibility study. *Health Education Research, 14*(1), 15–24.

Fletcher, S. W., Harris, R. P., Gonzalez, J. J., Degnan, D., Lannin, D. R., Strecher, V. J., et al. (1993). Increasing mammography utilization: A controlled study. *Journal of the National Cancer Institute, 85*(2), 112–120.

Gibbs, L., & Gambrill, E. (2002). Evidence-based practice: Counterarguments to objections. *Research on Social Work Practice,12*(3), 452–476.

Gilgun, J. F. (1994). Hand into glove: The grounded theory approach and social work practice research. In E. Sherman & W. J. Reid (Eds.), *Qualitative Research in Social Work* (pp. 115–125). New York: Columbia University Press.

Hoffman-Goetz, L., & Mills, S. L. (1997). Cultural barriers to cancer screening among African American women: A critical review of the qualitative literature. *Women's Health 3*(3/4), 183–201.

Howard, M. O., McMillen, C. J., & Pollio, D. E. (2003). Teaching evidence-based practice: Toward a new paradigm for social work education. *Research on Social Work Practice 13*(2), 234–259.

Lannin, D. R., Mathews, H. F., Mitchell, J., & Swanson, M. S. (2002). Impacting cultural attitudes in African American women to decrease breast cancer mortality. *The American Journal of Surgery, 184,* 418–423.

Lannin, D. R., Mathews, H. F., Mitchell, J., Swanson, M. S., Swanson, F. H., & Edwards, M. S. (1998). Influence of socioeconomic and cultural factors on racial differences in late-stage presentation of breast cancer. *Journal of the American Medical Association, 279*(22), 1801–1807.

Liebow, E. (1993). Tell them who I am: The lives of homeless women. New York: Free Press.

Mathews, H. F., Lannin, D. R., & Mitchell, J. P. (1994). Coming to terms with advanced breast cancer: Black women's narratives from eastern North Carolina. *Social Science & Medicine, 38*(6), 789–800.

Maxwell, J. A. (1996). *Qualitative research design.* Thousand Oaks, CA: Sage.

Myerhoff, B. (1978). *Number our days.* New York: Simon & Schuster, Inc.

Oktay, J. S. (2003). *The other breast cancer survivors: Daughters' stories.* New York: Haworth.

Oktay, J. S., & Walter, C. A. (1991). *Breast cancer in the life course: Women's experiences.* New York: Springer.

O'Malley, J. S., Earp, J.A.L., & Harris, R. P. (1997). Race and mammography use in two North Carolina counties. *American Journal of Public Health, 87*(5), 782–786.

Padgett, D. K. (1998). Qualitative *methods in social work research: Challenges and rewards.* Thousand Oaks, CA: Sage.

Reissman, C. K. (1994). Qualitative studies in social work research. Thousands Oaks, CA: Sage.

Rosen, A. (1994). Knowledge use in direct practice. *Social Service Review, 68,* 561–577.

Rosen, A. (1996). The scientific practitioner revisited: Some obstacles and precautions for fuller implementation in practice. *Social Work Research, 20,* 105–111.

Rosen, A., Proctor, E. K., & Staudt, M. (1999). Social work research and the quest for effective practice. *Social Work Research, 23,* 4–14.

Ruckdeschel, R., Earnshaw, P., & Firrek, A. (1994). The qualitative case study and evaluation: Issues, methods and examples. In E. Sherman & W. J. Reid (Eds.), *Qualitative Research in Social Work.* New York: Columbia University Press.

Sackett, D. L., Richardson, W. S., Rosenberg, W., & Haynes, R. B. (1997). *Evidence-based medicine: How to practice & teach EBM* (2nd ed.). New York: Churchill Livingstone.

Strauss, A., & Corbin, J. (1998). *Basics of qualitative research: Techniques and procedures for developing grounded theory* (2nd ed.). Thousand Oaks, CA: Sage.

Tessaro, I., Eng, E., & Smith, J. (1994). Breast cancer screening in older African American women: Qualitative research findings. *American Journal of Public Health Promotion, 8*(4), 286–293.

Urban, N., Anderson, G. L., & Peacock, S. (1994). Mammography screening: How important is cost as a barrier to use? *American Journal of Public Health, 84,* 50–55.

Viadro, C. I., Earp, J. L., & Altpeter, M. (1997). Designing a process evaluation for a comprehensive breast cancer screening intervention: Challenges and opportunities. *Evaluation and Program Planning, 20*(3), 237–249.

QUALITATIVE RESEARCH

78 *Cancer Prevention in Older Women*

Donna E. Hurdle

There is a long history of health promotion and prevention activities in the field of social work; however, the focus of social work practice, research, and professional literature in recent decades has been on treatment and rehabilitation. Although current social work practice textbooks describe prevention of psychosocial problems and promotion of adaptive functioning as one of the missions of social work, in actuality these activities have been very limited (Hepworth, Rooney, & Larsen, 2001). There is a strong need for increased social work activity in the area of health promotion as an emerging area of practice, particularly in the current managed care environment (Strom-Gottfried, 1997). There is also a foundation of social work literature in primary prevention that can guide these efforts.

Recent developments in the health care system, particularly in managed care, have contributed to a resurgence of interest and activity in health promotion and disease prevention. As cost containment has become a priority of managed care organizations and health providers, early identification of disease and maintaining wellness have emerged as useful means to that end. The disciplines of public health and nursing have taken a leading role in this emerging field; however, social workers have much to offer and must take a more visible role in service provision and development of professional literature. Social work education also needs to more clearly address health promotion as a practice modality and to teach students a variety of skills and interventions appropriate for this field of practice. This chapter will address the social work role in women's health promotion and a research study that I conducted on breast cancer prevention with older women.

SOCIAL WORK PREVENTION AND PROMOTION PRACTICE

Social work activity in the area of prevention first began as part of the settlement house movement at the end of the nineteenth century. Although settlement houses provided concrete services to meet the basic needs of poor immigrant communities, their major focus concerned reform efforts targeted to changing community conditions (Loavenbruch & Keys, 1987). These included sanitation, child labor, working conditions in factories, health, housing, and education. Settlement workers developed the first primary health clinics for children and families and provided classes to instruct community members on improved sanitation practices and the control of epidemic diseases, such as tuberculosis. The Henry Street Settlement in New York City developed the first visiting nurse program, which later became a separate agency when funded by the city government (Loavenbruch & Keys, 1987). These activities continued into the twentieth century, however, the tradition of individually focused casework, pioneered by the Charity Organization Societies, gradually became the prevalent methodology used by the profession and taught in its formal educational structures.

Despite a predominant focus on intervention, there continued to be advocates for prevention in the social work profession. Rapoport (1961) called for adaptations of practice, which would reach the healthy segment of the population and retard the incidence of social pathology. The federal community mental health act of 1963 and its subsequent amendments mandated consultation and education as part of the array of services provided to the populations in specific catchment areas by community mental health centers throughout the nation. However, only about 5% of staff time was ever devoted to this effort during the period of peak funding during the 1970s, and subsequent cutbacks have virtually eliminated this service (Bloom, 1987). A sampling of the social work literature in the late 1970s found that fewer than 3% of articles published between 1976 and 1980 related to preventive social work, and that those were reports of programs rather than theoretical or empirical papers (Nance, 1982, as cited in Bloom, 1987).

In the early 1980s, a new focus on health promotion and wellness care was described by then–Secretary of Health and Human Services Rich-ard Schweiker; however, no federal funding was devoted to this initiative (Bloom, 1987). In the social work profession, there was evidence of increased interest and activity in prevention in the 1980s. Several articles and books appeared in the literature during this period (Bloom, 1986; Germain, 1982; Levine, Allen-Meares, & Easton, 1987; Shannon, 1989), and the Council on Social Work Education published two monographs on prevention (Noble, 1981, as cited in Bloom, 1987).

In the 1990s, prevention activities have become more specialized, and social work attention has concerned HIV/AIDS prevention, substance abuse prevention, child abuse prevention, and other health issues. Bloom (1996) published a recent compilation of primary prevention practices that are applicable to a variety of prevention and promotion activities. In it, he defined primary prevention as "coordinated actions seeking to prevent predictable problems, to protect existing states of health and healthy functioning, and to promote desired potentialities in individuals and groups in their physical and sociocultural settings over time" (p. 2). Among the various types of prevention activities described are health promotion and disease prevention activities.

Health Promotion: An Emerging Health Field

Health promotion and disease prevention are clearly in the best interests of the general population, who can live more productive lives without the impact of debilitating disease and premature mortality. Research is now showing the tremendous impact that health promotion can make on reducing the incidence of many diseases. Approximately 75% of cancer deaths could be avoided by the elimination or minimization of cancer risk factors, such as smoking and high-fat diets (Lerman, Rimer, & Engstrom, 1989). For other diseases, such as HIV/AIDS, prevention is the only method of intervention, because a cure has still not been developed. *Healthy People 2000* and *Healthy People 2010*, the federal blueprints for the nation's health that were initially developed in 1990, devoted considerable attention to health promotion and disease prevention activities (Bowen, Urban, Carrell, & Kinne, 1993). However, as necessary as this field is, it is given less attention and funding than the treatment of disease; this is due to a variety of factors, including limited medical insurance reimbursement for prevention, physician training focused on disease treatment, and the structural bias of the medical/industrial complex (Bowen et al., 1993).

Currently, health promotion and disease prevention activities are more developed in some fields of health than others. Substantial activity occurs in HIV/AIDS prevention, teen pregnancy prevention, substance abuse prevention (particularly with youth), and smoking prevention. In the area of women's health, breast and cervical cancer prevention and early identification activities have been funded by the federal government for the last decade. Many studies have investigated the most useful education methods of encouraging women to use screening methods for breast and cervical cancer, which is currently the only method of prevention. The most effective methods appear to be those that use multiple strategies, including education, low-cost and accessible screening, the media, and mailed reminders to patients (Rimer, 1998). Health promotion and disease prevention have been shown to be effective with all age groups (Schweitzer et al., 1994). However, tailoring efforts to specific groups defined by ethnicity, socioeconomic status, or age is often necessary, because mass education efforts are more effective with educated and affluent persons than with traditionally underserved populations (Roetzheim et al., 1992).

Social Work Roles in Health Promotion with Women

Health issues for women have received less research attention from the health professions and less funding for clinical research than issues for men (Bowen et al., 1993). The social work profession parallels this situation: A survey of the social work literature found relatively few articles about women's health issues (Millner & Wideman, 1994). Given that most social workers and social work clients are female, this is an appalling finding. It is important that researchers correct this imbalance and study various ways to improve the health of U.S. women. In particular, "social work must expand its vision to focus on issues of health maintenance and disease prevention for women" (p. 168).

Many types of health promotion and disease prevention services are needed to improve women's health. In her discussion of women,

health care, and social work, Olson (1994) identified the following areas as being of priority for intervention: maternal and infant mortality and morbidity, cardiovascular disease, breast cancer, contraception and abortion services, and AIDS. In all of these areas, women are disproportionately or solely affected by the condition, there has been inadequate investigation into causation and treatment, and the incidence rates of the medical problem are higher in the United States than in other industrialized countries. Although greater attention is now being focused on women's health via federal initiatives such as the Office of Women's Health at the National Institutes of Health, the Women's Health Initiative research study, and a mandate for equal participation of women as subjects in clinical trials, it will be some time before substantial progress is made (Olson, 1994).

Social workers have a unique disciplinary perspective that can make a significant difference in health promotion activities. The profession's continuing focus on disadvantaged populations, its biopsychosocial ecological practice model, and its systems perspective (that includes the impact of environmental and social policy factors) will result in health promotion that is very comprehensive. Formulating health promotion as a process that is targeted not just toward individuals but also toward community and social policies broadens the type of services that will be developed. Looking at individual health in the context of family and community health leads to prevention interventions that include an emphasis on social support, building on strengths, decreasing stress, and considering the impact of the physical environment. One example of this social work perspective is Bloom's (1996) configural analysis for primary prevention practice, which includes increasing individual strengths, social supports, and physical environmental resources while decreasing individual limitations, social stresses, and physical environmental pressures. Another example is Hurdle's (2001) discussion of the critical importance of social support in women's health and health promotion.

To illustrate the social work role in health promotion, a description of one such intervention in women's health is described in the following section. This effort was a research study I undertook with the purpose of increasing the use of breast cancer screening by older women.

IMPROVING USE OF BREAST CANCER SCREENING BY HIGH-RISK WOMEN

The Critical Need for Services

Cancer is the second leading cause of death in American women, following heart disease, and breast cancer is the most frequently occurring cancer (Olson, 1994). It now affects one out of eight women, with a disproportionately higher incidence in older women. Whereas heart disease is the leading cause of death for all women, for subgroups of women it is cancer (malignant neoplasms were the leading cause of death for older women in 1991; Centers for Disease Control, 1994). Breast cancer was chosen as the focus for this health promotion effort, because it is predominantly a woman's disease, it is a leading killer of U.S. women, and its incidence has continued to rise over the last 30 years. Although breast cancer is curable if identified in the earliest stages, large groups of women do not take advantage of screening methods to identify the disease at early stages—particularly women of color and older women. Because the incidence of breast cancer increases as women age and older women are least likely to use screening methods, this is a lethal combination. This dynamic was the rationale for the present study.

The incidence of breast cancer has steadily risen in the last 20 years, including a 36% increase between 1973 and 1987 (Qualters, Lee, Smith, & Aubert, 1992). Older women are disproportionately affected, with half of all breast cancers occurring in women over 65 years of age; the incidence rate doubles in women between the ages of 40 and 65, and triples by the age of 75 years (Rimer et al., 1992). Although mortality rates have fallen slightly in recent years, largely because of greater screening efforts, they vary significantly by ethnic/racial and age groups. During the 1973 to 1989 period, deaths from breast cancer decreased for white women under 50 years of age but rose 5.4% for white women 50 years of age and older, 5.3% for black women under 50 years of age, and 21.9% for black women over 50 years of age (National Alliance of Breast Cancer Organizations, 1992). Between 1989 and 1992, mortality rates for Caucasian women declined by 5.5% but increased 2.6% for African American women (Smigel, 1995). Similarly, recent studies show that 5-year survival rates are 79% for white

women and 62% for black women (Eley et al., 1994). Native American women have also been found to have reduced survival rates in comparison with those of white women, 49% in contrast to 76% (AMC Cancer Research Center, 1994). Survival rates are also lower for uninsured women (Eley et al., 1994).

Breast cancer cannot yet be prevented, but the use of breast cancer screening methods, such as mammography, clinical breast examination, and breast self-examination, can greatly increase survival by identifying and treating the cancer in its early stages. Various methods have been developed to improve use of these screening methods (Champion, 1994; Lerman et al., 1992; Vernon, Laville, & Jackson, 1990). The American Cancer Society recommends that women between 40 and 50 years of age obtain biannual mammograms and that women over 50 years of age obtain yearly mammograms (Sienko, Osuch, Galinghouse, Rakowski, & Given, 1992). Breast exams by a medical professional are also recommended yearly for women over 40 years of age. Despite the recommendations of medical professionals, the use of breast cancer screening methods varies greatly by women's age, ethnicity, socioeconomic status, and insurance coverage (Polednak, Lane, & Burg, 1993). Women's use of mammography decreases as they age, as does their use of breast examination by a health professional (Hayward, Shapiro, Freeman, & Corey, 1988; Makuc, Fried, & Parsons, 1994). A 1990 study found that although 65% of American women had had a mammogram at some time, less than 30% of women aged 60 to 69 years of age, and less than 20% of women 70 and older, had ever had this test (Burg, Lane, & Polednak, 1990). Other studies have found that older women have less knowledge about and are less likely to perform breast self-examination (Dunbar, Begg, Yasko, & Bell, 1991; Millar & Millar, 1992).

Less educated women and those without health insurance also have significantly lower use of mammography and clinical exams (Makuc et al., 1994). The 1992 National Health Interview Survey found that only 35% of women with a high school education or less received mammography screening, in comparison with 53% of women with more education. Health insurance coverage also has a significant effect; only 19% of older women with Medicare only received a mammogram in 1992, in comparison with 44% of women who had Medicare plus supplemental insurance and 56% of those who received care from a health maintenance organization, or HMO (Makuc et al., 1994). Medicare currently covers mammography only every other year, despite the fact that the highest rates of breast cancer occur in women covered by Medicare.

Methodology

The purpose of this study was to assess the effectiveness of a gender-sensitive educational intervention designed to promote the use of breast cancer screening methods (mammography and breast self-examination) in senior women. The intervention consisted of two one-hour sessions, which were held one week apart and provided to older women in community-based settings, such as senior centers and residences. The focus was on promoting women's health, particularly breast health, and included brief mini-lectures interspersed with demonstration, activities, discussion, and use of audiovisual formats. A multisensory and participatory approach has been found to be useful in health promotion with seniors.

This study used a quasi-experimental design known as a nonequivalent control group design, which is appropriate for community-based interventions because there is no random assignment of subjects. A sample of senior women living in a northwestern U.S. city volunteered to participate in this study of breast cancer screening behaviors. No compensation was given to either the control or experimental groups who participated in the study.

Information about a given disease is important in changing preventive health behaviors, but the methods involved in teaching health education are equally, if not more, important. If the health education context, approach, and format are not appropriate for the learner, very little information about a particular disease or its prevention will be transmitted. Learning styles vary by gender and age, and educational methods have been developed for particular groups of learners. The learning styles of women are different from those of men and include a preference for applied learning, a collaborative learning environment, and a focus on subjective experience, connections, and relationships (Melamed & Devine, 1988). Feminist pedagogies have been developed that suggest a teaching style that actively engages students in the edu-cational process, with an emphasis on identifying and voicing their own views (Belenky, Clinchy, Goldberger, & Tarule, 1986; Maher, 1984). This approach is relevant to the provision of health education with women in community-based settings and provides a framework for more effective learning experiences.

Sample and Procedures

This study used a purposive, nonprobability sample of senior women living in the community. A total of 158 women between the ages of 54 and 94 years participated in the study; there were 126 women in the control group and 32 in the experimental group. Subjects were recruited from community-based organizations for seniors; the organizations chose whether to participate in the educational intervention (experimental group) or not (control group). Each member of both groups completed a survey on the health practices of older women, which included information about the subject's use of breast cancer screening methods and other health practices as well as demographic information. Subsequently, the experimental group received the educational intervention. Six months following the pretest, post-tests were mailed to all subjects, with stamped return envelopes. Any subjects failing to return their post-tests were sent reminder post cards. The return rate on the post-test was 62% for both the control and experimental groups. Only subjects completing both the pre- and post-test were included in the analysis of the effectiveness of the intervention.

Study Results

The sample for this study was predominantly Caucasian (73%); in women of color, the largest ethnic groups were Asian or Pacific Islander (9%), African American (7%), and Native American (6%). Most participants were between the ages of 66 and 75 years (56%), with 17% between 54 and 65, and 25% over 76. Most subjects were widowed (45%), whereas 27% were married, and 22% were divorced. Nearly equivalent groups of subjects had less than a high school education (23%), were high school graduates (29%), had some college (26%), or were college graduates (22%). Most subjects fell in the low (33%) or middle (31%) levels of socioeconomic status using Hollingshead's Two-

Factor Index of Social Position, and the remainder were in the low-medium (12%), medium-high (24%), and high categories (1%).

The older women in this sample were similar in some ways to those in national studies concerning the use of breast cancer screening by women in this age group, and they were different in others. Although the women in this sample reported higher levels of usage of breast cancer screening methods than those in national studies, there was a similar reduction in frequency of use to levels far below medical recommendations. A large majority of the subjects (89%) had had at least one mammogram; however, only 58% of the sample had had mammograms within the previous year. A large majority (82%) reported that they do perform breast self-examination. However, only 39% reported completing the exam each month as is recommended, and most (45%) reported performing it only three or four times a year.

With reference to subjects' use of screening methods by race and ethnicity, there was a statistically significant relationship between ethnicity and the recent use of mammography. More Caucasian women had had mammograms during the past year than had women of color. More Caucasian women also performed breast self-examination during the study period than did women of color. Both of these findings parallel the research literature on usage of breast cancer screening methods by ethnicity. Another consistency with national data was found for social status. A statistically significant relationship was found between socioeconomic status and breast cancer screening. National studies have also found that women of lower income levels use mammography less frequently than do women of higher incomes.

In comparing the results of the control and experimental groups on their use of breast cancer screening methods after the 6-month study period, I found that women in the experimental group used both mammography and breast self-examination more frequently than women in the control group. This difference was statistically significant at the $p > .05$ level. This finding indicates that the educational intervention was instrumental in encouraging senior women to use breast cancer screening methods.

Implications of the Study

Social workers can play an important role in health promotion efforts with older women. This study has shown that a gender-sensitive intervention, provided by a social worker in a community-based setting, was effective in encouraging older women to use breast cancer screening methods. This is a significant finding, because this approach can be readily used in community settings with senior women on a variety of health topics. It is cost effective, because existing staff can be trained to provide the information, thus eliminating the need for grant-funded programs with research assistants who perform the intervention only during a study. Previous research into the use of wellness education with seniors has found that programming in community senior centers can be effective in changing the health-related practices of seniors attending such programs for up to several years after the wellness classes were held (Lalonde & FallCreek, 1985; Lalonde, Hooyman, & Blumhagen, 1988). Peer role models have also been found to increase the effectiveness of health promotion in ethnic populations.

The limitations of this study include its limited representation of senior women due to the convenience sample, and the small number of women participating in the experimental group; however, this did not affect the statistical measures significantly. The subjects in the experimental group who completed the post-test were women of one ethnic group (Caucasian); therefore, to be consistent, only Caucasian women in the control group who completed the post-test were included. The effectiveness of the intervention can, therefore, only be considered for Caucasion women, which limits generalization about its effectiveness.

CONCLUSION

As social workers move into health promotion roles, they must become more familiar with various types of prevention methods. Evolving from the micro-macro dichotomy into a more fluid conceptualization of practice with different populations and communities based on intervention purpose would be helpful. In designing health promotion programs, social workers must be familiar with epidemiology studies and use them as guidance for determining which populations are most in need of services. The social work profession's investigation of the utility of prevention methods and its contribution to the emerging body of empirically based practice methods are also critical. Empirically based practice research in health-related prevention has been largely implemented by medical professionals; it is time for social workers to bring their unique perspective to this important field of practice. With these additions to the knowledge base, social work can take a more active role in providing health promotion services and in researching their effectiveness.

References

AMC Cancer Research Center. (1994, October). Native Americans and cancer. *The Quest for Answers*, p. 1.

American Cancer Society. (1994). *Cancer facts and figures—1994*. Atlanta, GA: Author.

Belenky, M. F., Clinchy, B. M., Goldberger, N. R., & Tarule, J. M. (1986). *Women's ways of knowing: The development of self, voice, and mind*. New York: Basic Books.

Bloom, M. (1987). Prevention. In A. Minahan, R. M. Becerra, S. Briar, C. J. Coulton, L. H. Ginsberg, J. G. Hopps, et al. (Eds.), *Encyclopedia of social work* (Vol. 2, pp. 556–561). Silver Spring, MD: National Association of Social Workers.

Bloom, M. (1996). *Primary prevention practices*. Thousand Oaks, CA: Sage.

Bowen, D. J., Urban, N., Carrell, D., & Kinne, S. (1993). Comparisons of strategies to prevent breast cancer mortality. *Journal of Social Issues, 49*, 35–59.

Burg, M., Lane, D. S., & Polednak, A. P. (1990). Age group differences in the use of breast cancer screening tests. *Journal of Aging and Health, 2*, 514–530.

Centers for Disease Control. (1994, February 11). Mortality surveillance system. *Monthly Vital Statistics Report, 42*(8), 4–9.

Champion, V. L. (1994). Strategies to increase mammography utilization. *Medical Care, 32*(2), 118–129.

Dunbar, J., Begg, L., Yasko, J., & Bell, S. (1991). Breast self-examination compliance among older high-risk women. *Patient Education and Counseling, 18*, 223–230.

Eley, J. W., Hill, H. A., Chen, V. W., Austin, D. F., Wesley, M. N., Muss, H. B., et al. (1994). Racial differences in survival from breast cancer: Results from the National Cancer Institute Black/White Cancer Survival Study. *Journal of the American Medical Association, 272*(12), 947–954.

Germain, C. B. (1982). Teaching primary prevention in social work: An ecological perspective. *Journal of Education for Social Work, 18*, 20–28.

Hayward, R. A., Shapiro, M. F., Freeman, H. E., & Corey, C. R. (1988). Who gets screened for cervical and breast cancer? Results from a new national study. *Archives of Internal Medicine, 148*, 1177–1181.

Hepworth, D., Rooney, R., & Larsen, J. (2001). *Direct social work practice: Theory and skills*. Pacific Grove, CA: Brooks/Cole.

Hurdle, D. E. (2001). Social support: A critical factor in women's health and health promotion. *Health & Social Work, 26*, 72–79.

Lalonde, B., & FallCreek, S. J. (1985). Outcome effectiveness of the Wallingford Wellness Project: A model health promotion program for the elderly. *Journal of Gerontological Social Work, 9*(1), 49–64.

Lalonde, B., Hooyman, N., & Blumhagen, J. (1988). Long-term outcome effectiveness of a health promotion program for the elderly: The Wallingford Wellness Project. *Journal of Gerontological Social Work, 13*(1/2), 95–111.

Lerman, C., Rimer, B., & Engstrom, P. F. (1989). Reducing avoidable cancer mortality through prevention and early detection regimens. *Cancer Research, 49*, 4955–4962.

Lerman, C., Ross, E., Boyce, A., Gorchov, A. M., McLaughlin, R., Rimer, B., et al. (1992). The impact of mailing psychoeducational materials to women with abnormal mammograms. *American Journal of Public Health, 82*, 729–730.

Levine, R. S., Allen-Meares, P., & Easton, F. (1987). Primary prevention and the educational preparation of school social workers. *Social Work in Education, 9*(3), 145–158.

Loavenbruch, G., & Keys, P. (1987). Settlements and neighborhood centers. In A. Minahan, R. M. Becerra, S. Briar, C. J. Coulton, L. H. Ginsberg, J. G. Hopps, et al. (Eds.), *Encyclopedia of social work* (Vol. 2, pp. 556–561). Silver Spring, MD: National Association of Social Workers.

Maher, F. (1984). Appropriate teaching methods for integrating women. In B. Spanier, A. Bloom, & D. Boroviak (Eds.), *Toward a balanced curriculum: A sourcebook for initiating gender integration projects*. Cambridge, MA: Schenkman.

Makuc, D. M., Fried, V. M., & Parsons, P. E. (1994, August 3). Health insurance and cancer screening among women. *Advance Data*. National Center for Health Statistics. Number 254.

Melamed, L., & Devine, I. (1988). Women and learning style: An exploratory study. In P. Tancred-Scherif (Ed.), *Feminist research: Prospect and retrospect*. Montreal: McGill-Queens University Press.

Millar, M. G., & Millar, R. V. (1992). Feelings and beliefs about breast cancer and breast self-examination among women in three age-groups. *Family and Community Health, 15*(3), 30–37.

Millner, L., & Wideman, E. (1994). Women's health issues: A review of the current literature in the social work journals, 1985–1992. *Social Work in Health Care, 19*, 145–172.

National Alliance of Breast Cancer Organizations. (1992, October). NCI breast cancer statistics released. *NABCO News*, p. 3.

Olson, M. M. (1994). Introduction: Reclaiming the "other"—Women, health care and social work. *Social Work in Health Care, 19*, 1–16.

Polednak, A. P., Lane, D. S., & Burg, M. (1993). Mammography use in Hispanic and Anglo visitors to community health centers. *Health Values, 17*(3), 42–48.

Qualters, J. R., Lee, N. C., Smith, R. A., & Aubert, R. E. (1992, April 24). Breast and cervical cancer surveillance, United States, 1973–1987. *Morbidity and Mortality Weekly Report: CDC Surveillance Summaries, 41*(2), 1–15.

Rapoport, L. (1961). The concept of prevention in social work. *Social Work, 6*, 3–12.

Rimer, B. (1998, May). Social and behavioral interventions in cancer prevention. Paper presented at Public Health in the 21st Century: Behavioral and Social Science Contributions conference, Atlanta, GA.

Rimer, B. K., Resch, N., King, E., Ross, E., Lerman, C., Boyce, A., et al. (1992). Multistrategy health education program to increase mammography use among women ages 65 and older. *Public Health Reports, 107*, 369–380.

Roetzheim, R. G., Van Durme, D. J., Brownlee, H. J., Herold, A. H., Pamies, R. J., Woodard, L., et al. (1992). Reverse targeting in a media-promoted breast care screening project. *Cancer, 70*, 1152–1158.

Schweitzer, S. O., Atchison, K. A., Lubben, J. E., Mayer-Oakes, S. A., DeJong, F. J., & Matthias, R. E. (1994). Health promotion and disease prevention for older adults: Opportunity for change or preaching to the converted? *American Journal of Preventive Medicine, 19*, 223–229.

Shannon, M. T. (1989). Health promotion and illness prevention: A biopsychosocial perspective. *Health & Social Work*, 32–40.

Sienko, D. G., Osuch, J. R., Galinghouse, C., Rakowski, V., & Given, B. (1992). The design and implementation of a community breast cancer screening program. *CA-A Cancer Journal for Clinicians, 42*(3), 163–175.

Smigel, K. (1995). Breast cancer death rates decline for white women. *Journal of the National Cancer Institute, 87*, 173.

Suarez, L., Nichols, D. C., & Brady, C. A. (1993). Use of peer role models to increase pap smear and mammogram screening in Mexican-American and Black women. *American Journal of Preventive Medicine, 9*(5), 290–296.

Strom-Gottfried, K. (1997). The implications of managed care for social work education. *Journal of Social Work Education, 33*, 7–18.

Vernon, S. W., Laville, E. A., & Jackson, G. L. (1990). Participation in breast screening programs: A review. *Social Science & Medicine, 30*, 1107–1118.

HOW FAMILY MEMBERS OF THE MENTALLY ILL VIEW MENTAL HEALTH PROFESSIONALS

79

A Focused Ethnography

Eric D. Johnson

Since the advent of deinstitutionalization over four decades ago, families with a seriously mentally ill member have been asked to take on increasing responsibilities for caregiving, as the primary locus of care shifted from the hospital to the community, and then professional community resources were faced with increasingly limited funds to do the job (Aviram, 1990; Bachrach, Talbott, & Meyerson, 1987). It has been estimated that approximately 40% of patients discharged from psychiatric units return to live with family members, and another 30% to 40% are in regular (e.g., weekly) contact with family members (Manderscheid & Sonnenschein, 1997).

In the early stages of deinstitutionalization, family care for people with serious mental illnesses was handicapped by a number of additional factors, including the influence of early theories of familial etiology of mental illness, limited information about the biological components and medical treatments for mental illness, and lack of organized support networks to aid families in caring for their mentally ill members and negotiating with the mental health system (Hatfield & Lefley, 1987). However, over the past two decades there has been a significant shift in understanding the process of mental illness and the family's role in this process, based largely on advances in medical technology (Torrey, Bowler, & Taylor, 1995; Whybrow, 1997), as well as follow-up research on the family etiology theories, which failed to demonstrate evidence that communication deviance *caused* mental illness (Goldstein, 1987).

A new conceptual framework emerged that used a *stress-diathesis* theory: An assumed genetic predisposition (diathesis) makes some people more vulnerable than others to breakdown under stress (Zubin, 1986). People with a genetic mental illness are seen as unable to process excessive environmental input (including overstimulating family or program environments) (Nuechterlein & Dawson, 1984). Life-course events are then viewed as triggers of a breakdown in functioning, rather than as formative of the illness (Nuechterlein et al., 1992), and these can be modified by social and environmental factors (e.g., social support system, family functioning, program modification) (Coyne & Downey, 1991; Goldstein, 1987).

This framework led to certain changes in thinking about families of the mentally ill and the development of psychoeducational approaches that sought to normalize families' experiences, provide educational input, and support the development of helpful coping strategies (Anderson, Reiss, & Hogarty, 1986; Bernheim & Lehman, 1985). Paralleling this development in the mental health profession was the rapid growth of the National Alliance for the Mentally Ill (NAMI), which has provided a strong national and regional support network of families and friends of people with serious mental illness (Hatfield, 1991; Lefley, 1996).

Although there has been a shift in the professional literature away from earlier theories of family communication patterns as the cause of mental illness, NAMI has been critical of psychoeducational programs that assume that mental health professionals have "the knowledge" and are imparting it to the families without sufficient attention to family views and contributions or recognition that unusual family characteristics might be the result of having to find ways of coping with the behaviors of a mentally ill person (Hatfield, 1991; Lefley, 1992). What seems clear from the accumulated literature is that living with and caring for a person with mental illness can have a tremendous impact on the family, and that the family has the potential for buffering some of the stressors on its mentally ill member (Lefley, 1996; Noh & Turner, 1987; Strachan, 1986).

There has been an increasing interest in the use of qualitative research methods for understanding families like these, because these methods allow for the description of experience and sense of meaning that the quantitative examination of family variables cannot capture (Ambert, Adler, Adler, & Detzner, 1995; Gilgun, Daly, & Handel, 1992; Rosenblatt & Fischer, 1993).

METHOD

The results reported here are part of a larger study of families of the seriously mentally ill (Johnson, 1998, 2000). For purposes of this study, a person considered to be seriously mentally ill was defined as someone who had had at least one previous hospitalization for a psychotic episode involving a mood or thought disorder as defined by the *DSM-IV* (American Psychiatric Association, 1994). The sample for this study consisted of referrals to the Family Support Project (FSP) in Mercer County, New Jersey, over a 3-year period. During this time, over 200 families were contacted by members of the FSP, and 180 families were interviewed and coded. All families had at least one member with a serious mental illness and were interviewed as close as possible to 6 months following hospitalization of the mentally ill member (IM). The IMs included 56% men and 44% women. Living situations were fairly evenly divided: 55% lived in the city and 45% in the suburbs; 60% lived with their families, and 40% lived elsewhere. The IMs were widely distributed by age ($M = 37$ years) and length of illness ($M = 13$ years), and most

were currently taking prescribed psychotropic medication (82%).

The families represented a cross-section of ethnic groups: European American (58%), African American (32%), and Hispanic American (10%). Socioeconomic status also was diverse: 39% upper-middle class (one or more family members with a professional job), 45% lower-middle class (one or more members with a blue-collar job), and 18% lower class (welfare or the IM's social security benefit providing the only income). The primary caregivers were mostly parents of the IMs (70%), with siblings (13%), spouses (6%), and adult children (8%) making up the rest of the sample. Most respondents were women (84%); they ranged in age from 25 to 80, but most were over 55 (62%; $M = 56$). Household and family size ranged broadly, with household size most often two to five people (70%), and family size most often four to eight people (72%). Referrals of families came from a wide variety of sources, including the community mental health center case management unit (16%), a clinician-led family support group (20%), outpatient clinics (23%), inpatient programs (12%), county jail system (10%), and the local NAMI chapter (19%).

Family members were interviewed about their experiences in managing the symptoms and behaviors accompanying mental illness, the meaning that the illness and their managing of it had for them, and their sense of competence in dealing with their IM and the mental health system. At least one first-order relative (parent, sibling, spouse, adult child) who was living with or was in frequent contact with the IM was interviewed using a semistructured interview schedule. Attempts were made to include as many family members as possible in each case. Family members were interviewed at length (interviews lasted at least 2 hours in each case) by me or by one of four staff members who comprised the FSP. All staff members had previous experience in working with the mentally ill and with family interviewing.

Quantitative aspects of the study, which are more fully described elsewhere (Johnson, 1998), found that both environmental stressors and illness-related stressors had significant negative effects on the community functioning of people with mental illness, but that this was buffered somewhat by general family functioning and was considerably buffered by the family's sense of competence in managing problems specifically related to the illness.

FINDINGS

As a part of the interview, family members were asked the question, "What would you like mental health professionals to know about you and your mentally ill family member?" In response to this, family members identified six major areas of concern. These categories, along with some defining needs, are presented here in order of the frequency with which they were mentioned. Following the list, each category is elaborated, with quotes from family members illustrating significant themes.

1. Professional communication
   a. More input to families from professionals
   b. Professionals receiving information from families
   c. Family inclusion in treatment planning
   d. More training for professionals
2. Community programs
   a. More continuity among programs
   b. More programs and better access to them
3. Housing and work issues
   a. Supervised housing
   b. Affordable housing
   c. Progressive independence
   d. Sheltered workshops and training programs
4. Case management
   a. More case managers
   b. More outreach and intensive services
5. Family support
   a. Information about the illness
   b. Help with problem solving
   c. Emotional support
   d. Respite care
   e. Information about services available
6. Hospitalization
   a. Commitment law problems
   b. Better rehabilitation programs
   c. More dual-diagnosis units
   d. Medication matching and monitoring

Professional Communication

In contrast to earlier reports of families' feeling blamed for the illness of their family member by mental health professionals, we rarely encountered a recent description of this behavior.

What we did frequently encounter, however, was the family members' experiences of being disregarded or dismissed as irrelevant by mental health professionals—this was expressed by families of all socioeconomic and ethnic groups. Family members' opinions or knowledge were rarely requested by mental health professionals in any settings, and they felt particularly disregarded by staff at the crisis center, staff at the hospitals, and psychiatrists in all settings. One father stated, "I tried to tell them about what I had observed with Abe. But they only seemed interested in making their own diagnosis—even though this was the first time any of them had ever seen him. There was a lot I could have told them, but they didn't seem to think my information was worth much."

Family members often felt excluded from access to mental health professionals, due to the invocation of confidentiality issues. However, in many cases, the mental health professional simply made an assumption about the need to keep information confidential, rather than discussing it with the IM. In other cases, the mental health professional had accepted at face value the IM's presentation of the family as negative. A mother noted, "When I tried to talk with the psychiatrist, she said she didn't think it would be a good idea, that Barbara wouldn't appreciate it and would object. I thought she'd talked it over with Barbara, but I later found out that they'd never discussed it."

In almost all cases, family members were attempting to provide information to the professional (e.g., lack of compliance with medication) or were looking for advice on how best to handle situations. Very rarely were they expecting release of confidential information. Nevertheless, they were frequently treated as intrusive busybodies or as people who merely coincidentally resided with the IM. A family member noted, "I wouldn't dream of trying to find out what Danielle talks about in therapy, even if she's saying things about me. All I want to do is be able to let the doctor know if there are problems or for him let me know how to help. But I get treated like I am trying to wreck her treatment rather than help her."

Of particular interest in this regard is the family's recognition of early warning signs of decompensation. In most families where the IMs illness was prolonged, the IM would behave in idiosyncratically characteristic ways in the early stages of decompensation: talking in a different manner, increasing pacing or other ritualistic behaviors, playing music louder, and so on. This information was rarely regarded by mental health personnel, who sometimes responded by suggesting that the family should be more accepting of the IM's individuality. One mother remarked, "Well, at the crisis center, they said, 'Lady, it seems like you're the one with the problem. I don't see any problem with him staying up late and playing the radio.' Why would I have gone to the crisis center, if my son was just playing the radio?"

Community Programs

In addition to the problem of limited program resources, family members noted that their IMs were frequently graduated from programs without adequate preparation for the next stage, sometimes due to the program's need to service additional numbers of clients. As a result, many of these patients subsequently relapsed and had to be rehospitalized after making this shift. This appeared to be a lack of attention to the IM's developmental needs for continuity in transitions. A father noted, "Families don't send their children off to college and tell them not to return, but the supervised housing program told Ed he had graduated and should go on to the unsupervised housing. They acted as if it were a sign of weakness to return and visit his old program. The few friends he had were in that program."

Similarly, people with mental illnesses are often *first* transitioned to a program that provides greater independence, and *then* provided help with activities of daily living skills. As one mother put it, "In the normal course of family life, we first learn new skills, then go out into the world to try them out. But they wanted to release Frankie from the hospital and send her to independent living, while enrolling her in a day program to learn how to live independently. What sense does that make?"

Lack of attention to basic family-oriented developmental needs has handicapped many professional programs. Like the confidentiality issue, it is frequently overlooked due to focus on the chronological, rather than socioemotional, age of the IM. One father put it this way: " 'Well,' they said, 'George is a big boy now. He has the right to refuse treatment.' " Physically,

he's a big boy, but he's still a little boy inside. Do you give your 5-year-old the right to refuse treatment?"

Case Management

Family members felt burdened by the expectation that they would provide housing and case management services for the IM. A particular difficulty in many families was lack of assignment of various aspects of these responsibilities to members of the nuclear and extended family available, so that the great burden of caregiving fell on one family member (most often the mother). Nevertheless, the shortage of case managers, and the tendency of case managers to close the case once the IM was connected with another service, was frustrating to family members. One mother said, "The case manager was very nice, but I could tell that she had way too many cases, and Henry was just another case. Once she got him an intake at the day treatment program, her job was done. But I knew he'd have trouble following through there, and sure enough, two months later I got to be the case manager again."

For many of the seriously mentally ill, case management is not a temporary need, and family members felt that the burden was left with them to provide for this ongoing need. In addition, staff turnover rates are high in community programs, and the mentally ill do not adapt well to this frequent change of contacts. Family members understand this; one noted, "I don't like to keep changing doctors or dentists myself, so why should Irene? She kept getting tired of changes at the clinic, and I don't blame her. But when you're poor, what can you do?"

Family Support

Families generally saw professionals in a positive light and appreciated input from them about medication issues (effects, side effects), some biological information about the illness (although many family members felt they were overloaded with technical information, which they could not process and act on), and help in problem-solving difficult management situations. One spouse said, "Well, the doctor really seemed to know what she was talking about, but it was pretty much over my head. I asked a question or two, but she looked impatient, like it was a stupid question or she didn't have time to answer. So after that, I just stopped asking."

Psychoeducational-format groups are helpful in this regard, provided that the professionals involved are not condescending in their approach to family members. However, many of these families indicated that they would be reluctant to join a support group. These families will need individual family help; this includes families of recent-onset patients, as well as those who are extremely cautious or awkward socially and may be embarrassed to discuss their difficulties outside the family. This may also be a necessary format for working with low-income or minority families, unless multifamily groups can be formed that specifically address their cultural issues and conceptions of the problem. A brother noted, "I went to the support group, and they were nice enough folks. But there were no other families of color in the group, and I just didn't feel right about speaking up. Maybe if I knew somebody else who had the problem, who would go with me . . . I don't know." Families require creative flexibility on the part of professionals to help them manage this difficult experience.

Hospitalization

Many families expressed concern about getting their IMs admitted to the hospital, particularly if the IM was not a voluntary commitment, because commitment laws are predicated on the IM's chronological, rather than functional, age. The issue of family members' recognition of early warning signs of decompensation is a good example of their frustration about not being heard, particularly at the crisis center or emergency room. Once the IM was admitted to the hospital, family members were allowed to visit but were rarely allowed to have input into the treatment protocol. They were contacted at the end of the hospitalization, when a discharge plan was being formulated. Some families were bold enough not to take the IM back without a written contract for program services or a sense that the IM was sufficiently stabilized, but most families felt inadequate and powerless to influence the decision of the judge or mental health professionals. A parent remembered, "When they got ready to discharge Julie, that was the first time I heard from the staff at the hospital. They insisted that I should take her home and didn't seem too concerned about my objections. Well,

what could I do? I couldn't say, 'No, I won't take my own daughter.' "

IMPLICATIONS FOR PRACTICE

Despite superficial attention to the biopsychosocial model of human functioning in the *DSM-IV*, it appears that the professional mental health community has become overinvested in a medical model of illness as an intraperson biological phenomenon that seemingly exists without a social context. Although there is significant research in many areas of physical illness that suggests that family interventions can be helpful (McDaniel, Hepworth, & Doherty, 1992; Rolland, 1994), many mental health professionals continue to overlook a rich resource for improving the community functioning of people with mental illness by not including family members' information and insights into the problem.

As an alternative paradigm, the partnership model (which is described more fully elsewhere; see Johnson, 2001) is intended to correct this problem by understanding the patient, the family, and the mental health providers as a triangular partnership team. Like any team, if the members are working together, impressive things can be achieved; but if one of the team members is omitted from the game plan, it is difficult to be successful. Worse, if two of the team members are working at cross-purposes, the results are likely to be ineffective at best, and possibly disastrous. When the IM starts to decompensate, family members tend to blame the professionals, professionals tend to blame the family, and everyone tends to blame the patient. To prevent this from happening, it is imperative that each of the three team components be regarded as an *equal partner* in planning and in executing the plan. If mental health professionals see treatment as something they do *to* or even *for* the patient, they operate with a sense of noblesse oblige that provides them with a feeling of superiority that makes cooperation as a team impossible, even when the intentions are good. To be truly effective in managing a problem as difficult as mental illness, all team members must have respect for the contributions of the other members.

Family members' answers to the question, "What would you like mental health professionals to know?" emphasize the importance of shared goals for the partnership team, and the importance of the way in which these goals are defined. Just as things look different from the perspective of each person in a family, so the triangle looks different from each corner. Because the experiences of people with mental illness are outside the experiences of most of us, it takes considerable effort to appreciate how scary it must feel to not be able to limit and control your thoughts or actions. It is also difficult for those in positions of power to appreciate the experience of powerlessness. Because mental health professionals are often in the position of making decisions about hospitalization, treatment protocol, admission to programs, and so on, it is sometimes difficult for them to appreciate the helpless feelings of family members who wish to aid their IM but are told that they are too intrusive in the program or too protective of the IM. Mental health professionals will *never* have the power that the family has for a person with a serious mental illness. Not to make use of that power is not only ineffective; it is foolish. The therapeutic job for mental health clinicians in the partnership model, therefore, is to enhance and use the competence of the family to help its own member. There is ample evidence to suggest that family members possess this competence, but mental health professionals will be unable to use it, unless their expertise is listened to and respected. The results of this study highlight important avenues for cooperation between members of the partnership team.

FUTURE DIRECTIONS

Results of this and other recent studies indicate that the functioning of people in the community with serious mental illness is strongly impacted by the negative effects of both environmental and illness-related strains, but that these can be significantly buffered by how the family perceives the problem and helps the IM to manage the illness. Possibilities for improved family satisfaction and IM functioning through the support and development of family sense of competence are considerable and achievable by using the resources of the patient, family, self-help supports in the community, and the mental health community in a partnership.

To achieve this vision, funders of mental health services need to work collaboratively with consumer groups and with NAMI to design plans that can be tried in specific situations. If the effort is made to coordinate efforts from the top down, planning is likely to be effective. However, to date, many grassroots efforts to involve family members have met with very limited success because of resistance or inertia in the larger system of mental health providers or funders.

Pilot projects developed for specific locales should include both qualitative and quantitative research components that allow administrators to assess the relative success of the project, both to insure ongoing funding and to see which elements can be replicated successfully. In the current economic climate, it is important that mental health services be provided that are both meaningful and efficiently delivered. This will require some reconceptualization by funders and administrators as well as mental health providers. If mental health professionals can step out of the box of previously defined services and create services that incorporate all three elements of the partnership team, they are likely to find that the end results are more satisfying for them, also.

References

Ambert, A. M., Adler, P. A., Adler, P., & Detzner, D. F. (1995). Understanding and evaluating qualitative research. *Journal of Marriage and the Family, 57,* 879–893.

American Psychiatric Association. (1994). *Diagnostic and statistical manual of mental disorders* (4th ed.). Washington, DC: Author.

Anderson, C. M., Reiss, D. J., & Hogarty, G. E. (1986). *Schizophrenia and the family.* New York: Guilford.

Aviram, U. (1990). Community care of the seriously mentally ill: Continuing problems and current issues. *Community Mental Health Journal, 26,* 69–88.

Bachrach, L. L., Talbott, J. A., & Meyerson, A. T. (1987). The chronic psychiatric patient as a "difficult" patient: A conceptual analysis. In A. T. Meyerson (Ed.), *New directions for mental health services: Vol. 33. Barriers to treating the chronic mentally ill.* San Francisco: Jossey-Bass.

Bernheim, K. F., & Lehman, A. F. (1985). *Working with families of the mentally ill.* New York: Norton.

Coyne, J. C., & Downey, G. (1991). Social factors and psychopathology: Stress, social support, and coping processes. *Annual Review of Psychology, 42,* 401–425.

Gilgun, J. F., Daly, K., & Handel, G. (Eds.). (1992).

Qualitative methods in family research. Newbury Park, CA: Sage.

Goldstein, M. J. (1987). Psychosocial issues. *Schizophrenia Bulletin, 13,* 157–171.

Hatfield, A. B. (1991). The National Alliance for the Mentally Ill: A decade later. *Community Mental Health Journal, 27,* 95–103.

Hatfield, A. B., & Lefley, H. P. (Eds.). (1987). *Families of the mentally ill: Coping and adaptation.* New York: Guilford.

Johnson, E. D. (1998). The effect of family functioning and family sense of competence on people with mental illness. *Family Relations, 47,* 443–451.

Johnson, E. D. (2000). Differences among families coping with serious mental illness: A qualitative analysis. *American Journal of Orthopsychiatry, 70,* 126–134.

Johnson, E. D. (2001). The partnership model: Working with families of people with serious mental illness. In M. MacFarlane (Ed.), *Family therapy and mental health: Innovations in theory and practice* (pp. 27–53). New York: Haworth Clinical Practice Press.

Lefley, H. P. (1992). Expressed emotion: Conceptual, clinical, and social policy issues. *Hospital and Community Psychiatry, 43,* 591–598.

Lefley, H. P. (1996). *Family caregiving in mental illness.* Thousand Oaks, CA: Sage.

Manderscheid, R. W., & Sonnenschein, M.A. (Eds.). (1997). *Mental health, United States, 1996.* Washington, DC: U.S. Department of Health and Human Services, Substance Abuse and Mental Health Services Administration.

McDaniel, S. H., Hepworth, J., & Doherty, W. (1992). *Medical family therapy: A biopsychosocial approach to families with health problems.* New York: Basic Books.

Noh, S., & Turner, R. J. (1987). Living with psychiatric patients: Implications for the mental health of family members. *Social Science and Medicine, 25,* 263–271.

Nuechterlein, K. H., & Dawson, M. E. (1984). A heuristic vulnerability/stress model of schizophrenic episodes. *Schizophrenia Bulletin, 10,* 300–311.

Nuechterlein, K. H., Dawson, M. E., Gitlin, M., Ventura, J., Goldstein, M. J., Snyder, K. S., et al. (1992). Developmental processes in schizophrenic disorders: Longitudinal studies of vulnerability and stress. *Schizophrenia Bulletin, 18,* 387–424.

Rolland, J. S. (1994). *Families, illness, and disability: An integrative treatment model.* New York: Basic Books.

Rosenblatt, P. C., & Fischer, L. R. (1993). Qualitative family research. In P. G. Boss, W. J. Doherty, R. LaRossa, W. R. Schumm, & S. K. Steinmetz (Eds.), *Sourcebook of family theories and methods: A contextual approach* (pp. 167–177). New York: Plenum.

Strachan, A. M. (1986). Family intervention for the rehabilitation of schizophrenia: Toward protection and coping. *Schizophrenia Bulletin, 12,* 678–698.

Torrey, E. F., Bowler, A. E., & Taylor, E. H. (1995). *Schizophrenia and manic depressive disorder: The biological roots of mental illness as revealed by the landmark study of identical twins.* New York: Basic Books.

Whybrow, P. C. (1997). *A mood apart: Depression, mania, and other afflictions of the self.* New York: HarperCollins.

Zubin, J. (1986). Models for the aetiology of schizophrenia. In G. D. Burrows, T. R. Norman, & G. Rubinstein (Eds.), *Handbook of studies on schizophrenia. Part I: Epidemiology, aetiology, and clinical features* (pp. 97–104). New York: Elsevier Science Publishers.

DEATH ON A DAILY BASIS

80

Integrating Research and Practice in Support Groups for ICU Nurses in Southern Brazil

William Gomes, Ciommara R. S. Beninca, & Sherri McCarthy

As noted in the keynote address at a recent Brazilian Psychological Society Convention (Gomes, 2003), psychological research in Brazil has followed a somewhat different path than psychological research in the United States. Until the last few decades, clinical psychologists in Brazil were trained in medical schools, generally by physicians, and Freudian psychoanalysis was the common mode of both research and practice for psychologists in Brazil. At the same time, developments in educational psychology were strongly influenced by the French tradition. In fact, the first psychology lab in Brazil was founded by Alfred Binet.

During the last two decades, graduate programs at federal universities have been preparing doctoral students to conduct more quantitative, outcome-based types of psychological research; but qualitative, phenomenological forms of data collection, case studies, and descriptive research are still the most common types used by Brazilian practitioners, generally quite effectively. This chapter describes a recent intervention to reduce stress in members of the nursing staff of an intensive care unit (ICU) in southern Brazil and its outcome for the nurses. The methodology of the study was derived from the phenomenological tradition of theory and research in psychology common in Brazil.

PHENOMENOLOGICAL THEORY AND PSYCHOLOGICAL PRACTICE

Spielberg (1982) defines phenomenology as a reliance on direct experience to examine the essence of a specific event. Merleau-Ponty (1971) explains it as the direct conscious awareness of life in an existential sense. Lanigan (1992) points out that communication of phenomenological experiences allows individuals to establish new connections between themselves and the people and events in their immediate environment, and hence to reframe their perceptions and redefine their interactions. Giorgi (1985) argues that analysis of phenomenological descriptions of events is the true basis of all worthwhile psychological research.

As suggested by these authors, an intuitive understanding of direct sensations, feelings, and experiences is the basis of self-understanding. Because self-understanding is what psychologists often work to help their clients attain, viewing phenomenological process as the heart of psychology seems to be a valid, logical premise. Furthermore, objectively analyzing and reframing perceptions and experiences to mediate feelings, expressions, and actions is the essential humanistic and cognitive therapeutic strategy that allows clients to adapt to unpleasant or undesired conditions and feelings. Mediating direct perceptions through communication with others to clarify, adjust, and understand one's life experiences is key to effective group and individual therapies. This phenomenological understanding of consciousness and individual reframing of experience is an essential underlying element of virtually all forms of humanistic, client-centered, and even rational-emotive and cognitive-behavioral therapies in use by practitioners (Gomes, 1998), although it is such a basic element that the literature often takes it for granted and fails to address it. Thus, a research methodology that allows for the systematic and sequential organization of a client's direct conscious experiences and sensations related to a particular event and a particular context is essential in psychology. Furthermore, a treatment is not likely to succeed that does not allow for these direct individual experiences and does not enable clients to describe, analyze, and interpret them. Mediating and transforming potentially painful events and maladaptive behaviors rooted in perceptions of these events is the goal of effective psychotherapy.

This is true of both individual and group forms of therapy. Grossman and Silverstein (1993) and Vinogradov and Yalom (1992) point out, in research specifically related to developing coping skills in hospital workers, that effective group therapy relies on combining strategies that enable participants to systematically reflect on their daily experiences and collectively agree on effective coping strategies. This social reframing of events appears to be the key to effective functioning of the psychological support groups that allow hospital staff who deal with death, grief, and bereavement daily to establish and maintain healthy coping skills.

RESEARCH ON DEATH AND DYING

Many psychologists (including Boemer, Rossi, & Nastari, 1989; Figueirado & Turato, 1995; and Spencer, 1994) have defended the necessity of offering health care workers—especially those who work in extremely stressful environments and frequently see death in the course of their work—psychological support to enhance the quality of their own lives. Even from the pragmatic perspective of industrial/organizational psychologists this is warranted, because employees who are under high levels of stress are less likely to work effectively and efficiently and may transfer their own anxiety to the colleagues and clients in their work environments (Ribiero, Baraldi, & Silva, 1998). Obviously, this is not a good situation in a hospital ICU, where skill and efficiency need to be combined with calm and nurturing public relations. Providing support to enhance the coping skills of hospital workers in these conditions is essential. Psychologists on staff in public hospitals should offer such services to health care workers routinely.

Death, dying, grief, and bereavement did not become a legitimate area of research in psychology until the 1970s, when Kübler-Ross's (1969, 1970, 1975, 1978) work with terminally ill patients brought it to the attention of mental health professionals as an important area in need of attention. It is a bit ironic that the one experience we can assume every human being shares, the one behavior we will all engage in and are likely to witness periodically throughout life, was among the latest to attract attention in our field (McCarthy, 1988), especially because philosophers have long noted it as a defining event for humanity. The capacity to accept the inevitability of death is the complex, multifaceted process that makes us uniquely human and allows us to transcend individual pleasures and view life as worthwhile in a long-term, historical, and cultural sense (Feifel, 1959; May, 1976). It may be, in some sense, the source of art and philosophy (Ariès, 1989; Beck, 1987; Morin, 1997; Zeigler, 1977); at the very least, coming to terms with our mortality is what separates us from the animal kingdom and allows us to give meaning to our lives. Furthermore, experiences with death, loss, and separation are defining elements in individual psychological development and influence the occurrence of depression and experiences with mental illness throughout life, as Bowlby's (1969, 1973, 1980) work clearly showed.

Perhaps the "What elephant?" approach to death in our discipline (and in Western society in general, as noted by Kastenbaum and Aisenberg, 1983) is simply a reflection of how difficult it is for humans to cope with the concept. Whether by the prospect of one's own death or by the death of someone close to one, defense mechanisms are triggered. Denial, suppression, repression, regression, and escape are called into play. We compartmentalize (Speer, 1974). We become depressed (Alves & Goody, 1997). We displace our anxiety into psychosomatic illnesses, or we escape with alcohol and drugs, prescription or otherwise. The well-documented tendency of nurses and other hospital staff to suffer from a variety of health-related problems such as fatigue, headaches, irritability, and hypertension and to be at risk for substance abuse (García, 1989) is likely a reflection of the stress associated with attempting to cope with death on a daily basis. Post-traumatic stress disorder symptoms may also reflect this difficulty for the human psyche.

Despite the slow start, by the late 1970s, a fair amount of research and treatment in psychology was devoted to thanatology and grief counseling. The University of Minnesota opened a Center for Death Education Research, and several professional journals were founded, including *Omega, Journal of Death and Dying, Suicide and Life-Threatening Behavior, Hospice Journal, Journal of Palliative Care,* and *Death Studies.* Research on death and death education in Brazil began nearly 20 years later, originating primarily in clinical programs and medical schools at the federal universities in Rio de Janeiro and São Paulo (Lucia & Gavião, 2001; Neves, 2001).

History, philosophy, and causal speculations aside, it has been documented in Brazil that hospital workers tend to use relatively primitive coping strategies such as escape and displacement unless helped to do otherwise (Menzeis, 1969), and that, as a result, both their personal and professional lives are negatively affected. Job burnout, personal crises, and workplace errors are common manifestations of stress in this group (Mallet, Price, Jurs, & Slenker, 1991; Miranda, Assis, Sposito, Araújo, & Delacoleta, 2001). Using what we know about facilitating effective coping with death and learning more about how to improve the process is essential. Because the mental state of staff affects patients and the workplace in general (Kovács, 1992; Santos, Carvalho, Mania, & Rech, 2001), it is an important concern for hospital and industrial/organizational psychologists (Carvalho, 1994; Leitão, 1993) as well as for all therapists and mental health professionals who seek to assist clients with problems. It is especially critical in support group settings among hospital workers (Lewis, 1977; Mandel, 1981; Murphy, 1986; Murray, 1974; Wise, 1974). As the work of Kübler-Ross (1969, 1975, 1978, 1996, 1998) and others (Bowlby, 1969, 1973, 1980; McCarthy, 1988, 1993) has shown, death is a uniquely felt and individually defined life event for each person who experiences the phenomenon. It is best researched and treated in a phenomenological manner, as illustrated in this study. Allowing clients to define, experience, discuss in light of other research, and reframe their individual perceptions of stressful events in supportive and nonthreatening environments is key to improving individual mental health as well as expanding knowledge in the area of grief and bereavement.

A BRIEF HISTORY OF CRITICAL CARE NURSING IN BRAZIL

ICUs in hospitals first became common in the United States during the late 1950s, due to rapid advances in medical technology. In Brazil, this development was delayed by nearly 20 years and occurred somewhat differently (Coelho, 1996). Such units, which now exist in nearly all hospitals in Brazil, are dedicated to preserving life at any cost for victims of accidents or other health conditions that threaten life. The latest medical technology is available to an interdisciplinary team that includes medical doctors from a variety of specialties, nurses, nursing assistants, paramedics, respiratory therapists, physical therapists, occupational therapists, speech pathologists, nutritionists, pharmacists, psychologists, and social workers. Those who work in intensive care units in Brazil must be specially trained and certified by the Brazilian Council of Medicine (Di Biagi, 1993). The staff-to-patient ratio is low in these units and the success rate is high; three of four patients admitted to ICUs survive the traumas that resulted in their admission (Sebastiani, 1999). Despite this, the burnout rate of ICU staff members is very high. The increased responsibility for patient survival and specific technical skills required puts workers at high risk for stress-related disorders (Laperta & Duarte, 1996; Rivetti, 1993; Silva, 1998). And the sense of failure and impotence staff members feel when a patient dies (Keyes & Hofling, 1985)—combined with the rapid pace and sense of immediacy, which allows no time for reflection (Barreto, 1993; Laufert, 1997)—increases the risk for stress-related illness and substance abuse (García, 1989). Another factor that increases stress is the perceived hierarchy in the medical work environment, with nurses feeling that the doctors are superior and constantly striving to maintain a cool, professional image, which requires constant impression management (Boemer et al., 1989; Hartmann, 1998; Pitta, 1991). In a work environment that demands constant attention (Spencer, 1994) and often requires staff to mask their true feelings for the benefit of patients (Alves & Godley, 1997), colleagues, or themselves (Ribeiro et al., 1998), it is no wonder that Menzies (1969) found in an extensive 3-year study that workers use defense mechanisms ineffectively, demonstrate immature and maladaptive coping strategies, and are emotionally overtaxed. It is also not surprising that Pitta (1991) concluded that it is difficult if not impossible for these workers to handle stress without psychological intervention and support.

HYPOTHESES AND DESIGN CONSIDERATIONS

The study described here was grounded in the basic information and framework just described. It was hypothesized that, because of the hierarchical nature of hospital social structure, relatively homogenous support groups including only members of relatively equal professional status would be most effective and would allow for the most open expression among members. Because, as Mello (1994) and others have noted, the employees with the least professional training and preparation are those most likely to have direct contact with terminal patients and thus to experience the most stressful conditions with the least preparation, the group presented here as an example is comprised primarily of nursing assistants. Phenomenological theory dictates that individual phenomena, as uniquely experienced and communicated by individuals, should comprise the basis of both psychological research and practice, so a design to allow for this was incorporated. Because context is also an important determinant of both effectiveness and transferability of group material, all research and treatment occurred at the hospital, in or near the ICU. Furthermore, because some of the research just cited noted that health care workers are likely to use rudimentary defense mechanisms and immature coping strategies, the design allowed for a comfortable distancing of potentially painful direct experiences. Group members were assisting the psychologist in examining data gathered in their workplace from observed behaviors and interviews.

The research and treatment occurred in a relatively seamless manner. During the first phase, the psychologist conducted a series of structured interviews with 10 ICU staff members on the jobsite and completed 15 systematic observations of approximately one hour each. During the second phase, 12 employees participating in a support group were asked to assist the psychologist with her research by discussing and critiquing the content of the interviews and observations during their group meetings. During the final phase, structured interviews, systematic obser-

vations, and other assessments of worker stress levels were used to determine the effectiveness of the treatment. Thus, the phenomenological experiences of the clients became the content of both the research and the treatment in a pure researcher–practitioner therapeutic design.

METHOD

Participants

Those who participated in the study were 22 nursing assistants employed in an ICU unit at a public hospital in a small city (population approximately 150,000) in southern Brazil. Each participant either completed a structured interview about his or her experience while working in the ICU or participated in a support group mediated by a trained psychologist. Specific information about subjects appears in Table 80.1.

Average age of the two males and eight females interviewed was 31 years. Most had worked in intensive care nursing for less than 4 years. The content of the interviews was discussed during three sessions of a support group comprised of two males and ten females. Most members of the support group had worked in intensive care nursing longer than members of the interview group, although the majority had also been working in the ICU for 4 years or less. Average age of group members was 31 years.

Procedure

As described previously, the data collected from the interviewed participants served as the basis for treatment. Support group discussions fo-

TABLE 80.1 Interview Participants

Gender	Age	Years at ICU
P1F	25	1
P2M	27	1
P3F	21	2
P4M	21	2
P5F	25	3
P6F	37	2
P7F	41	10
P8F	47	14
P9F	23	1
P10F	40	2

TABLE 80.2 Group Participants

Gender	Age	Years at ICU
P3F	21	2
P6F	37	2
P8F	47	14
P11M	22	2
P12F	42	4
P13F	28	4
P14F	34	8
P15M	40	11
P16F	19	1
P17F	37	2
P18F	21	7
P19F	25	3

cused on the information collected during systematic observations and scripted interviews. Observations followed research guidelines set forth by Patton (1990), including written accounts of setting, activities, people present, social situations, verbal exchange, expressions and nonverbal tone, and significant events on 15 different occasions in the ICU. The format for scripted interviews and for evaluation of qualitative data was developed according to qualitative research guidelines described in Creswell (1994), Gomes (1987, 1988), Lincoln and Gruber (1985), and Newman and Benz (1998). In line with appropriate analysis of phenomenological research, descriptive data was reduced to key elements and interpreted by both the clients and the psychologist researcher–practitioner. This process is depicted in Table 80.3.

Following data collection, the content of the observations and interviews was brought to groups for discussion. The content for discussion was derived by a method of identifying the themes that occurred most frequently in observations and interviews and those that elicited the most emotionally loaded reactions from staff during observations and interviews as evidenced by language, speech patterns, and nonverbal cues. These themes were then organized topically to guide three weekly support group sessions. Thematic reduction from interview and observation data used to structure group encounters appears in Table 80.4.

Results

The content of the interviews determined group content. Complete transcripts and analysis of all interview text, as well as detailed observational descriptions and outcome measures, are available (see Beninca, 2003), but for the sake of brevity, only the previously noted summary of selected topics and one sample discussion are presented here. The sample discussion shown in Box 80.1 was transcribed from the third session, when group members talked about their feelings about facing death of patients. It is worth noting that the research critique role of group members facilitated an immediate transition to a topic other support groups typically avoid due to the defense mechanisms and immature coping strategies characteristic of workers in an ICU environment, as noted by other researchers.

Because the process did encourage reflection and develop positive peer support, coping strategies were enhanced for all participants. Group members spontaneously suggested and discussed many positive strategies for reducing stress, practiced these suggestions, and shared the results in subsequent group meetings. Work environment improved, absenteeism and reported difficulties decreased, and systematic observations confirmed the success of the intervention.

Responses to questions in follow-up interviews also verified that group members were feeling more relaxed, less threatened by and less personally responsible for patient deaths, and less preoccupied. Healthier coping strategies were described, and members attributed their improvements in attitude to the group experiences, noting that the camaraderie and the sense that they were not isolated in their fears and feelings, as well as the constructive suggestions offered by coworkers, were responsible for their improved attitudes.

One month after support group sessions, subsequent observations and interviews—combined with group member evaluations of the process and workplace outcome measures such as absenteeism, employee turnover, health complaints, and employee error rates—were used to assess results of the intervention. According to all dimensions measured, the outcome of this phenomenologically derived group intervention and research process was a success.

IMPLICATIONS FOR PRACTICE-BASED RESEARCH

Researcher–practitioner models, considered an ideal practice mode for psychologists by many, are phenomenological in nature. A structure for

TABLE 80.3 Three-Step Phenomenological Design

Step	Focus	Instruments and Materials	Analysis	Phenomenological Results
1	Gathering of experiential (phenomenological) data in context	ICU observations Interviews	Description Observation protocols Transcriptions of interviews Reduction Thematic specification Interpretation Comprehensive analysis in context	Description
2	Group's discussion	Phenomenological description from Step 1	Description Group's discussion Reduction Thematic specification by group's participant Interpretation Group evaluation of process benefits	Reduction
3	Researchers' phenomenological analyses	Materials from Steps 1 and 2	Description Researchers' critical understanding of the whole process Reduction Defining crucial points of the experience Interpretation Critical comparison of present experiences of group to other data and group experience	Interpretation

research and practice, as illustrated by the case described here, offers many advantages. From a treatment perspective, dealing directly with actual experiences in grief support groups rather than simply educating group members about the stages of dying, and offering suggestions and as-

suming the role of an outsider educating those who are learning from their experiences daily, are powerful means of facilitating self-reflection and building healthy coping strategies. Using discussion of observational and interview data collected on the work site from others is an ap-

TABLE 80.4 Themes for Group Discussion

First Session: Characteristics of Working in ICU	Second Session: ICU Patients and Their Families	Third Session: Deaths in the ICU	Fourth Session: Group Experience Evaluation
• Professionalism • Team work • Isolation	• Nurse and patient relations • Nurse and patient's family relations • Nurse and family relations	• Facing death on a daily basis • Coping strategies	

Box 80.1 Phenomenological Reduction of Experience Facing Death: Group Transcript

P3F: I think that . . . the more difficult is not the death itself, but it's when a patient takes your hand and says, "Please help me; I cannot take this pain." I think that one feels very impotent facing it. Or when a patient says, "Let me go; I don't want stay here anymore." What can you say to them?

[Group reflection]

Group facilitator: What to say? That is the point.

P3F: I don't know what to say, I don't know what to do. . . . I am tired of saying to them, "Hold on just a little bit more, you're going to make it!" when we know that they probably won't make it. What do you say when you have no expectations left? I don't know what else to do with this, because you create an expectation and there's hope for you and the patient and then, before you know it, the patient dies.

P12F: I think that these situations are harder then death. . . . And it is harder to watch the suffering of a living patient that is with us every day.

P16F: Sometimes we think, "Oh, he died well, he rested!" It's odd to cheer for someone's death, but we do.

P12F: Mrs. C has to rest. She can even die with me! . . . I don't have the heart to be there, holding her myself. . . . And she says, "The real help that I need right now is to let me die!"

Group Facilitator: P3F pointed out that she feels she is lying to herself and the dying patient when she says, "No, you're not going to die."

P6F: We don't have anything else to say. We have to lie.

P12F: The patient says, "Will I leave the hospital?" Of course you will. . . . Will she, in the state that she is in?

P3F: Why prolong all this suffering if, in the end, the only propect is death?

P6F: Normally, the ones who are supposed to heal don't last long afterwards anyway."

P17F: It's as if the doctors say, "That one can die, but this one can't!"

P12F: Well, for how long can a doctor prolong one's suffering? When can we say that there is nothing else to do, that we should let someone die? . . . I don't feel well treating those who are on do-not-resuscitate orders. If the heart stops, stop trying to help." Because if it is "if stop, stop," will I keep investing? If it is "if stop, stop," take him out of here and put someone else in his place for me to help! No, he stays there. . . . We do what they tell us to do. But then I can feel relieved because I've done what I was told to and it wasn't my decision. It's not on me.

P3F: The problem is: you feel powerless, you can't do a thing.

propriate means of distancing the material from participants. As research helpers, those in helping professions are able to quickly go to the heart of issues that concern them without the direct threat that may exist if questions directly related to personal experiences are incorporated to lead them there.

This type of group preparation by psychologists—data gathering in context—is likely far more valuable than time devoted to reading and handouts in preparation for more traditional death education models for ICU staff support groups that are currently used in Brazilian hospitals. Even if a bit of the Hawthorne effect is responsible for the group success, success is success regardless. As famous writer Aldous Huxley once noted, it is amazing that someone without a strong background in psychological research can be a good practical psychologist, and perhaps even more surprising that someone with a strong research background can be a good practical psychologist. But the methodology described here supports both enterprises. The success of groups conducted following this model may be viewed as a sufficient end, but it is also worth noting that data gathered in this way are extremely valuable. This qualitative data are of the same type that Kübler-Ross used to begin her research on death and dying many years ago and are the purest and most useful form for use in death counseling. Organizing ICU support groups by first observing and interviewing staff members, then asking others to analyze and interpret the research in support group settings, results in a continuous, current, and contextual database for use by both hospital psychologists and other researchers. It is efficient as well as valuable and is a recommended practice for all practitioners who work in the area of grief and bereavement counseling with health care professionals.[1]

Note

1. The authors would like to thank Nat Pallone and Al Roberts for the opportunity to share this valuable strategy with other psychologists and to apologize for pirating Nat's e-mail epithet from Huxley for use, a quote that seemed so appropriate here.

References

Alves, R. N., & Godoy, S. A. F. (1997). Reflexões sobre a morte e a AIDS na rotina de Enfermagem. *Psicologia em Estudo, 2*(3), 79–91.

Ariès, P. (1989). *O Homem diante da morte*. Rio de Janeiro, Brazil: Francisco Alves.

Barreto, S. M. (1993). *Rotinas em Terapia Intensiva*. Porto Alegre, Brazil: Artes Médicas.

Beck, C. L. C. (1995). *O processo de viver, adoecer e morrer: Reflexões com familiares de pacientes internados em uma unidade de terapia intensiva*. Dissertação de Mestrado não-publicada, Curso de Mestrado em Assistência de Enfermagem, Universidade Federal de Santa Catarina, Florianópolis.

Beninca, C. R. S. (2003). *Apoio psicologia a enfermagem diante da morte: Estudo fenomeologia*. Dissertacao de Doutora nao-publicada, Curso de Doutora em Psicologia, Universidade Federal do Rio do Sul, Porto Alegre, Brazil.

Boemer, M. R. (1986). *A Morte e o morrer*. São Paulo, Brazil: Cortez.

Boemer, M. R., Rossi, L. R. G., & Nastari, R. R. (1989). A idéia de morte em Unidade de Terapia Intensiva: Análise de depoimentos. *Revista Gaúcha de Enfermagem, 10*(2).

Boemer, M. R., Veiga, E. V., Mendes, M. M. R., & Valle, E. R. M. (1991). O tema da morte: Uma proposta de educação. *Revista Gaúcha de Enfermagem, 12*(1), 26–32.

Bowlby, J. (1969). *Attachment and Loss: Vol. 1. Attachment*. London: Hogarth.

Bowlby, J. (1973). *Attachment and Loss: Vol. 2. Separation*. London: Hogarth.

Bowlby, J. (1980). *Attachment and Loss: Vol. 3. Loss, sadness and depression*. Harmondsworth, England: Penguin.

Bromberg, M. H. P. F., Kovács, M. J., Carvalho, M. M. M. J., & Carvalho, V. A. (1996). *Vida e morte: Laços de existência*. São Paulo: Casa do Psicólogo.

Carvalho, M. V. B. de. (1994). O preparo do professor de enfermagem, ensinando e refletindo com o aluno a lidar com a morte de pacientes terminais [Resumos]. Em Associação Brasileira de Enfermagem (Org.), *Anais, 46° Congresso Brasileiro de Enfermagem* (p. 26). Porto Alegre, Brazil: Seção RS.

Coelho, C. D. (1996). Humanizando a terapia intensiva. *Revista Realidade Hospitalar, 2*, 10–11.

Creswell, J. W. (1994). *Research design: Qualitative versus quantitative approaches*. London: Sage.

Di Biagi, T. M. (1993). Lidando com o paciente terminal e seus familiares. Em H. B. C. Chiatonne & M. Andreis (Orgs.), *Os limites da vida* (pp. 38–40). Simpósio conduzido pelo Serviço de Psicologia Hospitalar da Santa Casa, São Paulo, Brazil.

Feifel, H. (1959). *The meaning of death*. New York: McGraw-Hill.

Figueiredo, R. M., & Turato, E. R. (1995). A enfermagem diante do paciente com AIDS e a morte. *Jornal Brasileiro de Psiquiatria, 44*, 641–647.

García, J. C. (1989). As Ciências Sociais em Medicina.

Em E. D. Nunes (Org.). *Juan Cesar García/ ABRASCO* (pp. 62–63). São Paulo, Brazil: Cortez.

Giorgi, A. (1985). Sketch of a psychological phenomenological method. In A. Giori (Ed.), *Phenomenology and psychological research* (pp. 8–22). Pittsburgh, PA: Duquesne University Press.

Gomes, W. B. (1987). As aplicações sociais da pesquisa qualitativa. *Psicologia: Reflexão e Crítica, 2,* 3–12.

Gomes, W. B. (1988). A experiência retrospectiva de estar em psicoterapia: Um estudo empírico fenomenológico. *Psicologia: Teoria e Pesquisa, 4*(3), 187–206.

Gomes, W. B. (1998). A entrevista fenomenológica e o estudo da experiência consciente. Em W. B. Gomes (Org.), *Fenomenologia e Pesquisa em Psicologia* (pp. 19–44). Porto Alegre, Brazil: Ed. Universidade Federal do Rio Grande do Sul.

Gomes, W. B. (2003, May). Keynote Address at the Annual Meeting of the Brazilian Psychological Society, Joa Passoa, PN, Brazil.

Grossman, A. H., & Silverstein, C. (1993). Facilitating support groups for professionals working with people with AIDS. *Social Work, 38*(2), 144–151.

Hartmann, J. B. (1998). Saúde e doença na perspectiva dos profissionais de saúde no hospital. *Psico—USF, 3*(2), 59–74.

Kastenbaum, R., & Aisenberg, R. (1983). *Psicologia da Morte.* São Paulo, Brazil: Pioneira.

Keyes, J. J., & Hofling, C. K. (1985). *Conceitos básicos em enfermagem psiquiátrica.* Rio de Janeiro, Brazil: Interamericana.

Kovács, M. J. (1987). O Medo da morte: Uma abordagem multidimensional. *Boletim de Psicologia, 37*(87), 58–62.

Kovács, M. J. (1992). *Morte e Desenvolvimento Humano.* São Paulo, Brazil: Casa do Psicólogo.

Kübler-Ross, E. (1969). *On death and dying.* New York: Macmillan.

Kübler-Ross, E. (1975). *Death: The final stage of growth.* Englewood Cliffs, NJ: Prentice Hall.

Kübler-Ross, E. (1978). *To live until we say goodbye.* Englewood Cliffs, NJ: Prentice Hall.

Kübler-Ross, E. (1996). *Morte: estágio final da evolução.* Rio de Janeiro, Brazil: Record.

Kübler-Ross, E. (1998). *Sobre a morte e o morrer.* São Paulo, Brazil: Martins Fontes.

Lanigan, R. L. (1992). *Phenomenology of communication.* Pittsburgh, PA: Duquesne University Press.

Lanigan, R. L. (1997). *Capta versus Data*: Método e evidência em comunicologia. *Psicologia: Reflexão e Crítica, 10*(1), 17–45.

Laperta, M. C. M. T., & Duarte, M. S. Z. (1996). *Percepções e necessidades dos pacientes, familiares e equipes na Unidade de Terapia Intensiva—Um estudo qualitativo.* Monografia de Especialização não-publicada, Curso de Especialização em Psi-

cologia Hospitalar, Instituto Sedes Sapientiae, São Paulo, Brazil.

Laufert, L. (1997a). O desgaste profissional: Uma revisão da literatura e implicações para a enfermeira. *Revista Gaúcha de Enfermagem, 18*(2), 83–93.

Laufert, L. (1997b). O desgaste profissional: Estudo empírico com enfermeiras que trabalham em hospitais. *Revista Gaúcha de Enfermagem, 18*(2), 133–144.

Leitão, M. S. (1993). *O psicólogo e o hospital.* Porto Alegre, Brazil: Sagra Luzzatto.

Lewis, F. M. (1977, December). A time to live and a time to die: An instructional drama. *Nursing Outlook,* 762–765.

Lincoln, Y. S., & Guba, E. G. (1985). *Naturalistic inquiry.* Beverly Hills, CA: Sage.

Lucia, M. C. S., & Gavião, A .C. D. (2001). Novas abordagens em Psicologia hospitalar: Teoria dos Campos e escuta psicanalítica a equipes de enfermagem [Resumos]. Em Sociedade Brasileira de Psicologia (Org.), *Resumos e Comunicações Científicas* (p. 281). Rio de Janeiro, Brazil: SBP.

Mallett, K., Price, J. H., Jurs, S. G., & Slenker, S. (1991). Relationship among burnout, death anxiety, and social support in hospice and critical care nurses. *Psychological Reports, 68,* 1347–1359.

Mandel, H. R. (1981, June). Nurses' feelings about working with the dying. *American Journal of Nursing,* 1194–1197.

May, R. (1976). *Psicologia existencial* (pp. 67–82). Porto Alegre: Brazil Ed. Globo.

McCarthy, S. (1988). *A death in the family.* Vancouver, British Columbia, Canada: International Self-Counsel.

McCarthy, S. (1993, April). Death in our schools. Workshop at the annual meeting of the American Educational Research Association, Atlanta, GA.

Mello, C. M. M. (1994). *Divisão Social do Trabalho de Enfermagem.* São Paulo, Brazil: Cortez.

Menzies, I. E. P. (1969). El funcionamiento de los sistemas sociales como defensa contra la ansiedad. Em I.E.P. Menzies & E. Jacques (Org.), *Los sistemas sociales como defensa contra la ansiedad* (pp. 53–125). Buenos Aires, Argentina: Hormé.

Merleau-Ponty, M. (1971). *Fenomenologia da percepção.* (R. di Piero, trad.). Rio de Janeiro. Brazil: Livraria Freitas Bastos. (Originalmente publicado em francês, 1945.)

Miranda, F. M. L., Assis, F. M. V., Sposito, L. S., Araújo, R. R., & Delacoleta, M. F. (2001). O stress entre enfermeiros de um hospital universitário [Resumos]. Em Sociedade Brasileira de Psicologia (Org.), *Resumos e Comunicações Científicas* (p. 278). Rio de Janeiro, Brazil: SBP.

Morin, E. (1997). *O Homem e a morte.* Rio de Janeiro, Brazil: Imago.

Murphy, P. A. (1986). Reduction in nurses' death anxiety following a death awareness workshop. *Journal of Continuing Education in Nursing, 17*(4), 115–118.

Murray, P. (1974). Death education and its effect on the death anxiety level of nurses. *Psychological Reports, 35,* 1251.

Neves, F. S. (2001). Grupos de investigação em função terapêutica (GIFT)—Uma experiência psicanalítica na enfermagem dos Instituto Central do Hospital das Clínicas, FMUSP [Resumos]. Em Sociedade Brasileira de Psicologia (Org.), *Resumos e Comunicações Científicas* (p. 282). Rio de Janeiro, Brazil: SBP.

Newman, I., & Benz, C. R. (1998). *Qualitative versus quantitative research methodology: Exploring the interactive continuum.* Carbondale: Southern Illinois University Press.

Patton, M. Q. (1990). *Qualitative evaluation methods.* Beverly Hills, CA: Sage.

Pitta, A. (1991). *Hospital: Dor e morte como ofício.* São Paulo, Brazil: HUCITEC.

Ribeiro, M. C., Baraldi, S., & Silva, M. J. P. (1998). A Percepção da equipe de enfermagem em situação de morte: ritual do preparo do corpo "pós-morte." *Revista da Escola de Enfermagem da USP, 32*(2), 117–123.

Rivetti, L. A. (1993). Fatores estressantes do exercício profissional. Em H. B. C. Chiatonne & M. Andreis (Orgs.), *Os Limites da Vida* (pp. 41–42). Simpósio conduzido pelo Serviço de Psicologia Hospitalar da Santa Casa, São Paulo.

Santos, A. N. A., Carvalho, F. T., Mania, V. M., & Rech, T. (2001). Sou enfermeira. Meu paciente morreu. E agora? *Revista da Sociedade de Psicologia do Rio Grande do Sul, 1*(1), 7–11.

Sebastiani, R. W. (1999). Atendimento psicológico no centro de terapia intensiva. Em W. A. Angerami-Camon, F. A. R. Trucharte, R. B. Knijnik, & R. W. Sebastiani (Eds.), *Psicologia Hospitalar: Teoria e Prática* (pp. 29–71). São Paulo, Brazil: Pioneira.

Silva, C. O. (1998). Trabalho e subjetividade no hospital geral. *Psicologia Ciência e Profissão, 18*(2), 2633.

Speer, G. M. (1974). Learning about death. *Perspectives in Psychiatric Care, 12,* 70–73.

Spencer, L. (1994). How do nurses deal with their own grief when a patient dies on an intensive care unit, and what help can be given to enable them to overcome their grief effectively? *Journal of Advanced Nursing, 19,* 1141–1150.

Spielberg, H. (1982). *The phenomenological movement* (2 vols., 3rd ed., rev.). The Hague, The Netherlands: Martinus Nijhoff.

Vinogradov, S., & Yalom, I. D. (1992). *Manual de psicoterapia de grupo.* Porto Alegre, Brazuil: Artes Médicas.

Wise, D. J. (1974). Learning about dying. *Nursing Outlook, 22*(1), 42–44.

Ziegler, J. (1977). *Os vivos e a morte.* Rio de Janeiro, Brazil: Zahar.

FAMILY STATUS AND SOUP KITCHEN USE

81 *Some Policy Considerations Based on Qualitative Research Findings*

Harris Chaiklin & Marc Lipton

There have always been soup kitchens, but they usually do not surge in growth or get much attention until the economy is in decline. Their recent expansion only partly follows the historical trend. Contributing factors have been a recession, our productive economy's changing nature, lack of housing, deinstitutionalization, the cutback in federal support programs, and the failure to make up for these cuts at the state and local levels. Over the last 20 years, soup kitchen use has increased, even when economic conditions were good.

Historically and in the present, soup kitchen use is closely related to being homeless. Although not all soup kitchen users are homeless, those who are homeless get most of their food at soup kitchens. About 75% of the homeless have no family relations (Bassuk, 1984). The question this chapter is concerned with is whether this holds true for soup kitchen users.

It is becoming increasingly difficult to obtain services for the dispossessed. Housing, especially in large cities, is expensive and in short supply. The expansion of low-income housing is slowing down, and maintenance funds for existing public housing are shrinking. Low-priced centrally located rooming houses and hotels are scarce, and deinstitutionalization has put additional pressure on social welfare resources (Hartman, 1984).

Several of the megatrends identified by Naisbitt (1982) provide a way of summing up pressures that have allowed soup kitchens to flourish. One of these is the move from centralization to decentralization. There is resistance to enacting federal legislation that will apply uniformly across the country. National phenomena will have to be handled on a local basis. When it comes to helping the disadvantaged, this means that change will be slow.

There is a drift away from institutional help to self-help. People no longer believe that government can help them. The growth of the soup kitchen is an example of self-help at its best. The majority of them are staffed by lay citizens who prepare and serve food.

Two other elements support the move to decentralization and self-help. These are the shift from representative to participatory democracy and the change from hierarchies to networking (Naisbitt, 1982). People want to be involved in determining their fate. We are moving from a homogenized society to one of great diversity. This heterogeneity helps to create a situation in which the uniformity that is required by policy is difficult to achieve at any level.

As with any tension issue in society, trying to understand the soup kitchen is clouded by controversy. Questions about the family aspect of soup kitchen use are often dismissed as irrelevant to what is deemed to be an overwhelming immediate pressing need to feed people and to find a way to get rid of soup kitchens, because they represent a failure of our society.

THE SURVEY

These data were part of a survey undertaken for the Baltimore City Health Department in the summer of 1983.[1] It was a survey in the classic sense of the word. No hypotheses were being tested. The data were collected to illuminate the problem and to provide a basis for change. A survey is held to the same technical standards as research in its sampling and data collection procedures. The distinction between a survey and research lies in aim rather than technique. Any survey could become research simply through conceptualizing the data, even on an ex post facto basis.

Because the aim of a survey is to deal with problems, this inevitably raises the question of who defines something as a problem. Long ago, Willard Waller (1936) pointed out that an essential element in understanding why any issue is considered a social problem lies in finding where there is a conflict of values. One may be against poverty; there is also a limit as to how much one is willing to raise taxes to alleviate this. The Baltimore City Health Department wanted data to use for planning services.

PROCEDURE

The sample was developed by first identifying the number of soup kitchens in Baltimore. This was easier said than done. Starting with a list obtained from the Maryland Food Bank, we identified 31 soup kitchens before the study was over. The kitchens fell into three rough categories. Three large kitchens were responsible for about 60% of all meals fed. At least 10% of the users of the large kitchens were interviewed.

Of the 31 kitchens identified, interviews were done in 17, there were 7 refusals, and 7 kitchens either closed before they could be reached or opened too late to be included in the study. The refusals were concentrated in the mission kitchens, so only three of eight mission kitchens were sampled. These were small kitchens that usually fed only those living there, and all were run by fundamentalist groups that seemed suspicious of anything even remotely connected with government. The church-run soup kitchen refusals were for reasons similar to those given for the mission refusals. The final sample of 271 was approximately 15% of the population.

INTERVIEWING

In a survey, the major methodological problems lie in getting accurate interviews and sampling. In the present study, the interview was designed to maximize response. Only clear, simple objective questions were asked, and interviewers were trained before they entered the field. A review of the literature on self-reporting had indicated that even the most distressed people could give accurate answers to appropriately phrased objective questions (Chaiklin, 1983, pp. 22–29). All interviews were voluntary, and once initiated, fewer than a half-dozen interviews were not completed. Initial refusal rates ran about 40%, but these dropped to a steady 20% once the interviewers, who were graduate students in social work, gained confidence. Refusal rates were highest in the large central city kitchens where the users represented a more varied and distressed population.

Interviewers were instructed to ask every fifth person in line for an interview. If this person refused, the interviewer was to count off five more persons and ask again. Although this sample was not random, the population was homogeneous enough to make the data useful for planning purposes.

FINDINGS

Because the aim was to provide a picture of the user, data are presented in terms of modal categories. In a survey, the data are valuable for their descriptive powers, so no statistical tests were used.

Profile

In the summer of 1983, the typical soup kitchen user in Baltimore was male, African American, and under age 40, and had been born in Baltimore. He was single, had no children, lived alone, and was not a veteran. He did not finish high school, had few job skills, and was in Class V as measured by Hollingshead's two-factor index (Hollingshead & Redlich, 1958). He was unemployed (88%) but had been attached to the labor market (72% of those interviewed indicated that they had held one job for 2 years or longer). The typical soup kitchen user tended to feel that he had physical or emotional limitations in his ability to work. There were also some strengths. The typical user was not isolated and tended to report contact with children (70%), family (70%), and friends (79%). He also was likely to have some income (59%), usually from a government program. Despite this, the typical soup kitchen patron seemed to have few alternatives in the world, evidenced by his dependence on the kitchen for food. Such individuals tended to know where they would sleep on a given night, but many would spend the night either on a street or in a mission.

Service Use

Service use is high and shows the distress of these people. Over half (51%) said that they needed help from a service agency but 69% said they were not getting help. In the previous 10 years, 43% of the sample had been inpatients in medical hospitals, and 28% had been inpatients in mental hospitals. Alcoholism played an even larger role than mental illness, with 13% currently using such services and 17% saying that they needed them. An additional 11% said they did not know. Judging by the frequency with which alcohol was detected on the breath of interviewees and the fact that kitchens do not let in "messy drunks," it is our estimate that perhaps 67% of the soup kitchen population was involved with alcohol overuse. Soup kitchen use, therefore, appeared to be a reflection of either untreated alcoholism or treatment without the necessary social supports. However, alcoholism and soup kitchens are usually considered separately when policy related to service planning is made.

Family Status and Service Use

When family status was considered in relation to service use, those who reported being married were less likely to have been in medical or mental hospitals and less likely to have been using alcoholism clinics. They were also less likely to say that they needed to be treated in a medical outpatient clinic and less likely to say that they needed help from a social agency. The tendency of those who were married to have more positive social characteristics was carried over in their tendency to be healthier than what was reflected in the modal characteristics in the sample.

Those who reported being separated were more likely to say that they needed to go to a medical outpatient clinic and were more likely to

be getting help from a social agency. Here, too, the tendency of those who were separated to be from disadvantaged racial and social categories was reflected in a tendency to indicate that they needed help or were receiving help. Middle-aged African Americans reported high levels of physical health service use and need.

The widowed differed from the modal categories on so many characteristics that they can be said to constitute a distinctly separate category. They were more likely to have been in a medical hospital in the last 10 years but less likely to have been in a mental hospital. They were more likely to have used a medical outpatient clinic in the last 10 years and less likely to say that they needed a psychiatric outpatient clinic. They were more likely to be taking medication for a physical problem and less likely to be taking medication for an emotional problem. They were less likely to be getting help from a social agency and more likely to say that they needed it. The widowed were thus more likely to be physically sick and less likely to be involved with emotional illness. This is consistent with the social characteristics of older soup kitchen users. There were many females in the category.

The divorced were more likely than the mode to have been inpatients in medical hospitals and more likely to say that they need outpatient treatment in a medical clinic. This seemed to be a function of age.

Those who were single did not differ on any modal categories. Their greater numbers in the soup kitchen population tended to conceal the importance of family status as a variable for understanding soup kitchen users and planning services for them. Those who indicated having ever been in any kind of family arrangement were older, more likely to be women, and more likely to be physically sick and have great needs. When someone from a family used a soup kitchen, it meant that either the family had been shattered or that there was severe stress in the family relationship. When someone who had some kind of marital status used a soup kitchen, he or she represented a category of persons who were in greater relative need than those who said that they were single.

All soup kitchen users had great needs, but those who had created families seemed at more immediate risk of becoming institutionalized. Mental illness was the most probable cause, but it was doubtful that such a person would be able to stay in a hospital long enough to get the help that was needed, and outpatient facilities were inadequate. An important element in making deinstitutionalization finally take off occurred when state and local governments realized that this was a way to federalize the cost of caring for a significant share of the dependent population. Unfortunately, the community mental health centers that were supposed to accompany deinstitutionalization were never built in sufficient numbers. While this policy struggle continues, many of those who are affected by the lack of needed services eat in soup kitchens and sleep in shelters or on the streets.

This conclusion is supported by a look at selected behavioral characteristics on a mental-status-by-observation estimate done on each interviewee after the interview (Johnson, Snibbe, & Evans, 1975, Chapter 3). In only two characteristics, "dirty clothing" (52%) and "appears depressed" (51%) were negative feature characteristics and modal characteristics, but the diagnostic indicators in all other characteristics greatly exceeded the proportions found in the general population. The physical descriptors which had high rates were "looking unkempt," "poor posture," and "sadness." In short, from the perspective of the interviewers, this was a group of people who did not look good and who manifested a depressed air. In addition, a significant subgroup was anxious, angry, and agitated. There were few happy-go-lucky, irresponsible poor people using soup kitchens.

Marital status stood out as an important factor. Those who were married were less likely to have dirty clothing, more likely to manifest anxiety, and more likely to have angry facial expressions. They were less likely to have agitated body movements and less likely to be suspicious. But anxiety and anger were noted in far greater proportion than in the other categories. We do not want to make too many interpretations based on the 13 married people in the sample, but we should like to note that the positive features presented here, of looking better in terms of dress and seeming to be better put together, were consistent with the married persons' more positive social characteristics and pattern of service usage. Their anxiety and anger raised the possibility that they were suffering in a different way.

Those who were separated were more likely than the mode to have dirty clothing, less likely to manifest anxiety, and more likely to have sad facial expressions and agitated body movements, and to appear depressed. This, too, was consistent with prior differences. Their negative social characteristics and greater use of medical facilities marked those who were separated as a disadvantaged group who did not look well and who seemed depressed.

The widowed were more likely than the mode to have dirty clothing and less likely to have slumped posture or rigid posture, to manifest anxiety, to have sad facial expressions, or to be suspicious. This was consistent with the prior picture of the widowed as being old, poor, and sick but not making much use of mental health services.

The divorced were more likely than the mode to have slumped posture and angry facial expressions. This is consistent with being poor and not having good physical health. The single did not differ from the mode on any characteristic. They reflected the predominate view contained in the description of the sample's modal categories.

Interviewer's Estimates of Service Need

The interviewers were asked to estimate the need for service in the areas of interest to the Health Department. They concluded that 43% of soup kitchen users interviewed needed mental health services, 38% needed alcohol abuse treatment services, 8% needed drug abuse treatment services, and 5% needed mental retardation services. These estimates reflected the circumstances that make the greatest contribution to the soup kitchen population.

A methodological note on these estimates concerns the willingness of the interviewers to reach diagnostic conclusions. Even though the interviewers were social work students, they consistently underestimated the needs of the soup kitchen users whom they interviewed. This statement is based on the conclusions of the first author, who conducted about 5% of the interviews. Even though this was stressed in the interviewers' training, and the first author personally reviewed the coding of each schedule with the interviewer, it was hard for the interviewers to make judgments, because their socialization in the social work profession in an antidiagnostic era left them feeling like therapists but unwilling to make judgments.

In terms of difference from the modal categories, the married were less likely to be seen as needing services for alcohol abuse. The separated did not differ on any modal categories. The widowed were seen as less likely than the mode to need mental and alcohol abuse services. The divorced were seen as more likely to need alcohol abuse services. And the single did not differ from the mode in any respect. This patterning was more or less consistent with the self-reports. In terms of the interviewers' estimates for need of service, family status continued to distinguish between subcategories of soup kitchen users.

We also ran similar analyses of the service needs of those who had contact with family and with friends. There were no important differences between the categories or from the mode. When these categories were refined so that we compared the 27 (10%) isolates with the 244 who reported being in contact with someone, important differences appear. For example, 56% of the isolates but only 26% of those with contact reported living in a mission or on the street. These people tended not to have founded families, reported less use of services, and looked worse in the mental-status-by-observation estimates. Also, interviewers were more likely to see them as needing help for emotional problems.

It appeared that people who have families and have some contact with them probably can be helped to reestablish these ties on a stable basis and use them in supportive ways if they are provided proper material and service help. Those people who are isolated and have reached the point of living on the street or in missions are going to require outreach services and help over a long period of time if they are going to lead useful lives.

DISCUSSION

Although we question whether soup kitchens are the instrument of choice to feed the destitute, they are there, and people use them. Family status and contact with family have been shown to differentiate between categories of soup kitchen users. This information needs to be taken into account in planning services for soup kitchen users. We do not think any restrictions should be placed on those who want to use soup kitchens, but we do think that health and welfare services should establish outreach services at soup kitchens and offer to interview people to see if they qualify for needed services.

POLICY CONSIDERATIONS

Even though these data were collected 20 years ago, we have not seen anything that indicates a major change in the nature of the soup kitchen population or the conclusions that can be drawn from this study. Researchers and scholars continue to pay attention to homelessness and not to soup kitchens. There has been an increase in the number of women and children using soup kitchens, but the pattern of problems is not very different (Biggerstaff, Morris, & Nichols-Casebolt, 2002; Glasser, 1988). When soup kitchens are studied, the tendency is to look at specific problems or critiques, and almost no attention is paid to the users' family relationships (Littrell & Beck, 2000; Magura, Nwakeze, Rosenblum, & Joseph, 2000; Muller, 1987; Nwakeze, Magura, & Rosenblum, 2002; Nwakeze, Magura, Rosenblum, & Joseph, 2000; Nwakeze, Magura, Rosenblum, & Joseph, 2003; Schilling, Elbassel, & Gilbert, 1992; Stein, 1989).

Soup kitchen users have extraordinary rates of physical illness, mental illness, and alcoholism. Those who indicate that they have created a family are different from those who say that they are single. Those with a family status are older and sicker than those who are single. There are distinct differences between the categories of family status.

What can be done about this situation? We are specifically concerned about the question of family policy and what appear to be impediments to making such policy. At the most general level, a lot of concern is expressed, but little seems to be done concretely, except that more private groups open soup kitchens, and shelters and cities reluctantly drag behind. It is claimed that the public sector is devoid of money for such programs and that there should be reliance on the private sector. This seems to be an old story in the United States. The only difference appears to be that, in the past, concern in both the public and private sectors was more focused and effective. For example, a classic well-organized and well-financed effort was Sollenberger's (1911) survey of 1,000 homeless men. During the Depression, Abbott (1940) complained about the unparalleled way in which all segments of society hung on the idea that the private sector could handle the Depression. Efforts by Abbott and others finally brought governmental involvement at all levels.

There are other differences between the users of soup kitchens in the first half of the twentieth century and those who have used them in the last 50 years. Today's poor are less likely to be hobos. They are more likely to be African American and to come from a segment of society that hasn't dropped through the safety net; they never were in it. They are much more likely to be sick physically and emotionally. These are people who reflect the depths of misery. Hamburger (1983) went into a single occupancy hotel and turned on his tape recorder and produced a book that sears the soul. McQuaide (1983) lamented that the only way some people can get into state hospitals is to be arrested (as some have been advised by professionals).

Our historical tendency is to rely on the private sector and to respond only when there is a crisis that involves significant segments of our society and makes it difficult to respond to the current need. The social welfare and social work establishment was totally unprepared to deal with changes brought about by the Personal Responsibility and Work Opportunity Reconciliation Act of 1996, otherwise known as welfare reform (Stoesz, 2000).

If it is so difficult to think in terms of programs for individuals, it is doubly difficult to think of approaching these issues from a family perspective. All other industrial countries have child or family allowances, and most have mandated maternity benefits. Our culture has seen to it that disincentives toward handling problems on a family basis are built into our entire structure of health and welfare services. There are several characteristics of our public-tax-supported treatment system that serve as disincentives to emphasis on the family as the unit of focus.

Reimbursement

The major services provided to our alcoholic and mentally ill citizens are from one of three primary providers: (a) the freestanding community mental health or alcoholism program, (b) a mental health or alcoholism outpatient program associated with a medical hospital, and (c) inpatient alcoholism or mental health services provided by

designated units in medical hospitals or in state-operated psychiatric facilities. An examination of the fiscal incentives available to these programs for providing family therapy underscores why so few services are made available. There are three primary forms of reimbursement or fiscal support available to these institutions: patient fees, third-party reimbursement, and grant funding from the state agency responsible for the administration of mental health and alcoholism programs.

Freestanding programs receive such grants, charge patient fees on a sliding fee scale, receive per diem reimbursements from Medicaid for those clients who are enrolled, and also bill private insurance carriers. However, very little incentive is made available by these payers to encourage the providers to deliver family therapy. The per diem reimbursement from Medicaid remains the same whether the agency provides individual or family therapy. Few patients have money to pay, and those who do are charged no more if they have been provided family or individual assistance. Although some private insurance carriers such as Blue Cross/Blue Shield do set a higher relative value scale assignment for family therapy than for individual therapy, the difference is so small (as are the number of people with such coverage) that the differential rate of pay is not an adequate incentive to redirect services to a family model of care. Grant funding provided from a single state or city agency (although often requiring that supported programs specify that family therapy will be provided) does not hold programs accountable to levels of such treatment, nor is grant support withheld when agreed-on levels of care are defined but are not provided. Reimbursement available to the second category of programs, the hospital-based outpatient clinics, is identical to that of the freestanding programs. There is no fiscal incentive for providing family intervention.

For the inpatient providers—both medical hospitals and state mental hospitals—not only are incentives to provide family therapy lacking, but the system also provides some strong disincentives to involving the family in the client care plan. First, state facilities supported by state general funds do not provide any fiscal incentives for family therapy. Acute care medical hospitals with designated psychiatric or alcoholism treatment units are provided reimbursement based on a per diem rate that is established by a state health cost review commission or similar agency. For an inpatient facility to emphasize family therapy is costly. They cannot do it if they are not paid.

Further aggravating these disincentives is the DRG (diagnostic related groups) reimbursement mechanism for Medicare and Medicaid. The DRG system provides reimbursement to hospitals based on a preestablished amount for each diagnostic category. For a hospital to make a profit, length of stay below the average on which the DRG reimbursement was calculated must be attained, or on-the-unit costs must be drastically reduced. Clearly, this prospective form of reimbursement represents a strong disincentive to family involvement in inpatient treatment.

The Accountability Game and Family Intervention

Questions such as "Who is the real patient?" set the stage for a treatment system designed to serve the individual, not the family. Also, not surprisingly, accountability for services rendered follows the reimbursement system. Federal, state, and private agencies that allocate grant funds for hospital-based and freestanding programs and are responsible for holding programs accountable may be philosophically supportive of family intervention strategies, but these agencies have become wary of programs that attempt to count family members and ancillary patient involvement as documented service output. Documentation of family involvement is too often viewed by such funding sources as the program's effort to cover up for underuse and to pad service output. Cost effectiveness cannot be the only criterion by which programs are judged (Chaiklin, 1970).

CONCLUSION

The way to overcome the resistance to seeing the family aspect of important social problems is to begin using what we know. Rather than talk in the abstract of influencing social policy, specific proposals should be made. Monroney (1980) sounded a theme important to such an approach when he suggested that we stop thinking of the family and the state in terms of a dichotomy and start thinking of the family as a social institution

that needs support. He wrote, "The essence of these policies and services is a commitment to the principle that families and other social institutions need to interact in providing supports and services to individuals and groups" (p. 13). Without such supports and services, the family cycle of poverty will never be broken.

Our democracy is built on protecting individual political rights. This has not proved an effective basis for meeting social need. The laws dealing with the public welfare are individual and categorical. Thus, a person is helped either because he or she qualifies as an individual or because he or she belongs to a category. This often means that only part of a family can get help.

Finally, this chapter demonstrates that where the aim is to get information that has immediate use for planning and delivering services, the traditional survey has continued value. The quality of the data is the same as that in a research project. Usually, however, a survey can be formulated, executed, analyzed, and written up in less time than formal research. Social welfare agencies do not do enough research. Perhaps a return to the survey will help overcome this problem, because the data collected will be of immediate use to the agency.

Through the first three decades of the twentieth century, there was no area of U.S. life or problems that wasn't the subject of a survey. There were probably 4,000 surveys done during this period. So many surveys were done and so many people were involved that it became known as a social movement. Soup kitchen users need the continued attention that program-oriented surveys will bring.[2]

Notes

1. At that time, Marc Lipton was Assistant Commissioner for Mental Health, Mental Retardation, and Addictions.

2. This chapter is a revision of a paper presented at the National Conference on Family Relations, San Francisco, October 20, 1984.

References

Abbott, E. (1940). *Public assistance*. Chicago: University of Chicago Press.

Bassuk, E. L. (1984). The homelessness problem. *Scientific American, 251*(1), 40–45.

Biggerstaff, M. A., Morris, P. M., & Nichols-Casebolt, A. (2002). Living on the edge: Examination of people attending food pantries and soup kitchens. *Social Work, 47*(3), 267–277.

Chaiklin, H. (1970). Evaluation research and the planning-programming-budgeting system. In E. Schwartz (Ed.), *Planning programming budgeting systems and social welfare* (pp. 27–34). Chicago: University of Chicago School of Social Service Administration.

Chaiklin, H. (1983). *The service needs of soup kitchen users.* Baltimore: Baltimore City Health Department.

Denny, L. (2003, May 4). Pantries face bare shelves and higher demand. *New York Times,* p. 6.

Glasser, I. (1988). *More than bread: Ethnography of a soup kitchen.* Tuscaloosa: University of Alabama Press.

Hamburger, R. (1983). *All the lonely people.* New Haven, CT: Tickner and Fields.

Hartman, C. (1984). Shelter and community. *Society, 21*(3), 18–27.

Hollingshead, A. B., & Redlich, F. C. (1958). *Social class and mental illness: A community study.* New York: Wiley.

Johnson, C. W., Snibbe, J. R., & Evans, L. A. (1975). *Basic psychopathology: A programmed text.* New York: Spectrum.

Littrell, J., & Beck, E. (2000). Do inner-city African-American males exhibit "bad attitudes" toward work? *Journal of Sociology and Social Welfare, 27*(2), 3–23.

Magura, S., Nwakeze, P. C., Rosenblum, A., & Joseph, H. (2000). Substance misuse and related diseases in a soup kitchen population. *Substance Abuse & Misuse, 35*(4), 551–583.

McQuaide, S. (1983). Human service cutbacks and the mental health of the poor. *Social Casework, 64*(8), 497–499.

Monroney, R. F. (1980). *Families, social services, and social policy: The issue of shared responsibility.* Washington, DC: Government Printing Office.

Muller, J. (1987). The soup kitchen: A critique of self-help. *Community Development Journal, 22*(1), 36–45.

Naisbitt, J. (1982). *Megatrends.* New York: Warner.

Nwakeze, P., Magura, S., & Rosenblum, A. (2002). Drug problem recognition, desire for help, and treatment readiness in a soup kitchen population. *Substance Abuse & Misuse, 37*(3), 291–313.

Nwakeze, P. C., Magura, S., Rosenblum, A., & Joseph, H. (2000). Service outcomes of peer consumer advocacy for soup kitchen guests. *Journal of Social Service Research, 27*(2), 19–38.

Nwakeze, P. C., Magura, S., Rosenblum, A., & Joseph, H. (2003). Homelessness, substance misuse, and access to public entitlements in a soup kitchen population. *Substance Abuse & Misuse, 38*(3–6), 645–669.

Schilling, R. F., Elbassel, N., & Gilbert, L. (1992). Drug use and AIDS risks in a soup kitchen population. *Social Work, 37*(4), 353–358.

Sollenberger, A. W. (1911). *One thousand homeless men.* New York: Russell Sage Foundation.

Stein, M. (1989). Gratitude and attitude: A note on emotional welfare. *Social Psychology Quarterly, 52*(3), 242–248.

Stoesz, D. (2000). *A poverty of imagination: Bootstrap capitalism, sequel to welfare reform.* Madison: University of Wisconsin Press.

Waller, W. (1936). Social problems and the mores. *American Sociological Review, 1,* 922–933.

SECTION IX
Practice-Based Quantitative Research Exemplars

82

A COGNITIVE-BEHAVIORAL APPROACH TO SUICIDE RISK REDUCTION IN CRISIS INTERVENTION

Marjorie E. Weishaar

Working with suicidal patients can be anxiety-provoking for even the most experienced clinician because of the perceived responsibility for another person's life, the difficulty predicting the likelihood and timing of an individual's suicide based on population models, and the particular reliance on the therapy relationship when collaboration may be difficult.

Suicide is the 11th leading cause of death overall in the United States (Minino, Arias, Kochanek, Murphy, & Smith, 2002). Among adolescents, it accounts for a greater proportion of deaths than for the nation as a whole (McIntosh, 2000). Despite these facts, there is a paucity of well-designed research on treatments to reduce *suicidality* (i.e., suicide, suicide attempts, and suicide ideation; Linehan, 1997). Clinicians need empirically validated treatments or will continue to rely on methods that are unproven and perhaps ineffective. This chapter presents a summary of the research literature on randomized controlled trials to reduce suicide risk, descriptions of cognitive-behavioral treatments that have demonstrated efficacy, and guidelines for implementing cognitive and behavioral interventions with suicidal individuals.

KEY CONCEPTS AND DATABASES

The low base rate of suicide makes it statistically unpredictable on an individual basis, particularly because the database is limited primarily to cross-sectional studies (Clark & Fawcett, 1992). Despite the apparent differences between those who suicide and those who attempt it repeatedly (Clark & Fawcett, 1992; Linehan, 1986, 1993a), those who contemplate and attempt suicide are the available groups to study and reasonable proxies. Attempting suicide remains one of the most powerful risk factors for eventual suicide (Fawcett et al., 1990; Goldstein, Black, Nasrallah, & Winokur, 1991; Harris & Barraclough, 1997; Steer, Beck, Garrison, & Lester, 1988). A history of nonfatal attempts confers an elevated risk for eventual suicide that is five to six times greater than that for the general population (Clark & Fawcett, 1992). Similarly, reducing suicide ideation is presumed to break a pathway to overt suicidal behavior (Dieserud, Roysamb, Ekeberg, & Kraft, 2001). Much suicide research has focused on reducing the clinical (e.g., depression) and cognitive (e.g., hopelessness, poor problem solving; see Weishaar, 1996, for a review) risk factors associated with suicide. As Shea (1999) points out, a risk factor of a large sample does not accurately predict the chance of imminent suicide for an individual client, but knowledge of risk factors alerts the clinician to suspect increased risk and directs specific lines of questioning to assess risk for that client. Thus, research on treatments to reduce suicide risk targets suicide attempts and other parasuicidal behavior, suicide ideation and intent, and risk factors associated with suicide.

Suicide research has developed several assessment tools that are also very useful clinically, such as the Scale for Suicide Ideation (SSI; Beck, Kovacs, & Weissman, 1979; Beck & Steer, 1991); the Suicide Intent Scale (SIS; Beck, Schuyler, & Herman, 1974); the Beck Hopelessness Scale (BHS; Beck, Weissman, Lester, & Trexler, 1974); and various forms of the Reasons for Living Inventory (Jobes & Mann, 1999; Linehan, Goodstein, Nielson, & Chiles, 1983; Westefeld, Cardin, & Deaton, 1992). These assessment tools can structure a clinical interview to determine a particular individual's risk. A person's suicide risk should never be based on a score from a single scale.

Suicide intent, the intensity and pervasiveness of one's wish to die (Beck, 1986), is a key concept in working with suicidal individuals. High intent distinguishes suicide attempts from other *parasuicidal behavior* (i.e., intentional, acute self-injury with or without suicidal intent; Linehan, Armstrong, Suarez, Allmon, & Heard, 1991). Suicide intent cannot be inferred by the lethality of the attempt unless the patient has an accurate conception of the lethality of his or her chosen means (Beck, Beck, & Kovacs, 1975). That means the clinician has to ask the person how much he or she wished to die. In addition to self-report, which might be less than candid, questions on the SIS identify behavioral markers that indicate intent, such as having taken precautions against being discovered (Beck & Lester, 1976; Beck, Steer, & Trexler, 1989).

Suicide ideation is a target in both outcome studies and clinical treatments because it is a precursor to suicidal behavior. It is especially important for clinicians treating outpatients to ask about ideation at its worst point, for that is most closely linked to eventual suicide (Beck, Brown, Steer, Dahlsgaard, & Grisham, 1999). It is likely that for inpatients, the time of hospitalization is the worst point. Understanding the frequency, duration, power, and context of the suicidal thoughts, as well as the attitudes, purpose, and planning concerning an attempt, guides treatment. For example, someone who has thoughts of suicide when drinking alcohol might receive therapy that treats substance abuse as well as suicide. Someone who is shocked or dismayed by suicidal thoughts is more likely to collaborate with the therapist to challenge them than is someone who is comforted by images of death or convinced that suicide is the only solution to problems.

METHODOLOGICAL ISSUES AND RESEARCH LIMITATIONS

A number of methodological issues have hampered clinical research on suicide. Many suicidal individuals are screened out of or dropped from studies in which suicidality is a comorbidity because of risk-averse criteria. For example, 90% of suicide victims have had a psychiatric or substance abuse disorder, but there are few clinical trials aimed at treating psychopathology or substance abuse that also address suicidality (Fisher, Pearson, Kim, & Reynolds, 2002). Further, in studies of suicidal persons, *high-risk* subjects (i.e., those with a history of attempts, those who suffer mood disorders with concurrent ideation, and those abusing alcohol episodically with concurrent ideation; Maris, Berman, Maltsberger, & Yufit, 1992) are also often excluded for reasons of perceived liability to individual researchers and institutions (Fisher et al., 2002). Thus, one limitation on suicide research has been a reluctance to test treatments for suicidality with randomized clinical trials.

The notion of a control group raises issues for randomized clinical trials in suicide research because a no-treatment control group is unethical. The common solution is the treatment as usual (TAU) control group. However, TAU means different things in different studies, and sometimes even within the same study if some patients return to their primary-care physician while others are given referrals, phone contact, or lesser forms of follow-up. In some recent studies, all patients received more monitoring and more intensive care than would be available outside the study (Fisher et al., 2002). This is called enriched care plus treatment as usual and is the control condition for the current studies by Beck (2002). This EC+TAU condition provides more safety for research participants and is an effort to improve the standard of treatment across practice settings, as well as to reduce attrition from studies. However, there may be treatment effects from this control condition that reduce the power to detect differences between the control group and the experimental group (Fisher et al., 2002).

Difficulty detecting treatment effects due to small sample sizes has plagued randomized controlled trials (Arensman et al., 2001; Fisher et al., 2002; Hawton et al., 1998; Linehan, 1997; Rudd, 2000). Large, multisite studies are recommended in order to have sufficient statistical power to show treatment effects. Other methodological issues have been poor definitions of treatments and how they were applied, lack of standard measures of outcome, lack of information on whether treatment resulted in changes in the targets of treatment (e.g., improved problem solving, emotion regulation, or interpersonal skills; Arensman et al., 2001), and limited follow-up monitoring to evaluate lasting change (Rudd, 2000).

TREATMENT OUTCOME STUDIES TO REDUCE SUICIDE RISK

Recent reviews of the literature (Hawton et al., 1998; Linehan, 1997; Rudd, 2000; Rudd, Joiner, & Rajab, 2001) have identified only 16 randomized or controlled studies of psychotherapeutic treatments for suicide; 14 of them are short-term, and 2 are long-term. Four of the brief (less than 1 year) studies investigated the effectiveness of some intensive follow-up and crisis support in addition to TAU. The outcomes of these studies were generally negative. The remaining 10 studies were some variety of cognitive-behavior therapy (CBT), and all had a core component of problem-solving therapy. (Since those reviews, Guthrie and colleagues, 2001, et al., found that a brief psychodynamic treatment significantly reduced suicide ideation and repeated attempts at 6-month follow-up.) Eight of the 10 CBT studies reported decreases in psychological risk factors for suicidal behavior such as suicide ideation, hopelessness, and depression. Two of the studies (McLeavey, Daly, Ludgate, & Murray, 1994; Salkovskis, Atha, & Storer, 1990) found significant decreases in the frequency of suicide attempts. In the Salkovskis et al. (1990) study of high-risk attempters, the treatment group improved significantly more than the TAU control group in terms of depression, hopelessness, suicide ideation, and target problems at the end of treatment and at 1-year follow-up. The difference in frequency of repeat attempts between treatment and control groups was found at 6-month follow-up but not at 1 year. In the McLeavey et al. (1994) study, which excluded high-risk patients, the reduction in suicide attempts persisted to 12 months after treatment. Thus, brief psychological interventions can be successful in reducing subsequent suicidal behaviors, at least over the short term.

The two long-term studies yielded mixed results. Allard, Marshall, and Plante (1992) examined the role of intensive follow-up across several therapeutic modalities but did not test a specific psychotherapy. Methodological problems compromised the results. In contrast, Linehan and colleagues (1991) tested a very specific form of CBT, dialectical behavior therapy (DBT; Linehan, 1993a, 1993b), to treat parasuicidal behavior in women with borderline personality disorder. After 1 year of treatment, those receiving DBT had fewer incidences of parasuicide, less medically severe parasuicides, fewer inpatient psychiatric days, and a greater chance of remaining in therapy than those in the TAU control group. No between-group differences were found on measures of depression, hopelessness, suicide ideation, reasons for living, or the proportion of parasuicides classified as suicide attempts by the subjects. The superiority of DBT for reducing parasuicidal acts was maintained throughout the 1-year follow-up but not during the 18- to 24-month follow-up (Linehan, Heard, & Armstrong, 1993). Nevertheless, DBT was successful in reducing parasuicidal behavior in a group of severely dysfunctional, chronically suicidal subjects with limited use of hospitalization, thus demonstrating that outpatient treatment of high-risk patients can be safe and effective.

The emergence of CBT as an efficacious modality for the treatment of suicide risk highlights the role of skills training, particularly problem solving. DBT conceptualizes parasuicidal behaviors as maladaptive attempts at problem solving, the primary problem being unbearable emotional distress (Linehan, 1993a). The problem-solving training used in CBT studies is represented by the work of Nezu, Nezu, and Perri (1989) and by Hawton and Kirk (1989), for example. Linehan has a manualized treatment for DBT (Linehan, 1993a, 1993b) that targets suicidal behaviors, therapy-interfering behaviors, skills acquisition (e.g., mindfulness, interpersonal skills), emotion regulation and distress tolerance, post-traumatic stress, self-respect, and individual goals. Short-term adaptations of DBT have been used in studies that did not find significant differences in suicide attempts at the end of treatment, but some of these are preliminary or pilot studies (Evans et al., 1999; Koerner & Linehan, 2000; Rathus & Miller, 2002).

Based on a review of the treatment outcome literature, particularly the success of DBT, and an investigation of personality types and suicidal behavior (Rudd, Ellis, Rajab, & Wehrly, 2000), it has been argued that patients with severe personality pathology and *chronic suicidality* (i.e., unremittingly high suicide ideation, frequent threats of suicide, and difficulty articulating reasons for living; Linehan, 1999) require intensive treatment, closer follow-up monitoring to ensure treatment compliance, treatments to address specific skill deficits, such as CBT, and long-term treatment (Rudd et al., 2000). Short-term CBT appears effective in reducing suicide ideation, depression, and hopelessness in periods up to 1 year (Rudd, 2000). However, a study is currently under way to see whether short-term cognitive therapy immediately following an attempt can effectively reduce suicide attempts in a group of attempters (73% have made more than one attempt) who also have psychiatric and/or substance disorders and significant Axis II pathology (Beck, 2002).

As part of a large-scale investigation, Beck (2002) recently completed preliminary studies of a cognitive therapy treatment for suicidal behavior in a sample of urban, minority suicide attempters who are socially and economically disadvantaged and who present with serious psychopathology. Participants were recruited at the time of their hospitalization for a suicide attempt but were treated on an outpatient basis. The 10-week treatment included cognitive therapy for depression, hopelessness, and substance abuse, as well as cognitive and behavioral interventions specifically for suicidal behavior, including problem solving and focusing on the problem associated with their attempt. The primary outcome variables were the number and timing of suicide attempts following the index attempt, for the risk of a repeat attempt is highest within 3 years of an index attempt (Hawton & Fagg, 1988; Morris, Kovacs, Beck, & Wolffe, 1974). A secondary goal was to determine if cognitive therapy immediately following a suicide attempt reduces the severity of the risk factors depression, hopelessness, and suicide ideation.

Preliminary results show that patients who received cognitive therapy had decreases in depression that were significantly greater than the control group and significantly fewer hospitalizations. To date, it appears that the cognitive therapy intervention reduces the frequency of subsequent suicide attempts and prolongs the time before an individual makes another suicide attempt (Beck, 2002). Patients will be followed for 2 years.

MOVEMENT TOWARD THE DEVELOPMENT OF PRACTICE GUIDELINES

Practice guidelines are available for the legal and clinical care of suicidal patients (Bongar, 2002; Bongar, Maris, Berman, & Litman, 1992; Bongar et al., 1998). Among the clinical guidelines are lists of suicide risk variables, both acute and chronic, as determined by longitudinal studies (Beck, Brown, Berchick, Stewart, & Steer, 1990; Beck, Steer, Kovacs, & Garrison, 1985; Fawcett et al., 1990; Goldstein et al., 1991). Outpatient practice guidelines based on the research literature are presented by Rudd and his colleagues (Rudd, Joiner, Jobes, & King, 1999). Linehan (1999) also presents guidelines for treating chronically suicidal patients. In addition to these standardized guidelines for clinical care, Maltsberger (1986) identifies specific components necessary in formulating one's clinical judgment of suicide risk.

A study of imminent risk based on data from therapists who lost patients to suicide identifies three factors in a suicide crisis: (a) a precipitating event, (b) one or more intense affective states other than depression, and (c) at least one of three behavioral patterns, namely, speech or actions suggesting suicide, deterioration in social or occupational functioning, and increased substance abuse (Hendin, Maltsberger, Lipschitz, Haas, & Kyle, 2001).

Manualized treatments for suicide risk may be thought of as developments toward treatment guidelines when the therapies have demonstrated efficacy. Linehan's manual for DBT (Linehan, 1993a, 1993b), the cognitive-behavioral formulation by Rudd et al. (2001), and Choosing to Live (Ellis & Newman, 1996), which is part of Beck's research protocol, document cognitive-behavioral strategies to reduce suicide risk.

STEPS FOR USING CBT PRACTICE GUIDELINES

In CBT, suicidal behavior is viewed as a maladaptive coping behavior. Regardless of theoretical differences, all forms of CBT for suicide are active, directive, and problem focused. The following steps in assessing and treating suicidal thoughts and behavior are drawn from Beck's cognitive therapy. Throughout the CBT treatment literature, the quality of the therapy relationship is emphasized, so although these steps are presented in a formulaic manner, they are applied with great sensitivity, for the goals are to first understand the patient's view before challenging it and to build collaboration during a very stressful experience. The reader is referred to Shea's (1999) book on interviewing suicidal patients for more guidance.

Acute or Immediate Goals

1. Eliminate access to lethal means and assess need for hospitalization, type of therapy needed (e.g., Does the family need therapy?), presence of clinical risk factors.
2. Intervention begins with assessment: assess suicide ideation, intent, purpose of attempt, and hopelessness.
3. Reduce hopelessness and shake rigid conclusions that things cannot improve. Convey that hopelessness is a viewpoint and not an accurate reflection of the facts. Get a list of all the things the patient feels hopeless about. Are these situational stressors or indicative of a core belief (e.g., "I am a loser.")? Reduce cognitive distortions that complicate the picture.
4. Examine reasons for living and reasons for dying. Tip the balance in favor of living by undermining reasons for dying now and bolstering reasons for living (e.g., ask for details of positive reasons for living, add to the list). Make sure the patient considers consequences of dying for self and others. Reduce distortions that romanticize death. Make a list of deterrents in addition to positive reasons for living.
5. Assess the person's attitude toward suicide ideation and situations in which it occurs. If an attempt has been made, do a behavioral or functional analysis of the situation, thoughts, and emotions that preceded the attempt. Identify alternative thoughts and behaviors. Get descriptions of all other attempts and plans for future attempts.
6. Assess the patient's sense of control over ideation or action. In what situations are the controls effective or ineffective? What types of self-control strategies does the patient utilize?
7. What coping skills or psychological buffers does the patient have (e.g., coping beliefs, reasons for living, frustration tolerance, positive feelings of competence, ability to use distraction or to dispute suicidal ideas, ability to utilize social supports)?
8. Assess problem-solving skills and cognitive deficits that might interfere with problem solving (e.g., rigid or dichotomous thinking).
9. Construct a suicide emergency kit as early as possible. This is a written plan, which the patient can carry, to save oneself when having suicide ideation. It can be elaborated as therapy progresses. An example of a kit for a depressed, suicidal person appears in Table 82.1. The purpose of distraction from suicidal thoughts is to break the focus on negative thinking. Suicidal thoughts can be challenged with the help of the therapist, but not all patients are able to dispute them early in treatment without help. As therapy progresses, the patient can write negative thoughts with their rebuttals on the card along with the suicide emergency kit.

Short-Term to Long-Term Goals

1. Teach skills to identify and modify thoughts leading to suicidal behavior. Examine thoughts and beliefs logically and with behavioral experiments such as asking family members how they would feel if the person died rather than mind reading or assuming what others think.
2. Teach problem-solving skills and reduce cognitive distortions that interfere with each step. Start with problems associated with a suicide attempt, hopelessness, or suicide ideation. The steps in problem solving are as follows:
   a. Accepting problems as a normal part of life.
   b. Properly defining the problem.
   c. Generating alternative solutions.
   d. Anticipating the consequences (for self and others) of various courses of action.
   e. Considering the advantages and disadvantages ("pros and cons") of each alternative.
   f. Choosing an alternative to try first and withholding judgment about its success until it has been given an adequate trial.
   g. Evaluating the outcome with reasonable criteria (e.g., achieving degrees of success, doing a behavior correctly, but there being an outcome out of one's control).

TABLE 82.1 Suicide Emergency Kit

1. Recognize that the thoughts you are having are part of depression. (Note: Substitute whatever the patient identifies as his or her affective state—anxiety, anger.)

2. Recognize that the thoughts go away when you feel better.

3. You have had these thoughts x (patient supplies the number) times before and they have gone away.

4. These thoughts are time-limited and should not be responded to.

5. It is important not to act on these thoughts because they are part of depression (anxiety, anger, frustration, loneliness).

6. Do not focus on losses in the past or imagine losses in the future.

7. Focus on activities and distractions, the more active the better.

List of activities (Note: This list should be individualized for each person. Consider activities to do with other people or alone, daytime or nighttime. Add to the list as therapy progresses): walk or play with the dog, call Laura or Rick, shoot pool with Danny or another friend, visit Diana, call my therapist.

h. Tolerating the anxiety and frustration that are part of solving problems.

2. Reduce other cognitive risk factors that might predispose the patient to future suicidal episodes. These include the following:

a. Hopelessness: View hopelessness as a point of view and not an accurate reflection of the situation. List all the problems making the patient hopeless. Reduce cognitive distortions to clearly define problems. Share optimism about finding solutions. Do problem-solving training and skills training (e.g., communication skills, assertiveness, frustration tolerance) to implement solutions.

b. Impulsivity: Teach the patient to do a functional or behavioral analysis to see the process by which he or she loses control. Review the steps in problem solving. Identify lower levels of emotion. Break all-or-nothing thinking. Use relaxation, "time-out," or a "waiting period" to postpone action.

c. Low self-concept: Is the negative view of oneself about specific flaws, or is it global? Is rigid thinking operating? Focus on success experiences and positive qualities. Reframe negative labels such as "sensitive" or "dependent."

d. Dysfunctional assumptions: Gather evidence that supports the dysfunctional belief and that challenges the belief. Look for distortions, inaccuracies, and biases in evidence that support the negative assump-

tion. What would you like to, realistically, believe? Gather evidence for that positive assumption.

e. Cognitive rigidity: Treat beliefs as hypotheses to be tested and test them logically and with safe behavioral experiments. Build a continuum between extreme points of view and use "shades of gray" or percentages to break rigid judgments if dichotomous thinking is operating. Brainstorm solutions for someone else's problems. Role-play with role reversal to increase flexibility in generating alternatives. Look for exceptions to the client's rules.

f. View of suicide as desirable: List the reasons for dying and solutions. List the reasons for living. List the advantages and disadvantages of suicide relative to other solutions. Correct cognitive distortions and misinformation about the perceived advantages of dying.

3. Construct coping cards to deal with suicide ideation and relapse. An example of a coping card appears in Table 82.2.

CONCLUSION

The research literature on randomized controlled trials of psychotherapeutic treatments to reduce suicidality supports the use of CBT. Both short-term treatments and long-term therapies em-

TABLE 82.2 Coping Card

1. Warning signs for my suicidality
   a. I feel different, defective
   b. I feel overwhelmed; everything seems to be a problem
   c. I get very self-critical ("I'm a failure. I can't do anything right.")

2. My plan for dealing with suicidal thoughts (like Suicide Emergency Kit)
   a. Call friends—list names and numbers
   b. Exercise—"crunches," running, dancing, step aerobics
   c. Relax with a shower or listen to music (e.g., Stevie Wonder, Beatles)
   d. Read therapy notes and see how far I've come since the worst point

3. List my reasons to live
   a. What were my reasons to live when I was happier? Might they be true in the future? What new reasons to live have I found?
   b. Write a positive statement that rings true: "It would be a shame to kill myself today if I were to feel better in the future."

4. Write my old beliefs and new ideas that contradict them.
   a. Old idea: My life will never get better. New idea: I'm learning new things in therapy to change.
   b. Old idea: I'm a failure. New idea: On any given day, I'm a partial success and a partial failure at anything I try. The idea is to find what I like to do.
   c. Old idea: I am a burden to my family and friends. New idea: My family says they will never get over it if I die. My friends say they depend on me just like I depend on them.
   d. Old idea: I'm a loser. New idea: If I die, I'll never know what it feels like to win something. I don't want to lose my chances, my life.

---

phasize problem solving as a key component. Cognitive risk factors may be conceived of as both acute and chronic. Therefore, therapy should target these risk factors throughout treatment, even after the suicidal crisis has passed. If not, they could well predispose the individual to future suicidal episodes.

References

Allard, R., Marshall, M., & Plante, M. (1992). Intensive follow-up does not decrease the risk of repeat suicide attempts. *Suicide and Life-Threatening Behavior, 22,* 303–314.

Arensman, E., Townsend, E., Hawton, K., Bremner, S., Feldman, E., Goldney, R., Gunnell, D., Hazell, P., Van Heeringen, K., House, A., Owens, D., Sakinofsky, I., & Traskman-Bendz, L. (2001). Psychosocial and pharmacological treatment of patients following deliberate self-harm: The methodological issues involved in evaluating effectiveness. *Suicide and Life-Threatening Behavior, 31,* 169–180.

Beck, A. T. (1986). Hopelessness as a predictor of eventual suicide. *Annals of the New York Academy of Sciences, 487,* 90–96.

Beck, A. T. (2002, December). *An early cognitive intervention for suicide attempters.* Paper presented at the first annual conference of Treatment and Research Advancements Association for Personality Disorders, Bethesda, Maryland.

Beck, A. T., Beck, R. W., & Kovacs, M. (1975). Classification of suicidal behaviors: I. Quantifying intent and medical lethality. *American Journal of Psychiatry, 132,* 285–287.

Beck, A. T., Brown, G., Berchick, R. J., Stewart, B. L., & Steer, R. A. (1990). Relationship between hopelessness and ultimate suicide: A replication with psychiatric outpatients. *American Journal of Psychiatry, 147,* 190–195.

Beck, A. T., Brown, G. K., Steer, R. A., Dahlsgaard, K. K., & Grisham, J. (1999). Suicide ideation at its worst point: A predictor of eventual suicide in psychiatric outpatients. *Suicide and Life-Threatening Behavior, 29,* 1–9.

Beck, A. T., Kovacs, M., & Weissman, A. (1979). Assessment of suicidal intention: The Scale for Suicide Ideation. *Journal of Consulting and Clinical Psychology, 47,* 343–352.

Beck, A. T., & Lester, D, (1976). Components of suicidal intent in completed and attempted suicides. *Journal of Psychology, 92,* 35–38.

Beck, A. T., Schuyler, D., & Herman, I. (1974). Development of suicidal intent scales. In A. T. Beck, H.C.P. Resnik, & D. Lettieri (Eds.), *The predic-*

tion of suicide (pp. 45–56). Bowie, MD: Charles Press.

Beck, A. T., & Steer, R. A. (1991). *Manual for the Beck Scale for Suicide Ideation.* San Antonio, TX: Psychological Corporation.

Beck, A. T., Steer, R.A., Kovacs, M., & Garrison, B. (1985). Hopelessness and eventual suicide: A ten-year prospective study of patients hospitalized with suicidal ideation. *American Journal of Psychiatry, 142,* 559–563.

Beck, A. T., Steer, R. A., & Trexler, L. D. (1989). Alcohol abuse and eventual suicide: A five to ten year prospective study of alcohol abusing suicide attempters. *Journal of Studies on Alcohol, 50,* 202–209.

Beck, A. T., Weissman, A., Lester, D., & Trexler, L. (1974). The measurement of pessimism: The Hopelessness Scale. *Journal of Consulting and Clinical Psychology, 42,* 861–865.

Bongar, B. (2002). *The suicidal patient: Clinical and legal standards of care* (2nd ed.). Washington, DC: American Psychological Association.

Bongar, B., Berman, A. L., Maris, R. W., Silverman, M. M., Harris, E. A., & Packman, W. L. (1998). *Risk management with suicidal patients.* New York: Guilford Press.

Bongar, B., Maris, R., Berman, A. L., & Litman, R. E. (1992). Outpatient standards of care and the suicidal patient. *Suicide and Life-Threatening Behavior, 22,* 453–478.

Clark, D., & Fawcett, J. (1992). An empirically based model of suicide risk assessment for patients with affective disorders. In D. Jacobs (Ed.), *Suicide in clinical practice* (pp. 55–73). Washington, DC: American Psychiatric Press.

Dieserud, G., Roysamb, E., Ekeberg, O., & Kraft, P. (2001). Toward an integrative model of suicide attempt: A cognitive psychological approach. *Suicide and Life-Threatening Behavior, 31,* 153–168.

Ellis, T. E., & Newman, C. F. (1996). *Choosing to live: How to defeat suicide through cognitive therapy.* Oakland, CA: New Harbinger Publications.

Evans, K., Tyrer, P., Catalan, J., Schmidt, U., Davidson, K., Dent, J., Tata, P., Thornton, S., Barber, J., & Thompson, S. (1999). Manual-assisted cognitive-behavioural therapy (MACT): A randomized controlled trial of a brief intervention with bibliotherapy in the treatment of recurrent deliberate self-harm. *Psychological Medicine, 29,* 19–25.

Fawcett, J., Schefter, W. A., Fogg, L., Clark, D. C., Young, M. A., Hedeker, D., & Gibbons, R. (1990). Time-related predictors of suicide in major affective disorder. *American Journal of Psychiatry, 147,* 1189–1194.

Fisher, C. B., Pearson, J. L., Kim, S., & Reynolds, C. F. (2002). Ethical issues in including suicidal individuals in clinical research. *IRB: Ethics and Human Research, 24*(4), 9–14.

Goldstein, R. B., Black, D. W., Nasrallah, A., & Winokur, G. (1991). The prediction of suicide: Sensitivity, specificity, and predictive value of a multivariate model applied to suicide among 1906 patients with affective disorders. *Archives of General Psychiatry, 48,* 418–422.

Guthrie, E., Kapur, N., Mackway-Jones, K., Chew-Graham, C., Moorey, J., Mendel, E., Marino-Francis, F., Sanderson, S., Turpin, C., Broddy, G., & Tomenson, B. (2001). Randomised controlled trial of brief psychological intervention after deliberate self-poisoning. *British Medical Journal, 323,* 1–5.

Harris, E. C., & Barraclough, B. (1997). Suicide as an outcome for mental disorders: A meta-analysis. *British Journal of Psychiatry, 170,* 205–228.

Hawton, K., Arensman, E., Townsend, E., Bremner, S., Feldman, E., Goldney, R., Gunnell, D., Hazell, P., Van Heeringen, K., House, A., Owens, D., Sakinofsky, I., & Traksman-Bendz, L. (1998). Deliberate self-harm: Systematic review of efficacy of psychosocial and pharmacological treatments in preventing repetition. *British Medical Journal, 317,* 441–447.

Hawton, K., & Fagg, J. (1988). Suicide, and other causes of death, following attempted suicide. *British Journal of Psychiatry, 152,* 359–366.

Hawton, K., & Kirk, J. W. (1989). Problem solving. In K. Hawton, P. M. Salkovskis, J. Kirk, & D. M. Clark (Eds.), *Cognitive behaviour therapy for psychiatric problems: A practical guide* (pp. 406–426). Oxford: Oxford University Press.

Hendin, H., Maltsberger, J. T., Lipschitz, A., Haas, A. P., & Kyle, J. (2001). Recognizing and responding to a suicide crisis. *Suicide and Life-Threatening Behavior, 31,* 115–128.

Jobes, D. A., & Mann, R. E. (1999). Reasons for living versus reasons for dying: Examining the internal debate of suicide. *Suicide and Life-Threatening Behavior, 29,* 97–104.

Koerner, K., & Linehan, M. M. (2002). Dialectical Behavior Therapy for patients with borderline personality disorder. *Psychiatric Clinics of North America, 23,* 151–167.

Linehan, M. M. (1986). Suicidal people: One population or two? In J. J. Mann & M. Stanley (Eds.), *Annals of the New York Academy of Sciences: The psychobiology of suicidal behavior* (pp. 16–33). New York: New York Academy of Sciences.

Linehan, M. M. (1993a). *Cognitive behavioral treatment of borderline personality disorder.* New York: Guilford Press.

Linehan, M. M. (1993b). *Skills training manual for treating borderline personality disorder.* New York: Guilford Press.

Linehan, M. M. (1997). Behavioral treatments of suicidal behaviors: Definitional obfuscation and treatment outcomes. In D. M. Stoff & J. J. Mann (Eds.), *Annals of the New York Academy of Sciences: The neurobiology of suicide from the bench to the clinic* (pp. 302–328). New York: New York Academy of Sciences.

Linehan, M. M. (1999). Standard protocol for assessing and treating suicidal behaviors for patients in treatment. In D. G. Jacobs (Ed.), *The Harvard Medical School guide to suicide assessment and intervention* (pp. 146–187). San Francisco: Jossey-Bass.

Linehan, M. M., Armstrong, H. E., Suarez, A., Allmon, D., & Heard, H. (1991). Cognitive-behavioral treatment of chronically parasuicidal borderline patients. *Archives of General Psychiatry, 48,* 1060–1064.

Linehan, M. M., Goodstein, J. L., Nielson, S. L., & Chiles, J. A. (1983). Reasons for staying alive when you are thinking of killing yourself: The Reasons for Living Inventory. *Journal of Consulting and Clinical Psychology, 51,* 276–286.

Linehan, M. M., Heard, H., L., & Armstrong, H. E. (1993). Naturalistic follow-up of a behavioral treatment for chronically parasuicidal borderline patients. *Archives of General Psychiatry, 50,* 971–974.

Maltsberger, J. T. (1986). *Suicide risk: The formulation of clinical judgment.* New York: New York University Press.

Maris, R. W., Berman, A. L., Maltsberger, J. T. & Yufit, R. I. (Eds.), (1992). *Assessment and prediction of suicide.* New York: Guilford Press.

McIntosh, J. L. (2000). Epidemiology of adolescent suicde in the United States. In R. W. Maris, S. S. Canetto, J. L. McIntosh, & M. M. Silverman (Eds.), *Review of suicidology 2000* (pp. 3–33). New York: Guilford Press.

McLeavey, B. C., Daly, R. J., Ludgate, J. W., & Murray, C. M. (1994). Interpersonal problem-solving skills training in the treatment of self-poisoning patients. *Suicide and Life-Threatening Behavior, 24,* 382–394.

Minino, A. M., Arias, E., Kochanek, K. D., Murphy, S. L., & Smith, B. L. (2002). *Deaths: Final data for 2000.* National Vital Statistics Reports, 50(15). Hyattsville, MD: National Center for Health Statistics.

Morris, J. B., Kovacs, M., Beck, A. T., & Wolffe, A. (1974). Notes toward an epidemiology of urban suicide. *Comprehensive Psychology, 15,* 537–547.

Nezu, A. M., Nezu, C. M., & Perri, M. G. (1989). *Problem-solving therapy for depression: Theory, research, and clinical guidelines.* New York: Wiley.

Rathus, J. H., & Miller, A. L. (2002). Dialectical Behavior Therapy adapted for suicidal adolescents. *Suicide and Life-Threatening Behavior, 32,* 146–157.

Rudd, M. D. (2000). Integrating science into the practice of clinical suicidology: A review of the psychotherapy literature and a research agenda for the future. In R. W. Maris, S. S. Canetto, J. L. McIntosh, & M. M. Silverman (Eds.), *Review of Suicidology 2000* (pp. 47–83). New York: Guilford Press.

Rudd, M. D., Ellis, T. E., Rajab, M. H., & Wehrly, T. (2000). Personality types and suicidal behavior: An exploratory study. *Suicide and Life-Threatening Behavior, 30,* 199–212.

Rudd, M. D., Joiner, T. E., Jobes, D. A., & King, C. A. (1999). The outpatient treatment of suicidality: An integration of science and recognition of its limitations. *Professional Psychology: Research and Practice, 30,* 437–446.

Rudd, M. D., Joiner, T., & Rajab, M. H. (2001). *Treating suicidal behavior: An effective, time-limited approach.* New York: Guilford Press.

Salkovskis, P. M., Atha, C., & Storer, D. (1990). Cognitive-behavioral problem solving in the treatment of patients who repeatedly attempt suicide: A controlled trial. *British Journal of Psychiatry, 157,* 871–876.

Shea, S. C. (1999). *The practical art of suicide assessment: A guide for mental health professionals and substance abuse counselors.* New York: Wiley.

Steer, R. A., Beck, A. T., Garrison, B., & Lester, D. (1988). Eventual suicide in interrupted and uninterrupted attempters. A challenge to the cry-for-help hypothesis. *Suicide and Life-Threatening Behavior, 18,* 119–128.

Weishaar, M. E. (1996). Cognitive risk factors in suicide. In P. M. Salkovskis (Ed.), *Frontiers of cognitive therapy* (pp. 226–249). New York: Guilford Press.

Westefeld, J. S., Cardin, D., & Deaton, W. L. (1992). Development of the College Student Reasons for Living Inventory. *Suicide and Life-Threatening Behavior, 22,* 442–452.

EFFECTS OF RESTORATIVE JUSTICE ON FEAR OF REVICTIMIZATION

83

A Meta-Analysis Using Hierarchical Generalized Linear Models

Mona M. Williams-Hayes & William R. Nugent

Social scientists have begun to systematically organize and analyze data for major social concerns. It is vital that this type of comprehensive integration be employed and referred to in order to move a field of study and practice forward. Meta-analyses have been used to evaluate such issues as effective juvenile justice interventions and outcomes for children sexually abused (Lipsey, 1995; Rind, Bauserman, & Tromovich, 1998, respectively).

Professionals should make informed decisions about the types of intervention to apply in practice by understanding what the *entire* body of research seems to suggest. Meta-analyses can use findings presented at conferences, in program evaluations, or in peer-reviewed journals. Whether or not research findings are published is relevant but not problematic because all the findings can be analyzed to determine if the variation across "studies" is systematic or random. If the variation in findings across studies is systematic, the factors related to the variation can be tested to see whether they account for any or all of the variation. An example of a factor that may explain some of the systematic variation is the methodological quality of a study. More familiar moderating variables, such as respondent age or gender, can also be predicted. Some advantages of conducting a meta-analysis include an increase in statistical power, depth, and breadth because it includes all research, and the ability to predict variables that contribute to sys-

tematic variation (Cohen, 1988; Glass, 1977). There may be some limitations to specific meta-analyses such as the violation of important independence assumptions or having to collapse categories because of differences in how researchers measured variables (Williams-Hayes, 2002).

A meta-analysis can be performed in a number of ways (see Latimer, Dowden, & Muise, 2001, for a review). This particular study used Hierarchial Generalized Linear Models (HGLMs) with a logit link function to evaluate the effectiveness of restorative justice on fearfulness. The general purpose of this study was to conduct a meta-analysis of the research on the effects that two prominent forms of restorative justice (victim-offender mediation and family group conferencing) have on fear of revictimization and to determine the factors, if any, that explained variability across studies in magnitude of effect sizes (Williams-Hayes & Nugent, in press). If significant across-study variability existed, as was expected, then several potential explanatory variables were investigated to determine if the variability was explained by their presence.

RESTORATIVE JUSTICE

Restorative justice is an approach to justice that is in contrast to traditional, retributive justice. It is a humanistic approach to justice whereby the victim and offender meet to discuss how each was affected by the crime. This type of justice holds the offender accountable while offering support and fairness to the victim (Bradshaw & Umbreit, 1998; Zehr, 1997). Preferably, and in the case of this research, the victims and offenders meet face-to-face to negotiate reparations with the offender. The two most common expressions of restorative justice are victim-offender mediation (VOM) and family group conferencing (FGC). For detailed descriptions of approaches to restorative justice, refer to Presser and Van Voorhis (2002) or Umbreit (2000).

FEAR OF (RE)VICTIMIZATION

Fear of criminal victimization can be debilitating both physiologically and psychologically and may differ demographically (Williams-Hayes & Nugent, in press). For example, the elderly have higher rates of victimization fear than do younger people, especially those who have histories of prior victimization (Bazargan, 1994; Borooah & Carcach, 1997; Parker & Ray, 1990; Pogrebin & Pijoan, 1978). People who feel fearful may experience a myriad of symptoms (Table 83.1; for an overview, see Williams-Hayes & Nugent, in press). Victims are likely to fear being revictimized (Bradshaw & Umbreit, 1998; Vacha & McLaughlin, 2000; Zehr & Umbreit, 1982), but nonvictims are also afraid of crime.

The following three hypotheses were tested in this study:

1. Participants in restorative justice will report less fear of revictimization than participants in control groups.
2. There will be larger effect sizes for adolescent offenders than for adult offenders.
3. Effect sizes will vary systematically as a function of methodological quality scores, and studies that used comparison groups will report larger effect sizes.

These hypotheses were based on the literature. Because the victim can ask the offender questions directly about the victimization, the victim often sees that it was a random crime and also recognizes that the offender is a human being; the level of fear was hypothesized to thus be reduced. Further, it is common to find a discussion in the literature of the merit of rehabil-

TABLE 83.1 Symptoms of Victimization or Fear of Victimization

Category of Outcome	Specific Outcomes
Psychological	Depression
	Symptoms of PTSD
	Anxiety
	Sleep disturbances
	Psychosomatic illnesses
Physiological	Gynecological problems
	Gastrointestinal complaints
	Rheumatoid arthritis
	Immune ailments or changes
Behavioral	Keeping firearms loaded and accessible
	Abandoning regular/ healthy coping skills (e.g., increased tobacco smoking)
	Avoid leaving home after dark

itating adolescents when advocating prevention or treatment. Developmentally, adolescents are often viewed as more amendable to "change" or treatment. Therefore, studies of juvenile offenders may be more likely to report more positive results on outcomes than studies of adult offenders. Finally, erroneous information derived from the limitations of studies can lead to poor decisions. For example, if only white respondents complete a survey, the ability to generalize to other racial or ethnic populations is greatly reduced. Few researchers are able to assert a causal relationship because of the low internal validity of the design of their study. Better designed inquiry enables researchers to draw more accurate inferences of causality. Nugent, Williams, and Umbreit (in press) developed a scale to evaluate the methodological rigor of a study. The scale is composed of 12 questions and produces scores that can range from 0 to 12 in the total score metric, and 0 to 1 in the mean score metric. Higher scores on this scale were indicative of a more rigorous study in terms of the creation of comparison groups that were initially statistically equivalent. Consistent with the approach used by Nugent and colleagues (in press) in a prior meta-analysis, scores on this scale in the current meta-analysis were put into the mean score metric.

METHOD

Sample of Studies

The literature was reviewed to identify studies evaluating the outcomes of VOM and/or FGC for juveniles and/or adults during the formal existence of both programs, from the 1970s and onward. In the spring of 2002, research was conducted through the University of Tennessee's library catalog (Table 83.2).

Inclusion Criteria

To be included in this meta-analysis, a study had to have (a) used either juvenile and/or adult samples; (b) implied the use of either VOM or

TABLE 83.2 Search Engines and Descriptors

Type of Search	Descriptors
Article First	a
ERIC	a
E-subscribe	a
First Search	a
General Reference Center Gold	a
JSTOR	a
Papers First	a
PsychInfo	a
Social Science Abstracts	a
Digital Dissertations and Theses	a
NCJRS	a
Proquest (1980–present)	a
Internet (Google search engine)	b
Contacted authors/institutions	b

[a] Victim-offender mediation; victim-offender reconciliation program; mediation; family group conferencing; restorative justice; and various combinations of names of researchers in the field of restorative justice (e.g., Mark Umbreit).
[b] Evaluations of victim-offender mediation; assessments of victim-offender mediation; evaluations of family group conferencing; and assessments of family group conferencing.

FGC; (c) indicated that offenders and victims experienced a face-to-face meeting rather than indirect negotiation; and (d) focused on criminal as opposed to civil offenses.

Coding the Studies

Variables were coded in analyses as follows. The age of offender was coded as a dichotomous variable, with "juvenile" coded 0, and "adult" coded 1. This coding made juveniles the reference category. The mean score on the methodological quality scale (discussed earlier) represented the methodological rigor of a study. Finally, if a study included a comparison group, it was coded 0; otherwise it was coded 1. This coding scheme was analogous to the use of indicator or dummy variables to identify cases with missing values on a particular variable (Cohen & Cohen, 1983) and was used in an effort to determine if the explicit use of comparison groups was related to the magnitude of the obtained effect size.

Analysis

This meta-analysis used HGLMs with a logit link function, making the analysis analogous to logistic regression. The program HGLM version 4 was used. All outcomes analyzed in the meta-analysis were dichotomous. The binomial HGLM is appropriate for such data (Bryk, Raudenbush, & Congdon, 1996). It is analogous to logistic regression models in that a binary outcome (a person is still fearful of revictimization or is not still fearful) can be predicted from one or more independent variables. In addition to this method, a binary logistic regression was used, as well as ordinary least squares (OLS). There would be greater confidence in the results if the different analyses converged. If the results did not converge, further hypotheses could be developed to explore whether the findings were an artifact of the type of statistical method used. This can be considered a cautious approach to data analysis.

RESULTS

Using the inclusion criteria discussed earlier, a total of nine studies were identified as appropriate for this meta-analysis, with a total of 22 effect sizes. Of the nine studies, only three (33%)

were located in peer-reviewed journals. The remaining six studies were program evaluations. Of the nine studies, three were FGC studies.

A preliminary analysis of the data set indicated that there were few effect sizes in some "cells" representing specific combinations of levels of independent variables. Agresti (1996) refers to this situation as "sparse" data and shows how such data can lead to biased estimates of regression coefficients and odds ratios. A plot of effect sizes plotted by the type of restorative justice (VOM, FGC, or comparison group) was created for studies conducted with adult offenders to illustrate some of these sparse data (Figure 83.1). Figure 83.1 shows that there were only two data points for studies conducted with adult offenders. No data point could be displayed for FGC because there were no studies for this combination of independent variables. In addition to the age-of-offender variable, the comparison group variable (i.e., whether or not a study utilized a comparison group) also had few effect sizes for some combinations of independent variables. Because of the possibility of erroneous results arising from the sparse numbers of effect sizes for several combinations of values of categorical independent variables, it was decided *not* to include these variables in analyses.[1] For these reasons, hypothesis 2 and part of hypothesis 3 were not tested.

The results of fitting an unconditional HGLM to the data from studies that investigated levels of fearfulness suggested that there was significant variation across groups in magnitude of effect sizes (estimated parameter variance $\alpha^2 = .61$, $x^2[21] = 132.4$, $p < .001$). These results suggested that there was systematic variation across groups in fear of revictimization, and that an HGLM with predictors should be fitted to the data.

Therefore, an HGLM with the following predictors was fitted to the data: type of justice and the methodological quality of each study. The results suggested that this model accounted for more than two thirds of the significant variation (70%) across groups in magnitude of the effect sizes (estimated residual parameter variance = $\alpha^2 = .18$, $x^2[18] = 38.7$, $p = .003$). Results further suggested that there was significant residual systematic variation across groups. After controlling for all included explanatory variables, victims who participated in VOM were significantly less fearful of revictimization than were those who did not participate in restorative justice ($\beta = -1.07$, $t[18] = -3.55$, $p = .003$). These results suggested that the odds of VOM participants reporting themselves still fearful of revictimization were only .34 as great as the odds of nonparticipants reporting they were still fearful. Victims who participated in FGC also reported significantly less fear of revictimization than did victims who did not participate in restorative justice ($\beta = -1.32$, $t[18] = -4.10$, $p = .001$). These results suggested that the odds of FGC participants reporting their continuing fear of revictimization were only .27 as great as the odds of nonparticipants reporting that they were still fearful. When the level of fearfulness of revictimization of victims who had participated in VOM was directly compared with the level of fearfulness of revictimization of those who participated in FGC, the results suggested that there was not a significant difference between the impact of these two approaches to restorative justice on this outcome ($\beta = -0.25$, $t[18] = -0.74$, $p = .469$).

The variable indicating the methodological quality of a study was not significantly associated with the level of fearfulness outcome after controlling for all included explanatory variables ($\beta = 0.57$, $t[18] = 1.99$, $p = .062$). These results were inconsistent with hypothesis 3. Data from all nine studies were used, even though four of the studies did not have comparison groups. To evaluate whether the results could have been an

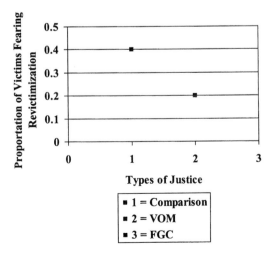

FIGURE 83.1 Effect sizes for fearfulness with adult offenders.

artifact of the method of analysis, another analysis was performed excluding effect sizes from studies without comparison groups. This more conservative approach suggested that whereas the VOM and methodological score effects were the same, FGC effects on fearfulness were not significantly different from the control group ($\beta = -.45$, $t[12] = -1.39$, $p = .189$). Extreme caution must be used, however, because only one FGC study was represented in this analysis. In another effort to determine whether or not findings were an artifact of the type of analysis performed, binary logistic regression and OLS were also used. Results from the binary regression and the OLS suggested that there was a significant difference in the level of fearfulness between groups, with treatment groups reporting less fear ($\beta = -1.21$, Wald $= 63.12$, $p < -.05$, $\beta = -.15$, $t = -3.40$, $p = .003$, respectively). The convergence of these analyses corroborates the reduced levels of fearfulness after participating in restorative justice.

DISCUSSION

Limitations of Study

All findings must be interpreted cautiously because of the following limitations of this meta-analysis: the number of effect sizes, the violation of an important independence assumption, low statistical power, and the parameters of selection criteria. Specific examples of how these problems may have affected the results of this meta-analysis are provided in the following discussion.

Hypothesis 2 and part of hypothesis 3 were not tested because of problems with sparse data. These omitted variables may have accounted for some of the remaining systematic variation in outcomes, a discrepancy that perhaps could have been overcome if those variables had been included in the HGLM. Further, inclusion of these omitted variables may have changed the results of data analyses and suggested substantively different conclusions. Second, if there were relatively few effect sizes for a specific approach to justice, such as FGC, and it was compared with other approaches to justice, such as VOM, then those few effect sizes representing FGC might have given a poor and inaccurate representation of the outcomes associated with FGC. Results from one study or effect size regarding a form of justice cannot be generalized.

This meta-analysis often included multiple effect sizes from a single study, a common practice in meta-analyses (Glass, McGraw, & Smith, 1981). To ensure that there was the maximum statistical power possible, effect sizes for each "category" were used. For instance, if a single study included fear effect sizes for both property and violent crimes, then both effect sizes were used, with each treated as an independent effect size. The results of this meta-analysis could, at least to some extent, be an artifact of complex interdependencies between the multiple effect sizes from the same studies (Glass et al., 1981). Finally, although the literature search was arguably exhaustive, the paucity of effect sizes means that statistical power was low.

Recommendations

Practice

Restorative justice appears to be a promising intervention for victims of crime in terms of reducing levels of fearfulness of revictimization. If lower levels of fearfulness are indeed found, then the quality of life for victims is enhanced. These findings have implications for the professional community, too. Medical professionals equipped with knowledge about potentially effective treatments can make referrals, such as to a community restorative justice program. Likewise, restorative justice practitioners can assess psychological and somatic complaints and make referrals to mental health and medical, respectively. Finally, practitioners should fully disclose to participants the potential benefits and limits of such an approach to justice.

Research

This meta-analysis needs to be replicated when additional studies and effect sizes are available. Future research should include the use of more comparison groups, preferably through random assignment. Few studies used random assignment, and without it causal relationships cannot be easily determined. Research should also begin evaluating differential effects. There is a paucity of studies reporting outcomes on adults. More programs need to test the effects of adult participation. The literature suggests that fear of victimization differs across the life span. Knowing if this form of brief intervention is effective with populations of different ages is vital. Similarly, data need to be gathered to evaluate the effectiveness with either gender and with different racial or ethnic groups. This meta-analysis could not consider either demographic variable because much research has not reported participant gender or race. Finally, researchers should disseminate their findings in various venues to reach multidisciplinary practitioners. Clients may reap the benefits of having all their caregivers know about the potentially positive effects of restorative justice.

Notes

1. One study used three sites, two used a mixture of adults and juveniles, and one used a sample of only juveniles.

2. When analyses included all potential explanatory variables, the results were very different, with some parameter estimates quite large. The relatively large parameter estimates were consistent with the likelihood of bias introduced by the sparse data in some cells, as described by Agresti (1996). These results are not reported here.

References

References marked with an asterisk indicate studies included in the first analysis of the meta-analysis.

References marked with a double asterisk indicate studies included in the second analysis of the meta-analysis.

Agresti, A. (1996). *An introduction to categorical data analysis*. New York: Wiley.

Bazargan, M. (1994). The effects of health, environmental, and socio-psychological variables on fear of crime and its consequences among urban black elderly individuals. *International Journal on Aging and Human Development, 38*, 99–115.

Borooah, V. K., & Carcach, C. A. (1997). Crime and fear: Evidence from Australia. *British Journal of Criminology, 37*, 635–657.

Bradshaw, W., & Umbreit, M. S. (1998, summer). Crime victims meet juvenile offenders: Contributing factors to victim satisfaction with mediated dialogue. *Juvenile and Family Court Journal*, 17–24.

Bryk, A., Raudenbush, S., & Congdon, R. (1996). *Hierarchical linear and nonlinear modeling with the HLM/2L and HLM/3L programs*. Chicago: Scientific Software International.

Cohen, J. (1988). *Statistical power analysis for the behavioral sciences* (2nd ed.). Hillsdale, NJ: Erlbaum.

Cohen, J., & Cohen, P. (1983). *Applied multiple regression/correlation analysis for the behavioral sciences* (2nd ed.). Hillsdale, NJ: Erlbaum.

**Davis, R. C., Tilchane, M., & Grayson, D. (1980).

Mediation and arbitration as alternatives to prosecution in felony arrest cases: An evaluation of the Brooklyn dispute resolution center. New York: VERA Institute of Justice.

Glass, G. V. (1977). Integrating findings: The meta-analysis of research. *Review of Research in Education, 5*, 351–379.

Glass, G., McGraw, B., & Smith, M. L. (1981). *Meta-analysis in social research*. Beverly Hills, CA: Sage.

*Hayes, H., Prenzler, T., & Wortley, R. (1998). *Making amends: Final evaluation of the Queensland community conferencing pilot*. Brisbane, Australia: Griffith University, Centre for Crime Policy and Public Safety, School of Criminology and Criminal Justice.

Herbert, T. B., & Cohen, S. (1993). Depression and immunity: A meta-analytic review. *Psychological Bulletin, 113*, 472–486.

Latimer, J., Dowden, C., & Muise, D. (2001). *The effectiveness of restorative justice practices: A meta-analysis*. Research and Statistics Division, Department of Justice Canada.

Lipsey, M. W. (1995). What do we learn from 400 research studies on the effectiveness of treatment with juvenile delinquents? In J. McGuire (Ed.), *Reducing reoffending: Guidelines from research and practice*. New York: Wiley.

**McCold, P., & Wachtel, T. (1998). *Restorative policing experiment: The Bethlehem Pennsylvania police family group conferencing project*. Pipersville, PA: Community Service Foundation.

Nugent, W. R., Williams, M., & Umbreit, M. S. (in press). Participation in victim-offender mediation and the prevalence of subsequent delinquent behavior: A meta-analysis. *Utah Law Review*.

Parker, K. D., & Ray, M. C. (1990). Fear of crime: An assessment of related factors. *Sociological Spectrum, 10*, 29–40.

Pogrebin, M., & Pijoan, G. N. (1978). The fear of crime by the elderly: Issues and consequences. *Journal of Sociology and Social Welfare, 5*, 856–862.

Presser, L., & Van Voorhis, P. (2002). Values and evaluation: Assessing processes and outcomes of restorative justice programs. *Crime and Delinquency, 48*, 162–188.

Rind, B., Bauserman, R., & Tromovich, P. (1998). A meta-analytic examination of assumed properties of child sexual abuse using college samples. *Psychological Bulletin, 124*, 22–53.

*Strang, H., Barnes, G. C., Braithwaite, J., & Sherman, L. W. (1999). *Experiments in restorative policing: A progress report on the Canberra Reintegrative Shaming Experiments (RISE)*. Australian Federal Policy and Australian National University.

*Umbreit, M. S. (1991, August). Minnesota mediation

center produced positive results. *Corrections Today*, 192–196.

**Umbreit, M. S. (1993). Juvenile offenders meet their victims: The impact of mediation in Albuquerque, New Mexico. *Family and Conciliation Courts Review, 31*, 90–100.

*Umbreit, M. S. (1994). Crime victims confront their offenders: The impact of a Minneapolis mediation program. *Research on Social Work Practice, 4*, 435–447.

**Umbreit, M. S. (1995). *Mediation of criminal conflict: An assessment of programs in four Canadian provinces*. St. Paul. Center for Restorative Justice and Mediation, School of Social Work, University of Minnesota.

Umbreit, M. S. (2000). *The handbook of victim offender mediation: An essential guide to practice and research.* San Francisco: Jossey-Bass.

**Umbreit, M. S., & Roberts, A. W. (1996). *Mediation of criminal conflict in England: An assessment of services in Coverty and Leeds*. Center for Restorative Justice and Mediation, School of Social Work, University of Minnesota.

Vacha, E. F., & McLaughlin, T. F. (2000). The impact of poverty, fear of crime, and crime victimization on keeping firearms for protection and unsafe gun-storage practices: A review and analysis with policy recommendations. *Urban Education, 35*, 496–512.

Williams-Hayes, M. M. (2002). *The effectiveness of restorative justice: A meta-analysis.* Unpublished doctoral dissertation, University of Tennessee.

Williams-Hayes, M., & Nugent, W. (in press). Effects of restorative justice on fear of revictimization.

Zehr. H. (1997, December). Restorative justice: The concept. *Corrections Today*, 68–70.

Zehr, H., & Umbreit, M. (1982). Victim offender reconciliation: An incarceration substitute? *Federal Probation, 46*, 63–68.

FACTORS ASSOCIATED WITH CRIME ON THE CASINO FLOOR

84

Implications of Secondary Data Analysis

Gerard LaSalle

Americans love to gamble, so concluded a congressionally funded national task force in 1998, studying the impact of gambling in the United States (National Gambling Impact Study Commission Report, 1999). All but two states (Utah and Hawaii) have some form of legalized wagering. Advocates look to gambling as an economic elixir for communities; opponents counter that these benefits exact punishing social costs,

including an increase in crime. Numerous studies have examined the casino-crime relationship and have produced mixed results. Some studies have confirmed that casinos have no direct effect on serious crime (Albanese, 1985, 1999), whereas others have either reached opposite conclusions (Grinols, Mustard, Dilley, 1999; Hakim & Buck, 1989; Friedman, Hakim, & Weinblatt, 1989) or reflected that certain crimes rose while others decreased (Giacopassi & Stitt, 1993).

These studies typically seek to measure the community impact of casinos by using aggregate Uniform Crime Report (UCR) statistics. Such studies are usually undertaken when communities are seeking to introduce casino gambling and want data on what economic and social impacts they can anticipate. By looking at locations where such gambling has been legalized and comparing the pre- and postcasino crime data, elected administrators believe they are better equipped to make a correct decision on whether to permit casinos in their communities. Since gambling is "big business," proponents argue that when the casino crime data are controlled for the increase in the tourist population ("boomtown effect"), casinos have no additive effect on crime. By contrast, adversaries claim their analysis of similar crime data suggests that the incidence of crime has risen, causing more police, health, and other community services to be taxed.

Prior to the completion of the current study, no recorded studies examining the casino-crime relationship have focused on the victim on the casino floor. Additionally, this study is distinguished by two important elements. One, it is strictly limited to examining reported crime in the actual gaming area, the area containing the largest concentration of hotel guests in proximity of potential offenders. Second, it answers the who, what, where, when, and how questions regarding casino patrons as victims. Victimization by "place" and victimization by "method" are always critical components of victim studies.

By empirically looking at the frequency of offenses, the demographics of the victim, and the type of crimes committed on the casino floor, this study aims to fill this void in the knowledge base, thus helping policy makers to be more responsive to the safety needs of casino patrons. Using the routine activities theory, data were analyzed for reported casino floor crime for all 12 casinos in Atlantic City, New Jersey, for 1999 and 2000. This chapter presents a quantitative and qualitative examination of one of the many hypotheses addressed by this larger study. Specifically, what is the most prevalent crime committed on the casino floor? What methods have the casinos employed in combating this crime, and how have industry officials explained its nature and extent? In terms of predatory crime, is the casino floor a patron's safest bet? The 7,908

reported incidents represent the total universe of UCR Part 1 crimes committed on the casino floor for 1999 and 2000.

THEORETICAL FRAMEWORK

The routine activities theory first espoused by Cohen and Felson in 1979 has received much empirical attention. It is grounded in the necessity of three elements to converge for a crime to occur: (a) motivated offenders, (b) suitable targets, and (c) the absence of capable guardians. Cohen and Felson attempted to explain crime trends by examining the "routine activities" of everyday life and how these activities created criminal opportunities. They included in their definition of "routine activities" leisure time spent away from home. They deemphasized characteristics of the offenders and, in fact, assumed criminal inclination as a given. Offenders were anyone predisposed to committing a crime who was drawn to the more visible target, either through a flash of money or an appearance that invites attack. The ease of access to either a building or a person also would render a target more suitable. Suitable targets, they said, can be an object (purse, car, wallet) or a human (for personal attack). Target selection is governed by the probability of success of completing the crime, as well as the value of the fruits of the crime. The third element of Cohen and Felson's theory focused on "guardianship." In addition to the victims acting as guardians, capable guardians were either police, family members, friends, or mechanical security devices that would frustrate a criminal attack and protect a target or alert security.

EMPIRICAL EXAMINATIONS OF ROUTINE ACTIVITIES THEORY

Empirically, the routine activities approach has received wide support. Analyzing the National Crime Victimization Survey, Miethe, Stafford, and Long (1987) found routine activities had a direct effect on property victimization. Stahura noted (1988) that routine activities also had a direct effect on arson rates. Outside-of-home victimization has also been well documented. Sampson and Woodredge (1987) and Kennedy and Forde (1990) reported high rates of victimization for youth out at night. Lasley and Rosenbaum (1988) found multiple victimization associated with high alcohol consumption and "partying" on Friday or Saturday night. Miethe, Stafford, and Sloane (1990) determined that generally those who left their homes for evening activity were more likely to be victimized. Hollinger and Dabney (1999) concluded that motivated offenders and absence of capable guardians significantly affected motor vehicle thefts at major shopping malls.

LITERATURE REVIEW

The effect of tourism is a major topic that has been examined in assessing the impact of casinos on crime in communities. Much of this literature points to the burgeoning tourist population that contributes to crime rather than specifically labeling casinos as the cause (Miller & Schwartz, 1998). A second element that is often discussed is how behavior patterns of tourists themselves enhance the likelihood of their victimization. Specifically, they carry portable wealth, are unknown in the community, and, as temporary visitors, are unfamiliar with the surrounding community (Chesney-Lind & Lind, 1986).

Tourism studies of the impact of casinos in Illinois, California, Colorado, Connecticut, Minnesota, Wisconsin, and Mississippi (Margolis, 1997) and Indiana (Wilson, 2001) all concluded that there was no statistically significant increase in crime by itself, or when the population was adjusted to include tourists. Similarly, Reuter (1997) examined the impact of 20 casino cities in the United States for the Greater Baltimore Committee that was considering the legalization of casino gambling in Maryland. He concluded that casinos had a minimal effect on crime.

Gambling and the Elderly

Certain empirical studies have confirmed an increase in the number of senior citizens who gamble. By surveying activity directors for elderly facilities in Omaha and Nebraska, McNeilly and Burke (2001) found that casino gambling was the most frequented day trip activity for the elderly. A University of Chicago National Opinion Research Center study from February 1999 determined that since 1974, the largest increase in gamblers has been for those aged 65 and older. Kennedy (1999) found that re-

garding gambling, the elderly were disproportionately represented, and in that group "women tend to play the slots and veg out, sometimes for hours." The elderly are also beginning to appear in greater numbers at treatment programs for disordered gambling. The executive director for the Compulsive Gambling Center in Baltimore notes that slot machines are preferred by seniors; slot machines allow them to play for hours unintimidated by face-to-face competition and without needing to learn the mechanics of a new game.

A profile of the casino resort vacationer (Morrison, Braunlich, Liping, & O'Leary, 1996), compared with beach, ski, and country resort vacationers, found that those favoring casino vacations were considerably older (one-fourth of the casino vacationers were 65 or older) and more likely to be female. Additionally, they participated in fewer activities outside of the casino; for them the main attraction was gambling. They typically spent less time in rooms or other available casino hotel activities; a significant number of patrons were retired.

Effect of Casinos in Atlantic City

Studies specific to Atlantic City, New Jersey, generally have examined the tourism and crime relationship. Albanese (1985), commenting on reports of a rise in crime in Atlantic City, noted that these studies suffered from serious methodological flaws by not controlling for the rise in population of tourists to the casinos. When he examined other data on index crimes from 1978 to 1982 in Atlantic City, and compared it with data for the entire state, controlling for tourism, he found that the increase in the crime rate was not attributable to casinos.

Friedman et al. (1989) reported that crime in adjacent communities and non-toll routes to Philadelphia and New York City rose significantly after casinos came to Atlantic City. Curran and Scarpitti (1991), after comparing Atlantic City index crimes with those in the rest of the state, ascertained that legalized gambling did not result in significant increases of index crime rates in Atlantic City. More specifically, by looking at the Atlantic City police department reports, they found that most crimes within close proximity of the casino hotels victimized non–community residents. Their data from the police department's Casino/Hotel Investigations Unit combined crimes on the casino grounds and the casino floor and refined the work of Albanese and others "by distinguishing between casino-based and community crime in Atlantic City." They presented a frequency table from 1985 to 1989 that indicated that on average there were over 8,000 thefts reported attributable to the casinos, this number having been achieved by aggregating all casino-related crime. That is, if a larceny was reported in the actual gaming area, in an elevator, in a hotel room, or within close proximity of the hotel, it was reported as casino related. These researchers did not disaggregate casino floor crime in their reporting or their illustrative tables. In fact, from their data, there is no way to distinguish if the hotel itself was the victim of an attempted larceny by unscrupulous patrons using bogus chips or other devious schemes to victimize the hotel.

THE CURRENT STUDY

This study examined the victimization risk of patrons at the 12 Atlantic City casinos. Since 1995, Atlantic City has averaged approximately 9 million bus passenger visitors per year and approximately 34 million visitors (Pollock, 2001). Casino settings have not been the focus of any victimization studies.

As with the bar studies mentioned earlier, casinos offer a similar environment and perhaps even more opportunity for victimization. Specifically, casinos are open and free to the public, and whereas some bars and clubs can either charge an entrance fee (cover) or require patrons to be suitably dressed, no such constraint exists for entrance to the casino floor, except the age requirement of 21. Patrons at bars may carry cash, but it is not always required because most bars accept credit card payment. The amount actually carried by a club patron for an evening's entertainment probably is less than what a patron carries to a casino.

Casinos attract an influx of tourists, who usually are carrying significant sums of cash, thus making them more alluring to offenders. This increases their target attractiveness, as would an ostentatious display of jewelry for an evening out on the town. However, the transportation of cash to the casino is not at issue because patrons can either obtain cash from the many automated teller machines on the casino floor or draw down on established lines of credit. All modes of transportation to the casino are protected by secured parking areas or provide for the immediate discharge of passengers at the casino front doors.

Offenders at casinos enjoy anonymity and are in close proximity, often side by side, with their potential victims on the casino floor. The casino floor provides an ideal environment for direct physical contact to steal or injure. Typically, most patrons who are wagering are not near any guardian who may have accompanied them to the casino.

If family members or other casino patrons who could serve as potential guardians are nearby, they often are engaged in gambling activities and are less watchful than they would be in a less busy area. This convergence of suitable targets, motivated offenders, and a potential strain or inadequate resource commitment by the casinos (a figurative absence) of capable guardians fulfills the necessary requirements for victimization to occur consistent with the routine activities theory.

The source of the data was each casino's investigation report, which is its crime-reporting document for all crimes committed on the casino floor. These reports revealed that approximately 4,085 crimes in 1999 and 3,823 crimes in 2000 were reported as Part 1 offenses of the Uniform Crime Reports. Crimes included in Part 1 include murder, rape, robbery, aggravated assault, burglary, larceny (theft), motor vehicle theft, and arson. These reports are a rich source of information on the victim-crime relationship. They contain biographical details about the victim (race, age, gender); the time, day, and date the crime occurred; the location on the casino floor where the crime occurred; the type of crime; the type of injury, if any, associated with the crime; the purpose of the visit (gambling, business, pleasure, convention); the victim's residence; and whether the victim had previously been victimized in Atlantic City. Analysis was based on the total population of reported crimes ($n = 7,908$).

Excluded from the index offenses were motor vehicle theft and arson. Additionally, reported incidents where the casino was the intended victim were not counted. Such incidents include patron attempts to use bogus casino chips, attempts to illegally circumvent proper payout by using cheating devices, or employee collusion with a player to defraud the casino by according the player an unfair advantage.

Drawing upon the information contained in the casino investigation crime report, which tells us that a patron has been the victim of a criminal offense while engaged in leisure activity (gambling); the sample's demographic characteristics (gender, age, race); temporal characteristics (time, day, month, year); spatial characteristics (location of victimization, type of wagering activity); the value and type of property stolen; injury sustained (serious, minor); the patron's residence (Atlantic City, Atlantic County, in-state, out-of-state); the reason for the patron's visit to Atlantic City (gambling, vacation, business, or a combination); and whether the patron was previously victimized at the casino.

FINDINGS

These findings are part of a larger study that is currently in progress seeking to examine not only the crime of choice at the casinos but whether victims vary by age and gender and whether the type of play (slot machines or table games) and the location of the casino (near or away from the boardwalk) influence the risk of victimization. Reported here are the data for one of the independent variables (crime type), as well as discussion with security officials for Trump properties, which represents 4 of the 12 casinos in Atlantic City.

In New Jersey, for the years 1999 and 2000, personal theft represented the most frequent crime—approximately 60% of all reported crimes. If motor vehicle theft is added, the percentage increases to 71% of all reported index crimes (Crime in New Jersey, Uniform Crime Report, 2000). The data specific to the casinos were consistent with that for all of New Jersey. As Tables 84.1 and 84.2 clearly illustrate, theft was the crime of choice for all the casinos. Trump officials believed that a more in-depth analysis would reveal that the thefts were moneys stolen from a patron's purse or coin cup and that patrons usually tend to be less vigilant

while engaged in play. Consistent with the general literature on the elderly noted earlier, as well as the routine activities theory (suitable targets element), the findings indicate that most victims are over 62, with a gradual rise to the 70s. With regard to the victim profile, 78% of the victims were females for both years.

Unexpectedly, the data demonstrated that most crime occurred between October and December, not June and August, the typical vacationing months, and the time of year that contingent shore communities in close proximity to Atlantic City are burgeoning with vacationers. Casino officials suggested some alternative explanations. October is the peak convention season for Atlantic City, and beginning shortly after Labor Day and into the end of September, at the culmination of the Miss America pageant, the total casino staff is downsized with the release of summer seasonal employees; this includes security staff.

Additionally, the casino bus companies are driven by incentive. Because of the general dwindling of attendance at the casino during this period, the casinos "sweeten the incentives" by offering greater amounts of monetary vouchers for casino visitors. Where during the summer months the casinos may return to each bus rider a $5 voucher, in October that amount escalates to $15 because business is slower. The crime spike is consistent with the routine activities theory, as fewer capable guardians are available.

A preliminary review of other data by injury reveals that less than 1% involved an injury to the patron. Overwhelmingly, 98% of the victims reported that they sustained no injury, attesting to the safety of the casino floor as it relates to all types of crime except theft. As indicated previously, the type of theft that occurs usually is possible because of the stealth of the offender and the inattention of the victimized patron.

TABLE 84.1 Frequency Distribution for All Casinos in 2000 by Crime Type

Crime Type	Frequency	Percent	Cumulative Frequency	Cumulative Percent
Robbery	1	0.03	1	0.03
Aggravated assault	5	0.13	6	0.16
Larceny	3,817	99.84	3,823	100.00

TABLE 84.2 Frequency Distribution for All Casinos in 1999 by Crime Type

Crime Type	Frequency	Percent	Cumulative Frequency	Cumulative Percent
Robbery	5	0.12	5	0.12
Aggravated assault	4	0.10	9	0.22
Larceny	4,076	99.78	4,085	100.00

THE THEFT PROFILE

The ingenuity of the offender often surpasses the shield of casino patrons who are somewhat vigilant and themselves act as guardians. Specifically, working in teams, offenders would distract a slot player by pointing to currency on the floor near the player (previously placed there by the team) and asking about ownership. When the patron leaned over to retrieve the money, the other offender would steal either the cup or the purse. In another instance, the potential thief used a jacket over his arm and backed up to a woman's purse, covering it with his jacket. Slowly he walked away with the purse, but he was caught on camera. When confronted by a guard, the offender engaged in a violent confrontation, which escalated the theft to a robbery charge; he was sentenced to incarceration.

Perhaps the most ingenious theft scheme took place in the women's rest room. The stalls in the rest room were first equipped with hooks on which hang purses. When women were attending to their garments, a thief in the next stall would reach over and steal their purse. After a series of thefts, casino security removed the purse hooks. Shortly thereafter, all the hooks were replaced, but not by the hotel. Apparently, the thief was not going to permit a target hardening by security to thwart such a scheme. It was not until the hotel plugged the hooks that the scheme disappeared. Experienced security observers are attuned to a typical thieving profile—a profile not of race, gender, or age, but one of movement. Typical slot players move up and down the slot machine aisles with their eyes fixed on the machine displays, such as fruit rows, numerals, or other glitzy icons located slightly above eye level. Offenders, on the other hand, walk up and down the aisles, looking downward toward the areas where patrons would typically place their purses or a coin when not engaged in play. This predatory body language alerts physical security on the floor and video surveillance security to a potential crime hazard.

Casinos are constantly trying to identify theft profiles and patterns. Barlow and Kauzlarich (2002) reported, however, that some thieves strive to remain generalists rather than become specialists. When thieves "have a line," they specialize in theft of certain merchandise or a particular type of theft—picking pockets, forgery, or con games. Thieves who remain generalists believe that having a specialty jeopardizes their anonymity and increases the chance of arousing suspicion. Generally, amateur thieves are distinguished from professionals by their likelihood of arrest and conviction, the potential financial proceeds of a theft, the technical skill required for success, and the fencing arrangement. This seems consistent with Sutherland's Professional *Thief*, who spoke about the highly technical skills needed and how they are learned, the careful planning required, and the prohibition of specializing in a type of theft. Based on the casino crime data of this study, where the average theft is usually of purses and coin cups averaging less than $100, it is apparent that the casino floor environment is for the amateur.

POLICY IMPLICATIONS

It is anticipated that the future findings of the study will point to the areas of greatest vulnerability for each casino. By identifying the demographics of the victim, as well as the location of victimization, greater generalizability of the data will be realized. Ideally, these findings will result in industrywide policy changes or initiatives directed by the state to provide better protection for its wagering public. As certain aspects of casino security are regulated by the state, which sets minimum security standards and requires casinos to arrange their facilities to promote security, the data may point to areas of vulnerability on the casino floor. Specifically, if the data were to suggest that most crimes occur in the slot machine area, on specific days, and at particular times, best-practice security strategies should employ an increase in guardians at those "hot spot" areas to deter offenses. Perhaps local ordinances could be enhanced to strengthen antiloitering laws or to increase penalties for crimes committed within casinos.

By examining all the illustrative graphics in tandem, one can conclude that theft of elderly women is the victim profile for casino floor crime. If further investigation reveals that most patrons travel to Atlantic City on public or private bus transportation, the state, via these companies, can institute initiatives in the form of video presentations or literature to educate casino patrons to be more vigilant with their possessions.

If the data reflect that the rate of victimization varies by casino, discussion with casino executives may result in a better policy to "environment out" potential areas of victimization. Conversely, if comparisons with other area casinos or major tourist attractions reveal that the Atlantic City casino floor is indeed a safe environment, as a preliminary analysis seems to suggest, then perhaps the New Jersey regulatory and casino security strategies can become a paradigm for the entire industry.

It is hoped that this study will enlighten casino administrators and sensitize them to the security requirements of their patrons. At the same time, it can provide empirical data to support important policy changes by the state.

References

Albanese, J. (1985). The effect of casino gambling on crime. *Federal Probation, 49*(2), 39–44.

Albanese, J. (1999). Casino gambling and white-collar crime: An examination of the empirical evidence. *Report for the American Gaming Association.*

Chesney-Lind, M., & Lind, I. Y. (1986). Visitors as victims: Crimes against tourists in Hawaii. *Annals of Tourism Research, 13,* 167–191.

Cohen, L., & Felson, M. (1979). Social change and crime rate trends: A routine activity approach. *American Sociological Review, 44,* 588–608.

Curran, D., & Scarpitti, F. (1991). Crime in Atlantic City: Do casinos make a difference? *Deviant Behavior, 12,* 431–439.

Faggiani, D., & Owens, M. G. (1999). Robbery of older adults: A descriptive analysis using the National Incident Based Reporting System. *Justice Research and Policy, 1*(1), 97–117.

Friedman, J., Hakim, S., & Weinblatt, J. (1989). Casino gambling as a "growth pole" strategy and its effect on crime. *Journal of Regional Science, 29,* 615–623.

Giacopassi, D., & Stitt, B. G. (1993). Assessing the impact of casino gambling on crime in Mississippi. *American Journal of Criminal Justice, 18,* 117–131.

Giacopassi, D. J., Stitt, B. G., and Nichols, M. (2000). Including tourists in crime rate calculations for new casino jurisdictions: What difference does it make? *American Journal of Criminal Justice, 24,* 203–215.

Grinols, E. L., Mustard, D. B., & Dilley, C. H. (1999). Casinos and crime. *Inside Illinois, 12*(13), 1–34.

Hakim, S., & Buck, A. J. (1989). Do casinos enhance crime? *Journal of Criminal Justice, 17,* 409–416.

Hollinger, R. C., & Dabney, D. A. (1999). Motor vehicle theft at the shopping centre: An application of the routine activities approach. *Security Journal, 12*(1), 63–78.

Kennedy, J. (1999, May 24). Gambling away the golden years. *Christianity Today,* pp. 41–47.

Kennedy, L. W., & Forde, D. R. (1990). Risky lifestyles and dangerous results: Routine activities and exposure to crime. *Sociology and Social Research, 74,* 208–211.

Lasley, J. R., & Rosenbaum, J. L. (1988). Routine activities and multiple personal victimization. *Sociology and Social Research, 73,* 47–50.

Margolis, J. (1997). Casinos and crime: An analysis of the evidence. *Report prepared for the American Gaming Association.*

McNielly, D. P., & Burke, W. J. (2001). Gambling as a social activity of older adults. *International Journal of Aging and Human Development, 52,* 19–28.

Miethe, T. D., Stafford, M. C., & Long, J. S. (1987). Routine activities: Lifestyle and victimization. *American Sociological Review, 52,* 184–194.

Miethe, T. D., Stafford, M., & Sloane, D. (1990). Lifestyle changes and risks of criminal victimization. *Journal of Quantitative Criminology, 6,* 357–376.

Miller, W. J., & Schwartz, M. D. (1998). Casino gambling and street crime. *Annals of the American Academy of Political and Social Science, 556,* 124–137.

Morrison, A. M., Braunlich, C. G., Liping, A. C., & O'Leary, J. T. (1996). A profile of the casino resort vacationer. *Journal of Tourism Research 35*(2), 55–61.

National Gambling Impact Study Commission Report. (1999). Washington, DC.

Ochrym, R. G. (1988). Street crime in Atlantic City,

New Jersey: An empirical analysis. *Nevada Review of Business and Economics, 12,* 2–7.

Ochrym, R. G. (1990). Street crime, tourism, and casinos: An empirical comparison. *Journal of Gambling Studies, 6*(2), 127–138.

Pizam, A., Tarlow, P. E., & Bloom, J. (1997). Making tourists feel safe: Whose responsibility is it? *Journal of Travel Research, 36*(1), 23–28.

Pollock, M. (2001). Six-year trend: Line vs. charter bus passengers. *Gaming Industry Oserver, 6*(3), 7.

Reuter, P. (1997). The impact of casinos on crime and other social problems: An analysis of recent experiences. *Report for the Greater Baltimore Committee.*

Sampson, R. J., & Wooldredge, J. D. (1987). Linking the micro and macro level dimensions of lifestyle routine activity and opportunity model of predatory victimization. *Journal of Quantitative Criminology, 3,* 371–393.

Stahura, J. M., & Hollinger, R. C. (1988). A routine activities approach to suburban arson rates. *Sociological Spectrum, 8,* 349–369.

Wilson, J. M. (2001). Riverboat gambling and crime in Indiana: An empirical investigation. *Crime and Delinquency, 47,* 610–640.

85

HOMICIDES OF OLDER WOMEN IN NEW YORK CITY

A Profile Based on Secondary Data Analysis

Patricia Brownell & Jacquelin Berman

Dramatic news stories of domestic violence homicides rivet the attention of newspaper readers daily:

- A young pregnant woman disappears and is found washed up on a beach months later with her baby attached to the umbilical cord. After the police learn that her husband had been having an affair with another woman, he becomes the primary suspect.
- A man stalks his estranged wife when she returns home from work after picking up their 2-year-old child. He shoots her dead while she holds their son in her arms.
- A young model, on the brink of success in her career, is shot in the face and killed by her ex-fiancé, who then commits suicide.

News stories about murdered older women are also horrifying, although they seldom appear on the front page or as a lead story on evening television:

- A recent retiree is murdered by her granddaughter, a crack-cocaine addict, because she finally says no to her granddaughter's demands for money.
- An elderly widow is murdered by a son described by neighbors as "just a bad person" while her young granddaughter, for whom

she was the primary caregiver, sleeps in an adjacent room.

- An elderly mother visits her institutionalized mentally ill adult daughter every week, until a street thug murders her in a botched robbery attempt. It takes a detective 5 years to identify the woman's killer.
- A 70-year-old man, despondent over his ill health, murders his wife of 50 years and then kills himself.

Just as news stories of murders involving older women victims are relegated to the back pages of newspapers, research involving murders of women has focused on younger victims. Certainly the specter of young women stalked and brutally murdered by loved ones or predatory strangers is terrible. However, the murder of older women—while not of childbearing age or at the beginning of their careers—is a tragic phenomenon that may reflect the continued vulnerability of women to abuse and violence in midlife and old age. As a hidden facet of violence against women, it is a social problem that deserves greater attention than it has received to date. For practitioners, researchers, and lawmakers concerned about elder abuse, it represents the ultimate expression of physical abuse. From this perspective, homicides of older women and elder abuse femicides are synonymous and will be used interchangeably in this chapter.

The objectives of this study on homicides of older women in New York City include identifying and better understanding the circumstances under which older women may become elder abuse homicide victims, the profiles of these homicides, and factors associated with them. The data set of 1,663 identified femicide victims dating from 1990 to 1997 was collected by a New York City Department of Health (DOH) research team, headed by Susan Wilt, assistant commissioner, Office of Health Promotion and Disease Prevention. Of the 1,663 femicides in the DOH data set, 315, or 19%, involved women aged 50 and older. The New York City Department for the Aging became a partner in the study discussed here because the agency believed that if more could be learned about these elder abuse femicides, more effective preventive measures could be planned and implemented with aging and law enforcement service networks.

Although attention was given to those cases involving intimate perpetrators, the study also examined homicides committed by strangers and unknown perpetrators. It developed a profile of victims and perpetrators related to elder abuse femicides involving older women who are victims of both stranger and intimate felony crimes. This is consistent with the definition of elder abuse, which includes all crimes against older adults, that is used in the literature (Yin, 1985), as well as in the Older Americans Act and the New York City Department for the Aging Elderly Crime Victims Resource Center.

NEED FOR RESEARCH ON HOMICIDES INVOLVING OLDER WOMEN AS VICTIMS

Homicides of older women have not been systematically studied to date (Cohen, 1999). Examples of key researchers who have integrated homicide research with younger intimate partner abuse culminating in homicide include Campbell (1995); Block, Donahue, and Block (2001); and Petee, Weaver, Corzine, Huff-Corzine, and Wittekind (2001). Interdisciplinary research efforts such as those supported by the Homicide Research Working Group (Petee & Corzine, 2002) can lead to fruitful cross-discipline knowledge building. Application of the findings to program planning and development of prevention and intervention strategies can save lives and improve safety for vulnerable populations of older women.

BACKGROUND AND SIGNIFICANCE

Estimates of the percentage of older Americans mistreated by family members range from 4% to 10% (Brownell, 2002; Thomas, 2002). These estimates address the issue of elder abuse (generally characterized as financial, physical, and psychological mistreatment), but there are few studies to date on homicides of older women. One reason may be because most homicide research to date has been undertaken by sociologists and criminologists, and not gerontologists. With the growing interest in research on older women by gerontologists and social workers, this situation is beginning to change (Wolf, 1999).

Most recently, Soos (1999) explored the issue of what he termed *gray murders*, a current topic of interest among elder abuse specialists who are concerned about the mistreatment of elder patients in nursing homes and health care settings. Gray murders are homicides disguised by perpetrators to look like natural deaths; this excludes assisted suicides that are planned by dying patients in partnership with medical personnel. The most infamous perpetrator of gray murders in recent history is the physician who murdered over 200 older female patients in England by lethal injection before he attempted to forge a victim's will and was apprehended. The focus of the study discussed here is different, in that these subjects' deaths have been ruled unambiguously as homicides by the New York City Examiner's Office.

Although the total number of reported homicides of older women in the New York City study is relatively small for the age groups examined (approximately 315 cases), it was felt to be sufficient to develop a preliminary profile of older female victims and their perpetrators, and to provide important information on homicides of older women and ultimately how to prevent them. A decision was made to include female victims who were 50 years or older at the time of their murder. In domestic violence homicide research, the focus is on younger women of childbearing age. Women in their 50s and older do not fit into this category and for the purposes of this study are considered older women.

OLDER WOMEN ABUSE VICTIMS

Studies to date suggest that the majority of elder abuse victims are women and their perpetrators are male (Brownell, 1998; Brownell, Berman, & Salamone, 1999). However, attempts to study the link between domestic violence and elder abuse, including a focus on female victims, have been limited (Penhale, 1999). Studies of homicide and the elderly are also rare. According to the Bureau of Justice Statistics (BJS, 2000), only about 5% percent of all homicides committed between 1975 and 1999 were of persons 65 years and older. Older males were more likely than older females of the same age to be homicide victims.

These statistics do not reflect the fact that most older females are killed by members of the opposite sex and that elderly females were more likely than elderly males to be killed by an elderly offender (BJS, 2000). Because males represent the majority of homicide victims, little of the research on homicide focuses on elderly femicides (Browne & Williams, 1993). One notable exception is the work of Campbell (1981, 1986, 1992, 1995). Campbell notes that the dynamics of homicides involving women are different than those involving men. Most women are killed by members of the opposite sex; most are killed by intimates; and of those, the majority of victims have been abused prior to the homicide (Campbell, 1995). Homicide perpetrated against a spouse followed by the suicide of the perpetrator is another form of homicide involving predominately female victims (Campbell, 1995; Cohen, 1999). Campbell's groundbreaking research on domestic violence-related homicides has focused on younger victims of spouse or partner abuse.

Other studies have found that homicides involving male perpetrators against their female partners are often precipitated by jealousy or serious threats by the victims to end the relationship. According to Koss et al. (1994), "The theme of male control—or the perceived loss of control via female independence, 'disobedience,' or attempts at autonomy—resurfaces in indepth studies of partner homicide" (p. 28). Brandl (2000) also explores this theme in her important work on elder spouse abuse.

HOMICIDES OF OLDER WOMEN

No published studies to date have focused specifically on homicides involving older women victims until the current study discussed in this chapter. As a result, important questions remain unanswered. Are older women most likely to be killed by a partner or spouse, other family members or acquaintances, or predatory strangers? How likely is it that perpetrators of homicides of older women are apprehended, given the greater isolation of older women in their communities? What is the race or ethnicity of older female victims and their perpetrators?

According to Campbell (1995), homicide is the leading cause of death of younger African American women. Since 1940, homicides have increased for both African American and European American women. An emergent interest in elder abuse in minority populations has generated a growing number of research projects (Tataro, 1997). However, the race or ethnicity of older female homicide victims has not been addressed until this study.

DISTINCTIONS BETWEEN HOMICIDES COMMITTED BY STRANGERS AND BY INTIMATES OR KNOWN PERPETRATORS

This data set included homicides of older women perpetrated by intimates and acquaintances and by strangers and unknown perpetrators. Homicide research typically includes these categories of perpetrators. One study of violent victimization of the elderly, utilizing the National Crime Victimization Survey and the Comparative Homicide File, examined lethal and nonlethal incidences of violent victimization against the elderly (Bachman, 1993). The study found that equal proportions of elderly homicide victims were killed by strangers, acquaintances, and relatives. The pattern differed depending on whether the victim was over or under the age of 65: Those younger than 65 were more likely to be killed by an acquaintance during an altercation.

Two important studies have been conducted to date on homicides involving older people: one that examined data on homicide cases involving elderly offenders in Chicago from 1965 to 1981, and another that examined elderly homicides committed by elderly offenders in Cuyahoga County, Ohio, from 1970 to 1983 (Kratcoski, 1992). In both studies the perpetrators and victims were overwhelmingly men. Alcohol appeared to play a role in the homicides for both perpetrator and victim, and homicide coupled with suicide of the perpetrator suggested that failing health and dementia could play a role in some homicides involving elderly spouses.

A subsequent study of homicide-suicide cases involving elderly spouses found that the homicides were virtually always carried out against unwilling female spouses or partners by male spouses or partners (Cohen, 1999). Homicide-suicides have been identified as a problem involving elderly victims and perpetrators (Holinger, 1987). Because homicide-suicide perpetrators who are elderly are often caregivers of ill or demented partners or spouses, this phenomenon is considered preventable with timely intervention (Flynn, 2000).

RESEARCH DESIGN

To learn more about homicides of older women, a descriptive study was undertaken to examine the variables related to homicides involving women aged 50 and older in New York City. The analysis was done on a subset of cases that were part of a secondary data set. The entire data set included cases of homicides of women aged 18 and older in New York City from 1990 to 1997. Of primary interest for the New York City Department of Health (DOH) study was a trend analysis of younger female domestic violence fatalities. Wilt and her team analyzed the homicides of women aged 18 to 49 years in relation to patterns of domestic and stranger violence. Variables examined in the study were race or ethnicity of the victim; circumstances of homicides, including method of femicide, location, toxicology of the victim, living arrangement with the alleged perpetrators and others; relationship with the alleged perpetrator; motive for homicide; and gender, age, and race or ethnicity of the alleged perpetrator. In the study discussed in this chapter, the homicides of older women (at least 50 years of age) were analyzed and compared with those of younger femicide victims (49 years or younger) in the DOH data set.

RESEARCH METHODOLOGY

The study represented a secondary data analysis using data from two sources: crime scene data from the Medical Examiner's Office and autopsy data from the Medical Examiner's Office. Data on the homicides were collected from Medical Examiner's Office records by the New York City DOH/Office of Health Promotion and Disease Prevention. All information related to the identity of victims remained strictly confidential as required by laws and regulations governing DOH record files and by federal and state laws governing protection of human subjects.

A total of 315 women aged 50 and older who were murdered in New York City between 1991 and 1997 were included in the study population. Criteria for inclusion in the study included the following: (a) the victim was 50 years or older; (b) the deceased was identified as a homicide victim by the New York City Medical Examiner's Office; (c) the homicide occurred between 1991 and 1997 in New York City; and (d) the victim resided in one of the five boroughs of New York City. Data from the Medical Examiner's reports were abstracted, coded, and entered by the DOH, and the SPSS data file was made available to the New York City Department of the Aging and Fordham University.

Descriptive statistics were used to describe

the victims and the circumstances surrounding the homicide events, as well as to make between-group and within-group comparisons related to age and other sociodemographic characteristics of victims and relationship to perpetrators, if known. Analyses were conducted for: (a) different ethnic and racial groups; (b) intimate and stranger perpetrators; (c) younger and older age groups; and (d) geographic areas in which femicides are committed. Missing data on perpetrators were handled through the development of a category, unknown perpetrator, which was analyzed separately from categories that included intimate or known perpetrator and stranger perpetrator.

RESEARCH FINDINGS

Profile of Victims

Of the 315 older female homicide victims, the majority were Black non-Hispanic (40%) and White non-Hispanic (38%), followed by Hispanic (19%), Asian (2%), and other (1%) (Table 85.1). The ages of victims ranged from 50 to 99, with a median age of 65, a mean age of 66.5, and a modal age of 50. Although the largest category of victims fell into the 50 to 59 age range, the oldest-old group of victims was the most disproportionate in comparison to the general population (Table 85.2).

Circumstances of Homicides of Older Women

The methods of homicides of older women in the study included the use of knives, guns, bludgeon instruments, strangling, asphyxiation, burning, and pushing. Of the older women homicides studied, most victims were stabbed (30%), shot (20%), or bludgeoned (18%). Of the rest, 15% were strangled, 4% were asphyxiated, and

TABLE 85.2 Comparison to Total NYC Population 60+ Female Population (1990 Census)

Age Group	% of 60+ Population	% of 60+ Victims
60–64	23	20
65–74	41	32
75–84	27	33
85+	9	15
Total	100	100

12% were killed by other means, including burning, pushing, and being exposed to smoke inhalation (Table 85.3). The majority of older female homicides (74%) occurred inside the victim's home (Table 85.4). Most victims did not reside with their perpetrators (51%), and an additional 3% possibly resided with their perpetrator. Only 14% of victims lived with their alleged perpetrator, and for 32% of homicides involving older women, living arrangements between victim and perpetrator were unknown.

Profile of Alleged Perpetrators

The ages of the alleged perpetrators ranged from 9 to 95 years, for the 70 perpetrators for whom the ages were known. For the 163 cases where gender of the alleged perpetrator was known, 90% were males, and 10% were females. For those cases where the race or ethnicity of the perpetrator was known, 39% were Black non-Hispanic, 30% were White non-Hispanic, 24%

TABLE 85.1 Race/Ethnicity of Victims

Race/Ethnicity	Number	Percent
Black non-Hispanic	126	40
White non-Hispanic	121	38
Hispanic	57	19
Asian	7	2
Other	4	1
Total	315	100

TABLE 85.3 Methods of Older Female Homicides

Method	Number	Percent
Knife	95	30
Gun	63	20
Bludgeon	57	18
Strangle	48	15
Asphyxiate	14	4
Other*	38	12
Total	315	100

*Burned; pushed; Happyland (a social club where a spurned suitor set a fire to kill his former girlfriend inside and caused the death of other patrons); smoke inhalation.

TABLE 85.4 Location of Older Women Homicides

Location	Number	Percent
Inside victim's home	232	74
Outside victim's home	83	26
Total	315	100

were Hispanic, 5% were Asian, and 2% were other. The relationships between the alleged perpetrator and victim were identified for 149 femicides. Husbands and boyfriends represented the largest category of perpetrators (26%), followed by adult children (19%, of which 79% were sons and 21% were daughters). The remaining categories of perpetrators were strangers (17%), other relatives (16%), acquaintances (9%), and other (12%; Table 85.5).

COMPARISON BETWEEN YOUNGER AND OLDER FEMALE HOMICIDE VICTIMS

In comparison with younger victims (under 50 years of age), older female homicide victims were more likely to live alone; more likely to be killed at home; less likely to be shot and more likely to be bludgeoned; more likely to be killed for financial reasons; more likely to be killed by an adult child or a grandchild; and less likely to be killed by a boyfriend. An analysis of age cohorts within the older victim data set demonstrated that the profile of homicides for young-old victims (50 to 64 years) more closely resembled the homicides involving younger vic-

TABLE 85.5 Relationship of Alleged Perpetrator to Victim

Relationship to Victim	Number	Percent
Husband/boyfriend	38	26
Son	22	15
Daughter	6	4
Stranger	26	17
Acquaintance	14	9
Other relative	25	17
Other	18	12
Total	149	100

tims than the old (65 to 74 years), the old-old (75 to 84 years), and the very old (85 years and older).

The young-old victims were more likely to be murdered by a spouse or partner, were more likely to be shot, and were more likely to be Black. Very old victims were more likely to be killed by younger family members (other than a spouse or partner) and were more likely to be White. Exceptions stood out. The oldest perpetrator was 95 years old: he bludgeoned and stabbed his 85-year-old girlfriend to death in her apartment, which he did not share.

DISCUSSION

This study was conducted to learn more about homicides involving older women victims and to sensitize professionals who come into contact with elder abuse victims to the correlates and prior abuse or crime patterns of older women homicides. One objective of the study was to increase the safety of older women in the community by identifying correlates of homicides involving older women victims that law enforcement agents, social workers, health practitioners, and other helping professionals can use to develop prevention and intervention strategies, and that researchers can use in designing additional studies. The researchers believe that emphasis must be placed on integrating social work, gerontology, public health, substance abuse prevention and treatment, and criminal justice knowledge and fields of practice.

One source of information on past history of abuse as reported to law enforcement could be a retrospective analysis of police complaint reports for homicides of older women (Rothman, 2000). Even crime reports on victims involving stranger perpetrators can suggest lifestyle or environmental risks to an elder victim that existed prior to the homicide event. Few significant studies to date have used police complaint reports to assess patterns of family violence. Two notable exceptions are Magnitude and Patterns of Family and Intimate Behavior in Atlanta, Georgia, 1984 (Saltzman et al., 1990) and *Family Crimes Against the Elderly: Elder Abuse and the Criminal Justice System* (Brownell, 1988).

Police reports can provide useful information, from a criminal justice perspective, on violence against older women who were ultimately murdered. They also can be useful in building a bridge between the fields of gerontology, social work, criminal justice, and sociology. Collaboration among law enforcement, health, and aging service systems to conduct a retrospective study of complaint reports filed over time for older femicide victims prior to the homicide event can yield important information on risk factors and red flags that can trigger lifesaving crisis interventions.

The development of a risk typology is beyond the scope of the current study. However, it is hoped that findings of this study can lead to the development of preliminary ideas about risk factors associated with crimes against older women by both intimates and strangers that lead to homicide. This, in turn, can lead to the development of a better understanding of what services might be needed to prevent homicides of older women, whether perpetrated by intimates, acquaintances, strangers, or unknown assailants, and how social workers, law enforcement, health and mental health professionals, and district attorneys can work together more effectively in this effort.

References

Bachman, R. (1993). The double edged sword of violent victimization against the elderly: Patterns of family and stranger perpetration. *Journal of Elder Abuse and Neglect, 5*(4), 59–76.

Block, C. R., Devitt, C. O., Donahue, E. R., & Block, R. (2001). Are there types of intimate partner homicide? In P. H. Blackman, V. L. Leggett, & J. P. Jarvis (Eds.), *The diversity of homicide: Proceedings of the 2000 annual meeting of the Homicide Working Group* (pp. 92–111). Washington, DC: Federal Bureau of Investigation.

Brandl, B. (2000). Power and control: Understanding domestic violence in later life. *Generations: Abuse and Neglect of Older People, 24*(11), 39–45.

Browne, A., & Williams, K. R. (1993). Gender, intimacy and lethal violence: Trends from 1976 through 1987. *Gender and Society, 7*, 78–98.

Brownell, P. (1998). *Family crimes against the elderly: Elder abuse and the criminal justice system.* New York: Garland.

Brownell, P. (2002). Elder abuse. In A. J. Roberts & G. J. Greene (Eds.), *Social workers' desk reference* (pp. 723–727). New York: Oxford University Press.

Brownell, P., Berman, J., & Salamone, A. (1999). Mental health and criminal justice issues among perpetrators of elder abuse. *Journal of Elder Abuse and Neglect, 11*(4), 81–94.

Bureau of Justice Statistics. (2000). Homicide trends in the U.S.: Eldercide [Online]. http://www.ojp.usdoj.gov/bjs/homicide/elders.htm

Campbell, J. C. (1981). Misogyny and homicide of women. *Advances in Nursing Science, 3*(2), 67–85.

Campbell, J. C. (1986). Assessment of risk of homicide for battered women. *Advances in Nursing Science, 8*(4), 36–51.

Campbell, J. C. (1992). "If I can't have you, no one can": Power and control in homicide of female partners. In J. Radford & D. Russell (Eds.), *Femicide: The politics of women killing* (pp. 99–113). New York: Twayne.

Campbell, J. C. (1995). Prediction of homicide of and by battered women. In J. C. Campbell (Ed.), *Assessing dangerousness: Violence by sexual offenders, batterers, and child abusers* (pp. 96–113). Newbury Park, CA: Sage.

Cohen, D. (1999). Elderly homicide/suicide: Depression turned deadly or elder abuse? *Nexus, 4*(3), 1–7.

Durfee, M. J., Gellert, G. A., & Tildon-Durfee, D. (1996). Reporting of child abuse–related deaths is inadequate. In A. E. Sadler (Ed.), *Current controversies* (pp. 101–105). San Diego, CA: Greenhaven Press.

Flynn, E. E. (2000). Elders as perpetrators. In M. B. Rothman, B. D. Dunlop, & P. Entzel (Eds.), *Elders, crime, and the criminal justice system* (pp. 43–83). New York: Springer.

Holinger, P. C. (1987). *Violent deaths in the United States: An epidemiology study of suicide, homicide, and accidents.* New York: Guilford Press.

Koss, M. P., Goodman, L. A., Browne, A., Fitzgerald, L. F., Keita, G. P., & Russo, N. F. (1994). *No safe haven: Male violence against women at home, and in the community.* Washington, DC: American Psychological Association.

Kratcoski, P. (1992). An analysis of cases involving elderly homicide victims and offenders. In E. C. Viano (Ed.), *Critical issues in victimology: International perspectives* (pp. 87–95). New York: Springer.

Penhale, B. (1999). Bruises on the soul: Older women, domestic violence, and elder abuse. *Journal of Elder Abuse and Neglect, 11*(1), 1–22.

Petee, T. A., & Corzine, G. S. (2002). Editors' introduction. *Homicide Studies, 6*(1), 3–5.

Petee, T. A., Weaver, G. S., Corzine, J., Huff-Corzine, L., & Wittekind, J. (2001). Victim-offender relationships and the situational context of homicide. In P. H. Blackman, V. L. Leggett, & J. P. Jarvis (Eds.), *The diversity of homicide: Proceedings of the 2000 annual meeting of the Homicide Research Working Group* (pp. 117–128). Washington, DC: Federal Bureau of Investigation.

Podnieks, E. (1992). Emerging themes from a follow-up study of Canadian victims of elder abuse. *Journal of Elder Abuse and Neglect, 4*, 59–111.

Rothman, M. (2000). Family crimes against the elderly: Elder abuse and the criminal justice system [book review]. *Journal of Elder Abuse and Neglect, 12*(2), 110–113.

Saltzman, et al. (1990). Magnitude and patterns of family and intimate behavior in Atlanta, Georgia, 1985.

Soos, J. N. (1999). Gray murders: Undetected homicides of the elderly. *Nexus, 2*(2), 1–32.

Tatara, T. (1997). Introduction: special issue elder abuse in minority populations. *Journal of Elder Abuse and Neglect, 9*(2) 1–4.

Thomas, C. (2000). The first national study on elder abuse and neglect: Contrast with results from other studies. *Journal of Elder Abuse and Neglect, 12*(1), 1–14.

U.S. House of Representatives. (1990). *Testimony on elder abuse.* Washington, DC: Government Printing Office.

Wolf, R. S. (1999). *Research agenda: A research agenda on abuse of older persons and persons with disabilities.* Washington, DC: National Center on Elder Abuse.

Yin, P. (1985). *Victimization and the aged.* Springfield, IL: Thomas C. Charles.

86   EFFECTIVE OUTCOMES MANAGEMENT AT DEVEREUX

Howard A. Savin

DEVEREUX

Devereux is a provider organization consisting of more than 50 behavioral health care treatment programs predominantly serving children and adolescents in 12 states and the District of Columbia (DC). Nearly 8 years ago, Devereux began its efforts to develop a coherent, quality-focused, and data-driven organization. This undertaking was faced with numerous challenges, not least a geographically dispersed and clinically diverse provider network. This chapter will summarize how Devereux designed and implemented a quality improvement infrastructure incorporating empirically based practice guidelines and an effective outcomes-based management system. Five developmental stages will be described: (a) assessing the organization's current status and planning for buy-in, (b) initiat-

ing data collection, (c) ensuring data integrity, (d) utilizing data to manage outcomes, and (e) system evolution. True to the spirit of continuous quality improvement (QI), our quality quest and interrelated outcomes management initiative is an ongoing work in progress. Its development has been previously chronicled (Savin, 2000) and expansively presented (Savin & Kiesling, 2000).

Devereux's organization consists of 15 discrete behavioral health care operations in 12 states and DC that evolved fairly autonomously during the 82 years that preceded the initiative described in this chapter. The client population served is largely from the public sector and divided between children and adolescents (approximately 80%) and adults. Roughly 60% of the clients receive mental health services, with the balance being supported by developmental disability programs. From the outset, caring and commitment to client welfare was high, and talented clinicians and administrators were on staff. However, 8 years ago, there were neither systemic standards, goals, or benchmarks guiding clinical operations, nor available information technology to drive programmatic accountability.

These conditions are not unique. Just recently, in April 2002, the National Academy of Science recognized the need to improve the quality of behavioral health care. Despite numerous system reforms, quality initiatives, alternative payment schemes, and the like, the committee concluded, "What is perhaps most disturbing is the absence of real progress toward restructuring health care systems to address both quality and cost concerns, or toward applying advances in information technology to improve administrative and clinical processes." In the continuing quest for quality, Devereux set out to establish a model of care that addresses these issues. The first challenge the clinical affairs team had to tackle was how to facilitate movement of a geographically dispersed and clinically diverse provider network into a coherent, quality-focused, and data-driven organization.

It has frequently been noted that provider entities such as ours are increasingly expected to address more complex and challenging behavior problems, including severe aggression, property destruction, substance abuse, and sexual disorders with both mental health and developmentally disabled clients. Furthermore, functional outcomes for programs working with such populations have never been clearly established, and burdensome regulations often impact the efficacy of behavior modification interventions (Spreat & Jampol, 1997).

Heightening this dilemma, Hans Strupp (1996), a renowned researcher and historian on the effectiveness of psychological treatment, has found a paucity of scientific data over the past 100-plus years to substantiate the benefits of psychotherapeutic endeavors. In the current era of cost containment and performance-based contracting, it became ever more critical to aggressively pursue challenge number two: to gauge consumer and payer interests related to the achievement of short- and long-term clinical objectives and to concretely track progress through treatment and beyond.

To meet these challenges, it was essential to establish a structure that supported change and improvement. Thus, Devereux launched a thoughtful organization-wide continuous QI initiative. Its goals were to enable grassroots ownership and dynamic refinement of the systemic initiatives listed earlier in this chapter. The establishment of a relevant and enduring commitment to the QI process as the organization's managerial philosophy, with an integrally related outcomes management component, proved to be a daunting challenge. Large, older, or decentralized organizations like ours tend to pride themselves on their history of survival, uniqueness, and autonomy. Thus, pervasive institutional inertia, often reinforced by a decade or more of failed quality initiatives, stood out as the most critical and essential point of entry.

The design and implementation of the QI infrastructure required 2 years of focused effort and incorporated five developmental stages: (a) assessing the organization's current status and planning for buy-in, (b) initiating data collection, (c) ensuring data integrity, (d) utilizing data to manage outcomes, and (e) system evolution.

Devereux's organizational journey continues to be both challenging and rewarding. We are committed to sharing our findings and experiences with fellow providers in the belief that it may be possible to hasten and broaden each other's learning curves.

STAGE 1: ASSESSING THE ORGANIZATION'S CURRENT STATUS AND PLANNING FOR BUY-IN

With the overarching goal of reducing variability in clinical operations and improving quality of care, a needs assessment was undertaken. This process involved visits to each treatment center to survey programs and interview executive directors, clinical directors, and staff responsible for quality assurance oversight. The initial task was to identify resources and anticipate barriers to compliance with an organization-wide initiative.

Resources were subsequently reviewed with regard to personnel, outcomes studies, existing indicators, and information systems (IS) capacity. Two or three centers had psychologists or psychiatrists conducting independent symptom reduction studies, virtually every program was engaged in satisfaction surveys of their own devise, and a number of Devereux's treatment centers were accredited by the Joint Commission on Accreditation of Hospital Organizations (JCAHO) and thus made some use of quality indicators (e.g., length of stay, planned versus against medical advice [AMA] discharges, medication errors). Furthermore, detailed intake information on each client was available, but each center had its own clinical record system, and almost all clinical records were in manual form. Information technology was quite primitive and highly variable, although a wide area network (WAN) was about to be rolled out, and money had been budgeted to adopt financial, human resources, administrative, and clinical and case management software over the next 3 years. In short, a wealth of data was being collected, but there was no logical or efficient means to analyze this information and learn from it.

Although staff at all levels sincerely believed in the quality of their program's services, they were not necessarily ready to subject themselves to corporate scrutiny and feared the overlay of yet another set of unwanted or potentially irrelevant senior management requirements. Early-stage, conceptual buy-in was achieved by invoking the mantra of managed care readiness. That is, agreement readily existed as to the need to look more like one organization and to be crisper in such areas as credentialing, record keeping, the structure and functioning of quality management (QM) committees, and the generation of meaningful outcome studies. This receptivity was attributed to survival motivation. Accordingly, movement toward this type of organizational efficiency was rightfully perceived as enabling our behavioral health care programs to remain viable in today's organized health care marketplace.

Necessary enabling conditions for the quality infrastructure included the development of quality improvement coordinator (QIC) roles at the treatment center level, regional QICs (RQICs), and a national QIC (NQIC). The QICs were charged with responsibility for dissemination of and compliance with our newly developed clinical quality standards, for conducting monthly QM committee meetings with a standing agenda, and for generating both the monthly minutes and a quarterly (now monthly) Quality Indicator Report. The RQICs were directed to assess the capabilities and need for training among the QICs, survey the QICs as to key issues at their center, including barriers to buy-in, and communicate with and educate QICs re-

garding corporate QI initiatives. Most important, treatment centers needed to be educated about the rationale for, nature of, and methodology for conducting outcome studies while concurrently grasping the operational virtues, or payoff, for embracing the QI program. Fortunately, there were some quick wins in the form of commendations following site visits by regulators and payers.

To facilitate buy-in and to demonstrate "walking the talk," an internal national QI newsletter was created. The newsletter served to share ideas and systems, highlight accomplishments, and offer tips and educational advice. Related to this, a recognition and celebration system was launched that included dedication of a quarterly issue of Devereux's market-oriented newsletter, *Networkings*, to feature laudatory QM team projects, annual presentation of the most outstanding team project to the board of trustees, a variety of QI innovation awards, and the subsequent development of a QI bulletin board on the Intranet.

STAGE 2: INITIATING DATA COLLECTION

In order for QI to occur, programs needed information regarding the efficiency and effectiveness of their processes and services. For that they had to gather data in some organized, systematic fashion. The Devereux Scales of Mental Disorders (DSMD), as refined, redesigned, and standardized by Naglieri, LeBuffe, and Pfeiffer (1994), had been in general use within the organization for a number of years. This instrument can serve as an excellent functional outcomes assessment tool for mental health populations under age 21, but it was not being used to its fullest potential. The scales measure the presence of specific challenging behaviors indicative of various diagnoses such as depression, conduct disorder, anxiety, and autism. Similarly, the Adaptive Behavior Scale (ABS; Nihira, Leland, & Lambert, 1993), which measures independent functioning, physical and mental development, social adjustment, and personal adjustment, was in some use as a behavioral assessment instrument in work with mentally retarded and developmentally disabled clients. Systemwide training was initiated that addressed the desirability of multiyear outcome studies versus "snapshots," how to properly administer and score targeted outcomes instruments, how to design and use satisfaction surveys, and the determination of appropriate data collection points. Consultations addressed distinctions between process measures and clinical outcomes such as symptom reduction and functional gains, at both discharge and postdischarge.

Benchmarking using process indicators was a goal of the outcomes initiative. As previously stated, a number of our centers were JCAHO accredited and thereby familiar with quality indicator reporting. With the goal of best practice and organizational relevance, the entire quality team undertook a year of refinement and review of this area under the direction of the national QI coordinator. This resulted in the creation of the Devereux Quality Indicator Report. The first revised report incorporated 8 functions represented by 15 indicators. It has since been refined and streamlined. Table 86.1 represents the most current version of the Quality Indicator Report. The report's success was validated by both internal acceptance and several publishers' requests to include it in best-practice compendiums (Devereux, 1997; Kiesling & Lee, 1998).

To succeed, the indicators had to be clearly and concisely defined, clinically relevant, meaningful to stakeholders, and inexpensive to purchase and/or complete. Over the course of the

postimplementation year, the QI team was able to establish a basis for valid and reliable reporting standards that would permit apples-to-apples interpretations across various centers and regions. The advent of this report enabled our centers to begin quarterly reporting with the resulting capability of intracenter benchmarking and organizational trend analysis.

STAGE 3: ENSURING DATA INTEGRITY

The major objectives of this stage were to reduce procedural variance and to develop systematic analyses. Following initial in-service training in such outcomes measurement tools as the Devereux Quality Indicator Report, DSMD, and ABS, it became painfully clear that centers were not all marching to the beat of the same drum. Compounding matters, most of our centers were working from a manual, paper-based approach in the clinical and programmatic area. This resulted in the generation of both sloppy and unusable data due to inconsistent data collection and over- or underreporting. Attempts to aggregate information at the national level on just one indicator of care, sentinel events (those events or incidents that the Joint Commission on Ac-

TABLE 86.1 Devereux Quality Indicator Report—Functions and Indices

Functions	Indicator(s)
Individual rights and organizational ethics	1. Informed consent is obtained prior to administration of psychoactive medication.
Continuum of care	2. Discharge placement will demonstrate discharge planning for individuals requiring continuing care.
Care of the individual/treatment	3. Treatment effectiveness based on specific outcome measurement.
	4. The number of facility-administered medication errors.
	5. Use of behavior management techniques/special treatment procedures.
Management of human resources	6. Staff injury rate.
	7. Staff credentialing.
Surveillance prevention and control of infection	8. Communicable illness/reportable infectious disease rate.
Management of the core environment	9. Risk events.

creditation of Healthcare Organizations defines as reportable Sentinel Events [e.g., suicide, loss of limb or function, rape]), resulted in the generation of different numbers at the center, regional, and national levels.

Corrective action involved initial migration toward databases; in-depth education both at semiannual organization-wide QM meetings and at the individual centers with regard to appropriate administration and scoring of behavior rating scales, such as the DSMD and ABS; and development and refinement of operational definitions for indicators, populations, and time frames. The RQICs were directed to continuously follow up in this area, and a research psychologist from the corporate clinical department (Devereux's Institute of Clinical Training and Research) was made routinely available to consult with the centers in the areas of research design and data analysis.

STAGE 4: UTILIZING DATA TO MANAGE OUTCOMES

Tools and systems were now in place to accurately monitor program processes and individual client progress from both clinical and functional vantage points. Overall, efforts stressed fidelity of data and methods of data collection. A concerted educational approach was used to promote methods for aggregating data at both program and organizational levels, to stress the importance of providing feedback to all stakeholders, and to reinforce the overarching objective of using all outcomes data (e.g., including satisfaction surveys, functional assessments, behavior rating scales, indicator reports) to learn and improve. Until 2 years ago, the focus was directed primarily at clinical services to the exclusion of other operational areas. To remedy this state of affairs, Devereux adopted a Balanced Scorecard (BSC), a strategic measurement and tracking tool that gauges operational performance based on key indicators within several domains of an organization (e.g., human resources, finance, marketing, and clinical services).

The BSC "translates an organization's mission and strategy into a comprehensive set of performance measures that provides the framework for a strategic measurement and management system" (Kaplan & Norton, 1996, p. 18). The method has been adopted by many leading Fortune 500 organizations to align and focus strategic initiatives. This concept offered Devereux the ideal combination of strategic, quality, and operational planning and has come to embody our commitment to QI as its management style. The BSC "rolls up" and allows an organization's corporate team to focus on major themes, while capturing creativity, responsiveness, and adaptation at the individual program level. It is also engineered to ensure balance by reflecting that an organization is developing its human resources and financial capability while enhancing its clinical programs.

Devereux's clinical affairs team identified three key performance measures, known as metrics, for the BSC to dynamically reflect the safety, sufficiency, and effectiveness of programmatic services. These metrics, major reportable events (MREs), positive discharge percent, and site visit scores, are defined in Table 86.2 Major reportable events are serious incidents involving clients or staff that result in either injury, illness, or property destruction. As such, the rate of MREs serves as a good indicator of program stability and safety. Positive discharge was chosen to reflect successful outcome of care. The metric of site visit scores measures the program's demonstrated ability to equal or exceed targeted operational standards. Each of these metrics quantifies a program's performance in key functional areas.

For example, Figure 86.1 illustrates the progressive decline in reportable risk events over a 2-year period. This is determined to be the result

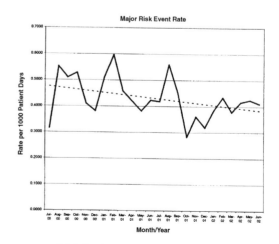

FIGURE 86.1 Utilizing the balanced scorecard for program improvement.

TABLE 86.2 Devereux's Balanced Scorecard Clinical Metrics

Critical Success Factors	Metric	Annual Target	Rationale
Highest quality programs	MREs per census		This accountability measure is utilized to indicate a stable treatment environment with limited risk opportunity for clients. The target was established based on aggregate MRE data reported by the centers in Categories 1–10 for the past year with the expectation that, as centers improve, their program utilization rate.
Market-Responsive Programs	% positive discharges		This measure was selected as it indicates clinical program effectiveness based on the clients' ability to function in a less restrictive setting after discharge. The target for mental health programs was established based on aggregate data reported by the centers for FY 2002 with the expectation that, as centers improve their program utilization rate, they continue to achieve positive outcomes.
	% community integration		This measure has been selected to measure the goal of MR programs. The goal of these programs is to achieve a greater "normalcy" for the MR clients; therefore the integration with the community is an appropriate measurement.
	Site Score Visit:	Clinical Operational/ residential Education	Site visit scores represent operational processes and educational programs per established internal standards. The target was established based on the scoring tool's measures of compliance as an achievable goal for which to strive.
Innovation	ICTR innovation		As ICTR's goal is to support 85% of its expenses within 5 years, this metric will measure progress toward this outcome.

of an organization-wide pursuit of an increasingly safe and stable setting of care as measured by an MRE metric of .50 events per 1,000 client days or less.

During this same period, greater emphasis was placed on compliance with practice guidelines and an increased focus on movement toward comprehensive program models. It seems logical to expect improvements in programming to be correlated with successful outcomes of care. The impact of this movement on the percentage of individuals with a positive outcome at discharge is routinely tracked. Positive outcomes in our mental health programs are defined by the percentage of discharges to less restrictive settings of care. Center MH, one of the largest treatment centers in the Northeast working with children and adolescents with emotional and behavioral disorders, mirrors and in some cases exceeds Devereux's overall strong performance in this area in Figure 86.2

In a related manner, positive outcomes in our programs for mentally retarded and developmentally disabled clients is indicated by the percentage of clients moved into more integrated community settings. Center MR, a large suburban center composed of residential, group home, and therapeutic foster care programs for the full spectrum of children and adolescents with mental retardation and developmental disabilities, performs equally well on this comparable metric for its population.

The advent of these metrics has allowed Devereux to establish and monitor the attainment of

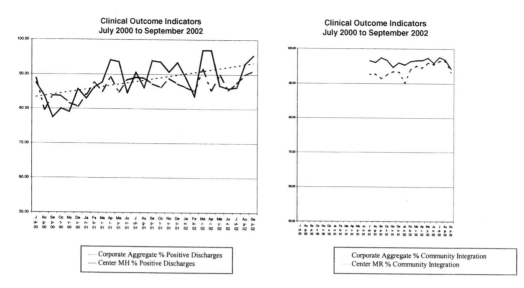

FIGURE 86.2 Benchmarking balanced scorecard metrics.

organizational goals while concurrently guiding the improvement process at the individual program or center level. Refinement and evolution of BSC measures continue. More recently, Devereux has implemented an "innovation" metric to assess the organization's return on investment for clinical or programmatic research and development activities.

STAGE 5: SYSTEM EVOLUTION

Efforts in this last stage were directed at natural selection of indicators and processes, database development, evolution of the outcomes management system, and the introduction of outside expertise into the Outcomes Initiative. Before proceeding, it had to be determined that buy-in had generally occurred—at least with the organization's executive directors. Additionally, the QI team needed to be confident that basic concepts and techniques had been grasped and that most centers were more than grudgingly compliant with data collection and reporting requirements.

Next, we convened work groups to revisit key components of the Outcomes Initiative. Revisiting allowed stakeholders to experience empowerment with regard to the ability to continuously modify standards and protocols in an unending quest to make systemic improve-

ments. For instance, the first iteration of Devereux's Quality Indicator Report consisted of 24 indicators. By October 1997, the number of indicators had been whittled to 15, with definitions tightened and data collection formulas made more relevant from our broad organizational perspective. Similarly, corporate and center QI staff began to design larger and more sophisticated outcomes initiatives, such as our first national satisfaction survey, and to aggregate data by affinity groups of like treatment programs across the organization (e.g., mental health child and adolescent programs, programs for mentally retarded and developmentally disabled adults). At the same time, information systems expertise was accessed to aid in the development of a number of Microsoft Access databases. This enhanced the integrity and scope of data collection for such purposes as quality indicator reporting and aggregation of programwide outcomes.

Although programmatic evaluation had been encapsulated within routine processes, data collection at the individual client level was typically done within the confines of a particular study rather than as part of the daily routine. Individual processes were measured and analyzed, but their relation to one another and to the program as a whole was not well understood. The time had come to "raise the bar" to the next level of sophistication. This involved establishing linkages between various individual and programmatic structural components to form an integrated outcomes system.

The Clinical Accountability Model (CAM) integrates many of the clinical quality standards developed in the field over the past quarter of a century while simultaneously taking full advantage of the power and efficiency of clinical informatics (Savin, 2002). The CAM encompasses an empirically based and yet flexible clinical work flow that supports effective clinical practice and continuous quality improvement. It is based on three key values: (a) implementation of empirically based practice (EBP), (b) commitment to continuous quality improvement, and (c) client-centered and family-focused services.

The first element of CAM requires that programs identify current practice standards. To achieve that end, Devereux embarked on a model program initiative to examine the structure and content of individual treatment programs. Each center was asked to operationally define its model of care in a document that outlines the essential program components (Table 86.3).

The rationale for this exercise is that sound, effective clinical treatment must begin with a guiding philosophy that clearly articulates conceptual beliefs regarding the treatment needs of the population served. This philosophy provides the basis for all decision making and ties together the various components of the model.

The next step involves specifying the *program content*, that is, the description of the program components. These components should be empirically based. This support may be derived from peer-reviewed literature or by persuasive outcome data. Empirically based practice helps to assure that services provided are effective and equitable (i.e., quality of services does not vary based on such factors as geographic locale or the academic background of key staff). Empirically based practice is the cornerstone of clinical accountability and is made manifest in Devereux's practice guidelines.

The clinical accountability model ensures that provider behavior is consistent with practice guidelines. This assurance begins with the provider groups articulating a set of guiding values and a theory of change that are incorporated in practice guidelines. These guidelines then determine the client dimensions that are critical to positive outcome. For example, treatment foster care (Chamberlain, 2002), an empirically supported practice, includes as an essential component of treatment the development of recreational interests and skills. This EBP component then becomes a client dimension. The clinical accountability model then requires that this dimension be assessed for each client along with the identification of needs and strengths. These needs and strengths must then be addressed in the clinical formulation for the client and ultimately reflected in the treatment plan. By specifying relevant dimensions, requiring assessment of those dimensions, and then requiring that the treatment plan incorporate assessment findings, the clinical accountability model can effect a rapprochement between EBP and the individual provider's daily practice.

To ensure its relevance and appropriateness, the CAM must continually evolve in response to both new information and the changing needs of consumers. The existing QM infrastructure ensures proactive program improvement based on ongoing monitoring and evaluation of programs. To enrich this process, Devereux developed an automated clinical core record. By maintaining client and treatment information data in the same database, this system enables the separation of outcomes by client and service variables. This, in turn, supports meaningful clinical QI efforts by identifying factors that contribute to or interfere with positive outcomes. Ultimately, adoption of automated clinical accountability systems could help behavioral health care providers, such as Devereux, to cross the quality chasm in one giant leap.

CONCLUSION

A continuous QI climate has been cultivated at Devereux. It continues to pulsate and evolve. The adoption of the BSC, along with the program models initiative related to our CAM, should result in improvements in targeted organizational outcomes—safety, stability, and effectiveness of care. Having created demand for more tools and techniques, we have undertaken the development of a sophisticated clinical and case management information system that will ultimately allow us to gather all relevant client data on a real-time basis. This information system will permit internal and external benchmarking of programs and an unlimited range of outcomes research. The journey continues.

TABLE 86.3 Model of Care Template

Characteristic/ Component	Description
Philosophy of treatment	1. Describes population 2. Identifies focus of treatment 3. Identifies beliefs about treatment needs
Mission Statement	
Program Objectives	1. Objectives lead to accomplishment of mission 2. Objectives identify core components of the treatment model 3. Objectives are measurable 4. Objectives describe the relationship to appropriate area of functioning
Program Components	
Admission	1. Describes criteria for inclusion/exclusion 2. Identifies special populations
Assessment	1. Identifies specific measures 2. Describes how staff are trained in administration 3. Assessments are linked to relevant areas of functioning 4. Provides clinical formulation of strengths and need statements 5. Describes method to ensure integrity of implementation of the assessments 6. Describes method of formative evaluation of the overall assessment process
Treatment Components	
Residential	1. Describes curriculum in use 2. Describes instructional methods 3. Describes methods for monitoring progress and evidences that monitoring leads to necessary treatment plan revision 4. Describes motivational elements of the treatment environment 5. Describes related staff training required to implement curriculum 6. Describes method to monitor staff implementation of curriculum
Ancillary components	1. Challenging behavior/crisis management 2. Family involvement/parent training 3. Transition/maintenance of treatment gains 4. Inclusion 5. Monitoring process and evidence that monitoring leads to necessary treatment plan revision
Education/vocation	1. Describes curriculum in use 2. Describes instructional methods 3. Describes methods for monitoring progress and evidences that monitoring leads to necessary treatment plan revision 4. Describes motivational elements of the treatment environment 5. Describes related staff training needed to implement the curriculum 6. Describes method to monitor staff implementation of the curriculum

ACKNOWLEDGMENT Requests for further information should be directed to Howard A. Savin, Ph.D., at hsavin@devereux.org. Thanks and recognition are given to Susan Soldivera-Kiesling for assistance in compiling data and for her abiding commitment and contributions to Devereux's Outcomes Initiative.

References

Chamberlain, P. (2002). Treatment foster care. In B. J. Burns & K. Hoagwood (Eds.), *Community treatment for youth: Evidenced-based interventions for severe emotional and behavioral disorders* (pp. 117–138). New York: Oxford University Press.

Devereux. (1997). The indicator report. In M. A. Freeman (Ed.), *High performance behavior healthcare: The breakthrough innovation sourcebook and mutual consultation guide* (pp. 59–61). Tiburon, CA: CentraLink.

Kaplan, R. S., & Norton, D. P. (1996). Strategic learning and the balanced scorecard. *Strategy and Leadership, 24,* 18.

Kiesling, S. S., & Lee, B. (1998). The indicator report. *Behavioral Healthcare Tomorrow, 7*(3), 49–50.

Naglieri, J. A., LeBuffe, P. A., & Pfeiffer, S. L. (1994). *The Devereux Scales of Mental Disorders.* San Antonio, TX: Psychological Corporation.

Nihira, K., Leland, H., & Lambert, N. (1993). *AAMR Adaptive Behavior Scales—Residential and Community* (2nd ed.). Austin, TX: PRO-ED.

Savin, H. A. (2000). Designing an effective outcomes management system: A case study. *Education and Treatment of Children, 23,* 48–59.

Savin, H. A. (2002). *The development and implementation of a clinical accountability model in behavioral healthcare.* [Available from CMHC, cmhcsystems.com, 800-434-CMHC]

Savin, H. A., & Kiesling, S. S. (2000). *Accountable systems of behavioral health care: A provider's guide.* San Francisco: Jossey-Bass.

Spreat, S., & Jampol, R. C. (1997). Residential services for children and adolescents. In R. T. Ammerman & M. Hersen (Eds.), *Handbook of prevention and treatment with children and adolescents: Intervention in the real world context* (pp. 106–133). New York: Wiley.

Strupp, H. H. (1996). The tripartite model and the consumer reports study. *American Psychologist, 51,* 1017–1024.

87

DEVELOPING TREATMENT PROGRAMS FOR DRUG COURTS AND EVALUATING EFFECTIVENESS

Sherri McCarthy & Thomas Franklin Waters

OVERVIEW

Court-mandated treatment delivered through drug court models is a natural venue for practice-based research. The data already routinely collected by criminal justice agencies and the behavioral control exerted by court sanctions simplify the research process while creating special challenges for therapists. According to DeAngelis (2001), psychologists have vastly underestimated the impact we can have in the area of substance abuse treatment. As rehabilitative measures such as drug courts are implemented by court systems internationally, this statement appears well-founded. There is a need for trained substance abuse counselors who can work within court systems. This is an important area for forensic psychologists to familiarize themselves with, especially in rural areas. Drug courts are effective models for delivering treatment for substance abuse and are also appropriate venues for practice-based research. Psychologists should be involved not only in delivering treatment but also in planning and evaluation of drug court models. Each drug court will have unique needs based on location, agency, and clients that must be considered in planning. For evaluation of success, a phenomenological approach to research that combines quantitative and qualitative data is optimum. This chapter provides a historical overview of drug courts in the United States and offers suggestions and guidelines to psychologists involved in planning, delivering, and evaluating treatment in drug courts. Two examples of planning, one of a juvenile drug court and one of a DUI court, are provided for consideration.

Drug courts are becoming increasingly common venues for dealing with those arrested for offenses related to substance abuse in the United States because they prove to be efficient, effective, and less costly than incarceration. More than a decade has passed since the first drug court model was established in the United States. Dade County, Florida, implemented the model in 1989 as a diversionary program for offenders facing charges of simple drug possession.

Several states have begun to legally mandate treatment as part of sentencing for drug-related cases, but this procedure often differs from drug court models. The mandated treatment is often not funded or overseen by the court. Offenders may be unable to afford treatment and must rely on whatever managed care system, if any, is available through state welfare indigent care coverage. From both a cost and a treatment perspective, this is not optimal, especially in rural areas, where there is a severe shortage of psychologists, substance abuse counselors, and detoxification units. The current national average for substance abuse treatment through managed care is a stay of 3.8 days for detoxification, followed by 10 daily sessions and 16 follow-up sessions (K. Yeager, personal communication, May 10, 2003). For those in rural areas, the detoxi-

fication and treatment generally occur in another city, offering high costs but little in the way of assistance to offenders when they return to their homes and to the conditions that trigger and exacerbate their problems. Treatment through a drug court model allows for continuing long-term counseling in the community, generally 1 or more years in duration, and assistance with the triggers and issues that are responsible for abuse. Cost is lower and benefits are higher because success is often correlated with time in treatment and with cultural and contextual factors in the therapeutic milieu. This is clearly a preferable model.

A drug court is a special judicial body given the responsibility to handle cases involving drug-addicted offenders through an extensive supervision and treatment program. Drug court utilizes a case management team approach, typically composed of the presiding judge, the prosecutor, the defense counsel, a psychologist and/or substance abuse treatment specialist, a vocational counselor, a probation officer, education specialists, and community leaders (Belenko, 1996). Drug courts attempt to motivate offenders to overcome their substance abuse problems and reconnect to the community as productive citizens. In addition, these courts are intended to ensure consistency in judicial decision making, enhance the coordination of community agencies and resources, and increase the cost-effectiveness of sentencing and maintenance for those convicted of minor drug-related crimes. Such courts have expanded recently into the juvenile justice system and also include programs to rehabilitate repeat offenders of DUI laws.

Since the implementation of the first U.S. drug court, over 150,000 offenders have participated in or are currently involved with treatment in similar programs. The current number of active drug courts in the United States exceeds 400, with over 200 more in various stages of implementation and development. More than 100,000 participants have graduated from drug court programs (Hora, Schma, & Rosenthal, 1999; Robinson, 2001). Research on these programs suggests that 73% of the participants have retained and/or obtained suitable employment after completion of the program, that 71% complete the program, and that other positive benefits to society, which would not be realized if offenders were simply incarcerated, result (Cooper, 1997). Over 750 drug-free babies have been born to drug court participants in the last decade. Over 3,500 participants have regained custody of their children, and over 4,500 are again able to make child support payments (Belenko, 1998; Lewis, 1998; Peters, 1996, 1999). Recidivism appears to be lower for drug court participants than for those who receive other types of sentencing (Deschenes, Turner, & Greenwood, 1995). The model appears to have many advantages from a social perspective, as well as from a cost-benefit perspective. It also appears to provide a useful arena for partnerships between psychologists and the courts (Foxhall, 2001). Because of the funding mechanisms in place for criminal justice agencies and the public demand to see outcomes of rehabilitation programs, it is imperative that psychologists be involved in the planning, implementation, data collection, and evaluation of drug and alcohol treatment programs administered by the courts, as well as in the treatment of offenders. This chapter provides guidelines for developing and evaluating such programs. Another chapter by the same authors in this handbook includes a report of a study of the effectiveness of an adult drug court program currently in operation in southwestern Arizona conducted according to the principles outlined here.

A PSYCHOLOGICAL PERSPECTIVE ON DRUG COURT TREATMENT

Although many psychologists have often seen forced, or coerced, treatment as less than optimal, research suggests that, in the case of substance abuse offenders, there may be benefits. For example, beyond a 90-day threshold, treatment outcomes appear to improve in direct relation to the time spent in treatment, with 1 year generally found to be the minimum effective duration for treatment. Over 60% of those who enter treatment through drug court models are still in treatment after 1 year (Belenko, 1998) compared with only 10% of those who voluntarily participate in substance abuse treatment programs. Clients who remain in treatment for extended periods apparently overcome much of the initial resistance coercion creates, as research on the outcomes of many U.S. drug courts shows success despite initial perceptions of coercion on the part of participants. This is especially true when continued individual and group counseling is mandated in the treatment program (Satel, 2001). Thus, from a psychological perspective, drug court models that keep clients in treatment with qualified clinicians for a duration of over 1 year, whether or not the initial entry is viewed as coerced, are likely to show success. Cognitive-behavioral therapy appears to be an especially useful approach with recovering addicts (Spurgeon, McCarthy, & Waters, 1999) and is often the treatment of choice in drug court programs.

Assisting recovered addicts in dealing with cues to prevent relapse is also critical from a psychological perspective (Foxhall, 2001). Therefore, a drug court model that includes extensive focus on a relapse prevention plan is likely to assist in client success. Because "triggers," or people, places, things, and events that have become associated with drug use through classical conditioning (Spurgeon et al., 1999), can also lead to relapse, long-term programs that establish new habits, social networks, and living arrangements are likely to demonstrate more success. Goal setting and the increased self-efficacy and sense of personal control that arise from meeting goals are also likely to be important to treatment success. Certainly there is evidence that a variety of variables influence success rates, including (a) drug history, (b) history of physical or social abuse, (c) family of origin alcohol or substance abuse, (d) length of abstinence, (e) employment status, (f) social support system/access to services, (g) religious affiliation, and (h) cultural cohort variables related to age and ethnicity. The type of treatment (group or individual; cognitive behavioral or psychodynamic) and length of treatment are also related to success rates.

Long-term individual therapy utilizing a cognitive behavioral approach seems to show evidence of being the most effective treatment strategy overall, especially when combined with goal setting and social support, which leads to improved self-efficacy. Education, job satisfaction, economic improvement, and stable family relationships and friendships are also correlated with success. For optimum success, an effective drug court model should combine all these forms of support. Psychologists should have an important role in designing and delivering services for criminal justice agencies and courts that develop drug courts. By the very nature of the relationship that ensues, practice-based research and research-based practice go hand in hand in such collaborations.

CONSIDERATIONS FOR PLANNING SUCCESSFUL TREATMENT IN DRUG COURTS

When developing a drug court treatment model, it is important to focus on the unique characteristics and needs of the area, agencies, and clients the court will serve. There is not, unfortunately, one "best" decision tree for all courts. Each must be approached as a unique entity, and ongoing research must influence treatment and operations. There are several important questions to consider in planning effective drug court treatment programs. Questions focused on potential clients include the following:

1. What are the characteristics of the population to be treated?
2. What languages and cultural orientations are most common?
3. What is the average age of clients?
4. What is the average socioeconomic status?
5. What types of use patterns are most frequent?
6. Which substances are generally abused?
7. What types of assessment tools are most appropriate?

Other related questions may also be important, and it may be that some areas will not have common patterns evident among clients. In our experience, however, this is not the case. When drug courts are integrated into communities, the clients they serve often have common characteristics, problems, and use patterns.

Questions focused on planning and implementation include the following:

1. What types and sources of funding are available to staff and administer treatment and data collection?
2. What is the level of training of the staff in the agency who work directly with clients?
3. What is the common organizational philosophy toward clients—is punishment or rehabilitation favored?
4. What types of training, resources, and services for staff will facilitate effective psychological treatment?
5. How can available community resources and services best be coordinated to serve in substance abuse treatment?
6. How will decisions be made, in an ongoing and systematic way, to improve treatment?

Who will be responsible for these decisions—that is, a community board, the judge, the interdisciplinary team?
7. How can the community best be apprised of and involved with treatment?

It may be necessary to collect preliminary data and conduct focus groups in order to answer these questions. It is also necessary to address how data will continue to be collected throughout the program. Questions focused on continuous data collection and reporting include:

1. Who will be the audience for the data?
2. Who will analyze the data and determine results?
3. What types of evidence will the local voters understand and prefer to see?
4. What criteria are demanded by the funding agencies?
5. What mechanisms are already in place that can provide data?
6. How reliable and valid will the data that are routinely collected be?
7. What types of issues related to confidentiality (or, in the case of minors, parent and family rights) may influence how data are collected?

All these questions must be answered before initiating a treatment program. Because the answers are likely to be very different depending on location and the agencies involved, psychologists working in such programs need to be true research–practitioners and may be well advised to utilize a phenomenological approach, tempered by careful examination of quantitative data from other, similar programs, during the planning stages. Be aware that each program will function somewhat differently and require unique procedures, and utilize available data to make decisions concerning which treatment modalities and data collection procedures are most appropriate. Two examples based on our experience follow for psychologists involved in developing, working in, and evaluating drug court programs.

Example One: Planning and Evaluating Treatment Within a Juvenile Drug Court

This example is based on a plan devised for a drug court implemented within a juvenile probation agency in the southwestern United States. The process began by setting specific goals in collaboration with judges and agency directors. A research model with several data-generating activities was then planned. The overall goal was to determine the effectiveness of juvenile drug court from three perspectives: implementation, process, and outcomes.

Overall, the evaluation plan sought to determine if program objectives were met by determining the impact of participation on the target population. This was to be accomplished by assessing whether graduation from drug court had any long-term effect (beyond 1 year) on participants' use of drugs and criminal activities and by determining if differences in other, related dimensions existed between graduates of drug court treatment programs and other youths who had been arrested for possession and/or use of illegal substances assigned to the same agency but had not participated in drug court treatment.

A relatively simple quasi-experimental design could assess to what extent, if any, substance abuse counseling caused the desired changes in participants, but this traditional assessment model was not considered optimal for several reasons. Implementation, process, and outcome are all important segments to examine from a phenomenological perspective. Key questions need to be answered even before determining and delivering treatment. These questions address characteristics of the target population: Who are the youths in the agency's charge? What were they arrested for? What is the common family structure they experience, including socioeconomic considerations, parent education, culture, and language? What are their prior arrest records like? What is the level of severity of substance abuse among members of this group?

Once these questions are answered, a treatment strategy that will reach this target population needs to be developed and implemented. Implementation must then be assessed. The primary objective of assessing implementation and process is to determine the extent to which the operationalized version of drug court treatment within a particular agency resembles the original design and intent. Gathering data about the common attitudes and practices of staff and the organizational philosophy and climate is important to this dimension of assessment. Additionally, when problems are identified and changes are introduced, such as staff training or policy revisions, do such changes achieve the desired

effect? This must also be determined and, because this is an ongoing process to improve treatment, also will effect results.

Process must be addressed. Because of the multiple influences, regulations, and procedures in effect in criminal justice agencies, it is impossible to implement a "clean" comparative experimental design. Instead, each agency program must be studied as an individual entity. Questions addressing process for the particular agency presented here as an example included the following:

1. How many juveniles were screened for the program? How many were accepted? How many were turned down? What patterns or reasons influenced this selection of subjects?
2. What types of treatment services are routinely provided for participants with specific characteristics, such as mental health issues and drug use? What is the average length of time the services are provided? What is the level of family involvement?
3. What ancillary services, if any, are provided to participants or their families?
4. What is the frequency of drug testing during each phase? Are drug tests given on a random basis? For what types of drugs are the participants being tested? What are the results?
5. Who is graduating from the program? Are there common characteristics of participants who successfully complete the program compared with those who do not? If so, what are these?
6. Who is being terminated from the program? What are the reasons for termination? During what phase of the program are participants generally terminated?
7. What sanctions are being given to the participants? What are the reasons for the sanctions? What are the incentives being given to the participants? What are the percentages of incentive versus sanctions being given to the participants?
8. Do school attendance and progress improve during the program? If so, what programs or services provided by schools may also be influencing the outcome? Are learning disabilities or problems identified and addressed during the program?
9. What is the level of judicial supervision? How many court hearings do the participants attend?

10. Is information communicated effectively among the team members?
11. What fees are assessed to the participants? What fees did the participants pay?
12. How does the drug court process compare with historical methods of treating juvenile substance abusers? What is the cost of the program in comparison to other methods?

Process evaluation should answer questions such as these and provide important data for interpreting results. It should also indicate any gaps in the treatment program. These gaps might include additional treatment services needed; cultural diversity issues; gender issues; political or community issues surrounding the drug court team; and parental or peer concerns. Evaluation should also indicate the strengths of the program and identify which participants with specific characteristics benefit most from the program. Process evaluation is used throughout planning and implementation as a learning tool to guide and refine the program in a direction that will increase its effectiveness. Process evaluation incorporates both qualitative and quantitative tools, strategies, and reports, which include:

1. Summary of referrals or screening to program.
2. Summary of declines to program.
3. Summary of participant demographics.
4. Summary of community demographics.
5. Summary of participant offense history, adjudication, and hearing data.
6. Summary of activity hours and program levels or phases.
7. Summary of treatment completed.
8. Summary of sanctions completed.
9. Summary of adjudications in the program.
10. Summary of detention days served by participants in program.
11. Summary of drug type testing of participants.
12. Summary of completion and expulsion rates.
13. Summary of rearrest history and detention days served by graduates and nongraduates from the program.

This list was compiled from accessible records and existing agency reports that provided relevant information. Another consideration of process evaluation is how to define, measure, and establish program success. Setting outcome objectives that are in line with the expectations of local constituents of the agency, political climate, and realistic treatment success rates is necessary. The following outcome objectives were identified as indicators of success for the drug court treatment program within this agency:

1. The juvenile drug court program will reduce commitments and out-of-home placements of substance abusing juveniles by 20% over a 2-year period.
2. Juvenile drug court graduates will show a 60% improvement in school attendance and academic performance as measured by passing grades.
3. 75% of the participants will successfully complete the drug court program.
4. 75% of the juvenile drug court graduates will remain drug and crime free for more than 1 year after graduation.
5. 75% of graduates' families will report improved family relations.
6. 75% of graduates' parents or guardians will report improved awareness of parenting skills and substance abuse issues.
7. Graduates will report a 30% increase in vocational readiness according to interviews.

Data to assess these outcomes were generated in several ways. Observations were utilized extensively. Program activities and pre-post interviews of program staff, participants, and family members of participants were recorded and reviewed. Data on drug testing, attendance at counseling sessions, school records, use of referral services, program compliance, and use of sanctions for all youths within the jurisdiction of the agency were collected and reviewed. The impact of drug court treatment on agency resources such as costs, jail space, human resources, and time was also assessed and compared with previous years.

Local, state, and federal criminal justice databases were utilized to compare outcomes for adolescents who completed drug court treatment with those of other defendants. In addition, follow-up interviews were conducted with all participants at 6-month and 1-year intervals after completion of drug court. Participation in follow-up community support groups for all drug participants for 1 year following completion of treatment was also tracked.

A matrix identifying the major data elements

needed for the evaluation, where the data were located, and the person responsible for the data was developed and implemented by the agency. Information and data were reviewed quarterly. The quarterly reports were reviewed with the Drug Court Advisory Board, and alterations to the program were based on the board's recommendations. Annual reports were compiled and shared with the public.

All strategies for gathering quantitative and qualitative data on the target population were monitored to ensure reliability and validity. All instruments used in treatment and data collection complied with Drug Office protocols and were appropriate to age, gender, sexual orientation, language, culture, literacy, disability, and racial or ethnic characteristics of the participants. All interaction with the target population was conducted in the appropriate language and cultural context.

Before beginning treatment and data collection, focus group meetings were conducted with members of the target population and/or their advocates to obtain input into the design and implementation of the evaluation plan. Quarterly meetings were held with members of the target population and/or their advocates to share evaluation progress reports and to discuss other issues and concerns related to the progress of the project.

The strategy presented here for measuring the overall effectiveness of cognitive-behavioral substance abuse treatment with adolescents provided information to enhance drug court operations and contributed to the growing body of knowledge concerning the effectiveness of drug courts and of cognitive-behavioral treatments within substance abuse counseling. The planning related to developing, implementing, and evaluating this juvenile drug court is presented here to consider as a model for psychologists conducting and assessing other such programs.

Example Two: Planning Enhancements for a DUI Court–Mandated Treatment Program

Unlike the previous example, which created and assessed a program, this example summarizes a modification of cognitive-behavioral treatment strategies and training materials to meet the needs of specific cultural groups within an existing program. Many of the offenders referred to a DUI court in Arizona were not fluent in En-

glish and were from Native American or Mexican American cultural backgrounds. The design described in this example used a single-site integrated evaluation model to determine the effectiveness of culturally appropriate treatment strategies in a court-mandated DUI treatment program from multiple perspectives: (a) meeting requirements of the Government Performance and Results Act (GPRA), (b) implementation, (c) process, and (d) outcomes. The design addressed these questions:

1. Does the treatment meet GPRA requirements?
2. Does the treatment meet specified goals and objectives?
3. Does the delivery of treatment function as designed?
4. Does the treatment achieve its desired outcomes?
5. Do culturally appropriate enhancements to treatment have a positive impact on the targeted population?

All strategies for gathering quantitative and qualitative data on the target population were monitored to ensure reliability and validity. Many of the data collection mechanisms already in place within the agency were determined to be appropriate. These were not altered. Instruments consistent with SAMHSA and CSAT protocols, appropriate to age, gender, sexual orientation, language, culture, literacy, disability, and racial or ethnic characteristics of the target population, were selected. All counseling, evaluation, and other interaction with the target population was conducted in the appropriate language and cultural context for participants. Mexican American and Native American counselors were included in developing the treatment plans.

During the enhancement-planning phase, focus group meetings were conducted with members of the target population and/or their advocates to share evaluation progress reports and to discuss other issues and concerns. This input was used to refine the practice-based research design. In addition, the project evaluator participated in all technical assistance and training activities designed to support GPRA and other evaluation requirements and met monthly with the project steering committee to provide progress reports. These interim evaluation findings were used to improve the quality of the enhancements and to ensure that the project met targeted goals and objectives.

As in the previous example, data were collected for each piece of the integration model (implementation, process, and outcomes). The same types of reports and criminal justice databases as those described in the previous example were utilized except for school and family records, because this intervention involved adults. In addition, because the majority of participants were Mexican American or Native American, multicultural treatment strategies, especially those that had proved successful with these particular groups, were adopted. Data obtained from structured interviews with DUI court graduates, staff, and providers were utilized to capture additional information concerning the perceived impact of the proposed enhancements on the DUI court experience. Finally, specific objectives to measure success were identified. These are depicted in Table 87.1.

As in the previous example, it is important to note how selection and implementation of treatment strategies, treatment process, and treatment outcomes were evaluated in a relatively seamless structure, uniquely designed for the particular agency and situation in which practice-based research occurred.

SUMMARY AND CONCLUSIONS

Treatment for substance abuse delivered within drug court models appears to have promising results, despite initial concerns about coercive treatment. The extended length of treatment and the influence of behavioral control on developing new habit patterns exercised within this environment seem to enhance success rates, provided treatment programs are overseen by psychologists who integrate practice-based research and evaluation into practice. A phenomenological approach to combining qualitative and quantitative data, as described here, is among the best methods to incorporate (De Souza, Gomes, & McCarthy, 2003) in the practice-based research that ideally characterizes effective drug court treatment programs. The two examples provided here are intended to serve as models for other substance abuse treatment programs integrated into criminal justice agencies. As more psychologists become involved and gather data on success rates, identify useful practices for specific populations, develop screening and assessment tools, and train probation officers and other agency personnel in effective cognitive behavioral techniques, it is likely that the benefit of drug court treatment programs, from both societal and cost-

TABLE 87.1 Objectives to Assess Success

Objective	Contact	Status
1. Revise current assessment procedures to address the target population in terms of cultural values, norms, traditions, and identity.	_____	_____
2. Revise current curriculum to address the target population in terms of cultural values, norms, traditions, and identity.	_____	_____
3. Provide case management services for Native American clients.	_____	_____
4. Provide counseling services for Native American clients.	_____	_____
5. Develop a Native America DUI court.	_____	_____
6. Provide case management services for Spanish-speaking clients.	_____	_____
7. Provide counseling services for Spanish-speaking clients.	_____	_____
8. Develop a Spanish-speaking DUI court.	_____	_____
9. Develop resource libraries of multicultural counseling strategies.	_____	_____
10. Include the target population in the planning, implementation, and maintenance of a culturally sensitive and competent DUI court program through involvement in the steering committee.	_____	_____
11. Develop an alumni group for the target population.	_____	_____
12. Increase the availability of age/gender/culturally specific programming for the target population.	_____	_____
13. Data collection, tracking, and integration of justice and treatment information on the target population will be expanded.	_____	_____

benefit perspectives, will continue to be recognized. The involvement of trained psychologists who competently integrate research and practice, however, is necessary for these programs to succeed.

ACKNOWLEDGMENT The authors would like to thank the Arizona Consortia of Substance Abuse Treatment and Research, Northern Arizona University–Yuma, the University of Arizona, the Arizona Department of Juvenile Corrections, and Maricopa County and Yuma County criminal justice agencies for their support and assistance with the projects described in this chapter. Results of the Yuma County Juvenile Drug Court outcomes assessment were presented as part of symposia on adolescent psychology and the courts chaired by Claudio Hutz, Ph.D., at the 2004 Congress of the International Union of Applied Psychology in Beijing, China.

References

Belenko, S. (1996). *Comparative models of treatment delivery in drug courts.* Washington, DC: Sentencing Project.

Belenko, S. (1998). Research on drug courts: A critical review. *National Drug Court Institute Review,* 1(1), 1–42.

Cooper, C. (1997). *Drug court survey report: Executive summary.* Washington, DC: American University.

DeAngelis, T. (2001). Substance abuse treatment: An untapped opportunity. *Monitor on Psychology,* 32(6), 24–25.

Deschenes, E. P., Turner, S., & Greenwood, P. W. (1995). Drug court or probation? An experimental evaluation of Maricopa County's drug court. *Justice System Journal, 18*(10), 55–73.

De Souza, M., Gomes, W., & McCarthy, S. (2003). *Reversible relationship between quantitative and qualitative data in self-consciousness research: A normative semiotic model for the phenomenological dialogue between data and capta.* Manuscript submitted for publication. Universidade Federal do Rio do Sul, Porto Alegre, RS, Brazil.

Foxhall, K. (2001). Preventing relapse. *Monitor on Psychology,* 32(6), 46–47.

Hora, P. F., Schma, W. G., & Rosenthal, T. A. (1999). Therapeutic jurisprudence and the drug court movement: Revolutionizing the criminal justice system's response to drug abuse and crime in America. *Notre Dame Law Review, 74*(2), 7–14.

Lewis, D. C. (1998). New studies find drug courts and drug treatment of prisoners, paroles and teens cut crime and drug use. *Physician Leadership on National Drug Policy, 10.*

Peters, R. (1996). Evaluating drug court programs: An overview of issues and alternative strategies [Online]. Available: http://gurukul.ucc.american.edu/justice/justb6.htm

Peters, R. (1999). *Current drug court evaluation results.* Paper presented at the National Association of Drug Court Professionals Fifth Annual Training Conference. Miami Beach, Florida.

Robinson, K. (2001). Research update: Reports on recent drug court research. *National Drug Court Institute Review, 3*(1), 121–134.

Satel, S. (2001). Drug treatment: The case for coercion. *National Drug Court Institute Review, 3*(1), 1–58.

Spurgeon, A., McCarthy, S., & Waters, T. (1999). Developing a substance abuse relapse indicator questionnaire for adults on intensive probation: A pilot study. *Journal of Offender Rehabilitation.*

88 APPLICATION OF LOGIC MODELS IN RURAL PROGRAM DEVELOPMENT

Paul Longo

In 1998 the Appalachian Partnership for Welfare Reform (APWR) was established as a collaborative, applied-research, and technical-assistance program funded by the Ohio Department of Job and Family Services (ODJFS) and administered by the Institute for Local Government Administration and Rural Development (ILGARD) at Ohio University's Voinovich Center for Leadership and Public Affairs. After five years as a grant-funded project focused on implementing policy changes in the areas of public assistance administration and workforce development at the county level in Ohio Appalachia, the APWR became a statewide technical assistance contract between the ODJFS Office of Family Stability (OFS) and ILGARD focused on strengthening performance measurement and accountability structures throughout the state of Ohio. The primary aim of APWR was to help enhance administrative infrastructure and capacity among the 29 APWR county agency partners implementing welfare reform throughout Ohio Appalachia. Among our principle activities, developing evaluation and performance measurement capacity was one of the APWR's biggest and most interesting challenges. This chapter describes the historical and social context of the APWR and outlines the Ongoing Performance Measurement and Management (OPM&M) framework that we used to develop processes intended to enhance evaluation capacity in this Central Appalachian setting. We also present one of the central features of the OPM&M framework, the Performance Blueprint, an integrated, nonlinear logic model that can be used as both an evaluation and a planning tool. In Chapter 89 we continue our discussion of the Performance Blueprint by focusing on some of

the unique features that allow it to support the development of technically useful and culturally appropriate evaluation processes that, in turn, can be driven by meaningful data, guided by a collaborative form of local self-determination, and legitimized by the universally applicable demand for accountability. We also share some feedback describing how the OPM&M framework and the Performance Blueprint have been instrumental in documenting success, identifying needs, learning from service delivery, and in general building individual and organizational *performance measurement literacy*, the name we have given to the constellation of skills and competencies that we have found to be fundamental for practitioners wishing to establish and nourish outcomes-based or performance-based practices.

The OPM&M framework, developed initially for APWR county partners situated throughout Ohio Appalachia, is as much a planning tool as it is an evaluation tool in that it aims to link strategic planning and performance measurement into a coherent and purposeful learning culture. It is not a coincidence that the OPM&M model was developed, piloted, and refined in many of the most economically distressed counties in the Appalachian Region. When economic resources are scarce, as they are in this Ohio section of central Appalachia, other forms of capital and creativity can and do take their place. The OPM&M framework, a work in progress, is an expression of this sort of ingenuity; it consists of both technically sound evaluation theory and practice and endogenous expressions of the innovation, persistence, and stewardship that characterize the public agencies throughout

Ohio Appalachia that contribute to and are generally served by ILGARD.

Since its inception in 1965, the Appalachian Regional Commission (ARC) has officially designated 29 of Ohio's 88 counties as Appalachian counties.[1] These counties represent 7% of the 410 counties that make up the nation's Appalachian Region, a 200,000-square-mile area that follows the contour of the Appalachian Mountains from northern Mississippi to southern New York.[2] According to the ARC, about 23 million people live in the Appalachian Region; 42 percent of the region's population is rural, compared with 20 percent of the national population. At the time of the establishment of the ARC, one in three Appalachians lived in poverty, as documented by Michael Harrington's book *The Other America* (1962). In recent years, though poverty has been on the decline in southern and northern parts of Appalachia, serious economic problems persists in the central Appalachian region that encompasses West Virginia, southeast Ohio, and parts of Pennsylvania and Kentucky (Sarnoff, 2003). In Sarnoff's view, central Appalachia,

while having moved from its 1960 era level of poverty (more due to public benefits than to industry) still lags behind the rest of the country economically, much as it did at Harrington's writing. Therefore, Central Appalachia has, for the most part, not entered the mainstream of America, and is, instead, still very much the 'other' America." (Sarnoff, 2003, p. 136)

When the APWR[3] was established in 1998 to provide technical assistance to the 29 county agencies as well as the state and local governments that serve Appalachian Ohioans living within this portion of central Appalachia and eligible for public benefits, the State of Ohio was 1 year into the implementation of its innovative Ohio Works First (OWF) Strategy. To implement the OWF, all 88 counties' human services agencies, now referred to as County Department of Job and Family Services (CDJFS), were required, on behalf of their county commissioners, to engage in a separate community-based strategic planning process and to prepare an individual Community Plan for Welfare Reform. The authorizing legislation, Ohio House Bill 408, stipulated that each planning document and process incorporate an outcomes-based performance measurement system to determine the strategies

for funding the OWF implementation. Consequently, in addition to providing various others types of technical assistance and applied research, the APWR began addressing the planning and evaluation needs of the 29 Appalachian CDJFS partners in relation to the Community Plans for Welfare Reform.

The APWR provided varying degrees of planning facilitation and technical assistance to approximately two thirds of the Appalachian CDJFS partners. Subsequently, the APWR developed additional capacity-building products and services grounded in this initial exposure to partners' needs and existing resources in relation to strategic planning and performance measurement. In five instances the APWR was asked to return to a CDJFS in order to revitalize and augment the county's Community Plan for Welfare Reform (Longo 2001b; see also Longo & Howe, 1999). Growing interest in these techniques led to the development of a more comprehensive framework for linking performance measurement and strategic planning called, as mentioned earlier, the Ongoing Performance Measurement and Management model, components of which are embedded in the following APWR products and services: Community-Based Welfare-Reform Strategic Planning, Ongoing Plan Management (OPM), Performance-Based Contract Management, Performance-Based Outcomes Management, Workforce Investment Act (WIA) Construction Kit, and the Social Marketing Initiative. These can be viewed at http://www.ilgard.ohiou.edu/apwr/.

The OPM&M model addresses capacity-building needs in the following four phases:

1. Visioning and revisioning—In this ongoing phase the community's assets and needs are assessed or reassessed in relation to federal and state outcome expectations; the community's desired and required outcomes are affirmed or reaffirmed; and appropriate strategic planning-evaluation strategies are envisioned or reenvisioned, including the establishment of evaluation criteria and corresponding informational baselines.

2. Performing—In this ongoing phase the "performance" of both strategists and their strategies is the focal point. Internally and externally oriented activities are set or reset in motion and viewed as the "performance" to be monitored and learned from.

3. Measuring—In this ongoing phase "perfor-

mance" is assessed, gauged, or otherwise *measured*. The focus is on the efficiency and effectiveness of the strategies, services, and activities *performed*, which includes the narrow scope of *performance measures* in relation to clients and/or customers targeted and reached as well as the broader scope of community-wide and agency-wide *outcome measures*.

4. Learning—In this ongoing phase performance measurement and evaluation information is used to make decisions, to identify the need for adjustments or changes. In the OPM&M model this focus on use, consistent with Patton's framework of utilization-focused evaluation (1997), is formalized and consists of regularly scheduled and open quarterly meetings, which we sometimes call "information festivals." The lessons learned and accompanying decision-making process, based on available and shared quantitative and qualitative evidence, naturally lead back to the visioning and re-visioning phase of the OPM&M cycle.

The OPM&M model, in part, is rooted in "theory-based" or "theory of change–based" evaluation traditions (Chen & Rossi, 1983; Connell & Kubisch, 1998; see also Patton, 1997, pp. 215–238). Accordingly, OPM&M revolves around an expanded and innovative logic model, called the Performance Blueprint, which in turn is used as both a planning and an evaluation tool.[4] The Performance Blueprint, depicted in Figure 88.1, is supported by (a) an anthropological orientation (Longo, 2001a; Longo & Miewald, 2000); (b) a social marketing orientation (Brown, 1997; Bryant, Lindenberger, Brown, Kent, Schreiber, Bustillo, & Walker-Canright, 2001; Lefebvre & Flora, 1988; Sutton, Balch, & Lefebure, 1995); and (c) Mark Friedman's Four-Quadrant Approach to Performance Measurement (Friedman, 1997; Friedman, DeLapp, & Watson, 2000). These enhancements have helped the Performance Blueprint exceed limitations often cited with regard to the use of logic models, most of which focus on how the logic model amounts to little more than a "Procrustean bed" (Stufflebeam, 2001, p. 39) that pays little or no attention to the underlying sociocultural and political variables associated with the program's "context" or "environment" (Fisher, 2001; Freddolino, Naegeli, Storoschuk, Neal, & Pasquarella, 1998; Perrin, 1998; EVALTALK, 2002).

In addition to the traditional elements encompassed by most standard logic models (e.g., United Way of America, 1996: inputs, activities, outputs, and outcomes), the Performance Blueprint also requires the identification and inclusion of direct and indirect beneficiaries (clients, customers, information users, etc.), as well as the direct and indirect service providers (providers, vendors, and collaborators). Moreover, by incorporating Friedman's Four-Quadrant Approach, the Performance Blueprint also offers a transparent strategy for identifying and prioritizing four types of performance measures as-

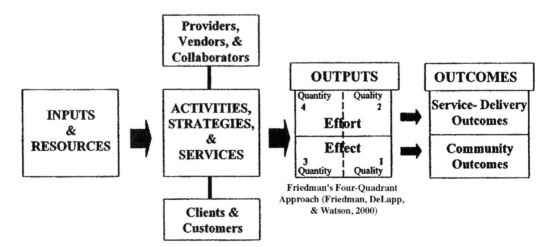

FIGURE 88.1 The Performance Blueprint.

sociated with a program's *effort*-related outputs and its *effect*-related outputs, each of which is further divided into quantity (individual counts) and quality (rate and percentages). The Performance Blueprint will be discussed in greater detail in Part II.

The Performance Blueprint offers practitioners a disciplined way of identifying and mapping strategic thought that, in turn, allows them to situate themselves in both actual and potential performance situations. Accordingly, once all of the required information has been inserted into the Performance Blueprint's component and shared, practitioners, stakeholders, and beneficiaries can engage in descriptive and prescriptive problem-solving activities while remaining grounded in the realities that surround them. What follows is an annotated and interrelated outline of the individual components that constitute the Performance Blueprint as depicted in Figure 88.1.

Inputs. Inputs are the resources needed to develop deliberate efforts intended to achieve desired outcomes. There are both material and nonmaterial inputs. Material inputs include funding, personnel, volunteers, equipment, and infrastructure. Nonmaterial inputs include leadership, vision, clearly formulated and measurable goals, strategies, strategic planning, a commitment to performance measurement, competence, realistic yet challenging performance targets, appropriate technology, interorganizational collaboration, and stakeholder involvement. Inputs also include the economic, social, and cultural capital of the community (the historical context) that may affect project success. Stated as a question, inputs can be understood as follows: What kind of hard and soft resources are already available or needed for service providers and collaborators (a) to have desired impacts on their clients, customers, and the community in which they live as well as (b) to construct an organizational culture that values efficiency, equity, and learning?

Activities, Strategies, and Services. These refer to all operational elements of what is essentially the "effort," that is to say, the program, the initiative, the project, and so forth. Activities, strategies, and services are expected first and foremost to benefit the customer and then the service-providing organization. The "effort" expresses the hope that inputs can be converted into results. However, since this does not always happen automatically, coincidentally, or accidentally, the underlying assumptions and strategies that are expected to drive the "effort" must be articulated explicitly, executed experimentally, and tied directly to performance measures that will look for evidence of efficiency, equity, and effectiveness. Stated as a question, then, activities, strategies, and services can be understood as follows: What sort of deliberate "effort" is necessary so that service providers know (a) what it means to deliver services effectively, that is, for the benefit of clients and customers, and (b) what it means to work collaboratively and efficiently with other service providers, that is, for the benefit of improving service delivery?

Providers, Vendors, and Collaborators. Paid and nonpaid personnel are required to develop and evaluate strategies, implement plans, provide services, manage and measure performance, and so forth. Stated as a question, providers, vendors, and collaborators can be understood as follows: Who directly or indirectly provides services to or otherwise comes in direct or indirect contact with clients and customers for the purpose of achieving or approximating desired results?

Clients and Customers. Clients and customers are the targeted beneficiaries of the effort. Their "performance," having come into contact with service providers or products associated with the effort, dramatizes the effectiveness, semieffectiveness, or ineffectiveness of the "effort." Also included in this component are the intended consumers of the evaluation information generated by the effort's performance measurement system. Stated as a question, clients and customers can be understood as follows: Who is served or otherwise influenced by the "effort," that is, the given set of activities, strategies, and/or services?

Outputs. Herein lies one of the most important distinctions of the Performance Blueprint, one that might even be considered controversial by some. Outputs in this model are narrower in scope and scale than are outcomes. They refer to specific impacts that service providers actually have on the clients or customers who are actually reached. In this sense, outputs are associated with a subset of the larger population to which outcomes are linked. The "performance" of service providers is gauged by examining their outputs, in terms of how efficiently and equitably (as judged by measures of effort) and how effectively (as judged by measures of effect) they are able to reach and satisfy their clients' or customers' needs and to what extent successes and gains along these lines can be associated with the attainment or at least the approximation of the overall desired outcomes of the community. Stated as a question, output measures of effort can be understood as follows: How will efficiency and equity of service delivery be measured? Likewise, output measures of effect can be understood as follows: How will the program's effectiveness be measured, that is, the impact on clients and customers in terms of desired changes in knowledge, attitude, behavior, and status?

Outcomes. Consistent with Friedman's effect-effort distinction, community outcomes (effect-related) represent what it takes to attain or approximate improvements that the entire community desires for its well-being and livability, whereas service-delivery outcomes (effort-related) refer to what the service-providing organization needs to do in order to express its social commitment to accountability, efficiency, and equity. Community outcomes encompass the community's entire population and/or its environmental conditions as indicated by measures of social justice, economic prosperity, health, education, safety, recreation, aesthetics, and so forth. Service-delivery outcomes include the organization's public intention to use resources wisely and to manage operations rigorously and transparently. Stated as a question, community outcomes can be understood as follows: What overarching impact on the entire community is the effort expected to have? Similarly, service-delivery outcomes can be understood as follows: What are the overarching operational goals and organizational commitments of the program?

The relational framework and accompanying terminology of OPM&M's Performance Blueprint has helped the APWR service-delivery team in our effort to build the evaluation capacities of our customers and partners throughout Appalachia Ohio by promoting the notion of ongoing performance measurement in ways that are consistent with the emerging accountability paradigm and its accompanying forms of strategic thought. Since 1998 the APWR has embraced the definition of performance measurement crafted by the U.S. General Accounting Office (1998).[5] This definition, which compares and contrasts performance measurement and program evaluation, has been helpful in explaining the implications of and further developments

recently associated with the Government Performance and Results Act (GPRA) of 1993.[6] We have attempted to operationalize performance measurement in the OPM&M approach by focusing on the following four characteristics: that performance measurement entails (a) systematically collecting and strategically using performance information (b) on an ongoing basis (c) in an intra- and interorganizational fashion (d) for a variety of internal and external purposes. Each of these four considerations merits further explanation.

1. Systematically collecting and strategically using performance information. . . .

   Within this consideration we stress the need to use a shared logic model and a single set of common terms so that all stakeholders can adopt a pragmatic, rigorous, and defensible approach to decision making. The Performance Blueprint, to be explored later in this chapter, offers this kind of pragmatic framework. As practitioners and trainees gradually become more familiar with the Performance Blueprint and, in particular, the logical interconnectedness of the components that constitute it, we have found that their performance measurement literacy increases. This will be discussed in greater detail later.

2. . . . on an ongoing basis . . .

   The OPM&M model is essentially cyclical, that is, visioning and revisioning, performing, measuring, and learning; it encompasses both planning and evaluation practices. Dusenbury (2000) makes the point that "strategic planning is a continuous process that requires constant feedback about how the current strategies are working . . . performance measurement provides the feedback that keeps the strategic plan on target" (p. 1). Figure 88.2 illustrates what Dusenbury calls the Circle of Strategic Planning and Performance Measurement.

3. . . . in an intra- and interorganizational fashion . . . In this consideration we call attention to the often-underestimated and misunderstood, yet crucial, role that "collaboration" plays in planning, evaluating, and performance measurement. Himmelman (1996) defines collaboration specifically for this context. According to Himmelman, collaboration involves exchanging information, altering activities, sharing resources, and en-

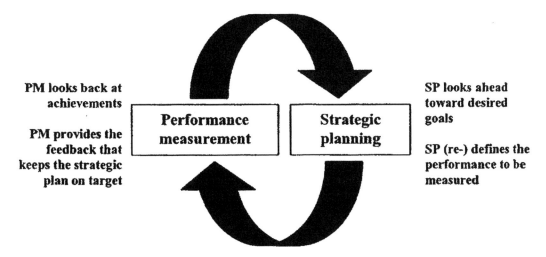

PM looks back at achievements

PM provides the feedback that keeps the strategic plan on target

SP looks ahead toward desired goals

SP (re-) defines the performance to be measured

FIGURE 88.2 Dusenbury's Circle of Strategic Planning (SP) and Performance Measurement (PM).

hancing the capacity of another for mutual benefit and to achieve a common purpose. Figure 88.3 represents Himmelman's definition by identifying how networking, cooperation, and coordination are the building blocks of collaboration. Himmelman's distinctions have been particularly useful for operationalizing how primary service pro-

viders, vendors, and other kinds of collaborators propose to work together and for assessing how they do work together.

4. . . . for a variety of internal and external purposes.

Given this broad definition and our pragmatic perspective, performance measurement can ren-

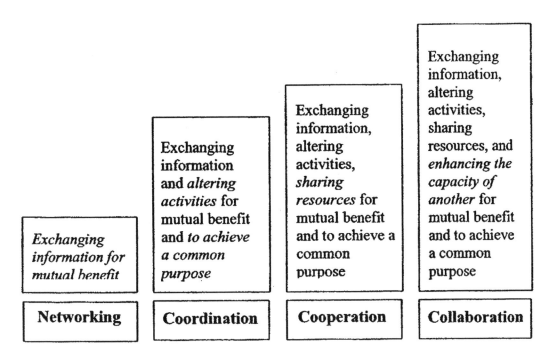

FIGURE 88.3 Himmelman's building blocks of collaboration.

der many benefits. In addition to complying in a narrow sense with federal and state laws and regulations, other benefits include the following:

- Contribute to improved organizational performance
- Clarify performance expectations
- Define success
- Communicate organization's goals and results
- Enhance local self-determination
- Reduce uncertainty
- Provide a mechanism to make decisions even when some information is lacking
- Apportion resources in an evidence-based fashion
- Control public education and public relations
- Market successful programs
- Foster accountability

Following these principles, the APWR service-delivery team has used the OPM&M framework and, in particular, the Performance Blueprint to promote the establishment and institutionalization of technical and cultural practices that support ongoing performance measurement in job and family-related human service agencies throughout Ohio Appalachia and to some extent throughout the state of Ohio.[7] As stated earlier, the APWR is a partnership established between the Ohio Department of Job and Family Services in its supervisory role, the 29 Appalachian County Departments of Job and Family Services, and ILGARD at Ohio University. The OPM&M framework is a product of that partnership that has been crafted and revised over time by contributing APWR partners, other human services administrators, public servants, and community leaders. It is impossible to gauge the exact value or to characterize the impact of the OPM&M framework; however, the majority of county directors and their colleagues have consistently expressed their support by citing numerous instances in which the framework and related techniques have helped them manage more efficiently and provide services more effectively to individuals and families who live in a section of this country that has been called "the *other* America."

In Chapter 89 we will continue this discussion by focusing on a few specific features of the Performance Blueprint that enable practitioners to facilitate processes whereby meaningful short-range and long-range performance mea-

sures can be developed in relation to state, regional, and local performance mandates. We will also discuss feedback from users of APWR's products in greater depth to illustrate the utility and customizability of the Performance Blueprint. Finally, we will outline the core competencies that we believe practitioners need to have in order to systematically collect and strategically use performance information, a skill set that we call *performance measurement literacy*.

Notes

1. By means of the Appalachian Regional Development Act of 1965, Congress established the ARC to support economic and social development in the Appalachian Region. The 29 Appalachian counties of Ohio are Adams, Athens, Belmont, Brown, Carroll, Clermont, Columbiana, Coshocton, Gallia, Guernsey, Harrison, Highland, Hocking, Holmes, Jackson, Jefferson, Lawrence, Meigs, Monroe, Morgan, Muskingum, Noble, Perry, Pike, Ross, Scioto, Tuscarawas, Vinton, and Washington.

2. The entire Appalachian Region includes all of West Virginia and parts of 12 other states: Alabama, Georgia, Kentucky, Maryland, Mississippi, New York, North Carolina, Ohio, Pennsylvania, South Carolina, Tennessee, and Virginia.

3. Core staff funded by the APWR project include a project manager, a data analyst, two senior research associates, and an outcome evaluator/performance measurement specialist, the position held by the author.

4. Logic models are visual depictions of what a program can be expected to produce and how it goes about producing it. I would argue that logic models, as used in this context, compellingly exemplify what Paulston (2000) calls "social cartography," that is, mapping ways of seeing social and educational change. In addition to "maps" and "strategy maps," logic models have also been called "results chains," "outcome-sequence charts," and so forth. In our current context, Wholey (1979) is one of the first to make use of the device and the term. See also Hatry (1999), Julian, Jones, & Deyo (1995), Julian (1997), McLaughlin and Jordan (1999), Plantz, Greenway, & Hendricks (1997), United Way of America (1996), and Wholey (1979, 1997).

5. According to the GAO, performance measurement is the ongoing monitoring and reporting of program accomplishments, particularly progress toward preestablished goals. It is typically conducted by program or agency management. Performance measures may address the type or level of program activities conducted (activities), the direct products and services delivered by a program (outputs), and/or the results of those products and services (outcomes). A program may be any activity, project, function, or policy that

has an identifiable purpose or set of objectives. Performance measurement focuses on whether a program has achieved its objectives, expressed as measurable performance standards. Because of its ongoing nature, performance measurement can serve as an early warning system to management and as a vehicle for improving accountability to the public.

6. The GPRA of 1993 requires federal agencies to develop strategic plans describing their overall goals and objectives, annual performance plans containing quantifiable measures of their progress, and performance reports describing their success in meeting those standards and measures. One of the five initiatives on the Bush administration's President's Management Agenda is "budget and performance integration." This initiative builds on GPRA 1993 and previous efforts to identify program goals and performance measures and to link them with the budget process. The president's FY 2003 budget was the first to include explicit assessments of program performance.

7. The APWR service-delivery team has also provided OPM&M-related technical assistance and training for statewide outcome management applications to the Outcome Management Unit, within the Bureau of Program Integration and Coordination of the Office of Family Stability (OFS) in the Ohio Department of Job and Family Services (ODJFS). Similar forms of technical assistance, consultation, and facilitation related to central-office-wide strategic planning are also being offered by APWR to OFS.

References

Brown, C. A. (1997). Anthropology and social marketing: A powerful combination. *Practicing Anthropology, 19*(4), 27–29.

Bryant, C., Lindenberger, J., Brown, C., Kent, E., Schreiber, J. M., Bustillo, M., & Walker-Canright, M. A social marketing approach to increasing enrollment in a public health program: A case study of the Texas WIC program. *Human Organization, 60,* 234–246.

Chen, H. T., & Rossi, P. (1983). Evaluating with sense: The theory-driven approach. *Evaluation Review, 7,* 283–302.

Connell, J. P., & Kubisch, A. C. (1998). Applying a theories of change approach to the design and evaluation of comprehensive community initiatives: Progress, prospects, and problems. In K. Fulbright-Anderson, A. C. Kubisch, & J. P. Connell (Eds.), *New approaches to evaluating community initiatives: Theory, measurement, and analysis* (Vol. 2). Washington, DC: Aspen Institute.

Dusenbury, P. (2000). *Governing for results: Fourth report of the Urban Institute's governing-for-results and accountability project.* Washington DC: Urban Institute Press.

EVALTALK Listserve Communications. (2002). #0300–33,-40,-42,-43,-55,-62,-64,-72,-76. American Evaluation Association Discussion List, EVALTALK@BAMA.UA.EDU.

Fisher, R. L. (2001). The sea change in nonprofit human services: A critical assessment of outcomes measurement. *Families in Society: The Journal of Contemporary Human Services, 82,* 561–568.

Freddolino, P. P., Naegeli, M., Storoschuk, S., Neal, S., & Pasquarella, J. M. (1998, November). *It's a great idea, but . . . Barriers to the use of program logic models in the real world of program activities.* Paper presented at the meeting of the American Evaluation Association, Chicago.

Friedman, M. A. (1997). *Guide to developing and using performance measures in results-based budgeting* [On-line]. Available: http://www.financeproject.org/measures.html.

Friedman, M. A., DeLapp, L., & Watson, S. (2000). *The results and performance accountability implementation guide* [On-line]. Available: www.raguide.org.

Harrington, M. (1962). *The other America.* New York: Macmillan.

Hatry, H. P. (1999). *Performance measurement: Getting results.* Washington, DC: Urban Institute Press.

Himmelman, A. (1996). On the theory and practice of transformational collaboration: Collaboration as a bridge from social service to social justice. In C. Huxham (Ed.), *Creating Collaborative Advantage.* London: Sage.

Julian, D. (1997). The utilization of the logic model as a system level planning and evaluation device. *Evaluation and Program Planning, 20,* 251–257.

Julian, D. A., Jones, A., & Deyo. (1995). Open systems evaluation and the logic model: Program planning and evaluation tools. *Evaluation and Program Planning, 18*(4), 333–341.

Lefebvre, R. C., & Flora, J. A. (1988). Social marketing and public health intervention. *Health Education Quarterly, 15,* 299–315.

Longo, P. (2001a, November). *Building on a firm foundation: An anthropological application of performance measurement utilization in rural Appalachia.* Paper presented at the conference of the American Evaluation Association, St. Louis, Missouri.

Longo, P. (2001b, November). *Performance measurement utilized and institutionalized in rural Appalachia in the context of welfare reform.* Paper presented at the conference of the American Evaluation Association, St. Louis, Missouri.

Longo, P., & Howe, S. (1999, September). *Community plan management handbook: A guide for revising and managing a community plan.* Athens:

Ohio University, Institute for Local Government Administration and Rural Development.

Longo, P., & Miewald, C. (2000, June). *Addressing multiculturalism in program evaluation: Focus on collaborative evaluation of county-level welfare reform in the context of Ohio Appalachia.* Paper presented at the 20th annual conference of the Ohio Program Evaluation Group, Columbus, Ohio.

McLaughlin, J. A., & Jordan, G. B. (1999). Logic models: A tool for telling your program's performance story. *Evaluation and Program Planning, 22,* 65–72.

Patton, M. (1997). *Utilization-focused evaluation.* Thousand Oaks, CA: Sage.

Paulston, R. G. (2000). *Social cartography: Mapping ways of seeing social and educational change.* New York: Garland.

Perrin, P. (1998). Effective use and misuse of performance measurement. *American Journal of Evaluation, 19,* 367–379.

Plantz, M. C., Greenway, M. T., & Hendricks, M. (1997). Outcome measurement: Showing results in the nonprofit sector. *New Directions for Evaluation, 75,* 15–30.

Sarnoff, S. (2003). "Central Appalachia—Still the other America." *Journal of Poverty, 7*(1&2), 123–139.

Stufflebeam, D. L. (2001). Evaluation models. *New Directions for Evaluation, 89,* 8–98.

Sutton, S., Balch, G., & Lefebvre, R. (1995). Strategic questions for consumer-based health communications. *Public Health Reports, 110,* 725–733.

United Way of America. (1996). *Measuring program outcomes: A practical approach.* Alexandria, VA: Author.

U.S. General Accounting Office. (1998, April). *Performance measurement and evaluation: Definitions and relationships* (Publication No. GAO/GGD 98–26). Washington, DC.

Wholey, J. (1979). *Evaluation: Promise and performance.* Washington DC: Urban Institute Press.

Wholey, J. (1997). Trends in performance measurement: Challenges for evaluators. In E. Chelimsky & W. Shadish (Eds.), *Evaluation for the 21st century.* Thousand Oaks, CA: Sage.

89

AMPLIFYING PERFORMANCE MEASUREMENT LITERACY

Reflections from the Appalachian Partnership for Welfare Reform

Paul Longo

In Chapter 88 we introduced the Performance Blueprint, another illustration of which is presented here as Figure 89.1 for the reader's convenience. As previously discussed, logic models have been identified throughout the literature on program evaluation and performance measurement as a helpful, albeit relatively limited, tool for better understanding, managing, and

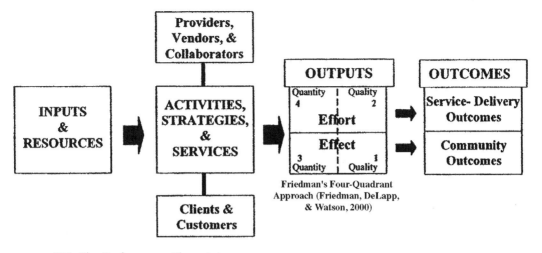

FIGURE 89.1 The Performance Blueprint.

documenting the performance of programs and the investments that go into them. Properly used, the heuristic power of logic models is capable of granting all the program's stakeholders (i.e., benefactors, beneficiaries, designers, implementers, service providers, and so forth) a standing invitation to compare the program's actual performance with its projected, desired, or even potential performance. The Performance Blueprint, which we claim is an enhanced, nonlinear logic model, is incorporated into many of the products and services that the Appalachian Partnership for Welfare Reform (APWR) offered to the 29 Appalachian County Departments of Job and Family Services (CDJFS) and continues to offer to the Columbus-based Office of Family Stability within the Columbus-based Ohio Department of Job and Family Services (ODJFS). By means of the APWR's annual performance assessment process, we learned that the majority of our clients, who use the Performance Blueprint in one way or another as a tool for systematically collecting and strategically using meaningful performance information, view it not only as a way to marshal important program-related evidence for a variety of purposes but also as a way to promote stakeholder involvement and engender a more productive and collegial type of collaboration.[1]

In Chapter 88 we opened the discussion of two critical distinctions that the APWR service-delivery team makes when presenting the Performance Blueprint in training, technical assistance, or consultation situations: the output-

outcome distinction and the effort-effect distinction. The latter distinction between effort and effect, based on Friedman's Four-Quadrant Approach (1997; see also Friedman, DeLapp, & Watson, 2000), makes it possible to identify two types of direct outputs: those associated with the "performance" of program personnel and those associated with the "performance" of the program's clients and/or customers once they have come in contact with the program. By parallel extension, it is also possible to identify two types of outcomes, service-delivery outcomes and community outcomes, which help to guide the program and to express the broader impact of the program on (a) the community in which the clients and/or customers live and (b) the service-providing organization's capacity to manage its resources and to improve service delivery on a continual and accountable basis.

By associating Friedman's Four-Quadrant Approach with outputs, the Performance Blueprint also offers a transparent strategy for identifying and prioritizing four distinct yet inter-related types of performance measures connected with a program's *effort*-related operational outputs and its *effect*-related productive outputs, each of which is further divided into quantity (individual counts) and quality (rate and percentages). It should be pointed out that Friedman's schematic does not make use of a standard, four-part logic model (e.g., inputs, activities, outputs, and outcomes). Rather, in his Four-Quadrant Approach to organizing program performance measures, as depicted in Figure

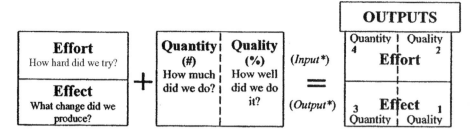

FIGURE 89.2 Friedman's Four-Quadrant Approach to program performance measures.

89.2, Freidman associates measures of effort with "input" (i.e., process or service delivered) and measures of effect with "output" (i.e., product or client condition achieved). For all practical purposes, Friedman uses the Four-Quadrant Approach as a self-contained logic model or strategy map; the Performance Blueprint, on the other hand, embeds the schematic into the more traditional, linear logic-model sequence, opening up the Performance Blueprint to accommodate more of the real-world complexities that permeate programs. The insertion of this dynamic schematic into the Performance Blueprint—as a way of organizing outputs—creates a ripple effect on the other components before and after its placement.

In Friedman's view, which assumes that the reader is a program staff person, measures of effort answer the question, How hard did we try? Measures of effect, then, answer the question, What changes did we produce? As already mentioned, for each of these types of measures there is an additional pair of questions that helps to distinguish between *quantity* (How much did we do?) and *quality* (How well did we do it?), where "quantity" will usually represent a number and "quality" a percentage or a rate of some sort. In this way Friedman's schematic gives stakeholders a powerful opportunity to understand how to develop logical and transparent criteria that, in turn, make it possible to prioritize and rank the four distinct types of measures: (a) measures of the quality of the effect, (b) measures of the quality of the effort, (c) measures of the quantity of the effect, and (d) measures of the quantity of effort. A very revealing set of mathematical relationships emerges when the appropriate information is placed into the appropriate quadrant. This chapter is not the proper context in which to elaborate on these mathematical phenomena; however, it must be pointed

out that, without such foundational information (i.e., the correct denominator) as that which is contained in the fourth-priority quadrant (e.g., number of people served), it would be impossible to achieve any accuracy in calculating any first-priority quadrant information (e.g., the percentage of targeted or reached clients who actually benefited in any sort of sustainable way).

As mentioned, the effort-effect distinction has a ripple effect on the logic and, therefore, potential usefulness of the entire Performance Blueprint. Figure 89.3 attempts to characterize this effect by tracing a dotted line that runs through the entire Performance Blueprint, virtually applying the same distinction to inputs, activities/strategies, and outcomes. Trainees and practitioners have found this feature useful because it helps to point out that performance measures of effort reflect the "performance" of service providers, collaborators, and vendors, whereas performance measures of effect reflect the "performance" of reached clients and customers. Similarly, as outputs can be labeled and categorized into measures of effort and measures of effect, so, too, can outcomes be similarly labeled and categorized—and prioritized accordingly. Take, for instance, a program manager who sees a funding opportunity sent out by a government agency or a foundation that emphasizes the importance of achieving one kind of community outcome or another. The request for proposal might also include language expressing the funder's organizational commitment to accountability, performance measurement, and outcome management. This kind of internally oriented organizational and programmatic priority falls squarely within the scope of the program's "effort." Using the effort-effect distinction that runs throughout the Performance Blueprint, the program manager and/or grant proposal writer could legitimately identify and label such an

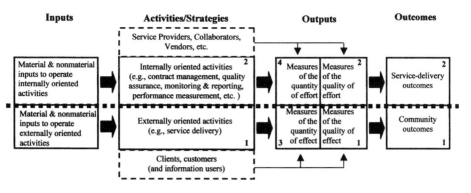

FIGURE 89.3 How the effort-effect distinction echoes throughout the Performance Blueprint.

organizational commitment on the part of the funder as the service-delivery outcome of the proposed program. Achieving that would necessarily require the development and operationalization of a set of "internally oriented" strategies and activities, including the development of some sort of performance measurement system, so as to produce any number of tangible, effort-related outputs to guide and periodically assess the performance of the program personnel in charge of executing this strategy. Measures of effort could include such items as the number or percentage of projects being tracked; the number of reports produced by the performance measurement system; the number of press releases produced by the performance measurement system; the number of executive decisions made based on data generated by the performance measurement system; measures of the fiscal and/or social return on investment; and so on. Above all, funding must be set aside from the very beginning for this kind of service-delivery outcome to work its way into the operational fabric of the program; for it ever to become a measurably achievable or "approximate-able" outcome; for some sort of performance measurement system to be designed, tested, implemented, maintained, and used; and for it to be able to produce meaningful and useful results (outputs). In the real world, examples as cut-and-dried as this are rare; however, we have found that the effort-effect distinction helps to shed light on both planning and evaluation. The Performance Blueprint can help identify these components and, more important, the linkages that relate and prioritize them.

On a practical note, it has often become necessary for the APWR service-delivery team to use separate blank Performance Blueprints to characterize large or thematically grouped strategies because it is usually impossible to characterize an entire program or organization using a single Performance Blueprint. Whenever possible, however, it is also recommended that a master Performance Blueprint be developed and posted publicly, using abbreviations and other shorthand techniques to create a single, "big-picture" image of the entire program so that stakeholders can remain informed of the program's progress in terms of outcome achievement or approximation. We have developed and are now testing a Microsoft Access database tool to accompany the Performance Blueprint that will allow practitioners to enter and update information, to create useful reports, and, in general, to help stakeholders visualize and critically understand the internal and external workings of programs that claim to convert resources into outcomes.

The same effort-effect distinction helps to sort out those outcomes that are more operational (and therefore more internally oriented) from those that are more productive, in terms of making a difference in the community (and therefore more externally oriented). Figure 89.4 attempts to illustrate the extension of these output categories so as to draw the distinction between service-delivery outcomes and community outcomes.

The Performance Blueprint has no beginning or end; in fact, the ability to make use of the Performance Blueprint in a left-to-right, right-to-left, bidirectional, convergent, or divergent fashion depending on the emergent needs at any given time is one of the *performance measurement literacy* competencies we hope to see

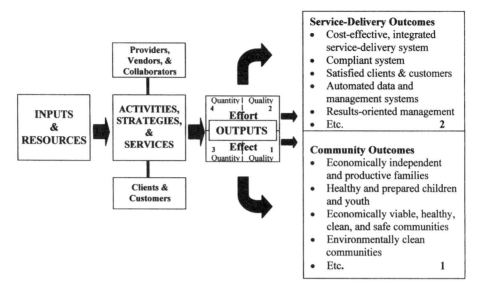

FIGURE 89.4 Outcomes as Extensions of Effort-Related and Effect-Related Outputs

emerge in users. This will be addressed in greater detail below. Nevertheless, in general training or consultation situations we do occasionally suggest that novice users can begin navigating their way through the Performance Blueprint in the following six-step sequence, essentially starting with outcomes and ending with inputs and resources in a right-to-left fashion:

1. Organize, collect, and chart outcomes. In this step one would begin with an exhaustive review of the applicable top-down (federal and state expected, required, mandated) and bottom-up (desired by the local community) outcomes. Some outcome statements may be clearly articulated, itemized, and possibly quantified statements; others may be very broadly or even universally stated; still others are disguised fragments partially embedded in the funder's mission or vision statement. At any rate, they all need to be gathered into a single list and then sorted into community outcomes or service-delivery outcomes. If there is any need to target an outcome, for example, the county's unemployment will drop to 2%, that too can be done at this point, as long as there are sufficient baseline and/or trend data to authenticate the targeted value in a realistically challenging manner.

2. Identify targeted populations (clients, cus-

tomers, consumers, etc.). With a clearer idea of the general direction in which the initiative is headed, this would be an opportune time to identify the population(s) targeted for product or service intervention. Target populations include not only the intended beneficiaries of the service strategies (clients, customers; primary, secondary, tertiary; etc.) but also the "users" of the performance-measurement information (consumers: decision makers, managers, public, etc.) for reporting and marketing purposes.

3. Define the results that clients or customers can expect in terms of output "effects." From the clients' and/or customers' point of view, consider how they can or must benefit from the program, classify these as effect-related outputs, and anticipate that from these considerations measures of effect will begin to emerge. In particular, ask what clients and/or customers can expect to learn or what they need to know (knowledge); what values they can expect or need to embody/reflect (attitude); what skill sets they can expect to or need to perform (behavior); and also what sorts of pivotal changes need to take place in their lives or in the organizational or environmental context in which they are situated (status).

4. Determine which activities, strategies, and services are needed to achieve Step 3 (in-

cluding an ongoing measurement *system*) and identify who will initiate, execute, provide, and/or monitor these efforts. Having formulated a more concrete idea of who needs to benefit and more or less how, in relation to broader aims, begin strategizing, that is, begin crafting strategies, proposed action steps, product lines, services, and so forth that would be likely to bring about the desired changes in knowledge, attitude, behavior, and/or status for the targeted clients and/or customers. Also, for each strategy, identify who executes it, who implements it, and who monitors it. These strategies—stated in a way that also identifies primary program personnel—may need to be prioritized or grouped thematically or otherwise structured to facilitate their assessment periodically. After all, the performance of these strategies is only hoped to be effective for clients or customers and efficiently executed by program personnel; collecting and using information directly and explicitly tied to their operationalization will be the real test of their efficacy.

5. Define and set the performance measures to assess the "effects" and "efforts" in relation to the chosen activities, strategies, and services. Given the preceding steps, determine the quantity and quality of the services to be delivered, how well the strategies must perform, and how well activities must be executed. Distinguish between effect-related and effort-related performance measures, and set targets when appropriate.

6. Use available resources and find additional needed resources. Obviously, it does not always work this way. Typically, funding becomes available, and this funding comes with strings attached. These strings are usually tied to goals and performance standards that force the organization to embark on unanticipated "activities." We recommend an approach that is somewhere between the ideal and the real. However, practitioners can take control by determining first what the priorities are, who needs to be served, why they need to be served, how well they need to be served, and then, finally, finding the resources to do the job.

Post-training feedback from APWR clients who have been exposed to the OPM&M model in general or the Performance Blueprint in particular has consistently provided evidence that users experience gains in their individual and organizational evaluation capacity, that is, *performance measurement literacy*.[2] By performance measurement literacy we mean the capacity of individuals and organizations to obtain, interpret, and understand performance measurement information and the competence to use such information to benefit clients, service delivery, and the entire community (see also Longo, 2002). As illustrated and exemplified in Figure 89.5, performance measurement literacy encompasses a wide range of *technical* and *cultural* competencies associated with both the *systematic collection* and *strategic utilization* of information; recall the operational definition of performance measurement outlined in Chapter 88. Beyond the acquisition of performance measurement literacy, there is no substitute for inclusive, representative, and collaborative stakeholder involvement (Burke, 1998; Clegg & Associates, Inc., & Organizational Research Services, Inc., 1999; Fetterman, 2001; Gaventa, Creed, & Morrissey, 1998; Preskill & Torres, 2000). When these are coupled, however, the resulting set of performance measurement practices is more likely to become institutionalized and to contribute to the attainment of sustainable outcomes.

County-, regional-, and state-level human services personnel exposed to APWR training incorporating the Performance Blueprint have described their evaluation-capacity gains in multiple ways. Given the opportunity to characterize their individual and organizational evaluation-capacity strengths and weaknesses in terms of the four performance measurement literacy skill sets depicted in Figure 89.5, APWR clients typically indicate that in their jobs they are most frequently called upon to exercise skills associated with Set 1 (i.e., technical/statistical skills in the systematic collection of performance information). In other words, they generally do little more than collect information that then more often than not disappears before having much operational value and local applicability. The performance measurement literacy construct has helped APWR clients identify two important needs: the need for organizational/cultural skills in relation to both collecting and using performance information, and the need for both technical/statistical and organizational/cultural skills in the general area of strategically using performance information. Our view is that successes

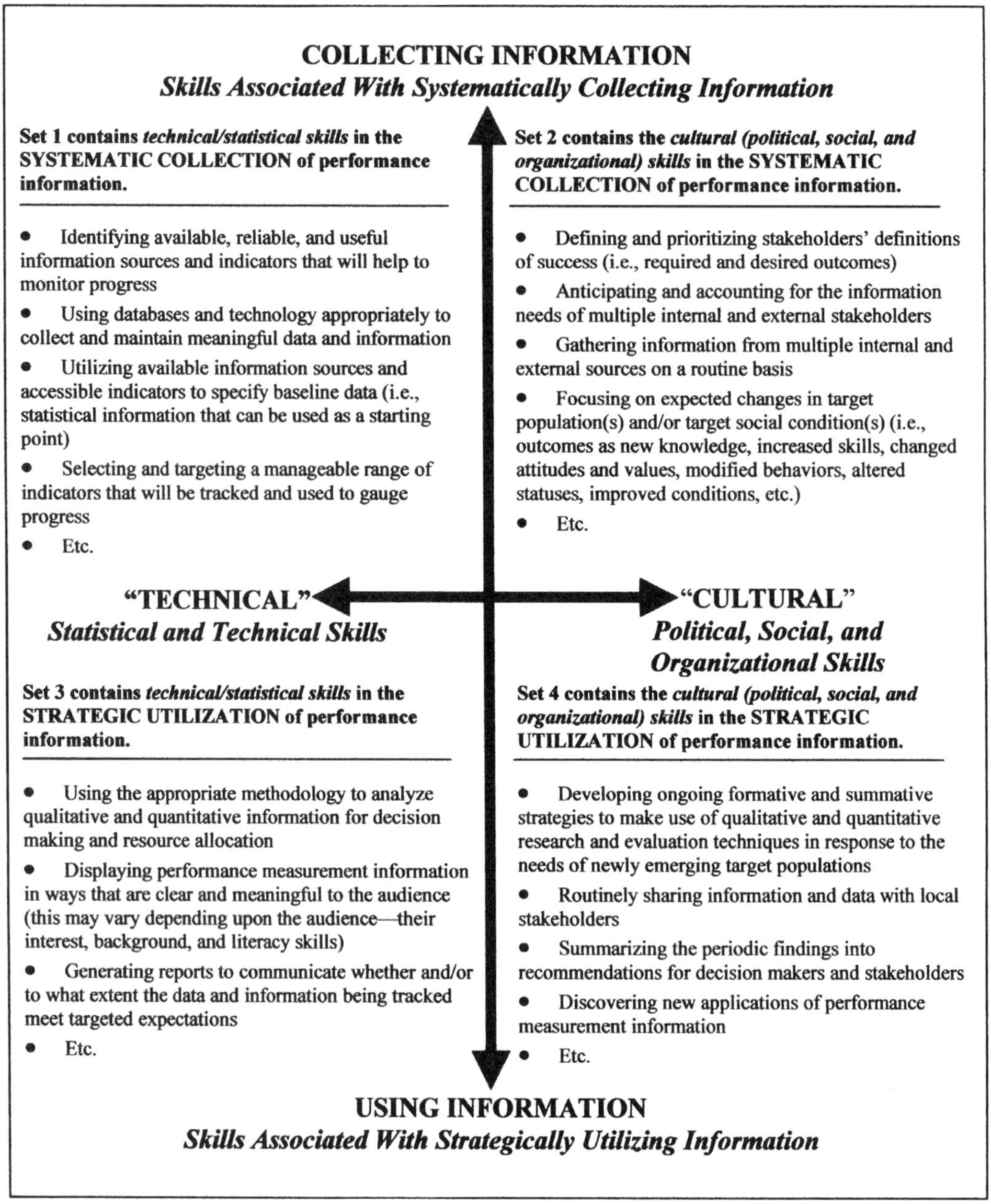

COLLECTING INFORMATION
Skills Associated With Systematically Collecting Information

Set 1 contains *technical/statistical skills* in the SYSTEMATIC COLLECTION of performance information.

- Identifying available, reliable, and useful information sources and indicators that will help to monitor progress
- Using databases and technology appropriately to collect and maintain meaningful data and information
- Utilizing available information sources and accessible indicators to specify baseline data (i.e., statistical information that can be used as a starting point)
- Selecting and targeting a manageable range of indicators that will be tracked and used to gauge progress
- Etc.

Set 2 contains the *cultural (political, social, and organizational) skills* in the SYSTEMATIC COLLECTION of performance information.

- Defining and prioritizing stakeholders' definitions of success (i.e., required and desired outcomes)
- Anticipating and accounting for the information needs of multiple internal and external stakeholders
- Gathering information from multiple internal and external sources on a routine basis
- Focusing on expected changes in target population(s) and/or target social condition(s) (i.e., outcomes as new knowledge, increased skills, changed attitudes and values, modified behaviors, altered statuses, improved conditions, etc.)
- Etc.

"TECHNICAL"
Statistical and Technical Skills

"CULTURAL"
Political, Social, and Organizational Skills

Set 3 contains *technical/statistical skills* in the STRATEGIC UTILIZATION of performance information.

- Using the appropriate methodology to analyze qualitative and quantitative information for decision making and resource allocation
- Displaying performance measurement information in ways that are clear and meaningful to the audience (this may vary depending upon the audience—their interest, background, and literacy skills)
- Generating reports to communicate whether and/or to what extent the data and information being tracked meet targeted expectations
- Etc.

Set 4 contains the *cultural (political, social, and organizational) skills* in the STRATEGIC UTILIZATION of performance information.

- Developing ongoing formative and summative strategies to make use of qualitative and quantitative research and evaluation techniques in response to the needs of newly emerging target populations
- Routinely sharing information and data with local stakeholders
- Summarizing the periodic findings into recommendations for decision makers and stakeholders
- Discovering new applications of performance measurement information
- Etc.

USING INFORMATION
Skills Associated With Strategically Utilizing Information

FIGURE 89.5 The Four-skill set of performance measurement literacy.

along either of these two lines already resonate with current efforts aimed at building and cultivating learning organizations and/or evaluation cultures (Davidson, 2001; Wenger, 1998; Trochim, 1999; Longo, 2001; Longo & Miewald, 2000). This sort of development has begun to occur throughout Ohio Appalachia because of the undeniable diffusion of a more comprehen-

sive notion of accountability that emphasizes not only the importance of traditional "top-down" accountability requirements, which have fostered and perpetuated a superficial attitude of compliance, but also the importance of the emergent "bottom-up" and localized forms of accountability, whose requirements are helping public managers understand the potential, multifaceted utility of establishing meaningful performance measurement systems. Establishing useful performance measurement systems at the local level requires a reconceptualization of traditional notions of leadership because the need for these systems in the first place is part of a much broader cultural reform that has begun to embrace ethical values that heretofore have been largely overlooked. The performance measurement literacy construct, like the notion evaluation capacity building (ECB), can play a role in energizing and nourishing this cultural reform, of which it is a product. It offers a way to reframe the public discourse needed to accelerate the development of new, technically and culturally appropriate evaluation customs that revolve around explicitly articulated, communally constructed, and logical evaluation criteria.

Some APWR clients have reported that using the Performance Blueprint to institute or enhance performance measurement practices has resulted in unexpected gains in intra- and interorganizational collaboration. In the 2002 annual performance assessment, which included an online survey of all APWR partners and beneficiaries, respondents ranked APWR's performance-based contract management training series highest in terms of "enhancing intra- and interorganizational collaboration." Their supporting, open-ended remarks pointed to the Performance Blueprint's consistent language and its unique capacity to distinguish between effort and effect as well as outputs and outcomes as clarifying and useful features in relation to promoting stakeholder buy-in and sustainability of active involvement.

One individual, who uses the Performance Blueprint to manage contracts for two Ohio Appalachian County Departments of Job and Family Services, made the following statement, which highlights many of his colleagues' comments:

In both counties, we have adopted the methods and terminology of the APWR manual. We constantly refer to the manual as a guide for our contract management. The manual has been extremely effective. It helps to have a comprehensive plan for contract management as described in the manual. The directors then know exactly where we're going with the process. And contract providers know "up front" what the expectations of the [agency] are. There are few "surprises" in regard to performance expectations and measurements that emerge after a contract is signed.

Another respondent, an assistant county administrator in an Appalachian county, reported that "the information and techniques learned during the training helped us to greatly improve our contracting process." He also mentioned that in contrast to the "haphazard" contracting and monitoring system of the past, his agency now has

a contracting process, monitoring system, and contract template that give us better control over the services we are purchasing. . . . Thanks to the training we can now better manage the contractors since all requirements are clearly spelled out in the document.

The value of the Performance Blueprint has begun to become evident by virtue of the fact that a small but growing number of county agencies, and to some extent state supervising units, have begun to institute practices amounting to changes in their standard operating procedures and, in turn, their organizational cultures. Some of this is due to the technical mechanics and features embedded within the Performance Blueprint that allow it to operate as both a planning and an evaluation tool. However, in and of themselves, tools are lifeless, inactive objects and, therefore, incapable of making a difference. People in organizational settings must use appropriately customized yet standardizable tools to make any kind of sustainable difference, whether that means purposefully maintaining a value or adding value by bringing about a change or managing transitions that are already set in motion by other changes. For this reason, as we present the Performance Blueprint as a tool, we also present the holistic performance measurement literacy construct as an assortment of skills aligned with the multitude of tasks associated with instituting performance measurement practices. These tools were developed to facilitate a better understanding of the differences between measures of effort and measures of effect, the scope of outputs and the scope of outcomes, and the technical and cultural skills needed to collect and use performance information.

The OPM&M framework, including the Performance Blueprint and the performance measurement literacy construct, emerged not from the America of plentiful resources but from the *other* America. As we have intended to suggest, the public administrators and managers with whom we have worked for more than 5 years have demonstrated that, though Ohio Appalachia may, in fact, lack certain kinds of resources, there is no scarcity of other, equally important, kinds of resources. The commitment to innovation, ingenuity, and stewardship that characterizes the public servants throughout this Ohio section of central Appalachia, especially the directors of County Departments of Job and Family Services, is on call 24 hours a day, 7 days a week, because the public servants, like the public whom they serve, have been forced to do much more with much less. The OPM&M framework, to the degree that it might be applicable elsewhere for the benefit of those being served as well as those doing the serving, is a product of Appalachian Ohio creativity and generosity.

Notes

1. The annual APWR performance assessments are available at http://www.ilgard.ohiou.edu/apwr/.

2. Our concept of *performance measurement literacy* should be understood in relation to what Baizerman and coeditors call the "evaluation capacity building (ECB) process," which they define as "the intentional work to continuously create and sustain overall organizational processes that make quality evaluation and its uses routine" (Baizerman, Compton, & Stockdill, 2002, p. 1). Their broader definition of ECB is indicative of an even closer relationship to OPM&M's operational definition of performance measurement; ECB is "a context-dependent, intentional action system of guided processes and practices for bringing about and sustaining a state of affairs in which quality program evaluation and its appropriate uses are ordinary and ongoing practices within and/ or between one or more organizations/programs/ sites" (Stockdill, Baizerman, & Compton, 2002, p. 8). M. Baizerman, D. W. Compton, and S. H. Stockdill are the editors of the Spring 2002 issue of *New Directions for Evaluation* entitled "The Art, Craft, and Science of Evaluation Capacity Building."

References

Baizerman, M., Compton, D. W., & Stockdill, S. H. (2002). The art, craft, and science of evaluation capacity building [Editors' notes]. *New Directions for Evaluation, 93*, 1.

Burke, B. (1998). Evaluating for a change: Reflections on participatory methodology. *New Directions for Evaluation, 80*, 43–56.

Clegg and Associates, Inc., and Organizational Research Services, Inc. (1999). *Outcomes for suc-*

cess. 2000 Edition. Seattle, WA: The Evaluation Forum.

Davidson, E. J. (2001, November). *Mainstreaming evaluation into an organization's "learning culture."* Paper presented at the American Evaluation Association Conference, St. Louis, Missouri, [On-line]. Avaliable: (http://unix.cc.wmich.edu/ ~jdavidso).

Fetterman, D. M. (2001). *Foundations of empowerment evaluation.* Thousand Oaks, CA: Sage.

Friedman, M. A. (1997). *Guide to developing and using performance measures in results-based budgeting* [On-line]. Available: http://www. financeproject.org/measures.html.

Friedman, M. A., DeLapp, L., & Watson, S. (2000). *The results and performance accountability implementation guide* [On-line]. Available: www. raguide.org.

Gaventa, J., Creed, V., & Morrissey, J. (1998). Scaled up: Participatory monitoring and evaluation of a federal empowerment program. *New Directions for Evaluation, 80*, 81–94.

Longo, P. (2001, November). *Building on a firm foundation: An anthropological application of performance measurement utilization in rural Appalachia.* Paper presented at the conference of the American Evaluation Association, St. Louis, Missouri.

Longo, P. (2002, November). *The Performance Blueprint, an integrated logic model developed to enhance performance measurement literacy: The case of performance-based contract management.* Paper presented at the annual conference of the American Evaluation Association. Washington, DC.

Longo, P., & Miewald, C. (2000, June). *Addressing multiculturalism in program evaluation: Focus on collaborative evaluation of county-level welfare reform in the context of Ohio Appalachia.* Paper presented at the 20th annual conference of the Ohio Program Evaluation Group, Columbus, Ohio.

Preskill, H., & Torres, R. T. (2000). The learning dimension of evaluation use. *New Directions for Evaluation, 88*, 25–37.

Stockdill, S. H., Baizerman, M., & Compton, D. W. (2002). Toward a definition of the ECB [Evaluation Capacity Building] process: A conversation with the ECB literature. *New Directions for Evaluation, 93*, 7–25.

Trochim, W.M.K. (1999). *Research methods knowledge base* (2nd ed.) [On-line]: Available: http:// trochim.human.cornell.edu).

Wenger, E. (1998). *Communities of practice: Learning, meaning, and identity.* New York: Cambridge University Press.

HIV PREVENTION

90

Evidenced-Based Practice With Infrastructure Support

Sarah J. Lewis & Ellen Goldstein

There are approximately 850,000 to 950,000 people living with HIV in the United States, and the Centers for Disease Control (CDC, 2002) estimates that there are 40,000 new HIV infections each year. There are no promising cures or vaccines to date, and success with a vaccine is defined as a meager 30% effectiveness. These facts alone make the case that effective prevention of infection should be a major priority.

The educated, white, gay community that was first hit by HIV in the early 1980s started to build a knowledge base about the condition and its causes. Grassroots community-based organizations came together to share knowledge about what worked and what did not work in supporting men to change their behavior and adopt safer sex practices. This empowered group recognized that sharing information about care and prevention with one another was imperative to reduce HIV (Indyk, Belville, Lachapelle, Gordon, & Dewart, 1993). HIV prevention research started in the mid-1980s to assess the effectiveness of behavioral and social interventions to reduce the risk of HIV infection (Office of Technology Assessment, 1996). There is an impressive list of well-designed interventions using several theoretical frameworks that have been found to be effective with various at-risk populations (National Institutes of Health, 1997).

OPERATIONAL DEFINITION OF EVIDENCED-BASED PRACTICE

Rosen and Proctor claim that evidenced-based practice has "empirically demonstrated links to the desired outcome" (2002, p. 744). It is important to parse this definition to have a clear understanding of evidenced-based practice. "Empirically" means that information has been collected in a systematic way. "Demonstrated links to the desired outcome" implies that the intervention either caused or is at least correlated to change in the condition being tested. As one can imagine, many interventions can be considered empirically based under this definition, but not all of those interventions are of the same caliber. There must be some standard set for what empirical means before agreement can be reached about whether or not practice can be deemed "evidenced based."

Model programs in HIV prevention are interventions that have been tested and retested using randomized clinical trials and found to be effective. These model programs are listed in a database that has strict inclusion criteria and can be thought of as the "gold standard" of evidenced-based practice. Many other programs that the community has developed also may be effective, but those programs have not been rigorously evaluated because of limited resources, and therefore are not included in the database.

DATABASES OF MODEL PROGRAMS

The Prevention Research Synthesis (PRS) project, otherwise known as the Compendium of HIV Prevention Interventions with Evidence of Effectiveness, was launched in 1996 and is another database of evidenced-based studies. The intention of this database is to systematically review how different factors are associated with intervention effectiveness. Inclusion criteria for PRS are as follows: The program must be based on a completed study using pre-post design; the design must include a control groups; the study must be evaluated by quantitative methods; and, significantly, less risky behavior or significantly more protective behavior must be found following the intervention. The rigor of each study is identified, as well as the magnitude of the results (Sogolow et al., 1998). Interventions included within the compendium have been tested on several populations: heterosexual adults, women, high-risk youth, incarcerated persons, injection drug users, and men who have sex with men. The Web site for the PRS project is http://www.cdc.gov/hiv/projects/rep/default.htm.

The difference between evidenced-based HIV prevention and many other conditions that may be presented elsewhere in this text is that most funders of HIV prevention services require the use of either model programs or, at minimum, evidenced-based interventions. This inevitably leads to a greater investment in model program dissemination by researchers, as well as a stronger incentive within community-based AIDS service organizations to attempt to utilize model programs. In the case of implementation, however, willingness is not always equated with ability.

CONCERNS ABOUT IMPLEMENTATION OF EVIDENCED-BASED PROGRAMS

There are some legitimate concerns about strict adherence to model programs in HIV prevention. Even though the primary outcome—"HIV risk reduction"—is consistent across all populations, the layers of conditions leading to high-risk behavior may be very different. One piece of the intervention may be deemed appropriate for the population being served by the prevention worker, but other pieces may be deemed inappropriate. For example, the area may be rural, whereas the model program may have been tested in an urban setting, or the population may be culturally different from the study sample. A successful adaptation of an intervention would maintain the core elements of the program while modifying contextual elements. The question then becomes, How much of the model program can be modified and still be considered the model

program? How robust is the program-to-agency or practitioner influence?

The problem is that interventions are tested as a package. The manual from introduction to conclusion makes up the contents of the package. No one knows, unless it is tested, whether a program is effective because of a specific part of an intervention, the interaction of several parts, or the succession of one component after another. Therefore, in an ideal situation, the model program should be used in its entirety.

Ideal situations are rare in life, however, and even rarer in AIDS service organizations with limited budgets. The CDC recognizes this reality and has attempted to minimize the difficulty in transferring model program technology into community-based organizations. There are two major difficulties with technology transfer: the language difference between intervention researchers and community practitioners, and the need to adapt the model program to the community-based agency. Several steps are necessary to go from intervention study to community-based intervention program.

Diffusion of technology first requires an investment by the researcher to translate the intervention study into a usable community product, as well as ongoing support to guide the agency in its adoption efforts (Kelly et al., (2000). Interestingly enough, this step goes back to funding. The researchers must have more than a moral obligation to disseminate their results. Instead, they should be compensated for disseminating results to practitioners because more team members are required. To successfully disseminate the intervention, team members require different skills than those required by the team members who create and evaluate the intervention model. Dissemination has to involve more than conference appearances and articles in top-tiered journals to which practitioners probably will not have access. Many researchers working in HIV prevention have made this commitment and have contributed to a growing body of "community-friendly" interventions in which community-based organizations have access not only to manuals, videos, CD-ROMs, and so forth, but also to the original research team. This translation into community-friendly interventions, however, still is not enough. Community-based agencies have to be able to find the intervention and then determine whether the intervention meets their programming needs and whether or not adapting the program is feasible for their organization.

To accommodate this step the CDC has funded the Diffusion of Effective Behavioral Interventions (DEBI) Project. The goal of this project is to develop and coordinate a national-level strategy to provide high-quality training, technical assistance, and other capacity-building activities to diffuse science-based HIV interventions to state- and community-level HIV programs (Collins, 2002). There are six key guiding principles to the DEBI Project:

1. Diffusion design must be tailored to both agencies adopting the model program, and the model program itself must be considered;
2. Organizational characteristics of most community-based organizations are positive factors;
3. Combination of manuals, training, and technical assistance is most effective;
4. Successful transfer of technology must consider access, cost, resistance, and public attitudes;
5. Just the use of the program concept (based on explanatory theory and interventive theory) is a valid outcome and can be linked to program improvement; and
6. Internal validity is easy to focus on and control in a study (independent variables strongly linked to dependent variables); however, external validity (generalizability) remains relatively unexplored.

Rogers's (1983, 1995) diffusion of innovation theory purports that "diffusion is the process by which an innovation is communicated through certain channels over time among the members of a social system" (Rogers, 1995, p. 5). In other words, it takes time before an intervention is adopted; it is not an instantaneous process. Community readiness and capacity, staff training, cost, adaptation, fidelity, and sustainability are some key model program dissemination issues (Neumann & Sogolow, 2000).

STEPS FOR DESIGNING AND IMPLEMENTING EFFECTIVE PROGRAMS

For the practitioner, deciding to use a model program is done through a series of stages. The first step is the establishment of need, which is often done through a community planning board and/or the local health department. A needs assessment would address both the populations that need the program (i.e., heterosexuals, intravenous drug users, men who have sex with men, high-risk youth) and the specific HIV prevention need of the local population (i.e., basic information, behavior change, safer behavior maintenance). Once it has been established that there is need for HIV prevention services within a population, a community-based organization or the health department moves into the second step, which is program planning.

Program planning is a critical stage that is made up of several steps and determines whether an evidenced-based program will be implemented. The program planner must first find funding for any potential program, and that funding will often set the parameters for the size and type of program. The parameters of the funding should be consistent with the agency mission and basic philosophy as well as with the need that has been established.

The next step for the program planner is to meet with key agency staff to brainstorm for types of programs or to attempt to establish what the staff is envisioning for the program. It is important to obtain staff buy-in early in the process. The program staff will often be the frontline practitioners who have to implement the program. If they do not believe in the program, they probably will not follow it.

The program planner must then go to one of the model program databases such as the Compendium of HIV Prevention Interventions with Evidence of Effectiveness with a list of what is known about the program needs so far: key elements about the population, agency setting, budget, and general philosophy. It helps at this point if the program planner is familiar with the basic theories on which most HIV interventions are based: health beliefs model, reasoned action, transtheoretical model of behavior change, social learning theory, and social cognitive theory. This not only allows the program planner to translate the needs assessment into program components but also gives her or him some idea of what to look for in a model program. Each model program in the compendium is theory driven, and it is helpful to be able to recognize which theory is congruent with agency philosophy and community needs.

The first step in searching the compendium is to consider the elements of the population in need that were identified in the needs assessment and through brainstorming with staff. The next step is to go through each of the model programs and see if any appear to meet the needs of the population. An example of this is the successful adaptation of a program evaluated on white gay men in a non-epicenter city by an agency working with African American adult women in housing projects. What the two populations shared was a tight-knit community that revolved around popular opinion leaders, a core element of the intervention.

Additionally, one must consider elements such as agency, capacity, and community norms in assessing the interventions. Conveniently, the compendium includes two important tables in its appendix. In the first table, one can cross-reference the program with population, agency setting, duration of intervention, and level of intervention (i.e., individual, group, or community). The second table gives a listing of all programs that have CDC support for materials production, technical assistance, and training. The next step is to determine if the agency can adopt the entire program or if the program needs to be adapted to the specific needs of the agency.

Once an intervention is chosen from the compendium, the agency program planner contacts the CDC for the intervention package. This package includes all the videos, forms, and other possible props for the intervention; it also includes technical assistance for implementation. Each intervention has technical assistance for agency personnel who are attempting to either adopt the intervention as a whole or adapt to agency needs. Technical assistance comes in the form of highly explicit, detailed guidance approved by the original researchers, in addition to ongoing support through the Behavioral and Social Science Volunteer (BSSV) program developed by the American Psychological Association and funded by the CDC as well as other CDC-funded programs.

When the community-based agency is implementing the program, it is important to continually assess fidelity to the core elements of the model program. Staff training is essential, as is process evaluation to track implementation issues.

Each intervention package includes an exten-sive built-in evaluation plan. It is important to evaluate all programs, even model programs. When the model program is adapted to fit an agency, it becomes even more important to test for effectiveness. If an agency decides not to adopt a model program but would still like to have technical assistance to develop an evaluation plan for either an existing program or a program that is currently being developed, that is available as well. The BSSV offers technical assistance to AIDS education providers through a volunteer researcher network. The BSSV contacts a researcher who is located in the same geographic area as the agency that is willing to provide time and limited project support.

CASE ILLUSTRATION

CARES, Inc., is an AIDS service organization that provides case management and other services for people with HIV in Hempstead County, a mid-metropolitan area in the Northeast. HIV education was never offered because the organization's mission stated that it provides "compassionate comprehensive social services for the HIV positive population of Hempstead County." More and more, however, CARES recognized that it is important to provide HIV education and risk reduction services to those infected with sexually transmitted diseases (STDs) because there is such high comorbidity, and there is a good chance that many individuals in the STD clinic population are also positive for HIV. The planning board of Hempstead County agreed with the CARES agency and made prevention with the STD population a priority. The program planner at CARES now had to find a program that was appropriate for both the high-risk population and the agency.

The program planner worked closely with the social worker and nurses at the local STD clinic to brainstorm about what kind of intervention they would like to see at the clinic. They thought about the time each client spends in the clinic and the opportunity to intervene, about the clinic population, about staff time, and space for an intervention. They concluded the following:

• Peer influence was important, and a group setting might be best.
• Education was important; however, discussion

about what was being learned was equally important.

- There was a small room off the waiting room, and the intervention could happen there.
- Each person usually had about a 20-minute wait from the time he or she checked in with the nurse until seeing the doctor, and that might be the perfect time to have the intervention.
- There were three doctors at the clinic, which meant there were usually about nine people in the waiting room most of the time.

The intervention specialist took these facts to the HIV compendium to see if there were any programs that met the criteria, and she found the Video Opportunities for Innovative Condom Education and Safer Sex (VOICES/VOCES). The intervention appeared to be perfect except that it had been tested only on men. To find out more, the program planner found the citation for the original article describing the intervention (O'Donnell, O'Donnell, San Doval, Duran, & Labes, 1998) and got a copy of it from the library. The program planner found that the researcher had her contact information in the compendium and called him after reading the article. Dr. O'Donnell, the original researcher, informed the program planner that she could call the DEBI Project and receive the intervention package, as well as assistance in adapting the program to fit both men and women.

The staff at the DEBI Project sent the program planner the intervention package and put her in touch with the BSSV program to arrange for technical assistance with program adaptation and implementation. After making some gender changes in the intervention, it was important to also make changes in the evaluation. The BSSV volunteer helped CARES to develop an additional evaluation instrument and gave the organization some ideas about keeping a database of evaluation results. In this way, the program was constantly monitored and also evaluated over time.

CONCLUSION

Evidenced-based practice in HIV prevention has become the norm. For years the field of social work has dreamed about and referred to the bridge that connects researchers and practitioners. The CDC, with the help of many dedicated behavioral researchers, community practitioners, and empowered consumers, has built the bridge. Evidenced-based practice needs infrastructure to support it. Diffusion of new technology must be carefully planned and executed; it is not something that just happens. Evidenced-based interventions that sit on library shelves gathering dust and not impacting practice are a waste of valuable resources. Researchers must make their effective interventions user-friendly, flexible, and affordable, and practitioners must increase their knowledge of basic behavioral science and participate in the technology transfer by seeking out effective interventions.

References

Centers for Disease Control. (1996). *Replication of effective HIV behavioral interventions* [Announcement 627]. Atlanta, GA: Author.

Centers for Disease Control. (1998). *Technology translation and transfer of effective HIV prevention interventions.* [Announcement 99089]. Atlanta, GA: Author.

Centers for Disease Control. (1999). *Technology translation and transfer of effective HIV prevention interventions* [Announcement 99089]. Atlanta, GA: Author.

Centers for Disease Control and Prevention, HIV/AIDS Prevention Research Synthesis Project. (1999). *Compendium of HIV prevention interventions with evidence of effectiveness.* Atlanta, GA: Author.

Centers for Disease Control and Prevention. (2002). Primary and secondary syphillis among men who have sex with men—New York City, 2001. *Morbidity and Mortality Weekly Report, 51*(38), 853–856.

Collins, C. (2002, December). Diffusion of effective behavioral interventions. Presentation at the Behavioral and Social Scientist Volunteer Training, New Orleans, Louisiana.

Indyk, D., Belville, R., Lachapelle, S., Gordon, G., & Dewart, T. (1993). A community-based approach to HIV case management: Systematizing the unmanageable. *Social Work, 38*, 380–387.

Kelly, J. A., Somlai, A. M., DiFranceisco, W. J., Otto-Salaj, L. L., McAuliffe, T. L., Hackl, K. L., Heckman, T. G., Holtgrave, D. R., & Rompa, D. (2000). Bridging the gap between the science and service of HIV prevention: Transferring effective research-based HIV prevention interventions to community AIDS service providers. *American Journal of Public Health, 90*, 1082–1088.

National Institutes of Health. (1997). Interventions to prevent HIV risk behaviors. *NIH Consensus Statement, 15* (2), 1–41.

Neumann, M. S., & Sogolow, E. D. (2000). Replicating effective programs: HIV/AIDS prevention technology transfer. *AIDS Education and Prevention, 12*(Suppl. A), 35–48.

O'Donnell, L., O'Donnell, C. R., San Doval, A., Duran, R., & Labes, T. (1998). Reductions in STD infections subsequent to an STD clinic visit: Using video-based patient education to supplement provider interactions. *Sexually Transmitted Diseases, 20,* 161–168.

Office of Technology Assessment. (1996). *The effectiveness of AIDS prevention efforts: A state-of-the-science report.* Washington, DC: American Psychological Association Office on AIDS.

Prevention Technology Transfer. *AIDS Education and Prevention, 12* (Suppl. A), 35–48.

Rogers, E. M. (1983). *Diffusion of innovations.* New York: Free Press.

Rogers, E. M. (1995). *Diffusion of innovations* (4th ed.). New York: Free Press.

Rosen, A., & Proctor, E. K. (2002). Standards for evidence-based social work practice: The role of replicable and appropriate interventions, outcomes, and practice guidelines. In A. R. Roberts & G. J. Greene (Eds.), *Social worker's desk reference* (pp. 743–747). New York: Oxford University Press.

Sogolow, E. D., Kay, L., Semaan, S., Mullen, P., Johnson, W., Neumann, M., & Norman, L. (1998). Development of an HIV intervention studies database for providers and researchers. World AIDS Conference, 12894 [Abstract No. 43242].

91

COMMUNITY REINTEGRATION PRERELEASE RESEARCH EXEMPLAR

Applying Theory to Practice-Based Research

Harris Chaiklin

Practice theory explains behavior and suggests interventions to maintain or change it. This chapter will show how data from the Community Reintegration Project, a prison prerelease program, were used to explicate the intervention component in practice theory. The practice concerned helping offenders prepare for release from prison. The program was designed to identify needs, to facilitate family and other social connections, and, where appropriate, to make referrals to community resources.

The aim was not to develop new theory but to make existing theory useful for practice. Tallman (2002) says that theory and not data provides a rationale for intervention and that data are not the basis for "building a cumulative body of knowledge" (p. 228). This does not mean the data are irrelevant, but, as Merton (1957) says, the abstractions of middle-range theory "are close enough to observed data to be incorporated in propositions that permit empirical testing" (p. 39). Middle-range practice theory helps avoid what Mills (1959) called "abstracted empiricism" and the rejection of rationality in dealing with human affairs.

Using this way to build knowledge for practice may be an antidote to what has happened to sociology, the source of so much practice knowledge. Berger (2002) says it has come to value "methods over content" and has been transformed into "an instrument of ideological advocacy" (p. 27). This diminishes the hope that it can help to improve the human condition.

THE COMMUNITY REINTEGRATION PROJECT

The Community Reintegration Project was funded by the Maryland Governor's Commission on Law Enforcement and the Administration of Justice. The grant was made to the Division of Correction, which subcontracted it to the University Of Maryland School of Social Work.[1] It ran from September 1971 to June 1973 and was conducted at the Maryland Division of Correction Camp Center in Jessup, Maryland (Chaiklin, 1973).

On-site project staff included a program director, who was a master's degree social worker and an ex-offender, a research associate, a university field instructor, and 10 student interns. Of these only the on-site director, the data associate who was a graduate student, did not have job protection when the project ended.

THE PROGRAM

The program was built around the idea that individual and family services were to be reality based. Men were to be readied for release by helping them make appropriate connections to family and community agencies. Our aim was to relate to offenders in ways that built trust so that their personal and material needs could accurately be identified and met. There was no effort to create new practice principles or a new agency. Rather, the goal was to show that corrections can and should function like any other social agency. The aim was to leave behind a set of procedures that could be used by classification officers, social workers, and other correctional personnel.

To qualify, a man had to be within 90 days of release and had to agree that family members or significant others could be contacted. Referrals could be self-made or from any other correction personnel. All participation was voluntary, and the men were told that participation in the program would not be useful in any way in influencing the prison in its decisions. As a matter of practicality, it was decided to serve men who were mainly from the Baltimore-Annapolis area.

For the most part there was great cooperation between institutional personnel at the Camp Center and project personnel. The most serious impediment came because the division could not keep its promise that on referral the man would have his release date. Without this, coordination between the offender, his family, and community agencies was difficult. Initially it took almost 2 months after parole was granted to process a man's papers and determine a release date. The addition of an institutionally based parole officer later reduced this time to 2 weeks.

This blip did not affect the program's theoretical orientation to practice. It did reduce the number of men who could be served. The time lag meant staff had to put extra effort into keeping it clear that participation in the program was neutral as far as positive or negative recommendations concerning parole, and what happened to the man in the institution.

OPERATIONALIZING THE SOCIAL IN PRACTICE

The social worker is a specialist in social, emotional, and cultural reality. This requires a broad definition of social practice. The social worker does the following:

1. Works at the nexus of physical, psychological, social, and cultural factors that influence behavior
2. Works with or at least takes account of all problems
   a. What led person to behave this way?
      (1) Assumes multi-causality

3. Sees the problem in the place where it happens or at least takes account of the situation
4. Works with individual, family, group, or community
5. Knows the community and its resources
6. Coordinates delivery of services
7. Meets need without requiring attitude change (Chaiklin, 1978, p. 476)

In working with a man, the worker was not to get involved in looking for deeper meanings to behavior, to establish a psychotherapeutic relationship, or to try to correct possible miscarriages of justice. If there were needs in any of these areas, referral was to be made to an appropriate resource.

DATA SYSTEM

Records were designed to reflect project philosophy. With the research associate, Harald Lohn, taking the lead, a reality-oriented computer-based data system was developed. Any process recording the interns did was for educational purposes and was not a part of the permanent project record. All data in the system pertained to information needed for administrative or practice reasons, and no data were collected for research purposes.

The core of the system identified physical, mental, social, legal, and financial problems. There were subcategories for specific problems, for example, alcoholism, employment, housing, and income management (Chaiklin, 1978).[2]

Understanding and using the data system required continuous training and monitoring. Some workers saw it as another "bothersome" educational requirement. Others saw using data forms as a cold, impersonal, inflexible approach that was unable to capture the richness of the client-worker relationship.

Although the need for efficient data systems is well known, numerous agencies, especially in the public sector, continue to have trouble meeting what are often mandated data requirements. One of the major accomplishments of this project was to demonstrate that it is possible to keep records current without an excessive expenditure of money or administrative time.

PROJECT FUNCTIONING

We gave full service to 213 men. We had contact with more men than this, but some rejected the project after one or two contacts, and some suddenly were transferred, were released, or "escaped." Initially members of the prison staff were skeptical of the family focus and said that neither the offenders nor their families were interested in each other. As the project began to function, this idea quickly changed.

Many questioned whether services would be available. We quickly demonstrated that when men were referred to appropriate services, with a professional referral and a good summary, there were services available. By the end of the project the opposite complaint was being made— that we were getting more than our fair share.

One element in making the referral process work so well was the preparation of a community resource manual, which contained a description of services, phone numbers, intake workers' names, intake policy, and other information relevant to referral. Such manuals used to be a standard part of social work practice; their discontinuance is a loss.

Implementing the data system encountered some resistance from field instructors and interns. The need for instant accountability was upsetting. While we eventually overcame the resistance to the data system, the resistance that was encountered highlights learning and practice issues that are relevant today. In many agencies face sheet information is collected in a ritualistic manner and is often inaccurate. In this project a basic assumption was that before one can be effective as a caseworker, fundamental social facts must be accurate and organized.

FINDINGS

There were no surprises in the men's social profile. Their average age was 31 years, 67% were Black, 55% were not married, and 62% were Protestant. On Hollingshead's two-factor Index of Social Position, 55% were in the lowest social class, 60% had little or no job skills, and 47% did not go beyond junior high school (Hollingshead & Redlich, 1958). About 50% of the men reported that they were employed at the time of incarceration, and about 75% said that they had not been able to hold a job for more than 2 years.

This social profile corresponded to the general population at the Camp Center. These occupational and educational characteristics indicate how difficult it is for some people to maintain a stable attachment to society. Even though almost half of the men were employed at the time of their offense, it was not enough to deter them from committing. It is not just that the jobs do not pay well. To retain a job, many other social supports need to be in place. Many programs put the stress on having a man get a job. As our program evolved, we began to put more emphasis on the factors that would help a man keep his job.

For example, we helped the men learn how to handle money. This involved such things as opening bank accounts and avoiding the pitfalls of credit card debt. This was difficult because people in prison usually have no acceptable personal identification. Interns had experiences with banks refusing to cash State of Maryland checks that men received from their accounts on release, even though the interns offered to cover the checks from their own accounts. In such circumstances men are forced to cash checks in bars or at check cashing services, which exact a heavy service fee.

As we began to make contact with community agencies, we found that much repetitious explanation was needed because intake workers were rotated or numerous individuals handled incoming requests. We met with the agencies concerned, and a liaison system was developed where personnel were designated to handle or channel all requests coming from the project. Among the more important of these liaisons were with Social Security, the Department of Social Services, Legal Aid, the U.S. Department of Labor Wage and Hour Contract Division, and the State Office of Consumer Protection.

The Social Security experience illustrates what liaisons can accomplish. Some men needed only a few quarters to qualify for minimum benefits. There were 6 men with multiple Social Security numbers and 18 men with no numbers. When the Social Security Administration has to handle account problems on an individual basis, it is expensive and time-consuming to search through the more than 40 million records. It readily agreed to appoint a liaison and even wanted to service the whole system. The Corrections Division said it did not have enough money to make a special run of their computer to locate the men who either had multiple numbers or no numbers.

Problems with Social Security can create major disruption in a person's life. A few men had a valid record that had been misplaced. Men who had no number had immediate problems in that when they were referred to work-release jobs,

they were turned down. We made a special effort to place men on work release when they were within a few quarters of qualifying for minimum benefits.

In sum, when appropriate referrals were made, services were available to prisoners preparing for release. Lack of resources or the refusal of an agency to give service was a minor problem. Many agencies do not serve incarcerated offenders simply because they are not asked. Offenders and their families can get help with their problems if they are helped to find appropriate services. As short as services are, many agencies have a service capability that is not utilized because suitable requests are not made. Accurate social facts are a necessary requisite to developing effective prerelease programming.

CASE EXAMPLE

This was a large and complex project. A case example can convey what happened without presenting a full statistical report. We called this man Legion, from Mark 5:9, which says, "My name is Legion: for we are many." Legion is a typical offender, a human being with strengths and failings.[3] He is about 25 years old. The following are pertinent social facts about him.

Offense Record

1. Breaking and entering
2. Larceny
3. Shoplifting
4. Atrocious assault
5. Violation of parole
6. Possession of narcotics

Family Structure

Legion's father has been absent since Legion was 4 years old. Legion was 7 when he last saw his father. Legion's mother is on welfare and is an alcoholic. The family includes 11 children: 8 at home, 1 married and doing well, and 2 (including client) in jail. There are minor problems involving almost all the other children. There are at least three different fathers for the children.

Individual Functioning

Lack of stability dominates Legion's life. He is personable, articulate, and good-looking and makes an excellent initial impression. His dependency and impulsivity are so close to the surface that he seldom sustains any relationship or activity for long. When he was about 10, he began missing school and hanging around with older boys. By age 13, he had been introduced to heroin and eventually had a habit that he claims cost him $125 a day. Although Legion finished high school during one of his incarcerations and received some subsequent technical training, he was never able to hold a job for any length of time. He has no support from his family, and he has made no connections to work. Drugs rule his life.

Family Process

Legion's family lives in a five-room house in a dilapidated and crime-ridden part of Baltimore. Without Legion, nine people live in this tiny row house. The mother is not able to manage herself or her children. When she has money, she drinks. She escapes from home as often as possible by visiting a female friend. When, after much effort, the worker saw Legion's mother and told him, he asked, "Was she high?"

Legion's mother handles the problems in her life by denial and escape. She said that she had no awareness that her son was involved with drugs. Legion said his drug activities are so well known that narcotics officers call him by his first name.

Casework Process

Legion was a willing participant in all activities. During a sociodrama session he expressed a strong interest in going to school and improving vocational skills he already had. This became the focus of several later group sessions and was the starting point in the casework relationship.

In sociodrama Legion "played" obtaining college applications and filling them out, making application and being interviewed for scholarship aid, and dealing with landlords. The latter was particularly important because Legion feared returning to his old neighborhood. Drugs would be a constant temptation.

His mother did not see herself as emotionally supporting Legion's plans. Her only comment when this was discussed with her was that she would provide him with a place to stay and something to eat. In individual sessions Legion showed great desire to follow through on his

plans, but he always asked for a lot of help. Vocational Rehabilitation was contacted and agreed to pay his room rent so that he could live away from home.

At the same time a referral was made to Model Cities, which agreed to pay Legion's first semester's tuition of approximately $200. All this took place while the application to college was in process. A special furlough was arranged so that Legion could take a placement test. On the basis of the test and a completed application the college offered a scholarship of $225 and a job at the school to further supplement the financial aid.

Legion committed a minor infraction during this period and was transferred to another institution in the camp system. This meant the worker had to travel to visit him. In addition, he was released from this institution on a Christmas commutation, and this threw his job and rental plans out of kilter. Extra contact with the landlord was necessary, and a referral had to be made to the Department of Social Services for emergency assistance and food stamps.

For 6 weeks after his release Legion lived at home. He reported great discomfort over this arrangement. During this time the worker saw him weekly either to help him ventilate feelings or to help make arrangements for housing, school, and welfare.

Legion started school, and the worker continued to see him about adjustment difficulties he was having. He needed tutoring in math. The worker provided this and helped him with summer job plans, conditions of a lease, and general problems in living. Toward the end of the school year Legion found that he could not afford the apartment he had rented, and he returned home. He began associating more with drug users and indicates that he had "fired" a few times.

Follow-up Interview

Legion's case was closed in the middle of May because the project ended. He was having trouble in school, was living at home again, and had no clear summer job plans. He would prefer not to be in this position. Like many offenders, he will not do much without help. In August we did a follow-up taped interview. Some excerpts follow:

The first program I became involved with was the Seven Step Program. I really felt I had combated narcotics to a certain extent myself but I still wanted to involve myself in this self-help program. . . . At the time I was in this program I came in contact also with the Community Reintegration Program.

I really don't know what made me so interested in the program. Most people might say that, well, it was a way out. I really don't think that I was looking for a way out. I was looking for help. I knew that I was due for release, and the Community Reintegration Project itself sounded to be the exact thing that I needed for helping me with my problems. Besides, at that time I was interested in going to college. I really didn't know at this time that CRP could help me, but I soon found out. I believe that my worker and me started the sort of relationship that every so-called convict and social worker should have because it seems to me that is the only way that there can possibly be any understanding between the two and the program. Even though—— was a white social worker, there wasn't any kind of hostile feelings toward him as a person. As far as my understanding was concerned, as far as the way I feel about it—a person is a person, especially when someone is trying to help—when both are trying to help each other.

Once I had gotten into the program, me and—— worked together to see that I got entered into college. . . . In all our efforts everything seemed to work out well. I did everything possible to find out whether or not I could make it in a college atmosphere. We had two groups dealing with the situation and also had students in so that we could have a rap session concerning college affairs. . . . It really influenced me a lot as far as going to college was concerned. I really thought that I wanted to make it on the outside in a college atmosphere.

I remember the occasions when I was released from incarceration before. Most of the times I was released I really didn't have enough money in my pocket for a day or more. I really hated the system itself for the fact that I wasn't being offered the help that I really needed. I really think that getting a person the money he needs to make it within his community is a very important thing. It seems as though most of the guys feel the same way.

It seems as though the system itself feels that, well, after a guy has spent a certain amount of time in jail, I guess they feel that they can just, you know, throw him back out on the street with no money in his pocket, no place to stay, no job, no means of income and expect him to make it or expect him to stay out of trouble with the law, but it really cannot be done in that particular manner. That is why I speak so much about the program itself because, like, it seems the program did everything possible to make sure that a person coming home from an institution was able to return to that community and start some kind of means of successful living. During the time of my release, money was given to me through the program itself and, as I previously stated, from the Department of Social Services.

One of the main things that really gets to me—whenever I do go to look for a job and that is when, you know, you go into the office and find out that you can't get it because something or another might be affecting your life, like say, for instance, the fact that I have a criminal record, a very long criminal record. Well, with the help of the program it seems as though this criminal record was unnoticed by most employers. But the minute that I was alone and didn't have the help of the program, it seems as though this record was noticed to the point where I was refused a certain position that I did qualify for. . . . I applied for jobs in fields I was qualified for and was refused a position for some reason or another. I didn't have a program to back me up and speak for me as a person. During the time that I was involved with the program I remember many occasions where the program itself made many doors open up.

Like, you know, most of the difficulty came after I left the program. The program itself made it understandable to me from the jump that I had to do something for myself, which is true, you know, as far as any program in itself is concerned. The person involved in the program has to do something for himself in order to have the program do something for him. Okay, I'll agree with that statement to some-extent—only to the extent that sometimes, you know, like even though I might want to do I can't do. Why? Because like, say, for instance, I'm really down and out—I've got a burden on my shoulders, something bothering me, you know. The program helped lift the burden off my shoulders by the discussions that we used to have and, you know, how it was. It was really helping me to get out and, you know, strive for the kind of work I wanted to do. As far as I see, most programs don't do that. . . . You just can't set up a program for jobs or something like that and expect to just leave the person, you know, helpless and defenseless after you done put him on his feet.

Summary

When Legion was seen at follow-up, he was slowly drifting into the state that would once again see him in prison. He had come partway. He had been out of prison, at that point, longer than at any time since he was 16. Even though it was difficult, he found that he could go to college and that people were interested in helping him.

This, then, is Legion. He poignantly illustrates that men can be prepared for release without a stupendous investment in time, money, and personnel. In terms of the theoretical aim of the project, he shows what can be done by concentrating on the social aspect of behavior. Legion and the many like him are difficult to work with. They do not trust easily. They are living a revolving-door life in which they come to feel that their only friends are in prison. They seldom are consistent with their facts. They handle their inner hurt and insecurity by denying that they need help and refusing to ask for it in the traditional way. Great skill is needed to work with these men. Once they trust that they have a true choice, many remember it and begin to accept service, sometimes after months have passed. Legion and his compatriots need to be approached in a way that reflects an understanding of their behavior.

Going to jail is usually the end product of a long and progressive dissociation from society. If correctional programming is to have any effect, it must include an understanding of how to help a man fit into society once he has served his time. This requires contact with the man's family and community social agencies both while he is in jail and after he is released.

DISCUSSION

This chapter was designed to illustrate the role of theory and theory development in practice. That this project was conducted 30 years ago reflects another characteristic of theory. Its propositions are timeless and considered to hold until proven otherwise. There is a continued need for socially based prerelease services. A high proportion of current prisoners have problems that indicate they will need help both while in prison and when they are released. Within 3 years of their release, more than 50% of these men are back in prison (Langan & Levin, 2002).

Prison inmates have higher rates than comparable groups in the general population of physical illness, mental illness, and learning, speech, vision, and hearing problems. They also suffer higher rates of physical injury (Hammett, Roberts, & Kennedy, 2001; Maruschak & Beck, 2001). In 1998 it was estimated that there were 283,800 incarcerated mentally ill offenders, and only 60% of these received any treatment (Ditton, 1999). Comparable figures for social, financial, and legal problems are not easily available, but it is a reasonable assumption that rates in

these areas are also higher than in the general population. If people about to be released from prison do not get the services they need, it will only add further to an already large criminal justice bill.

The increase in the prison population and men serving short terms and a decline in the use of parole have brought a renewed interest in release planning (Austin, 2001; Hagan & Coleman, 2001; La Vigne & Krachnowski, 2003; Lynch & Sabol, 2001; Petersilia, 2001; Seiter, 2002; Travis, 2000; Travis & Petersilia, 2001; Travis, Solomon, & Waul, 2001). Even though the literature often addresses developing comprehensive programs, it is just as often targeted at specific problems such as job training, education, or drug treatment (Austin, 2001; Hagan & Coleman, 2001; Lynch & Sabol, 2001). The literature tends to retain an orientation to treatment rather than viewing reentry as mainly a reality-oriented social service. There are some imaginative proposals, such as one to include victims in the reentry process (Herman & Wasserman, 2001). In Maryland one small program, the Maryland Re-Entry Partnership, in Baltimore, strives to be comprehensive. In 2001 it served 125 of the 4,411 prisoners who were released to Baltimore (La Vigne & Krachnowski, 2003). Most Maryland programs concentrate on release projects related to drug addiction (Taxman, 1998; Taxman & Cronin, 2000; Taxman, Cronin, Moline, Douglas, & Rosenmerkle, 2001; Taxman, Reedy, Klem, & Silverman, 2002; Taxman & Soule, 1999). In recognition of the need for greater attention to reentry, in 2002 the Justice Department, in collaboration with other agencies, made $100 million available for the Serious and Violent Offender Reentry Initiative.

CONCLUSION

This chapter has emphasized the role of theory in practice. It showed how theory helps guide and control practice. In turn, the data generated in this practice can be used to develop further theoretical propositions that can be tested to advance practice.

The basic strategy was to start with a practical problem, prisoner reentry. Then, using a middle-range theory of the social, this was conceptualized as paying specific attention to the offender's social characteristics and relating to the offender in terms of reality-based straight talk. The other aspects of the offender's needs were not neglected. In turn, the findings were used to help contribute to making social theory more specific for practice. Going from a practical problem to theory and then back to the problem is a procedure advocated by Hans Zetterberg (1962).

Practitioners tend to avoid presenting their work in terms of the theory they are using. Many deny they are using theory, many say they are eclectic, and many say theory interferes with their ability to relate. This only means they are using whatever explanation suits them at the moment. Zetterberg (1963) provides a succinct answer to these positions: "To ask for an explanation in science is to ask for a theory" (p. 1). Professional practice is beyond the point where it can get by only by reference to the principles of art on which practice is based. More is demanded by way of explanation from those who fund the practice (Bailey, 1980). The aim is not to achieve perfection and absolute authoritativeness but to make things better than they were before (Lindblom & Cohen, 1979). The title of Polansky's (1986) article, "There Is Nothing So Practical as a Good Theory," provides an apt summary of what this chapter is about.

The work toward integrating the social into comprehensive diagnosis and treatment needs to go on. So far, efforts to develop classifications of social problems have not proved successful (Bahn, 1971; Karls & Wandrei, 1994). This is so because the systems developed have attempted to emulate the numerical systems used in physical and psychological diagnosis. For the present, attempts to develop such systems should concentrate on middle-range theory concepts.

In like manner, there is a need to emphasize social interaction skills in professional relationships. Most people who go to social workers or other professional helpers are not asking for psychotherapy. They are asking for help with concrete social problems. The demands of insurance reimbursement have forced many agencies into classifying many social problems as psychological problems in need of treatment. This adds to the expense of the service without meeting the need that brought the person to ask for help.

Finally, there is a need for practitioners to organize their practice so that they can access data for research purposes (Epstein & Blumenfield, 2001). For those who work in settings that have institutional review boards to approve research proposals, the ability to organize service records where all data collected are necessary for the service record and no special data are collected for research purposes facilitates the research process. When the organization of the records is guided by theory, it helps make the products of such practice research scientifically acceptable.

Notes

1. I wrote the original grant and was the project director. This arrangement was used because it facilitated employing project personnel and utilizing funds for student stipends. The university had more experience in employing people on grants and disbursing student stipends.

2. In keeping with project philosophy, if a client was identified as having an emotional problem that needed treatment, the instructions were to make an immediate referral and do what was necessary to facilitate the referral.

3. Details have been altered to protect identity.

References

Austin, J. (2001). Prisoner reentry: Current trends, practices, and issues. *Crime and Delinquency, 47,* 314–335.

Bahn, A. K. (1971). A multi-disciplinary psychosocial classification scheme. *American Journal of Orthopsychiatry, 41,* 830–838.

Bailey, J. (1980). *Ideas and intervention.* London: Routledge and Kegan Paul.

Berger, P. L. (2002). Whatever happened to sociology? *First Things, 126,* 27–29.

Chaiklin, H. (1973). *Community Reintegration Project.* Baltimore: University of Maryland School of Social Work and Community Planning.

Chaiklin, H. (1978). Role and utilization of the social worker in clinical practice. In G. U. Balis, L. Wurmser, E. McDaniel, & R. G. Grenell (Eds.), *The psychiatric foundations of medicine: Psychiatric clinical skills in medical practice* (Vol. 5, pp. 475–481). Boston: Butterworth.

Ditton, P. M. (1999). *Mental health and treatment of inmates and probationers.* Washington, DC: U.S. Department of Justice.

Epstein, I., & Blumenfield, S. (Eds.). (2001). *Clinical data-mining in practice-based research: Social work in hospital settings.* New York: Haworth Social Work Practice Press.

Hagan, J., & Coleman, J. P. (2001). Returning captives of the American war on drugs: Issues of community and family reentry. *Crime and Delinquency, 47,* 352–368.

Hammett, T. M., Roberts, C., & Kennedy, S. (2001). Health-related issues in prisoner reentry. *Crime and Delinquency, 47*, 390–410.

Herman, S., & Wasserman, C. (2001). A role for victims in offender reentry. *Crime and Delinquency, 47*, 428–445.

Hollingshead, A. B., & Redlich, F. C. (1958). *Social class and mental illness: A community study.* New York: Wiley.

Karls, J. M., & Wandrei, K. E. (Eds.). (1994). *PIE manual: Person-in-environment system.* Washington, DC: National Association of Social Workers.

Langan, P. A., & Levin, D. J. (2002). *Recidivism of prisoners released in 1994.* Washington, DC: U.S. Department of Justice.

La Vigne, N., & Krachnowski, V. (2003). *A portrait of prisoner reentry in Maryland.* Washington, DC: Urban Institute Justice Policy Center.

Lindblom, C. E., & Cohen, D. K. (1979). *Usable knowledge.* New Haven, CT: Yale University Press.

Lynch, J. P., & Sabol, W. J. (2001). *Prisoner reentry in perspective.* Washington, DC: Urban Institute Justice Policy Center.

Maruschak, L. M., & Beck, A. J. (2001). *Medical problems of inmates, 1997.* Washinngton, DC: U.S. Department of Justice.

Merton, R. K. (1957). *Social theory and social structure.* Glencoe, IL: Free Press.

Mills, C. W. (1959). *The sociological imagination.* New York: Oxford University Press.

Petersilia, J. (2001). Prisoner reentry: Public safety and reintegration challenges. *Prison Journal, 81*, 360–375.

Polansky, N. A. (1986). There is nothing so practical as a good theory. *Child Welfare, 65*, 3–15.

Seiter, R. P. (2002). Prisoner reentry and the role of parole officers. *Federal Probation, 66*(3), 50–54.

Tallman, I. (2002). Aspirations and possibilities: Coming to terms with other people's reality. In S. K. Steinmetz & G. W. Peterson (Eds.), *Pioneering paths in the study of families: The lives and careers of family scholars* (pp. 215–237). New York: Haworth Press.

Taxman, F. S. (1998). *Reducing recidivism through a seamless system of care: Components of effective treatment, supervision, and transition services in the community.* College Park: University of Maryland Bureau of Governmental Research.

Taxman, F. S., & Cronin, J. (2000). *Break the cycle year 1: Process evaluation of Maryland's break the cycle: first year activities.* College Park: University of Maryland Bureau of Governmental Research.

Taxman, F. S., Cronin, J., Moline, K., Douglas, K., & Rosenmerkle, S. (2001). *Break the cycle year 2: Overview of offender and system issues in year 2 of implementation.* College Park: University of Maryland Bureau of Governmental Reasearch.

Taxman, F. S., Reedy, D. C., Klem, T., & Silverman, R. (2002). *Break the cycle year 3: Implementation.* College Park: University of Maryland Bureau of Governmental Research.

Taxman, F. S., & Soule, D. (1999). Graduated sanctions. *Prison Journal, 79*, 182–205.

Travis, J. (2000). *But they all come back.* National Institute of Justice [On-line]. Available: http://www.ncjrs.org/txtfiles1/nij/181413.txt.

Travis, J., & Petersilia, J. (2001). Reentry reconsidered: A new look at an old question. *Crime and Delinquency, 47*, 291–313.

Travis, J., Solomon, A. L., & Waul, M. (2001). *From prison to home: The dimensions and consequences of prisoner reentry.* Washington, DC: Urban Institute Justice Policy Center.

Zetterberg, H. L. (1962). *Social theory and social practice.* New York: Bedminster Press.

Zetterberg, H. L. (1963). *On theory and verification in sociology* (2nd ed.). New York: Bedminster Press.

PRINCIPLES, PRACTICES, AND FINDINGS OF THE ST. LOUIS CONUNDRUM

92

A Large-Scale Field Experiment With Antisocial Children

Ronald A. Feldman

The St. Louis Experiment represents perhaps the largest and most rigorous field experiment concerning group intervention to be found in the social work literature. The overarching objectives of this experiment were threefold. The first was to ascertain which of three group treatment methods was most effective at reducing the antisocial behavior of youths who took part in an 8-month intervention program. The second was to determine the respective impacts of two different modes of treatment group composition upon the behavior of referred and nonreferred youths who participated in the program. The third was to examine whether group workers with graduate training in social work were better able than group workers with no such training to generate changes in the behavior of the participating youths. The St. Louis Experiment also entailed a number of additional research objectives that are described in this chapter.

Funds from the National Institute of Mental Health permitted the design and implementation of an expansive field experiment that involved more than 1,000 boys ranging in age from 7 to 15 years: 324 in a 4-month pilot phase and 701 in two successive 8-month intervention and evaluation phases. Because of the study's complex experimental design and the intricate procedures needed to trace subjects' behavioral changes over time, the book that reports the study findings was titled *The St. Louis Conundrum* (Feldman, Caplinger, & Wodarski, 1983).

Reflecting the fact that the study reported decidedly positive behavioral outcomes for the subjects—an all too rare finding in the social work literature—the book was further subtitled *The Effective Treatment of Antisocial Youths*. Of special relevance for the present chapter are the overarching principles and research practices that guided the St. Louis Experiment. These evolved from the investigators' fundamental concerns about the quality of extant social work research regarding group interventions with antisocial youths.

RESEARCH DEFICITS, RESEARCH PRINCIPLES, AND RESEARCH PRACTICES

Only a few large-scale field experiments in the social work literature examine treatment interventions with antisocial youths. Even fewer investigate group-based interventions. Among the latter, virtually none employ multifactorial designs and stringent research methods like those typically found in the literatures of the social sciences and related professions. Extant publications regarding group work with antisocial youths tend to neglect many conceptual and methodological issues of importance. Yet, attention to such issues is imperative if one is to draw valid and reliable conclusions about the efficacy of group interventions and thereby generate research-based advances for group work practice. Therefore, in devising the St. Louis Experiment, we first identified key conceptual and methodological deficits in the existing research on social group work with antisocial youths and then generated corresponding research principles and practices that guided our study. These are described in the following sections.

Paucity of Field Experiments

Perhaps the foremost deficit of the extant social work literature is the marked dearth of experimental field research concerning group-based interventions. Only two content analyses of the social group work literature have been conducted in the last 15 years. Based on a review of publications in leading social work journals, Feldman (1987) found that only 10% of articles between 1975 and 1983 were based on empirical research or surveys. The vast preponderance of published articles consisted merely of descriptions of group work programs (48%) and, to a lesser extent, of restated practice principles, recommendations for expanding group work into various areas of practice, and appeals to strengthen the group work literature in one way or another. Of the empirical studies, very few employed statistical tests, control groups, baseline periods, or more than a score of subjects. Seven years later, Tolman and Molidor (1994) reviewed 54 group research studies published over a 10-year period in nine social work journals and in *Social Work Research and Abstracts*. Their analysis revealed that articles based on nonexperimental designs and quasi-experimental designs together exceeded those with experimental designs. The present author performed a more recent literature review in May 2003 by examining abstracts of 254 articles on group work research that appeared in *Social Work Abstracts* from 1977 through 2003. Fewer than a dozen publications employed a true experimental design, and none constituted a large-scale multifactorial field experiment. The sorry state of group work research and the corresponding need to strengthen the knowledge base of social group work practice motivated the author and colleagues to conduct the St. Louis Experiment. Our principal aim was to design and implement a *large-scale multifactorial field experiment with substantial numbers of subjects, a wide range of experimental variables and comparisons, and state-of-the-art data analysis techniques*.

Dysfunctional Treatment Group Composition

A major barrier to effective group work with antisocial youths is the fact that nearly all treatment programs tend to cluster groups of referred youths together for intervention purposes. Yet a persuasive literature demonstrates that this mode of group composition poses significant barriers to effective treatment. Among them are selective reinforcement of deviant behavior by the antisocial members of the "treatment" group, modeling of antisocial behavior by one's antisocial peers, affective ties formed among the antisocial peers, and stigmatization due to one's association with antisocial peers (for a more detailed discussion, see Feldman et al., 1983, pp. 16–36). Therefore, in a major departure from the typical group work paradigm, the St. Louis Experiment sought to *treat selected antisocial youths in small groups consisting of prosocial peers*. To accomplish this, we studied 60 activity groups at a community center. In 22 of these groups, one or two boys who had been referred to our program due to antisocial behavior were incorporated into an activity group where *none* of the other members were known to have engaged in significant antisocial behavior.

Dearth of Comparison Groups

Only a handful of group intervention studies build comparison groups into their research design. Because the St. Louis Experiment primarily studied treatment interventions in "mixed" groups consisting of prosocial youths and one or two antisocial peers, it was deemed necessary to investigate the effects of like interventions in comparison groups populated entirely by putatively antisocial youths who had been referred to our program. Accordingly, two main categories of subjects were studied in the St. Louis Experiment: antisocial youths in mixed groups (i.e., groups where all but one or two referred members were prosocial youths) and antisocial youths in referred groups (i.e., groups where all the members had been referred because of antisocial behavior). The latter mode of treatment group composition is the norm in mental health programs. Importantly, however, because we had introduced antisocial boys into "mixed" groups of prosocial peers, it also was essential to examine behavioral outcomes for the prosocial, or nonreferred, members of these groups. Was it possible, for instance, that they would become antisocial as a result of prolonged exposure to one or two antisocial peers? Would the "bad apples" in the group spoil the good ones? Therefore, comparison groups consisting solely of prosocial, or nonreferred, boys also were formed in the St. Louis Experiment. As a result, two additional categories of subjects were studied: prosocial, or nonreferred, boys treated in mixed groups; and prosocial boys treated in groups consisting solely of prosocial peers. Altogether, then, for purposes of comparison, *four categories of youths were studied* in the course of the St. Louis Experiment. In concert with other independent variables described here, this yielded the multifactorial research design depicted in Table 92.1.

Few Comparisons of Treatment Methods

Most group intervention studies examine merely a single treatment modality. However, the effects of that modality seldom are contrasted with those for an alternative method of group treatment or, especially, with comparison groups that receive minimal or no treatment. Therefore, the St. Louis Experiment sought to examine the effects of traditional group work by contrasting them with the outcomes for a second treatment method, namely, behavioral group work. Moreover, the findings for youths treated by traditional group work and behavioral group work were contrasted with those for youths placed in comparison groups that received minimal or no treatment. (Detailed descriptions of these three group modalities are reported elsewhere; see Feldman & Wodarski, 1975.) Hence, the St. Louis Experiment employed a *research design that compared the findings for two group treatment methods and, in turn, contrasted them with the outcomes for minimal-treatment groups.*

Paucity of Comparisons Among Differing Treatment Agents

Very few studies compare the treatment outcomes generated by trained social workers with those produced by other intervention agents. This is regrettable insofar as many comparison studies suggest that untrained intervention agents fare as well as or better than trained mental health professionals. This may be attributable to substandard professional education, but it is equally or more likely that the failure to employ rigorous research methods hinders investigators'

TABLE 92.1 Research Design Implemented for the St. Louis Experiment by Leader Training, Treatment Method, and Mode of Group Composition (total n = 701 subjects and 60 groups)

Group Composition	Experienced Leaders			Inexperienced Leaders			Total
	Behavioral Method	Traditional Method	Minimal Method	Behavioral Method	Traditional Method	Minimal Method	
Referred	Ss = 61	Ss = 41	Ss = 37	Ss = 34	Ss = 25	Ss = 39	Ss = 237
	Gs = 6	Gs = 4	Gs = 4	Gs = 4	Gs = 3	Gs = 4	Gs = 25
Mixed	Ss = 55	Ss = 50	Ss = 44	Ss = 30	Ss = 61	Ss = 50	Ss = 290
	Gs = 4	Gs = 4	Gs = 3	Gs = 4	Gs = 4	Gs = 3	Gs = 22
	(5)	(5)	(4)	(4)	(4)	(4)	(26)
Nonreferred	Ss = 38	Ss = 22	Ss = 14	Ss = 40	Ss = 30	Ss = 30	Ss = 174
	Gs = 3	Gs = 2	Gs = 2	Gs = 2	Gs = 2	Gs = 2	Gs = 13
Total	Ss = 154	Ss = 113	Ss = 95	Ss = 104	Ss = 116	Ss = 119	Ss = 701
	Gs = 13	Gs = 10	Gs = 9	Gs = 10	Gs = 9	Gs = 9	Gs = 60

Ss= Number of subjects per cell; Gs = number of groups per cell; () = number of referred subjects assigned to each group category.

efforts to unearth real differences between the treatment efficacy of trained social workers and intervention agents who lack social work education. Therefore, the St. Louis Experiment *examined the differential treatment effectiveness of two types of group intervention agents:* social work students who were in their second year of graduate education and intervention agents who had no graduate training in social work or any other mental health profession. Consequently, as seen in Table 92.1, the St. Louis Experiment employed a 3 × 3 × 2 factorial design where three major sets of variables were studied: mode of group composition (referred groups vs. non-referred groups vs. mixed, or integrated, groups); group treatment method (behavioral group work method vs. traditional group work method vs. minimal group method); and extent of group leader's experience with social work education (experienced vs. inexperienced).

Infrequent Use of Random Assignment Procedures

A major deficit of the social work literature inheres in the fact that relatively few studies assign subjects and experimental conditions on a random basis. This is especially the case in group work research. Therefore, the St. Louis Experiment *employed random assignment procedures for all major components of the research.* After stratification by age, all referred subjects were assigned randomly to a treatment method and to either a mixed group or a referred group. Likewise, each group worker's treatment method (behavioral, traditional, or minimal) and mode of group composition (referred, nonreferred, or mixed) was assigned on a random basis.

Deficient Implementation of the Treatment Variable

When treatment studies fail to report positive outcomes, it is nearly always concluded that the intervention was not effective. In fact, however, many such studies report negative findings merely because the treatment interventions never were implemented faithfully. Often treatment programs are not implemented properly or fully because of inadequate funding, poor supervision, or critical deficiencies that are wholly independent of the treatment method's particular merits. It is virtually impossible to determine

what accounts for the failure of an intervention method unless the research can ascertain to what extent, if at all, the prescribed interventions actually were implemented with integrity. If the expected intervention was not implemented properly, it hardly can be concluded that its effects were evaluated adequately. To address this concern, at periodic intervals throughout the research program trained nonparticipant observers completed a checklist that enabled them to indicate which one of the three group treatment methods was actually being implemented by the group worker. Importantly, the observers never were informed about the particular objectives of the research program. Nor were they told that differing treatment methods had been assigned to the various groups participating in the study. This practice permitted *assessment of the extent to which the key independent variables (i.e., each group treatment method) actually were implemented.*

Undue Emphasis on Dichotomous Behavioral Measures

Most research on antisocial youths categorizes their behaviors dichotomously. Examples include such common designations as "delinquent" versus "nondelinquent" and "oppositional" versus "nonoppositional." This trend is linked integrally with the predominance of *DSM* nosological systems for the diagnosis and categorization of behavior disorders (see, e.g., Dziegielewski, 2002). Such a system inevitably relegates one's diagnostic status to a dichotomous nominal-order category in which the individual either "does" or "does not" exhibit a given behavior disorder such as "conduct disorder," "affective disorder," or "schizophrenia." Yet it clearly is the case that an individual seldom manifests a particular type of behavior disorder consistently and invariably. A youth's delinquent behavior represents but a mere fraction of his or her overall behavior pattern. Very few individuals are unambiguously and always "delinquent" or "nondelinquent." Nearly all youths engage in some form of delinquent activity at one time or another, and virtually no youths engage in delinquent activity all of the time. Likewise, it cannot properly be said that any particular youth's behavior is entirely antisocial or, for that matter, entirely prosocial. Dichotomous behavioral measures are inadequate for representing an individual's actual behavior profile.

As a result, they often yield misleading information about changes in a youth's behavior over the course of treatment. This is especially so when a given target behavior occurs at a very low base rate, as in the case of serious assault or homicide.

Therefore, rather than employ dichotomous measures of subjects' behavior, the St. Louis Experiment introduced *interval measures that examine the subjects' proportionate behavioral profiles*. Most research on antisocial youths focuses exclusively on deviant behavior and therefore neglects to examine as well their conventional or prosocial behavior. To avert this bias *three* types of behavior were studied concurrently in the St. Louis Experiment. *Prosocial behavior* was defined operationally as any action by a group member that was directed toward completion of a peer group's tasks or activities. *Antisocial behavior* was defined as any action that disrupts, hurts, or annoys other members, or that otherwise prevents them from participating in the group's tasks or activities. *Nonsocial behavior* was defined as any action that is not directed toward completion of a group's tasks or activities but does not interfere with another youth's participation in them. By studying all three of these behaviors, it was possible to analyze each subject's overall behavior pattern and to calculate his proportionate behavioral profile at any particular juncture of the research program.

Failure to Employ Nonparticipant Observers

In field research the least biased reports concerning subjects' behavior are likely to come from highly trained nonparticipant observers. Yet most social work research evaluates subjects' behavior change by means of data acquired from the two parties who are least likely to provide unbiased reports, namely, the subjects themselves and the intervention agents charged with delivering treatment. This is a significant deficit of the research literature in social work. To address it, the St. Louis Experiment trained nonparticipant observers to employ a 10-second summated partition sampling system that classified each subject's actual behavior into one of the three previously described categories, that is, prosocial, antisocial, or nonsocial. Behavioral observations were made throughout each group meeting and in a fixed order every 10 seconds

for one of the subjects, then for another, and so on until all the youths had been observed. This procedure was repeated for the full duration of each group session. In each instance, the first behavioral act that was observed for the target youth during the requisite 10-second period was rated as either prosocial, nonsocial, or antisocial by marking a box labeled, respectively, as either "P," "N," or "A." All observations for each subject were tabulated after each group meeting. Consequently, it was possible to *determine the proportion of each youth's behavior profile that was either prosocial, nonsocial, or antisocial* during a given group meeting and throughout the entire course of the treatment program.

Deficient Efforts to Maximize Observer Reliability

Even in studies where nonparticipant observers are employed, efforts to maximize their accuracy and reliability are limited. Accordingly, to minimize potential expectation biases in the St. Louis Experiment, nonparticipant observers never were informed about the hypothesized changes for any experimental condition or any given subject. Likewise, to enhance the probability of consistent agreement among observers, they took part in training and biweekly testing with videotapes throughout the program. Each training session was completed when all observers could agree reliably on behavioral coding with their colleagues and an expert judge at a level of .90 or above. Hence, an integral practice employed throughout the St. Louis Experiment was implementation of a *nonparticipant observation system that entailed regular and ongoing checks for accuracy and reliability*.

Failure to Employ Baseline Periods

There are few examples of baseline periods in group work research. Yet, to properly assess the longitudinal effects of treatment, it is essential to establish an adequate baseline period during which there are few, if any, efforts by group workers to effectuate treatment. Consistent with this principle, no group worker in the St. Louis Experiment was trained in any treatment method until an 8-week baseline period had been concluded. During the baseline period, and throughout the remainder of the program, the nonparticipant observers recorded data regarding the subjects' behavior as described earlier. Hence, a key feature of the St. Louis Experiment entailed *implementation of an extensive baseline period during which group workers were not able to implement any given treatment method.*

Dearth of Multiple Time Series Data Analyses

In group work research where subjects' behavior is measured more than a single time, pretest and post-test measures typically are employed. Although this permits summative conclusions regarding the ultimate outcomes of a treatment program, it does not enable researchers to evaluate varying changes in the subjects' behavior as they occur over time. Correspondingly, it is not possible to gain an informed understanding of the varying dynamics of individual and group change as treatment progresses. Therefore, to facilitate longitudinal analysis of subjects' behavior change in the St. Louis Experiment, we *employed multiple time series data analyses.* Four successive time periods were examined. The first, or pretest, period lasted for approximately 8 weeks. It constituted a baseline period during which, as noted, no treatment efforts were attempted. Thereafter, the treatment program was divided into three successive time periods (respectively, T1, T2, and T3), each lasting approximately 8 weeks. Proportionate behavioral profiles for each group member were calculated for each of the above periods merely by averaging the relevant figures for the total number of group meetings observed within that period. This procedure enabled the research team to acquire continuous records of the respective proportions of prosocial, nonsocial, and antisocial behavior exhibited by each youth and, as described later, to do so for each activity group that took part in the study. Even more, it enabled us to conduct survivor analyses and end point analyses. These yielded informative findings about the differing behavior profiles of youths who either continued in treatment through completion of the program or, instead, dropped out prior to its conclusion.

Failure to Acquire Group-Level Data

Perhaps the most paradoxical deficit of the group work literature is the fact that very few studies provide data about the behavioral characteristics of treatment groups themselves. Yet it is virtually impossible to advance the knowledge base of social group work without measuring and learning about differences that emerge over time *within* treatment groups. Therefore, besides measuring behavior change on the part of individual youths, the St. Louis Experiment also *measured attributes of the activity groups* in which subjects participated. For instance, by averaging the reported figures for individuals' prosocial, nonsocial, and antisocial behavior (see earlier discussion), it was possible to generate estimates of the proportionate extent to which each activity group exhibited these behaviors either at a given meeting or over the course of time. Likewise, as described later, it was possible to determine the extent of each activity group's normative integration, functional integration, and interpersonal integration at any point in time. In concert with multiple time series data analyses and cross-lag analyses, these measures also enabled the research team to *longitudinally examine the internal dynamics of the various treatment groups as they evolved* over time. This capability enabled the St. Louis Experiment to substantially address one of the most perplexing deficits in the literature of social group work.

Limited Use of Multiple Measures and Multiple Judges

Typically, social work research employs merely one or two measures to evaluate subjects' behavior. Moreover, the requisite data tend to be collected from merely a single set of respondents such as the subjects themselves or their intervention agents. To enhance the reliability and utility of research findings from the St. Louis Experiment, it was deemed advisable to employ multiple assessment measures and to acquire data from multiple sources. Accordingly, many different measures were utilized to gather data about the subjects' behavior.

• Behavior Checklist for Professional Workers. Referral agents for the St. Louis Experiment were asked to respond to each of 13 checklist questions by estimating the average number of times that a youth exhibited specific types of prosocial, nonsocial, or antisocial behavior during a 1-week period. These data enabled us to determine whether a referred youth met our entrance criterion (namely, 21 antisocial acts per week) for enrollment in the research.

- Behavior Checklist for Parents. This instrument was similar to the one completed by referral agents.
- Behavior Checklist for Group Workers. This instrument was similar to the one completed by referral agents and the subjects' parents.
- Behavior Checklist for Youths. This instrument was similar to the one completed by referral agents, the subjects' parents, and group workers.
- Observational Data. As described earlier, throughout the St. Louis Experiment proportionate measures of the subjects' prosocial, nonsocial, and antisocial behavior in activity groups were derived from data collected by trained nonparticipant observers.
- Jesness Inventory, Manifest Aggression Subscale. This is a standardized measure that examines self-reported aggressive behavior on the part of youths (Jesness, Derisi, McCormick, & Wedge, 1972).
- Normative Integration. The research team also measured each individual youth's normative integration into his activity group. This construct refers to the extent to which a youth adheres to basic norms shared by the peer group. Analogously, we measured the normative integration of each activity group, that is, the degree of consensus among members concerning group-relevant behaviors. Group workers and nonparticipant observers were asked to fill out pretest and post-test forms designed to assess the extent to which each group member adhered to the basic behavioral norms of the group. Specifically, respondents were asked to indicate how frequently each member adheres to the norms that most of the other members seem to follow. Possible response categories were 0%, 25%, 50%, 75%, and 100% of the time. Based on these responses, a subject's mean normative integration score could range from 1.0 to 5.0, with a higher score representing a greater degree of normative integration. Likewise, to determine the extent of normative integration for a particular activity group, a mean score was calculated for all of the group's members.
- Interpersonal Integration. Interpersonal integration refers to that mode of social integration which is based on the extent of reciprocal liking among the members of a group. Accordingly, a youth's interpersonal integration into his activity group reflects the extent to which he likes others in the group and is liked by them. This construct was operationalized by creating a grid with the name of each group member on both axes and then asking the group workers and nonparticipant observers to indicate how much each person listed along one axis likes each person listed along the other axis. A 5-point scale was utilized, with response categories ranging from "likes very much" to "dislikes very much." The mean interpersonal integration score for any group member could vary from a low of 1.0 to a high of 5.0. Likewise, an interpersonal integration score for the group could be calculated by averaging the scores for all of the group's members.
- Functional Integration. An individual's functional integration into a peer group refers to the extent to which he contributes effectively toward key group goals pertaining to goal attainment, pattern maintenance, and external relations. An activity group's functional integration refers to the extent to which group members effectively perform these three functions and, also, the extent to which responsibility for their performance is distributed among the members in an equitable and complementary fashion. To operationalize this construct, a complex coding procedure was devised (see Feldman et al., 1983, pp. 87–88). Using this procedure, it was possible not only to estimate the extent to which individual members contribute functionally to their activity group but also to gauge the extent to which the group is functionally integrated at various stages of the treatment process.
- Social Power. To measure the pretest and post-test social power of each youth, group workers and nonparticpant observers were asked to respond to a single question: "How effective is he [the youth] at getting other members in the group to do what he wants?" A 5-point scale, ranging from "very ineffective" to "very effective," was used. A higher score indicates greater social power.

Clearly, then, the St. Louis Experiment *employed multiple measures* to assess the behaviors and statuses of each boy who took part in the program. Moreover, *data were acquired from multiple respondents*, including referral agents, parents, group workers, nonparticipant observers, and the youths themselves. This enabled the research team to evaluate the subjects' behavior in varying social contexts and to compare similarities and differences among the respondents' ratings over time. The schedule for administration of these research instruments is depicted in Table 92.2.

Rudimentary Data Analysis Methods

The data analysis methods employed in much of the group work literature are simplistic and inadequate to the tasks at hand. In contrast, the intricacies of the St. Louis Experiment required the *application of elaborate univariate and multivariate data analysis procedures*. For example, we employed arcsine transformations of all proportionate behavioral scores for subjects to meet customary requirements for the statistical analysis of percentage and proportionate data. Besides conventional univariate analyses, multivariate analyses of the data were performed by means of composite measures that distinguished between the referred and nonreferred samples. Typically, these combined information from each of the five basic self-report instruments employed during the research (mean manifest aggression scores, absolute frequencies of antisocial behavior, and proportionate mean inci-

dences of antisocial, nonsocial, and prosocial behavior). Differences between the two samples were ascertained by means of standardized discriminant analyses. By averaging the discriminant scores for all cases within a particular group, it was then possible to derive group centroids, or statistical means, for the multiple measures defining a discriminant function and to succinctly depict complex multivariate findings in graphic fashion.

By employing analyses of covariance to assess pretest-post-test behavior changes among the subjects, we were able to avoid certain analytic problems associated with classical experimental designs. Pretest data were employed as the concomitant variable in the analysis of covariance to partial out that portion of variance in the subjects' scores that can be predicted from pretest scores. Moreover, reliability-corrected analyses of covariance were employed to adjust for differences in the subjects' pretest behavioral profiles and to subsequently determine pretest-post-test behavioral gains on their part.

In sum, then, the St. Louis Experiment employed numerous methodological advances. These include a multifactorial design; randomized assignment of group workers, subjects, and treatment methods; comparison groups for the main independent variables; a no-intervention baseline period; trained nonparticipant observers who were tested for reliability on a biweekly ba-

TABLE 92.2 Schedule for Administration of Research Instruments, by Respondents and Time Period

	Respondents				
Time Period	Referral Agents	Parents	Group Leaders	Children	Observers
Intake	1	1			
Baseline*			1,3,4,5,6	1,2	3,4,5,6,7,8
T1					7,8
T2					7,8
T3	1	1	1,3,4,5,6	1,2	3,4,5,6,7,8
Follow-up**	1	1			

Research instruments: 1, behavioral inventory; 2, Jesness inventory, manifest aggression subscale; 3, normative integration index, individual and group; 4, interpersonal integration index, individual and group; 5, functional integration index, individual and group; 6, social power index, individual and group; 7, behavioral ratings; 8, report of treatment method.

* Approximately 8 weeks after first group session; thereafter, approximately 8 weeks transpired between successive treatment periods.

** Approximately 1 year following termination of treatment.

sis; a multiple time series research design; measures that account for subjects' prosocial and nonsocial behavior, as well as their antisocial behavior and, further, that report each subject's proportionate behavioral profile; multiple independent judges, including referral agents, group workers, parents, nonparticipant observers, and the participating youths themselves; measures of the extent to which the treatment variable actually was implemented; a blind intake criterion applied by two sets of independent judges; a standard measure of manifest aggression; arcsine transformations of proportionate data; reliability-corrected analyses of covariance that adjust for differences in the subjects' pretest behavioral profiles; multiple discriminant analyses; and, end point, dropout, and survivor analyses. Although the research design could not guard against all possible threats, it did permit numerous conclusions to be drawn from the data with considerably greater assurance than usually is the case for field studies of group work with antisocial youths.

SELECTED RESEARCH FINDINGS OF THE ST. LOUIS EXPERIMENT

The research practices employed during the St. Louis Experiment permitted the examination of interrelationships among a wide range of variables. Because highly detailed reports appear elsewhere (Feldman et al., 1983; Feldman, 1992), only selected research findings are summarized here.

Effects of Social Work Education

A central research finding for social work pertains to the clear superiority of experienced group workers (i.e., intervention agents who had graduate social work training) vis-à-vis inexperienced group workers. End point data acquired by the nonparticipant observers revealed that boys who were treated by experienced workers benefited considerably more from the program than did boys who were treated by inexperienced workers. The former exhibited marked reductions in proportionate antisocial ($M = -3.1\%$, $p < .001$) and nonsocial ($M = -1.9\%$), $p < .001$) behavior. By the end of treatment, 96.7% of these boys' observed behavior was prosocial. This represents a substantial upturn in prosocial

behavior ($M = +5.0\%$, $p < .001$) from their mean pretreatment incidence. At the end of treatment, merely 2.4% of their behavior was antisocial. By contrast, about 6.9% of the behavior of boys with inexperienced group workers was antisocial at end point. This is nearly three times the incidence for boys with experienced workers. Equally important, 83.2% of the latter boys exhibited prosocial gains during the program, whereas only 54.7% of the former did. Further, longitudinal analyses demonstrate that the experienced workers were able to bring about more rapid declines in the boys' antisocial behavior (that is, during the T1 period) and to sustain them over time. In comparison, boys who were treated by inexperienced group workers displayed negative behavioral outcomes, especially if they quit the program prior to its scheduled conclusion.

Effects of Treatment Method

In contrast with the findings for group workers' educational experience, the particular method of group treatment employed had little or no impact on the subjects' behavior. The behavioral method promoted significantly better outcomes than traditional group work ($p < .001$) but it fared no better than the minimal-treatment method ($p < .79$). Overall, experienced group workers achieved positive outcomes regardless of which treatment method they applied, whereas inexperienced workers had relatively negative outcomes, especially when they tried to implement traditional group work.

Effects of Group Composition

Findings about the effects of treatment group composition were, in general, in the expected direction. Thus, whereas the observed antisocial behavior of referred boys in unmixed groups actually increased somewhat over time, antisocial behavior declined significantly among their referred peers in mixed groups. At end point, 5.7% of the observed behavior for the former boys was antisocial, and barely half of them (50.9%) displayed any discernible decline in antisocial behavior. By contrast, only 3.2% of the end point behavior of the latter boys was antisocial, and 91.3% of them had achieved a decline in antisocial behavior! In fact, by end point the behavior patterns of the referred boys in mixed groups differed very little from those of the nonreferred members in their groups. Furthermore, no significant differences were found between the end point behavioral profiles of the nonreferred boys in mixed groups and the nonreferred boys in unmixed groups. Hence, it appears that the behavior of the former boys was not affected adversely by sustained group interaction with one or two antisocial youths.

The treatment potential of mixed groups is demonstrated further by the fact that referred boys in these groups achieved noteworthy gains in prosocial behavior even when they were led by inexperienced workers. Although they did not benefit as much as referred boys in mixed groups led by experienced workers, they nonetheless improved markedly. Hence, the therapeutic strengths of mixed groups evidently compensate in large part for the deficits of inexperienced workers. The validity of this supposition is further supported by the finding that referred youths fared especially poorly when treated in unmixed groups led by inexperienced workers. At end point, 9.1% of their behavior was antisocial; this represents a significant increase in antisocial behavior from baseline ($M = +3.6\%$, $p < .01$). Hence, the combined salutary impact of social work education and mixed treatment groups surpasses the separate treatment benefits of either variable alone.

CONCLUSION

Additional findings of the St. Louis Experiment demonstrate how the behavior of subjects tends to change over the course of treatment, how this alters the nature of their treatment group's "behavioral composition," and, in turn, how the latter enhances the group's potency as a change agent. Related findings show how various modes of group integration change over time and how continuance or discontinuance of subjects can have unanticipated positive and negative effects on their outcomes. Although only selected findings of the St. Louis Experiment are reported here, they demonstrate clearly how rigorous multifaceted field experiments can greatly facilitate the analysis of client behavior change and the advancement of social work practice.

ACKNOWLEDGMENT The research on which this chapter is based was funded by the Center for Studies of Crime and Delinquency, National Institute of Mental Health (Grant No. MH18813). The writer is especially grateful to John S. Wodarski and Timothy E. Caplinger, with whom he coauthored *The St. Louis Conundrum: The Effective Treatment of Antisocial Youths* (Englewood Cliffs, NJ: Prentice-Hall, 1983).

References

Dziegielewski, S. F. (2002). *DSM-IV-TR in action.* New York: Wiley.

Feldman, R. A. (1987). "Group work knowledge and research: A two-decade comparison. In S. D. Rose & R. A. Feldman (Eds.), *Research in social group work* (pp. 7–14). New York: Haworth Press.

Feldman, R. A. (1992). The St. Louis Experiment: Effective treatment of antisocial youths in prosocial peer groups. In J. McCord & R. E. Tremblay (Eds.), *Preventing antisocial behavior: Interventions from birth through adolescence* (pp. 233–252). New York: Guilford Press.

Feldman, R. A., Caplinger, T. E., & Wodarski, J. S. (1983). *The St. Louis conundrum: The effective treatment of antisocial youths.* Englewood Cliffs, NJ: Prentice-Hall.

Feldman, R. A., & Wodarski, J. S. (1975). *Contemporary approaches to group treatment.* San Francisco: Jossey-Bass.

Jesness, C. F., Derisi, W. J., McCormick, P., & Wedge, R. F. (1972). *The Youth Center Research Project.* Sacramento, CA: California Youth Authority.

Tolman, R. M., & Molidor, C. E. (1994). A decade of social group work research: Trends in methodology, theory, and program development. *Research on Social Work Practice, 4,* 142–159.

93

MEASURING POLICE AND CITIZEN PERCEPTIONS OF POLICE POWER IN NEWARK, NEW JERSEY

Gina Robertiello

In the 40 or so years of research on police behavior, serious questions have been raised about the "public relations" problems police have had when confronting the general public. This research has allowed police to come to appreciate how some of their everyday routines are in need of revision. Research of the past 15 years, for example, demonstrates that random patrol has a limited effect on crime, and that the general public is a critical dimension in the reporting and detecting of criminal behavior. In the wake of these more recent investigations into the impact of police work on public safety, the idea is that a "partnership" needs to be forged between the public and police if more effective and fruitful relationships are to grow.

For this particular research project, I was interested in examining whether citizens were cooperative, understanding, and supportive of police and had perceptions similar to those of police. My assumption was that although contextual and demographic variables may be expected to influence the outcome of an encounter, police and citizens felt similarly regarding the impact of these factors. In addition, my hypothesis was that citizens would be supportive of particular police action due to efforts to improve police-community relations. Based on research examining the relationship between police and the public, findings suggest the two groups have begun to demonstrate high levels of cooperation during encounters. For example, civilian-police academies are gaining momentum, which shows a willingness on the part of citizens and police to get to know each other. Police-sponsored programs such as DARE and COP have also helped

present police as a much more reasonable, accessible, and trusted dimension of the community. Further, there is an understanding by administrators that police-citizen relationships are critical to effective police work. Thus, police work does seem to be forging a closer relationship with the public, and we should expect that the police will receive a greater sense of trust from the public. Consequently, I theorized that these efforts would lead to a convergence in beliefs on the part of police and citizens.

I attempted to measure and compare perceptions and attitudes about police power via the utilization of a survey instrument administered to police officers and citizens in the city of Newark, New Jersey. This area was chosen because Newark, a densely populated city that has a racially and ethically diverse population and a high crime rate, has experienced numerous altercations between police and the public. It is also unique in that it has demonstrated innovation in experimentation despite its problems.

Survey research was used in this study; this method is good for descriptive, explanatory, and exploratory research purposes. Standardized techniques were implemented through the application of a questionnaire, which I developed in consultation with numerous sources.

IDENTIFYING AND OVERCOMING PROBLEMS AND OBSTACLES TO MEASURING OUTCOMES

Unfortunately, Newark (at the time of survey administration) was infamous for its rating as the most dangerous city in the United States (Morgan, Morgan, & Quitno, 1997). Thus, my advisory committee—concerned for my physical safety—asked that the surveys not be administered door-to-door but in a public place. As a result, I administered the surveys at various locations on the streets of Newark. To obtain the citizen sample, I used the Yahoo Yellow Pages on the Internet and printed out a list of all delis, hardware stores, and grocery stores in Newark (including their addresses). Then I used the resources at the Newark Public Library to obtain a map of the city and the published 1990 census data (the most recent census information at the time) to identify the tracts that Newark was divided into. Tracts are small areas, usually with a population of 3,000 to 6,000 people, into which certain large cities have been subdivided for statistical and local administrative purposes. Using this census information, I examined each of Newark's four wards and each tract within the wards. After examining over 98 tracts for demographic characteristics, I attempted to choose one predominantly "White," "Hispanic," and "Black" area in each ward. Once I found a tract with the acceptable characteristics, I referred to the list of stores to determine which were located in the tract selected. The surveys were administered by asking patrons of the store to complete the questionnaire either before or after they completed their shopping. Some were administered to individuals walking in the vicinity of the store.

Based on the demographic characteristics of each tract, I found that there were predominantly Black areas in all wards (and most tracts) in Newark. Whites and Hispanics constituted the majority of the population in only a few tracts. There were no tracts in the West or South districts where Whites represented the majority of the population. However, I did find predominantly White areas in the North and East districts. Unfortunately, even in the areas labeled "Hispanic" and "White," the majority of the persons who shopped, worked, and/or lived in the area and filled out the survey did not always fit the expected characteristics for that particular area. There were more Blacks in all the tracts regardless of the census information. A validity threat to the census information is that the data were dated (census data are updated every 10 years), and so the racial and ethnic makeup of the tracts may have changed over time. In ad-

dition, with administration conducted in this fashion, there was no guarantee of obtaining a representative sample. Regardless of these potential problems, I administered the surveys in person in each of the chosen tracts and obtained a sample of Newark residents and workers. This method was useful because my safety was preserved. I also obtained access to most of the residents in the area and ended up with a diverse population to analyze.

The use of surveys provided the best method for collecting the original data and describing a population that was too large to observe directly, while still providing me with a cover of safety. It was easier for persons to discuss the sensitive topic of racial attitudes in a survey as opposed to face-to-face interviews. Although the census data were a bit dated, this method allowed me to conduct my research on the streets of Newark as planned. To avoid some of the obstacles that can arise during administration in this fashion, it is suggested that the researcher construct clear questions in consultation with experts in the field of criminal justice, such as police officers and professionals who conduct research on this topic regularly. In addition, the researcher should obtain the most recent demographic data on the population to be studied, even if it means delaying the administration for a while.

Obtaining honest responses often becomes a problem, especially if perceptions of the police, by citizens, are negative. Thus, some threats to validity may have developed during the course of this investigation. Unfortunately, some citizens may be unwilling to report how they believe police will behave because they are embarrassed by their lack of knowledge of the law or their stand on crime. They may also fear reporting their own prejudgments against police or persons of a certain racial or ethnic background. Thus, a researcher must attempt to design surveys that appear as innocuous as possible. In addition, it is important to assure respondents that none of the responses will be used against them and that there are no wrong answers to the survey questions.

While administering to the citizen sample, I ran into a few problems in each tract. There were many refusals to complete the survey fully simply because of its length. However, some people felt obligated to fill out the survey and had a hard time saying no when asked. Based on the comments I received, I realized the survey should have been shorter. I would have had an easier time getting responses if I asked fewer questions.

In general, once persons realized the survey was about perceptions and opinions of police, they wanted to fill it out. Most respondents completed the survey after they finished shopping. Some were concerned they would somehow get into trouble or feared being classified as racist. It was also difficult to obtain responses from a Black area with a White person administering the surveys. Some citizens walked right past the table before they could even be asked to fill out the survey. In addition, some respondents only spoke Spanish. Thus, I ran into trouble regarding response rate, honesty, and consent.

In the Hispanic area in particular, a concern was the language barrier. To counteract this problem, the Hispanic student assisting me translated two of the surveys for a Hispanic couple, demonstrating a frisk rather than explaining it. For future studies, I would suggest preparing a translated version of a survey if the researcher knows there will be Spanish-speaking respondents in the sample.

As for the honesty issue, most citizen respondents did not even read the consent form as they signed it, and they asked no questions. However, the police officer respondents were very concerned about being identified, and some refused to sign the consent form. Unfortunately, I needed to obtain consent from respondents because this research was originally conducted as part of my doctoral dissertation, and my committee members at Rutgers University wanted verification of my work, and the institutional review board (IRB) required informed consent. To meet these requirements, I had the respondents sign the consent form and then separated the front page from the rest of the survey in front of them so they realized they could not be identified. I hoped this would ease their minds and improve the likelihood of honest responses.

Another problem was related to safety. There was a significant amount of drug activity in some of the tracts, even during the survey administration. In one particularly "hot" drug area, a mother was selling drugs with her child in plain view on the street. Some dealers even wanted to fill out the survey; they demonstrated a strong hate for the police. Amusingly, the Newark police stopped by and asked what I was

doing because I stood out as the only white person in a minority area.

The weather was cold at the time of administration of some of the surveys, and some respondents asked to take their surveys home to fill out and requested that they be picked up later in the day at their homes. Because I had to leave this tract by 3:00 p.m. due to safety concerns, I agreed. I was not expecting to get these surveys back, but some were obtained. For future studies on similar populations, I would suggest daytime administration in warm weather, as well as administration in an area that is familiar to the researcher; this would allow the researcher to fit in more easily, thus protecting his or her safety and increasing the response rate. I realized that the Saturday administration was successful because more people were available and willing to fill out the surveys. In addition, as the surveys are being filled out, the respondents should be monitored to ensure that they understand the format and do not leave questions blank. I used this technique, which helped to alleviate the problem of incomplete surveys.

The police officer sample was not as problematic to obtain, although it did introduce different challenges. Because I had established rapport with the Newark police department and had been granted permission from the chief (who sent out a memo to all bureau commanders asking for full cooperation), a high response rate was obtained. In addition, the police officer surveys were administered at roll calls, allowing many to be completed at once. I was also able to establish the best time to administer surveys. For example, doing so on weekday mornings increased the response rate because more officers were present at that time.

However, studies of police may demonstrate a reluctance to divulge officers' own perceptions of what they will do in certain situations. Another problem involves the likelihood of a Hawthorne effect, or reactivity, where respondents may feel the need to respond in the "correct" manner to specific questions. This may be demonstrated through responses that are "by the book" and always legal. Officers may be afraid to answer sincerely because they believe that their behaviors may be illegal or discriminatory. I tried to compensate for this problem by using a self-administered questionnaire and consent forms that were separated from the surveys in front of each officer (to demonstrate anonymity). In addition, I had the assistance of a few "gatekeepers" who vouched for my presence. I also hand-delivered the surveys, met with officers before and after the administration, made eye contact with the officers, and in general maintained a friendly rapport with the Newark police department. I found refusal rates to be much lower when I politely asked officers to fill out the surveys. Based on the study results, this technique was successful; many officers were willing to admit that they expected to intrude differently based on specific demographic and situational characteristics.

Consequently, the survey was self-administered, allowing *police* to establish their perceptions of behavior anonymously. I found that a self-administered survey was more likely to enhance confidentiality because no interviewer is present. The method also allowed *citizens* to be completely candid when describing their perceptions of police power without fear of repercussions. If their perceptions were negative, the use of the anonymous survey allowed uncomfortable questions to be posed while leading to the collection of trustworthy responses. In fact, Kavanaugh (1994) found that officers were willing to admit to illegal acts if data were gathered in a noninvasive manner. Further, most people enjoy talking about themselves and their feelings and behavior, especially if they feel they can "change the world" by being frank.

In all districts, supervising officers helped out immensely by vouching for me. Most surveys were administered at roll call, and some were left with officers to return the next day. Although some surveys were lost in the shuffle, this approach did allow them enough time to really think about their responses. In addition, the letter from the chief was most helpful in gaining access to the respondents.

However, there were a few problems with the administration of the police surveys. In contrast to the citizen sample, some officers started the survey and never completed it, and some officers walked away with the surveys and did not return them. Most officers were reluctant to sign the consent form because they felt it was not confidential. After reading the consent form and seeing others sign it, other officers complied. Some asked who was going to read the results. Some signed the consent form as "X," and others made up names because they were concerned about being identified or experiencing repercussions. I noticed many officers were unwilling to

record demographics for fear of identification. When officers refused to sign their names, I was prohibited by my IRB requirements from doing any follow-up. Although this problem can be seen as a validity threat, these responses may have been more honest because the officers knew they could not be identified.

Although this survey was created with the assistance of Newark officers, some officers still thought the survey was unrealistic, too long, too negative, too broad, and too racial. Because street scenarios are not so simple, there was no way I could cover every type of encounter. For example, some officers mentioned specific problems with the three levels of intrusiveness. They had problems with the terms *frisk* and *crime scene*. Officer 148 said, "My life means more to me than anything else—a bulge could be a gun." Officer 42 said, "The 'bulge' question was vague—could appear to be a weapon" (I intended to suggest exactly this, without stating it outright). Officer 44 said, "A pat down should be done for weapons only—not the search of a suspect." Officer 150 said, "You're not supposed to frisk people unless you have probable cause." That is what the law says, and it is what this officer follows. Other officers responded differently; some were more liberal in their perceptions, and others were more conservative. Thus, regardless of the complaints, I obtained the data I was looking for. A researcher evaluating street behavior needs to set limits. Many confrontations depend on factors the survey did not or could not cover. Because of time constraints, it is necessary to place restrictions on the depth of the questions and stay focused on the important issues being examined or the hypotheses being tested.

Regardless of the potential limitations of this research, I was able to get most of the officers to confide in me. The overall consensus I found through this study was that one's own environment and how one was raised governed the actions that would be taken in the field. Some officers expressed how clothing worn by people the police are dealing with had nothing to do with how they reacted to certain situations. The officers admitted that, although training helped a lot, they mostly relied on their instincts. Officer 30 said, "Actions taken by police officers are based on instinct and body language: glance, switching direction, walking other ways. A good officer would read this and act accordingly, but his actions are correct only about 60% of the time." Officer 31 said, "I treat others as I expect to be treated," and Officer 39 said, "Police officers are trained not to look at color, or religion, and do the job only." Officer 40 said, "I approach anyone to get to know him. I only detain if there is good reason (evidence of something)." He continued, "Everyone gets asked what they have in their possession, and I frisk most people in the wrong neighborhood for my own safety."

To overcome administration problems, I utilized numerous pretests (see next section), which helped me to exclude confusing, misleading, double-barreled, and suggestive questions. Once I revamped the scenarios after the pretesting, I found that even though some of the questions posed appeared to demonstrate discrimination by police, officers and citizens still indicated they or the police would treat certain persons or situations differently. These pretest findings demonstrated that respondents would be honest when filling out the questionnaires, further supporting the contention that the potential problem of reactivity was overcome. However, to attempt to counteract any prejudices, the questionnaire scenario characteristics varied, and the ordering of the characteristics was alternated to eliminate any response sets. Further, the more sensitive questions (based on racial issues) were placed in the middle of a section to make the characteristic appear more innocuous. To eliminate legal or ethical complications, participation in this study was completely voluntary. I obtained participants' informed consent, and there was no penalty for refusing to cooperate. In addition, participants were given my contact information for future questions, problems, or comments.

SELECTING ITEMS FOR MEASURING OUTCOMES

It is frequently necessary to include insiders on a research advisory committee and to discuss findings with these insiders to ensure that they are presented in a way that will be accepted and used before moving to publication. Thus, as mentioned earlier, the survey was pretested numerous times in an attempt to eliminate threats to validity.

In the first pretest, responses were gathered from 22 subjects who tested the instrument to create the scenarios and uncover any obvious problems before administration to the study population. Next, 10 officers (who were not included in the actual study) were surveyed. They were questioned regarding the stability of the measurement of perceptions of police power, enabling me to eliminate questions that were unclear or repetitive. A sample questionnaire was also administered to 12 Rutgers University students in a research methods course. I also interviewed a focus group with 5 Newark police officers to obtain their opinions and add their expertise to the proposed survey. The officers assisted in further developing the research instrument and in creating "realistic" street scenarios that would be easy for officers and citizens to understand. The results of the interviews demonstrated some important themes and helped guide me in selecting "items" (i.e., scenarios and particular demographic and situational characteristics) for the survey.

The final pretest of the survey instrument was conducted on the streets of South Orange, New Jersey, and allowed me to solidify the exact items and scenarios that would be included on the final survey. It was determined that demographic and situational characteristics (contextual variables) would be useful to include on the survey. Thus, questions on the race, age, income, gender, ethnicity and marital status of respondent were incorporated. In addition, it was determined that time of day and dress, race, area, and demeanor of subject(s) would be included on the survey to examine whether these situational factors influenced perceptions of what police would do. Further, comparisons between police and citizen perceptions as well as comparisons among police and among citizens were considered useful. Finally, questions on the level of support citizens had in their attitudes about specific police actions as presented in the vignettes were thought to be important to include. Thus, items on whether the public supported specific police actions and whether citizens believed police *should* be allowed to use certain behavior were integrated into the survey.

TOOLS

A variety of situations can occur on the street between police and citizens; thus I used a rating scale to determine the range of police intervention in a citizen's life from (a) a search and seizure initiated on probable cause to (b) a stop and frisk initiated on reasonable suspicion to (c) encounters where police and citizens are only engaging in verbal interaction on the street. Encounters of the third type normally occur without constitutional implications, and they may involve an approach and interview or inquiry.

By comparing the responses to posed scenarios by police officers to responses by citizens, an analysis of the level of convergence was determined. I developed a new tool by creating a numerical scale. A numerical value was assigned to each level of intrusiveness in increasing order (1–3) and the scores were compared with each other (among and between groups) to obtain a general overview of the differences in perceptions of the police and the public. Different situational factors were assessed to determine which led to the perception that a higher level of interference would be used (according to police and citizens). Data were coded as received and entered into Statistical Package for the Social Sciences (SPSS) to analyze. Descriptive statistics were used to assess the mean and frequencies, and cross-tabulations were used to compare the situational and demographic characteristics of respondents to the perceptions of the levels of intrusiveness that would be used. Finally, chi-square tests were done to determine whether differences between the groups were statistically significant.

Vignettes

Scenarios are devices for ordering perceptions about future and plausible future states in terms of variables that define the future in a consistent manner. They are best for long-range forecasting and uncertain situations. As scenarios are generated, specific strategic alternatives are developed to address the environments outlined in each scenario (Venable, Ma, Ginter, & Duncan, 1993). Scenario analysis is an alternative to conventional forecasting and is better suited to an environment with numerous uncertainties. (Thus, the streets of Newark would qualify.)

Utilizing scenarios in this specific study allowed me to examine every possible variation of a few variables and to select a few plausible scenarios from the set. In this study, police and citizens were asked to evaluate each issue, and responses were converted into a 3-point numerical scale. A score of 1 corresponded to the lowest level of interference, and a score of 3 corresponded to the highest level of interference. The

mean score for each scenario was used to plot issues as to their impact. In addition, a "vignette" was utilized to examine how various dimensions influence perceptions of the respondent. Vignettes are short descriptions that can be beneficial at illustrating behavior without making a specific statement (Thurman, Lam, & Rossi, 1988). Vignettes approximate the "real world" and thus increase external validity (Keppel, 1973). Other researchers have been successful with this technique. For example, in a study of mental illness, researchers used vignettes by illustrating feelings of depression with behavior rather than directly asking if the individual was "frequently depressed" (Thurman et al., 1988). In another example, 16 vignettes were used to describe separate types of police conduct. There were three dimensions (race, record, and mode of coercion) and three levels, (e.g., race can include White, Black, Hispanic). Their random combination generated 27 vignettes (Riksheim & Chermak, 1993). The authors used characteristics and created dummy variables for each characteristic, leaving one category characteristic as a reference. Russell and Gray (1992) used the scenario method by asking subjects to report how they would behave in each of several described situations. Because this method was successful for others, I decided to employ a similar format. However, to utilize these vignettes efficiently, respondents must read each "case" and then assess how they feel about the issue. They can be asked to read the hypothetical vignette and estimate their likelihood of performing the activity described (Elis & Simpson, 1995). Respondents may be asked to rate sentences (too high or too low) via a hypothetical scenario describing various crimes, criminal offenses, and prison sentences (Miller, Rossi, & Simpson, 1986).

In this particular survey, respondents were asked to rate the level of intrusiveness of police behavior that they believed would be used by police officers regardless of the law. Variability within and between subjects of the population was measured to assess the degree to which agreement existed in ratings. An assessment of the extent to which segments of the general population and the criminal justice system were alike in the degree to which they discriminated among different elements of information when they form seriousness judgments was then determined (Miller, 1984). The vignette surveys allowed me to consider many aspects of a situation without making unreasonable demands on the respondents.

DISCUSSION

The goal of this research was to develop a definitive picture of how police and citizens viewed the typical encounter and to determine how contextual variables such as demographic and situational characteristics were expected to influence the handling and outcomes of encounters. I wanted to gather this honest information in a way that protected the safety of the researcher, controlled for problems, and overcame as many obstacles as possible. The research was also aimed at developing an understanding of the preferences of the police and public in order to improve relations between the two groups and make police more responsive to the needs of the community. The analysis of these findings helped me determine the degree to which different members of the population were alike in the way they discriminated among elements of information. By measuring police perceptions of their power and authority on the street in comparison to citizen perceptions of police power, it was possible to discover the extent of the variation of opinions between the police and the public regarding police officer response tactics. The results also provided data on social definitions of behavior (the perceived level of seriousness of intrusions and the differences in ratings of intrusiveness). Because the questionnaire was closed-ended, answers were more structured and coding was simplified.

By creating a second and third section of the survey instrument for citizens only, I was able to determine the power citizens believed an officer should be able to use, and of what behavior they were supportive. For these sections, within-group differences were examined (i.e., differences among race-gender, age, income, marital status, and ethnicity), as well as situational factors that appeared to influence support for particular police action.

CONCLUSIONS

This research was timely and had important implications. Based on the results gathered via the survey instrument, it was determined that, with a little creativity, research on the streets of a dangerous community could be gathered honestly. In addition, it was determined that police officers were a bit more trusting of researchers than portrayed in the media. The long-range goals of this research were met. I was able to determine what citizens expected from the police, develop theories on how to increase compliance rates, and create suggestions to develop better police training to meet citizen expectations. In addition, this research was successful in educating police on the implications of encounters through citizens' eyes.

Specific results of the research demonstrated that although the age, ethnicity, and marital status of police officer were not statistically significant factors influencing police perceptions, race, gender, and income were. Income was not a statistically significant factor influencing citizen perceptions, but gender, ethnicity, race, age, marital status, and the combined factors of gender/race and gender/ethnicity were. The hypothesis that there would be no between-group differences was rejected, and the hypothesis that citizens were supportive of police was also rejected. In conclusion, some factors influenced perceptions of the level of intrusiveness that would be used. In addition, more between-group than within-group differences were discovered. Although the actual results of this research project are important, the premier issue is that I was able to obtain these results with a little imagination and resourcefulness.

To demonstrate the success of this mission, it is important to look at the response rate. Of the 500 surveys copied and administered, 169 police officer surveys were administered: (157 completed, 12 incomplete, 15 refusals). There were 331 citizens surveys administered (29 incomplete, 302 completed, 91 refusals). Thus, a total of 459 surveys were completed by police or citizens. I was able to convert these results into a viable dissertation and successfully obtained my Ph.D. based on my presentation of the findings.

References

Black, D., & Reiss, A. J. (1970). Police control of juveniles. *American Sociological Review, 35,* 63–77.

Elis, L. A., & Simpson, S. A. (1995). Informal sanction threats and corporate crime. *Journal of Research in Crime and Delinquency, 32,* 399–424.

Kavanaugh, J. (1994). *The occurrence of resisting arrest in arrest encounters: A study of police-citizen violence.* Ann Arbor, MI: University Microfilms International.

Keppel, G. (1973). *Design and analysis.* Englewood Cliffs, NJ: Prentice-Hall.

LaFave, W. R. (1965). *Arrest: The decision to take a suspect into custody.* Boston, MA: Little, Brown.

Miller, J. L. (1984). *Normative consensus in judgments of prison sentences: Popular and selected criminal justice system perceptions of fair punishments for convicted.* Ann Arbor, MI: University Microfilms International.

Miller, J. L., Rossi, P. H., & Simpson, J. E. (1986). Perceptions of justice: Race and gender differences in judgments of appropriate prison sentences. *Law and Society Review, 20,* 313–334.

Miller, L. S., & Braswell, M. C. (1992). Police perceptions of ethical decision-making. *American Journal of Police,* 11(4), 27–45.

Morgan, K. O., Morgan, S., & Quitno, N. (1997). *City Crime Rankings: Crime in metropolitan America* (3rd ed.). Lawrence, KS: Quitno Press.

Mylonas, A. D. (1973). *Perceptions of police power.* South Hackensack, NJ: Fred B. Rothman.

Riksheim, E., & Chermak, S. (1993). Causes of police behavior revised. *Journal of Criminal Justice, 21,* 353–382.

Russell, P. A., & Gray, C. D. (1992). Prejudice against a pro-gay man in an everyday situation: A scenario study. *Journal of Applied Social Psychology, 22,* 1676–1687.

Skolnick, J. H., & Bayley, D. H. (1986). *The new blue line.* New York: The Free Press.

Sykes, R. E., & Brent, E. E. (1983). *Policing: A social behaviorist perspective.* New Brunswick, NJ: Rutgers University Press.

Thurman, Q. C., Lam, J. A., & Rossi, P. H. (1988). Sorting out the cuckoo's nest: A factorial survey applied to the study of popular conceptions of mental illness. *Sociological Quarterly, 29,* 565–588.

Venable, J. M, Ma, Q. L., Ginter, P. M., & Duncan, W. J. (1993). The use of scenario analysis in local public health departments: Alternative futures for strategic planning. *Public Health Reports, 108,* 701–710.

THE ROLE OF FAMILIES IN BUFFERING STRESS IN PERSONS WITH MENTAL ILLNESS

94

A Correlational Study

Eric D. Johnson

Work with people with serious mental illness and their families provides an excellent forum for examining the importance of two reciprocal processes: practice-based research and evidence-based practice. As a way of providing a focus for the study discussed in this chapter, a brief history of the relationship between practice and research with this population is provided.

FAMILY INTERVENTIONS WITH FAMILIES OF THE MENTALLY ILL

The beginnings of family therapy in the United States, in the early 1950s, involved families with schizophrenic members, most of whom were interviewed in the context of the ill member's hospitalization. Based on earlier psychodynamic ideas like the *schizophrenogenic mother*, many of these early family therapy pioneers speculated that family communication and affiliation dynamics were responsible for causing schizophrenic symptoms (Bateson, Jackson, Haley, & Weakland, 1956; Wynne & Singer, 1963). However, these observations were based on small samples and tended to make assumptions about the family interaction that failed to take into account the possibility of a biological illness process, as well as the influences of the illness and hospital contexts. These theories were subsequently tested in research studies during the 1960s and were found wanting. Those studies concluded that the theories of family etiology of mental illness failed to produce any variables that could be clearly linked to the development of schizophrenia (Meissner, 1970). However, long before these theories had been adequately tested, therapeutic interventions based on them were already taking place, often to the detriment of families of the mentally ill, who felt blamed by family therapists for causing their family member's illness (Hatfield & Lefley, 1987).

In light of this research information, in the 1970s the focus of attention shifted to examining the course, rather than the cause, of serious mental illness. British researchers developed the concept of *expressed emotion* (EE) and found that high EE levels (especially negative emotion) of family members correlated with patient relapse or rehospitalization (Brown, Birley, & Wing, 1972; Vaughn & Leff, 1981). They concluded that people with schizophrenia may be especially sensitive to too much stimulus (physical or emotional) and seem to function best in environments that are structured, not extremely complex or demanding, and neutrally stimulating (Brown et al., 1972; Wing, 1978). These findings suggested that steps could be taken by families to lessen the likelihood of relapse (Miklowitz et al., 1989). However, in the late 1970s, a grassroots organization of professionals and family members developed into the National Alliance for the Mentally Ill (NAMI). This organization has been critical of the EE studies, feeling that they continue to "blame" families for mental illness, and suggesting that "unusual" family characteristics might be the *result* of having to cope with a family member who behaves in unusual ways (Hatfield, 1991; Lefley, 1992).

In the 1980s, clinicians began to develop the possibilities suggested by the EE researchers into a new approach to helping families with a mentally ill member. This new approach sought to avoid blaming and attempted to lower emotional expression through the use of a "psychoeducational" methodology (Anderson, Reiss, & Hogarty, 1986; Bernheim & Lehman, 1985). The approach was based on a *stress-diathesis* theory: Some people have a genetic predisposition (diathesis), which makes them more likely to break down under stress. If the vulnerability is a heart condition, these people are more likely than others to have a heart attack under stressful conditions. If the vulnerability is a biological mental condition, they are more likely to have a psychotic breakdown under stressful conditions (Zubin, 1986). The focus of psychoeducational approaches has been to help normalize the experience of the family, avoid reference to family etiology, identify biological and genetic influence factors, provide information about medication use, and train family members in reducing emotional expression while dealing with problematic situations. This has usually been done in a group format, through either all-day workshops or an ongoing series of topic-focused meetings (Lefley, 1996; Miklowitz & Hooley, 1998).

Research in the field of mental illness has called attention to the issues of caregiving for people with serious mental illness, as well as the impact (often referred to as *family burden*) on family caregivers (Goldstein, 1987; Lefley 1996; Solomon & Draine, 1995). Although there appears to be a growing consensus that the family system has the potential for buffering the negative effects of chronic illnesses generally (Ross, Mirowsky, & Goldstein, 1990; Walsh, 1996), there is relatively little empirical evidence that identifies particular family characteristics that can aid in coping with a chronic disability like mental illness (Hatfield & Lefley, 1987; Spaniol, Zipple, & Lockwood, 1992). Furthermore, much of the focus in research on families of the mentally ill has been on features such as *communication deviance* and EE with considerably less attention paid to positive family functioning, coping skills, or satisfaction and their relation to successful adaptation (Kanter, Lamb, & Loeper, 1987; Lefley, 1992).

Starting from a standpoint of family strengths, the present study assessed the influence of both family resources and family interpretation on the functional adaptation of the ill member, and the ability of these family variables to buffer strains (i.e., ongoing stressors) common in the lives of people with mental illness who are living in the community. This was undertaken in an attempt to provide information about further directions that clinicians might take to improve the lives of the seriously mentally ill and their families.

THEORETICAL BASIS: FAMILY CRISIS THEORY

Since Reuben Hill (1949) introduced what has come to be known as the ABCX Model of assessing family crisis, most theory and research in the area of family coping has centered around his four basic components: a precipitating "event" (A), the family's resources for coping (B), the family's interpretation of the event (C), and the family's response (X). Other family theorists have subsequently expanded on Hill's ideas to incorporate levels of influence and complexities of interaction. Since 1980, most writers have emphasized the systemic nature of adaptation to ongoing stressful situations rather than the adjustment to a single crisis, which Hill had described. With the resulting emphasis on feedback loops, the "pileup" of stress inducing components, and the reciprocal interactions of the component parts, these enhancements represent a significant departure from the static causal model originally proposed by Hill. Of the current models, the Double ABCX Model of McCubbin and colleagues (McCubbin & Patterson, 1983) is still the dominant version and the most researched. The Double ABCX Model was revised in the late 1980s to the Family Adjustment and Adaptation Response Model (FAAR) (Patterson, 1989). This modification shifts the focus from negative outcomes to emphasize positive outcomes and elements of "resilience" in the face of ongoing stressors (McCubbin & McCubbin, 1988), but it is more heuristic than causal in its structure of reciprocal influence and feedback loops.

THE SOCIAL CONTEXT OF TREATMENT: DEINSTITUTIONALIZATION

During the same period in which these theories of family treatment and family stress and coping have developed, the mental health system in the United States has undergone a profound change, generally referred to as *deinstitutionalization* (Grob, 1987). Despite the positive rhetoric of the 1950s and 1960s, the conceptions of deinstitutionalization and community mental health care have turned out to be extremely naive (Bachrach, 1986). Since deinstitutionalization began, families of the seriously mentally ill have been asked to take on an increasingly heavy burden of responsibility for the care and management of their mentally ill member (Hatfield & Lefley, 1987). Approximately 40% of those discharged from psychiatric units are likely to return to live with family members, and another 30% to 40% are in regular (at least weekly) contact with family members (Manderscheid & Sonnenschein, 1997). Thus, information about significant components of the family/patient/illness interaction is likely to help a substantial percentage of persons with serious mental illness, as well as their caregivers.

THE RESEARCH PROBLEM

Following the theoretical structure of the Double ABCX Model, accumulated strains were examined for their impact on the adaptation level of persons with serious mental illness, while family resources and appraisal were examined for their possible buffering role in the stress process. In this study, exogenous variables of "illness-specific strains" (chronicity of the mental illness and substance abuse complications) and "nonspecific strains" (demographic and environmental family characteristics) were assessed for their potential negative impact on the functional level (adaptation to community living) of the ill family member (IM). In addition, two endogenous variables, "family functioning" (in general), and "family members' sense of competence" (in the specific context) were assessed for their potential positive impact on the functional level of the IM. In addition to the assessment of main effects, the intervening (family) variables were examined for their ability to mediate the negative impact of stressors on the IM. The dependent variable in this study was a complex variable reflecting the "functional level of adaptation" of the seriously mentally ill person who is currently living in the community.

METHODS

Population and Sample

The population of concern in this study consisted of families with a seriously mentally ill member currently living with them or in regular (at least weekly) contact. (For purposes of this study, *seriously mentally ill* was defined as someone who has had at least one previous hospitalization for a psychotic episode involving mood or thought disorder, as defined by the fourth edition of the *Diagnostic and Statistical Manual of Mental Disorders*; American Psychiatric Association, 1999.)

The sample for this study consisted of referrals to the Family Support Project (FSP) in Mercer County, New Jersey, over a 3-year period. During this time, more than 200 families were contacted by members of the FSP, and 180 families were interviewed and coded. Because it was not possible to construct a randomized design, it was a goal of the study to ensure that referrals came from a wide variety of sources, reflecting a balance of socioeconomic and ethnic representation. Sources of referral included the community mental health center case management unit (16%) and family support group (20%); outpatient clinics (23%); inpatient programs (12%); the county jail system (10%); and Alliance for the Mentally Ill (19%).

Procedure

At a point as close as possible to the time when the IM had been released from psychiatric hospitalization for 6 months, at least one first-order relative (parent, sibling, spouse, adult child) who was living with or in frequent contact with the IM was interviewed, using a semistructured interview schedule. Family members were interviewed at length (interviews lasted at least 2 hours in each case) by the author and/or one of four staff members who constituted the FSP. Attempts were made to include as many family members as possible in each case. In the case of multiple informants, a single summary score was derived for each of the variables.

Because limitations in cognitive abilities and literacy were anticipated among a substantial portion of the sample, self-report questionnaires were not utilized. All staff members had previous experience in working with the mentally ill and with family interviewing; thus ratings were based on staff assessments of family responses and interaction, after interrater reliability had been established.

Respondent Characteristics

Of the total sample of families ($N = 180$), the primary caregivers were mostly parents of the IM (70%), with siblings (13%), spouses (6%), and adult children (8%) making up the rest of the sample. Distribution of socioeconomic status (SES) included 39% upper-middle-class families (one or more family member with a professional job), 45% lower-middle class families (one or more member with a blue-collar job), and 16% lower-class families (welfare and/or the IM's Social Security providing the only income). Most of the respondents were women (84%); they ranged in age from 25 to 80, but most were over 55 (62%); $M = 56.5$. Household and family size ranged broadly, with family size most often 4 to 8 people (72%; $M = 5.7$), and household size most often 2 to 5 people (70%; $M = 3.3$). Respondent characteristics are summarized in Table 94.1

Patient Characteristics

The IM sample ($N = 180$) included 56% men and 44% women. They ranged in age from 20 to 70, with 26% in their 20's, 38% in their 30s, and 22% in their 40s; only 14% were over 50 ($M = 37.3$). The sample included 58% European American, 32% African American, and 10% Hispanic American patients. Only 23% of the IM sample failed to graduate from high school, and 42% had gone beyond high school in education. Most had never been married (62%), and only 12% were currently married. Their diagnoses included six categories: thought disorder (schizophrenia; 22%), mood disorder (manic-depressive; 10%), thought and mood disorder (schizoaffective; 29%), thought disorder and

TABLE 94.1 Characteristics of Respondents

Category	Percent	Category	Percent
Primary caregiver		**Age of caregiver**	
Parent	70	25–44	20
Sibling	13	45–54	18
Spouse	6	55–64	37
Adult child	8	65–80	25
SES of family		**Gender of caregiver**	
Upper middle	39	Female	84
Lower middle	45	Male	16
Lower	16		
Number in household		**Number in family**	
IP alone	18	1–3 people	16
2–3 people	44	4–5 people	36
4–5 people	26	6–8 people	36
6+ people	12	9+ people	12
Problem areas		**Problem areas**	
Neighborhood safety	30	Occupational stability	28
Physical health/disability	33	Loss of family members	15

substance abuse (24%), mood disorder and substance abuse (4%), and all three disorders (11%). The age of onset of the illness varied from 14 to 65, with 52% developing the illness by the age of 21 ($M = 24.1$). The number of hospitalizations ranged widely and was essentially evenly distributed ($M = 5.1$), as were the total period of hospitalization ($M = 18.7$ months) and the length of time the IM had experienced the illness ($M = 13.3$ years). Living situations were fairly evenly divided: 60% lived with their families, and 40% lived elsewhere; 56% lived in the city, 44% in the suburbs. Most of the IM population (82%) were currently taking prescribed psychotropic medication. Patient characteristics are summarized in Table 94.2

Measures

Ill Member Level of Adaptation

The instrument developed for this study consisted of 46 items, which together provided a way of assessing the IM's observable behavioral functioning in six important areas of family and community living: "self-care," "social functioning," "vocational functioning," "emotional stability," "symptoms," and "substance use." These items incorporated substantial features of

the Global Level of Functioning and Specific Level of Functioning assessment instruments developed by the National Institute of Mental Health (Carter & Newman, 1976). Each category was rated by the staff interviewer on a 9-point scale from low to high functioning, based on family members' evaluation of the IM's *current* functioning.

Family Functioning

Two established instruments were used to assess family functioning: the Clinical Rating Scale (Olson et al., 1985) and the Family Functioning Scale (Geismar, 1980). Both of these are direct-observation instruments that are derived from other instruments, which have a substantial history of use and verification. The Family Adaptability and Cohesion Evaluation Scale (FACES) of Olson and associates has been used in dozens of studies and has gone through several revisions since it was introduced in 1979 (Olson, 1986). The St. Paul Scale of Geismar and associates has been in use for several decades and has established both validity and reliability (Geismar, 1980; Camasso & Geismar, 1992). The Clinical Rating Scale (CRS) utilizes three dimensions: cohesion, adaptability/change, and com-

TABLE 94.2 Characteristics of IM Population

Category	Percent	Category	Percent
IM gender		**IM race**	
Female	44	European American	58
Male	56	African American	32
		Hispanic American	10
IM age		**IM education**	
20–29	26	< high school	23
30–39	38	H.S. graduate	35
40–49	22	H.S. +	31
50–70	14	B.A.(+)	11
IM marital status		**Psychotropic medications**	
Never married	62	Yes	82
Currently married	12	No	18
Previously married	26		
IM diagnosis		**IM diagnosis**	
Thought disorder	22	Thought and substance abuse	24
Mood disorder	10	Mood and substance abuse	4
Thought and mood disorder	29	All 3 disorders	11
IM location		**Living situation**	
Trenton	56	IM with family	60
Suburbs	44	IM elsewhere	40
Age of onset		**Length of illness**	
14–17	17	0–5 years	24
18–21	35	6–10 years	17
22–25	20	11–15 years	22
26–30	15	16–21 years	21
31–65	13	22–40 years	16
Number of hospitalizations		**Total period of hospitalization**	
1–2	26	1–3 months	21
3–4	22	4–9 months	20
5–8	23	10–18 months	21
9+	29	19–36 months	24
		37+ months	14

munication. It assesses functioning on Likert-style scales for cohesion and adaptability/change, in which midrange (moderate) scores are viewed as preferable to extreme scores. Communication is assessed on an interval-level scale from low to high facilitation. The Family Functioning Scale (FFS) utilizes four dimensions: family health-welfare, individual role competence, satisfaction, and conformity. It assesses functioning on a Likert-style scale from inadequate to adequate. Categories for both scales were adjusted to 9-point scales, rated by the staff interviewer based on family responses and interactions.

Family Members' Sense of Competence

The instrument developed for this study utilized the three-part frameworks developed by Kobasa (1979; Kobasa, Maddi, & Courington, 1981) and Antonovsky (1987, 1998). These elements were modified to be appropriate to the experience of living with the mentally ill and were organized into a brief (12-item) index. Family sense of competence is a construct composed of three dimensions, "evaluation of the past," "sense of competence in the present," and "challenge/threat of the future." Each category was rated by the staff interviewer on a 9-point scale, ranging from low to high, based on family members' responses to direct questions about these criteria.

Environmental Strain

Environmental or demographic strains are those that impact on the family and IM, independent of the IM's mental illness. The following categorical variables, identified in the literature as likely to impact on people with mental illness, were examined for their influence on the IM level of adaptation: status SES; environmental problems (neighborhood safety, family occupational stability, family physical health/disability); life-event changes (both positive and negative) in the past year; family (and household) size; location of residence; IM living with/away from family; age, race, and gender of the IM; age, gender, and family position of the primary caretaker; and family history of substance abuse.

Illness Strain

Illness-related strains are those conditions directly and specifically related to the course of the IM's mental illness—especially components of diagnosis, chronicity, severity, and substance use complications. The following categorical variables, identified in the literature as likely to impact on the IM's current level of adaptation, were examined: age at first hospitalization, number of hospitalizations, period of total hospitalization, length of time since the first hospitalization, psychiatric diagnosis, substance use history, previous mental health and substance use treatment services, and family history of mental illness.

RESULTS

IM Level of Adaptation

Psychometric properties of this developed instrument are described more fully elsewhere (Johnson, 2003). Through factor analysis, the IM level of adaptation index was reduced from 46 to 30 items (correlation = .990 with the original instrument). The revised index consisted of five factors, which roughly paralleled the categories of the original instrument. Reliability analysis for the revised index provided Cronbach's alpha = .953 for the total index, with a range from

.830 to .943 for the subcategories. Correlations among subcategories ranged from .294 to .632. Interrater reliabilities for the index ranged from .941 to .990. A single variable entitled "IM level of adaptation" (IMLA) was created by taking the average score on each of the 30 revised index items. This interval-level score was used as the dependent variable in subsequent analyses.

Family Functioning

Clinical Rating Scale

Index reliability analysis provided Cronbach's alpha = .884 for the total index, with a range from .710 to .879 for the subcategories. Correlations among subcategories ranged from .083 to .398. Interrater reliabilities for the index ranged from .552 to .930.

Family Functioning Scale

Index reliability analysis provided Cronbach's alpha = .946 for the total index, with a range from .858 to .939 for the subcategories. Correlation between the subcategories was .861. Interrater reliabilities for the index ranged from .763 to .989.

Factor analysis supported the three categories of the CRS but found the FFS to be essentially unidimensional. Both the CRS and the FFS had similar correlations with the IMLA (CRS = .373; FFS = .437); in addition, they had a moderately high correlation with each other (.684). It appears that the two scales are measuring somewhat different, but complementary, aspects of family functioning, and that family functioning is significantly related to the IMLA. Scores from the five subcategories of the CRS and FFS were combined into a single family functioning score, which had a higher correlation (.445) with the IMLA. Therefore, this interval-level score was used in subsequent analyses to represent the variable "family functioning" (FF).

Family Sense of Competence

Psychometric properties of this developed instrument are described more fully elsewhere (Johnson, 2003b). Through factor analysis, the family sense of competence index was reduced from 12 to 10 items (correlation = .989 with the original instrument). Reliability analysis for the revised index provided Cronbach's alpha = .853

for the total index, with a range from .686 to .843 for the subcategories. Correlations among subcategories ranged from .337 to .504. Inter-rater reliabilities for the index ranged from .830 to .951. The interval-level score used in subsequent analyses to represent the variable "family sense of competence" (SC) was determined by taking the average score on each of the 10 revised index items.

Exogenous (Strain) Variables

In contrast to the dependent variable and the two endogenous variables just described, all of which relied on assessment instruments that utilized interval-level scales, the two exogenous variables in this study were formed from combinations of nominal and ordinal level categorical variables. Those variables that demonstrated sufficient differentiation among categories in a one-way ANOVA, and were statistically significant at the $p < .05$ level when entered into a simultaneous multiple regression, were recoded to represent ordinal rankings from low (1) to high (3 or 4) strain, as reflected in IMLA mean scores.

Environmental Strain

Five of the 10 variables examined reached significance. These included (a) changes in the past year, with greater numbers of negative changes demonstrating a stronger negative correlation with the IMLA; (b) problem areas (neighborhood safety, family occupational stability, family health/disability), with greater numbers of problems demonstrating a stronger negative correlation; (c) socioeconomic status, with lower SES demonstrating a stronger negative correlation; (d) family size, with larger family size demonstrating a stronger negative correlation; and (e) gender and race. Neither gender nor race separately was a significant predictor of the IMLA. When combined, however, they differentiated the population into four groupings (with subsequent categories demonstrating a stronger negative correlation): European American women, European American men, minority women, and minority men. A single variable score for "environmental strain" (ES) was created by adding the scores (ranks) from each of these five variables. A greater score represented a greater accumulated strain.

Illness Strain

Four of the 10 variables examined reached significance. These variables included (a) number of hospitalizations, with a greater number demonstrating a stronger negative correlation with the IMLA; (b) total number of mental health services received, with a greater number demonstrating a stronger negative correlation; (c) substance use history, which differentiated the population into three groupings (with subsequent categories demonstrating a stronger negative correlation): no use, alcohol only, multiple drugs; (d) psychiatric diagnosis, which differentiated the population into four groupings (with subsequent categories demonstrating a stronger negative correlation): mood disorder (manic-depressive), mood and thought disorder (schizoaffective), thought disorder (schizophrenia), and dual disorders (substance abuse and psychiatric diagnosis). A single variable score for "illness strain" (IS) was created by adding the scores (ranks) from each of these four variables. A greater score represented a greater accumulated strain.

Relative Influences of the Independent Variables on the IMLA

Table 94.3 provides information on zero-order correlations between variables in the study. From the table, it can be seen that the independent variables demonstrate significant correlations with the dependent variable in the hypoth-

TABLE 94.3 Zero-Order Correlation Coefficients Between Variables

Independent Variable/ Dependent Variable	Correlation Coefficient
ES/IMLA	−.480
IS/IMLA	−.446
FF/IMLA	.445
SC/IMLA	.495
ES/FF	−.506
ES/SC	−.393
IS/FF	−.256
IS/SC	−.249
FF/SC	.528

ES = environmental strain; IS = illness strain; FF = family functioning; SC = family sense of competence; IMLA = ill member level of adaptation

esized directions, and that the exogenous (strain) variables impact in a negative way on the endogenous (family) variables, as well as on the IM.

However, while the correlation coefficients provide an important measure of the nature and strength of associations between individual variables, they fail to account for overlap of influence and possibilities of error. To provide a clearer assessment of multiple influence factors, the dependent variable was regressed on all four independent variables. In addition, the independent variables were standardized to assess interaction effects. The interaction of environmental strain and family sense of competence provided a significant addition to the model; no other interactions were found to approach significance. Table 94.4 provides information about the multiple regression model. All four independent variables were entered simultaneously (to best assess relative strengths of influence); the interaction effect was entered hierarchically.

The multiple regression analysis indicates that this model accounts for over 40% of the possible variance in the IMLA. The model as a whole is highly significant; its weakest part is clearly family functioning, which would have been eliminated in a "stepwise entry" analysis of the regression. Illness strain and family sense of competence emerge as the two strongest influences on the IMLA.

DISCUSSION

This study sought to test the premises of the Double ABCX/FAAR theory of stress and coping. It examined the relative negative influences of two forms of ongoing stressors (environmental strain and illness-related strain) on the functional adaptation of people with serious mental illness living in the community. In addition, it sought to assess the relative positive influences of two family variables (family functioning in general and family members' sense of competence in managing the problem of mental illness).

The Negative Influence of Strains on People With Mental Illness

Although a large number of environmental and illness-related stressors were examined in this study, less than half of them were significantly correlated with the IMLA. Within both ES and IS, the influence of any one factor was very limited and did not exhibit enough strength to be considered a separate variable. In support of the Double ABCX/FAAR theory, it appears that the "pileup" of elements produce a significant effect (cf. also Turner & Lloyd, 1995).

Nevertheless, when summated scores were created from the most significant components, both ES and IS were significant predictors of the IMLA, together accounting for over 20% of the variance in the dependent variable. The results of this study strongly suggest that without a buffering influence, the negative effects of environmental and illness-related problems will take a devastating toll on people with mental illness who are trying to function outside of the hospital environment.

TABLE 94.4 Multiple Regression Analysis for Variables Predicting IM Level of Adaptation

Variable	Regression Coefficient	Standard Error	Standardized Regression Coefficient	t-score	p-value
Environmental strain	−.088	.037	−.174	−2.38	.018
Illness strain	−.163	.044	−.243	−3.71	.000
Family functioning	.076	.049	.119	1.58	.115
Sense of competence	.418	.099	.307	4.22	.000
Interaction of ES and SC	−.192	.092	−.128	2.10	.038

Total model information: multiple $r = .649$; $R^2 = .421$; standard error = 1.17; F-score = 24.402; significance of F-score = .000.

The Positive Influence of Family on People With Mental Illness

As hypothesized, both family functioning (general) and family members' sense of competence (specific) were positively correlated with the ill member's level of adaptation to community living. However, the influence of FF on the IMLA changed dramatically in the multiple regression analysis; its influence in this study appeared to be largely mediated by SC, which proved to be the single most important contributor to the IMLA.

Recent literature in the stress and coping field has recognized the complexity of coping mechanisms, the difference between generalized and specific coping skills (Rosenberg, Schooler, Schoenbach, & Rosenberg, 1995), and the importance of using different coping patterns in different situations (Mattlin, Wethington, & Kessler, 1990; Solomon & Draine, 1995). The importance of perception in improving coping responses has been addressed in a number of recent articles on "hardiness," "competence," and "resilience" in the face of adversity (McCubbin, Thompson, Thompson, & Fromer, 1998; Ross, Mirowsky, & Goldstein, 1990; Walsh, 1996). In particular, research literature on families of the mentally ill has identified elements of "resilience" (Marsh et al., 1996) and "confidence" (Axelrod, Geismar, & Ross, 1994) as important for family members' personal coping, as well as tolerance for problematic behaviors of the ill family member.

The Mediating Influence of Family Variables

In addition to demonstrating significant negative direct effects of the strain variables and direct positive effects of the family variables on the IMLA, this study found a significant interaction effect between ES and SC. The strength of this interaction on the IMLA suggests a possible role for family sense of competence in affecting the impact of environmental strain on the IM, as well as having a powerful main effect. This impact was even more dramatic when the data were controlled for level of influence. At the lowest levels of SC, ES had a strong (and fairly consistent) negative correlation with the IMLA. This dropped sharply as levels of the SC rose and held through the upper levels. This finding suggests

a strong moderating influence for family sense of competence. It appears that, at the lowest levels of family functioning and limited perception of success, there is little that families can do to buffer the impact of environmental stressors on their family member. However, at even moderate levels of functioning and satisfaction with performance, there is a dramatic difference in the family's ability to buffer this impact and have a significant influence on the ill member's functioning. These differences were also found to vary by ethnic group and by SES, as reported in a recent article (Johnson, 1998).

With regard to illness-related stressors, the influence of the family variables was reasonably constant across levels of functioning and was quite limited. Although this suggests that there may be little that families can do to affect the course of the illness, the relatively weak correlation between IS and the family variables also provides evidence that family sense of competence is *not* a function of the illness history (i.e., family members do not merely become weary and discouraged over long periods of chronic recycling of the IM through the hospital and community mental health systems; nor do families necessarily appear to become more competent through time). This is consistent with the findings of Biegel and associates (Biegel, Milligan, Putnam, & Song, 1994), who investigated illness-related strains with reference to family burden.

Limitations of the Study

This was a cross-sectional study, using one extended interview. As such, it was affected by the limitations of all cross-sectional studies; it was only able to assess correlations in the relationships among the variables of concern. It would require a longitudinal design to assess whether, over time, changes in the various elements would actually predict change in the community functioning of people with mental illness.

In addition, the number of variables examined in this study was very limited. Although the combination of strain and family variables accounted for over 40% of the variance in the IMLA, the study did not include personal variables for the IM, programmatic variables for the mental health system, or developmental variables for either IM or family. All of these variables (and others) interact in very complex ways. Further research on the importance and inter-action of variables at different systemic levels (individual, family, and social) is needed.

Research into the lives of people with mental illness and their families will require increasingly specialized instruments, as those measures designed for the general population fail to adequately assess the differences found in these families. This necessitated the creation of indices specific to this study. Although these instruments demonstrated strong psychometric properties (to be reported in forthcoming articles), the further validation of these and other instruments for assessing problems and (especially) strengths in the IM, the family, and the mental health system is badly needed (Dworkin, 1992).

Implications of the Study for Evidence-Based Practice

This study has attempted to advance practice knowledge by examining the problem of the functional adaptation of people with serious mental illness living in the community, the identification of some major negative influences (strains) on the level of adaptation, the identification of some significant positive influences (supports) on the level of adaptation, and an understanding of how these interact. The goal of this research has been to better understand social and environmental sources of stress and support for the mentally ill that may be able to translate into clinically relevant interventions to improve life for people with serious mental illness and their families.

The findings of this study support those of other recent studies that have examined the importance of "competence," "mastery," or "sense of control," demonstrating that a sense of meaning and competence can have significant effects on psychological and physical outcomes, as well as a buffering effect on stress exposure (Mueser et al., 2002). This study has gone beyond the examination of personal competence/outcome to suggest that a family "atmosphere of competence" can contribute to the outcome of a vulnerable member. This has important implications for psychotherapeutic and psychoeducational work with families of the mentally ill, as well as other families with vulnerable members (Dyck, Hendryx, Short, Voss, & MacFarlane, 2002; Walsh, 1996).

A number of recent studies have documented the importance of family to the seriously mentally ill (Brekke & Mathiesen, 1995; Pitschel-Walz et al., 2001). Given the importance of family variables for IM functioning, and the necessity of family caretaking for many of the mentally ill in the community, it is important that mental health systems incorporate services for families of the mentally ill into the continuum of mental health care. Recent reviews of empirically supported interventions with families of the mentally ill strongly encourage family support efforts as aiding families in realizing and utilizing their sense of competence (Dixon et al., 2001; Marsh, 2001; Pinsoff & Wynn, 2000).

To date, the most successfully utilized form of family support in mental health settings has been the use of multifamily groups (with and without the IM present). The work of McFarlane and associates (McFarlane, Link, Dushay, Marchal, & Crilly, 1995) suggests that in the first year following hopitalization the most important intervention is psychoeducation about the illness. This aids family members by addressing illness attributions, knowledge as a form of "mastery," and specific coping behaviors to manage difficult times.

Moreover, the McFarlane group's 4-year follow-up research suggests that as families get past the critical first year reentry period, the experience of support may be more helpful than information in boosting the confidence and competence of family members. Many of the participants in the present study were unaware of other families struggling with the problem of mental illness and had no frame of reference on how they were doing. The provision of social support (or the availability of it) can be as helpful to the caregivers as their support is to the ill person.

However, Goldstein and Miklowitz (1995) point out that a significant percentage of families will not join a support group and will need individual family help; this includes families of recent-onset patients, as well as those who are extremely cautious or awkward socially and may be embarrassed to discuss their difficulties outside of the family. This may also be a necessary format for working with low-income or minority families, unless multifamily groups can be formed that specifically address their cultural issues and conceptions of the problem (Milstein, Guarnaccia, & Midlarsky, 1995).

The use of both psychoeducational and psychotherapeutic approaches, in individual family and multifamily settings, offers significant opportunities for increasing family members' sense of competence in managing the problem of mental illness. Along with self-help support groups, such as the Alliance for the Mentally Ill, these interventions show promise for improving the lives of both the mentally ill and their families. They are informed by the current state of research; in turn, they suggest future directions for additional research in this area, particularly the need for mental health professionals, family members, and persons with mental illness to work together in a partnership for improving services and making them more culturally and personally relevant (Johnson, 2001).

References

American Psychiatric Association. (1994). *Diagnostic and Statistical Manual of Mental Disorders* (4th ed.). Washington, DC: Author.

Anderson, C. M., Reiss, D. J., & Hogarty, G. E. (1986). *Schizophrenia and the family*. New York: Guilford Press.

Antonovsky, A. (1987). *Unraveling the mystery of health*. San Francisco: Jossey-Bass.

Antonovsky, A. (1998). The sense of coherence: An historical and future perspective. In H. I. McCubbin, E. A. Thompson, A. I. Thompson, & J. E. Fromer (Eds.), *Stress, coping, and health in families* (pp. 3–20). Thousand Oaks, CA: Sage.

Axelrod, J., Geismar, L. & Ross, R. (1994). Families of chronically mentally ill patients: Their structure, coping resources, and tolerance for deviant behavior. *Health and Social Work, 19,* 271–278.

Bachrach, L. L. (1986). Deinstitutionalization: What do the numbers mean? *Hospital and Community Psychiatry, 37,* 118–121.

Bateson, G., Jackson, D. D., Haley, J., & Weakland, J. (1956). Toward a theory of schizophrenia. *Behavioral Science, 1,* 251–264.

Bernheim, K. F., & Lehman, A. F. (1985). *Working with families of the mentally ill*. New York: Norton.

Biegel, D. E., Milligan, S. E., Putnam, P. L., & Song, L. Y. (1994). Predictors of burden among lower socioeconomic status caregivers of persons with chronic mental illness. *Community Mental Health Journal, 30,* 473–494.

Brekke, J. S., & Mathiesen, S. G. (1995). Effects of parental involvement on the functioning of noninstitutionalized adults with schizophrenia. *Psychiatric Services, 46,* 1149–1155.

Brown, G. W., Birley, J. L. T., & Wing, J. K. (1972). Influence of family life on the course of schizophrenic disorders: A replication. *British Journal of Psychiatry, 121,* 241–258.

Camasso, M. J., & Geismar, L. L. (1992). A multivariate approach to construct reliability and validity assessment: The case of family functioning. *Social Work Research and Abstracts, 28* (4), 16–26.

Carter, D. E., & Newman, F. L. (1976). *A client-oriented system of mental health service delivery and program management: A workbook and guide*. Washington, DC: National Institute of Mental Health.

Dixon, L., McFarlane, W. R., Lefley, H., Lucksted, A., Cohen, M., Falloon, I., Mueser, K., Miklowitz, D., Solomon, P., & Sondheimer, D. (2001). Evidence-based practices for services to families of people with psychiatric disabilities. *Psychiatric Services, 52,* 903–910.

Dworkin, R. J. (1992). *Researching persons with mental illness*. Newbury Park, CA: Sage.

Dyck, D. G., Hendryx, M. S., Short, R. A., Voss, W. D., & McFarlane, W. R. (2002). Service use among patients with schizophrenia in psychoeducational multiple-family group treatment. *Psychiatric Services, 53,* 749–754.

Ell, K. (1996). Social networks, social support, and coping with serious illness: The family connection. *Social Science and Medicine, 42,* 173–183.

Geismar, L. L. (1980). *Family and community functioning* (2nd ed.). Metuchen, NJ: Scarecrow Press.

Goldstein, M. J. (1987). Psychosocial issues. *Schizophrenia Bulletin, 13,* 157–171.

Goldstein, M. J., & Miklowitz, D. J. (1995). The effectiveness of psychoeducational family therapy in the treatment of schizophrenic disorders. *Journal of Marital and Family Therapy, 21,* 361–376.

Grob, G. N. (1987). The forging of mental health policy in America: World War II to new frontier. *Journal of the History of Medicine and Allied Sciences, 43,* 410–446.

Hatfield, A. B. (1991). The national alliance for the mentally ill: A decade later. *Community Mental Health Journal, 27,* 95–103.

Hatfield, A. B., & Lefley, H. P. (Eds.). (1987). *Families of the mentally ill: Coping and adaptation*. New York: Guilford Press.

Hill, R. (1949). *Families under stress*. New York: Harper and Row.

Johnson, E. D. (1998). The effect of family functioning and family sense of competence on people with mental illness. *Family Relations, 47,* 443–451.

Johnson, E. D. (2001). The partnership model: Working with families of people with serious mental illness. In M. MacFarlane (Ed.), *Family therapy and mental health: Innovations in theory and practice* (pp. 27–53). New York: Haworth Press.

Johnson, E. D. (2003a). The "Level of Adaptation Index for Persons with Serious Mental Illness": The development and psychometric properties of an index assessing the functional adaptation of people with serious mental illness living in the community. In submission.

Johnson, E. D. (2003b). The "Family Sense of Competence Index": The development and psychometric properties of an index for assessing family adaptation to chronic illness. In submission.

Kanter, J., Lamb, H. R., & Loeper, C. (1987). Expressed emotion in families: A critical review. *Hospital and Community Psychiatry, 38*, 374–380.

Kobasa, S. C. (1979). Stressful life events, personality, and health: An inquiry into hardiness. *Journal of Personality and Social Psychology, 37*, 1–11.

Kobasa, S. C., Maddi, S. R., & Courington, S. (1981). Personality and constitution as mediators in the stress-illness relationship. *Journal of Health and Social Behavior, 22*, 368–378.

Lefley, H. P. (1992). Expressed emotion: Conceptual, clinical, and social policy issues. *Hospital and Community Psychiatry, 43*, 591–598.

Lefley, H. P. (1996). *Family caregiving in mental illness.* Thousand Oaks, CA: Sage.

Manderscheid, R. W., & Sonnenschein, M. A. (Eds.). (1997). *Mental health, United States, 1996.* Washington, DC: Substance Abuse and Mental Health Services Administration, U.S. Department of Health and Human Services.

Marks, N. F. (1996). Caregiving across the lifespan: National prevalence and predictors. *Family Relations, 45*, 27–36.

Marsh, D. T. (2001). *A family-focused approach to serious mental illness: Empirically supported interventions.* Sarasota, FL: Professional Resource Press.

Marsh, D. T., Lefley, H. P., Evans-Rhodes, D., Ansell, V. I., Doerzbacher, B. M., LaBarbera, L., & Paluzzi, J. E. (1996). The family experience of mental illness: Evidence of resilience. *Psychiatric Rehabilitation Journal, 20*, 3–12.

Mattlin, J. A., Wethington, E., & Kessler, R. C. (1990). Situational determinants of coping and coping effectiveness. *Journal of Health and Social Behavior, 31*, 103–122.

McCubbin, H. I., & McCubbin, M. A. (1988). Typologies of resilient families: Emerging roles of social class and ethnicity. *Family Relations, 37*, 247–254.

McCubbin, H. I., & Patterson, J. M. (1983). The family stress process: The double ABCX model of adjustment and adaptation. In H. I. McCubbin, M. B. Sussman, & J. M. Patterson (Eds.), *Social stress and the family* (pp. 7–38). New York: Haworth Press.

McCubbin, H. I., Thompson, E. A., Thompson, A. I., & Fromer, J. E., (Eds.). (1998). *Stress, coping, and health in families.* Thousand Oaks, CA: Sage.

McFarlane, W. R., Link, B., Dushay, R., Marchal, J., & Crilly, J. (1995). Psychoeducational multiple family groups: Four-year relapse outcome in schizophrenia. *Family Process, 34*, 127–144.

Meissner, W. W. (1970). Thinking about the family: Psychiatric aspects. In N. W. Ackerman (Ed.), *Family process* (pp. 131–170). New York: Basic Books.

Miklowitz, D. J., Goldstein, M. J., Doane, J. A., Nuechterlein, K. H., Strachan, A. M., Snyder, K. S., & Magana-Amato, A. (1989). Is expressed emotion an index of a transactional process? I. Parents' affective style. *Family Process, 28*, 153–168.

Miklowitz, D. J., & Hooley, J. M. (1998). Developing family psychoeducational treatments for patients with bipolar and other severe psychiatric disorders. *Journal of Marital and Family Therapy, 24*, 419–435.

Milstein, G., Guarnaccia, P. J., & Midlarsky, E. (1995). Ethnic differences in the interpretation of mental illness: Perspectives of caregivers. *Research in Community and Mental Health, 8*, 155–178.

Mueser, K. T., Corrigan, P. W., Hilton, D. W., Tanzman, B., Schaub, A., Gingerich, S., Essock, S. M., Tarrier, N., Morey, B., Vogel-Scibilia, S., & Herz, M. I. (2002). Illness management and recovery: A review of the research. *Psychiatric Services, 53*, 1272–1284.

Olson, D. H. (1986). Circumplex model VII: Validation studies and FACES III. *Family Process, 25*, 337–351.

Olson, D. H., McCubbin, H. I., Barnes, H., Larsen, A., Muxen, M., &. Wilson, M. (1985). *Family inventories* (Rev. ed.). St. Paul, MN: Family Social Science, University of Minnesota.

Patterson, J. M. (1989). The family stress model: The family adjustment and adaptation response. In C. N. Ramsey (Ed.), *Family systems in medicine* (pp. 95–118). New York: Guilford Press.

Pinsoff, W., & Wynn, L. (Eds.). (2000). *Family therapy effectiveness: Current research and theory.* Washington, DC: American Association for Marriage and Family Therapy.

Pitschel-Walz, G., Leucht, S., Bauml, J., Kissling, W., & Engel, R. (2001). The effect of family interventions on relapse and rehospitalization in schizophrenia: A meta-analysis. *Schizophrenia Bulletin, 27*, 73–92.

Rosenberg, M., Schooler, C., Schoenbach, C., & Rosenberg, F. (1995). Global self-esteem and specific self-esteem: Different concepts, different outcomes. *American Sociological Review, 60*, 141–156.

Ross, C. E., Mirowsky, J., & Goldstein, K. (1990). The impact of the family on health: The decade in review. *Journal of Marriage and the Family, 52*, 1059–1078.

Solomon, P., & Draine, J. (1995). Subjective burden among family members of mentally ill adults:

Relation to stress, coping, and adaptation. *American Journal of Orthopsychiatry, 65,* 419–427.

Spaniol, L., Zipple, A. M., & Lockwood, D. (1992). The role of the family in psychiatric rehabilitation. *Schizophrenia Bulletin, 18,* 341–347.

Turner, R. J., & Lloyd, D. A. (1995). Lifetime traumas and mental health: The significance of cumulative adversity. *Journal of Health and Social Behavior, 36,* 360–376.

Vaughn, C. E., & Leff, J. P. (1981). Patterns of emotional response in relatives of schizophrenic patients. *Schizophrenia Bulletin, 7,* 43–44.

Walsh, F. (1996). The concept of family resilience: Crisis and challenge. *Family Process, 35,* 261–281.

Wing, J. K. (1978). Social influences on the course of schizophrenia. In L. C. Wynne, R. L. Cromwell, & S. Matthysse (Eds.), *The nature of schizophrenia: New approaches to research and treatment* (pp. 599–616). New York: Wiley.

Wynne, L. C., & Singer, M. T. (1963). Thought disorder and family relations of schizophrenics. *Archives of General Psychiatry, 9,* 191–206.

Zubin, J. (1986). Models for the aetiology of schizophrenia. In G. D. Burrows, T. R. Norman, & G. Rubinstein (Eds.), *Handbook of studies on schizophrenia. Part I: Epidemiology, aetiology and clinical features* (pp. 97–104). New York: Elsevier Science.

COGNITIVE REHABILITATION AND NEURONAL PLASTICITY

95 *Research on the Effectiveness of Quantitative EEG Biofeedback*

Kirtley Thornton

The rehabilitation and understanding of brain function has been the focus of academic and federal research for decades. Significant advances in the understanding of neuronal plasticity and the retraining of damaged neurons in the brain have been made in the past decade as a result of practice-based research. These developments have led to significantly greater progress in the improvement of cognitive function than had previously been obtained with improvements in auditory memory functioning in learning disabled children, averaging 378% after only 20 hours of treatment.

The population addressed by these efforts includes special education students, brain-damaged subjects, and aging patients. The federal government has spent $350 billion over a 20-year period on special education programs (U.S. Department of Education), which were designed to improve the cognitive functioning of the special education child. According to the Brain Injury Association of America, millions of dollars have been spent on cognitive rehabilitation intervention programs, which are directed toward the 5.3 million individuals who have experienced a brain trauma due to car accidents, falls, strokes, and so forth.

Assessment precedes rehabilitation, because improvement cannot be measured unless there is a pretreatment measure. The initial assessment impetus was from the outside of the brain and employed neuropsychological and educational measures, which focus on ability and achievement levels. A more recent approach has focused on the inside—the physical parameters of brain function such as blood flow, electrical activity, oxygen consumption, and a host of other modern medical diagnostic techniques. The most recent direction of the research has begun to bring these two areas together and has examined the relationship between cognitive function and the physical response of the brain— the classic mind-body problem. This new focus will become the future of the research in this area.

There are two main subject populations in the rehabilitation area. The first is the special education child. Interventions have employed psychoeducational methods, such as the Orton-Gillingham method, phonics training, stimulation programs, and direct instruction. These programs, by and large, have produced limited changes in achievement levels and no changes in basic abilities, but they continue to be used on a widespread basis. The second is the brain-injured subject, for whom interventions have employed cognitive rehabilitation. These programs have used cognitive exercises and strategy-based and computer-based rehabilitation programs and have also produced disappointing results. The current chapter focuses on the application of quantitative EEG (QEEG) biofeedback, resulting in improved neuropsychological functioning. Thornton's patent, when used with brain-injured clients, usually changes the value of deficient EEG signals for particular cognitive tasks. Follow-up studies 1 month and 12 months after QEEG biofeedback treatment seem to confirm the positive outcomes with this innovative approach.

INDIRECT METHODS

Fast-Forward Research

One of the few studies that attempted to relate psychoeducational interventions to physical measurements is that by Temple et al. (2003), who studied 20 dyslexic children aged 8 to 12 years. Their subjects' brains were scanned (while the subjects performed a simple rhyming task) using functional magnetic resonance imaging (fMRI) before and after participation in the 8-week training program focusing on auditory processing and oral language training. A control group of 12 children with normal reading abilities also had their brains scanned but did not participate in the training. The treatment group showed increased activity in multiple areas (left temporoparietal cortex and left inferior frontal gyrus), which corresponded to increases in oral language ability. The training employed the fast-forward computer program for an average of thirty 84-minute sessions grouped in periods of 100 minutes a day for 28 days. Significant improvements were noted in word identification, word attack, and passage comprehension, as well as language measures of receptive and expressive speech and rapid naming. Long-term follow-up of the subjects has not been completed to date.

Cognitive Rehabilitation

Cognitive rehabilitation for memory disorders has focused with different methods of interventions on different groups of patients and has obtained variable results. Specific techniques such as method of loci, cognitive strategies, and visualization have shown different degrees of effectiveness. Researchers have noted that these methods face the problem of continuation of the approach by the subject. Franzen and Haut's (1991) review concluded that it may be possible to positively intervene, but our confidence in such a statement should be tempered with caution. The researchers focused on the methodological problems in the research literature.

Lack of success in memory improvement has been documented by Van Dam, Brinkerink-Carlier, and Kok (1986; $N = 108$), who obtained no significant effect using visual and verbal embellishment techniques. Ryan and Ruff (1988) obtained an average improvement of 2% to 5% after treatment, and their control group improved equally. Steingass, Bobring, Burgart, Sartory, and Schugens (1994) employed an 18-

session memory and attention program to improve memory functioning in recovering alcoholics and found no difference between the experimental and control groups.

Strategy Training

The more successful interventions have employed strategies to obtain their results. Best, Hamlett, & Davis (1992) demonstrated with a group of elderly subjects the effect of strategy training (visualizing, mnemonics; 9 $N = 55$, mean age of 82) and found increases on higher prose (immediate recall, 38%; delayed recall, 77%). Grafman (1984) employed the PQRST technique (preview, question, read, study, test) with subjects with brain injury and was able to obtain improvement in 40% of the patients on 50% of the 14 memory tests employed.

Berg, Koning-Haanstra, and Deelman (1991), in a long-term follow-up study, employed a strategy training, drill, and practice and obtained a positive effect on objective memory measures at 4-month follow-up, although there was no sustained effect at 4 years. Wilson (1991; $N = 43$) studied the long-term improvement of memory in severe memory disorders. About 30% of the subjects showed an improvement in memory as assessed by a standardized measure. A small number had deteriorated, and 60% showed little or no change after leaving the rehabilitation clinic (5 to 10 years later). About 88% of the subjects admitted to still having memory problems.

Malec and Questad (1983) reported in a single case study the improvement of prose memory (logical memory of Wechsler Memory Scale) in a brain-injured individual. The subjects underwent approximately 50 sessions of training in visual imagery and semantic elaboration in a word recall task. Generalization to the logical memory task indicated a 53% improvement on short-term recall and 15% improvement on long-term recall.

DIRECT METHODS

Stimulation

Direct methods, which rely on physical interventions to change the underlying physical response of the brain, include increasing blood flow, changing electrical patterns, and direct physical stimulation of the brain. Hayes, Warrier, Nichol, Zecker, & Kraus (2003) have demonstrated that a physical intervention with commercially available programs can improve cortical processing of auditory information and behavioral improvement effects. The study examined children aged 8 to 12 and provided 8 weeks of training consisting of 35 to 40 one-hour sessions. The findings argue for the plasticity of cortical areas and demonstrate genuine changes in cortical responses to sounds with training.

EEG Biofeedback: Operant Conditioning

The most impressive results have been obtained with an operant conditioning approach to the electrophysiology of the brain. During the past two decades the digitization and quantification of the classical analog EEG signal have allowed researchers to expand their knowledge of the functional operation of the brain. Classical operant conditioning methodology (reward-inhibit of spontaneous behavior) has been successfully employed in terms of changing the electrical patterns.

The EEG signal is divided into four bandwidths, which reflect the number of sine waves per second (or hertz). Present definitions of bandwidths include delta (0–4 Hz), theta (4–8 Hz), alpha (8–13 Hz), and beta (anything greater than 13 Hz). A visual representation of these waveforms is presented in Figure 95.1. Developmentally, delta and theta decrease in amplitudes, whereas alpha and beta increase. Beta is associated with an active, thinking brain; alpha, with a relaxed brain; theta and delta, with an inactive brain. The standard 10–20 system places the electrodes in standard locations on the head (Figure 95.2). Once the EEG signal has been digitized and the information stored on a hard disk, a number of variables can be mathematically generated, analyzed, and compared with a normative reference group for different conditions (eyes closed, activation conditions). There are two general classes of variables. The first involves the type of activity at a particular location and can include the magnitude of a particular frequency across a period of time (an epoch), relative power of a frequency (total microvolts of a particular frequency divided by the total microvolts produced at a location), and others such as peak frequency, peak amplitude, and sym-

Beta

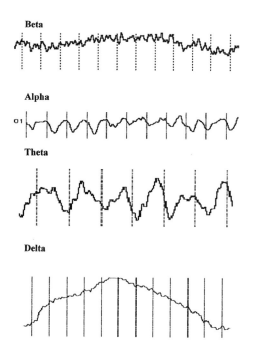

Alpha

o1

Theta

Delta

FIGURE 95.1 Bandwidths.

metry. The second class involves the connection patterns between two locations, and are designated as coherence and phase and mathematically represented as numerical values between 0 and 100. Figure 95.3 presents a visual example of the coherence relationships. Figure 95.4 presents a visual example of the phase relationship. Phase is calculated during the first milliseconds of the recording of an epoch and ceases when an amplitude match is obtained.

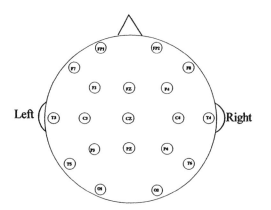

FIGURE 95.2 Standard nomenclature for positions in the 10–20 system.

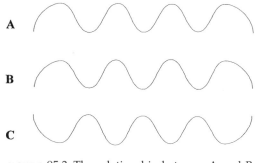

A

B

C

FIGURE 95.3 The relationship between A and B present a high-coherence relationship. The relationship between B and C presents a low-coherence relationship.

Classical databases have focused on obtaining norms for the eyes-closed condition (Thatcher, Krause, & Hrybyk, 1986) and have yielded high discriminant values (.90 and above) in differentiating normal individuals from brain-injured individuals in three cross-validation samples (Thatcher, Walker, Gerson, & Geisler, 1989).

Discriminant analysis with QEEG variables has yielded impressive results. For dyslexic and normal readers the theta activity in the temporal lobes was the main discriminating variable between the two groups (Galin et al., 1992). Children with a poor or very poor educational evaluation had more delta in left frontal and temporal areas (F3, F7, and T3; Harmony et al., 1990). A discriminant analysis using the theta values showed 85% correct classification in the children with attention deficit disorder (ADD)

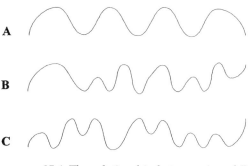

A

B

C

FIGURE 95.4 The relationship between A and B represents a high-phase relationship. The relationship between B and C represents a low-phase relationship. Phase is calculated according to when an amplitude match is obtained.

Listen to Paragraphs

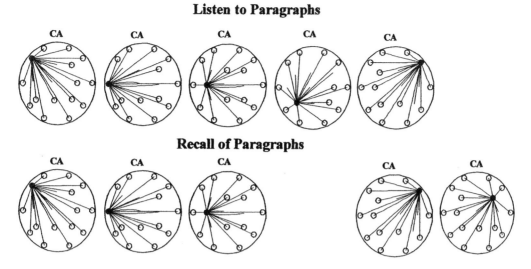

FIGURE 95.5 Relationship between QEEG variables and recall ability during input and immediate silent recall conditions (CA-coherence alpha).

and 78% in children with a good evaluation (Chabot, Merkin, Wood, Davenport, and Serfontein, 1996). EEG abnormalities have been found to predict later delinquency (Mednick, 1981) and have been found in delinquent adults (Williams, 1969).

Several rehabilitation efforts (Lubar & Lubar, 1984; Tansey, 1991; Othmer & Othmer, 1992; Linden, 1996; Thompson & Thompson, 1998) have been directed toward the specific clinical problems of ADD and learning disability. The results have indicated improvement in cognitive functioning in terms of IQ scores (average of 15 points) and school performance (as well as attitudinal and behavioral changes). However, the specific link between successful cognitive task performance and QEEG variables is inferred from the improvement and not demonstrated empirically. The locations employed have focused predominantly on the C3-Cz positions (sensorimotor strip), have augmented beta magnitude activity (13–21 Hz), and have inhibited theta magnitude activity (4–8 Hz) under nontask conditions. Improvements were noted in social interaction, decreased use of medication, and improvement in academic functioning and on standardized tests. The total sample size for the four studies was 155. Tansey (1993) documented stability of EEG functioning and academic functioning in a 10-year follow-up of a boy who was classified as hyperactive/perceptually impaired.

Lubar demonstrated stability of gains in a 10-year follow-up study (Lubar, Swartwood, Swartwood, & Timmerman, 1995).

Thornton investigated the QEEG correlates of 18 cognitive tasks to understand the relationship between neuropsychological functioning and the QEEG variables under activation conditions. A normative database for auditory memory was developed, and the QEEG variables that correlated with successful auditory memory were identified (Thornton 2000). Figure 95.5 presents the variables (measured at time of input and immediate 30-second silent recall) that correlated with subsequent total auditory recall ability (combination of immediate and 30-minute delayed recall scores; $N = 57$ adults over age 14). In the figures a solid black circle represents a site of origin of a generator for that frequency. This method of generator analysis was employed for statistical and conceptual reasons. A generator is analogous to a flashlight beam spreading its frequency to the other brain locations. An examination of the figures indicates that successful recall is correlated with almost the same variables (coherence alpha) during the input as during the immediate recall condition, with the exception of the right frontal (F4) location (immediate recall) and left posterior (P3) location (input stage).

The role of the right frontal location in recall had previously been argued to be important to the hemispheric encoding/retrieval asymmetry

(HERA) pattern model (Tulving, Markowitsch, Fergus, Craik, & Houle, 1996), which asserts that the "right frontal lobes are more involved than left in episodic memory retrieval" (p. 71). The QEEG variables in this study confirm this assertion but also underscore the importance of left hemisphere coherence alpha activity. Mazoyer et al. (1993) had previously demonstrated in a positron emission tomography (PET; blood flow) study the important role of the T3 and F7 location in the storage of auditory information. The QEEG variables represent a validation of these results from a different physical measurement. The combination of the PET studies and Thornton's (2000) QEEG study presents an integration of neuropsychology, neuroanatomy, the QEEG, and cognitive neuroscience in developing a complete understanding of the functioning of auditory memory.

The development of the database and knowledge of the effective QEEG parameters of a cognitive function allow for an evaluation of an individual to indicate exactly which electrophysiological variable is not functioning within the normal range. Once this information is obtained, it is a relatively easy matter to design protocols that attempt to change the value of the deficient EEG signal for a particular cognitive task. Thornton (2000c, 2002d) has employed this approach with learning disabled, brain-injured (structurally damaged [hematoma, stereotaxic surgery on left temporal lobe] and nonstructurally damaged) individuals and a normal population ($N = 10$) for auditory memory tasks and obtained results averaging around 100% for these groups. An important change from previous interventions is the addition of training under relevant task conditions. For example, a subject who demonstrates deficit coherence alpha values during auditory memory tasks is trained during auditory memory conditions (i.e., listening to audiotapes). The control group ($N = 15$) did not demonstrate any significant gains in memory. It is important to note that not only did the memory abilities improve but the relevant electrophysiological variable remained improved in the subjects retested from 1 month to 1 year later, thus indicating both stability of results and relevance of the QEEG variable.

Unpublished data with nine learning disabled subjects have indicated an average improvement of 378% in auditory memory abilities (average of thirty to forty 30-minute sessions) and generalization of improvements to reading memory of 250% in one learning disabled child. Additional auditory memory improvements of 110% ($N = 7$) with brain injuries occurring during auto accidents, 63% ($N = 2$) with structural damage to the brain (hematomas, stereotaxic surgery of left temporal lobe), and 130% ($N = 3$) with normal subjects (no history of brain injury, learning problems) have also been obtained. Generalization of improvement in cognitive function is an important consideration in any rehabilitation program. Thornton's modification of the standard EEG biofeedback protocol has been able to demonstrate generalization to auditory memory of 110% even when reading memory issues were addressed in one brain-injured subject. In a reading disabled subject, left posterior beta activity was the focus of the interventions for thirty 30-minute sessions. Follow-up evaluation (6 months post-treatment) on a standardized computerized achievement and aptitude battery (with reported minimal practice effects) indicated increases of grade levels of 5.2 in reading comprehension, 5.3 in science, 6.4 in social studies, and 2.4 in reading. On nationally standardized testing (CT, 1 year post-treatment) there were increases in grade levels of 3.7 in language expression, 6.1 in math computation, 2.4 in math concepts and applications, and 2.1 in study skills. Thus improvement of a specific electrophysiological variable may have diffuse cognitive effects.

The 18 cognitive tasks involved in the original research included visual and auditory attention, eyes closed, memory for auditory information (paragraphs and word lists), reading material, visual information, names of faces, and autobiographical information. Additional cognitive tasks involved abilities for spelling, mathematics (multiplication, internal spatial addition of two-digit numbers), pronunciation of nonsense words, problem solving (Raven's matrices), visualization, a "to-do" list, where objects are located, and the emotions of love, happiness, and sadness. The identification of the electrophysiological correlates of the emotional states may allow for effective interventions for emotional disorders with the EEG biofeedback. In addition to the critical difference from previous research in this area of employing activation conditions, the frequency range of the data collected was extended from the traditional 32 Hz to 64 Hz. Previously the frequencies above 32 Hz had generally been considered muscle artifact, except for references to the gamma band

(40 Hz). The inclusion of this frequency range resulted in a number of significant and relevant findings for many of the cognitive tasks. In particular, it appears to be the critically affected bandwidth in the brain-injured individual (Thornton, 2002a).

Published articles in peer-reviewed journals have addressed visual memory (Thornton, 2002b), reading memory (Thornton, 2002c), why the brain-damaged subject cannot recall auditory information (Thornton, 2002a), and discriminating between normal and brain-injured individuals under both the eyes-closed (Thornton, 1999) and activation conditions (Thornton, 2000b).

The change in approach of improving cognitive functioning from the outside with psychoeducational methods to the inside with direct interventions on the physical functioning of the brain represents a paradigm shift in the field and potentially could change how the present educational system functions.

References

Berg, I. J., Koning-Haanstra, M., & Deelman, B. G. (1991). Long-term effects of memory rehabilitation: A controlled study. *Neuropsychological Rehabilitation, 1* (2), 97–111.

Best, D. L., Hamlett, K. W., & Davis, S. W. (1992). Memory complaint and memory performance in the elderly: The effects of memory-skills training and expectancy change. *Applied Cognitive Psychology, 6,* 405–417.

Birsh, J. (1999). *Multisensory teaching of basic language skills.* Baltimore: Brookes.

Brody, N. (1992). *Intelligence.* San Diego, CA: Academic Press.

Chabot, R. J., Merkin, H., Wood, L. M., Davenport, T. L., & Serfontein, G. (1996). Sensitivity and specificity of QEEG in children with attention deficit or specific developmental learning disorders. *Clinical Electroencephalography, 27,* 26–33.

Clark, A. (1988). *Dyslexia: Theory and practice of remedial instruction.* Timonium, MD: York Press.

Foorman, B. R., Francis, D. J., Winikates, D., Mehta, P., Schatschneider, C., & Fletcher, J. M. (1997). Early interventions for children with reading disabilities. *Scientific Studies of Reading, 1,* 255–276.

Franzen, M.D., & Haut, M. W. (1991). The psychological treatment of memory impairment: A review of empirical studies. *Neuropsychological Review, 2,* 29–63.

Galin, D., Raz, J., Fein, G., Johnstone, J., Herron, J., & Yingling, C. (1992). EEG spectra in dyslexic and normal readers during oral and silent reading. *Electroencephalography and Clinical Neurophysiology, 82,* 87–101.

Glisky, E. L., & Schacter, D. (1986). Remediation of organic memory disorders: Current status and future prospects. *Journal of Head Trauma Rehabilitation, 1* (3), 54–63.

Grafman, J. (1984). Memory assessment and remediation in brain-injured patients: From theory to practice. In B. A. Edelstein & E. T. Couture (eds.), *Behavioral assessment and treatment of the traumatically brain-damaged* (pp. 151–189). New York: Plenum.

Hardt, J. V, & Kamiya, J. (1978). Anxiety change through EEG alpha feedback seen only in high anxiety subjects. *Science, 201,* 79–81.

Harmony, T., Hinojosa, G., Marosi, E., Becker, J., Rodriguez, M., Reyes, A., & Rocha, C. (1990). Correlation between EEG spectral parameters and an educational evaluation. *International Journal of Neuroscience, 54,* 147–155.

Hayes, E. A., Warrier, C. M., Nichol, T. G., Zecker, S. G., & Kraus, N. (2003). Neural plasticity following auditory training in children with learning problems. *Clinical Neurophysiology,* In press, 1–12.

Linden, M., Habib, T., & Radojevic, V. (1996). A controlled study of the effects of EEG biofeedback on cognition and behavior of children with attention deficit disorder and learning disabilities. *Biofeedback and Self Regulation, 21* (1).

Lubar, J. F., Swartwood, M. O., Swartwood, J. N., & Timmerman, D. L. (1995). Quantitative EEG and auditory even-related potentials in the evaluation of attention deficit/hyperactivity disorder: Effects of methylphenidate and implications of neurofeedback training. *Journal of Psychoeducational Assessment.* (Monograph Series Advances in Psychoeducational Assessment) Assessment of Attention Deficit/Hyperactivity Disorders, 143–204.

Lubar, J. O., & Lubar, J. F. (1984). Electroencephalographic biofeedback of SMR and beta for treatment of attention deficit disorders in a clinical setting. *Biofeedback and Self-Regulation, 9* (1), 1–23.

Lyon, G. R., & Moats, L. C. (1988). Critical issues in the instruction of learning disabled. *Journal of Consulting and Clinical Psychology, 56,* 830–835.

Malec, J., & Questad, K. (1983). Rehabilitation of memory after craniocerebral trauma: A case report. *Arch. Phys Med Rehabil, 64,* 436–438.

Mazoyer, B. M., Tzourio, N., Frank, V., Syrota, A., Murayama, N., Levrier, O., Salamon, G., Dehaene, S., Cohen, L., & Mehler, J. (1993). The cortical representation of speech. *Journal of Cognitive Neuroscience, 5,* 467–479.

McKinlay, W. W. (1992). Achieving generalization of memory training. *Brain Injury, 6,* 107–112.

Mednick, S. (1981). EEG predicts later delinquency. *Criminology, 19*, 219–229.

Oakland, T., Black, J., et al. (1998). An evaluation of the dyslexia training program: A multisensory method for promoting reading in students with reading disabilities. *Journal of Learning Disabilities, 31*, 140–150.

Olson, R. K, Wise, B., Ring, J., & Johnson, M. (1997). Computer based remedial training in phoneme awareness and phonological decoding: Effects on the posttraining development of word recognition. *Scientific Studies of Reading, 1*, 235–253.

Othmer, S., & Othmer, S. F. (1992). EEG biofeedback training for hyperactivity, attention deficit disorder, specific learning disability, and other disorders. Handout. EEG Spectrum 16100 Ventura Blvd., Ste 100, Encino, CA.

Ryan, T. V., & Ruff, R. M. (1988). The efficacy of structure memory retraining in a group comparison of head trauma patients. *Archives of Clinical Neuropsychology, 3*, 165–179.

Steingass, H. P., Bobring, K. H., Burgart, F., Sartory, G., & Schugens, M. (1994). Memory training in alcoholics. *Neuropsychological Rehabilitation, 4*, 49–63.

Tansey, M. (1993). Ten year stability of EEG biofeedback results for a 10 year old hyperactive boy who failed in a class for the perceptually impaired. *Biofeedback and Self-Regulation, 18*, 33–44.

Tansey, M. Wechsler (WISC-R). (1991). Changes following treatment of learning disabilities via EEG biofeedback training in a private practice setting. *Australian Journal of Psychology, 43*, 147–153.

Temple, E., Deutsch, G. K, Poldrack, R. A., Miller, S. L, Merzenich, M. M., & Gabrieli, J. D. (2003). Neural deficits in children with dyslexia ameliorated by behavioral remediation: Evidence from functional MRI. *Proc. Natl. Acad. Sci. USA, 100*, 2860–2865.

Thatcher, R. W., Krause, P. J., & Hrybyk, M. (1986). Cortico-cortical associations and EEG coherence: A two-compartmental model. *Electroencephalography and Clinical Neurophysiology*, 123–143.

Thatcher, R. W., Walker, R. A., Gerson, I., & Geisler, F. H. (1989). EEG discriminant analysis of mild head trauma. *Electroencephalography and Clinical Neurophysiology, 73*, 94–10.

Thompson, L., & Thompson, M. (1998). Neurofeedback combined with training in metacognitive strategies: Effectiveness in students with ADD. *Applied Psychophysiology and Biofeedback, 23*, 243–263.

Thornton, K. (1999). Exploratory investigation into mild brain injury and discriminant analysis with high frequency bands (32–64 Hz). *Brain Injury, 13*, 477–484.

Thornton, K. (2000a). Electrophysiology of auditory memory of paragraphs. *Journal of Neurotherapy, 4* (3), 45–72.

Thornton, K. (2000b). Exploratory analysis: Mild head injury, discriminant analysis with high frequency bands (32–64 Hz) under attentional activation conditions and does time heal? *Journal of Neurotherapy, 3* (3–4), 1–11.

Thornton, K. (2000c). Improvement/rehabilitation of memory functioning in brain injured subjects with neurotherapy/EEG biofeedback. *Journal of Head Trauma Rehabilitation, 15*, 1285–1296.

Thornton, K. (2002a). Electrophysiology of the reasons the brain damaged subject can't recall what they hear. *Archives of Clinical Neuropsychology, 17*, 1–17.

Thornton, K. (2002b). Electrophysiology of visual memory for Korean characters. *Current Psychology, 21*, 85–108.

Thornton, K. (2002c). Electrophysiology (QEEG) of effective reading memory: Towards a generator/activation theory of the mind. *Journal of Neurotherapy, 6*(3), 37–66.

Thornton, K. (2002d). Rehabilitation of memory functioning with EEG biofeedback. *Neurorehabilitation, 17* (1), 69–81.

Tulving, E., Markowitsch, H. J., Fergus, I. M., Craik, R. H., & Houle, S. (1996). Novelty and familiarity activations in pet studies of memory encoding and retrieval. *Cerebral Cortex, 6* (1), 71–79.

Van Dam, G., Brinkerink-Carlier, M., & Kok, I. (1986). Influence of visual and verbal embellishment on free recall of the paragraphs of a text. *American Journal of Psychology, 99*, 103–110.

Van Den Bos, L., Siegel, D. Bakker, D., & Share. (1994). *Current directions in dyslexia research.* Lisse: Swets and Zeitlinger.

Williams, D. (1969). Neural factors related to habitual aggression: Consideration of differences between those habitual aggressive and others who have committed crimes of violence. *Brain, 92*, 503–520.

Wilson, B. (1991). Long-term prognosis of patients with severe memory disorders. *Neuropsychological Rehabilitation, 1*, 117–134.

SECTION X

Establishing, Monitoring, and Maintaining Quality and Operational Improvement

96 FRAMEWORK FOR INSTITUTIONALIZING QUALITY ASSURANCE

Diana R. Silimperi, Tisna Veldhuyzen van Zanten, & Lynne Miller Franco

THE IMPORTANCE OF INSTITUTIONALIZING QUALITY ASSURANCE IN HEALTH CARE PRACTICE

The quest for quality of health care services has become a focal point for many health care systems, fueled in part by growing costs of medical care, concerns about medical safety, issues of choice and access to services for different population groups, and patient satisfaction. No longer is there a need to convince policymakers and health professionals about the importance of quality health care. In fact, in some developing countries, health sector reforms are mandating measures to improve the quality of health care through performance contracts that include patient satisfaction and quality measurements, or regulatory mechanisms such as accreditation (Pan American Health Organization and Quality Assurance Project (draft 2003). Our experience in a wide range of health care organizations and countries has often shown that the critical question is not so much a technical one—how to do quality improvement activities—but rather how to establish and maintain quality assurance (QA) as an integral, sustainable part of a health care practice or system.

The QA Project[1] developed a framework for the institutionalization of QA based on more than 10 years of experience in developing countries and a review of the literature in organizational development and sustainability (Baldridge National Quality Program, 2001; Bartleson et al., 1998; Brown, 1995; Gnecco, 1999; Hermida, 1999; Jennings et al., 1994; Kinney et al., 1997; O'Malley, 1998; Øvretveit, 1994; Penland, 1997; Powell, 1995; Preston et al., 1995; Renzi, 1996; Shortell et al., 1998; Shortell et al., 1998; Wagner et al., 1997). This framework is both a conceptual model and an operational tool to help health care practices improve and sustain quality health care. It combines the key components of QA with a clear delineation of the essential elements and the process of institutionalization (Franco et al., 2002; Massoud et al., 2001; Silimperi et al., 2002). The framework contains, at its core, three functional QA activities: defining quality, measuring quality, and improving quality. Thus, it underscores the importance of building ongoing measurement and assessment in a health care practice, to measure improvement as well as to monitor the development of QA elements needed to sustain QA systems in the organization. The framework can be applied at both the macrolevel (health systems) and microlevel (individual facility or practice). This chapter describes the essential elements as well as the process needed to institutionalize QA in a health practice or system. Case examples from developing counties are included to illustrate how the framework can be used. The chapter concludes with a discussion about the utilization of the framework to institutionalize specific quality improvements, as well as a quality improvement approach such as a learning collaborative in a health practice or organization.

CORE QA ACTIVITIES: THE QA TRIANGLE

The QA Project's approach to achieving quality health care services encompasses three core QA activities or functions (see Figure 96.1): defining quality, measuring quality, and improving quality. (To stress the central theme of quality, the abbreviations of core activities in the QA Triangle start with Q and are followed by the action: Defining quality is QD, measuring quality is QM, and improving quality is QI.) These three activities work synergistically to ensure quality care as an outcome of the system, and together they encompass a range of mutually supportive QA methodologies and techniques. Although one may focus quality efforts in a core activity area, in fact, no core activity is sufficient on its own to improve and maintain quality. It is the interaction and synergy of all three that facilitate and sustain quality health care. Each core activity encompasses a group of interrelated activities.

Defining Quality

QD includes actions to define quality, the development of expectations or standards of quality, as well as designing systems for quality. As seen in Table 96.1, standards can be developed

TABLE 96.1 Taxonomy of Health System Standards

System Components	Categories	
	Administrative	Technical
Input	Administrative policies Rules and regulations Qualifications*	Job descriptions* Specifications*
Process	Standard operating procedures	Algorithms Clinical pathways Clinical practice guidelines Procedures Protocols Standing orders
Outcome	Expected results*	Health outcomes

*Can be found in either category.
Source: Ashton, 2001b.

for inputs, processes, or outcomes; they may be clinical or administrative (Ashton, 2001b). A good standard is reliable, realistic, valid, clear, and measurable. It is best to make standards explicit to assure that all practitioners are operating with the same expectations of care. Clinical practice guidelines (e.g., for treatment of pregnancy-induced hypertension, or for integrated case management of common childhood illnesses) are common examples of standards and should be based on the best scientific evidence available. However, the range of standards needed in a health care organization is quite diverse, ranging from clinical practice guidelines to protocols for infection prevention and from administrative procedures for patient consent to job descriptions.

Undertaking an inventory of standards is a useful preparatory step for health care staff who are interested in institutionalizing QA within their practices. Examining the evidence substantiating clinical practice standards (see Table 96.2) may be a second key step in determining if the standards need revision. If standards don't exist, they must be designed or adapted from existing standards. Although standards are context spe-

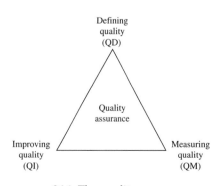

FIGURE 96.1 The quality assurance triangle.

TABLE 96.2 Coding System for the Hierarchy of Evidence

Level of Evidence	Description
I	Well-designed randomized control trials
II-1a	Well-designed control trials with pseudorandomization
II-1b	Well-designed control trials with no randomization
II-2a	Well-designed cohort (prospective) study with concurrent controls
II-2b	Well-designed cohort (prospective) study with historical controls
II-2c	Well-designed cohort (retrospective) study with concurrent controls
II-3	Well-designed cohort (retrospective) study
III	Large differences from comparisons between times or places or both, with and without intervention (in some cases this may be equivalent to Level II or I)
IV	Opinions of respected authorities based on clinical experience, descriptive studies, and reports of expert committees

Source: NHS, 1996.

cific, internationally accepted standards are often a good starting point for developing local standards. Many times, even when national standards exist, they must be refined or made operational for practical use in a specific health care practice.

For standards to be used they need to be communicated and accessible. Health practices should develop plans and systems for communicating standards to those who will use them, including a mechanism to reach new employees and to share revisions or updates in standards previously communicated.

QD encompasses more than the development of standards. For a system of care to be providing care according to agreed-on standards, all processes must be designed to meet these standards, including standards aimed at meeting the needs of the clients. Quality systems and standards may be designed to address the various dimensions of quality shown in Table 96.3.

Measuring Quality

QM consists of quantifying the current level of performance or compliance with expected standards, including standards regarding patient satisfaction. (Ashton, 2001a; Bouchet, 2000). To measure quality, one needs to develop and use indicators related to performance or quality standards; this has proved to be one of the most difficult tasks for health care organizations. Most practitioners need some assistance to develop indicators that are simple, measurable, accurate, reliable, feasible, and timely. Furthermore, the act of collecting and analyzing indicator data takes time and resources, resources that may not have been considered during the budget planning cycle of the health organization or practice. Whenever possible, quality indicators should be included in existing information systems, but routine monitoring may not be able to capture the specific performance data needed for measuring compliance with quality standards or measuring changes based on improvement interventions.

A variety of approaches may be used to measure quality, including self-assessment, routine quality monitoring, special studies and periodic assessments such as audits, or data collected through supervisory visits. Direct observation, simulations, chart reviews, and interviews with providers and clients can all be used to collect the data. The purpose and use of the measurement data will determine the best, most efficient methodology. However, the poor quality of clinical records in many developing countries makes chart reviews less useful than expected; thus, improving the content and quality of recording

TABLE 96.3 Dimensions of Quality

Technical performance
Access to services
Effectiveness of care
Efficiency of service delivery
Interpersonal relations
Continuity of services
Safety
Physical infrastructure and comfort
Choice of services

is often a critical first step prior to the introduction of a monitoring system or other quality measurements of performance.

The use of run charts to regularly collect indicator information over time (often monthly) is key in Quality Improvement to measure the impact of changes or improvement interventions on the process one is attempting to improve. It is important to focus and be realistic about what data can be regularly collected at a facility level. A simple performance-monitoring system, with a limited number of indicators related to the improvement goal, is usually very effective. Standards should be discussed, indicators identified, and a measurement strategy developed with full participation of the team in charge of making improvements or collecting data.

Improving Quality

Not surprisingly, QM leads directly to the identification of areas for QI. Quality Improvement refers to the application of methods and tools to close the gap between current and expected levels of quality by understanding and addressing system deficiencies (as well as enhancing strengths) to improve or in some cases redesign health care processes (Massoud et al., 2001). As noted previously, QM is also essential in the Quality Improvement process, to evaluate whether or not changes made to improve quality actually result in improvement.

A spectrum of Quality Improvement approaches exists (see Figure 96.2), from individual problem solving to process improvement (Massoud et al., 2001), with variations in time, resources, and complexity required. Nonetheless, every approach shares in common the four steps to Quality Improvement shown in Figure 96.3. Inherent in Quality Improvement is Step 4: Test

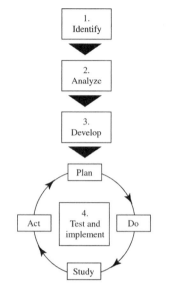

1. Identify	Determine what to improve
2. Analyze	Understand the problem
3. Develop	Hypothesize about what changes will improve the problem
4. Test and implement	Test the hypothesized solution to see if it yields improvement; on the basis of the results, to abandon, modify, or implement the solution

FIGURE 96.3 Four steps to quality improvement. Source: Massoud et al., 2001.

and implement, which incorporates Shewhart's cycle for learning and improvement, the plan-do-study-act cycle (PDSA), as depicted in Figure 96.4.

In essence, this cycle, which is built on local testing of small improvements, is the essence of operations research. However, quality management has extended the research cycle to include action based on the results learned. The PDSA cycle thus promotes continuous improvement as hypotheses are created, tested, revised, and implemented, only to be adapted in the next cycle of learning.

South Africa Country Example—Accreditation

When initiating QA, there is no single right activity to start; any one of the core activities can serve as a starting point; likewise, it is possible to start several simultaneously. Some QA ap-

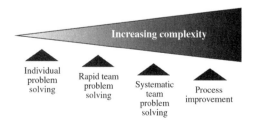

FIGURE 96.2 Spectrum of approaches to quality improvement.

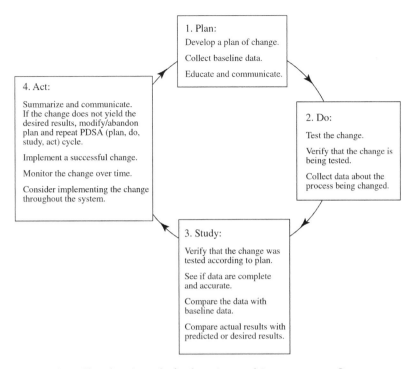

FIGURE 96.4 Shewhart's cycle for learning and improvement. Sources: Massoud et al., 2001; Shewhart, 1931.

proaches such as collaborative improvement, or accreditation, especially as it is practiced in developing countries, contain all three core QA activities. For example, in South Africa, the accreditation standards of care (QD) for hospitals were first developed by the Council for Health Service Accreditation of Southern Africa (COHSASA). The standards were then disseminated and published. Every hospital participating in the accreditation process receives a copy of the standards. The accreditation process includes an educational survey in which the hospital's current operations and practices are evaluated against the accreditation standards and criteria (QM). The hospital then receives feedback about its performance and is supported with technical assistance to make improvements (QI). During the period of quality improvement interventions, the hospital may continuously measure its performance. The accreditation surveyors then perform the formal quality measurement and determine the institution's score. Score and related findings will be reviewed by the accreditation board, which will determine the hospital's accreditation status. Accreditation

thus includes QD, QM, and QI, as well as being a regulatory approach to quality health care (Whittaker, 1999).

THE PARTICULAR ROLE OF PRACTICE-BASED ASSESSMENT AND MEASUREMENT IN QA

QM consists of explicitly quantifying the current level of performance or compliance with expected standards, including patient satisfaction. The use of data to assess quality of care and to test changes is one of the underlying principles of QA. QA promotes decision making on the basis of accurate and timely data rather than assumptions. Measurement provides data to guide improvement activities, to verify that an improvement is reaching its intended results, or to ensure that levels of quality are being maintained. It involves defining indicators and developing or adapting information systems or special studies to collect data on performance according to standards, as well as analyzing and interpreting the results.

Practice-based activities related to QM include the collection and analysis of data on adherence to established standards through supervisory assessments, self- or peer assessment, continuous quality monitoring, and special studies or periodic assessments, such as audits. Measuring client satisfaction is one important form of quality assessment that is often neglected. There are a wide range of assessment, monitoring, and evaluative approaches which can be used to measure quality. The type of QM most appropriate for a health care practice will depend on characteristics of the organization, the purpose of measurement, and resources available, as well as take into account the strengths and weaknesses of various measurement methods (see Table 96.4).

Furthermore, measurement provides a potent form of feedback on performance and, as such, can be an intervention to stimulate improvement. When directed feedback is coupled with measurement of performance (especially performance according to evidence-based standards), it can be a powerful stimulant to behavior change and improvement.

Eritrea Country Example—Quality Assessment

In Eritrea, the QA Project and the Ministry of Health performed an interactive assessment of current case management practices in the care of hospitalized children with serious infections and severe malnutrition. The assessment sections corresponded to international guidelines for care of children at first referral level hospitals developed by the World Health Organization (WHO) (World Health Organization, Department of Child and Adolescent Health and Development, 2000). The assessment methodology purposefully incorporated use of the new guidelines in an "open book" format, to introduce the standards and orient providers to the guide for their later use. Direct observations of client encounters, record reviews (of current and past charts), client and provider structured interviews, client and caretaker exit interviews, inspection, and physical inventories were all used in the assessment, which was conducted over a 2- to 3-day period at each site. The assessment exercise not only provided useful data in terms of current practices but also was used to introduce the new case management guidelines, provide immediate onsite feedback and assistance, and identify pri-

ority improvement areas. Immediate onsite feedback was given during the assessment and at the conclusion, in a more structured format. Improvement teams and initial quick-fix improvements were identified and an improvement action plan agreed upon. In this way, the assessment also served to initiate QI.

One of the potential drawbacks with broad assessments, especially if performed by outside teams, is that the findings are not used to stimulate, specific and needed improvements. In Eritrea, this was avoided by incorporating immediate feedback of findings along with agreement on improvements and assignment of actions.

Sustaining the Use of Data for Measurement and Improvement

The challenge facing many health care practices and organizations is not necessarily the use of data for incidental and targeted improvements. What is more challenging is to ensure that data are used regularly and consistently throughout the practice or organization to assess quality or measure performance according to standards, and then use it to make continuous improvement.

The institutionalization framework can be applied to assess where on the continuum of institutionalizing measurement and monitoring an organization finds itself and can help guide options for continued development. An organization that has institutionalized QA will use data consistently to measure its performance and to take actions accordingly. To help health care practices reach that goal of institutionalizing QA, there are some important ways in which measurement and data can be incorporated into health care practices. They follow.

- Involve clinic staff in the collection of data
- Use data and performance results to identify successful practices, to focus on priority health issues, and to document and share improvements with all involved
- Document improvements through the measurement of performance
- Build on what is learned through measurement to be successful
- Disseminate results through diffusion and collaborative learning of best practices
- Illustrate measurement results on time series run charts or other graphic displays of date
- Display data and results for all staff to see

TABLE 96.4 Measurement Strategy and Approach Methods

Strategy/Approach/Methods	Strengths	Weaknesses/Cautions
A. Facilitative supervision	—Obtains data on performance through observation, interview, and record review —Identifies problems —Provides feedback to providers on their performance and psychic rewards —Can provide coaching to team problem solving —Can improve health worker motivation and interest	—Human and financial resources (e.g., for transport) is required —Supervisory standards, capacity development, and supervision of supervisors are also needed —Training of supervisors in supervisory skills as well as technical content is needed for effectiveness —Adequate time spent in each supervised location is needed
B. Routine health information system (HIS)	—Data collected routinely; few added costs	—Routine health information systems (HIS) usually collects data on outputs and diagnoses —Routine HIS has difficulty collecting data on the details of the process of clinical care or on many outcomes of care —Commonly collected and sent to headquarters without examination or use in facility or organization where collected; dissociation between data collection and analysis/use —Data on self-assessment of performance may not be valid
C. Self or peer assessment	—Low cost —Empowers health workers to be accountable to themselves for quality of care —Reinforces standards —Complements supervision —Essential for teams to assess impact of their improvement efforts —Usually leads to improvement or performance over time even if self-reported data is not accurate	—Data should not be used for assessing absolute level of performance
D. Special studies	—Provides needed information once or on ad hoc basis; thus can be more cost-effective (e.g., DHS surveys)	—Not available on a routine basis —May be costly since outside or routine; may be seen as research, with little direct application to facility

Ecudor Country Example—Sharing Data on Compliance with Standards

As part of a QA intervention to improve compliance with maternal and child care standards in hospitals in Ecudor, data on monthly compliance with the standards are posted in each hospital's public areas for staff and clients to see. Monthly staff discussions of the trends in compliance with standards have generated collective "self-supervision," creating the opportunity to discuss causes for problems and practical interventions and heightening awareness among staff of their role in quality improvement (Hermida, 2002).

A FRAMEWORK FOR INSTITUTIONALIZING QUALITY ASSURANCE

The core QA activities, represented by the QA triangle (see Figure 96.1), are the heart of any effort to institutionalize quality care. It is the continuous application of these activities that will ensure high-quality health care over time. The institutionalization model (see Figure 96.5) contains the QA triangle at its center, with eight essential elements or building blocks necessary to support and ensure sustainable implementation of these core QA activities over time. The model's elements are similar to focal areas noted in other quality audit frameworks (Øvretveit, 1994; Wagner, DeBakker, & Groenewegen,

1999). These eight essential elements can be grouped in three categories: (a) the internal enabling environment, internal to the organization or system (comprised of the essential elements of leadership, policy, core values, and resources); (b) organizing for quality (structure); and (c) support functions (containing the essential elements of capacity building, communication and information, and rewarding quality).

The Internal Enabling Environment

An internal environment conducive to initiating, expanding, and sustaining QA is necessary to institutionalize QA. Such a supportive and facilitative environment is comprised of (a) *policies* that support, guide, and reinforce QA; (b) *leadership* that sets priorities, promotes learning, and cares about its staff; (c) *core* organizational *values* that emphasize respect, quality, and continued improvement; and (d) adequate *resources* allocated for the implementation of QA activities. The full impact of the internal enabling environment is achieved only through the synergy created among all four of these elements.

Organizing for Quality

Institutionalization requires a clear delineation of roles, responsibilities, and accountability for the implementation of QA activities. We refer to this organization for implementing QA as the

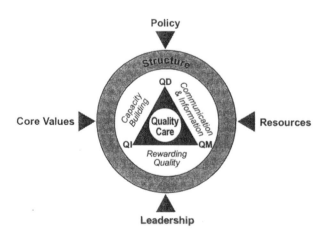

FIGURE 96.5 Model for the institutionalization of quality assurance.

essential element, *structure*. However, in this context structure should not be equated with an organization chart or reporting relationships. Instead, it refers to the mapping out of responsibilities and accountability for QA in the organization, including oversight, coordination, and implementation of QA activities.

Support Functions

Several essential elements are needed to support sustained implementation of QA and improved quality of care. Three critical support functions are (a) *capacity building* in QA, such as training, supervision, and coaching for health care providers and managers; (b) *information and communication* for the purposes of sharing, learning, and advocating for quality; and (c) *rewarding* and recognizing individual and team efforts to improve quality. These three categories are represented in Figure 96.5 as a series of overlapping concentric circles that work together. At the center is quality health care, the desired outcome of QA. Surrounding the center is the triangle of core QA technical activities for improving the quality of care: QD, QM, and QI. The impact of these core QA activities will depend on an enabling environment that encourages a culture of quality and facilitates continued implementation of QA, an appropriate organizational structure for effective QA implementation, and the presence and adequacy of support services. Developing a culture of quality requires all eight essential elements. Selecting where to begin depends on the status of each essential element.

Although each category of elements is important unto itself, it is the combination of all eight elements that facilitates and ensures institutionalization of QA. This model and the ensuing discussion of essential elements focus on those elements that operate within the organization's sphere of influence. At the same time, we recognize that every health care organization operates in a larger environment that influences its ability to implement QA. For example, some health care organizations approach the institutionalization of QA within a stable institutional context, whereas others operate in systems undergoing reform. External environmental factors create both constraints and opportunities for assuring quality and institutionalizing QA. Health sector reforms focused on decentralization or

new financing mechanisms may provide opportunities for QA to contribute to better health outcomes. By the same token, external factors can negatively affect the institutionalization of QA, as is sometimes the case with civil service policies or resource flow to the health sector based on the country's financial situation. Although this model recognizes the influence of external factors, it focuses on the more important role that the categories of essential elements have in the institutionalization of QA.

The Phases of Institutionalizing QA

The institutionalization model presents a rather static depiction of what should be in place when QA is institutionalized. However, in reality, institutionalization is a process. This process can be described as a passage through a series of phases, between an initial state of pre-awareness of QA and the end state of maturity. The QA Project has identified four main transitional phases: awareness, experiential (see Figure 96.6), expansion, and consolidation. The phases and their descriptions were derived from QA Project experience in developing country health systems and are consistent with concepts in the organizational development literature (Brown, 1995; Gnecco, 1999; Hermida, 1999; Renzi, 1996; Wagner et al., 1999; Project Report, 2000). The characteristics, strategies, and activities depicted for each phase are illustrative and are not meant to be prescriptive.

Although institutionalization is a continuum, subdividing it into four distinct phases helps to map out the process that organizations are likely to experience. Such a road map can assist health care organizations to assess their own level of QA development and to make decisions (human resource, financial, and technical) on how best to further their organization's advancement toward incorporating QA as part of day-to-day operations.

The phases of institutionalization reflect the degree of organizational commitment and capacity to do QA and the extent to which QA activities are implemented within the organization. Figure 96.6 depicts the phases an organization passes through as it moves toward QA maturity, when QA is formally and philosophically integrated into the way the organization functions. Although the figure depicts progress through the phases as linear, different reasons may cause

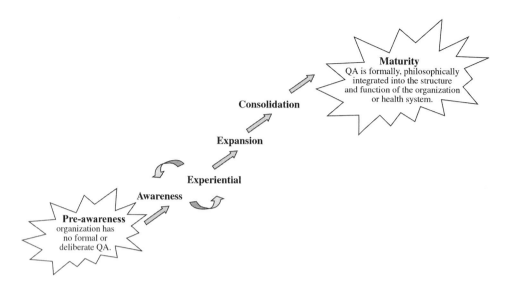

FIGURE 96.6 The phases of institutionalizing quality assurance.

actual progress to stall or revert to an earlier phase. Furthermore, some phases (e.g., awareness and experiential) often occur simultaneously or in an iterative fashion, as suggested by the curved arrows.

Table 96.5 lists the characteristics, strategies, and indications of readiness to progress for each phase. Organizational leaders and managers can use this table to determine their organization's location on the institutionalization continuum, either as a whole or at the level of each essential element. The description of potential strategies and activities in each phase provides guidance for planning how to most efficiently move toward QA maturity by helping leaders visualize where the organization should go and how to get there.

USING THE FRAMEWORK: CASE STUDIES FROM DEVELOPING COUNTRIES

Morocco

The Ministry of Health in Morocco is decentralizing and has begun to transfer responsibilities for monitoring quality of public health services to the regional level. Two regions have gained significant experience with QA over the past 7 years, each building capacity in QA among health professionals and improving targeted services in select health centers. One region has focused efforts on building basic capac-

ity for QA among all health professionals and on experimenting with different forms of QI. The other region has added focused accreditation as an additional axis of intervention. As part of the decentralization effort, both regions are developing strategic plans for the next 5 years. They independently have reached the conclusion that they want to deepen their analysis of advancement of QA, to make good choices for the future and safeguard their gains. To do this, both regions have used the institutionalization framework.

The steps they are undertaking follow:

- *Development of a vision for quality of care:* As part of the strategic planning process, each region developed a clear vision describing the quality of care they seek to provide to the population. The vision refers to the dimensions of quality and includes a focus on satisfying their clients. The vision was developed by the regional management team and is being circulated for feedback and comments among provincial and district health managers.
- *Analysis of the status of institutionalization of QA:* Using the framework, a questionnaire has been developed to enable all health care providers and managers to state their opinion with regard to the phase of institutionalization in which they believe their region is. The questionnaire uses the elements of the

TABLE 96.5 Institutionalization Phases: Characteristics, Strategies, and Indications of Readiness to Progress

Phase	Illustrative Characteristics	Potential Strategies or Activities	Indications of Readiness to Progress
Awareness	Decision makers become conscious of need to systematically address improvements in quality of care	Demonstrate need for improvements (using quality data, community surveys, media) Create QA awareness through formal and informal benchmarking Communicate to stakeholders that there cannot be improvement without some change.	Deliberate decision by the organization to explore QA as a mechanism to improve quality of care
Experiential	Organization tries QA approaches to learn and document that QA leads to improved care	Implement small-scale QA activities or experiments Develop mechanisms for diffusion of QA results and lessons learned	Leadership support for formal decision to develop an organizational strategy for QA
Expansion	Organization strategically expands QA activities in scale and scope Organization increases its capacity to conduct QA activities	Develop strategy for QA expansion (e.g., define priorities, set goals, plan implementation) Build capacity and develop leadership for QA Share results and innovation	Existence of demonstrated improvements in quality as a result of QA activities Consensus among decision makers that QA merits continuation
Consolidation	Organization simultaneously strengthens and anchors existing QA activities into routine operations, while addressing lagging or missing activities	Identify missing essential elements or lagging QA activities and take corrective action Enhance coordination of QA strategy and activities Support establishment of a learning environment	Full implementation of a balanced set of QA activities, integrated into routine responsibilities throughout the organization

framework, thus allowing detailed feedback for each of the elements of the framework. The questionnaire is being administered in each of the health centers where staff have been trained in applying QA tools in the region.

- *Documentation of achievements to date:* This is an important step. Documentation provides an objective measure of quality, allows for better understanding of the results, opens the way to share the results to other health centers, and provides a basis to analyze future direction and priorities. Each improvement must be documented and a plan for dissemination and scale-up developed.
- *Articulation of strategic directions:* These are framed using health information data to determine public health priorities, coupled with client satisfaction surveys. The strategic directions for improvements are directly linked to quality of care, public health priorities, and morbidity and mortality data.
- *Development of institutionalization plan:* In conjunction with the priorities for improvement, the analysis of the status of institutionalization identifies the phase of development of each element. The regional management team is using this data to prepare a detailed plan for continued institutionalization of QA.

The process to develop a strategic institutionalization plan for QA in these two regions in Morocco is ongoing. This experience underscores the importance of integrating QA planning and activities into the planning and monitoring of priority health activities of the institution or health practice so that QA becomes functionally integrated into existing processes and structures. Thus, a reflection on the status and future directions for institutionalization of QA goes hand-in-hand with an analysis and decisions on public health priorities.

Zambia

Zambia has introduced and invested significant effort in QA since 1993. In fall 2002, a review of the status of institutionalization of QA was completed, using the framework and the questionnaire mentioned above. The review, done by a representative sample of QA-trained health staff from the national, provincial, and clinic level, analyzed the advancement of each element

of the framework and formulated recommendations on where investments in strengthening QA in the country should be made. Health staff identified four elements that needed strengthening (i.e., policy, core values, information and communication, and rewarding quality), they then formulated recommendations to be submitted to the Central Board of Health.

The Zambian health staff determined that one of the main ways they could support QA would be to integrate and harmonize their work with QA tasks. For example, when they set a standard, they should encourage routine monitoring of performance related to that standard until enough time has passed to assure that performance will be maintained. The staff realized that a baseline and one after-measure would not be sufficient to demonstrate true improvement. The Zambians agreed that when routine monitoring showed that compliance with the standard has been established, they could turn to intermittent spot checks to judge whether performance was sustained. They also recommended that, when possible, HMIS indicators can be used to monitor performance according to the new standard. Finally, the health staff suggested whenever there is a desire to introduce new monitors, or methods of improvement, health care managers were encouraged to work with local QA people to harmonize approaches.

MOVING FORWARD: SCALING UP AND SUSTAINING QUALITY IMPROVEMENTS IN A HEALTH CARE PRACTICE

We conclude this chapter with a discussion of how the framework can also be used by a health care practice to plan and monitor the institutionalization of a specific improvement (or a package of improvements), as well as to institutionalize improvement methodology (such as collaborative improvement approach).

The Relationship Between Scaling Up, Sustaining Improvements, and the Phases of Institutionalization

Quite simply, scaling up is an attribute of the expansion phase of institutionalization. Expansion is not limited to geographic spread or numerical increases but also includes increased scope (e.g., spread of an improvement to other departments in a facility or to other topics). Other characteristics of this phase—such as increasing organizational capacity to undertake the improvement or diffusing innovation—help to prepare the way for sustaining the improvement. However, expansion does not assure sustainability. It is during the consolidation phase of institutionalization that sustainability is most directly addressed. Without consolidation, improvement will be short-lived, because it is during this phase that resources for the improvement are aligned with policies supporting the improvement, and systems for documentation, sharing, and advocacy are operating more or less routinely. Similarly, leadership's commitment to the improvement is evidenced by its commitment of resources and staff time.

How to Use the Framework to Institutionalize Specific Improvements

We suggest that the essential elements needed to institutionalize QA are the same ones needed to institutionalize a specific improvement (a package of changes underlying improvement, or even an improvement approach such as a learning and improvement collaborator).

The internal enabling environment will of course play an integral role in institutionalizing any specific improvement. The leadership must be convinced to sustain the human, material, and financial resources needed and to encourage the staff to devote their efforts to the improvement. Policy can support the continuation of key activities or sanction sustained changes in roles, responsibilities, or scopes of practice and can allocate needed resources. Of course, resources, human and material, are necessary to sustain improvements. Documented, measurable improvement results can be useful in convincing decision makers or stakeholders to continue supporting the specific improvement, including the costs of measurement. Core values, especially among management and staff continuing to implement the improvement activities, must be in concert with the values espoused by the initial improvement teams, or else practitioners may be loath to continue.

Just as a structure is needed to implement and support QA, it is needed to support the continuity of any successful improvement. Clear identification of roles, responsibilities, oversight, and coordination is essential for continuing specific improvements, including those implemented by collaboratives. Coordination between multiple improvement efforts becomes critical.

Support functions are the linchpins in the framework to institutionalize improvement. Systems for building and sustaining the necessary technical and QA capacity to implement the improvement are critical, especially given the inevitability of staff turnover and attrition. Likewise, mechanisms to reach and sensitize new leaders and policymakers must be developed. Collaborative improvement intrinsically incorporates the recording of improvements, sharing of results, and use of lessons learned, but as collaboratives expand and less testing takes place, there may be a tendency to decrease sharing and learning. Thus, attention to the essential element of information and communication remains vital to sustain any improvement. Internal recognition as a reward for quality happens automatically as results are shared between colleagues, but recognition by leaders and those not involved in the improvement can also be a reward. Finally, external recognition systems may be useful, especially to boost sustained improvement results.

Thus, it is rather easy to see that the essential elements have equal utility when seeking to institutionalize a particular improvement or package of changes, as well as to institutionalize a process of improvement (such as a collaborative that incorporates all three QA activities).

In a similar way, the phases of institutionalizing QA apply to institutionalizing a specific or collaborative improvement. The awareness phase is similar to the demonstration or prototype phase of an improvement effort on the pre-work phase of a collaborative, the period when the idea of a need for change enters the health care practice. The experiential phase mirrors the start-up phase of any improvement or the demonstrative phase of a collaborative. The characteristics and strategies of the expansion phase for institutionalizing QA are quite applicable to expanding a specific improvement similar to those of the expansion phase of a collaborative developing a specific expansion strategy, delineating clear roles and responsibilities for implementing the expansion, and of course building the capacity among leaders and implementers. Organizational capacity must also be enhanced to support more complicated logistics and management needed for expansion.

To reach consolidation for a particular improvement on a collaborative, the changes needed for improvement activities must be incorporated into routine operations within each participating facility. Furthermore, every participating facility should be implementing the tested improvements with a similar range of effectiveness, as evidenced by their run chart results. Thus, during this phase, the most useful strategies will address lagging or missing components of the change or improvement package, or direct attention to energizing those sites lagging in implementation, documentation, or reporting.

Finally, maturity—the state of sustained quality of care and a culture of quality—includes the sustainability of particular improvements, as well as the QA activities that are the foundation of those improvements. At maturity, the improvement (and the collaborative) will have become part of routine activities, appropriately incorporated into scopes of work, supported by policy and leaders, with sufficient resources routinely identified and incorporated into operating budgets so that resources are consistently available. Mechanisms are in place to continuously build the needed capacity, perhaps even starting in preservice training. Documentation and the sharing of lessons learned are routine, as is the collection of quantifiable data regarding performance related to the improvement.

SUMMARY

The QA triangle illustrates three core QA functions or activities. As we discussed, when a health care practice or organization decides to begin QA efforts, it can begin with any one of the core activities or with any combination. There is no single best way to start QA. Likewise, there are many paths to strengthen and ultimately sustain QA. The framework seeks to provide some guidance, a road map to health care practices and practitioners interested in institutionalizing QA in order to sustain quality.

In summary, the framework and related self-assessment and monitoring tools not only are useful for institutionalizing QA, but also can be used by health care practitioners to sustain specific improvements (or a package of improvements) in a health care practice or organization.

ACKNOWLEDGMENT This chapter is largely based on the Quality Assurance Project monographs "Sustaining Quality of Healthcare: Institutionalization of Quality Assurance" (Franco et al., 2002) and "A Modern Paradigm for Improving Healthcare Quality" (Massoud et al., 2001), as well as the article "A Framework for Institutionalizing Quality Assurance" (Silimperi et al., 2002).

Note

1. The work to develop this framework was carried out as part of the work of the Quality Assurance Project implemented by the University Research Co., LLC, funded by the United States Agency for International Development, contract number HRN-C-00-96-90013.

The Quality Assurance Project (QA Project) is funded by the U.S. Agency for International Development (USAID) under contract number GPH-C-00-02-00004-00. The project provides comprehensive, leading-edge technical expertise in the design, management, and implementation of quality assurance and workforce improvement in developing countries.

References

Ashton, J. (2001a). Monitoring the quality of hospital care. *Health manager's guide.* Bethesda, MD: Published for USAID by the Quality Assurance Project.

Ashton, J. (2001b). *Taxonomy of health system standards.* Bethesda, MD: Published for USAID by the Quality Assurance Project.

Baldrige National Quality Program. (2001). *Health care criteria for performance excellence.* Gaithersburg, MD: Author.

Bartleson, J. D., Anshus, A. L., Halvorson, A. M., Kamath, J. R., Johnson, T. J., & Herman, J. S. (1998). Benchmarking the communication of continuous improvement activities. *Quality Management in Health Care, 6,* 43–51.

Bouchet, B. (2000). Monitoring the quality of primary care. *Health manager's guide.* Bethesda, MD: Published for USAID by the Quality Assurance Project.

Brown, L. D. (1995). Lessons learned in institutionalization of quality assurance programs: An international perspective. *International Journal for Quality in Health Care, 7*(4), 419–425.

Franco, L. M., Silimperi, D. R., Veldhuyzen van Zanten, T., MacAulay, C., Askov, K., et al. (2002). Sustaining quality of healthcare: Institutionalization of quality assurance. *QA Monograph Series, 2*(1). Bethesda, MD: Published for USAID by the Quality Assurance Project.

Gnecco, T. (1999). Making a commitment to quality development of the quality assurance program in Chile: 1991–1999. *International Journal for Quality in Health Care, 11,* 443–445.

Hermida, J. (1999). The road to institutionalizing quality assurance in Ecuador in an environment of health sector reform. *International Journal for Quality in Health Care, 11*, 447–450.

Hermida, J., & Robalino, M. E. (2002). Increasing compliance with maternal and child care quality standards in Ecuador. *International Journal for Quality in Health Care, 14*(Suppl.), 25–34.

Jennings, K., & Westfall, F. (1994). A survey-based benchmarking approach for health care using the Baldrige quality criteria. *Joint Commission Journal on Quality Improvement, 20*(9), 500–509.

Kinney, C. F., & Gift, M. S. (1997). Building a framework for multiple improvement initiatives. *Joint Commission Journal on Quality Improvement, 23*, 407–423.

Massoud, R., Askov, K., Reinke, J., Franco, L. M., Bornstein, T., Knebel, E., et al. (2001). A modern paradigm for improving healthcare quality. *QA Monograph Series 1*(1). Bethesda: Published for USAID by the Quality Assurance Project.

O'Malley, S. (1998). Building a culture that supports change. *Quality Letter for Healthcare Leaders, 10*, 2–9.

Øvretveit, J. (1994). A comparison of approaches to health service quality in the UK, USA, and Sweden and of the use of organizational audit frameworks. *European Journal of Public Health, 4*, 46–54.

Pan American Health Organization and Quality Assurance Project (2003). Maximizing quality of care through health sector reform: The role of quality assurance strategies. Bethesda: Published for USAID by the Quality Assurance Project.

Penland, T. (1997). A model to create "organizational readiness" for the successful implementation of quality management systems. *International Journal for Quality in Health Care, 9*, 69–72.

Powell, T. C. (1995). Total quality management as competitive advantage: A review and empirical study. *Strategic Management Journal, 16*, 15–37.

Preston, A. P., Saunders, I. W., O'Sullivan, D., Garrigan, E., & Rice, J. (1995). Effective hospital leadership for quality: Theory and practice. *Australian Health Review, 18*, 91–110.

Quality Assurance Project. (2000). Institutionalization of quality assurance. *Project Report*. Bethesda, MD: Published for USAID by the Quality Assurance Project.

Renzi, M. (1996). An integrated tool kit for institutional development. *Public Administration and Development, 16*, 469–483.

Shewhart, W. (1931). *The economic control of quality of manufactured products*. New York: D. Van Nostrand Co. Reprinted by the American Society of Quality Control. (1980).

Shortell, S. M, Bennett, C. L., & Byck, G. R. (1998). Assessing the impact of continuous quality improvement on clinical practice: What will it take to accelerate programs? *Milbank Quarterly, 76*, 593–624.

Shortell, S. M., O'Brien, J. L., Carman, J. M., Foster, R. W., Hughes, E. F., Boerstler, H., et al. (1995). Assessing the impact of continuous quality improvement/total quality management: Concept versus implementation. *Health Services Research, 30*, 377–401.

Silimperi, D. R., Franco, L. M., Veldhuyzen van Zanten, T., & MacAulay, C. (2002). A framework for institutionalizing quality assurance. *International Journal for Quality in Health Care, 14* (Suppl.), 67–73.

Wagner, C., DeBakker, D. H., & Groenewegen, P. P. (1999), A measuring instrument for evaluation of quality systems. *International Journal for Quality in Health Care, 11*, 119–130.

Westphal, J. D., Gulati, R., & Shortell, S. M. (1997). Customization or conformity? An institutional and network perspective on the content and consequences of TQM adoption. *Administrative Science Quarterly, 42*, 366–394.

Whittaker, S. (1999). Quality improvement in South Africa: The COHSASA accreditation initiative. *2A Brief 8*(2). Bethesda, MD: Published for USAID by the Quality Assurance Project, 21–24.

APPLICATION OF QUALITY MANAGEMENT METHODS FOR PREVENTING AN ADVERSE EVENT

The Case of Falls in Hospitals

97

Catherine Grenier-Sennelier & Etienne Minvielle

Many prevention strategies are, naturally, approached from clinical and statistical perspectives. Clinical and organizational strategies, care effectiveness, and the risks or benefits of preventive measures are often not well defined, but the efficacy of these programs also depends in many ways on management and organizational processes. First, different causes of the occurrence of an adverse event can be the result of organizational dysfunctions (e.g., lack of coordination among caregivers). Second, implementation of preventive measures requires management skills regarding availability, affordability, and acceptability of procedures to prevent these adverse events, for which clinicians are rarely trained. Preventive measures must eventually be taken by others who help to manage the adverse event when it unfortunately occurs. For this reason, all levels of prevention and risk management must be considered, from primary prevention (targeting risk factors to prevent occurrence of disease or injury), to secondary prevention (targeting subclinical disease through early identification and treatment), to tertiary prevention (aiming at established disease or injury to ameliorate progression and maximize function for the person affected). In this context, continuous quality improvement (CQI) or total quality management can enhance clinical outcomes through management channels, enriching prevention program effects. We define CQI as "an ongoing process whereby top management takes whatever steps necessary to enable everyone in the organization, in the course of performing all duties, to establish and achieve standards which meet or exceed the needs and expectations of their customer" (Miller, 1996). The aim of this chapter is to test the value of a quality improvement approach in the specific case of falls prevention.

Falls are common among elderly hospital inpatients of any countries (Dargent-Molina & Bréart, 1995; K. Morse, 1996; Rubinstein, Josephon, & Robbins, 1994). Their consequences are serious, with 1.3 to 14% of patients sustaining fractures (Baker & Harvey, 1985; De Vincenzo & Watkins, 1987; J. M. Morse, Prewse, Morrow, & Federsperl, 1985). Psychological effects such as fear of falling, anxiety and depression, and loss of confidence compound patient problems (Vetter & Ford, 1989). Falls by inpatients are also associated with a greater chance of unplanned readmissions and of discharge to nursing homes (Bates, Pruess, Souney, & Platt, 1995). Therefore, the occurrence of falls often represents a turning point in the clinical course of elderly persons, in addition to increased costs to the system.

The prevention of falls remains a challenging issue (Tinetti et al., 1994). Many clinical characteristics (including use of particular medications, muscle weakness, postural hypotension, and poor vision) increase the incidence of falls occurring at home or outdoors (Hindmarsh &

Estes, 1989) and contribute to the possibility of a fatality. Moreover, in the specific context of hospital, falls are often perceived by physicians and nurses as an unavoidable consequence of encouraging patients to regain mobility shortly after an acute illness.

In October 1996, a study entitled Programme d'Amélioration de la Qualité (Quality Improvement Program) was commenced to prevent falls in the National Rehabilitation Hospital of Saint-Maurice (France). This project was sponsored by the French Ministry of Health and the National Agency for Accreditation, as a national research and demonstration program. The medical and rehabilitation unit was chosen for this program because of its relatively high frequency of falls, due to its patient characteristics over many years.

A CQI program was implemented in two distinct phases: Phase 1, an accurate enumeration and assessment of falls, viewed as undesirable events appearing during the process of care; and Phase 2, development and diffusion of a set of recommendations for preventing the falls. The goal of the study was to evaluate the effects of CQI on prevention strategies. Using this study design, we are able to report on the benefits of using CQI in designing a prevention program.

METHOD

The two phases were conducted at the National Rehabilitation Hospital of Saint Maurice in the eastern suburbs of Paris, a 400-bed rehabilitation, reeducation, and follow-up hospital with both inpatient and outpatient services. During Phase 1, the medical and rehabilitation unit was the pilot unit of the study. This unit had 100 beds in five wards. In 1995, the bed occupation rate was 84%, the average length of stay was 36 days (standard deviation 15 days), and its patients were mainly elderly persons with a mean age of 76.0 years (standard deviation 20.3 years). Most of the patients returned home (73%), whereas 8% were discharged to long-term care. There were 575 patients accounting for 860 admissions.

Phase 1: Assessment of Falls

The general principles of CQI require acknowledgment and assessment of the undesirable falling event as a process, in which the decomposi-

tion of an activity occurs in several steps. A fall was defined, according to Oliver, Britton, Seed, Martin, and Hopper, as "all situations in which a patient suddenly and involuntarily came to rest upon the ground or surface lower than his original station" (1997).

For assessing falls, we combined two types of studies: (a) a retrospective survey to quantify the number of falls and (b) a prospective study to identify the causes of falls. The first survey was undertaken in 1996. It included all patients admitted to the unit during 1995 ($N = 575$). Data were collected from the falls register, an administrative database in which all professionals have to declare falls, from the hospital medical information system, and from the patients' medical records. From the hospital medical information system, we obtained a list of the 575 inpatients admitted to the unit in 1995. We then recorded the patients who were the subject of a declaration in the administrative register and began to collect the set of data described below. At the end, we reviewed the medical records of the 575 patients to complete the data set and to compare the different sources of data. Eleven patients were excluded due to lack of information about their identities or because their medical records were not obtained, leaving a sample of 564 patients (which accounts for 822 admissions).

Using the previously mentioned approach, the following data were collected:

- Patients' characteristics: age, gender, pathology (principal diagnosis of hospitalization), and dependence
- Place and time of each fall
- Consequences of the falls (e.g., fractures, cranial trauma, soft tissue injuries, anxiety, depression, fear of falling, loss of confidence)

The falls were the unit of analysis. Patients who fell more than once were included in several data sets. Data obtained during this retrospective study allowed us to quantify the number of falls and to observe the quality of the falls register's account (by comparison of the number of these accounts and the number of falls noted in the patient's medical record). However, they did not allow us to analyze the specific circumstances of each fall's occurrence and thus to understand the causes of the falls. No existing records (even individual patient records) were found to provide detailed descriptions of factors leading to the falls.

Therefore, we developed a prospective qualitative study that ran from August to December 1996. This study was based on interviews with patients who fell and aimed to identify causes of falls. For each fall ($N = 59$), our procedure was the same: (a) Within 48 hours of each fall, and after explaining the study and promising anonymity, we requested the patient's consent to be interviewed; (b) we reviewed the patients' medical records and then interviewed them, their neighbors, members of the attending staff, and others who were present at the time of the falls in order to understand fully how they occurred; and (c) we created a typology of the etiologies of falls using this material, based on the analysis of 53 cases (we were not able to identify causes for 6 cases in which patients had been found on floor). One fall could have more than one etiology. For each case, two observers analyzed the data, to consider the number and the types of etiologies and to determine the main etiology. The observers started with a list of individual etiologies well-known in the literature, but they also considered the possibility of system failures as mentioned in the CQI literature (Deming, 1986). The number of cases analyzed ($N = 53$) was determined by the principle of saturation of categories; that is, we had to analyze sufficient new cases until we had found again the same etiologies for each category (Strauss & Corbin, 1998). After 42 cases, no new etiologies were identified; the last 11 cases analyzed proved that all causes were already defined. Comparison of the analyses of the two observers showed seven cases of discordance that they reexamined together to obtain consensus.

Phase 2: Developing and Implementing Recommendations

According to the principles of CQI, actions for improving a phenomenon must be deduced from the first step (assessment of the phenomenon). We created a focus group to develop a set of recommendations derived from the results of the assessment of falls and their etiologies. This focus group was composed of care professionals: two nurses, two physicians, the unit's head nurse, the financial director, and the medical director. The group's work, which began in December 1996, was based on the results of Phase 1, combined with group members' own empirical experiences of the phenomenon and a review of the existing literature. The group produced recommendations by informal consensus, covering primary, secondary, and tertiary prevention of falls, as defined above. An initial version was submitted to a panel of two physicians, four nurses (from the unit), and two members of the administrative staff. Comments given in return led to production of a revised version, which was presented to the advisory committee and senior hospital management in June 1997.

The next step was to implement these recommendations in the pilot unit and also in the three other units of the hospital in which patients had experienced falls. These three units have an overall capacity of 120 beds and are also specialized in rehabilitation care but admit younger patients (mean age 54 years, range 23 to 81 years). Adaptations due to the specific context of each unit required one meeting with the staff of each unit. The hospital's nursing committee also played a major role by scheduling different meetings in which these recommendations were explained to 21 nurses who worked in these three units. We decided to maintain the same set of recommendations and to allow some of them to be developed further to fit the specific context of each unit.

Finally, an impact study of this prevention program was conducted in 1998. Rates for falls (number of falls occurring during the year per number of patients hospitalized during the same year), fallers (number of patients who fell during the year per number of patients hospitalized during the same year), and multifallers (number of patients who fell more than once during the year per number of patients hospitalized during the same year) were assessed from the administrative register and the hospital medical information system. These rates were compared for the years 1995 and 1998.

Statistical analysis was performed with SPSS. Association between the occurrence of falls and patients' characteristics, and comparisons on the time scales of falls, fallers, and multifallers were analyzed by $\chi2$ and Fisher's exact tests. Continuous variables were analyzed by Student's two-sample t-tests. For all statistical tests, $p < 0.05$ was considered significant.

RESULTS

Phase 1: Assessment of Falls

Definition of the Process

Referring an event or an activity to a process in this specific case required choosing between ei-

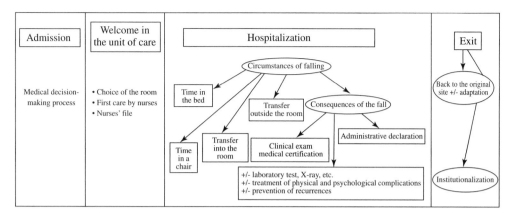

FIGURE 97.1 Overall process of care during hospitalization.

ther the clinical phases (prevention, diagnosis, treatment) or the overall process of care during the patient's hospitalization. According to CQI, we choose the latter because of its ability to describe the concrete phases of the patient's care, developing a longitudinal reading of the phenomena (see Figure 97.1).

Characteristics of Fallers

Of 564 people admitted to the unit in 1995, 103 were victims of falls (18.3%), accounting for 245 falls entered in the medical records. Compared with the 195 falls recorded in the falls register, this number points to a 20.4% underreporting rate. As shown in Table 97.1, patients with at least one fall during their hospitalization differed significantly from nonfallers ($N = 461$): They were older, had experienced longer hospital stays, included more men, had more neurological causes of hospitalization, and were more

likely to be institutionalized at discharge (see Table 97.2). Most falls occurred at the end of the week (20% on Fridays alone). The daily distribution also showed three peaks of frequency (10 A.M., 1 P.M., and 7 P.M.). The location of falls was most often the bedroom or contiguous spaces (for example, the bathroom) or during transfer.

In terms of consequences, the administrative falls report recorded a fracture rate of 5%, whereas patient medical records found it to be 10%. This difference is explained, in part, by the

TABLE 97.1 Comparison of Age and Length of Hospital Stay: Fallers and Nonfallers

| | Patients | | |
	Victims of falls ($N = 103$)	Nonfallers ($N = 461$)	p value
Mean age (years)	79.6	75.8	<0.01
Mean length of stay (days)	51.3	33.0	<0.001

TABLE 97.2 Comparison of Qualitative Variables: Fallers and Nonfallers

| | Patients | | |
	Victims of falls (%)	Nonfallers (%)	p
Gender			
Male	44 (42.6)	140 (30.4)	<0.01
Female	59 (57.4)	321 (69.6)	
Neurological pathology[1]			
Yes	44 (44)	46 (10)	<0.0001
No	57 (56)	412 (90)	
Institutionalization after hospitalization			
Yes	14 (17.5)	18 (5)	<0.0001
No	66 (82.5)	337 (95)	

[1] Data missing due to the poor quality of medical records

fact that the falls register did not contain information on subsequent clinical consequences.

Etiology of Falls

The etiologies of falls were identified from the prospective study. For the 53 documented falls, we identified 111 etiologies, which correspond to a mean of 2.1 etiologies (range 1 to 4) per fall. In 35 cases of falls (66%), specific circumstances appeared to be associated with the occurrence of the fall (e.g., the patient's foot caught the phone wire; the opening or closing of the elevator door; lack of assistance for toileting during the postprandial period; lack of coordination between the transfer of patients and floor cleaning). It is difficult to evaluate the exact interaction between individuals and organizational factors with respect to the causes of falls, but the analysis of each case by two observers showed four types of interaction: 22 cases in which organizational factors were considered the main cause (11 of these were combined with individual factors), and 31 cases in which individual factors were considered the main cause (13 of these were combined with organizational factors).

From these facts, we built a typology consisting of two categories of causes: One addressed individual factors, and the other, organizational features. As we have already mentioned, these two categories of causes were not mutually exclusive in explaining falls; they were interdependent. Table 97.3 lists these two sets of factors and gives the number for which the factor was considered the main cause. Thus, we structured recommendations based on both the individual and organizational cause categories.

Phase 2: Elaborating and Implementing Recommendations

A set of recommendations was defined at the beginning of 1997. It contained both clinical measures and organizational aspects, as follows:

1. Implement procedures upon the patient's arrival in the care unit.
2. Develop a medical score in order to evaluate the risk of falls.
3. Discuss with patients and their families the risk of falls, emphasizing organizational aspects of daily activities.
4. Implement procedures concerning the transfer of patients, allowing for better coordination among staff members of the different units.
5. Implement new procedures concerning the internal organization of the unit (for example, one procedure should specify the need for regular analysis of falls).
6. Improve the use of information systems with regard to the description of falls (patient file and falls register).

These recommendations were disseminated in the pilot unit during summer 1997 and to the three other units during October 1997. Most of them were components of an awareness campaign addressed to patients and their families. For instance, we demonstrated one recommendation concerning the patient's arrival (Recommendation 1) in its full form:

- Allow sufficient time for completion of the reception phase. Admission is a major phase in the patient's care, which requires time; it is an actual part of the care process.
- Estimate on admission (within 24 hours) the patient's self-sufficiency and risk of falling (using the list of characteristics and the mobility score listed in Recommendation 2).
- Verify the patient's needs (e.g., glasses, suitable shoes, toilet case).

Implementation of these recommendations was carried out during the second half of 1997. Although we had no formal strategy, we were aware of removing several barriers to this implementation. This is not to say that this project did not experience problems. As in most hospitals, the information systems were not able to provide the required data without some difficulties. The same people were repeatedly involved in the project efforts, and it was sometimes difficult to get the right people together and to develop ownership of the project. However, the project also reinforced known key factors for success. Shortell et al. (1995) and Gillies et al. (2000) defined four types of barriers to success: (a) structural, (b) cultural, (c) technical, and (d) strategic. We had to deal with different situations related to each of these, as described in the following sections.

TABLE 97.3 A Typology of the Causes of Falls

	No. of cases in which the factor is	
Cause of falls	Identified as a cause	Considered the main cause
Individual factors	69	31
Medical pathology (e.g., agitation, hypotension)	15	7
Dependence (e.g., mobility, visual impairment)	23	12
Related to treatment (e.g., opiates, sedatives)	31	12
Organizational factors	42	22
Dependent on use of equipment	7	4
Table on wheels	1	0
Misuse of physical restraints	3	3
Walker	3	1
Linked to the structure of the hospital	10	5
Telephone cords	3	3
Use of elevator and automatic fire doors	3	2
Bad position of handrails	4	0
Lack of assistance	13	10
Walking without cane in treatment of disease by baths	3	1
Operation of firebreak doors without accompanying caregiver	7	6
Wet floor	3	3
Poor perception of risk (no assistance for improving mobility)	8	2
Poor coordination of patient/professional care (unanswered call, misunderstanding concerning need for assistance)	4	1
All factors	111	53

Structural Dimension

Larger hospitals find that size inhibits effective interaction and communication. In our study, the pilot unit was composed of five wards, and the three other units were not in the same building. The focus group, composed of people working in these different units, and the nurse manager meetings allowed us to develop more of a cross-functional approach that cut across units.

The existing information system was also not useful for producing data that we could use to analyze the causes of falls. For this reason, we developed a specific qualitative and prospective study. However, we never tested the possibility of developing a system that could allow for a routine assessment procedure in all care units. This would stipulate the need for specific analyses of falls but would also require prolonging the program to a point when there would be no more specific support. Therefore, we are currently developing a risk assessment tool that could be used to promote prevention programs for patients at high risk of falling.

Cultural Dimension

Organizational and psychological barriers exist among hospital units, limiting the extent to which people are willing to participate in cross-unit projects. For this reason, integrating members of each unit has been a key factor in the successful development and implementation of recommendations with respect to daily activity. In addition, documentation of falls was not seen as punishment oriented: Identification of systems failures helps to reinforce a team-oriented approach more than an individual one.

Technical Dimension

The lack of physicians' and managers' involvement is an important barrier to the implemen-

888 SECTION X • ESTABLISHING, MONITORING, AND MAINTAINING QUALITY

tation of recommendations. In our study, both clinicians and management were involved in a coordinated approach, which is essential given the importance of the individual patient factors and the environment. The term *coordination* is often just a word; rifts among physicians, other caregivers, and administrative groups—rather than a real coordinated approach—are often revealed. In our experience, several factors were essential for providing a concrete sense of a coordinated approach: the quality improvement rule, which defines the event; the multidisciplinary character of the program expressed in the composition of each group; and the institutional incentive given by the organization's support of the program.

Strategic Dimension

A major strategic barrier is that there is often no linkage between quality improvement plans and the strategic plans of a unit. The presentation of the recommendations to senior hospital management and the presence of two members of the administrative staff in the focus group helped to link this project to the strategic goals of this hospital. Moreover, we presented this project several times to the board and the director of this hospital, to diffuse knowledge of our activities in the hospital community.

DISCUSSION

This study was conducted in a French medical and rehabilitation unit with a specific case mix and its own style of management. However, we note that our population of fallers had characteristics similar to those reported in the literature: more men (Morgan, Mathison, Rice, & Clemmer, 1985), longer length of stay (Sehested & Severin-Nielson, 1977), predominance of neurological pathologies (Bates et al., 1995; Blake et al., 1988; Deming, 1986; Gillies et al., 2000; Hindmarsh & Estes, 1989; Morgan et al., 1985; J. M. Morse et al., 1985; Oliver et al., 1997; Sehested & Severin-Nielson, 1977; Shortell et al., 1995; Strauss & Corbin, 1998; Tinetti et al., 1994; Vetter & Ford, 1989), and higher degree of dependency (Tinetti, Liv, & Claus, 1993). The conditions surrounding the occurrence of falls also confirmed findings in the literature, that is, more falls at the end of the week (Bates et al., 1995; Deming, 1986; Gillies et al., 2000; Hind-

marsh & Estes, 1989; Morgan et al., 1985; J. M. Morse et al., 1985; Oliver et al., 1997; Sehested & Severin-Nielson, 1977; Shortell et al., 1995; Strauss & Corbin, 1998; Tinetti et al., 1994; Vetter & Ford, 1989), which can be explained by the psychological consequences of staying in the hospital over the weekend. Falls occur more frequently after eating, especially among the elderly, perhaps due to postprandial orthostatic hypotension (Vaitkevicius, Esserwein, Maynard, O'Connor, & Fleg, 1991). We also observed that falls happened disproportionately after lunch, when caregivers were not readily available and patients went to the toilet or for a nap. Finally, falls occurred most frequently in the bedroom, toilet, and bathroom.

Limits of the Study

From a methodological perspective, one can argue that it would have been better to study the occurrence and the etiology of falls from the same sample, and that a case-control study would have been a better method for the comparison between fallers and nonfallers. Moreover, the results do not demonstrate the real impact of this prevention program on the occurrence of falls. These results have been limited to a quantitative analysis of falls, based on the data in the falls register, and showed the following:

1. A significant decrease of the rate of falls between 1995 and 1996 (44.6% to 36.3%; $p < 0.01$), 1997 and 1998 (40.7% to 31.0%; $p < 0.001$), and between 1995 and 1998 (44.6% to 31.0%; $p = 0.0001$).
2. Analysis of the rates for fallers does not show any significant trend.
3. If we focus on the multifallers, the decrease of their rate between 1997 and 1998 (7.7% to 3.8%; $p = 0.01$), and also between 1995 and 1998 (6.9% to 3.8%; $p = 0.03$) is significant.

From the different phases of the quality improvement program, results suggest the following:

1. An initial decrease in the number of falls in 1996, linked to the announcement of the program.
2. An increase in the number of reported falls in 1997. Positive presentations, including

clear communication on the medical aspects of the phenomenon, the need for systematic recording along with a precise definition, and limiting blame and legal implications for unit personnel seem to have led to improved awareness and recording.
3. A decline of falls in 1998 linked with implementation of recommendations.

Even if these results suggest a positive impact of such a program, they must be interpreted with great caution: Variables for case mix should be controlled, the time period should be given more emphasis when interpreting the results regarding the historical trend in the occurrence of falls, and no evidence is given on changes in professional practice as a result of the prevention strategy. All these limitations have been noted, and a statistical program, including follow-up of the different rates from 1999 to 2004 and development of a valid medical score in order to evaluate the risk of falls (Recommendation 2), has been established.

Empirical Findings of a Practice-Based Research

Given these limitations, our main objective was to understand the role of CQI in improving a fall prevention strategy in a rehabilitation hospital. Taking this into consideration, this study showed that quality management methods provide three ways of improving organizational processes to prevent falls:

1. Identification of the organizational causes in addition to the clinical ones
2. Development of methods for promoting implementation of the recommendations by all stakeholders
3. Introduction of a vision of risk management

Using accepted CQI principles and techniques, we identified all causes of falls. This approach helped us to identify situations in which there was high risk due to clinical and organizational factors. By comparison, the literature (on falls) focuses mainly on clinical etiologies and rarely mentions organizational causes. Sehested and Severin-Nielson (1977) discussed some external causes, and Tinetti et al. (1994) examined extrinsic factors. Thus, this study is unique in its merging of clinical and organizational perspec-

tives and emphasizes the benefits of elucidating and formalizing the links between the organization of work and the risk of occurrence of falls. It helps to point out organizational factors involved in the occurrence of this adverse event, a key point in the prevention of any risks (Reason, 1997).

It is well documented that the diffusion of any corrective actions requires not only clear definitions and recommendations but also consideration of alternative strategies for implementation, as we mentioned above. We tested integrated quality management methods and derived principles for managing the development and implementation of clinical and organizational recommendations among diverse stakeholders.

The development of pragmatic risk assessment tools is certainly a first step for preventing falls. The objective of zero falls is unrealistic. CQI methods and, more broadly, risk-management strategies reinforce this view and stress the need for distinguishing avoidable and unavoidable occurrences of undesirable events and outcomes. This view suggests that, because some falls are unavoidable, it is more reasonable to consider that actions for primary and secondary prevention must be complemented by actions of tertiary prevention to minimize consequences when the undesirable event occurs. This explains why some of the recommendations focus on clinical and organizational procedures after the occurrence of the fall.

Designing a New Approach for Preventing Adverse Events on the Basis of Empirical Findings

Regarding all of these findings, this study permits extension of existing CQI methods for designing and implementing a prevention program that may be incorporated directly into daily activity.

1. In addition to education and therapeutic principles applied by medical and other staff, organizational recommendations concerning the use of equipment, staff vigilance for patient safety, and the availability of information to the patient and family appear to be equally as important. The challenge is to raise awareness among hospital personnel of the problems of internal organization and

its impact on clinical events. It is also a way of directing inquiry into new areas (e.g., the managerial aspects of implementing clinical and organizational improvements).

2. By elaborating and implementing recommendations, CQI methods also give basic methods for a professional group to learn from an adverse event such as falls (U.K. Department of Health, 2000).

3. Finally, the study introduces acceptance of the concept of unavoidable falls and of the notion that falls are only partially preventable. The programs and recommendations do not aim to achieve an illusory objective of zero falls but instead are designed to eliminate avoidable falls and to minimize consequences of unavoidable falls.

More than a sum of techniques, CQI offers a new frame of analysis when prevention strategies can combine clinical and managerial components. Beyond semantic debates, CQI methods can help to introduce a vision of risk management. Further studies are needed to determine how these methods are able to direct inquiry into new areas for designing prevention strategies. All of them can help to eliminate combinations of individual and organizational errors (Krohn, Corrigan, & Donaldson, 2000).[1]

Note

1. We thank patients, nurses, and physicians and Isabelle Lombard, Catherine Jeny-Loeper, Marie-Christine Maillet-Gouret, Patrice Barberousse, Nadine Ribet-Reinhart, Jeanine Parlange, and Nadine Barbier, for their valuable contribution to this work. This study was funded by the National Agency for Accreditation and Evaluation in Health Care (ANAES).

References

Baker, S., & Harvey, A. (1985). Fall injuries in the elderly. *Clinics in Geriatric Medicine, 1,* 501–512.

Bates, D., Pruess, K., Souney, P., & Platt, R. (1995). Serious falls in hospitalized patients: Correlates and resource utilization. *American Journal of Medicine, 99,* 137–143.

Blake, A. J., Morgan, K., Bendall, M. J., Dalloss, H., Ebrahim, S. B., Arie, T. H., et al. (1988). Falls by elderly people at home: Prevalence and associated factors. *Age and Ageing, 17,* 365–372.

Dargent-Molina, P., & Bréart, G. (1995). [Epidemiology and trauma related to elderly patients' falls]. *Rev Epidemiol Sante Publique, 43,* 72–83.

Deming, W. E. (1986). *Out of crisis.* Cambridge, MA: Cambridge University Press.

De Vincenzo, D., & Watkins, S. (1987). Accidental falls in a rehabilitation setting. *Rehabilitation Nursing, 12*(5), 248–252.

Gillies, R. R., Reynolds, K. S. E., Shortell, S. M., Hughes, E. F. X., Budetti, P. P., Rademaker, A. W., et al. (2000). Implementing continuous quality improvement. In J. R. Kimberly & E. Minvielle (Eds.), *The quality imperative: Measurement and management of quality in healthcare* (pp. 79–100). London: Imperial College Press.

Hindmarsh, J. J., & Estes, E. J. (1989). Falls in older persons: Causes and interventions. *Archives of Internal Medicine, 149,* 2217–2222.

Krohn, L. T., Corrigan, J. M., & Donaldson, M. S. (Eds.). (2000). *To err is human: Building a safer health system.* Washington, DC: National Academy Press. Retrieved June 30, 2003, from http://www.nap.edu/books/0309068371/html/

Miller, W. J. (1996). A working definition for total quality management (TQM) researchers. *Journal of Quality Management, 1*(2), 149–159.

Morgan, R., Mathison, J. H., Rice, J. C., & Clemmer, D. I. (1985). Hospital falls: A persistent problem. *American Journal of Public Health, 75,* 775–777.

Morse, J. M., Prewse, M. D., Morrow, N., & Federsperl, G. (1985). A retrospective analysis of patient falls. *Canadian Journal of Public Health, 76,* 116–118.

Morse, K. (1996). *Preventing inpatient falls.* London: Sage.

Oliver, D., Britton, M., Seed, P., Martin, F. C., & Hopper, A. H. (1997). Development and evaluation of evidence based risk assessment tool (stratify) to predict which elderly inpatients will fall: Case-control and cohort studies. *British Medical Journal, 315,* 1049–1053.

Reason, J. (1997). *Managing the risks of organizational accidents.* Aldershot, Hampshire, England: Ashgate.

Rubinstein, L., Josephon, K., & Robbins, A. (1994). Falls in the nursing home. *Annals of Internal Medicine, 121,* 442–451.

Sehested, P., & Severin-Nielson, A. (1977). Falls by hospitalized elderly patients: Cause, prevention. *Geriatrics, 32*(4), 101–113.

Shortell, S. M., O'Brien, J. L., Carman, J. M., Foster, R. W., Hughes, E. F., Boerstler, H., et al. (1995). Assessing the impact of continuous quality improvement/total quality management: Concept versus implementation. *Health Services Research, 30*(2), 377–401.

Strauss, A., & Corbin, J. (1998). *Basics of qualitative research: Techniques and procedures of developing grounded theory.* London: Sage.

Tinetti, M. E., Baker, D. I., MacAvay, G., Claus, E. B., Garrett, P., Gottschalk, M., et al. (1994). A multifactorial intervention to reduce the risk of falling among elderly people living in the community. *New England Journal of Medicine, 331,* 821–827.

Tinetti, M. E., Liv, W. L., & Claus, E. B. (1993). Predictors and prognosis of inability to get up after falls among elderly persons. *Journal of the American Medical Association, 269*(1), 65–70.

U.K. Department of Health. (2000). *An organisation with a memory. Report of an expert group on learning from adverse events in the NHS,* *chaired by the Chief Medical Officer.* London: Author.

Vaitkevicius, P. V., Esserwein, D. M., Maynard, A. K., O'Connor, F. C., & Fleg, J. L. (1991). Frequency and importance of postprandial blood pressure reduction in elderly nursing home patients. *Annals of Internal Medicine, 115*(11), 865–870.

Vetter, N., & Ford, D. (1989). Anxiety and depression scores in elderly fallers. *International Journal of Geriatric Psychiatry, 4,* 158–163.

98 ESTABLISHMENT AND UTILIZATION OF BALANCED SCORECARDS

Kenneth R. Yeager

Whereas most for-profit organizations have adopted the use of strategic planning and balanced scorecards to achieve a competitive advantage in the marketplace, health care organizations have used strategic planning since the 1970s to help them meet the health needs of communities. This process has evolved over the past decade into a well-recognized and utilized management tool in health care organizations. The purpose of this chapter is to outline the strategic planning process, using a balanced scorecard to assist agencies and organizations in adapting to the ever-challenging and changing health care environment (Zuckerman, 2003). Despite the relatively simplistic approach presented in this chapter, it should be noted that some have experienced difficulty in applying this tool to centralized systems, which are frequently driven by multiple missions, have multiple practice applications, and sometimes exist in environments with multiple and competing political and programmatic goals (Chesley & Wenger, 1999).

The concept of managing strategy is essentially equal to the process of managing change. Frequently, managing change is as difficult as controlling the inertia of human nature to resist change. There are times when resistance to change outweighs ability of small agencies (and even large hospital facilities) to design and implement effective strategic planning. The organization's resistance to change is frequently overlooked as organizational leaders strive to develop strategic planning. This is a fatal error on the part of administration, because the implementation of strategic planning involves leadership, teamwork, and development of an organizational culture that includes a value for process change.

This chapter examines the process of developing and implementing a strategic plan using best practices and balanced scorecards to track implementation of an organization's goals and objectives. In this process, there are three overarching processes that serve as the framework for development and implementation of strategic planning. The overarching framework is as follows:

Phase 1. Building momentum: A 3- to 6-month period devoted to executive-level momentum building. *Focus:* Communication and examination of processes driving the need for change, establishment of a leadership team, and clarification of the organization's mission and vision (Kaplan & Norton, 1996).

Phase 2. Design and rollout: A 6-month period in which new strategies are examined, agreed on, and introduced at top levels in the organization. *Focus:* Design and implementation. Processes are designed to address organizational needs. Implementation plans are developed by direct practitioners and support staff. Balanced scorecards are used to visualize and document all implementation processes across the organization. Scorecards include the contributions of each department and team to the execution of the strategic plan (Kaplan & Norton, 1996).

Phase 3. Sustainable execution: A 12- to 24-month period in which strategies agreed upon by top administration, direct care staff, and support staff are integrated into the day-to-day work and culture of the organization. Balanced scorecards are used to educate individuals and to document progress toward established goals. Sustainable long-term results and short-term gains are generated and presented to staff in clear, concise goal statements.

Historically, strategic planning has been reserved for senior management, with the process requiring little to no input from the remainder of the organization. However, it is becoming increasingly clear that organizations expecting success are demonstrating a greater focus on the organizational-wide interest, support, and participation in strategic planning initiatives. The remainder of this chapter will focus on effective development of and communication regarding the implementation of a strategic plan developed by all staff. Emphasis will be placed on processes that facilitate staff acceptance of responsibility for execution of the strategic plan.

Application of the process will require certain shifts in previous thinking, defined as follows:

- Shift from administrative planning to planning by departments (the players are direct line staff)
- Shift from administrative view to a holistic view of the organization's strategy and measurements of success
- Continuous versus annual strategic planning and budgeting
- Shift from administrative to holistic approach to strategic planning processes and reporting
- Capitalizing on the potential of all organizational members
- Assuring the strategic plan is a living process undergoing frequent review, assessment, validation, and revision
- Establishment and broad communication of planning processes throughout the organization
- Taking steps to ensure that compensation and employee incentive are driven by the strategic plan

STEP-BY-STEP STRATEGIC PLANNING AND IMPLEMENTATION

Step 1: Analyzing the Situation

Establishing an understanding of the organization's current reality is extremely important to the development of a strategic plan, because the organization's current reality forms the foundation of all planning. Although it may be tempting to understate or underestimate the shortcomings of your agency, do not under any circumstances fall victim to this trap. Figure 98.1 outlines a visual process for conducting a strict inventory of the strengths and weaknesses and pros and cons of current programming and operations. All strategic plans must be realistic; unfortunately all too often it is a harsh reality when business digs the foundation for future growth. Reality must build the foundation for all future planning activities (Pink, McKillop, Schraa, & Preyra, 2001).

Step 2: Establishing Strategic Direction

Following a complete analysis of the organization's current reality, organizational leaders are now challenged to plot the course of the organization. Searching for the best fit between the organization's strengths and its ability to grow toward a particular area of new business can in-

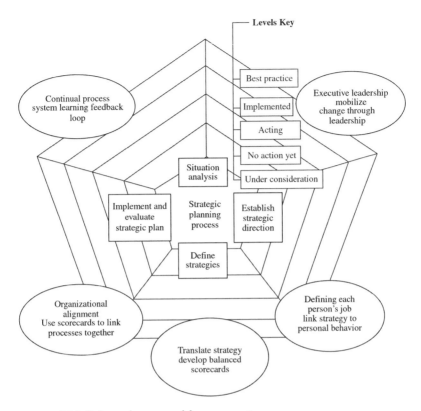

FIGURE 98.1 Balanced scorecard key concepts.

dicate the organization's strategic direction. This is the time to develop action plans, establish time lines and critical paths, assign ownership for action plans, identify resource requirements and budget requests, and link all of these to current and future operating plans (Curtright, Stolp-Smith, & Edell, 2000).

Step 3: Defining Strategies

Strategies are inseparable from planning and doing. Therefore, particular attention should be given to the identification of gaps in current efforts to achieve organizational goals. Efforts to identify new opportunities to accomplish organizational goals should close current gaps in service. Finally, supportive strategies for new initiatives should be considered (e.g., linking annual budgets to planning) (Rovinsky, 2002). For each strategy, organizational leadership must define the following:

- Major components of the action plan
- Resource requirements (for example, staffing patterns, budget, staffing skill level)

- Project ownership
- Barriers to implementation
- Technology requirements
- Estimated completion time frames
- Communication processes required

Step 4: Defining Each Person's Job

When the above activities have been completed, it is time to educate staff on the next steps of strategic development, to empower staff to assume an active role in the processes that have been put into action with their input, and to motivate those at all levels of the organization to implement and execute the chosen strategies (Fielden, 1999).

Step 5: Translating Strategy (Visualizing the Process)

The importance of communicating this process through a single communication tool that is easily identified, and on which progress can be tracked with a single glance, cannot be over-

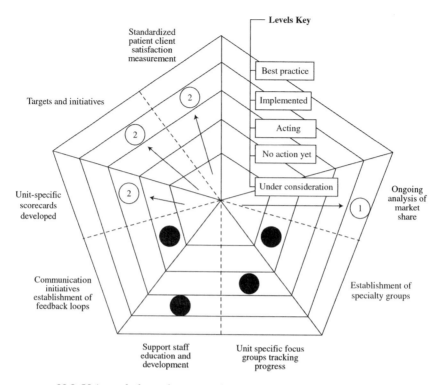

FIGURE 98.2 Using a balanced scorecard to document progress to strategic objectives.

stated. Figure 98.2 provides an example of a balanced scorecard designed to accomplish this process. Use the balanced scorecard to translate strategy into operational terms (Kaplan & Norton, 1997).

Step 6: Creating Organizational Alignment

In addition to the balanced scorecard's providing a strong communication component, the scorecard can be used to translate the organizational goals into organizational behaviors that are measurable and linked to specified business units and support units. Business-unit-specific goals can consist of acquiring new customers, addressing specific problem populations, increasing patient or client satisfaction, or increasing the patient's or client's satisfaction with the value of services received (Cleverley, 2001; Kaplan & Norton, 1997).

Step 7: Continuing the Process

When specific goals have been established, the next step becomes providing staff with clear or-

ganizational targets for each objective of the strategic plan. Targets are a tool for communication of progress toward organizational objectives and goals. Targets also provide reinforcement for desired organizational behavior. Therefore, targets should be clear, measurable, and to the point. This can be accomplished very simply by listing goals and specific targets as demonstrated below. For example:

Goal:	Measurement:
1. Acquisition of new customers	1. Maintenance of 53% of market share
2. Addressing of problem populations	2. Development of specialty treatment programming for difficult populations by July 1, 2004
3. Increased patient satisfaction	3. Increase in overall patient satisfaction to 71% 9s and 10s on 10-point scale

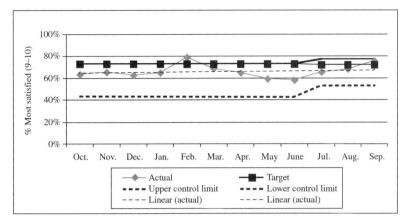

FIGURE 98.3 A demonstration of the use of control charts to track progress over time.

Figure 98.3 demonstrates the use of control charts to track progress over time.

The individual goals of the process are not the only continual process. Strategy is also a continual process. Scorecards assist with alignment of leadership and staff for the completion of strategic processes, including rollout and sustaining goals (Curtright, Stolp-Smith, & Edell, 2000). It is important to understand that plan development does not mean plan execution. A downfall of many organizations is failure to accurately implement the plan as designed. Strategic planning is not accomplished as easily as it is imagined. It is the responsibility of the leadership team to keep all strategic initiatives on track. Communication is an essential component of any strategic plan. Utilization of targets, control charts, and balanced scorecards will assist staff in understanding how close or far away from the organization's goal they are over a period of time (Cleverley, 2001; Kaplan & Norton, 1997).

True team behavior has not yet been developed. Additionally, the shared vision for the strategic plan has not been developed. The balanced scorecard assists with communicating the team plan and also with the current stage of implementation for each department as demonstrated in Figure 98.1. As seen in the example of the balanced score card, each strategic initiative is linked to the correlating organizational goal. The scorecard indicates the current progress of the initiative. Multiple departmental progress toward implementation of strategic goals can be displayed using color-coded or different-shaped indicators to identify specific

business performance. In addition, the scorecard can indicate the person or persons responsible for the initiative (Abrahamson, 2000; Bellenfant & Nelson, 2003).

Effective management uses scorecards to

- monitor progress
- motivate appropriate behavior
- communicate information
- establish accountabilities
- identify opportunities for improvement

Effective scorecards are

- concise
- balanced
- used to communicate strategy
- easy to understand
- dynamic

For the strategic plan to be effective, organizational leadership must (a) ensure that everyone understands the strategic plan and is demonstrating efforts to demonstrate organizational behaviors, actions aligned with the strategic plan; and (b) demonstrate leadership's commitment to a new form of management, one that is linked to a focused strategic plan. Leadership behaviors include holding frequent focused meetings reviewing the progress of each strategic initiative. Analysis must be understandable and visual in nature, hence the use of the scorecard or statistical control chart. The process will gain increasing credibility as all members of the organization, from direct care staff to board members, begin to identify movement in positive directions as a result of focused strategic planning and management of change (Cleverley, 2001; Gershon, 2003; Kaplan & Norton, 1997).

The organization's effectiveness in adapting to challenges in the environment includes the ability to respond quickly and demonstrate flexibility to ensure that budgeting, staffing, and resources are available to align the organization with the stated strategic plan. Process management or management by objective will assist with implementation of strategic planning. Effective strategic planning is functioning optimally when it is hardwired into management processes in the organization. Awareness of optimal functioning of the strategic plan comes as unit managers and line staff begin to ask questions reflecting the strategic plan, for example, "Have you seen the patient satisfaction data for this month?" Once the strategic plan has become a part of the organizational culture, the ability to manage strategy by management of change processes will have successfully been accomplished, providing the organization with the ability to adapt to the ever-changing world we live in (Gershon, 2003; Kaplan & Nelson, 1997).

References

Abrahamson, E. (2000, July/August). Change without pain. *Harvard Business Review, 78*(4), 75–78.

Bellenfant, W. L., & Nelson, M. J. (2002, October). Strategic planning: Looking beyond the next move. *Healthcare Financial Management, 56*(10), 62–67.

Chesley, J. A., & Wenger, M. S. (1999, Spring). Transforming an organization: Using models to foster a strategic conversation. *California Management Review, 41*(3), 54–74.

Cleverley, W. O. (2001, Spring). Financial dashboard reporting for the hospital industry. *Journal of Healthcare Finance, 27*(3), 30–40.

Curtright, J. W., Stolp-Smith, S. C., & Edell, E. S. (2000). Strategic performance management: Development of a performance measurement system at the Mayo Clinic. *Journal of Healthcare Management, 45*(1), 58–68.

Fielden, T. (1999). Pilot refines decision support. *InfoWorld, 21*(48), 77–78.

Gershon, H. J. (2003, January/February). Strategic positioning: Where does your organization stand? *Journal of Healthcare Management, 48,*(1), 12–14.

Kaplan, R. S., & Norton, D. P. (1996). *The balanced scorecard.* Boston: Harvard Business School Press.

Kaplan, R. S., & Norton, D. P. (1997). Why does business need a balanced scorecard? *Journal of Cost Management, 111*(3), 5–11.

Pink, G. H., McKillop, I., Schraa, E. G., & Preyra, C. (2001). Creating a balanced scorecard for a hospital system. *Journal of Health Care Finance, 27*(3), 1–19.

Rovinsky, M. (2002). *Healthcare financial management, 56*(1), 36–39.

Zuckerman, A. M. (2003). A call for better strategic planning. *Health Forum Journal, 46*(1), 25–30.

99

STRENGTHENING PRACTICE THROUGH RESULTS MANAGEMENT

Dennis K. Orthner & Gary L. Bowen

Evidence-based practice (EBP) does not operate in a vacuum. Typically, intervention practice models are built and sustained in an organizational or agency context. EBP is more likely to occur if the organization and its leadership are open to acquiring and using new information to improve agency practice. On the other hand, if the organization is not used to basing program decisions on empirical data, it will be much more difficult to use gathered evidence to plan programs or to optimize the delivery of client services.

In the language of Gambrill (1999), an organization that guides practice through authority-based systems of information—such as regulations requiring a specific practice model—will find it difficult to develop mechanisms or processes that base practice decisions on new evidence. In contrast, EBP requires leadership and staff openness to new ideas, a serious desire to improve client results or outcomes, and a planning process that uses new information to improve agency practices.

To successfully implement an EBP intervention system, the organizational context must assure the acquisition, management, and use of evidence to inform and update the prevailing practice model within the agency. This prevailing practice model, specified in the context of the agency's mission and its outcome objectives, depicts the path of influence between agency activities and intended client results. Unfortunately, in many cases current models are more implicit than explicit and focus more on what an agency *delivers* than on the intended *consequences* of its efforts. Such a lack of clearly defined practice models compromises practice accountability. This lack also limits an agency's probability of

achieving outcome objectives through modification of policies, programs, and direct practice interventions over time.

In this context, and on the basis of our consulting work with human service organizations over the last decade, we have developed a management planning model called *results management* (RM). RM attempts to promote a planning and information utilization process in human service organizations that encourages EBP and supports organizational learning.

This chapter describes the RM model and provides general practice guidelines for implementing a results-based perspective to serve as a foundation for EBP. We also offer guidelines for assessing human service intervention designs to determine if clear links are being made—or can be made—between current interventions and intended outcomes.

RESULTS MANAGEMENT

In simple terms, RM is a decision-management and resource-allocation strategy to map the path of influence between intervention activities and targeted outcomes. A key RM principle is planning with the intended results in mind (Covey, 1990). In other words, RM helps practitioners manage *results* rather than *activities*; it specifies program activities only after defining intended results. Intended results are then organized in the form of a logic model based on theory, empirical research, practice wisdom, and discussion with stakeholders at multiple levels.

Although regulations often partly drive agency programs, the specific nature and implementation of activities can vary. RM helps ensure the best fit between the activities or interventions undertaken and the intended results. RM assists agencies in redirecting their services toward clearly defined and anticipated results. The design and implementation of program activities should achieve results carefully scripted for the population served.

To achieve such design goals, we link specific short-term or *program results,* which are the direct consequence of interventions, with longer term *target results.* These anticipated target results then inform a clear practice or a logic model that determines the specific intervention activities we build into the program. This requires (a) a deliberate planning process, (b) a specific practice model or theory of change, (c) hypothesized direct links between intervention activities and results, (d) measurable indicators of activities and results, (e) a resource allocation strategy to ensure support of activities and results, (f) an organizational culture founded on innovation and accountability, and (g) decision tools to promote organizational learning and potential changes in the proposed practice model.

The Context

The need for RM arises from a variety of factors operating in human services today, including a shift toward program accountability and performance-based management. For example, the Government Performance and Results Act of 1993 (P.L. 103–62) requires federal agencies to define and monitor their outcomes through a strategic planning process. In addition, the United Way of America (1996) has developed resource materials to assist member agencies in developing logic models connecting program inputs to program outcomes.

In addition, evaluation scholars and program planners have shown a renewed interest in performance measurement (Hatry, 1999; Martin & Kettner, 1996; Newcomer, 1997). Stimulated in part by the efforts of the United Way of America, the use of logic models as integrative frameworks is becoming standard practice in the articulation of practice models and in program planning and evaluation (see, for example, Cooksy, Gill, & Kelly, 2001). The outcome–asset impact model (Reed & Brown, 2001) is a notable example of a planning and evaluation framework that shares many assumptions in common with RM.

A surge of interest in EBP among practice professionals—especially in the social work community—has occasioned the need for RM. In their discussion of standards for evidence-based social work practice, for example, Rosen and Proctor (2002) use EBP to describe the actions of practitioners who "select interventions on the basis of their empirically demonstrated links to the desired outcomes" (p. 743).

There are several important intersections between RM and EBP. First, EBP requires attention to the specific needs of a target client or participant population. Unless such needs are specified and measured as inputs into program interventions, it is difficult to build a measurable intervention model to address them. RM begins its management process by specifying the needs, problems, or challenges the practice model intends to address.

Second, EBP requires a clear theory of change with very specific, measurable links between implemented program activities and intended client outcomes. RM develops this theory of change for agency practice, and it makes the model explicit for purposes of program planning and evaluation.

Third, EBP requires a clear outcome orientation that specifies measures of results and operationalizes those measures. RM provides a detailed planning process, specifies results, and builds measurement strategies for both results (outcomes) and activities (interventions).

Fourth, EBP works best when it includes a feedback process from results to intervention, enabling modification of program activities to improve practice interventions. RM offers a staff and leadership review process that should help staff and evaluators monitor interventions, determine if they are indeed producing the intended outcomes, and decide which strategies are most likely to produce these outcomes.

Key Concepts

To understand how to build an RM strategy that accomplishes program objectives, it is necessary to define four central concepts: (a) client needs and challenges, (b) program activities, (c) program results, and (d) target results.

Client needs and challenges are inputs into the RM model. Client or participant needs consist of measurable, specific problems, concerns, or issues that may compromise the achievement of critical personal or relational objectives if left unaddressed. At a personal level, for instance, needs may involve the frequency of inappropriate behavior. At a relational level, needs may include the level of interpersonal conflict in the setting. At a community level, needs may comprise the reduction of youth violence. Whatever the level, it is important to understand and to clearly define the problems or challenges an agency intends to address, and to use such definitions as the foundation of a results-based model. It is also important to identify assets and strengths that may function as resources in responding to such needs and challenges.

Program activities are the measurable events or interventions employed by an agency to achieve specific program results. This could involve an educational activity or a specific clinical intervention designed to achieve an outcome for a specific category of persons. At a personal level, for example, a program activity might include parent training for mothers and fathers of children removed from the home due to neglect. At a community level, this could include a new after-school curriculum for youth at risk of dropping out of school. In many human service agencies, program activities, rather than the intended results, serve as the central focus of attention.

Program results are the short-term measurable benefits or outcomes achieved by individuals, families, communities, or organizations served directly by agencies or indirectly influenced by an agency's community-based efforts. An agency will take credit or be held accountable by its stakeholders for these direct or short-term outcomes. For example, because an agency provides financial services and education, clients participating in this training program should gain a better understanding of financial management strategies and make better future decisions regarding personal finances.

Target results include the longer term measurable benefits or outcomes achieved by individuals, families, communities, or organizations, which can be directly or indirectly tied to meeting client or participant needs and challenges. These are typically broader results; thus, no single agency or program can take direct credit when such programs meet expectations, nor will an agency assume total blame when they fall short of expectations. These results affect clients directly served by agencies as well as those only indirectly served. For example, family support programs partly influence the ability of military families in a community to manage the

pressures of frequent deployments (Orthner & Rose, 2003). However, many other service providers (and certainly the work organization) also play a role in how well these families adjust.

The more indirect the result of a program activity, the more likely that it is a target result. Target results take longer to achieve—they are a secondary rather than a primary product of program activities. In program design, a more important distinction is the direct link between program activities and the intended or actual program results (i.e., benefits or consequences) of those activities. For example, the target result for an after-school program may be to reduce dropout rates for participating children. But intervention activities are more likely to focus on the immediate program results of increasing school attendance, improving grades on homework assignments, and garnering more involvement of parents in school-related activities.

MANAGEMENT DESIGNS

Activity-Oriented Program Design

Traditional designs for human services programs have tended to be *activity oriented* rather than results driven (see Figure 99.1). This classical approach to human services focuses on personal, family, and community needs and on agency responses to these needs. However, this model often fails to clearly define results or to gather the evidence needed to promote EBP. The model expects results to occur, but it seldom measures those results because the focus is on the intervention activities themselves and how these activities respond to identifiable needs.

When using an activity-oriented approach to program planning and delivery, program designers typically list results that should occur if they are successful, but program staff rarely measure results or outcomes because their attention becomes overwhelmed by the activities. For example, we say that our programs help people transition more successfully or spend their money more wisely or reduce family stress, but we rarely ever link what we do to client results.

Unfortunately, the summary reports that many agencies are required to submit to their sponsors or stakeholders are consistent with this activity model of agency accountability. They place priority on program outputs (e.g., the number of people served or the number of

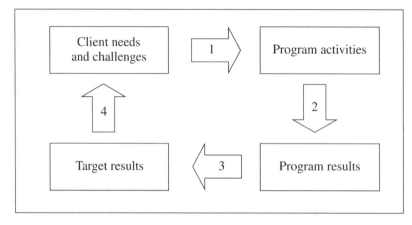

FIGURE 99.1 Activity-oriented design.

classes offered) rather than program results. Program outputs are really measures of whether an activity is occurring, not how well they benefit anyone, and include measures such as the number of programs and services delivered and the number of contacts or people served.

By endorsing such "activity accountability," program managers inadvertently help to keep agencies focused on activities rather than results. This is not to say that these program outputs are not important to record and to monitor over time; they are simply not sufficient as an accountability system for measuring program effectiveness. RM, in contrast, gives little attention to such program outputs and instead considers them program activity indicators.

Results-Oriented Program Design

The reliance on activities-oriented design is changing. For example, agencies supported by United Way increasingly report outcome indicators, rather than activity indicators, as measures to determine whether these agencies receive funding.

Results-oriented program designs such as RM are quite different from activity-oriented program designs (see Figure 99.2). Though the same factors are included in both design models, the RM model primarily focuses on results that must occur to meet client needs. Implemented program activities receive attention only after the path of intended results is clearly specified.

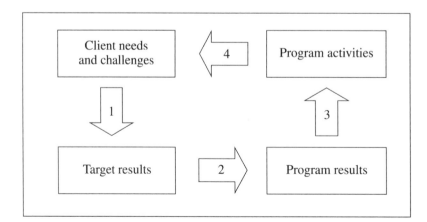

FIGURE 99.2 Results-oriented design.

Thus, this model directs activities toward such results and establishes measurable indicators, ensuring that results remain the focus and link to activities.

For example, if a program intends to teach parents the skills required for successful reunification with their children, it is important to go beyond just understanding their needs. Such a program must also measure whether parents have sufficient knowledge of their children's developmental requirements and the behavioral skills to manage their children without causing them physical or psychological harm.

For these results to occur, the program must first define the elements of successful parenting and then identify the factors, conditions, and events that support the desired result—in this case, reunification, child safety, and positive developmental outcomes for both children and parents. This approach results in intervention activities designed specifically to achieve these clearly defined program results. One aim of RM is to reduce the complexity of social interventions, to make explicit the proposed working of an intervention. This helps to define the theory of change behind an intervention and improves the practice guidelines and evaluability of the program model.

STEPS IN THE RESULTS MANAGEMENT PROCESS: WORKING WITH SCHOOL PRACTITIONERS

To illustrate how an agency would develop an RM process to become more effective in implementing and evaluating EBP, we will use an example from our own work: assisting in developing effective violence interventions in schools. In the school context, a number of evidence-based strategies exist for reducing the incidence of school violence (Bowen, Powers, Woolley, & Bowen, in press). During our consultation and evaluation of schools and communities, we have found RM principles and concepts helpful, particularly when working with school and community practitioners to select and monitor EBP strategies for reducing school violence.

Step 1: Gathering Evidence of Needs

The first step in the RM model gathers specific evidence of the problem, challenge, or need the intervention intends to target. Consistent with an RM framework, we begin the conversation by conducting a joint review of the presenting problem or situation, including the incidence of the problem. We often employ both administrative and survey data in our attempt to construct a baseline for the presenting problem and to gauge whether the problem and its indicators have been increasing, decreasing, or remaining stable over the previous several years. Sometimes, in the context of this discussion, we discover a redefinition of the nature of the problem; for instance, we may change our focus from overall school violence to aggression on school buses and during school events. This discussion intends to define the problem and the target needs very specifically.

Step 2: Defining Target Results

The second RM step is to clearly define the target results on the basis of what a successful intervention will achieve. In other words, the planning team should be able to say, "We will know we are successful when x (the end goal) is achieved." Furthermore, although some practitioners define baseline problem levels in negative terms, we ask practitioners to focus of the positive side of the problem; for instance, rather than examining incidents of school violence, we look for evidence of school safety.

In addition, we ask practitioners to define a performance standard—the desired result to be achieved during a specified time period. Target results can be framed in terms of knowledge, attitudes, or behavior, and to the extent that one of these results can be examined, we have found that behavioral result indicators are better indicators of success than knowledge or attitudes. In this example, a target result might include a specified number of weeks during the school year without reports of bus or event-related violent incidents.

Step 3: Specifying Program Results

At this point, we begin the third RM step, specifying program results. This critical step clearly identifies the path that leads to the identified target results. We believe most practitioners at this stage jump to defining the activities they want to undertake, without clearly defining what those activities need to achieve. To assist practitioners in slowing down and specifying program results, we ask the team to form a learning question: What would have to be different about this school's current functioning to increase school safety from its current level to our desired level?

In answering this question, we focus on specific knowledge, attitude, and behavior indicators. For example, we ask what students need to know, believe, or be able to do to close the performance gap. In addition, we ask the team to identify potential partners or allies the school should enlist to achieve the intended result. Such allies might include neighborhood leaders, parents, law enforcement officials, and teachers. For each partner or ally, we ask the participant group to specify what knowledge, attitudes, or behavior would be required, and we ask the group to estimate the current and desired levels of performance of these program results.

At this stage of the RM practice model, our emerging theory of how to influence the target result becomes exponentially more complex (see Figure 99.3). The complication arises because, for every target result, there are multiple program results or leverage points that increase the probability of achieving our end goal. This needs to be refined to create a manageable number of achievable program results. The role of the consultant at this stage is to share research and practice information about the factors that distinguish safe schools from unsafe schools, such as the level of student participation in extracurricular activities and the level of parent involve-

ment in the schools. This consultation should lead to refining the program results to a number both manageable and likely to have a high impact on achieving the target results.

Step 4: Proposing Evidence-Based Activities

After specifying target and program results, the practitioner group is ready for the fourth step in the RM process. It is now time to engage in a discussion of evidence-based strategies (program activities) that can directly influence the defined program results. For example, if constructive parent involvement at school events is an important program result, we examine the role of coaches or parent organizations in engaging positive parental involvement at these events. We also look at our science of practice in this area. For instance, we might turn to the Families and Schools Together (FAST) program to find strategies for developing parent–professional collaborative teams (McDonald, 2002). Developed by a social worker, Lynn McDonald, FAST has been endorsed by both the Office of Juvenile Justice and Delinquency Prevention and the Center for Substance Abuse Prevention as an evidence-based program for strengthening families (see McDonald, 2002, for additional details about FAST and a review of evaluation research supporting its effectiveness). For each critical program result, a specific activity or set of activities should exist to ensure achievement of that result. We agree with Rosen, Proctor, and Staudt's

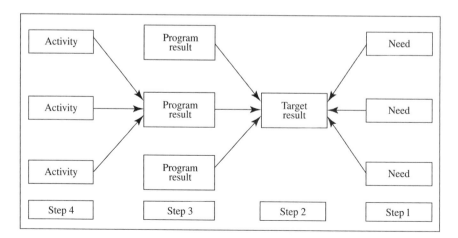

FIGURE 99.3 Illustrative results management program development model.

(2003) call for continued development of practice guidelines that link target outcomes with effective interventions.

Step 5: Reviewing Agency Capacity for Change

Finally, we examine changes required in the agency or system itself to ensure successful implementation and evaluation of the new practice model. This includes investigating the resources required to implement these new or expanded types of program activities, exploring organizational changes that will support these activities in achieving results, developing metrics to gauge progress and success, and executing an agreed-on implementation time line.

CONCLUSION

RM comprises a disciplined strategy for discovering and implementing an outcome-oriented and evidence-based program intervention practice model. RM attempts to open up the black box between program activities and target results. The aim is to identify and make explicit the critical processes that increase the likelihood that systematic program activities will achieve program-specific and longer term target results. Fully describing the links between interventions and results enables program staff, evaluators, or other stakeholders to clearly describe the underlying theory of change a given agency relies on to achieve client success. It is this theory of change that serves as the hypothesis for making program decisions and conducting evaluations.

Returning to the components described earlier in this chapter, the RM model promotes the unfolding of a carefully crafted outcomes-driven planning process and produces an EBP model with an explicit theory of change. This model offers what is needed in building and testing an evaluable program: hypothesized links between intervention activities and results and measurable indicators of activities and results. As intervention technology moves toward higher expectations for program success indicators, RM provides a useful strategy for developing measurable interventions and procedures for measuring those interventions.

Experience with this process also tells us that taking a team through RM is meaningful for those who participate in it. It often takes hidden assumptions and expectations out of the closet and into the open for exploration, manipulation, and refinement. The process usually reveals new potential pathways to success, and it creates opportunities to envision new ways of overcoming barriers and achieving results that everyone agrees are necessary. Whereas the process sometimes suggests that current strategies are unlikely to be effective, it can also identify program components with a high likelihood for success, and those that need redesigning to optimize their effectiveness.

Altogether, the RM model offers greater opportunities to incorporate evidence into practice design (Bowen, Richman, & Bowen, 2002) and assists in the testing of social interventions. First, using empirical and practice evidence to review potential program results can lead to longer-term target results. In addition, RM relies on evidence, developing intervention activities previously linked to the intended results. Finally, evidence from the new RM practice model is reviewed to substantiate or revise the intervention. This approach achieves the best results possible for the people served by the program. Ultimately, the success of any intervention comes when outcomes for people in need are achieved and agencies continue to refine their activities to better serve those who rely on them.

References

Bowen, G. L., Powers, J., Woolley, M. W., & Bowen, N. K. (in press). School violence. In L. A. Rapp-Paglicci, C. N. Dulmus, & J. S. Wodarski (Eds.), *Handbook of prevention interventions for children and adolescents*. New York: John Wiley.

Bowen, G. L., Richman, J. M., & Bowen, N. K. (2002). The school success profile: A results management approach to assessment and intervention planning. In A. R. Roberts & G. J. Greene (Eds.), *Social workers' desk reference* (pp. 787–793). New York: Oxford University Press.

Cooksy, L. J., Gill, P., & Kelly, P. A. (2001). The program logic model as an integrative framework for a multimethod evaluation. *Evaluation and Program Planning, 24,* 119–128.

Covey, S. (1990). *The 7 habits of highly effective people.* New York: Fireside.

Gambrill, E. (1999). Evidence-based practice: An alternative to authority-based practice. *Families in Society, 80*(4), 341–350.

Hatry, H. P. (1999). *Performance measurement: Getting results.* Washington, DC: Urban Institute Press.

Martin, L. L., & Kettner, P. M. (1996). *Measuring the performance of human services programs.* Thousand Oaks, CA: Sage.

McDonald, L. (2002). Evidence-based, family-strengthening strategies to reduce delinquency: FAST—Families and Schools Together. In A. R. Roberts & G. J. Greene (Eds.), *Social workers' desk reference* (pp. 717–722). New York: Oxford University Press.

Newcomer, K. E. (1997). Using performance measurement to improve programs. In K. E. Newcomer (Ed.), *Using performance measurement to improve public and nonprofit programs* (pp. 5–14). San Francisco: Jossey-Bass.

Orthner, D. K., & Rose, R. (2003). Dealing with the effects of absence: Deployment and adjustment to separation among military families. *Journal of Family & Consumer Science, 95*(1), 33–37.

Reed, C. S., & Brown, R. E. (2001). Outcome–asset impact model: Linking outcomes and assets. *Evaluation and Program Planning, 24,* 287–295.

Rosen, A., & Proctor, E. K. (2002). Standards for evidence-based social work practice: The role of replicable and appropriate interventions, outcomes, and practice guidelines. In A. R. Roberts & G. J. Greene (Eds.), *Social workers' desk reference* (pp. 743–747). New York: Oxford University Press.

Rosen, A., Proctor, E. K., & Staudt, M. (2003). Targets of change and interventions in social work: An empirically based prototype for developing practice guidelines. *Research on Social Work Practice, 13,* 208–233.

United Way of America. (1996). *Measuring program outcomes: A practical approach.* Alexandria, VA: Author.

100   MEASURING CLIENTS' PERCEPTION AS OUTCOME MEASUREMENT

Céline Mercier, Michel Landry, Marc Corbière, & Michel Perreault

In 1995, our team was developing a continuous quality improvement system for the Dollard-Cormier Center, a public substance abuse rehabilitation center located in Montreal (hereafter called "the agency"). One of the main concerns for the agency was that this system reflected its stakeholder-based orientation and its participative approach. In this perspective, the clients' input was to be a key dimension in the process of quality assessment, and their opinions should be considered in the future continuous quality improvement program.

In November of that year, *Consumer Reports* published an article entitled "Mental Health: Does Therapy Help?" (Mental Health, 1995; Seligman, 1995). This article reported the results of a survey conducted with the readers of the journal. Almost 7,000 of them answered 26 questions dealing with the types of problems they had encountered, how severe these problems were when they asked for help, whom they consulted, the type of treatment they received, how they felt at the current time, to what extent the therapy had helped them (from *has im-*

proved the situation a lot to *has worsened it*), in which domain, and how satisfied they were. This paper raised a controversy about the respective validity of two approaches (efficacy and effectiveness) for the outcome assessment of psychotherapy.

Some months later, a special issue of the *American Psychologist* was dedicated to "Outcome Assessment of Psychotherapy" (Vander-Bos, 1996). In that issue, Martin Seligman (1996), the author of the survey published in *Consumer Reports* (Mental Health, 1995), exposed his methodology at length and discussed its relevance and validity. Other papers also supported his point of view, while other authors raised serious concerns or denied any scientific validity to the retrospective approach. The main points under discussion in these papers were the validity of self-report measures and third-party or objective measures, the relative importance of external criteria to assess success or failure, and clients' perceptions.

This debate led our team to further study the issue of the validity of the clients' perception regarding the issue of the treatment. In the context of our mandate of developing client-centered quality indicators, the research questions were as follows: Should the input from the clients be limited to satisfaction? If one wants to know the clients' perception about the treatment results, why not ask them directly? What is the relevance and validity of such a procedure?

This chapter reports the results obtained with an instrument developed to assess treatment outcomes from the clients' perspective. These psychometric data bring some evidence regarding the relevance and validity of monitoring and evaluation practices that would take more into account the clients' experience with the treatment.

LITERATURE REVIEW

The literature review confirms that satisfaction remains the most current performance and quality indicator involving the client. Some satisfaction questionnaires include items dealing with satisfaction with treatment results. For example, the Client Satisfaction Questionnaire (CSQ-8) asks the respondent, "Have the services you received helped you to deal more effectively with your problems?" (Larsen, Attkisson, Hargreaves, & Nguyen, 1979, p. 201). The Service

Satisfaction Scale (SSS-30; Greenfield & Attkisson, 1989) contains a nine-item subscale named Perceived Outcome/Efficacy. This scale has items on satisfaction "with effects of services in helping relieve symptoms," "on well-being and preventing relapse," "in helping deal with problems," and "with contribution to achieving life goals" (p. 275). A subscale on "Efficacy" is also found in the Verona Service Satisfaction Scale, European version (VSSS-EU; Ruggeri et al., 2000).

In the literature on quality assurance and performance indicators, the changes in clinical status are considered as one main domain of interest. Very often, the clinician assesses these changes. As an example, one can refer to the Clinical Global Impression (CGI; Guy, 1976), in which one of the three global subscales asks the clinician to quote the patient's global improvement. However, it is very difficult to find in the literature a corresponding index that would cover the client's impression. An example of such an attempt is the consumer survey designed by Srebnik et al. (1997) to assess the quality of public mental health care. In that survey, four items ask clients to what extent they consider they have attained their work and education goals.

The Human Service Research Institute (HSRI) Evaluation Center (Mulkern, Leff, Green, & Newman, 1995) reviewed literature on performance indicators with a view of proposing a consumer-oriented mental health report card. Of the 26 monitoring systems they surveyed, only one identified as an indicator the "average score on consumer-rated effectiveness/change" (p. 39). However, there could be a growing interest for self-report outcome measures: In February 2001, a meeting was conducted involving the Federal Drug Administration (FDA) that addressed "Important Issues in Patient-Reported Outcomes Research" (MAPI Research Institute, 2001).

INSTRUMENT DEVELOPMENT

To measure the clients' assessment of the results of their treatment, we developed the Questionnaire on Perceived Changes. This questionnaire is structured around 19 life domains or skills in which changes can be expected. These domains were selected following a consultation (focus groups) with clients and practitioners. They include the seven dimensions covered in the Addiction Severity Index (ASI; Bergeron, Landry, Brochu, & Guyon, 1998; McLellan et al., 1992), the scale being used in the agency both for the initial clinical assessment and for follow-ups (short form). Examples of domains covered are medical status; legal status; psychological status; status of family and social relationships; employment or support status (from the ASI); nutrition and sleep; housing; emotional stability; problem solving; stress management and crisis management; self-image; and overall condition. The response choices on the Change Scale (Likert scale) are *a lot of improvement, some improvement, nothing changed, worse, don't know*, and *doesn't apply*.

An attribution scale was built to assess to what extent the perceived change was related to the participation in the agency program. Following the Perceived Changes Scale, this scale refers to the same domains with the question, "To what extent do you consider that changes in Domain X can be related to your participation in the (agency) program?" The possible answers are *entirely, partly, not at all, don't know*, and *doesn't apply* (the last one being used when the respondent did not perceive any change).

In terms of substance use, the agency gives greater importance to a harm reduction approach. In that perspective, the clients can choose as a goal (regarding their consumption) between total abstinence, abstinence from given substances, controlled consumption, or harm reduction. In the questionnaire, a multiple-choice item includes these four options, with the question, "What is your main goal regarding consumption?" The following item asks "To what extent did you reach your main goal regarding consumption (of substance abuse)?" with the choice of answers being 100%, 75%, 50%, 25%, or 0% ("My main goal was attained at 100%" and so on—Likert scale). The last items cover sociodemographic and relevant clinical information.[1]

RESEARCH STRATEGY AND METHODOLOGY

Data Collection

The Questionnaire on Perceived Changes was pretested as part of a telephone survey in which interviews were conducted with a randomized sample of 100 clients (Mercier & Landry, 1999). Another set of data was collected, taking advantage of a pre- and post-outcome study that was conducted with 228 clients. This offered the opportunity to compare results about changes from two strategies: differences between baseline and 6-month scores on a standardized scale (ASI) and clients' retrospective assessment.

Statistical Analyses

In search of some evidence about the validity of outcome indicators that would be based on clients' self-report of changes, analyses were conducted on the data to assess some of their psychometric properties. Construct validity was tested using exploratory factorial analysis, and reliability was assessed with Cronbach's alpha. Finally, some results on criterion validity could be obtained when the differences on ASI scores at baseline and 6-month follow-up were compared with the results from the Questionnaire of Perceived Changes (Pearson's correlations).

RESULTS

Study Population

The clients that participated in these studies were representative of the main characteristics of the agency's overall clientele: 66% of them were male, with an average age of 36 years. Half of them had a high school or greater level of education.

Factorial Analysis and Internal Consistency

When the exploratory factorial analysis was conducted, a three-factor solution emerged and 51.3% of the variance was explained. Factor 1 covered nine items (43.3% of variance) related to social and psychological domains; it was labeled "Self/Relationships." Factor 2 (4.4% of variance) brought together four items in relation to "Physical Health." Factor 3 (three items, 3.6% of variance) was related to "Living Conditions." Three items were deleted because they loaded on more than one factor.

The internal consistency (Cronbach's alpha) for the whole scale was 0.92. The alphas for the subscales were .91 (Factor 1), .68 (Factor 2), and .82 (Factor 3).

Concordance Between ASI Scores and Perceptions of Changes

Moderate correlations were found between the scores on the Questionnaire of Perceived Changes and the changes as measured with the ASI in the before-and-after design in the outcome study (see Table 100.1). One can observe that a greater difference between baseline and follow-up on the Alcohol Use and the Psychological Status subscales on the ASI corresponds to a higher score on the Questionnaire of Perceived Changes. The same trend is observed between changes in psychological status, as measured with the ASI, and the perceived change as measured with the Self/Relationships subscale. It is of interest that the highest correlations were found in the domains of alcohol use, drug use, and psychological status, domains on which most of the treatment activities were focused. The fact that the difference between the before-and-after measures on the ASI Employment/Support subscale was correlated with the Living Conditions subscale in the Questionnaire of Perceived Changes can be seen as a good indicator of face validity. On the other hand, the negative correlation between Psychological Status (ASI scale) and Physical Health (Questionnaire of Perceived Changes) is difficult to interpret.

Concordance Between Goal Attainment and Perception of Changes

At 6-month follow-up, lower scores (meaning improvement) on the Alcohol and Drug Use subscales were observed ($p < .001$) when either of the goals regarding substance consumption was perceived as attained. The level of improvement (difference between baseline and 6-month follow-up scores on Alcohol and Drug Use sub-scales) was also greater when the goals regarding consumption were considered as attained.

A correlation was found between the scores on ASI Alcohol and Drug Use subscales and the type of goal regarding consumption. The clients who identified abstinence (42%) as their goal had the lowest scores on these scales. The abstinence group was also the group that showed more improvement on the Alcohol and Drug Use subscales ($p < .001$).

DISCUSSION

The objective of this study was to generate some research evidence about the validity of measuring clients' perceptions of treatment results as an outcome indicator. Even if this study was not conceived as a validation study in the strictest sense, the preliminary results on the development of the Questionnaire on Perceived Changes are encouraging. Psychometric analyses have demonstrated that this questionnaire involves factors that are not only clinically sound but also present good internal consistency (global questionnaire and subscales based on the different factors). Tests of criterion validity (perceived changes compared with differences on before-and-after ASI scores) tend to support the hypothesis that clients' points of view are reliable and valid.

This type of indicator offers new opportunities for outcome studies. The scale allows for flexibility to evaluate the outcomes of interest for the clinicians or the clients. For instance, the clinician and the client can identify some rehabilitation goals (domains of expected changes or skills to be developed) at the beginning of the treatment and assess the level of changes some months later. Another strategy would be to dis-

TABLE 100.1 Correlations Between Differences on ASI Scores and Scores on Perceived Changes Scale

Perceived Change Scales	Self/Relationship	Physical Health	Living Conditions	Global
ASI scales:				
Alcohol use				0.20
Drug use	0.27		0.23	
Psychological status	0.28	−0.30		0.29
Employment/Support			0.32	

card some domains at follow-up, using the category *doesn't apply*. The Attribution scale allows collecting data on whom and what brings the observed changes, these changes being positive or negative.

The measurement of perceived changes represents a significant contribution to the issue of calibration (Sechrest, McKnight, & McKnight, 1996). This issue refers to the fact that a statistically significant change on a standardized scale doesn't necessarily translate into a significant change in real life. When the client reports the effects, one can assume more surely that the observed changes are of sufficient amplitude to have a real impact on his or her life, condition, or behaviors.

One of the main concerns regarding clients' evaluation of their treatment is the return to a prescientific world of subjective judgment and "ultimately, toward the loss of scientific credibility" (Mintz, Drake, & Crits-Christoph, 1996, p. 1084). This has to be taken into consideration, and self-report evaluations have to be accompanied by other methods of impact evaluations, such as experimental (efficacy) and quasi-experimental designs (effectiveness). However, outcome rating by clients improves the evaluation process with another source of data, in addition to evaluation by the clinician, the evaluator, a third party, or objective measures. This is especially relevant when "the changing and turbulent environment of health care now demands a broader vision" (Newman & Tejeda, 1996, p. 1048).

The issue of bias is particularly challenging when considering clients' self-reports on outcomes. Such measures could be particularly sensitive to positive bias in terms of social desirability and cognitive rationalization, given the amount of effort—the emotional investment and eventually the money—that the individual has devoted to the treatment. Detailed instructions, assurance of confidentiality (preferably anonymity), and reliance on other sources could limit the influence of these biases. Another limitation is the absence of baseline data, which prevents controlling for regression to the mean and for the ceiling effect.

CONCLUSION

The purpose of this chapter was to provide some evidence regarding a client-centered outcome in-

dicator that is valid, clinically relevant, and useful in assessing performance and quality. Clients' retrospective assessments of the changes they experienced following their treatment in a rehabilitation center for substance abusers were corroborated by before-and-after measures in relevant domains, such as substance use and psychological status.

These first results open quite exciting perspectives, both from the clinical and administrative points of view. At the clinical level, feedback to clinicians on their clients' perceptions could support treatment planning and clinical practices. The concept of perceived change could also impact directly on the treatment process. One can hypothesize that satisfaction with services and perception of positive changes could play a role in motivation, compliance, and retention in treatment.

The concept of perceived changes could be a critical component for an empowerment-oriented program. As Chamberlin (1997) stated, "When a person brings about actual change, he or she increases feeling of mastery and control. This in turn leads to further and more effective change" (pp. 45–46). From this perspective, asking the client about the changes that he or she can see in his or her life and taking this judgment into account could have a significant therapeutic effect.

The use of a measure of clients' perceptions about changes is most advantageous from an administrative standpoint because of its ease of use. As an outcome measure, it can be used for a program evaluation or in a quality improvement monitoring system. It offers the opportunity to monitor outcomes on a regular basis, at low cost, and it can be included in a large-scale satisfaction survey. It opens new research perspectives, such as the study of the relationships between treatment compliance and retention and between satisfaction and perceived improvement. Finally, it responds to the growth of the consumer movement and to the public policy support of citizens' participation in the management of the health system. Ultimately, asking clients about the effects of the treatment they receive could be, in itself, a quality indicator.[2]

Notes

1. This questionnaire is available (French and English versions) from the first author (Céline Mercier, 8000 Notre-Dame Ouest, Lachine, QC, CANADA

H8R 1H2, phone (514) 364-2282, ext. 2360, e-mail cmercier.crld@ssss.gouv.qc.ca).

2. The satisfaction survey and the secondary analyses were supported by a contract from the Montreal Health and Social Services Regional Board. The outcome study was conducted under a grant from Health Canada. We wish to thank practitioners, clients, and research assistants for their contribution to this study. A first draft of this chapter was presented at the Annual Conference of the American Evaluation Association, Washington, D.C., November 2002.

References

Bergeron, J., Landry, M., Brochu, S., & Guyon, L. (1998). Les études psychométriques autour de l'ASI/IGT [Psychometric studies regarding Addiction Severity Index]. In L. Guyon, M. Landry, S. Brochu, & J. Bergeron (Eds.), *L'évaluation des clientèles alcooliques et toxicomanes, l'ASI/IGT* (pp. 31–46). Quebec, Canada: Les Presses de l'Université Laval/De Boecke.

Chamberlin, J. (1997). A wording definition of empowerment. *Psychiatric Rehabilitation Journal, 20*(4), 43–46.

Greenfield, T. K., & Attkisson, C. (1989). Steps toward a multifactorial satisfaction scale for primary care and mental health services. *Evaluation and Program Planning, 12*, 271–278.

Guy, W. E. (1976). *Assessment manual for psychopharmacology* (Rev. ed.). Rockville, MD: U.S. Department of Health, Education, and Welfare; Public Health Service; Alcohol, Drug Abuse and Mental Health Administration; NIMH Psychopharmacology Branch, Division of Extramural Research Programs (DHEW Publ. No. ADM 76-338).

Larsen, D. L., Attkisson, C. C., Hargreaves, W. A., & Nguyen, T. D. (1979). Assessment of client/patient satisfaction in human service programs: Development of a general scale. *Evaluation and Program Planning, 2*, 197–207.

MAPI Research Institute. (2001). A decisive step towards the recognition of patient reported outcomes in clinical trials: Meeting with the FDA: February 16, 2001: Important issues in patient-reported outcomes (PROs) research. *QOL Newsletter, 26*, 24–25.

McLellan, A. T., Kushner, H., Metzger, D., Peters, R., Smith, I., Grissom, G., et al. (1992). The fifth edition of the Addiction Severity Index. *Journal of Substance Abuse Treatment, 9*, 199–213.

Mental health: Does therapy help? (1995, November). *Consumer Reports*, 734–739.

Mercier, C., & Landry, M. (1999). Comparaison entre le questionnaire auto-administré et l'entrevue téléphonique pour l'évaluation de la satisfaction [A comparison between a self-administered questionnaire and a telephone interview for assessment of satisfaction]. *Canadian Journal of Program Evaluation, 14*, 2, 105–118.

Mintz, J., Drake, R. E., & Crits-Christoph, P. (1996). Efficacy and effectiveness of psychotherapy: Two paradigms, one science. *American Psychologist, 51*(10), 1084–1085.

Mulkern, V., Leff, S., Green, R. S., & Newman, F. (1995). Section II: Performance indicators for a consumer: Oriented mental health report card: Literature review and analysis. In Center for Mental Health Services (Ed.), *Stakeholder perspectives on mental health performance indicators: Working papers prepared for the MHSIP Phase II Task Force on the Design of the Mental Health Component of a Healthcare Report Card* (pp. 1–75). Cambridge, MA: Evaluation Center at Human Service Research Institute.

Newman, F. L., & Tejeda, M. J. (1996). The need for research that is designed to support decision in the delivery of mental health services. *American Psychologist, 51*(10), 1040–1049.

Ruggeri, M., Lasalvia, A., Dall'Agnola, R., Wijngaarden, van B., Knudsen, H. C., Leese, M., et al. (2000). Development, internal consistency and reliability of the Verona Service Satisfaction Scale—European Version. In G. Thornicroft, T. Becker, M. Knapp, H. C. Knudsen, A. Schene, M. Tansella, et al. (Eds.), Reliable outcome measure for mental health service research in five European countries: The EPSILON Study. *British Journal of Psychiatry, 177*(Suppl. 39), 41–48.

Sechrest, L., McKnight, P., & McKnight, K. (1996). Calibration of measures for psychotherapy outcome studies. *American Psychologist, 51*(10), 1065–1071.

Seligman, M. E. P. (1995). The effectiveness of psychotherapy: The *Consumer Reports* study. *American Psychologist, 50*(12), 965–974.

Seligman, M. E. P. (1996). Science as an ally of practice. *American Psychologist, 51*(10), 1072–1080.

Srebnik, D., Hendryx, M., Stevenson, J., Caverly, S., Dyck, D. G., & Cauce, A. M. (1997). Development of outcome indicators for monitoring the quality of public mental health care. *Psychiatric Services, 48*(7), 903–909.

VanderBos, G. R. (Ed.). (1996). Outcome assessment of psychotherapy. (1996, October). [Special issue]. *American Psychologist, 51*, (10).

101 SOCIAL WORK ROLE IN DISEASE MANAGEMENT

Nancy Claiborne & Henry Vandenburgh

After World War II, developed countries shifted their emphasis of health from the absence of disease to curing diseases and minimizing effects of diseases. The goals then became the attainment of more effective lives for patients and the preservation of physical functioning and well-being. This formulation introduced quality of care theory (Lohr, 1988), which expanded the goals of health care to encompass improvement in quality of life and the preservation of physical and mental functioning. Quality of care theory is composed of three subconcepts: (a) the structure (type of delivery system), (b) the process (technical competence of the provider and the patient–provider relationship), and (c) outcomes (end results) of care. Large geographic variations in numbers of medical procedures, unnecessary surgeries, and mortality statistics in the United States concerned both practitioners and health analysts. Inadequate reporting, poor data collection, limited numbers of valid, diagnosis-based instruments, and the lack of national standards greatly hindered attempts to adequately measure outcomes and thus define quality. Standardizing practice and interventions as clinical practice guidelines through the Agency for Healthcare Research and Quality (AHRQ) has helped to delineate quality care and allows outcomes research methodology to be generalized to larger populations. Nineteen clinical practice guidelines, derived from rigorous studies, were developed from 1992 to 1996 with support from AHRQ (http://www.ahrq.gov/).

Disease-specific and general purpose instruments have also been developed to measure process and outcomes, two aspects of defining quality care. These instruments establish basic clinical and therapeutic data to be collected about patients at admission, during treatment, at discharge, and after treatment. Efforts in instrument development have focused on short, reliable, and valid instruments that can be administered so that individual patient and physician interaction can be compared (Health Outcomes Institute, 1992). Outcome management can therefore incorporate the process of care with results of outcomes measurement to achieve quality care (Ezell & McNeece, 1986; Gordon, 1991; Klein & Bloom, 1994; Pfeiffer, 1990; Theis, 1993). Researchers using this model propose that measures serve one or more of three purposes: discrimination, prediction, and evaluation (Kirshner & Guyatt, 1985). Discrimination measurements allow researchers to discriminate between potential treatments. Thus, providers are able to match patients to specific treatment elements and levels of services on a continuum-of-care model optimizing patient components. This model allows prediction of outcomes of a particular intervention with a particular patient. Finally, evaluation measurements demonstrate the level of treatment effectiveness (Lehmann, Fenton, Deutsch, Feldman, & Engelsmann, 1988; Rost, Burnam, & Smith, 1992), monitor medicine and practitioner patterns, and benchmark findings concerning clinical effectiveness within and across programs.

CARE COORDINATION MODELS AND DISEASE MANAGEMENT PROGRAMS

Driven by demands for cost containment, treatment effectiveness, and quality improvements, new health care delivery models providing greater precision in discrimination and prediction are now being developed. (Roper, 1997). They are derived from population-based care concepts emphasizing evidence-based health practices, disease prevention, proactive treatment, and follow-up objectives (Ellrodt et al., 1997; Hunter & Fairfield, 1997). Care coordination is one such delivery model that attempts to clinically manage and integrate necessary biopsychosocial interventions for specific high-risk populations of patients across an array of services, regardless of service location (Ellrodt et al., 1997; Hunter & Fairfield, 1997). The goals of care coordination are to ensure optimal medical management, enhance and support patient self-management, and eliminate barriers to efficient and effective utilization of health care services (Lorig et al., 1999; Naylor et al., 1999). Rosenbach and Young (2000) identify three models: a centralized team model in which team members located at a central office coordinate services for all patients, a regionalized model coordinating services only for patients identified within geographic boundaries, and a provider-based model coordinating care for all patients served by a specific provider entity (e.g., hospital or physician group). The goals are to prevent patient decline, facilitate patient access to resources, support adherence to medical treatment, and enhance restorative efforts (Simons, 1994).

Disease management programs are based on care coordination delivery models, targeting individuals with chronic illnesses, specifically chronic conditions that have empirically based practice guidelines. Interest in these programs has grown since 1997, as large integrated delivery systems and managed care companies announced improvements in medical outcomes and substantial cost reductions (Rauber, 1999). Disease management programs group patients by population, for example, individuals diagnosed with diabetes, asthma, depression, or heart diseases. An interdisciplinary team applies clinical practice guidelines to meet certain prescribed objectives (Katon et al., 1997). This requires a paradigm shift from individual practitioners treating episodes of illness to an interdisciplinary team coordinating essential services for patients during subacute and acute periods (Hunter & Fairfield, 1997). The clinical practice guidelines drive the preventive and acute interventions proven to provide effective outcomes. The team is typically composed of a primary care physician, the patient, and the care coordinator. Their efforts focus on controlling chronic conditions and preventing related complications. Individuals whose diseases are not controlled are at risk of immediate health problems, using more inpatient and emergency room services, develop-

ing comorbidities, and increasing the cost of care (Hunter & Fairfield, 1997; Keehn, Roglitz, & Bowden, 1994).

Disease management also requires data collection and an outcome tracking system, because patient feedback and objective medical data are used to ascertain what does and does not work. Quantitative outcome instruments and laboratory results measure individual patient changes over time. Treatment and progress also can be compared with national data on best practices and expected outcomes. Continuous quality improvement is central. The team can track the disease process over time, using available feedback to optimize patient recovery and prevent recurrence (Hunter & Fairfield, 1997).

Disease management programs are different from case management. Disease management is a prospective, disease-specific approach that emphasizes self-care education and practice guidelines, whereas case management applies to specific individuals with complex cases. Case management targets the high-risk, high-cost, multiple-problem individuals such as those with head injuries, AIDS, or dual diagnoses (e.g., developmental disability and a mental illness dual diagnosis, or alcoholism and a mental illness dual diagnosis). Both approaches are client centered and endeavor to coordinate resources across the health care delivery system rather than to provide separate services within a fragmented system (Ellrodt et al., 1997). The case manager and the disease management coordinator assess, plan, coordinate services, and monitor an individual's health needs (Berger, 1996). However, the disease management care coordinator is less likely to be engaged in protracted problem-solving activities. The case manager dedicates more time to each individual in an attempt to meet his or her complex health needs. Another major difference is that care coordination is designed to be a brief intervention, whereas case managers may work with patients for months or years.

LIMITATIONS OF DISEASE MANAGEMENT PROGRAMS

Disease management works when there is paradigmatic general knowledge of effective treatment in terms of measurable indicators and when implementation confers benefits that clearly exceed the cost of disease management programs. When nuanced intervention must be tailored to individual cases, disease management programs have less success. Similarly, if net economic benefits from disease management are small, it makes little sense to implement these programs. Thus, certain diseases for which only small marginal gains result are probably not worth placing under this regimen. Also, this new paradigm is most effective with those patients who have the intellectual and organizational skills to respond to instructions and take increasing control of their care in appropriate ways. If disease management is applied willy-nilly to persons who lack these skills, they may fall through the cracks or may even be stigmatized for their failure to comply. Accordingly, patients must be carefully assessed to see whether or not they are appropriate for disease management or a more stringent case management regimen.

USE OF SOCIAL WORKERS IN DISEASE MANAGEMENT PROGRAMS

The disease management program care coordinator proactively contacts the patient at identified intervals and focuses on disease education, adherence to medical regimen, and identification of unmet medical needs. Contact can be made in the physician's office, on the telephone, or via e-mail. Ideally, the patient is also an active participant. Program success depends on the patient's becoming an informed and empowered member of the health care team and adhering to a self-care regimen (Ellrodt et al., 1997). The practitioner, also the team leader, is expected to identify not only physical risks but also psychological and social risks affecting medical, cost, and quality-of-life outcomes. In *Healthy People 2010,* the Department of Health and Human Services (2000) has identified substantial gaps in the delivery of appropriate screening and counseling services related to health behaviors, specifically by physicians. Essential to treating undetected biopsychosocial problems (e.g., substance abuse, depression) is development and implementation of services identifying patients in need of services linked to appropriate follow-up services or counseling for identified at-risk individuals. Regulatory demands and health care reforms advocating insurance parity for behavioral health care place greater pressure on primary care facilities to provide additional psychosocial services.

Disease management programs are currently positioned in medical environments and have not routinely addressed the need for assessment and intervention in psychosocial areas affecting patients. The care coordinator in these settings is typically a nurse. However, after the initial experience of operating these programs, organizations are finding that the addition of social workers provides necessary services alleviating high utilization of the disease management care coordinator (Stern, Soule, Walker, & Vance, 2002). Social workers in disease management programs assess psychosocial stressors, mental health issues, long-term care needs, financial concerns, and caregiver issues. They facilitate access to appropriate services, facilitate patient self-care education and adherence, facilitate and advocate for entitlement services, assess and engage in the problem solving of psychosocial issues, facilitate linkages to community resources, and perform crisis intervention (Stern et al., 2002). Because disease management assesses the effectiveness of treatment interventions indicated by changes in patient quality of life, social work's ability to intervene in terms of personal and environmental factors may affect outcomes positively.

Social workers make critical contributions to disease management programs in the role of care coordinator or by assisting care coordinators, because they are the team members likely to be aware of current psychosocial and mental health factors affecting patients and their families. They have the training and skills to assist patients when patients are at acute and subacute levels of care, to help patients adapt to chronic disorders, and to effectively intervene when life stressors and impaired coping create problems such as depression, anxiety, impeded work performance, or diminished social functioning.

Social workers are also able to help patients become empowered team members. This includes developing patient self-awareness regarding health values, needs, and goals in order to make informed health decisions and judge the cost benefits of adopting a wide variety of health care recommendations, and enabling the patient to acquire problem-solving and communication skills and explore self-image issues and beliefs that direct behaviors and influence decisions (Parsons, Hernandez, & Jorgensen, 1988).

Social workers are specifically trained to consider diversity issues such as ethnicity, race, gender, sexual orientation, age, socioeconomic status, physical and mental conditions, and environmental differences in cultural, social, and historical contexts (Germain & Gitterman, 1996). Social workers' expertise in these arenas is essential to helping individual patients become active decision-making participants on disease management teams.

CASE ILLUSTRATION

Maria's health care is provided by her employer and administered by a managed care company, which has contracted with a private disease management company to manage her type II diabetes. She is one of several hundred thousand members of this managed care company diagnosed as having diabetes, and one of several thousand identified as needing a disease management program. Maria is a 56-year-old Hispanic woman, fluent in English and Spanish, living in a large city. She has been taking an oral diabetes medication for about 3 years. She had not seen her physician for 11 months but made an appointment with him after experiencing tingling and numbness in her feet. Following the American Diabetes Association's (ADA) standards of medical care (1998), he stabilized her glycemic levels (blood sugars) and noted that her lipid profile and blood pressure were within normal ranges. His examination of her feet revealed no lesions, and her medical history revealed that she is not a smoker. However, Maria had not undergone an examination for retinopathy in 2 years and received a referral for this. Also, the physician noted that she was overweight and needed to lose 50 pounds, and that she was not monitoring her blood glucose at home. Maria met with the physician's nurse for nutritional education and instruction on using the home glucose meter. The nurse educated Maria in the importance of monitoring blood glucose and trained her in the usage of the home meter. The nurse also gave Maria a brief nutritional instruction and pamphlets from the ADA.

During her current visit, her physician discovered that she has been experiencing neuropathy symptoms for several years. These symptoms only recently began to worry her. Laboratory results showed that her glycemic levels exceeded the normal range, and her blood pressure was elevated. She also expressed the belief that as long as she took the diabetes medication, she did not need to monitor her blood

levels, lose weight, or follow a diet. She also did not follow up on the eye exam referral. Her diabetes medication was adjusted and she was prescribed a beta-blocker for her elevated blood pressure. She was reminded of the importance of following her self-care regimen, including blood glucose monitoring and diet. She was instructed to make a follow-up appointment in 3 months.

Clinical practice guidelines for diabetes require that glycemic control be maintained. Thus, glycosylated hemoglobin laboratory test results of less than 7 inform the team and patient that the glycemic goal, the objective medical outcome, has been met. Outcome measures tend to be laboratory tests, such as glucose levels, lipid profiles, blood pressure levels, and body weight. These tests are conducted at least yearly in patients who have stable glycemic control and more frequently in those whose treatment has changed or who are not meeting glycemic goals. Thus, process outcomes identify expected benchmarks related to the frequency of laboratory tests. Process benchmarks also include the frequency of exams, such as foot and eye exams (ADA, 1998). Process measures become important when they have been strongly linked to clinical outcomes if those clinical outcomes do not immediately become apparent. Research on diabetes has demonstrated that intensive monitoring of glycemic control may be valuable for short-term control of the disease and for reducing the risk of developing as well as slowing the progression of diabetic retinopathy (blindness), nephropathy (liver damage), and neuropathy (the leading cause of diabetic amputations; Diabetes Control and Complications Trial Research Group, 1993).

When Maria failed to appear at her 3-month follow-up appointment, her physician referred her to the disease management company. The disease management model identifies patients who are at risk of high acuity on the basis of diagnosis, clinical deterioration, existing comorbidities, or social and psychological issues. Individual team members engage in educational and intervention processes with patients to improve these areas. Within a few weeks a disease management care coordinator contacted Maria by phone. The care coordinator found that there was no change in Maria's status. She had filled the beta-blocker prescription but stopped taking it because she did not like the way it made her feel. The care coordinator focused on assessing

Maria's understanding and adherence to her self-care regimen. The coordinator identified three major areas for education: glycemic monitoring, nutritional education, and medication adherence. They briefly discussed the importance for glycemic monitoring, and Maria was asked to test her blood levels with the glucose meter and report the results during the call, thus allowing the care coordinator to assess Maria's ability to use the machine. The care coordinator reinforced Maria's need to eat foods that help maintain glycemic control and highlighted dietary issues. They discussed Maria's need to continue with the medications to reduce risk for vascular related complications. The coordinator summarized the call and urged Maria to ask any questions. After answering her questions, a follow-up telephone call was scheduled. Three subsequent phone calls failed to change Maria's behavior with regard to taking the beta-blockers or her dietary intake. She was monitoring her glucose only intermittently. The care coordinator indicated that she would make a referral to the social worker so that Maria could receive additional support for making these difficult but important changes.

The licensed MSW-level social worker contacted Maria in a few days and conducted a targeted assessment. The social worker found Maria to be mentally alert. She had no apparent depression, substance abuse, or mental health issues, and her physical functioning was not impaired. However, she was experiencing a number of psychosocial stressors. Their discussion revealed that Maria was the sole support for her aging mother and two grandchildren in middle school. She had a close network of friends associated with her church but had disengaged from all social activities. Although Maria worked, her finances barely covered household expenses. In addition, her daily schedule allowed little time for leisure. By the time she arrived home from work via public transportation, she was occupied with meal preparations, ensuring that the children completed their homework, and caring for her mother, who recently suffered a stroke. Maria's mother needed help in bathing and dressing and was not able to leave the house. The stroke left her cognitively confused, requiring Maria to closely monitor her medication intake. The social worker focused first on Maria's nonadherence to the beta blockers. Maria was adherent with diabetes medication, indicating that she was not "in denial" about having a

chronic condition. She was not resisting being dependent on the diabetes medications. Both medications were accessible to her, as she utilized a mail order pharmacy that was reimbursable through her managed care company. Further discussion revealed that beta-blockers made her feel lethargic, which interfered with her family obligations. She also felt that the beta-blockers did not change her physical status and they were an additional cost she could not afford.

The social worker identified three areas for resource coordination. The first area was finances. Maria was assessed and found that she did not qualify for medication assistance. A community resource was then identified that would provide Maria with financial consultation services. The second area was caregiver issues. Maria was clearly experiencing stress related to the burden of being the sole caregiver to her physically and cognitively impaired mother, as well as to her grandchildren. Also, Maria's community's culture promoted taking care of one's family. The inability to do so might mean failure on her part. She was thus uneasy about asking others for help in caring for family members. The social worker identified acceptable community resources that coordinate home health care and respite services pertaining to her mother's care. The social worker also investigated the existence of appropriate community support groups, and suggested Maria talk with her priest to discover additional formal and informal support the church might offer. They also discussed ways Maria could engage in more leisure activities with her family and friends. Research shows that patients with diabetes can be placed at increased medical risk by dysfunction in family support, by depression, or by unmet social needs (Jacobson & Weinger, 1998). Effective interventions must consider each component of a patient's quality of life. Thus, the social worker targeted interventions toward caregiver relief, financial support, and social functioning.

The third area involved referring Maria to her physician to discuss the side effects she was experiencing from the beta-blockers. The social worker helped Maria identify the troubling symptoms and prepare written questions for the physician. This also helped Maria deal with her cultural concerns of showing respect and not challenging a person of authority. Such advanced preparation helps ensure that all of Maria's concerns are addressed by the physician during the brief office visit. This may also involve discussing negative feelings Maria has about her physician, how she is treated by the office staff, or her general satisfaction with the care she is receiving. Social workers have the ability to clarify patient complaints, thereby decreasing patient medical use by reducing emergency room visits, diagnostic procedures, and hospitalizations. In addition, social workers' skill in dealing with emotional issues can relieve the amount of time physicians spend in patient visits. This can save physicians' nonreimbursed time spent with patients and increase patient satisfaction.

Maria and the social worker engaged in several more telephone contacts. These focused on Maria's issues related to diet and weight loss. The major barrier was found to be the need for cultural sensitivity related to diet, weight loss, and diabetes self-management. Maria expressed particular distrust of her physician's nurse for giving her the impression that traditional foods were unhealthy and were considered against medical advice. Maria also felt that bad outcomes were inevitable because many Hispanics in her community had already experienced the chronic complications of diabetes. While reinforcing previous nutritional education, the social worker identified Hispanic diabetes cookbooks and Spanish-language diet information. Maria was also referred to a Spanish-speaking nutritionist for individual weight loss counseling. The social worker and Maria discussed ways in which Maria could share her knowledge about her culture with the physician's nurse. The social worker also shared cultural characteristics of Hispanic patients with the physician's nurse, offering to provide the office with Spanish-language pamphlets and cookbooks. To address Maria's belief in the inevitability of diabetes complications, she was informed about several programs sponsored by local hospitals and the local ADA chapter office. These programs featured Hispanic individuals who successfully maintain their glycemic levels and enjoy no diabetes complications.

Maria's caregiving burden was moderately relieved by using a home health agency and church support systems. She continues to feel financially pinched, but has received some help from the financial consultation she received. Although she attended a few diabetes programs, she did not participate in recommended support groups. However, she reactivated her social life. She also expressed feeling more confident about

getting her questions answered and needs met during physician visits, especially after her physician changed the type of beta-blocker prescribed for her elevated blood pressure. Her outcome measures were successfully achieved. Maria is adherent to all medication regimens, and her glycemic and blood pressure levels have been within acceptable ranges for 6 months. She followed through on her physician appointment, eye appointment, and nutritional counseling and has lost 12 pounds. Although she does not monitor her blood levels as often as recommended, she has increased the frequency.

Significantly for social workers, disease management incorporates preventive practices associated with specific diseases into patient care because they are ultimately the key to long-term control of chronic illnesses (Cooper & Clancy, 1998). Expected outcomes for the prevention component of disease management are the elimination of or, at least, the slow onset of a disorder, a reduction in comorbidity and relapse, and a general decrease in the disease burden for the individual. Therefore, social work intervention with an individual with diabetes focuses on secondary prevention including ongoing adherence to diet and blood monitoring; problem solving for community support; stress management; and counseling for family issues, depression, and substance abuse issues. Early intervention in these issues is likely to be cost beneficial by precluding increased medical severity (Jacobson & Weinger, 1998).

CONCLUSION

Disease management is a system of care coordination that stresses effective treatment according to up-to-date health management paradigms and patient compliance with clinical instructions derived from those paradigms. It can provide potent systems of intervention when effective treatment is fairly standard, indicators of pathology and improvement or decline are measurable, and economic benefits can be realized, compared with the costs of establishing and running programs. It cannot replace individualized case management, which should be used when patient or disease characteristics call for an individualized approach. Disease management offers opportunities for improvement of the health care delivery system, because of enhanced standardization of delivery of care according to best practices and more uniform patient response to clinical direction. It is a key part of implementing a more scientifically based, contemporary health care system.

References

American Diabetes Association. (1998). Clinical practice recommendations 1998. *Diabetes Care, 21*(Suppl. 1), 1–87.

Berger, C. S. (1996). Case management in health care. In C. D. Austin & R. W. McClelland (Eds.), *Perspectives on case management practice* (pp. 145–174. Milwaukee, WI: Families International.

Cooper, J. K., & Clancy, C. M. (1998). Health services research agenda for clinical preventive services. *American Journal of Preventive Medicine, 14,* 331–334.

Diabetes Control and Complications Trial Research Group. (1993). The effect of intensive treatment of diabetes on the development and progression of long-term complications in insulin-dependent diabetes mellitus. *New England Journal of Medicine, 329,* 977–986.

Ellrodt, G., Cook, D. J., Lee, J., Cho, M., Hunt, D., & Weingarten, S. (1997). Evidence-based disease management. *Journal of the American Medical Association, 278,* 1687–1692.

Ezell, M., & McNeece, C. A. (1986). Practice effectiveness: Research or rhetoric? *Social Work, 31*(5), 401–402.

Germain, C. B., & Gitterman, A. (1996). *The life model of social work practice: Advances in theory & practice* (2nd ed.). New York: Columbia University Press.

Gordon, K. H. (1991). Improving practice through illuminative evaluation. *Social Service Review, 65,* 365–378.

Health Outcomes Institute. (1993). *Health Outcomes Institute outcomes measurement instrumentation.* (Report No. Rev. 11/01/93). Bloomington, MN: Author.

Hunter, D. J., & Fairfield, G. (1997). Disease management. *British Medical Journal, 314,* 50–54.

Jacobson, A. M., & Weinger, K. (1998). Treating depression in diabetic patients: Is there an alternative to medications? *Annals of Internal Medicine, 129,* 656–657.

Katon, W., Von Koff, M., Lin, E., Unutzer, J., Simon, G., Walker, E., et al. (1997). Population-based care of depression: Effective disease management strategies to decrease prevalence. *General Hospital Psychiatry, 19,* 169–178.

Keehn, D. S., Roglitz, C., & Bowden, M. L. (1994). Impact of social work on recidivism and nonmedical complaints in the emergency department. In G. Rosenberg & A. Weissman (Eds.), *Social work in ambulatory care: New implications for health and social services* (pp. 65–75). New York: Haworth Press.

Kirshner, B., & Guyatt, G. H. (1985). A methodological framework for assessing health indices. *Journal of Chronic Disease, 38,* 27–36.

Klein, W. C., & Bloom, M. (1994). Is there an ethical responsibility to use practice methods with the best empirical evidence of effectiveness? In W. W. Hudson & P. S. Nurius (Eds.), *Controversial issues in social work research* (pp. 100–112). Needham Heights, MA: Allyn & Bacon.

Lehmann, H. E., Fenton, F. R., Deutsch, M., Feldman, S., & Engelsmann, F. (1988). An 11-year follow-up study of 110 depressed patients. *Acta Psychiatry Scandanavia, 78,* 57–65.

Lohr, K. N. (1988). Outcome measurement: Concepts and questions. *Inquiry, 25,* 37–50.

Lorig, K. R., Sobel, D. S., Stewart, A. L., Brown, B. W., Jr., Bandura, A., Ritter, P., et al. (1999). Evidence suggesting that a chronic disease self-management program can improve health status while reducing hospitalization: A randomized trial. *Medical Care, 37*(1), 5–14.

Naylor, M. D., Brooten, D., Campbell, R., Jacobsen, B. S., Mezey, M. D., Pauly, M. V., et al. (1999). Comprehensive discharge planning and home follow-up of hospitalized elders: A randomized clinical trial. *Journal of the American Medical Association, 281*(7), 613–620.

Parsons, J., Hernandez, S. H., & Jorgensen, J. D. (1988). Integrated practice: A framework for problem solving. *Social Work, 33*(5), 417–421.

Pfeiffer, S. I. (1990). An analysis of methodology in follow-up studies of adult inpatient psychiatric treatment. *Hospital and Community Psychiatry, 41,* 1315–1321.

Rauber, C. (1999, March 29). Disease management can be good for what ails patients and insurers. *Modern Healthcare, 29*(13), 48–54.

Roper, W. L. (1997). Outcomes and quality-related research in a changing health care environment. Agency for Health Care Policy and Research Publication No. 98-R054. Washington, DC: Department of Health and Human Services.

Rosenbach, M., & Young, C. (2000). *Care coordination in Medicaid managed care: A primer for states, managed care organizations, providers, and advocates.* Princeton, NJ: Center for Health Care Strategies, Inc.

Rost, K., Burnam, M. A., & Smith, G. R. (1993). Development of screeners for depressive disorders and substance disorder history. *Medical Care, 31,* 189–199.

Simons, J. (1994). Community-based care: The new social work paradigm. *Social Work in Health Care, 20*(1), 30–46.

Stern, P. M., Soule, D. S., Walker, D. R., & Vance, R. P. (2002). Social services in a disease management company. *Disease Management,* 5(1), 25–35.

Theis, G. A. (1993). Behavioral health care services: emerging concepts. *American Association of Preferred Provider Organizations,* 9-12.

U.S. Department of Health and Human Services. (2000). *Healthy People 2010.* Washington, DC: Government Printing Office.

102 ESTABLISHING BENCHMARK PROGRAMS WITHIN ADDICTIONS TREATMENT

Ronald J. Hunsicker

For over 50 years, the providers of addiction treatment have intermittently struggled with claiming their birthright as a legitimate provider of health care in the larger arena of health care providers and seeing themselves as outside or alongside the mainstream providers of health care. Although this vacillation between being in or being out has significant implications in a variety of areas, none can be more pronounced than the impact this has had on embracing the tools and practices adopted by other health care providers.

This seems especially pronounced in the area of *benchmarking.* While health care has moved toward established standards of care and standardized protocols, the addiction treatment providers have struggled to be recognized as providing treatment for a disease that is not an isolated tumor or organ but comes encapsulated in a very complex and complicated human being. This complicated and complex human being (not just the tumor or organ) needs the treatment attention. Although this is certainly true, it is also true that this argument has often been used to avoid examining and comparing the treatment processes of one provider against another.

As a trade association, the National Associa-

tion of Addiction Treatment Providers (NAATP) has been facilitating a discussion concerning having its members use a benchmarking process and then having that process spark dialogue with the larger health care industry so as to make use of the experience of examining a variety of health care processes. For NAATP, the discussion began at the board of directors level as individuals, interacting with one another, became curious about how others approached a variety of processes related to addiction treatment and how others achieved results from those processes. The key ingredient was the curiosity that emerged from this select group of providers.

Emerging out of this curious discussion was the formation of some basic, yet established, definitions. The addictions treatment field, like both the behavioral health care field and the larger health care field, has struggled to borrow techniques and applications from business and industry and to apply them in an authentic, non-artificial fashion to activities in addictions treatment. For NAATP, this was the key first step.

For nearly 2 years, time at almost every board meeting was allocated to working on definitions, approaches, and applications for what began as a nebulous discussion of something that was called *benchmarking* and emerged as something much less amorphous and far more critical to the ongoing future of the organization. Through those discussions, a consensus grew about what it was that NAATP was proposing to undertake. Although the literature is quite varied on definitions and applications of benchmarking, NAATP began to define what it was proposing in the following manner:

Benchmarking is a tool to help you improve your addiction treatment processes. Any aspect of addiction treatment and thus any process can be benchmarked.

Benchmarking is the process of identifying, understanding, and adapting outstanding addiction treatment practices from organizations anywhere to help your organization improve its delivery of addiction treatment.

Benchmarking is a highly respected practice. It is an activity that looks outward to find best practice and high performance in the addiction treatment universe and then measures actual business operations against those goals.

The initial interest on the part of NAATP was driven by curiosity about how others were able to achieve particular results from the various treatment processes. This approach was less threatening and at the same time seemed to have the most interest and added value for participants in this proposed effort. As the discussion moved forward, it became clear that they were talking about not only looking at processes in the abstract but also moving toward the identification of best practices or at least best particular processes. NAATP members found themselves looking for answers to the following questions: Who does this process or does an addiction treatment process well and has processes that are adaptable to my organization? Who is the most compatible for me to benchmark with?

NAATP board members believed that a benchmarking process would enable NAATP members to address the above questions and also that this information for addiction-specific organizations was currently not available. In 1998, NAATP launched its first annual benchmarking survey among its members. The NAATP board believed that health care organizations providing treatment for addictive disease disorders needed to have a way to measure their performance against each other to determine best practices and then to determine how those best practices

achieved given performance levels. Finally, it was hoped that by using the information gathered, the NAATP members would collectively improve their effectiveness and efficiency in delivering addiction treatment.

IDENTIFYING AND OVERCOMING PROBLEMS AND OBSTACLES

This chapter has already alluded to a number of systemic issues at work against this NAATP initiative. The very fact that this information was not available meant that there was no general model to draw upon, and there was very little experience among the member organizations with benchmarking in general. There were also the anticipated issues of who was going to collect the information, who was going to see the information, how members would know whether everyone was defining a particular process in the same way, and so on. Any attempt to engage in a process that had the potential to look like standardization was going to be met with resistance and skepticism.

At a second and more significant level was the issue of moving isolated providers of addiction treatment into some conversation with each other about what it was that they were delivering, how they delivered that treatment, and what the anticipated results of that treatment were. It was this level of discussion that held the most long-term benefits for benchmarking and for moving addiction treatment into a full partnership with other health care providers and within the national debate on improving the health of everyone.

Finally, the decision was made to only provide the results of this benchmarking process to those who had participated. Anyone who wanted to see the results (to really see how his or her organization's practices benchmarked with others) needed to participate and provide the information. Because NAATP did not have any other leverage to use for participation, this approach seemed to be the most workable. Now, some 6 years into the process, this same approach continues, and NAATP has found that it encourages participation and has increased the ownership of the process from the original board of directors to a substantial number of members of the association.

What NAATP had not anticipated as a potential obstacle was the use of the information. As the process has moved forward, it has been discovered that considerable time and energy needs to be invested in helping organizations move from receiving a reporting tool to implementation of the information—analyzing the information and using the information to establish targets to be measured in the next round of benchmark collecting.

SELECTING ITEMS TO BE INCLUDED IN THE BENCHMARK SURVEY

The board of directors of the NAATP is made up of chief executives of organizations delivering addiction treatment. Where better to begin than by asking the chief decision makers about what information would be helpful to them in examining and making decisions about their processes of delivering addiction treatment? This was also a way to continue the discussion about how addiction treatment was a collection of processes and that it was the identification of the various process components that was key to helping NAATP members look at what they did that was like what others did and what they did that was different from what others did.

These chief executives were then asked to submit (to a subcommittee appointed to launch this new service) those indicators and those processes that they would like to have included. The critical key questions that initiated this idea generation were as follows: What component process of your delivery system are you interested in examining in comparison to other members of NAATP? What information from your processes are you willing to share in such a survey?

The board members were committed to not only identifying the information that organizations wanted but also asking them to make a commitment in terms of what information they were willing to share via the established process. NAATP had members with some experience in sharing information via requested and mandated state and federal surveys, and it also had members who represented closely held private companies. The sharing of information was not a usual practice, and thus a new culture and expectation needed to be established.

Appendix A is the first benchmark survey instrument with the finalized data set questions or process questions that emerged out of this board-generated discussion. Because these were chief executives, they gravitated toward looking

at operational and financial operations, with clinical processes making up the third focus of the instrument.

In addition to the particular focus that emerged, these executives requested that the survey not exceed two typed pages. This reflected their own understanding of time and availability to complete the survey and the fact that many NAATP members had ignored requests for voluntary information in the past. The first survey instrument also reflected the overwhelming emphasis on inpatient or residential treatment activity, which was a reflection of the makeup of the board of directors and of the overall emphasis of NAATP at that time.

Appendixes B and C are examples of the evolutionary process the survey instrument has taken. Although it is clear that a core set of collection questions has remained constant, the instrument has been redesigned and aligned to reflect the reality of diversity in addiction treatment and in the membership of NAATP. A core value of this NAATP service is to keep as many questions as possible constant so that trend-line reports are possible, and at the same time to be responsive to the requests of participating members. As a result of this commitment, the instrument has crept well beyond two pages. To assist with this, for the past 2 years, members have been able to complete the survey on-line via the NAATP Web site (http://www.naatp.org). This has resulted in some shortening of the completion process. Some formula calculations are also built into the on-line version so that respondents need only plug in the raw numbers and the calculations are automatically made for them.

PRODUCTS

Having made the decision to move forward with the benchmarking effort, NAATP was also committed to providing the participating members with a product that would be viewed as value added for their membership. Having determined that this information was not available specifically for addiction treatment providers, it stood to reason that a tool that offers a snapshot look at various processes in addiction treatment delivery would be valued.

The benchmarking effort was viewed as a part of a much larger effort to encourage continuous improvement of the processes related to delivering addiction treatment and to identification of core and common processes associated with addiction treatment, so that best practices or best processes could be identified, examined, and learned from and ultimately the entire addiction treatment component of health care improved. On more individual levels, it meant having a tool to assist in focusing resources in target-specific processes and prioritizing areas that needed improvement.

The first benchmark effort resulted in a survey instrument that collected information in more than 50 processes related to addiction treatment. The product or tool that resulted was a comprehensive color report that graphed the results for each of the identified processes. Each process was on a separate page, with a bar graph showing the results for each respondent. The average and the standard deviation were also calculated.

This report was then provided to each participant in the collection process with a cover letter that identified that participant's bar graph number, which was constant on all pages of the report. This was done in response to the request for confidentiality, so that each participant knew which bar graph number represented that particular organization, but other agencies did not. However, all member organizations did know that they were being compared or benchmarked to other member agencies of the National Association of Addiction Treatment Providers.

This initial report provided the members with a professional prepared instrument that graphically took a great deal of information and displayed it in a useful and user-friendly environment. In a rather quick way, members were able to determine how they benchmarked with the other respondents, viewing their organizations in relation to the average and ascertaining where they were in relation to one or two standard deviations.

Appendixes D and E are two examples of this first report that graphically displayed the results of the information collected. By the middle of 1998, a process was in place to collect information, with a tool to report the collected data to the participants.

DISCUSSION

As with most initiated projects, the first year yielded a great many learnings for NAATP as a whole and for its participating members. From a nebulous idea and hours of discussion emerged a collection instrument and a results tool. Nevertheless, if the board of directors believed in continuous improvement (as board members hoped that all NAATP members did), then the board needed to also commit to continually seeking ways to improve and enhance this effort so as to always add value to member organizations.

Some of the immediate and ongoing learnings and thus dialogue points from this project have been as follows:

• There was an assumption made about the base level of terms and processes among addiction treatment providers that proved to be not true. The board discovered that what were expected to be commonly understood business terms and definitions were not uniform or understood by everyone.
• The board members discovered that levels of care or modules of treatment delivered may have the same nomenclature but are understood differently by different members. The lack of clear and accepted definitions for terms that has plagued the addictions treatment field surfaced again in this effort.
• The board discovered that common terms (such as *FTE, days in accounts receivable*) and some ratio calculations were calculated differently by different member organizations.

Because of these issues, a by-product of this effort was ongoing discussion about standard terms, the need to raise the level of business understanding among the NAATP members, and the need to have some core processes identified that were common to everyone and that would define the core business of delivering addiction treatment.

Perhaps the most energizing aspect of this project initiated in 1998 has been the growing participation rate and the efforts to mine the collected information for additional value. After the third year, trend-line reports could be produced for NAATP member organizations that had participated for a number of years. These reports displayed organization-specific information over the course of that organization's involvement, and this information could be superimposed over the overall average, and so on. All of this was based on the assumption that data alone are of limited value; however, relational data (benchmarking or trend lines) become information. Information is the key to any successful organization.

In addition to the trend-line reports, NAATP has also been able to generate custom reports that allow participants to compare themselves to most like organizations. Using any number of comparison lenses, NAATP offers participants an opportunity to look at themselves in comparison to other organizations that are most like them via revenue sources, size, and so on. With this additional product, the NAATP office has made numerous presentations to member organizations, to their executive management staff, to their boards, and so on, regarding the overall benchmark results and the custom reports.

Appendixes F, G, and H illustrate the trend-line reports and some examples of the custom reports that can be generated. Appendix I is the 2003 and most recent benchmark survey instrument. This illustrates the expansion of the instrument, the organization of the tool to reflect the diversity of membership, and also the attempt to build in common definitions and calculations so that information reported is as useful as possible.

CONCLUSION

A health care process or an addiction treatment process is best defined as any function in an or-ganization that enables the organization to successfully deliver its addiction treatment service. By viewing addiction treatment as a single process rather than looking at it as the sum of the component processes, NAATP has focused on differences as opposed to similarities. A simple analogy would be to look at an addiction treatment organization as a wheel and the individual processes as the spokes of the wheel.

Having just one or two spokes loose can make a wheel out of balance. The longer a wheel runs out of balance, the more damaging the effect to the organization. When the wheel on a cart becomes so unstable that its primary function fails, you would simply replace the wheel. And although you cannot replace your own organization, the purchasers of care can. Thus, paying attention to the individual processes and learning from what others are doing are key to keeping your wheel in balance. Benchmarking has proven to be one way to balance the wheel.

In 1998, the NAATP undertook a process not only to provide its members with information that was significantly absent but also to use that process to ratchet up the discussion about what addiction treatment is, what constitutes addiction treatment, and how this treatment should be viewed by the major purchasers of health care. On both fronts, this effort has substantially improved the information flow.

Appendix A

National Association of Addiction Treatment Providers (NAATP)
Data Set Collection Form
Provide the following information for the *most recent completed fiscal year*
for your organization
Please return this form to the **NAATP office** before **February 15, 1998**

All Information will be confidentially and strictly maintained at the NAATP Office

Do your offer an **Outpatient Detox** Program?	Yes	No
Percent (%) of patients who **AMA** from **Inpatient Detox**		
Percent (%) of patients who **AMA** from **Outpatient Detox** if applicable		
Dyou have any **Capitation Contracts?** **If yes, how many?**	Yes	No
ALOS for **Inpatient Detox**		
ALOS for residential (inpatient) Adult rehabilitations		
ALOS for residential (inpatient) Adolescent rehabilitation		
Average rate (%) of occupancy to total licensed beds		
Gross number of days in **A**ccounts **R**eceivable		
Total cost of Benefits as a percent (%) of total salary costs		
Total costs of Salaries as a percent (%) of total costs		
Primary **C**ounselor ratio to occupied bed		
Nursing (**RN only**) ratio to occupied bed		
Average **S**tarting **S**alary **for P**rimary **C**ounselor		
Average **S**tarting **S**alary **for R**egistered **N**urse		
Current Ratio = Current Assets / Current Liabilities		
Total **L**ong **T**erm **D**ebet / **T**otal **A**ssets		
Net In**P**atient **R**evenue per **day**		
Percent (%) of Gross Revenue received from: Medicare _____ Medicaid _____ Self Pay _____ Other _____		
Percentage (%) of your total revenue of operations from Outpatient operations		

NAATP contact Person _____

Program Name: _____

Address: _____

Appendix B

National Association of Addiction Treatment Providers

Data Set Collection Form—2000
Provide the following information for the *most recent completed fiscal year*
for your organization
Return this form to the **NAATP office** before *March 10, 2000*

All Information will be confidentially and strictly maintained at the NAATP Office

"Inpatient Activity"		
Do you offer an **inpatient detox** program?	YES	NO
Percent (%) of patients who leave **AMA** from **inpatient detox.**		
Average **LOS** for **inpatient detox**		
Average **LOS** for residential (inpatient) **adult rehabilitation**		
Average **LOS** for residential (inpatient) **adolescent rehabilitation**		
Average occupancy percentage **(average daily census/total licensed beds)**		
Number of days in **A**ccounts **R**eceivable (Total Gross Dollars receivable ÷ average daily gross revenue for past 90 days)		
Total cost of Benefits as a percent (%) of total salary costs		
Total cost of Salaries as a percent (%) of total **operating expenses**		
Clinical Staff turnover during the past fiscal year (show as a percent (%) of total clinical staff)		
Total FTE's per occupied bed		
Average **S**tarting **S**alary **for P**rimary **C**ounselor		
Average **S**tarting **S**alary **for R**egistered **N**urse		
Do you obtain **objective** Performance Measures on patients during or after Treatment?	YES	NO
If you answered **YES** to the above question, identify the instrument you use: **L12, ASI, PFIB, BASIS** etc., **Other** (List the actual instrument in the column to the right)		
"Out Patient Activity"		
Do you offer an **outpatient detox** program?	YES	NO
Percent (%) of patients who **AMA** from your **outpatient detox program**		
Average **LOS** for **Day Treatment**		
Average **LOS** for **Intensive Out Patient**		
How long does it take to "receive" outpatient services in your system? (Average length of time from first call/contact to first appointment in your system) Respond in hours		
Do you provide an *"Evening IOP"* Program?	YES	NO

Hours **open** and **providing** clinical services: **M-** **T-** **W-** **Th-** **F-** **Sa-** **Su-** (Total)	
Do you provide housing for persons in outpatient treatment?	**YES** **NO**
What are clinical productivity rates for your **primary outpatient counselors?** (Total billable hours ÷ total primary outpatient counselor FTE's) [Billable hours per week per outpatient counselor]	
Total **outpatient net revenue**/ total **outpatient FTE's [Net revenue dollars per outpatient FTE] Annual**	
Percentage of patients (**inpatient**) on psychotropic medications	
Percentage of patients (**outpatient**) on psychotropic medications	
Percentage of **patients** who have been **abstinent six (6) months** after discharge from **inpatient** treatment	
Percentage of **patients** who have been **abstinent six (6) months** after discharge from outpatient treatment	
Percent of **families/significant other** who participate in family treatment **(inpatients)**	
Percent of **families/significant other** who participate in family treatment **(outpatients)**	
Percentage of total inpatient admissions who were **discharged from any level of treatment,** from *your program,* within **thirty (30) days of** *this* admission	

Percent Discharge (all levels of care)
 	
                                                                     Male
                                                                     Female	

Percent (%) of patients who attend AA/NA meetings following discharge from treatment-
 	
                                                                     30 Days
                                                                     6 Months	

Percent (%) of Gross Revenue (from TOTAL operations) received from:
                                        Medicare————————
                                        Medicaid————————
                                        Self Pay————————
                                        Insurance————————
                                        Philanthropy————————
Other (includes State, County, etc funds
and block grants and other grants)————————————————
                                                        100%	

Percent (%) of **Gross Revenue (from inpatient operations)** received from: Medicare———————— Medicaid———————— Self Pay———————— Insurance———————— Philanthropy———————— Other (includes State, County, etc funds and block grants and other grants)———————————————— 100%	
Percent (%) of **Gross Revenue (from outpatient operations)** received from: Medicare———————— Medicaid———————— Self Pay———————— Insurance———————— Philanthropy———————— Other (includes State, County, etc funds and block grants and other grants)———————————————— 100%	
Percentage (%) of your total revenue of all operations from Outpatient operations	

1/20/2000

Benchmark Contact Person ——————————————————————————————————

Program Name and Address ——————————————————————————————————

Appendix C

National Association of Addiction Treatment Providers

Data Set Collection Form—2002
Provide the following information for the *most recent completed fiscal year*
for your organization
Return this form to the **NAATP office** before *April 3, 2002*

All Information will be confidentially and strictly maintained at the NAATP Office

"Inpatient Activity"	
Percent (%) of patients who leave **AMA** from **inpatient detoxification**	%
Average **LOS** for **inpatient detoxification**	Days
Average **LOS** for residential (inpatient) **adult rehabilitation PRIMARY TREATMENT)**	Days
Average **LOS** for residential *adult extended care treatment*	Days
Percent (%) of patients who leave **AMA** from adult inpatient rehabilitation treatment	%
Average **LOS** for residential (inpatient) **adolescent rehabilitation (PRIMARY TREATMENT)**	Days
Average **LOS** for residential *adolescent extended care treatment*	Days
Percent (%) of patient who leave **AMA** from adolescent rehabilitation treatment	%
Average occupancy percentage (**average daily census ÷ total licensed beds**)	%
Percent of **families/significant other** who participate in family treatment (**inpatients**)	%
Percentage of **patients** who report being **abstinent six (6) months** after discharge from **inpatient** treatment	%
Percentage of patients (**inpatient**) discharged on psychotropic medications	%
FTE per Equivalent Patient Days (see glossary for formula)	
Conversion Rate: Percentage of **actual admissions** vs. **scheduled admissions:** Actual admissions ÷ Scheduled Admissions	%
Percentage (%) of total *inpatient admissions* that were **first time** admissions into your system	%
Percentage (%) of inpatient admissions that were patients admitted within 30 days of inpatient discharge from *any* inpatient program.	%
Percentage of total inpatient admissions who were **discharged from any level of treatment,** from *your program*, within **thirty (30) days** of *this* **admission**	
"Out Patient Activity"	
Do you offer an **outpatient detoxification** program?	YES NO
Average Daily Census (ADC) in your outpatient detoxification program	

Percent (%) of patients who **AMA** from your **outpatient detoxification program**		%
Average **LOS** for **Day Treatment program**		
Average **LOS** for **Intensive Out Patient program**		
How long does it take to "receive" outpatient services in your system? (Average length of time from first call/contact to first appointment in your system) Respond in hours		**Hours**
Conversion Rate for Outpatient Services: Percentage of **actual admissions** to **outpatient services** : Actual Admissions ÷ Scheduled Admissions		%
Do you provide an *"Evening IOP"* Program?	**YES**	**NO**
Total hours **per week** offering **outpatient** clinical services:		**Hours**
What are clinical productivity rates for your **primary outpatient counselors?** (Total billable hours ÷ total primary outpatient counselor FTE's) [Billable hours per week per outpatient counselor]		
Total **outpatient revenue** ÷ **total outpatient FTE's** [revenue dollars per outpatient FTE] Annual		
Percentage of patients (**outpatient**) discharged on psychotropic medications		%
Percentage of **patients** who report being **abstinent six (6) months** after discharge from outpatient treatment		%
Percent of **families/significant other** who participate in family treatment **(outpatients)**		%
Combined/Total Activity		
Number of days in **A**ccounts **R**eceivable (Total Gross Dollars Receivable ÷ average daily gross revenue for last 90 days)		**Days**
Total cost of Benefits as a percent (%) of total salary costs		%
Total cost of Salaries as a percent (%) of total **operating expenses**		%
Percent of Operating Expense Budget spent on Marketing and PR activities		%
Do you obtain **objective** Performance Measures on patients during or after Treatment?	**Yes**	**No**
Percent Discharge (all levels of care) Male Female		 % %
Percent (%) of patients who attend 12-Step meetings following discharge from treatment- 30 Days 6 Months		 % %
Percent (%) Clinical Staff TURNOVER rate during the past fiscal year. (Clinical staff turnover (divided) by total number of clinical staff)		%

Percent (%) of Gross Revenue (from TOTAL operations) received from: 　　　　　　　　　　Medicare———— 　　　　　　　　　　Medicaid———— 　　　　　　　　　　Self Pay———— 　　　　　　　　　　Insurance———— 　　　　　　　　　　Philanthropy———— Other (includes State, County, etc funds and block grants and other grants)————————	TOTAL 100%
Percent (%) of Gross Revenue (from inpatient operations) received from: 　　　　　　　　　　Medicare———— 　　　　　　　　　　Medicaid———— 　　　　　　　　　　Self Pay———— 　　　　　　　　　　Insurance———— 　　　　　　　　　　Philanthropy———— Other (includes State, County, etc funds and block grants and other grants)————————	TOTAL 100%
Percent (%) of Gross Revenue (from outpatient operations) received from: 　　　　　　　　　　Medicare———— 　　　　　　　　　　Medicaid———— 　　　　　　　　　　Self Pay———— 　　　　　　　　　　Insurance———— 　　　　　　　　　　Philanthropy———— Other (includes State, County, etc funds and block grants and other grants)————————	TOTAL 100%
Rating of National Managed Care Organizations: Only rate the organizations you have had experience with. Us the (5 point) rating scale where **1** is the most negative and **5** is the most positive	
Ease of obtaining admission approval: 　**Magellan** 　**UBH** 　**Value Options** 　**Health Management Strategies (HMS)**	1　2　3　4　5 1　2　3　4　5 1　2　3　4　5 1　2　3　4　5
Promptness of Payment: 　**Magellan** 　**UBH** 　**Value Options** 　**Health Management Strategies (HMS**	1　2　3　4　5 1　2　3　4　5 1　2　3　4　5 1　2　3　4　5
Overall General Responsiveness to your concerns: 　**Magellan** 　**UBH** 　**Value Options** 　**Health Management Strategies (HMS)**	1　2　3　4　5 1　2　3　4　5 1　2　3　4　5 1　2　3　4　5
Percentage (%) of total revenue of all operations from Outpatient operations	
Are you Accredited by: Circle your response **JCAHO**　　　　**CARF**　　　　**Both**　　　　**Neither**	

1/20/2002

Benchmark Contact Person _____

Program/Organization Name _____

Address _____

City, State, Zip _____

Phone: _____

Email: _____

Appendix D

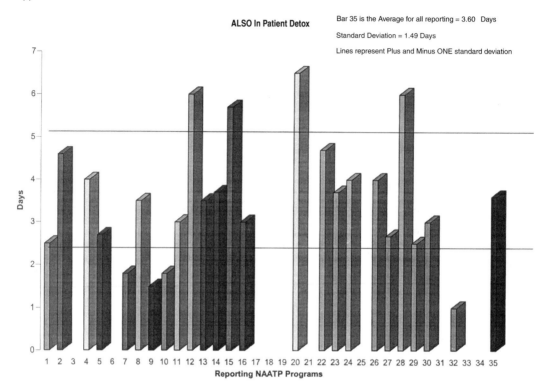

ALSO In Patient Detox

Bar 35 is the Average for all reporting = 3.60   Days

Standard Deviation = 1.49 Days

Lines represent Plus and Minus ONE standard deviation

Appendix E

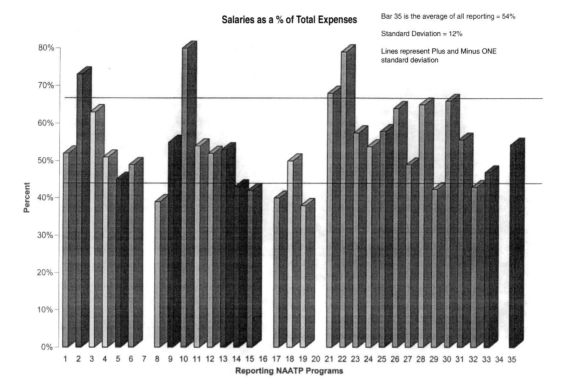

Salaries as a % of Total Expenses

Bar 35 is the average of all reporting = 54%

Standard Deviation = 12%

Lines represent Plus and Minus ONE standard deviation

Reporting NAATP Programs

Appendix F

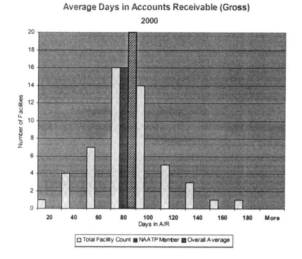

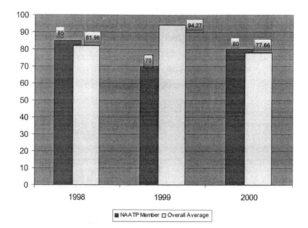

Appendix G

% Inpatient Detox AMA

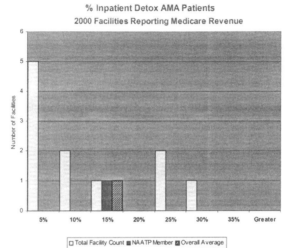

% Inpatient Detox AMA Patients
2000 Facilities Reporting Medicare Revenue

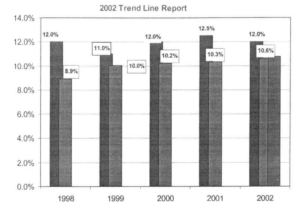

% Inpatient Detox AMA Patients
2002 Trend Line Report

Appendix H

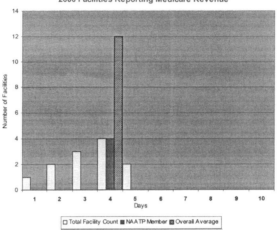

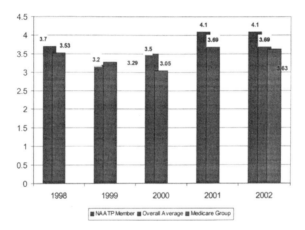

Appendix I

National Association of Addiction Treatment Providers

Data Set Collection Form—2003
Provide the following information for the *most recent completed fiscal year*
for your organization
Return this form to the **NAATP office** before *April 4, 2003*

All Information will be confidentially and strictly maintained at the NAATP Office

Inpatient Activity	
Percent (%) of patients who leave **AMA**(See Def #1 Below) from **inpatient detoxification**	%
Average **LOS**(See Def #2 Below) for **inpatient detoxification**	Days
Average **LOS**(See Def #2 Below) for residential (inpatient) **adult rehabilitation (PRIMARY TREATMENT)**	Days
Average **LOS**(See Def #2 Below) for residential *adult extended care treatment*	Days
Percent (%) of patients who leave **AMA**(See Def #1 Below) from adult inpatient rehabilitation treatment	%
Average **LOS**(See Def #2 Below) for residential (inpatient) **adolescent rehabilitation (PRIMARY TX)**	Days
Average **LOS**(See Def #2 Below) for residential *adolescent extended care treatment*	Days
Percent (%) of patient who leave **AMA**(See Def #1 Below) from adolescent rehabilitation treatment	%
Average occupancy percentage **(average daily census ÷ total licensed beds)**	%
Percent of **families/significant other** who participate in family treatment **(inpatients)**	%
Percent of patients **(inpatient adult only)** admitted on psychotropic–schedule 2—medications	%
Percentage of patients **(inpatient–adult only)** discharged on psychotropic–schedule 2—medications	%
FTE per Equivalent Patient Days (For Definition of FTE, see Def #3 Below) (for formula of "FTE per Equivalent Pt Days", see Attachment 1)	
Conversion Rate: Percentage of **actual admissions** vs. **scheduled admissions:** Actual admissions ÷ Scheduled Admissions	%
Percentage (%) of total *inpatient admissions* that were **first time** admissions into your system	%
Percentage (%) of inpatient admissions that were patients admitted within 30 days of inpatient discharge from *any* inpatient program.	%
Percentage of total inpatient admissions who were **discharged from any level of treatment,** from *your program*, within **thirty (30) days of** *this* **admission**	%

DEFINITIONS

1. **AMA = Against Medical Advice**
   Any discharge of a patient for any reason other than having completed the treatment process or meeting the treatment goals.

2. **Average LOS (Length of Stay)**
   Total patient days for a particular level of care ÷ Total admissions for this level of care

3. **FTE = Total organization salary hours paid ÷ 2080**

OutPatient Activity		
Do you offer an **outpatient detoxification** program?	**YES**	**NO**
Average Daily Census (ADC) in your outpatient detoxification program		
Percent (%) of patients who **AMA**(See Def #1 Below) from your **outpatient detoxification program**		%
Average **LOS**(See Def #2 Below) for **Day Treatment program**		
Average **LOS**(See Def #2 Below) for **Intensive Out Patient program**		
How long does it take to "receive" outpatient services in your system? (*Average* length of time from first call/contact to first appointment in your system) Respond in hours (Using a sample the average number of hours between first call/contact and actual appointment where service is delivered)		**Hours**
Conversion Rate for Outpatient Services: Percentage of **actual admissions** to **outpatient services**: Actual Admissions ÷ Scheduled Admissions		%
Do you provide an *"Evening IOP"* Program?	**YES**	**NO**
Total hours **per week** offering **outpatient** clinical services:		**Hours**
What are clinical productivity rates for your **primary outpatient counselors?** (Total billable hours ÷ total primary outpatient counselor FTE's) [Billable hours per week per outpatient counselor]		
Total **outpatient revenue ÷ total outpatient FTE's [revenue dollars per outpatient FTE] Annual** (See Def #3 Below re FTE) (Revenue = Gross revenue)		
Percentage of patients (**outpatient–adult only**) admitted on psychotropic–schedule 2—medications		%
Percentage of patients (**outpatient–adult only**) discharged on psychotropic–schedule 2—medications		%
Percent of **families/significant other** who participate in family treatment (**outpatients**)		%

DEFINITIONS

1. **AMA = Against Medical Advice**
   Any discharge of a patient for any reason other than having completed the treatment process or meeting the treatment goals.

2. **Average LOS (Length of Stay)**

Total patient days for a particular level of care ÷ Total admissions for this level of care

3. **FTE = Total organization salary hours paid ÷ 2080**

Combined/Total Activity	
Number of Days in **A**ccounts **R**eceivable (Total Gross Dollars Receivable ÷ average daily gross revenue for last 90 days)	**Days**
Total cost of Benefits as a percent (%) of total salary costs	%
Total cost of Salaries as a percent (%) of total **operating expenses**	%
Percent of Operating Expense Budget spent on Marketing and PR activities	%
Do you obtain **objective** Performance Measures on patients during or after Treatment?	**Yes** **No**
Percent Discharge (all levels of care) <div align="right">Male</div><div align="right">Female</div>	 % %
Percent (%) of patients who attend 12-Step meetings following discharge from treatment- <div align="right">30 Days</div><div align="right">6 Months</div>	 % %
Percent (%) Clinical Staff TURNOVER rate during the past fiscal year. (Clinical staff turnover (divided) by total number of clinical staff)	%
Percent (%) of **Gross Revenue (from *TOTAL* operations)** received from: <div align="right">Medicare</div><div align="right">Medicaid</div><div align="right">Self Pay</div><div align="right">Insurance</div><div align="right">Philanthropy</div>Other (includes State, County, etc funds and block grants and other grants)	 TOTAL 100%
Percent (%) of **Gross Revenue (from *INPATIENT* operations)** received from: <div align="right">Medicare</div><div align="right">Medicaid</div><div align="right">Self Pay</div><div align="right">Insurance</div><div align="right">Philanthropy</div>Other (includes State, County, etc funds and block grants and other grants)	 TOTAL 100%

Percent (%) of **Gross Revenue (from *OUTPATIENT* operations)** received from:	
Medicare	
Medicaid	
Self Pay	
Insurance	
Philanthropy	
Other (includes State, County, etc funds and block grants and other grants)	
	TOTAL 100%

Rating of National Managed Care Organizations					
Only rate the organizations you have had experience with. Use the (5 point) rating scale where **1** is the most negative and **5** is the most positive					
Ease of obtaining admission approval:					
Magellan	1	2	3	4	5
UBH	1	2	3	4	5
Value Options	1	2	3	4	5
Health Management Strategies (HMS)	1	2	3	4	5
Promptness of Payment:					
Magellan	1	2	3	4	5
UBH	1	2	3	4	5
Value Options	1	2	3	4	5
Health Management Strategies (HMS					
Overall General Responsiveness to your concerns:					
Magellan	1	2	3	4	5
UBH	1	2	3	4	5
Value Options	1	2	3	4	5
Health Management Strategies (HMS)	1	2	3	4	5
Percentage (%) of total gross revenue of all operations from Outpatient operations					
Are you Accredited by: Circle your response **JCAHO** **CARF** **Both** **Neither**					

1/20/2002

Benchmark Contact Person _____

Program/Organization Name _____

Address

_____

City, State, Zip

_____

Phone _____

Email _____

103 ESTABLISHMENT OF QUALITY PROGRAMMING

Helen P. Hartnett & Stephen A. Kapp

Historically, there has always been an extensive gap between practice and research. This is particularly true in organizational practice and administrative practice, where possible explanations range from the differences in methods to alternative sets of priorities: an emphasis on doing business as usual versus an emphasis on rigor and technique, or an emphasis on accountability versus evaluation and information utility. These priorities may exacerbate a difference between organizational roles and methods for evaluating, planning for, and maintaining programs. The gap between research and practice at the organizational level has the potential to maintain programs that operate on the basis of the status quo, either due to funding priorities or for the purpose of organizational survival. Ultimately, the welfare of people being served may not be at the forefront.

In this chapter, the authors briefly examine the literature related to administrative practice research, specifically, the discussion of evidence-based practice. In addition, an approach to administrative practice research is forwarded using program logic models as a foundation for integrating research and practice by defining, promoting, assessing, evaluating, and improving programs and service delivery. This material should be of interest to program managers interested in designing, implementing, maintaining, and evaluating programs with an eye toward the well-being of clients.

EVIDENCED-BASED PRACTICE

While debates are waged over evidence-based practice, one thing remains clear: Social work as a profession has an ethical mandate to create and maintain programs that provide viable services that address actual needs of clients. Evidence-based practice assists program and service managers in holding themselves accountable to that mandate. According to Macdonald (2001), the possibility for evidence-based practice to occur assumes the following: "First, an investment in good quality research. Secondly, access to reliable summaries of the available evidence. Thirdly, the ability of practitioners to make use in their assessments and intervention plans. Fourthly, the ability to implement or commission skills and services indicated by such summaries; and finally, the ability to review and carefully monitor the progress of individual cases" (p. 25).

In this framework, evidence-based practice also assumes a process of decision making that is overt, accountable, and based on careful consideration of valid and relevant information regarding the practices that promote the welfare of specified individuals, groups, and communities (Macdonald, 2001). Gambrill (2001) contends that involving clients and the use of evidence can improve outcomes by relying not only on what social workers believe should happen but also on what really works.

One central tenet of evidence-based practice is the inclusion of clients in the process; the process described later in this chapter provides this information loop. Additionally, as a profession, social work ethics and values require the use of the best available information for planning and evaluation purposes. Proctor (2002) not only calls for planning processes that incorporate sound research but also states that the implementation and operation of programs need to include a sound research plan. The ability of any program to provide the necessary feedback loop of research and practice is essential in assuring the quality of programs provided to clients. As the reader will see, the described process provides the opportunity to include human judgment and experience in the research equation, one of the oppositions to evidence-based practice (Gabor & Grinnell, 1994). Additionally, incorporating this model in the program design and implementation process provides a constant information and data source for administrators to contribute to the body of knowledge regarding best practices, thus reducing the gap between research and practice.

Organizational Context

The organizational context provides or impedes the ability to implement evidence-based practice as described above. Many organizations operate based on the need for survival, rather than on the need to improve or hone services (Brueggemann, 2002). This is often based on the realities of funders, public policy, and perceptions of the program. Ultimately, programs may succumb to a greater and more immediate pressure from those entities than from the clients served (Brueggemann, 2002). The result creates a gap in the process of evaluation, perhaps confusing it with accountability. For example, some programs may count numbers for funders (bed nights, service or contact hours) that in actuality have little to do with service quality. In addition, the information required by funders may contribute to the idea that research is not an essential or integral part of administrative practice. Thus, some organizations may collect and maintain evidence that is based on authority of external forces, rather than on sound practice utility. The end result may be the maintenance or creation of programs with little effectiveness for clients (Gambrill, 2001).

Meenaghan and Gibbons (2000, p. 138) contend that the political realities of nonprofit organizations require a balance between what is determined necessary information for key stakeholders and that of sound planning and evaluation. Often social service agencies are charged with improving the lives of client groups that may be seen as symbols of value by some external or internal stakeholders. As described by Yeager (2002), social workers are faced with new and challenging situations in which they are required to link multiple disciplines in an organizational context. Balancing all constituents in the process of evaluation and research is also a daunting task for many administrators. Thus, it becomes essential to use a reality-based approach in the nonprofit organization that improves the quality of evaluation and service delivery for clients while responding to needs of other constituents involved in the organization.

Administrative Practice Roles and Evidence-Based Practice

Rapp and Poertner (1992) state that, to respond to the needs of clients, social work administrators should practice from a client-centered approach. In doing so, administrators are not removed from, nor do they ignore, the experiences of clients or staff; instead they focus on these groups in the management, evaluation, and monitoring of any program. Coupled with this, Tripodi (1994) contends that administrators must be prepared to be research practitioners. These roles of the administrator (client-centered and research practitioner) require the ability to effectively plan, implement, and evaluate programs. Therefore, the use of evidence in the equation enhances good administrative practice. In addition, evidence-based administrative practice allows the organization to respond to the changing environment, a reality for nonprofits. Program logic models provide excellent tools for program managers to apply these principles in the interest of evidence-based practice. Logic models are intended to describe the theory behind programs. Originally, logic models were developed as tools to prepare programs for evaluations (Kapp, 1991; Wholey, 1983, 1994). More recent practice has discussed their implementation as a tool for specifying programs (Kapp, 2000; Savas, 1996) and practice research (Alter & Egan, 1997; Alter & Murty, 1997). This chapter describes an evidence-based practice approach to program management and assessment that includes the following steps: development of a program model, analysis of the model, identifying key information, and assessing and improving the program.

DEVELOPMENT AND REVIEW OF A LOGIC MODEL

One of the many strengths of the logic model is that is provides administrative and other practitioners with an outcome-oriented framework for thinking about program design, management, and performance emphasizing clients' well-being. An outcome-oriented program depiction helps to focus critical efforts on client benefits, including program design, program promotion, program evaluation, and accountability. In addition, the process of collecting information for model development and the review and revision of the model are very well suited to a public forum including multiple points of view—a critical element of evidence-based practice and good administrative practice. The logic model is a critical tool for targeting information that will be useful for monitoring and evaluating program performance.

Seeking Input for Model Development

The first step in model development is to acquire viewpoints of multiple contingencies about overall program functioning. There are a variety of methods for acquiring this information. We have conducted individual interviews (see Wholey, 1983), facilitated large group meetings at which each small group takes on an aspect of the model (i.e., resources, activities, program processes, and outcomes), and have had different contingents develop independent models. As much as possible, this process should be as inclusive as possible, including practitioners, administrators, funders, clients, community supporters, and so on. Although multiple data collection processes can be used, the end result is the presentation of a model depicting the intended program in a chart that reflects resources, activities, program processes, and outcomes. (Figure 103.1 presents a residential program logic model for juvenile offenders.)

Analysis and Review of the Program Model

When a model has been developed, it can be scrutinized for agreement among key stakeholders interested in the program's intended functioning. Often practitioners working with the same program have differing views on the program's primary outcomes. In our example (Figure 103.1), it is possible that residential staff may be focused on outcomes that emphasize program completion (Outcome 4.1), whereas family workers may be more attentive to maintaining a legal lifestyle (Outcome 5.3). Public reviews of a program logic model can help to illuminate these differences, highlight the implications of such a disagreement, and motivate opposing contingencies to develop workable

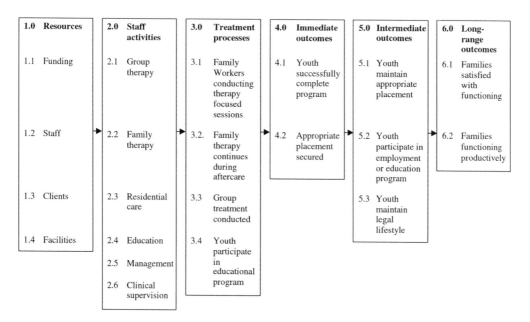

FIGURE 103.1 Residential treatment program logic model.

TABLE 103.1 Key Information Needs

Outcome	Indicator	Source
5.3 Youth maintain legal lifestyle	Percentage of youth without reported law violation at 3 and 12 months after discharge	Survey completed by program secretary with staff, youth, and family Reported quarterly by program database

resolutions between such conflicts. This process is often iterative, whereby different versions of compromises are reviewed or revised, with the end goal being the development of a model with which all parties can live.

Once an acceptable model has been constructed, a second type of review takes place. This type of review, referred to by Wholey (1983) as a plausibility analysis, challenges the stakeholders to scrutinize the model to determine if the underlying logic is sound. In other words, when these resources are devoted to these activities and processes, is it likely that the intended outcomes will be achieved? For example, in the context of our model it is possible that practitioners often focused on program processes (such as the finite elements of the implementation of group therapy) may see a need to shift their focus to the quality of aftercare services when they link the immediate service processes to intermediate outcomes. Although this process does not require the collection of information, this type of analysis can have a significant impact on a program's performance. It provides the ability to critically analyze the connection between service delivery and outcomes.

IDENTIFYING KEY PROGRAM INFORMATION NEEDS

A program model that has major stakeholder endorsement and has been approved as having a solid theoretical basis can serve as an excellent tool for linking information to program performance and practice. Other approaches to evaluation, especially those focusing on total quality management, offer prescriptive uses of information related to process and outcome (Yeager, 2002). In this case, program stakeholders are in-

structed to simply circle components of the model (resource, process, or outcome) for which performance information is needed. This is followed by the identification of possible indicators that can be pursued to assess a particular aspect. For example, staff may be very interested in Outcome 5.3, "Youth maintain legal lifestyle." Discussion would then focus on specific approaches to collecting information about this aspect of the program, which may include police records or self-report surveys or a collection of information from the youth, staff, and family (see Table 103.1). In essence, a program component from the program model is highlighted as the focus of needed information, a specific indicator is developed that would reflect program performance in the respective arena, and a data collection plan is detailed, enumerating the source of the information, the method of collection, and the frequency of collection and reporting.

The Development of a Program Improvement Plan

Historically, practice-based research has a dubious record when it comes to the utility of the information for the program's ongoing operation. Extensive agency-based research has been conducted; however, it is often not very influential in the arena of decision making and routine program operation. We have experience with program improvement plans that connect the program innovation with information sources for assessing ongoing performance. This integrated approach attempts to remove the distinction between ongoing program management and program evaluation by integrating the ongoing use of the information into the routine management of the program.

Program Assessment

The improvement initiative begins with a collaborative program assessment that, as before, is inclusive of all stakeholders with relevant information about and commitment to program performance. The assessment should include three sources of information: (a) systematically collected information (standardized instruments or data from an existing information system), (b) treatment documentation (information that is collected in the treatment process, such as routine treatment planning reports and documents), and (c) clinical or administrative wisdom (information and expertise that practitioners possess as a result of their function in the practice setting). Whereas a traditional research perspective may view the inclusion of such unconventional sources of information as heresy, these are included in this process for two reasons. Much in the practice world is not captured by conventional research methodologies, and to exclude this key information from the process of planning for future program or practice innovation may severely limit the viability of such efforts. In addition, such insights are ingrained in the practitioner's consciousness; hence, such knowledge should be recognized publicly, evaluated accordingly, and included in this process.

The process for program assessment is organized in a fashion similar to that of the logic model: resources, activities, processes, and outcomes. Individually, each participant develops his or her own point of view on the program, on the basis of his or her knowledge from the previously listed sources. Next, a roundtable discussion occurs, in which all interested parties share their knowledge about the program. After all points of view are aired, the focus moves toward judgment about the program: What is strong about the program? What parts of the program are opportunities for growth? And what are some suggestions for maximizing improvements?

Targeting a Program Outcome

Another critical step in the development of an improvement plan is the identification of a target outcome for the improvement process. A crucial outcome is chosen as a candidate for improvement based on the criticality of the outcome to the program, the need for improvement on this particular outcome, or both. A standard of performance is developed as a target representing effectiveness. The indicator, including the standard, for Outcome 5.1, "Youth maintain appropriate placement," could be that 75% of youth maintain their home placement 12 months after discharge. The rationale for setting the standard at that level could be based on previous research or previous experience with the program (clinical and administrative wisdom; Krill, 1990), or in the case in which there is no precedent for setting a standard, a level is developed on the basis of best estimates.

Development of the Improvement Plan

The heart of the program improvement plan is an initiative that is likely to move performance on the targeted outcome to the specified level of effectiveness. The initiative could include adding a new component, such as a new program or training component. The initiative could also involve organizing and investing new resources in an existing but underperforming component of a program.

Figure 103.2 illustrates a program improvement plan based on the development of aftercare services to support clients with reintegration into the community after discharge from the residential facility. The targeted outcome goal is for youth to maintain their home placement, as stated earlier. The objective—the heart of the initiative—is the development and implementation of a comprehensive aftercare program. The intervention column represents the steps that need to be conducted to implement this innovation. The column of indicators on the left side of the chart represents the information that can be used to monitor the implementation of the intervention steps. The column on the far right of the chart represents the support the intervention will require to be implemented. This chart allows the manager(s) of the intervention to design the innovation and develop a specific plan for its implementation.

Monitoring Implementation of the Plan

This chart also serves as the template for the development of a monitoring plan for this innovation. The monitoring plan is a deliberate strategy for using the information identified in the improvement plan to make sure that it is

Outcome goal: 75% of youth will remain in their family homes 6 months after discharge

⇑

Objective: Develop and implement comprehensive aftercare service

⇑

Indicator: ⟸	Intervention: ⟸	Support
Logic model and accompanying documentation exists.	Develop aftercare model.	Organizational endorsement and support of aftercare
Training curriculum is developed including manuals.	Develop training modules.	Management support of training and program changes
Family work and other treatment staff complete training.	Schedule and coordinate training. Train staff on aftercare service. Train family workers.	Treatment team participation in training and implementation
An implementation plan is documented with time lines and treatment staff signing off.	Train other treatment team members. Develop implementation plan with treatment teams. Schedule implementation of new procedures.	
Management and treatment staff team approve implementation dates.	Begin implementation. Monitor implementation.	

FIGURE 103.2 Program improvement plan.

implemented as intended and, if it is not, to make adjustments in a timely fashion and to assess its intended effect. The plan should specify the mechanisms for collecting the information as well as organizational entities for analyzing the data and making decisions. Although some programs striving for quality use a review process as outlined in Yeager (2002), this approach can enhance the plan, do, check, and act phases by customizing the monitoring process to fit the agency, client, and program capacity and need. As such, the act of monitoring is consistent with the agency resources and is more likely to occur in a timely and accurate fashion. In this case, a management and staff team would have biweekly meetings to keep abreast of the implementation, specifically looking at the indicators of implementation to make sure they are occurring as intended and, if not, making and implementing plans to accommodate changes. In addition, the team will develop a plan for collecting the outcome data and using that data to make decisions. The decisions focus on judging overall implementation of the plan and its success. For example, the outcome data might be reviewed at 6 months to assess whether the targeted outcome is changing and if adjustments need to be considered. There might also be an 18-month target date at which the team would review the

outcome data and determine if the improvement plan is having its intended effect. At this point, the team would decide whether to make a summative decision (which could include continuing the aftercare program as is or terminating the service) or to make a formative decision (which would include implementing program adjustments). This example of using a program logic model to specify and analyze the rationale of an intended service and as the basis for identifying key information (that can be used to develop a program improvement plan) provides a concrete method of integrating evidence-based practice in ongoing program management.

IMPLICATIONS FOR SOCIAL WORK ADMINISTRATIVE PRACTICE

Research and practice are often seen as separate activities. However, in the realm of administrative practice, this division is neither useful nor warranted. The use of information and evidence is a key component of administrative practice and is necessary for programs to respond to the needs of people and the changing politics of service delivery.

One of the many strengths of using the evidence-based practice framework in administrative practice is that it negates the distinction between research and practice. A sound administrator, one who practices from a client-centered orientation, should maintain an approach that builds on the organizational context and capacity. In doing so, it is necessary to respond to the needs of the many stakeholders involved in maintaining, using, and funding programs, be they workers, clients, or funding sources. Administrative practice that ignores or denies these groups may lead an organization focused on survival rather than on competent sound practice. Using the logic model and accompanying the processes as an information-based technique allows a means of integrating practice and research. This approach provides administrators, academics, clients, and other key stakeholders with the opportunity to design, manage, and improve programs with an understanding of the organizational context while maintaining the importance of client outcomes.

References

Alter, C., & Egan, M. (1997). Logic modeling: A tool for teaching critical thinking in social work practice. *Journal of Social Work Education, 33*(1), 85–102.

Alter, C., & Murty, S. (1997). Logic modeling: A tool for teaching practice evaluation. *Journal of Social Work Education, 33*(1), 103–117.

Brueggemann, W. G. (2002). *The practice of macro social work.* Belmont, CA: Brooks/Cole, Thomson Learning.

Gabor, P., & Grinnell, R. M., Jr. (1994). Debate 11: Should program decisions be based on empirical evidence of effectiveness? In W. Hudson & P. Nurius (Eds.), *Controversial issues in social work research* (pp. 142–154). Boston: Allyn & Bacon.

Gambrill, E. (2001). Social work: An authority-based profession. *Research on Social Work Practice, 11*(2), 166–175.

Kapp, S. (1991). Program improvement planning: Better client services through evaluation. *Research and Evaluation in Group Care, 2*(1), 22–23.

Kapp, S. (2000). Defining, promoting, and improving a model of school social work: The development of a tool for collaboration. *School Social Work Journal, 24*(2), 20–41.

Krill, D. (1990). *Practice wisdom: A guide for helping professionals.* Newbury Park, CA: Sage.

Macdonald, G. (2001). *Effective interventions for child abuse and neglect: An evidence-based approach to planning and evaluating interventions.* New York: Wiley.

Meenaghan, T. M., & Gibbons, W. E. (2000). *Generalist practice in larger settings: Knowledge and skill concepts.* Chicago: Lyceum Books.

Proctor, E. (2002). Social work, school violence, mental health, and drug abuse: A call for evidence-based practices. *Social Work Research, 26*(2), 67–69.

Rapp, C. A., & Poertner, J. (1992). *Social administration: A client-centered approach.* New York: Longman.

Savas, S. A. (1996). How do we propose to help children and families? In P. Pecora, W. R. Seelig, F. A. Zirps, et al. (Eds.), *Quality improvement and evaluation in child and family services: Managing into the next century* (pp. 37–52). Washington, DC: Child Welfare League of America.

Tripodi, T. (1994). Debate 10: Is the scientist–practitioner model appropriate for administrative practice? In W. W. Hudson & P. S. Nurius (Eds.), *Controversial issues in social work research* (pp. 128–141). Boston: Allyn & Bacon.

Wholey, J. (1983). *Evaluation and public management.* Boston: Little, Brown.

Wholey, J. S. (1994). Assessing the feasibility and likely usefulness of evaluation. In J. S. Wholey, H. Hatry, & K. E. Newcomer (Eds.), *Handbook of practical program evaluation* (pp. 15–39). San Francisco: Jossey-Bass.

EPILOGUE

Epilogue

THE CLINICAL UTILITY OF THERAPY RESEARCH

Bridging the Gap Between the Present and the Future

Peter E. Nathan

Evidence-based practices have thoroughly infused the activities, especially the therapeutic practices, of all members of the core mental health professions over the past decade. However, they have not until recently appeared to impact substantially on the broader array of healthcare and human services. The *Evidence-Based Practice Manual* reflects both of these welcome developments. In so doing, it lends support to the extremely encouraging view that empirically supported practices, including but by no means restricted either to mental health practices or mental health practitioners, have now extended their reach very widely. In eloquently portraying this very positive development in human services, including as it affects their social work, psychiatry, and other human services colleagues, the editors of this volume provide us with both an impressive portrait of the scope and reach of evidence-based practice today as well as a sense of the most promising models for successful utilization of new empirically supported practices tomorrow. Although I am loath to predict in the absence of data, I think I can confidently anticipate that this volume, which reflects an extraordinary diversity of current practices, will ultimately influence an even wider array of practices. For this we owe thanks to editors Al-

bert R. Roberts and Kenneth Yeager and their colleagues, for their clear-eyed view of the present and, as important, their prescient vision of the bright future in healthcare and human services.

OVERVIEW OF EPILOGUE

Despite the outpouring of research on counseling and psychotherapy over the past half century, the clinical activities of most counselors and psychotherapists remain largely untouched by it (Barlow, 1981; Kopta, Lueger, Saunders, & Howard, 1999; Nathan, Stuart, & Dolan, 2000). Various explanations have been offered to explain the low clinical utility of research on behavior change. Two of the most widely accepted include the impact of the long-standing debate about whether counseling and psychotherapy work and, if they do, which methods work best, and the effects of the continuing controversy over behavior change models, focused on the relative value of the efficacy model and the effectiveness model. If psychotherapy researchers, after more than fifty years, cannot agree on whether therapy works, whether one treatment works better than another, or even on how best to assess the worth of a given therapeutic strategy, the logic of the explanation goes, why should clinicians put much faith in the results of therapy research? This chapter looks carefully at the data, past and present, on these issues, in the effort to understand better why practitioners largely ignore findings from therapy research and how they might be induced not to do so in the future.

RESEARCH ON PSYCHOTHERAPY EFFICACY AND EFFECTIVENESS

Fundamental to the identification and dissemination of empirically supported or evidence-based treatments is the continuing controversy over which of two research models best captures the most salient differences among counseling and therapy techniques and procedures. The two models are called the *efficacy model* and the *effectiveness model*; they are discussed in detail in this section, then referred to frequently in what follows in the chapter. These two research models take substantially different views on the best way to study behavior change. Thus, if you believe strongly in the value of the efficacy model and depend on it to inform you about those treatments that achieve the most positive outcomes, you will be unlikely to be impressed by claims from researchers using the effectiveness model that they have identified empirically supported or evidence-based treatments. Similarly, if you think that only by means of effectiveness research can appropriate empirical support be marshaled in support of a behavior change technique, you will almost certainly be unimpressed by data on outcomes generated only by efficacy researchers. In truth, as this chapter suggests, neither model by itself captures the entirety of what makes a counseling or therapy approach worthwhile. For that reason, researchers have begun to try to integrate the two approaches in the effort to create a research model that will yield the broadest-base empirical support for the treatments it evaluates.

Psychotherapy efficacy research is concerned above all with *replication*, on the assumption that replicated psychotherapy outcome data are more likely to be valid. Efficacy studies contain a number of research elements that are not often found in effectiveness studies. Prominent among them is *inclusion of an appropriate control con-*

dition with which the experimental treatment can be compared, so that the impact of the experimental treatment can be determined as clearly as possible. For the same reason, efficacy research studies generally require *random assignment of subjects either to experimental or comparison/control treatments*, in the effort to ensure the absence of systematic, subject-based bias. Efficacy studies also *carefully describe the elements of the treatment provided*, to permit it to be replicated to the extent possible in subsequent studies. This quest for replication of treatment conditions, both within a study and between studies, has led to the widespread—and occasionally controversial—use of *treatment manuals*, which are designed to ensure that therapists conducting the intervention will be able to maintain therapeutic consistency. Finally, priority is given in efficacy studies to *diagnostically homogeneous groups of patients whose psychopathology is well defined* by reliable and valid measures of psychopathology, so the diagnostic groups that respond to the experimental treatment can be clearly specified.

Effectiveness research, by contrast, is concerned with the *feasibility of treatments in real-world settings*. Persons who need treatment, regardless of diagnosis, comorbid psychopathology, or duration of illness, can participate in effectiveness studies. Therapists in effectiveness studies are not usually trained to deliver the experimental treatment with the kind of consistency that is a hallmark of efficacy studies. Clinical considerations rather than the demands of the research design dictate choice of treatment method, as well as its frequency, duration, and means of outcome assessment. Although assignment of patients to treatments in effectiveness studies may be randomized, disguising the treatment to which the patient has been assigned is rarely feasible. Outcome assessments are often broadly defined, and may include such "soft" indices as changes in degree of disability, quality of life, or personality rather than targeted evaluations of symptoms by structured interviews.

Barlow (1996) succinctly differentiated efficacy and effectiveness studies as follows: *efficacy studies* yield "a systematic evaluation of the intervention in a controlled clinical research context. Considerations relevant to the internal validity of these conclusions are usually highlighted" (p. 1051); by contrast, *effectiveness studies* explore "the applicability and feasibility of the intervention in the local setting where the treatment is delivered" and are designed to "determine the generalizability of an intervention with established efficacy" (p. 1055).

Up to this time, most of the research that has led to identification of evidence-based treatments has been done according to the efficacy model. As what follows later in this chapter suggests, however, that research model preference may be changing.

COMMON FACTORS

All psychological treatments and counseling procedures share common elements that are responsible for a substantial amount of the treatment outcome variance. "Common factors" are thought to be responsible, at least in part, for the frequent finding that all psychosocial treatments in a study yield comparably positive outcomes. This effect has a lengthy history. Almost seven decades ago, psychologist Saul Rosenzweig first referred to the difficulty mental health professionals had distinguishing among the psychotherapies of the time in effectiveness. Rosenzweig (1936) reasoned that, if all psychotherapies affect patients equivalently, then, paraphrasing Lewis Carroll's Dodo Bird in *Alice in Wonderland* (1865, 1962), "All have won and all must have prizes." Even though more than sixty-five years separate the year of the Dodo Bird metaphor's birth from today, psychotherapy researchers still refer to Lewis Carroll's footrace when they want to make the point that many studies have suggested that most psychotherapies are pretty much interchangeable in effectiveness. In this section, we closely examine some of the so-called common factors responsible for this common research result.

Common factors are associated with *therapist, client or patient,* and *therapeutic process,* according to Lambert and Bergin's influential proposal (1994). They further envision three subfactors: (1) *support factors,* which include therapeutic alliance, catharsis, and therapist warmth; (2) *learning factors,* including corrective emotional experiences, insight, and feedback; and (3) *action factors,* like cognitive mastery, modeling, and behavioral regulation. Lambert and Bergen report that many of these factors and subfactors are associated positively with outcomes, regardless of specific therapeutic technique employed. Making the same point on completing a meta-analysis of components of

treatment hypothesized to be efficacious, Ahn and Wampold (2001) asserted that this investigation of the power of therapy techniques to affect outcomes had "provided no evidence that the specific ingredients of psychological treatments are responsible for the beneficial outcomes of counseling and psychotherapy" (p. 254). Wampold (2001) has taken the results of these and other studies to signify that outcome research has failed to demonstrate a significant relationship between specific therapeutic techniques and outcomes—and that common factors rather than specific therapy components are largely responsible for positive outcomes. Wampold's extensive research and writing on common factors, however, has also been strongly criticized; Deegear and Lawson (2003) summarize these criticisms, which center on a Wampold's failure to consider a number of the studies that do not support his views on the primacy of common factors in determining psychotherapy outcomes.

Beutler, Machado, and Neufeldt (1994) also affirmed the importance of common factors in counseling and psychotherapy outcomes. They emphasized therapist variables, which they see as extending from their demographic characteristics and sociocultural backgrounds to more subjective factors like values, attitudes, and beliefs. These factors may be quite specific to therapy (e.g., the therapist's role in the therapeutic relationship and his or her expectations for its success), as well as more distant from it (e.g., therapists' cultural attitudes and emotional well-being). Therapist variables reflecting therapy-specific states, including therapist's professional identity (Berman & Norton, 1985) and his or her therapeutic style and choice of interventions (Robinson, Berman, & Neimeyer, 1990), exert an especially strong impact on therapy outcomes according to this view. Therapist-specific factors like age and gender, by contrast, appear to affect outcomes much less (Zlotnick, Elkin, & Shea, 1998).

Patient variables have not generally predicted therapeutic outcomes (Luborsky & Diguer, 1995). Although Strupp (1973) and Orlinsky and Howard (1986) maintained that process variables—the strength of the therapeutic bond, the skillfulness of therapeutic interventions, and the duration of the therapeutic relationship—impact on outcomes, process research has proven difficult to carry out and its findings have been inconsistent.

THE CLINICAL UTILITY
OF OUTCOME RESEARCH:
A FIFTY-YEAR SURVEY

Hans Eysenck's landmark 1952 and 1960 evaluations of the effects of psychotherapy were distinguished from the few other such efforts of the time by his willingness to bring the scanty data then available to bear on the question, rather than relying on opinion and clinical judgment, and in so doing to reach an unpopular conclusion. In fact, Eysenck reached a very unpopular conclusion: that the psychotherapies in widest use at mid-century were largely ineffective. He also admitted that the inadequate methodologies of the studies on which he based his conclusions required him to qualify them.

In the early 1970s, a quarter of a century after the tumultuous professional response to Eysenck's unwelcome observations on the effects of psychotherapy, several comprehensive reviews of the therapy research literature of the time began to note some of the hard-won advances in the methodology of psychotherapy research and some of the encouraging findings on the efficacy of new therapies, especially the behavior therapies and cognitive behavior therapies. None of these reviews, however, acknowledged the failure of clinicians generally to utilize these findings, despite the fact that the clinical utility problem had long ago been discussed by Cronbach (1957) and Cohen (1965).

In 1970, Gendlin and Rychlak reiterated Eysenck's 20-year-old observations in a review of late 1960s research on therapeutic processes, lamenting the inadequacy of the research methods but recognizing the promise of the behavior therapies. In a review published a year later, Krasner (1971) observed that although behavior therapy had developed from experimental psychology laboratories, it had clearly been transformed even then into clinically effective behavior change procedures. A year later, the same rhetoric: Howard and Orlinsky (1972) took note of a series of promising therapeutic process studies, but also chose to ignore the unresponsiveness of practitioners to data that would appear to hold great interest for them. Similarly, in a review of behavioral treatments three years later, Bergin and Suinn (1975) chronicled accelerating advances in both therapy research methodology and the effectiveness of the behavioral and cognitive-behavioral treatments—and said nothing about the significance of these findings

for practitioners. In like fashion, three years hence, Gomes-Schwartz, Hadley, and Strupp (1978) made no mention of the problems of transfer from laboratory to consulting room, even while they commented favorably on contemporary research on outcomes of individual psychotherapy and behavior therapy.

Researchers finally began to confront the issue of the clinical utility of therapy research in the 1980s. One of the first to do so was Barlow (1981), writing in a special issue of the *Journal of Consulting and Clinical Psychology*. His observations were trenchant:

At present, clinical research has little or no influence on clinical practice. This state of affairs should be particularly distressing to a discipline whose goal over the last 30 years has been to produce professionals who would integrate the methods of science with clinical practice to produce new knowledge. (Barlow, 1981, p. 147)

Commenting on the results of a meta-analysis of 143 contemporary psychotherapy outcome studies, Shapiro and Shapiro (1982, 1983) drew the same conclusion. Even though the statistical conclusions from and internal validity of the studies used in the meta-analysis were "generally satisfactory," they felt their construct and external validity had been "severely limited by unrepresentativeness of clinical practice" (1983, p. 42). The same year and in the same vein, Rosenthal (1983) lamented the difference between the statistical and social importance of psychotherapy, going so far as to suggest a new statistical means to heighten the real-world usefulness of psychotherapy research findings. At exceptional variance to this consensus, Goldfried, Greenberg, and Marmar (1990) grandly concluded that "the development of methods for demonstrating clinical (in addition to statistical) significance (during the decade of the 1980s) has been one of the major advances in outcome research" (p. 661).

In the 1990s, therapy researchers have become even more concerned about clinical utility, as evidenced by their preoccupation with the meaning and significance of distinctions between efficacy and effectiveness research. Early in the decade, in a thoughtful review of contemporary psychotherapy outcome research, Persons (1991) raised questions about the external validity of efficacy research by observing that the designs of many earlier psychotherapy outcome studies appeared to her to be incompatible with the models of psychotherapy those studies were designed to evaluate. Persons assigned principal blame for this situation to the predominant efficacy model's expectation that assignment of patients to standardized treatments should be done by diagnosis rather than a theory-driven psychological assessment of each individual. Her solution to this problem of long-standing: "The case formulation approach to psychotherapy research," which requires development of an "assessment-plus-treatment protocol" based directly on the psychotherapeutic model itself.

The same year, Jacobson and Truax (1991) proposed to solve another common outcome research problem affecting clinical utility, the statistically significant pre- and post-therapy behavior change scores that are so often of little apparent clinical significance. Jacobson, Follette, and Revenstorf (1984) had previously operationalized clinically significant change as an individual's movement out of the range of the dysfunctional population or into the range of the functional population. Accordingly, Jacobson and Truax (1991) proposed to define clinically significant change according to this formulation. An example:

The level of functioning subsequent to therapy should fall within the range of the functional or normal population, where range is defined as within two standard deviations of the mean of that population. (p. 13)

In 1995, Ogles, Lambert, and Sawyer reanalyzed outcome data from the NIMH Treatment of Depression Collaborative Research Program (Elkin, 1994; Elkin et al., 1985, 1989) according to these criteria for assessing clinical significance. Although the initial analysis of the study's findings by Elkin and her colleagues in 1989 had revealed significant improvements in symptoms of depression following both psychological and pharmacological treatments, subsequent analyses revealed few statistically significant differences between treatment groups. Ogles and his colleagues hypothesized that reanalysis according to the 1991 Jacobson and Truax criteria would reveal clinically significant differences between conditions, and that is what they found, thereby confirming the therapeutic advantages of the psychological treatments for depression.

In 1994, a subsample of 180,000 subscribers to Consumer Reports was asked a series of ques-

tions about their experiences with mental health professionals, physicians, medications, and self-help groups, in the largest survey to date of mental health treatment outcomes. The survey's principal findings, reported in 1995, were that:

- Almost half of the respondents whose emotional state was "very poor" or "fairly poor" reported significant improvement following therapy.
- The longer psychotherapy lasted, the more it helped.
- Psychotherapy alone worked as well as combined psychotherapy and pharmacotherapy

Psychologist Martin Seligman, a consultant to the survey, reviewed its findings a year later, detailed its "methodological virtues and drawbacks," and proposed eight characteristics of efficacy studies that he thought differentiated them from effectiveness studies. Seligman (1995) concluded that the Consumer Reports survey "complements the (more traditional) efficacy method (so that) the best features of these two methods can be combined into a more ideal method that will best provide empirical validation of psychotherapy" (1995, p. 965).

A series of commentaries on Seligman's 1995 article that dealt largely with the real-world utility of efficacy research and the significance of the distinction between efficacy and effectiveness research appeared a year later. Goldfried and Wolfe (1996) proposed "a new outcome research paradigm that involves an active collaboration between researcher and practicing clinician" (p. 1007), which "individualizes the intervention on the basis of an initial assessment and case formulation" (1996, p. 1013). Hollon (1996) concluded that while efficacy studies "leave much to be desired," effectiveness designs are not a panacea, in large part because they cannot substitute "for the randomized controlled clinical trial when it comes to drawing causal inferences about whether psychotherapy (or any other treatment) actually works" (1996, pp. 1029–1030). Jacobson and Christensen (1996) found the Consumer Reports study to be so seriously flawed that they could draw few conclusions from it. Like Hollon (1996), they also believed that "the randomized clinical trial is as good a method for answering questions of effectiveness as it is for answering questions of efficacy," despite its limitations (1996, p. 1031). However, Howard and his colleagues (1996) suggested moving away from treatment-focused research altogether, in favor of "patient-focused research," which attempts to monitor an individual's progress over the course of treatment and provide feedback of this information to the practitioner, supervisor, or case manager.

Responding, Seligman (1996) acknowledged the validity of many of these criticisms of the *Consumer Reports* study but insisted that the study had nonetheless had significant value:

Both the experimental method (efficacy) and the observational method (effectiveness) answer complementary questions ... (although) efficacy studies ... cannot test long-term psychotherapy because long-term manuals cannot be written and patients cannot be randomized into two-year-long placebo controls, so the "empirical validation" of long-term therapy will likely come from effectiveness studies. (Seligman, 1996, p. 1072)

The 1990s witnessed additional advances in psychotherapy outcome research methodology, coupled with positive outcome results from several large-scale randomized clinical trials of behavioral and cognitive behavioral treatments for alcoholism, the mood disorders, and the anxiety disorders. Publication of practice guidelines for the treatment of a wide range of psychopathologic conditions by the American Psychiatric Association (e.g., 1993, 1994, 1995, 1996, 1997) and the Division of Clinical Psychology of the American Psychological Association (Chambless et al., 1996, 1998; Division 12, 1995) coincided with these positive developments. All were based in large part on research according to the efficacy model. The guidelines' appearance, in turn, generated predictably strong negative reactions from persons who questioned the clinical utility of the psychotherapy outcome research on which the guidelines were based (Nathan, 1998). Sol Garfield (1996), a well-known psychotherapy researcher, took especially strong exception to the initial list of "empirically validated treatments" published in 1995 by the Division 12 Task Force. Several of his concerns reflected doubts about the efficacy model, including the distortion to the psychotherapy process he believed manuals typically used in efficacy studies cause, as well as the incomparability of psychotherapy patients in efficacy studies and those in real-world psychotherapy settings.

Echoing similar sentiments in their 1999 *Annual Review of Psychology* chapter on contemporary psychotherapy research, Kopta, Lueger, Saunders, and Howard highlighted the continuing gap between clinical research and clinical practice. Suggesting that part of the problem might lie in the field's preference for randomized clinical trials (RCTs), they proposed instead "that this approach should be replaced by naturalistic designs, which can provide results more applicable to real clinical practice, therefore strengthening external validity" (p. 449). Effectiveness studies, of course, epitomize "naturalistic designs."

CURRENT EFFORTS TO INCREASE THE CLINICAL UTILITY OF THERAPY RESEARCH: INTEGRATING EFFICACY AND EFFECTIVENESS STUDIES

Four recent approaches—three experimental, one statistical—to the clinical utility problem, all designed to resolve the effectiveness/efficacy controversy, have recently been proposed. All presume that efficacy studies alone or effectiveness studies alone will never provide clinicians the help they require.

Norquist, Lebowitz, and Hyman (1999) put forth a proposal by which the National Institute of Mental Health (NIMH), which Hyman directed at the time, in consultation with basic scientists, advocates, and other federal agencies, would endeavor to bridge the gap between the two outcome research models (NAMHC Workgroup, 1999; Niederehe, Street, & Lebowitz, 1999; Norquist, Lebowitz, & Hyman, 1999). They label the models the *regulatory* (efficacy) *model* and the *public health* (effectiveness) *model*. The first is named for the detailed steps drug manufacturers must take to demonstrate the safety and efficacy of their new products to the Federal Food and Drug Administration (FDA), the second, for research designed to evaluate the effectiveness of clinical interventions as delivered in the community. Norquist and his colleagues envision a new research paradigm that will "combine the designs of traditional clinical and services research studies," thereby requiring compromises between the strict randomized designs of traditional clinical research and the more flexible observational designs of services research. Merging these designs will require NIMH "to bring together methodologists with expertise across these fields to delineate what we currently know and what we don't (because it is) quite likely that new methods and statistical analytic approaches will need to be developed to address studies in the mental health area" (1999, p. 6). To achieve the ambitious goals of the new paradigm, new methods and new statistical approaches will be required. New methods of grant review and a new research infrastructure to facilitate grant submission, review, and funding are also planned. While anticipating great things, including a quantum leap in the clinical utility of psychotherapy research, this new enterprise will founder unless the promised new methods and statistical procedures, which have yet to be developed, can in fact be brought into being.

The same year, Klein and Smith proposed establishment of "dedicated, multi-site efficacy/effectiveness clinics" to confront the conflicting demands of efficacy and effectiveness studies. The clinics would facilitate studies of process and outcome and help accumulate outcome norms for well-defined populations on such variables as diagnosis, economic status, history, and comorbidity. The near-term goal of the clinics would be to generate "a large volume of well-delineated patients who could be treated and studied and may have high comorbidity with medical, psychiatric, and substance abuse conditions" (1999, p. 5). More distant goals would include development of benchmarks for expected treatment outcomes for these distinct groups of patients by means of normative sampling, and generation of hypotheses the clinics would themselves ultimately be in a position to test. As with NIMH's new paradigm, however, Klein and Smith's proposal for efficacy/effectiveness clinics is long on enthusiasm, problem identification, and aspirations for change, shorter on concrete design, methodology, and details of statistical analyses. Although understandable, the relative lack of substance leaves the reader who appreciates some of the problems attendant upon integrating efficacy and effectiveness studies uncertain whether the integration these authors propose can actually be brought about.

Two years later, Rounsaville, Carroll, and Onken (2001a) outlined a *Stage Model of Behavioral Therapies Research*. The model, originally proposed by Onken, Blaine, and Battjes in 1997, details three sequential steps leading from an initial innovative clinical procedure through efficacy and then effectiveness testing.

Stage I consists of pilot/feasibility testing, manual writing, training program development, and adherence/competence measure development for new and untested treatments. . . . Stage II initially consists of

randomized clinical trials (RCTs) to evaluate efficacy of manualized and pilot-tested treatments which have shown promise or efficacy in earlier studies. Stage II research can also address mechanisms of action or effective components of treatment for those approaches with evidence of efficacy derived from RCTs. Stage III consists of studies to evaluate transportability of treatments for which efficacy has been demonstrated in at least two RCTs. Key Stage III research issues revolve around generalizability; implementation issues; cost effectiveness issues; and consumer/marketing issues. (Rounsaville, Carroll, & Onken, 2001a, pp. 133–134)

In a critique of this model, Kazdin (2001) acknowledged the "critically important goal" of developing treatments that can be used effectively by practitioners. At the same time, he emphasized the importance as well of addressing—and answering—crucial questions about "why and how new treatments work." In his view, the Stage Model as described by Rounsaville and his colleagues (2001a) does not address these questions.

Rounsaville, Carroll, and Onken (2001b) restated Kazdin's (2001) critique in terms of three major omissions: "(a) lack of emphasis on theory-driven components to stage model research; (b) failure to address the need for research on "what are the mechanisms through which therapy operates and under what conditions is therapy likely to be effective and why;" and (c) exclusive reliance on randomized clinical trials as the basis for evidence of efficacy/effectiveness of a treatment under study" (p. 152). Pointing to a number of their prior publications that showed that they share similar concerns and would want them included in this effort, these authors nonetheless conclude that "implicit in Kazdin's characterization and reaction to the stage model is a cut-and-dried, assembly-line view of the process," whereas they see it as "a tree, which has a directional, upward course, but a course that branches to catch the most light and to bear more than one fruit" (p. 154).

Although Shadish and his colleagues (Shadish et al., 1996, 1997, in press) take a very different starting-point from these three proposals for restructuring the experimental venue of therapy research to make it more practitioner-friendly, their meta-analyses of the psychotherapy outcome literature address a closely related set of issues and appear to arrive at conclusions very similar to those to which the authors of the three other proposals might ultimately come. Shadish and his associates used sophisticated random effects regression analyses to undertake secondary analyses of earlier meta-analyses that permitted them to ask whether therapy outcome studies ranging from less to more "clinically representative" differed in effectiveness according to a substantial array of outcome variables. They wanted to determine whether therapy evaluated by the efficacy research model and psychotherapy assessed for effectiveness research purposes differ in outcome: whether substantive differences in results reflect substantive differences in research methods.

Shadish's meta-analyses failed to reveal differences in therapeutic outcome as a function of where on the efficacy/effectiveness ("clinically representative") continuum a study fell. While these findings do not transform the real methodological differences between the efficacy/effectiveness research models into semantic ones, they do suggest that, in terms of one very important factor, clinical usefulness, the distinction may be more apparent than real.

RESEARCH ON CLINICAL UTILITY: PAST, PRESENT, AND FUTURE

The Past and the Present

Psychotherapy researchers in the 1950s and 1960s expressed only modest concern that the statistical significance of their findings was rarely accompanied by clinical significance. Surprisingly little was written during those years about the issue of clinical utility. Perhaps this reflected the primitive state, by current standards, of the psychotherapy research methodologies of the time: Psychotherapy research data during these years appears to have been wholly inadequate as bases for understanding or implementing treatment.

The 1970s witnessed marked advances in therapy research methods and the parallel emergence of promising behavioral and cognitive behavioral treatments. Despite these advances, not much was written about how those advances might augment clinical practice, suggesting that the issue of clinical utility had not engaged psychotherapy researchers. Perhaps that omission reflected caution in the face of the rapid changes affecting outcome research methodologies.

By the 1980s, however, researchers began to express concern about how rarely therapy research informed clinical practice. Continued enhancements in research methodology that enabled researchers for the first time reliably to assess the comparative efficacy of different therapies clearly played a role in the emergence of these concerns. Solutions to the clinical utility problem tended to focus on efforts to make the existing psychotherapy research model—the efficacy model—more relevant to clinical practice. A few prescient commentators suggested weighing the differing contributions of what today we differentiate as efficacy and effectiveness research, while others refocused the issue altogether by suggesting that emphasizing therapeutic techniques as prime determinants of outcome might have less ultimate payoff for practitioners than emphasizing factors common to all therapies.

Early in the decade of the 1990s, these concerns coalesced around the nature and significance of distinctions between therapy outcome studies that examine efficacy and generalizability, and those that examine effectiveness and feasibility. In this recent extended debate, some researchers suggested that modest improvements in efficacy research ought to be sufficient to fix the problem, even though partial efforts of this kind thus far have not been successful. Others concluded that emphasizing effectiveness studies represented the best solution, despite the randomization and control problems that solution engenders. Still others recommended a simultaneous tweaking of both models, to achieve an optimal mix of internal and external validity even though, both conceptually and experimentally, that solution would be difficult to bring about. Most recently, as we have noted, conceptually ambitious but modestly detailed proposals have been made to radically restructure institutions, including the NIMH, in order to facilitate integration of efficacy and effectiveness research.

The Future

Recent decades have witnessed clear, documented gains in therapy effectiveness. Behavioral and cognitive-behavioral treatments have become treatments of choice for the anxiety and mood disorders (Chambless & Ollendick, 2001; Roth & Fonagy, 1996) and cognitive-behavioral treatments for alcohol abuse, eating disorders, and other common psychopathologic conditions are also widely used and well-accepted. Marked advances in outcome research methodologies, including the recent emphasis on heuristically important distinctions between the effectiveness and efficacy research models, have also energized efforts to promote empirically supported treatments. Regretfully, despite these clear advances, there is general agreement that most of the theories and therapeutic approaches used by clinicians today remain unsupported empirically (Beutler, Williams, Wakefield, & Entwistle, 1995; Plante, Andersen, & Boccaccini, 1999). In contrast, research on new psychopharmacological agents utilizing randomized clinical trials strongly influences clinical decision-making, although it must be acknowledged that FDA requirements for proof of safety and efficacy certainly play a central role in this regard.

The continuing functional separation of therapy research and clinical practice prevents researchers and psychotherapists from benefiting mutually from their observations. Partly for this reason, concurrence between therapy researchers and clinicians on issues that represent obvious opportunities for it, like agreement that treatments with strong empirical support are more likely to be effective than those without it, has not taken place.

Deegear and Lawson (2003) have recently summarized the most common arguments for and against integrating the results of research on empirically supported treatments into clinical practice, weighed the evidence for the alternative view that common factors rather than techniques play the most important role in therapy outcomes, and suggested alternatives to exclusive emphasis on empirically supported treatments in teaching, learning, and practicing therapy. Those alternatives include (1) an emphasis on common factors rather than techniques, if it can be demonstrated that common factors are in fact more powerful determinants of therapy outcomes than technique differences; (2) technical eclecticism, which involves choosing the techniques that work best for the particular problem the patient brings to treatment; and (3) integration of common factors and technical eclecticism. Unfortunately, these alternatives present problems that are at least as significant as those associated with empirically supported treatments: There has not been agreement either on which common factors are most influential or on how to teach them. Similarly, there is not agreement on the specific techniques that ought to be used with specific patients, how to teach them, and when to apply them.

If there is a light at the end of the tunnel, it may be our intense preoccupation over the past several years with how to solve the efficacy/effectiveness paradox so as to achieve consensus on how best to identify evidence-based treatments. While a number of solutions to the paradox posed by internal and external validity have been proposed, none has yet proven ideal (Addis, 2002). Our view is that, within a shorter rather than a longer time, a solution will be found and the Dodo Bird metaphor will lose its currency. Exclusive endorsement of either the efficacy or the effectiveness research models alone will not do the job; efforts along those lines have not yielded much encouragement to date. Likewise, tinkering with both models simultaneously to achieve some optimal balance of the two does not seem to be the answer; experience does not suggest it will be. One must also entertain serious doubts about whether it will be possible to develop new conceptual and statistical methods to permit integration of the two models that NIMH and others envision. Instead, the most likely solution seems to be to take findings from the best efficacy studies and use them to design the most robust effectiveness studies. Then, in bootstrap fashion, alternating between the two approaches, meaningful and clinically relevant findings might well emerge. This back-and-forth variant of the Onken/Rounsaville/Carroll model makes the most sense to us, in large part because a reading of the literature suggests that is the means by which consensus is often reached on a pharmacological or psychological treatment that works.

Resolving the efficacy/effectiveness paradox is only the first step, albeit a big one, toward solution of the fundamental unresolved issue. When and how will counseling and psychotherapy researchers and clinicians feel comfortable enough with each other to be able to benefit from the kind of mutual interaction that has proven fruitful elsewhere? Perhaps when research on therapy outcomes seems close enough to actual clinical practice to enable practitioners to see themselves in the research psychotherapists and their patients in the research patients and the research environment in the real-world settings within which the effectiveness research takes place. Or perhaps when more psychotherapists in training receive training in empirically supported treatments (e.g., Addis, 2002; Crits-Christoph et al., 1995; Hays et al., 2002).

A recent report provides encouragement for the view that enhancement in the clinical utility of our therapy research efforts is not so far off. In it, Chorpita and his colleagues (2002) describe the large-scale implementation of empirically supported treatments for children in the State of Hawaii by the Hawaii Empirical Basis to Services Task Force, whose participants "included health administrators, parents of challenged children, clinical service providers, and academicians from the areas of psychology, psychiatry, nursing, and social work" (p. 167). Following a review of treatment efficacy, these findings "were extended through a systematic cataloguing of effectiveness parameters across more than one hundred treatment outcome studies" (p. 165). The effectiveness parameters included feasibility, generalizability, and cost and benefit.

This report is encouraging because a broad-based group of administrators, providers, consumers, and researchers were able to come together and agree on a set of treatments that met efficacy and effectiveness standards that could then be recommended to providers throughout an entire state as most useful to them and to their patients. Among the possible reasons for the apparent success of this effort may be that (1) much of the work was done by dedicated, committed volunteers who cared enough to do much of the work on their own time; (2) the effort was open to anyone with a stake in the system, so a diverse group of interested persons came together to develop the standards; (3) once the State of Hawaii recognized what the group had achieved, it decided to invest funds in the initiative, thereby making its dissemination and implementation possible. If it can be done in Hawaii, perhaps it can be done elsewhere!

References

Addis, M. E. (2002). Methods for disseminating research products and increasing evidence-based practice: Promises, obstacles, and future directions. *Clinical Psychology: Science and Practice*, 9, 367–378.

Ahn, H. & Wampold, B.E. (2001). Where oh where are the specific ingredients? A meta-analysis of component studies in counseling and psychotherapy. *Journal of Counseling Psychology*, 48, 251–257.

American Psychiatric Association. (1993). Practice guidelines for the treatment of major depressive disorder in adults. *American Psychiatric Association*, 150 (No. 4, Supplement), 1–26.

American Psychiatric Association. (1994a). *Diagnostic and Statistical Manual of Mental Disorders*, 4th edition. Washington, DC: American Psychiatric Association.

American Psychiatric Association. (1994b). Practice guideline for the treatment of patients with bipolar disorder. *American Journal of Psychiatry*, 151 (No. 12, Supplement), 1–36.

American Psychiatric Association. (1995). Practice guideline for the treatment of patients with substance use disorders: Alcohol, cocaine, opioids. *American Journal of Psychiatry*, 152 (No. 11, Supplement), 1–59.

American Psychiatric Association. (1996). Practice guideline for the treatment of patients with nicotine dependence. *American Journal of Psychiatry*, 153 (No. 10, Supplement), 1–31.

American Psychiatric Association. (1997). Practice guideline for the treatment of patients with schizophrenia. *American Journal of Psychiatry*, 154 (No. 4, Supplement), 1–63.

Barlow, D. H. (1981). On the relation of clinical research to clinical practice: Current issues. *Journal of Consulting and Clinical Psychology*, 49, 147–155.

Barlow, D. H. (1996). Health care policy, psychotherapy research, and the future of psychotherapy. *American Psychologist*, 51, 1050–1058.

Bergin, A. E. & Suinn, R. M. (1975). Individual psychotherapy and behavior therapy. In M. R. Rosenzweig & L. W. Porter (Eds.), *Annual review of psychology*, vol. 26 (pp. 509–556). Palo Alto, CA: Annual Reviews, Inc.

Berman, J. S. & Norton, N. C. (1985). Does professional training make a therapist more effective? *Psychological Bulletin*, 98, 401–407.

Beutler, L. E., Machado, P. P. P., & Neufeldt, S. A. (1994). Therapist variables. In A. E. Bergin & S. L. Garfield (Eds.), *Handbook of psychotherapy and behavior change*, 4th ed. (pp. 229–269). New York: Wiley.

Beutler, L. E., Williams, R. E., Wakefield, P. J., & Entwistle, S. R. (1995). Bridging scientist and practitioner perspectives in clinical psychology. *American Psychologist*, 50, 984–994.

Carroll, L. (1962). *Alice's adventures in wonderland*. Harmondsworth, Middlesex, England: Penguin Books (Original work published in 1865).

Chambless, D. L., Baker, M. J., et al. (1998). Update on empirically validated therapies, II. *The Clinical Psychologist*, 51, 3–16.

Chambless, D. L., Sanderson, W. C., et al. (1996). An update on empirically validated therapies. *The Clinical Psychologist*, 49, 5–18.

Chambless, D. L. & Ollendick, T. H. (2001). Empirically supported psychological interventions: Controversies and evidence. In S. T. Fiske, D. L. Schacter, & C. Zahn-Waxler (Eds.), *Annual review of psychology* (vol. 52) (pp. 685–716). Palo Alto, CA: Annual Review.

Chorpita, B. F., Yim, L. M., Donkervoet, J. C., Arensdorf, A., Amundsen, M. J., McGee, C., Serrano, A., Yates, A., Burns, J. A., & Morelli, P. (2002). Toward large-scale implementation of empirically supported treatments for children: A review and observation by the Hawaii Empirical Basis to Service Task Force. *Clinical Psychology: Science and Practice, 9*, 165–190.

Crits-Christoph, P., Frank, E., Chambless, D. L., Brody, C., & Karp, J. F. (1995). Training in empirically validated treatments: What are clinical psychology students learning? *Professional Psychology: Research and Practice, 26*, 514–522.

Cohen, J. (1965). Some statistical issues in psychological research. In B. Wolman (Ed.), *Handbook of clinical psychology.* New York: McGraw-Hill.

Cronbach, L. J. (1957). Two disciplines of scientific psychology. *American Psychologist, 12*, 671-684.

Deegear, J. & Lawson, D. M. (2003). The utility of empirically supported treatments. *Professional Psychology: Research and Practice, 34*, 271–277.

Division 12 Task Force. (1995). Training in and dissemination of empirically-validated psychological treatments: Report and recommendations. *The Clinical Psychologist, 48*, 3–23.

Elkin, I. (1994). The NIMH Treatment of Depression Collaborative Research Program: Where we began and where we are. In A. E. Bergin & S. L. Garfield (Eds.), *Handbook of psychotherapy and behavior change* (pp. 114–139). New York: Wiley.

Elkin, I., Parloff, M. B., Hadley, S. W., & Autry, J. H. (1985). NIMH Treatment of Depression Collaborative Treatment Program: Background and research plan. *Archives of General Psychiatry, 42*, 305–316.

Elkin, I., Shea, M. T., Watkins, J. T., Imber, S. D., Sotsky, S. M., Collins, J. F., Glass, D. R., Pilkonis, P. A., Leber, W. R., Docherty, J. P., Fiester, S. J., & Parloff, M. B. (1989). National Institute of Mental Health Treatment of Depression Collaborative Research Program: General effectiveness of treatments. *Archives of General Psychiatry, 46*, 971–982.

Eysenck, H. J. (1952). The effects of psychotherapy: An evaluation. *Journal of Consulting Psychology, 16*, 319–324.

Eysenck, H. J. (1960). *Behavior therapy and the neuroses.* Oxford: Pergamon Press.

Garfield, S. L. (1996). Some problems associated with "validated" forms of psychotherapy. *Clinical Psychology: Science and Practice, 3*, 218–229.

Gendlin, E. T. & Rychlak, J. F. (1970). Psychotherapeutic processes. In P. H. Mussen & M. R. Rosenzweig (Eds.), *Annual review of psychology,* vol. 21 (pp. 148–190). Palo Alto, CA: Annual Reviews, Inc.

Goldfried, M. R., Greenberg, L., & Marmar, C. (1990). Individual psychotherapy: Process and outcome. In M. R. Rosenzweig & L. W. Porter (Eds.), *An-nual review of psychology,* vol. 41 (pp. 659–688). Palo Alto, CA: Annual Reviews, Inc.

Goldfried, M. R. & Wolfe, B. E. (1996). Psychotherapy practice and research: Repairing a strained alliance. *American Psychologist, 51*, 1007–10016.

Gomes-Schwartz, B., Hadley, S. W., & Strupp, H. H. (1978). Individual psychotherapy and behavior therapy. In M. R. Rosenzweig & L. W. Porter (Eds.), *Annual review of psychology,* vol. 29 (pp. 435–472). Palo Alto, CA: Annual Reviews, Inc.

Hays, K. A., Rardin, D. K., Jarvis, P. A., Taylor, N. M., Moorman, A. S., & Armstead, C. D. (2002). An exploratory survey on empirically supported treatments: Implications for internship training. *Professional Psychology: Research and Practice, 33*, 207–211.

Hollon, S. D. (1996). The efficacy and effectiveness of psychotherapy relative to medications. *American Psychologist, 51*, 1025–1030.

Howard, K. I., Moras, K., Brill, P. L., Martinovich, Z., & Lutz, W. (1996). evaluation of psychotherapy: Efficacy, effectiveness, and patient progress. *American Psychologist, 51*, 1059–1064.

Howard, K. I. & Orlinsky, D. E. (1972). Psychotherapeutic processes. In P. H. Mussen & M. R. Rosenzweig (Eds.), *Annual review of psychology,* vol. 23 (pp. 615–668). Palo Alto, CA: Annual Reviews, Inc.

Jacobson, N. S. & Christensen, A. (1996). Studying the effectiveness of psychotherapy: How well can clinical trials do the job? *American Psychologist, 51*, 1031–1039.

Jacobson, N. S., Follette, W. C., & Revenstorf, D. (1984). Psychotherapy outcome research: Methods for reporting variability and evaluating clinical significance. *Behavior Therapy, 15*, 336–352.

Jacobson, N. S. & Truax, P. (1991). Clinical significance: A statistical approach to defining meaningful change in psychotherapy research. *Journal of Consulting and Clinical Psychology, 59*, 12–19.

Kazdin, A. E. (2001). Progression of therapy research and clinical application of treatment require better understanding of the change process. *Clinical Psychology: Science and Practice, 8*, 143–151.

Klein, D. F. & Smith, L. B. (1999). Organizational requirements for effective clinical effectiveness studies. *Prevention & Treatment, 2*, Article 0002a.

Kopta, S. M., Lueger, R. J., Saunders, S. M., & Howard, K. I. (1999). Individual psychotherapy outcome and process research: Challenges leading to greater turmoil or a positive transition? In J. T. Spence, J. M. Darley, & D. J. Foss (Eds.), *Annual review of psychology,* vol. 50 (pp. 441–470). Palo Alto, CA: Annual Reviews, Inc.

Krasner, L. (1971). Behavior therapy. In P. H. Mussen & M. R. Rosenzweig (Eds.), *Annual review of psychology*, vol. 22 (pp. 483–532). Palo Alto, CA: Annual Reviews, Inc.

Lambert, M. J. & Bergin, A. E. (1994). The effectiveness of psychotherapy. In S. L. Garfield & A. E. Bergin (Eds.), *Handbook of psychotherapy and behavior change*, 4th ed. (pp. 143–189). New York: Wiley.

Luborsky, L., & Diguer, L. (1995, June). *The psychotherapist as a neglected variable: The therapist's treatment effectiveness*. Paper presented at the meeting of the Society for Psychotherapy Research, Vancouver, Canada.

Nathan, P. E. (1998). Practice guidelines: Not yet ideal. *American Psychologist, 3*, 290–299.

Nathan, P. E., Stuart, S. P., & Dolan, S. L. (2000). Research on psychotherapy efficacy and effectiveness: Between Scylla and Charybdis? *Psychological Bulletin, 126*, 964–981.

National Advisory Mental Health Council (NAMHC) Workgroup. (1999). *Bridging science and service*. Washington, DC: National Institute of Mental Health.

Niederehe, G., Street, L. L., & Lebowitz, B. D. (1999). NIMH support for psychotherapy research: Opportunities and questions. *Prevention & Treatment, 2*, Article 0003a.

Norquist, G., Lebowitz, B., & Hyman, S. (1999). Expanding the frontier of treatment research. *Prevention & Treatment, 2*, Article 0001a.

Ogles, B. M., Lambert, M. J., & Sawyer, J. D. (1995). Clinical significance of the National Institute of Mental Health Treatment of Depression Collaborative Research Program data. *Journal of Consulting and Clinical Psychology, 63*, 321–326.

Onken, L. S., Blaine, J. D., & Battjes, R. (1997). Behavior therapy research: A conceptualization of a process. In S. W. Henngler & R. Amentos (Eds.), *Innovative approaches from difficult to treat populations* (pp. 477–485). Washington, DC: American Psychiatric Press.

Orlinsky, D. E. & Howard, K. I. (1986). Process and outcome in psychotherapy. In S. L. Garfield & A. E. Bergin (Eds.), *Handbook of psychotherapy and behavior change*, 3rd ed. New York: Wiley.

Persons, J. B. (1991). Psychotherapy outcome studies do not accurately represent current models of psychotherapy: A proposed remedy. *American Psychologist, 46*, 99–106.

Plante, T. G., Andersen, E. N., & Boccaccini, M. T. (1999). Empirically supported treatments and related contemporary changes in psychotherapy practice: What do clinical ABPPs think? *The Clinical Psychologist, 52*, 23–31.

Robinson, L. A., Berman, J. S. & Neimeyer, R. A. (1990). Psychotherapy for the treatment of depression: A comprehensive review of controlled outcome research. *Psychological Bulletin, 108*, 30–49.

Rosenthal, R. (1983). Assessing the statistical and social importance of the effects of psychotherapy. *Journal of Consulting and Clinical Psychology, 51*, 4–13.

Rosenzweig, S. (1936). Some implicit common factors in diverse methods in psychotherapy. *American Journal of Orthopsychiatry, 6*, 412–415.

Roth, A. D. & Fonagy, P. (1996). *What works for whom? A critical review of psychotherapy research*. New York: Guilford Press.

Rounsaville, B. J., Carroll, K. M., & Onken, L. S. (2001). A stage model of behavioral therapies research: Getting started and moving on from stage 1. *Clinical Psychology: Research and Practice, 8*, 133–142 (a).

Rounsaville, B. J., Carroll, K. M., & Onken, L. S. (2001). Methodological diversity and theory in the stage model: Reply to Kazdin. *Clinical Psychology: Science and Practice, 8*, 152–154 (b).

Seligman, M. E. P. (1995). The effectiveness of psychotherapy: The *Consumer Reports* study. *American Psychologist, 50*, 965–974.

Seligman, M. E. P. (1996). Science as an ally of practice. *American Psychologist, 51*,1072–1079.

Shadish, W. R., Matt, G. E., Navarro, A. M., & Phillips, G. (in press). The effects of psychological therapies in clinically representative conditions: A meta-analysis. *Psychological Bulletin*.

Shadish, W. R., Matt, G. E., Navarro, A. M., Siegle, G., Crist-Christoph, P. et al. (1997). Evidence that therapy works in clinically representative conditions. *Journal of Consulting and Clinical Psychology, 65*, 355–365.

Shadish, W. R., & Ragsdale, K. (1996). Random versus nonrandom assignment in controlled experiments: Do you get the same answer? *Journal of Consulting and Clinical Psychology, 64*, 1290–1305.

Shapiro, D. A. & Shapiro, D. (1982). Meta-analysis of comparative therapy outcome studies: A replication and refinement. *Psychological Bulletin, 92*, 581–604.

Shapiro, D. A. & Shapiro, D. (1983). Comparative therapy outcome research: Methodological implications of meta-analysis. *Journal of Consulting and Clinical Psychology, 51*, 42–53.

Strupp, H. H. (1973). *Psychotherapy: Clinical, research, and theoretical issues*. New York: Jason Aronson, Inc.

Wampold, B. E. (2001). *The great psychotherapy debate: Models, methods, and findings*. Mahwah, NJ: Erlbaum.

Zlotnick, C., Elkin, I., & Shea, M. T. (1998). Does the gender of a patient or the gender of a therapist affect the treatment of patients with major depression? *Journal of Consulting and Clinical Psychology, 1998*, 655–659.

INTERNET RESOURCES ON EVIDENCE-BASED PRACTICE AND RESEARCH IN HEALTH CARE AND HUMAN SERVICES

RESOURCES, GUIDELINES, AND TUTORIALS (LEARNING EBM)

- *Academic Center for Evidence-based Nursing (ACE):* ACE is part of The University of Texas Health Science Center at San Antonio School of Nursing and a companion entity to VERDICT (see below). As a center of excellence, its purpose is to advance cutting-edge, state-of-the-art, evidence-based nursing practice, research, and education within an interdisciplinary context. The goal is to turn research into action, improving health care and patient outcomes in the community, through evidence-based practice (EBP), research, and education. Contains some learning resources. **http://www.acestar.uthscsa.edu/**

- *Assessment, Crisis Intervention, and Trauma Treatment (ACT Model):* The ACT Intervention model is based on an integration of evidence-based assessment and treatment studies with persons in crisis and trauma. The ACT model presented on this website includes rapid assessment instruments, triage assessment, bio-psychosocial assessment, the 7-stage crisis intervention model, and the 10-step trauma assessment and treatment protocol.

http://www.crisisinterventionnetwork.com or **http://www.brief-treatment.oupjournals.org**

- *The Agency for Healthcare Research and Quality (AHRQ):* The United States premier evidence-based practice agency. To date, they have funded 13 Evidence-Based Practice Centers in the United States and Canada. AHRQ was established by the U.S. Congress and is the "lead agency charged with supporting research designed to improve the quality of healthcare, reduce its cost, improve patient safety, decrease medical errors, and broaden access to essential services. AHRQ sponsors and conducts research that provides evidence-based information on healthcare outcomes; quality; and cost, use, and access. The information helps healthcare decision makers—patients and clinicians, health system leaders, and policymakers—make more informed decisions and improve the quality of healthcare services." On the AHRQ site can be found full text documents on evidence reports, clinical practice guidelines, quick-reference guides, and consumer brochures. Since 1996, AHCPR has produced evidence reports. Available free of charge via **http://www.ahrq.gov**

- *Bandolier:* Evaluation of systematic reviews

and good quality evidence for health professionals. **http://www.jr2.ox.ac.uk/Bandolier**

- *Best Evidence:* This database of summaries of articles from the major medical journals, together with expert commentaries, is the CD-ROM equivalent of the combined ACP Journal Club and Evidence-Based Medicine output. Details of subscriptions are found at the BMJ site. **http://www.bmjpg.com/template.cfm?name=specjou_be#best_evidence**
- *BJM:* Full text of current issue, a searchable archive, collected resources, and access to Pubmed (public version of Medline) and Medline (password-controlled for BMA members). **http://www.bmj.com**
- *Campbell Collaboration:* A nonprofit international organization designed to assist persons in making well-informed decisions regarding the effects of interventions in the social, educational, criminology, and behavioral arenas. Objectives are to maintain, prepare, and disseminate systematic reviews of studies of interventions. **http://www.campbellcollaboration.org/index.html**
- *Centres of Health Evidence (CHE):* The principal task of CHE is to develop, package, disseminate, and present health care knowledge in ways that facilitate its optimum use. The website contains educational packets as introduction to EBP. **http://www.cche.net/about/**
- *CHID Online:* A database produced by health-related agencies of the Federal Government. This database provides titles, abstracts, and availability information for health information and health education resources. **http://chid.nih.gov/**
- *Clinical Evidence:* A database of clinical questions designed to help clinicians make evidence-based medicine part of their everyday practice. Hundreds of clinical questions cover the effects of treatments and interventions based on the best available research. Topics are selected to cover common or important clinical conditions seen in primary care or ambulatory settings. **http://www.ovid.com/products/clinical/clinicalevidence.cfm**
- *ClinicalTrials.gov:* The U.S. *National Institutes of Health*, through its *National Library of Medicine*, has developed *ClinicalTrials.gov* to provide patients, family members and members of the public with current information about clinical research studies. **http://clinicaltrials.gov/**
- *Cochrane Database:* Collection of databases specializing in evidence-based literature and systematic reviews. *NB Home access requires a Password—register on the NELH page to obtain a password. **http://nww.nelh.nhs.uk** (NHS) or **http://www.nelh.nhs.uk** (Home)*
- *Cochrane Database of Systematic Reviews:* A rapidly growing collection of regularly updated, systematic reviews of the effects of health care, maintained by contributors to the Cochrane Collaboration. New reviews are added with each issue of *The Cochrane Library*. Cochrane reviews are reviews mainly of randomized controlled trials. Evidence is included or excluded on the basis of explicit quality criteria to minimize bias. The Cochrane Database of Systematic Reviews is available on subscription only; the abstracts of Cochrane Reviews are available without charge and can be browsed or searched. **http://www.cochrane.org/cochrane/revabstr/mainindex.htm**
- *Cochrane Library:* A quarterly updated electronic database containing systematic reviews and other information that will assist in making diagnostic, treatment, and other health care decisions. The Cochrane Library consists of four main databases: The Cochrane Database of Systematic Reviews, The Database of Abstracts of Reviews of Effectiveness, The Cochrane Controlled Trials Register, and The Cochrane Review Methodology Database. **http://www.cochrane.org/cochrane/cdsr.htm**
- *Cochrane Library [Abstracts]:* This facility from Update Software allows you to search the abstracts of the Cochrane Database of Systematic Reviews. The full text of the reviews is only available through the Cochrane Library (see above). **http://www.update-software.com/abstracts/Default2.htm**
- *Consumer and Patient Health Information Section (CAPHIS):* A section of the Medical Library Association, an association of health information professionals with more than 5,000 individual and institution members. **http://www.caphis.mlanet.org/index.html**
- *CPB Infobase:* This website presents guidelines produced or endorsed in Canada by a national, provincial, or territorial medical or

health organization, professional society, government agency, or expert panel. **http:// www.cma.ca/cpgs**

- *Crisis Intervention, Co-morbidity Assessment, Domestic Violence Intervention, and Suicide Prevention network:* This website includes the latest abstracts on evidence-based practice articles as well as evidence-based practice handbooks published by Oxford University Press in New York. In addition, evidence-based rapid and triage assessment protocols, crisis intervention, drug treatment, and suicide prevention protocols are presented. **http://www.crisisintervention network.com**

- *Database of Abstracts of Reviews of Effectiveness:* DARE is a database of high-quality systematic research reviews of the effectiveness of health care interventions produced by the NHS Centre for Reviews and Dissemination at the University of York. **http://agatha. york.ac.uk/darehp.htm**

- *Evidence-Based Health Care—Latest Articles:* A list of the latest articles on evidence-based health care provided by the Evidence Based Resource Centre in New York. **http://www. ebmny.org/pubs.html**

- *Evidence-Based Medicine Reviews (EBMR):* Electronic information resource. Available via Ovid Online and on CD-ROM, this database from Ovid combines three EBM sources into a single, fully searchable database with links to MEDLINE® and Ovid full text journals. Sources covered include (1) the Cochrane Collaboration's Cochrane Database of Systematic Reviews, (2) Best Evidence, which consists of ACP Journal Club and Evidence-Based Medicine from the American College of Physicians and the BMJ Publishing Group, and (3) The Database of Abstracts of Reviews of Effectiveness, produced by the expert reviewers and information staff of the National Health Service's Centre for Reviews and Dissemination (NHS CRD). **http://www.ovid. com/products/clinical/ebmr.cfm**

- *Evidence Based Medicine Toolkit:* (University of Alberta): Provides [something left out here?—ed.]to be applied in the implementation of evidence-based practice, including calculators and electronic resources. **http://www .med.ualberta.ca/ebm/ebm.htm**

- Hardin Library for the Health Sciences (University of Iowa) A comprehensive electronic resource for medical evidence. This site pro-

vides database, search, decision, and technological support. **http://www.lib.uiowa.edu/ hardin/electron.html**

- *Health Information for the Consumer:* From the University of Pittsburgh Health Sciences Library System. **http://www.hsls.pitt.edu/ chi/**

- *Health Information for the Consumer: Drug Information* from the University of Pittsburgh. Includes links to other drug information websites. **http://www.hsls.pitt.edu/ guides/chi/druginformation.html**

- *Health Technology Advisory Committee Evaluation Reports:* Reports and issue briefs from the HTAC in Minnesota. **http://www .health.state.mn.us/htac/techrpts.htm**

- *Health Technology Assessment (HTA) Database:* The HTA Database, mounted by the NHS Centre for Reviews and Dissemination at the University of York, contains abstracts produced by INAHTA (International Network of Agencies for Health Technology Assessment) and other health care technology agencies. **http://agatha.york.ac.uk/htahp .htm**

- *Hospital Libraries Section of the Medical Library Association:* The Hospital Libraries Section of the Medical Library Association promotes and supports excellence in knowledge management and information resource development in the patient care and healthcare environment. **http://www.hls.mlanet .org/Organization/index.html**

- *InfoPOEMS:* Searchable database of POEMS (Patient Oriented Evidence that Matters) from the Journal of Family Practice. POEMS are summaries similar to ACP Journal Club articles in methodology and format, targeted at family practitioners. **http://www. infopoems.com**

- *JAMA—Rational Clinical Examination Series:* Provides framework for evaluation of examination of clinical evidence to be applied within evidence-based practice services. **http: //library.downstate.edu/resources/rce.htm**

- *JANCOC—Japanese informal network for the Cochrane Collaboration:* The first systematic workshop review, held in Tokyo, Japan, in December, 1995, with 28 practitioner researchers in attendance, including physicians, pharmacists, biostatisticians, and consumers, led to a Directory of Japanese Researchers. The Chairman of JANCOC is Dr. Kiichiro Tsutani, Professor of Clinical Pharmacology at the Tokyo Medical and Dental University. For further information go to the JANCOC home page or **www.cochrane. umin.ac.jp/Whats2.html**

- *Lab Tests Online:* "Designed to help you, as a patient or caregiver, to better understand the many clinical lab tests that are part of routine care as well as diagnosis and treatment of a broad range of conditions and diseases." **http://www.labtestsonline.org/site/ index.html**

- *Lamar Soutter Library Evidence-based Practice for Public Health Project:* Located at the University of Massachusetts, the purpose of this project is to examine the clinical EBM models and assess their effectiveness to the public health literature. The project will also identify any existing evidence-based projects in public health and assess their effectiveness. **http://library.umassmed.edu/ebpph/**

- *Making Research Count in the Personal Social Services:* A collaborative venture between six English universities (based at the University of East Anglia School of Social Work and Psychosocial Studies), offering staff in Local Authority Social Services Departments (and the NHS and voluntary organizations where joint schemes are running) the opportunity to work in partnership with their academic colleagues to develop evidence-based social work and social care practice, and to improve the dissemination of research. **http: //www.uea.ac.uk/swk/research/mrc/ welcome.htm**

- *MedlinePlus:* Provides quality health care information from the world's largest medical library, the National Library of Medicine at the National Institutes of Health. **http:// medlineplus.nlm.nih.gov/medlineplus/**

- *Middlesex University Teaching and Learning Resources for Evidence-based Practice, Center for Transcultural Studies in Health:* Focuses on traditional and nontraditional approaches to evidence based practice. **http://www.mdx .ac.uk/www/rctsh/ebp/main.htm**

- *National Guideline Clearinghouse:* The Agency for Healthcare Research and Quality (AHRQ), in partnership with the American Association of Health Plans (AAHP) and the American Medical Association (AMA), is sponsoring the National Guideline Clearinghouse (NGC). The NGC is a publicly available electronic repository for clinical practice guidelines and related materials that provides online access to guidelines. Recently, the Clearinghouse has added measures to the collection. *Note:* Only minimal criteria for quality are applied to guidelines listed in the Clearinghouse. **http://www.guideline.gov**

- *National Library of Medicine's Health Services/Technology Assessment Text (HSTAT):* This WWW resource contains the following collections: AHCPR Supported Guidelines, AHCPR Technology Assessments and Reviews, ATIS (HIV/AIDS Technical Information), NIH Warren G. Magnuson Clinical Research Studies, NIH Consensus Development Program, PHS Guide to Clinical Preventive Services (1989), and SAMHSA/CSAT Treatment Improvement Protocol (TIP). **http:// hstat.nlm.nih.gov**

- *National Research Register (NRR):* A register of ongoing and recently completed research projects funded by, or of interest to, the United Kingdom's National Health Service. The current release contains information on over 57,000 research projects, entries from the Medical Research Council's Clinical Trials Register, and details on reviews in progress collected by the NHS Centre for Reviews and Dissemination. **http://www.update -software.com/National/nrr-frame.html**

- *NettingtheEvidence:* Introduction to evidence-based practice on the Internet. Produced by Sheffield University. Searching option offers links to evidence-based health care sites, tips on searching, how to formulate a clinical question. **www.nettingtheevidence.org.uk**

- *NHS Economic Evaluation Database (NHS EED):* A database of structured abstracts of economic evaluations of health care interventions produced by the NHS Center for Reviews and Dissemination at the University of York. **http://agatha.york.ac.uk/nhsdhp.htm**

- *NOAH (New York Online Access to Health):* Seeks to provide high-quality full-text health information for consumers that is accurate, timely, relevant and unbiased. NOAH currently supports English and Spanish. **http:// www.noah-health.org/**

- *OMNI:* Searchable catalogue of quality health information available on the Internet. **http://omni.ac.uk**

- *Ovid Medline Tutorial:* Powerful tutorial for the construction and implementation of literature searches within the framework of evidence-based treatment. **http://library. downstate.edu/medtut/medtoc.htm**

- *PEDro—Physiotherapy Evidence Database:* An initiative of the Centre for Evidence-Based Physiotherapy (CEBP), PEDro is the Physiotherapy Evidence Database. It has been developed to give physiotherapists and others rapid access to bibliographic details and abstracts of randomized controlled trials in physiotherapy. Most trials on the database have been rated for quality to help to quickly discriminate between trials that are likely to be valid and interpretable and those that are not. **http://ptwww.cchs.usyd.edu.au/pedro/**
- *Population Index:* This bibliography is designed to cover the world's demographic and population literature, including books and other monographs, serial publications, journal articles, working papers, doctoral dissertations, and machine-readable data files. **http://opr.princeton.edu/popindex/**
- *Primary Care Clinical Practice Guidelines:* This site will include all guidelines, evidence-based, consensus, practice parameters, protocols, as well as other resources such as primary articles, integrative studies, meta-analysis, critically appraised topics, and review articles. Compiled by Peter Sam at the UCSF School of Medicine. **http://medicine.ucsf.edu/resources/guidelines/**
- PubMed Tutorial: Tutorial for the development and utilization of evidence based medicine searches.**http://www.library.health.ufl.edu/pubmed/PubMed2/**
- *RehabTrials.org:* A new website created by the nonprofit Kessler Medical Rehabilitation Research and Education Corporation (KMRREC) to promote, encourage, and support clinical trials in medical rehabilitation. **http://www.rehabtrials.org**
- *RxList:* The Internet drug index search for indications, symptoms, side effects, and drug interactions. Includes the "Top 200 Prescriptions." **http://www.rxlist.com/**
- *SUMSearch:* A single gateway that attempts to provide references to answer clinical questions around diagnosis, etiology, prognosis, and therapy (plus physical findings, adverse treatment effects, and screening/prevention) by searching only high-quality sources. SUMSearch always searches (1) Merck Manual, (2) MEDLINE, for review articles and editorials that have full texts available, (3) National Guideline Clearinghouse from the Agency for Health Care Policy and Research (AHCPR), (4) Database of Abstract of Re-

views of Effectiveness (DARE), and (5) MEDLINE for original research. Depending on the focus requested, SUMSearch will search PubMed with the highest sensitivity filters developed by Haynes et al. **http://SUMSearch.UTHSCSA.edu/cgi-bin/SUMSearch.exe**
- *SUNY Downstate Evidence-Based Medicine Course:* Provides resources including tutorial for the development of evidence based program development. **http://library.downstate.edu/ebm/toc.html**
- *Task Force on Community Preventive Services:* The Task Force on Community Preventive Services is an independent, non-federal Task Force and consists of 15 members, including a chair, appointed by the Director of CDC. The Task Force's membership is multi-disciplinary and includes perspectives representative of state and local health departments, managed care, academia, behavioral and social sciences, communications sciences, mental health, epidemiology, quantitative policy analysis, decision and cost-effectiveness analysis, information systems, primary care, and management and policy. **http://www.thecommunityguide.org**
- *Turning Research Into Practice (TRIP) Database:* This resource, hosted by the Centre for Research Support in Wales, aims to support those working in primary care. The database has 8,000 links covering resources at 28 different centers and allows both boolean searching (AND, OR, NOT) and truncation. **http://www.tripdatabase.com**
- *University of York NHS Centre for R&D:* Full text of most Effective Health Care and Effectiveness Matters publications and access to databases. Compiled by: Susan Merner, Librarian Poole Hospital NHS Trust. **http://www.york.ac.uk/inst/crd**
- *U.S. Preventive Services Task Force:* The Task Force was convened by the U.S. Public Health Service in 1984 to systematically review the evidence of effectiveness of a wide range of clinical preventive services, including screening tests, counseling, immunizations, and chemoprophylaxis. The Task Force is composed of 15 members and is closely affiliated with AHRQ. The Task Force publishes the Guide to Clinical Preventive Services. **http://www.ahrq.gov/clinic/uspstfab.htm**
- *Users' Guide to Evidence Based Practice:* Provides practical application advice for

evidence-based practice. **http://www.cche. net/usersguides/main.asp**

- *Veterans Evidence-Based Research Dissemination Implementation Center (VERDICT):* VERDICT's mission is to foster a knowledge-based health care system in which clinical, managerial, and policy decisions are based upon sound information from research findings. The multidisciplinary team addresses systematic implementation of evidence in clinical practice within the Veterans Health Administration, leading to integrated models of care and improved service, quality and efficiency. Learning resources include VERDICT Briefs. **http://verdict.uthscsa.edu/ verdict/default.htm**
- Widener University: Evaluating websites for evidence-based practice. **http://www2. widener.edu/Wolfgram-Memorial-Library/ webevaluation/webeval.htm**

EBM AND EBP BOOKS

- *Evidence-Based Practice Manual* / edited by Albert R. Roberts and Kenneth R. Yeager
- *Diagnostic Strategies for Common Medical Problems* / edited by Edgar R. Black
- *Evidence-Based Medicine: How to Practice and Teach EBM* / David L. Sackett
- *Evidence-Based Physical Diagnosis* / Steven McGee
- *How to Read a Paper: The Basics of Evidence-Based Medicine* / Trisha Greenhalgh
- *PDQ: Evidence-Based Principles and Practice* / Ann McKibbon
- *Social Workers' Desk Reference* / edited by Albert R. Roberts and Gilbert Greene
- *Users' Guides to the Medical Literature: Essentials of Evidence-Based Clinical Practice*
- *AMA Evidence-Based Medicine Working Group* / edited by Gordon Guyatt and Drummond Rennie

EBM CALCULATORS

- UBC Clinical Significance Calculator **http:// www.healthcare.ubc.ca/calc/clinsig.html**
- Stats Calculator from the University of Toronto **http://www.cebm.utoronto.ca/ practise/ca/statscal/**

CLINICAL TRIALS

- ClinicalTrials.gov **http://www.clinicaltrials .gov/**

EBM COMPLEMENTARY AND ALTERNATIVE MEDICINE

- Alternative Medicine Foundation: Examines alternative medicine approaches compatible with evidence-based practice. **http://www .amfoundation.org/**
- Complementary and Alternative Therapies (from Bandolier) **http://www.jr2.ox.ac.uk/ bandolier/booth/booths/altmed.html**

EVIDENCE-BASED CONSUMER HEALTH

- Ask NOAH about: Evidence-Based Medicine **http://www.noah-health.org/english/ebhc/ ebhc.html**
- Cochrane Collaboration Consumer Network **http://www.cochraneconsumer.com/**
- Crisis intervention, suicide prevention, and drug-induced psychosis facts and evidence-based assessment and treatment protocols. **http://www.crisisinterventionnetwork .com**
- Medline Plus **http://www.nlm.nih.gov/ medlineplus/**
- IntelliHealth **http://www.intelihealth.com/ IH/ihtIH/WSIHWOOD/408/408.html**
- Eccles Health Science Library's Health Brochures **http://medstat.med.utah.edu/library/ refdesk/24lang.html**—contains materials in 24 different languages.
- Massachusetts Health Promotion Clearinghouse **http://www.maclearinghouse.com/ catalog.htm**—contains materials in multiple languages.

EVIDENCE-BASED DRUG INFORMATION

- UNC Health Sciences Library: Drug Information: Provides resources to assist understanding of complex nature of medication management within evidence-based practice. **http://-**

www.hsl.unc.edu/lm/druginformation/
ebm.htm

EBM GERIATRICS

- Merck Institute of Aging and Health: Providing comprehensive approaches to evidence-based treatment within the practice of aging and health care. **http://www.miahonline .org/**

EBM GLOSSARIES

- Clinical Epidemiology Glossary **http://www. med.ualberta.ca/ebm/define.htm** (from Evidence Based Medicine Working Group)
- Glossary from SUNY Downstate's EBM tutorial **http://library.downstate.edu/ebm/glos .htm**
- Evidence-based Medicine Resource Center **http://www.ebmny.org/glossary.html**
- Medline Glossary **http://www.ebmny.org/ glossary.html**
- Duke Medical Center Library—Evidence-based Medicine (EBM) **http://www .mclibrary.duke.edu/respub/guides/ebm/ overview.html**
- Clinical Epidemiology and Evidence-based Medicine Glossary **http://www.vetmed.wsu. edu/courses-jmgay/GlossClinEpiEBM.htm**

EBM GUIDELINES

- U.S. Clinical Practice Guidelines **http://www .guidelines.gov/index.asp**
- Canadian Medical Association Clinical Guidelines **http://www.cma.ca/cma/common/start .do?lang=2**
- New Zealand Guidelines Group includes tools for guideline development and evidence-based health care practices and guidelines. **http:// www.nzgg.org.nz/tools.cfm**

EBM MENTAL HEALTH

- Centre for Evidence-Based Mental Health **http://cebmh.warne.ox.ac.uk/cebmh/**
- Evidence-Based Mental Health **http://ebmh .bmjjournals.com/**

- Centre for Evidence-Based Mental Health **http://www.psychiatry.ox.ac.uk/cebmh/ guidelines/**
- The Royal College of Psychiatrists **http:// www.rcpsych.ac.uk/cru/focus/access/ access12b.htm**
- Internet Mental Health **http://www .mentalhealth.com/p00.html**

EVIDENCE-BASED PRACTICE AND HUMAN SERVICES

- Evidence-Based Practice and the Evaluative Agenda: Providing tips and guidance and methods for application of evidence-based practice within human services. **http://www .sws.soton.ac.uk/rminded/SRS3/SRS37 .htm**
- Evidence-Based Practice in Social Work: Providing application of evidence-based practice protocols to the field of social work. Provides specific examples to evidence-based approaches in social work. **http://library.wustl .edu/subjects/sw/ebp.html**
- Secondary Data in Evidence-based Practice: Providing an overview of methodologies for analysis and application of secondary database research within a framework compatible with evidence-based practice. **http://www.lib .umich.edu/socwork/secondarydata.html**
- Center for Technology in Social Work Education and Practice (SWTECH) is located at the College of Social Work at the University of South Carolina. The center trains human service workers in the utilization of technology for practice; examines what technologies will benefit distance education and instructional technology endeavors of schools and colleges of social work; and consults with institutions of higher education and social service agencies on implementing communication/information technologies. **http://swtech .sc.edu/about.htm**
- Council on Social Work Education is a nonprofit organization that sets accreditation standards and oversees and monitors site teams approximately every seven years to determine compliance with the accreditation standards by all accredited baccalaureate and master's degree programs in social work.

Their long-standing goal for the past 50 years has been to promote high-quality standards in social work education throughout the United States. Each spring CSWE holds an annual conference with about 10 preconference faculty skills workshops, and numerous peer-reviewed presentations, panels, and poster sessions. The first two American universities to implement social work courses in evidence-based practice (EBP) were Columbia University and Washington University in St. Louis, Missouri. **www.cswe.org**

- HUSITA organization is an international association dedicated to the dissemination of information technology to human service professionals. It has a listserv, mailing list, and annual conferences. The owners of the listserve are Dr. Dick Schoech and Tom Hanna of the University of Texas at Arlington School of Social Work. **HUSITA@ LISTSERV.UTA.EDU**
- Formulating a Question and Effective Search Strategy: Powerful tool for development of effective evidence-based practice literature search. Provides basic and advance tips for literature searches. **http://www.lib.umich .edu/socwork/secondarydata.html#form**

EBM NURSING AND ALLIED HEALTH

- Centre for Evidence Based Nursing **http:// www.york.ac.uk/healthsciences/misc/ lksebn.htm**
- Evidence-Based Nursing **http://ebn .bmjjournals.com/**
- Evidence-Based Occupational Therapy **http:// www-fhs.mcmaster.ca/rehab/ebp/**
- Physiotherapy Evidence Database **http:// www.pedro.fhs.usyd.edu.au/**
- OT Seeker **http://www.otseeker.com/**

PREVENTION AND SCREENING

- The Agency for Healthcare Research and Quality (AHRQ) **http://www.ahcpr.gov/**
- Preventive Services **http://www.ahcpr.gov/ clinic/prevenix.htm**
- U.S. Preventive Services Task Force **http:// www.ahcpr.gov/clinic/uspstfix.htm**
- The Guide to Clinical Preventive Services **http://www.ahcpr.gov/clinic/cpsix.htm**
- Put Prevention Into Practice **http://www .ahcpr.gov/clinic/ppipix.htm**

EBM WEBSITES

- Canadian Centres for Health Evidence **http:// www.cche.net/che/home.asp**
- Bandolier Home Page **http://www.jr2.ox.ac .uk/bandolier/**
- Evidence-Based Medicine Resource Center **http://www.ebmny.org/index.html**
- ScHARR Netting the Evidence **http://www .sheffield.ac.uk/scharr/ir/netting/**
- University of Toronto's Centre for Evidence-Based Medicine **http://www.cebm.utoronto .ca/**
- JAMA Rational Clinical Examination Series **http://library.downstate.edu/resources/rce .htm**
- Mt. Sinai School of Medicine **http://www. mssm.edu/medicine/general-medicine/ ebm/**
- National Quality Measures Clearinghouse **http://www.qualitymeasures.ahrq.gov/**
- Consumer Assessment of Healthplans **http:// www.ahcpr.gov/qual/cahpsix.htm**
- Core Library for Evidence-Based Practice **http://www.shef.ac.uk/scharr/ir/core.html**
- Healthlinks: Evidence-Based Practice and Guidelines **http://healthlinks.washington. edu/clinical/guidelines.html**

PDA RESOURCES

- Ectopic Brain—General Resources for both PC and Palm **http://pbrain.hypermart.net/**
- MedRules—Diagnosis tools for Palm only **http://pbrain.hypermart.net/medrules. html**
- EBM Calculator **http://www.cebm.utoronto. ca/palm/ebmcalc/** Center for Health Evidence in Canada—Palm Only
- NNT Tables **http://www.cebm.utoronto.ca/ palm/nnt/download.htm** Center for Health Evidence in Canada—Palm Only
- Healthy Palmpilot **http://www. healthypalmpilot.com/** General Resources for Palm Only
- Pediatric Pilot Page **http://keepkidshealthy. com/pedipilot.html** Palm Only

- Medical Palm Webring—General Resources for both PC and Palm **http://library-downstate.edu/resources/ebm.htm**
- EBM Tools **http://www.healthypalmpilot. com/Research_Tools/Evidence_Based_**

Medicine/ Healthy Palmpilot—Evaluation guides and calculators for both PC and Palm
- Mobile EBM Guidelines for hand-held devices **http://www.ebm-guidelines.com/ mobile.html**

GLOSSARY

Compiled and Edited by Evelyn Roberts Levine

Abstinence (Detoxification) Orientation: An approach to opioid agonist therapy that views abstinence from all opioids and opioid agonists, including methadone, as the ultimate goal of therapy. A detoxification orientation among clinic staff has been linked to lower retention rates, more restrictive dosing and take-home privileges, and more punitive responses to illicit drug use.

Abstinence Orientation Scale: In 1998, Caplehorn and associates developed a 14-item scale that assesses a treatment provider's endorsement of statements reflective of an abstinence orientation toward opioid agonist therapy. The mean score across treatment providers at each clinic can be used as an indication of overall clinic philosophy. High Abstinence Orientation Scale clinic scores are predictive of poorer program retention and higher rates of illicit drug use among enrolled patients.

Abuser: A person or persons who inflict harm or threat of harm on another person. An abuser may be a family member, significant other, acquaintance, or opportunistic stranger. *See also Domestic Violence Typology, Elder Abuse,* and *Woman Battering Continuum.*

Accounting: The process of keeping and verifying accounts and records, usually of a monetary nature.

Acculturation: A complex social process that is initiated when members of one cultural group are exposed over an extended period of time to members of another cultural group. It refers to the adoption of the values, preferences, and behaviors of the host society.

Action Factors: Interactions between the therapist and client or patient including cognitive mastery modeling and behavioral regulation.

Activities, Strategies, and Services: These refer to all operational elements of what is essentially the "effort," that is to say, the program, the initiative, the project, and so forth. Activities, strategies, and services are expected first and foremost to benefit the customer and then the service-providing organization. The "effort" expresses the hope that inputs can be converted into results. However, since this does not always happen automatically, coincidentally, or accidentally, the underlying assumptions and strategies that are expected to drive the "effort" must be articulated explicitly, executed experimentally, and tied directly to performance measures that will look for evidence of efficiency, equity, and effectiveness.

Actuarial Test: Measures designed to predict risk of future violence. These measures are designed following retrospective research looking for factors associated with recidivism in specific offender populations.

Adjectival Scale: A scale in which the respondent must select one of a series of graded adjectives (e.g., Excellent / Very Good / Good / Fair / Poor).

Age-Specific Mortality Rate (ASMR): The *mortality rate* adjusted for the age of the sample. The number of deaths from a specific disease "X" in a specific age range "Y" divided by the total number of deaths in specific age range "Y". This rate allows you to age-adjust mortality rates for a given disease.

Agoraphobia: Agoraphobia ("fear of the marketplace" in Greek) is an anxiety disorder defined by intense fear of being placed in situations where no help is available should some incapacitating or embarrassing event occur. Frequently, agoraphobia is related to or associated with repeated panic attacks. If untreated, over long periods of time agoraphobia can lead to the individual's fear of leaving his or her home altogether.

Alpha: A frequency range in the EEG, defined as 8–13 Hertz per second.

Alternate Form Reliability: Also called parallel forms, this refers to the consistency of measurement between equivalent measurement tools. It is obtained by giving two different but equivalent forms of the same measure to the same group of clients. If there is no measurement error, clients should score the same on both measures, thus yielding a high correlation coefficient (Pearson's r).

AMA (Against Medical Advice): Any discharge of a patient for any reason other than having completed the treatment process or meeting the treatment goals. Discharges against medical advice have a strong probability of being readmitted for the same or related diagnosis within a brief period of time.

American Indian: Descendants of the aboriginal people of the Americas; these persons are often called Native Americans.

Annual Incidence: The *incidence* expressed in cases per year.

Anxiety: An emotional state characterized by fear-related beliefs and/or physiological arousal. Anxiety is an adaptive emotion when experienced and responded to in proportion to the triggering event(s). Anxiety disorders are characterized by inordinately high levels of anxiety connected with an inaccurate perception of danger. They are maintained by avoidant strategies that are intended to reduce or minimize the perceived threat but which ultimately serve to reinforce the fear-related beliefs and anxiety.

Anxiety Disorders: Anxiety disorders are defined by intense feelings of anxiety and tension in the absence or presence of "real danger." Symptoms associated with anxiety disorder frequently cause significant distress. Mild to moderate symptoms frequently interfere with daily activities. Sufferers of anxiety disorders may take extreme measures to avoid situations that provoke anxiety. The physical symptoms associated with anxiety are restlessness, irritability, disturbed sleep, muscle aches and pains, gastrointestinal distress, and difficulty concentrating.

Applied Research: Research designed to solve a specific problem. It may or may not be theory based.

Area under the Curve (AUC): The AUC is a statistical measure used in a ROC analysis. In assessing sexual offenders, it is the probability that the detection method will give a randomly selected violent person a higher score than a randomly selected nonviolent person. A perfect detection method would give an AUC score of 1.0 and test that was no better than chance would give an AUC score of 0.5.

Assessment: Process of systematically collecting, organizing, and interpreting data related to a client's functioning in order to determine the need for treatment, as well as treatment goals and intervention plan.

Auditing: The process of officially examining information to ensure that it is in order. Although usually focused on financial information, audits may also be conducted on working hours, services provided, and clients of services.

Authenticity: A qualitative research term that refers to the degree to which the research process has genuinely involved key stakeholders in the phenomenon under study in the actual research process and the degree to which the study has led to a benefit for these stakeholders. Authenticity is one of a number of factors used to judge the rigor or trustworthiness of a qualitative study.

Average Days in Accounts Receivable: This phrase indicates the amount of time passed from the point a bill is submitted to a payer group until the time the account is paid. Days in accounts receivable indicates the effectiveness of collection of payment for billed services. In general, average days in accounts receivable under 60 days is considered to be very good for medical detoxification.

Average LOS (Length of Stay): Total patient days for a particular level of care divided by the total admissions for this level of care. This is utilized to determine the optimal amount of hospitalization for a given diagnostic category and degree of severity weighed against risk of rehospitalization. Utilized as a quality indicator for most medical facilities in medical detoxification.

Axial Coding: The process of coding qualitative data around a single conceptual category and drawing connections between the conceptual category and relevant subcategories.

Balanced Scorecard: An evaluation device that specifies the criteria your organization will use to rate business performance in progress toward and attaining previously established and applied strategic planning. This tool provides an at-a-glance monitor for senior administrative leaders to monitor progress made toward implementation of organizational strategic plans and specifically defined targets for rollout and ongoing rating of performance on clearly defined organizational targets, objectives, and goals.

Baseline: An initial assessment of a program at a given time to be compared with another data point or assessment in the future (ideally with an intervention or "treatment" in between the two data points).

Behavioral Exchange: A technique used in cognitive-behavioral couples therapy in which the amount of day-to-day positive behaviors between partners are increased, ameliorating partners' focus on negative parts of the relationship.

Benchmark: The best-achieved outcome score, preferably risk-adjusted, among treatment groups.

Benchmarking: A term referring to the identification of standards for performance on a particular indicator. Performance data for a given organization are compared with data from similar organizations in order to guide decision making. In order to be valid and useful, benchmarking data need to be based on similar *measures* and methods. A term utilized to describe comparison of data between a group of data points for the purpose of determining relative value. It can be utilized as a method to measure or judge quality of services provided or as a point of reference when comparing like categories, e.g., diagnostic groupings. The process of comparing one's own performance on a specific measure against a like entity. The process of taking collected data from different organizations or from different programs of the same organization and displaying that data so as to demon-strate the relative relationship of one organization to another. Benchmarking does not so much indicate what the results should be as it does display what is actually measured and allows organizations to see themselves in relationship to the other organizations.

Best Practices: Best practices are those assessment, intervention, or evaluation practices identified by authoritative review groups, such as committees set up by professional organizations, as being most appropriate for routine use in service systems. Typically, such review groups examine available scientific evidence as well as professional consensus. Feasibility and cost may also be considered.

Beta: A frequency range in the EEG, defined as greater than 13 Hertz per second.

Bipolar Disorder / Manic Depression: A serious mood disorder that involves extreme mood swings or highs (mania) and lows (depression); sometimes termed manic-depressive psychosis.

Blinding: Keeping the participants (single blind) or the participants and the researcher (double blind) ignorant of which people are in which group in a study. This is done to reduce the possibility of *placebo* or *Hawthorne* effects.

Budget: An estimate or plan of income and expenditures. It is the organization's fiscal plan, usually developed for one year but, in some cases, longer or shorter periods of time.

Buffering: The process by which an intervening or mediating variable lessens the impact of an independent variable on the dependent variable. Generally considered a protective coping factor in stressful situations.

Build Capacity: Program staff members and participants learning to conduct their own evaluations (evaluation capacity) and enhancing their ability to operate their own programs (program capacity).

Building Momentum: A three- to six-month period devoted to the establishment of executive-level support for a given project. This process involves communication and examination of processes associated with and contributing to the need for change. Frequently the establishment of a leadership team is required, as is clarification of the organization's mission and vision.

Case-Based Reasoning: A knowledge-based application in which the demographics, services, and outcomes in thousands of cases are entered into a computer software application. Practitioners can then enter the circumstances of their existing case to see how similar cases were handled and review case outcomes. A case-based reasoning system stores both successful and unsuccessful cases. A problem-solving approach is taken in which case goals are specified as well as problems that are avoided. As new cases and their outcomes are entered into the software, these cases become integrated into the "memory" of cases that are used in future case analyses.

Case-Control Study: A research design in which people with a specific outcome (e.g., a disease or syndrome) are matched with people who do not have the outcome. This is usually done to determine if the groups differ with respect to the risk of exposure to a putative causal agent (e.g., the groups could be those with and without lung cancer, with the exposure being cigarette smoking; *Compare with Cohort Study*).

Case-Fatality Rate: The proportion of people with a disorder who die from it within a specific time frame. The number of deaths from a disorder in the time period divided by the number of people with the disorder. This number focuses only on those people who have the disorder and will be higher than the more general *mortality rate.*

Case Management: Coordination of services to help meet a patient's health care needs, usually when the patient requires multiple services from multiple providers. This term is also used to refer to coordination of care during and after a hospital stay.

Casino: A single room in each casino where gaming is conducted pursuant to the provisions of the New Jersey Casino Control Act.

Casino Security Employee: A person employed by a casino to provide physical security in the gaming area, simulcasting facility, or restricted casino area. It does not include any person who also provides physical security solely in any other part of the casino hotel.

CCTV: Closed Circuit Television System (CCTV), which makes a video and, if applicable, an audio recording of, and takes a still photo-graph of, any event capable of being monitored on the CCTV system.

C-DISC: The Computerized Diagnostic Interview Schedule for Children (C-DISC) is a computerized version of the NIMH DISC-IV, which is a highly structured diagnostic interview, designed to assess more than 30 psychiatric disorders occurring in children and adolescents, suitable for administration by trained lay (non-clinician) interviewers. The instrument has been in development since 1979, and various versions have been produced to match different classification systems. The current version of the DISC (National Institute of Mental Health [NIMH] DISC-IV), based on the DSM-IV and ICD-10, was released for field use in 1997. Although originally intended for large-scale epidemiological surveys of children, versions of the DISC have been used in clinical studies, in prevention/screening exercises, and as an aid to diagnosis in service settings. There are parallel versions of the instrument: the DISC-P for parents (or knowledgeable caretakers) of 6- to 17-year-olds, and the DISC-Y (for direct administration to children and youths aged 9–17).

Central Tendency: The property of a distribution that refers to the extent to which there is a convergence of observations at or around a limited set of values. Statistical indices of central tendency try to assess what are the average, typical, or most likely values; they include the mean, median, and mode.

Certified Public Accountant: One who has passed state examinations and received a certificate of professional competence in accounting and who has subscribed to the state's professional expectations for accountants.

Change Levers: Motivators of change, in this chapter, discussed in an organizational context.

Chronic Battering: Victims experience numerous severe abusive incidents during their marriage. The abuse is frequently inflicted when the batterer has been drinking heavily or has explosive anger toward the victim. The chronic pattern of victimization by their intimate partners lasts from several years to several decades, and often ends when the victim or perpetrator is permanently injured, hospitalized, arrested and detained, or dead. The injuries for these victims are usually extensive and include sprains, fractures, broken bones, cuts, and head injuries that often require emergency medical attention. *See also Woman Battering Continuum.*

Chronic Suicidality: Unremittingly high suicide ideation, frequent threats of suicide, and difficulty articulating reasons for living.

Client-Centered Administrative Practice: This term was developed by Rapp and Poertner in 1992 and refers to social work practice in managing, designing, and evaluating programs that keep the realities, knowledge, and needs of the recipients of services as central to effectiveness. Along with client concern, this form of practice considers the staff implementing the services as integral to effectiveness and success.

Clinical Practice Guidelines: Clinical practice guidelines are systematically developed statements designed to structure practitioner and service recipient decisions about appropriate service for specific problems, conditions, or populations. These guidelines prescribe how practitioners should assess and treat service recipients. Sometimes the guidelines are based on research findings. Sometimes, research is not available and, therefore, the guidelines are based on professional consensus. Professional organizations and governmental agencies have formulated practice guidelines for various conditions.

Clinical Relationship: The attitudes of a client and practitioner toward each other that develops from their personal characteristics and processes of interaction. It is widely considered to be a significant factor in the client's achievement of outcomes but is difficult to formally measure. At a basic level a positive clinical relationship should feature a bond between the parties characterized by some level of collaboration, agreement on goals, trust, and mutual comfort.

Clinical Theory: Clinical theories are systematic conceptual systems intended to explain, describe, or predict some circumscribed aspect of the empirical world pertaining to clinical practice. Such theories can purport to explain or describe a clinical problem, condition, or intervention. Theories are made up of constructs that are abstract terms representing key theoretical terms as well as propositions showing how these constructs are interrelated. These propositions may or may not have been examined in empirical research. The propositions of scientific clinical theories require empirical validation through the testing of corresponding hypotheses.

Clinical Wisdom: Clinical groups, including professional specialties, typically develop collective beliefs about their respective sphere of practice such as about the causes of typical problems or conditions seen in practice, or about which methods of assessment or intervention are most appropriate for particular problems, conditions, or populations. These beliefs emerge from the collective experience of the group; they are often codified in professional papers, manuals, and texts and are taught to new clinicians in formal training programs as well as supervision. Clinical wisdom is not verified through scientific research, but at times hypotheses derived from clinical wisdom are tested in scientific research.

Clustered Systems: Systems that use information about the provider to predetermine which information tools to present to the user. Presentation of a relevant drug database, for example, can be automated upon recognizing that a particular type of physician is logged on.

Cognitive Behavior Therapy (CBT): A form of psychotherapy that is largely present-centered and problem-oriented and which uses verbal procedures and behavioral experiments to examine and test the validity and utility of the client's perceptions and interpretations of events. A form of psychological therapy focusing on the modification of both cognitive processes and behavior. The primary focus is on current functioning and modification of maladaptive behaviors and thoughts while reinforcing positive behaviors and thoughts. CBT draws heavily on cognitive theory and research, as well as more traditional techniques of behavior modification. Therapy that involves training, discussion, and operant conditioning techniques to allow clients to recognize and change maladaptive behaviors, thoughts, attitudes, and beliefs. There are a variety of forms of CBT, but in the treatment of suicidality, they all emphasize rapid cognitive assessment and problem solving.

Cognitive Pretesting: One of many methods used to assess the thought processes of individuals responding to questionnaire items. In the current study, cognitive pretesting involved asking children questions while they answered prototype ESSP questions to determine if they understood and responded to questions as intended by the ESSP developers.

Cognitive Therapy: A form of psychotherapy used to help patients identify, challenge, and correct characteristic mistaken ideas and assumptions that lead to excessive emotional responses. In the case of anxiety disorders, patients often overestimate the probability of disastrous consequences. In cognitive therapy, patients are taught to recognize such overestimates and subject their probability estimate to logical scrutiny, leading them to reduce their estimate and hence their fears.

Cognizant Systems: Systems that use artificial intelligence to respond to clinical events, detect patterns, and determine which knowledge resources are most appropriate for problem solving. No such systems exist today.

Cohen's Kappa: A measure of the degree to which there is agreement between judges on how they rate a person or object.

Coherence: The average similarity between the waveforms of a particular band in two locations over the one-second period of time. Conceptualized as the strength/number of connections between two positions.

Cohort Study: Involves identification and selection of two groups (cohorts) of patients, one group that did receive the exposure/treatment of interest, and one group that did not, and then monitoring and evaluating these cohorts prospectively for the outcome of interest. A research design in which people who were exposed to a putative causal agent are compared to those not exposed, to determine if they differ with respect to the risk of some outcome (e.g., the groups could be smokers and nonsmokers, with the outcome being lung cancer). *See also Study Designs* and *Case-Control Study*.

Collaborative Evaluation: Approaches to evaluating social interventions developed by teams that include researchers, managers, and staff of agencies that serve families and children, consumers, providers of informal supports, and other stakeholders.

Collectivism: A type of social orientation held by a cultural group where deep value is placed on interdependent relationships within social groups. It is one end of an individualism-collectivism continuum onto which societies may be located.

Combined Systems: Systems that unite one or more components under a common interface. A combined drug prescription system, for example,

may include menus that allow the clinician to search for dosing details or patient advice handouts before generating prescriptions.

Common Cause Variation: Fluctuation caused by unknown factors resulting in a steady but random distribution of output around the average of the data. It is a measure of the process potential, providing indication of how well the process can perform when special cause variation is removed.

Community: As defined by Boudon and Bourricaud in 1989, physical communities consist of three elements: (1) a social network that is both resilient and flexible; (2) some symbolic ties to an object of identification; and (3) an identified group that is part of a larger society.

Community Context: The state of organization or order within the community at any given time.

Community or Collective Efficacy: The belief that the community will improve over time.

Community Outreach Specialist: A community outreach specialist (COS) serves a particular role in lay health advisor (LHA) programs. The COS serves as a liaison between the LHAs, the community advisors, and the people implementing the intervention (e.g., researchers or agency staff). The COS may also participate in training the LHAs, monitoring their work, providing ongoing training, and collecting information for use in a project evaluation.

Community Quality: The physical and social state of a community.

Comorbidity: The co-occurrence of two or more conditions with related etiology and/or mechanism of maintenance. The simultaneous appearance of two or more illnesses, such as the co-occurrence of schizophrenia and substance abuse or of alcohol dependence and depression. The association may reflect a causal relationship between one disorder and another or an underlying vulnerability to both disorders. The related decisions of what, when, and how to treat any one or more of the conditions must be considered within the context of the comorbid conditions. It is also possible for the appearance of the illnesses to be unrelated to any common etiology or vulnerability.

Compulsion: A pattern of attempts to neutralize or avoid the anxiety associated with obsessions in obsessive-compulsive disorder. A symptom of obsessive-compulsive disorder involving urges to perform stereotyped ritualistic behaviors to reduce distress associated with obsessions. The words *compulsion* and *ritual* are used interchangeably. Compulsions are negatively reinforced; the function of the compulsion is simply to decrease discomfort, not to provide enjoyment. Compulsions are most often overt behaviors, such as hand washing or seeking reassurance from religious professionals. Mental compulsions are also quite common and are characterized by mental processes intended to neutralize the anxiety or discomfort associated with obsessions. Examples include repeated checking, washing, excessive praying or confessing, needless ordering and arranging, or mentally "canceling out" intrusive thoughts.

Computer-Assisted Assessment: A client assessment approach that captures assessment information via a computer software application. Computer assessment systems can be administered prospectively with the client present or retrospectively after a client interview has taken place. One example is the Client Assessment System (CAS), developed by Walter Hudson and Paula Nurius. CAS allows the client to conduct the assessment independently by keying in responses to a preset list of standardized assessment instruments. The program also scores the assessment and integrates with case management software for use by the case manager.

Computer-Assisted Personal Interviews (CAPI): A computer-assisted personal interview (CAPI) is similar to a computer-assisted telephone interview (CATI), in which a computer software program facilitates the interview process. The primary difference between a CATI and a CAPI is that the interview is conducted face-to-face, with the computer screen visible to the client or respondent.

Computer-Assisted Telephone Interviews (CATI): A computer-assisted telephone interview is a computer software program that facilitates the interview process. An interviewer follows prompts provided by the software and displayed on the computer screen to ask questions and record responses. One advantage to a CATI system is that it eliminates a separate data entry step.

Concept Map: A concept map depicts the structure of knowledge about any phenomenon of interest such as a program, organization, public policy, process or content domain. Concept maps provide guidance for evaluators to ensure that data collection is focused on key facets and relationships in the theory of the program or its implementation. The knowledge portrayed in concept maps is context-dependent. Different maps containing the same concepts convey different meanings depending upon the hierarchical relationships, linking descriptors, and arrangement of individual concepts. Related terms are logic models, systems dynamics, and implementation analysis.

Concept Paper: A short document (three to five pages) that summarizes a proposed project or research/evaluation study. The paper highlights the concepts underlying the project or study, rather than specific, technical details. The concept paper should focus on the rationale or need for the project/study, its purpose as well as its significance, and provide a limited description of the methods.

Concordant Items: The number of items upon which raters agree.

Conduct Disorder: The overriding feature of conduct disorder is a persistent pattern of behavior in which the rights of others and age-appropriate social norms are violated. This diagnosis is reached if the child demonstrates at least 3 of 15 symptoms within the past 12 months, with at least 1 symptom present within the past 6 months, and experiences impaired functioning. The symptoms of conduct disorder fall into four main groupings: (1) aggressive conduct that causes or threatens physical harm to other people or animals, (2) nonaggressive conduct that causes property loss or damage, (3) deceitfulness or theft, and (4) serious violations of rules (APA, 2000).

Confidence Interval (CI): The range of numerical values in which we can be confident (to a computed probability, such as 90% or 95%) that the population value being estimated will be found. Confidence intervals indicate the strength of evidence; where confidence intervals are wide, they indicate less precise estimates of effect.

Conjoint Therapy: Treatment that involves at least one family member in addition to the identified client.

Consensus: Substantial agreement measured by the degree of consensus that has been achieved by asking participants to agree that they can live with and support the concept both internally and externally.

Consistency/Absolute Agreement: Terminology used by SPSS to represent two different forms of the interclass correlation coefficient (ICC). Like a Pearson's r, if consistency is used, the judges' ratings can vary in a consistent manner. Absolute agreement takes into account the magnitude of the agreement, that is, how closely the judges rate the same object.

Construct: Typically used to indicate a feature of experience, behavior, etc., that has been theoretically defined and empirically measured, typically through use of several more narrowly defined variables. Higher-order general constructs may incorporate a number of lower-order specific constructs. For example, depending upon results of empirical testing of proposed quality/appropriateness items in a consumer survey, "relationship with provider" may be defined and measured as a higher-order construct incorporating more specific constructs of "responsiveness," "recovery orientation," etc.

Construct Validity: Construct validity is the highest form of validity and assures that the tool measures the client behaviors that are under assessment. This type of validity is concerned with the degree of measurement of a theoretical construct or trait.

Content Validity: Content validity refers to the evaluation of items on a measure to determine if the content contained in the items relates to and is representative of the domain that the measure seeks to examine.

Context-Sensitive Systems: Systems that are "aware" of the clinical context, allowing more efficient use of all context-compatible information systems that may be combined under a common interface. The context includes at least five elements: patient, practitioner, problem, procedure, and policy. A context-sensitive drug prescription support system, for example, would allow the user to view a laboratory result in one software application, then immediately switch to a drug database where a search for drug dosing modifications can be made based on prior knowledge of the patient's age and primary medical problems.

Contextualized: A qualitative research term that refers to taking into consideration salient aspects of a setting, such as environmental factors, interpersonal relationships, prevailing social and political structures, and/or cultural values and beliefs when investigating, describing, or analyzing a phenomenon or experience.

Contingency Management (CM): CM refers to a broad group of behavioral interventions that structure the client's environment in such a way as to encourage change. This is accomplished by setting specific, objective behavioral goals and specific, objective consequences for meeting or not meeting these goals. CM is most effective when initial behavioral goals are small and relatively easy to achieve, and consequences are provided as immediately following the demonstration of the behavioral goal as possible.

Continuous Quality Improvement: The routine collection and use of information gleaned from a program's development, implementation, and/or evaluation to improve program operations and to better achieve desired outcomes.

Control Chart: A graphical tool for monitoring changes that occur within a process, by distinguishing variation that is inherent in the process (common cause) from variation that yields a change to the process (special cause). This change may be a single point or a series of points in time—each a signal that something is different from what was previously observed and measured.

Control Group (Concurrent): A comparison group enrolled at the same time as the experimental group and treated exactly the same way, with the exception of not receiving the intervention being studied.

Control Group (Historical): A comparison group composed of people for whom data already exist (e.g., patients who were seen before a new treatment was introduced).

Coping: Adjusting; adapting; successfully meeting a challenge.

Coping Mechanisms: All the ways, both conscious and unconscious, that a person uses in adjusting to environmental demands without altering his goals or purposes.

Core: The term is used for a relatively small number of people who play a critical role in sustaining the transmission of sexually transmitted diseases in a population. Definitions vary, but they generally include people who have several sexual partners while infected and who thus transmit their infection to more than one other person.

Cost-Benefit Analysis: Converts effects into the same monetary terms as the costs and compares them.

Counterfactual: The empirical estimate of what would have happened to a client if an intervention had been withheld. The counterfactual condition can be achieved through the use of a no-treatment control group, a matched comparison group, or pre-intervention outcome estimates of a treated group.

Coupled: Systems automatically link knowledge to observations, given a specific clinical event. A coupled drug prescription system, for example, would alert the clinician to alternative, potentially cheaper, interventions just before a prescription is generated.

Covariance: The variation in a given variable that is associated with the variation in one or more other variables. For example, annual income has a great deal of variation, as has education. Education and income also co-vary, meaning that a low or high value in one is associated with a low or high value in the other.

Criminal Justice: The institution that deals with criminal violations of the law and processes alleged offenders. It includes police, courts, probation and parole, juvenile justice, and correctional agencies.

Crisis: An acute disruption of psychological homeostasis in which one's usual coping methods fail and there exists evidence of distress and functional impairment. The subjective reaction to a stressful life event or pileup of stressors that compromises the individual's stability and ability to cope or function. The main cause of a crisis is an intensely stressful, traumatic, or hazardous event, but two other conditions are also necessary: (1) the individual's perception of the event as the cause of considerable upset and/or disruption; and (2) the individual's inability to resolve the disruption by previously used coping methods. An event or situation that is experienced as distressing and challenging of human adaptive abilities and resources.

Crisis Assessment: An objective appraisal based on validated scales or measures of a cli-

ent's perception of present situational or acute stressors in terms of personal threat, ability to cope, and barriers to action, as well as type of aid needed from the crisis counselor.

Crisis Intervention: A therapeutic interaction that seeks to decrease perceived psychological trauma by increasing perceived coping efficacy. It is a timely and brief intervention that focuses on helping to mobilize the resources of those differentially affected.

Criterion validity: Criterion validity refers to the correspondence between a measurement of a variable and a measurement derived from some external standard thought to have established validity. The external standard can occur concurrently (concurrent validity) or in the future (predictive validity). Validity of a measure refers to the correspondence between the measure and how the property measured actually occurs in the empirical world. The extent to which a measure relates to an external criterion. Research is done to establish the correlations (relationships) between scores on the measure and the outcomes of the external criteria.

Critical Appraisal: Methods of critical thinking used to arrive at a key question: *How good (strong) is the evidence for that?* In the evaluation of evidence for use in the practice of clinical medicine, inquiring about and understanding the impact of evidence from clinical observations, laboratory results, scientific literature, or other sources (after answering the question *What is the evidence for that?*).

Critical Friend: An evaluator who believes in the program aims but is critical in a way that is helpful and constructive, helping define terms, clarify relationships, questioning underlying assumptions, helping to make the program theory explicit, and other activities that help program staff members and participants critically examine their goals and the strategies they implement to accomplish those goals.

Critical Thinking: The disciplined ability and desire to assess evidence. An active effort to seek a breadth of contradicting as well as confirming information, to make objective judgments on the basis of well-supported reasons as a guide to belief and action, and to monitor one's thinking while doing so (metacognition). The thought processes necessary and appropriate for critical thinking depend on the knowledge domain (e.g., scientific, mathematical, historical, anthropological, economic, philosophical, moral). Critical thinking demonstrates universal criteria: clarity, accuracy, precision, consistency, relevance, sound empirical evidence, good reasons, depth, breadth, and fairness.

Cronbach's Alpha: A measurement of internal consistency reliability with a numerical range from 1.0–0. Alpha values lower than .60–.70 are considered too weak to use except for clinical practice. Lower alpha values may be acceptable if the purpose is research rather than clinical practice.

Cross-Sectional Survey: A research design in which all of the data are collected at one time.

Culture: A social phenomenon that refers to a set of beliefs, values, attitudes, and behavioral preferences that are shared by a group of people (Barnouw, 1985). It is communicated from one generation to another or to new arrivals in a host society through socialization practices.

Current Best Evidence: As applied by the medical field, this term means to use the current best evidence in making decisions about patient care. Assessment and treatment decisions are based on empirical evidence from research studies that are published in professional literature. Current best evidence requires the use of diagnostic criteria and instruments to develop a clinical assessment and treatment plan. See chapters 2–5 in this volume for detailed discussions of best evidence and expert consensus models used in medicine and public health.

Curvilinear relationship: A relationship in which scores on either extreme represent the same concept. For example, in the FACES clients who score on either end of the spectrum are dysfunctional, and clients who score in the middle are functional.

Data: Isolated collected measures that only indicate the actual measurement of a particular activity. For instance, the Average Length of Stay is measured data. Data also constitutes the raw observations associated with health interventions (e.g., physical examination, laboratory tests, treatment results, etc.).

Data Mining: *See Expert Systems.*

Deception: In the context of research, deception refers to withholding informed consent from research participants. Deception may occur along a continuum from participants not being made aware that research is taking place to participants not being fully informed about the nature of the research project. Deception is sometimes justified in qualitative research when the method is required to elicit authentic responses about a significant problem or phenomenon when no other method would lead to this information. Deception is not justified in clinical trials of treatments. International ethics guidelines now demand that participants be made aware that the clinical trial involves the possibility of receiving a placebo (fake treatment).

Decision Analysis: Refers to analyzing a clinical decision under conditions of uncertainty through the application of explicit, quantitative methods that numerically measure prognoses, treatment effects, and patient values.

Decision Support Systems: A computer-based software application designed to help professionals make complex decisions effectively, often in a "what-if" question format. A decision support system retrieves and records the information linked to a decision. It includes a database of case information, including the information considered critical to making a decision and some kind of statistical modeling technique that determines the decision process. The software program compares the current case of interest to its database of cases and can respond with "what if" scenarios based on available case information.

Deinstitutionalization: The process, begun in the 1950s, of moving mentally ill and mentally disabled people out of institutional settings and into community living arrangements. Although originally conceived as a way of reintegrating these persons into society, it has been used economically to justify the closing of many institutions, without commensurate funds being provided in the community settings.

Delta: A frequency range in the EEG, defined as 0–4 Hertz per second.

Depression: A mood disorder involving disturbances in emotion (excessive sadness), behavior (apathy and loss of interest in usual activities), cognition (distorted thoughts of hopelessness and low self-esteem), and body function (fatigue, loss of appetite). Symptoms extend into many parts of an individual's life and include lack of interest in daily activities, decreased motivation, feelings of worthlessness, and sometimes suicidal thoughts.

Descriptive Statistics: Statistical indices that are derived from measures that are observed on each member of the reference population or sample. As an example, defining the mean grade point average of the freshman class as a descriptive statistic implies that the mean GPA has been calculated from the GPA of each and every member of the freshman class.

Desensitization Phase: Fourth phase of EMDR where bilateral eye movements are used to activate the neural network, which typically results in the client recalling the target image and experiencing a sequence of emotions. In this phase, EMDR can be effective in minimizing or eliminating the blockage experienced through the client's traumatized neural networking system.

Design and Rollout: A six-month process in which new strategies are examined, agreed upon, and introduced at top levels of an organization. Processes are designed to address organizational needs. Within this process implementation plans are developed and implemented by direct-care practitioners across the organization.

Detained: May begin with a stop on the street by a law enforcement officer, a request by the police officer for the citizen to identify himself, and an explanation of what the suspect was doing. If probable cause exists, then the suspect may be required to stand by while the officer investigates him, searches him, or asks witnesses to identify him. Sometimes alleged lawbreakers are temporarily detained in police lockups or county detention centers pending a bail hearing before a magistrate.

Developmental Validity: A quality of an item, scale, or instrument that focuses on the degree to which it can be read, comprehended, and responded to in the intended way by respondents in the targeted age range or developmental stage. Developmental validity, like other kinds of validity, is concerned with how well items, scales, or instruments actually measure what they are intended to measure.

Dialogue: Discussing why a person assigned a specific rating to an activity during the stocktaking step.

Diffusion and Dissemination: Diffusion is the process by which an idea or practice becomes adopted by a growing number of people in a population. In some instances dissemination is considered synonymous with diffusion. Alternatively, dissemination can be considered a situation in which diffusion is actively encouraged.

Diffusion of Innovation: This is a process by which a particular innovation is communicated through certain channels over time among the members of a social system. This process results in social change also known as an alteration in the structure and function of a social system.

Dimension: Used in a nontechnical sense to refer to an aspect or component of a broader concept or domain, as in a dimension of performance or dimensions of access. In some cases, as with aspects of quality/appropriateness from the perspective of consumers, proposed dimensions may also meet the more technical criteria of *constructs*.

Disequalibrium: An emotional state that may be characterized by confusing emotions, somatic complaints, and erratic behavior. The severe emotional discomfort experienced by the person in crisis propels him or her toward action that will reduce the subjective discomfort.

Dispersion: The property of a distribution that refers to the heterogeneity of values or the degree to which there is variability in a distribution. Indices of dispersion include the variance, standard deviation, and range. As an example, there is relatively low variation in I.Q. among graduate students in physics at a major university compared to the variation in I.Q. among a group of passengers in a subway in New York City.

Domain: A group of issues, elements, or components that have some important aspects in common. For example, "access to service" is a domain; "timeliness of receipt of service" is a component or *dimension* of access. An area of individual functioning (e.g., communication, independent living, etc.).

Domestic Violence Typology: A framework for classifying information into specific categories or ideal types of woman battering that contribute to understanding the phenomenon of domestic violence. *Also see Woman Battering Continuum.*

Double ABCX Model: A model of family stress and coping, developed by Hamilton

McCubbin and associates, that focuses on the interaction of a pileup of stressors (AA), present and past family resources (BB), and present and past family interpretation/appraisal process (CC) to produce the resultant level of family adaptation (XX).

Drill Down Analysis: Examination of the data within a particular case to determine potential contributing factors to the occurrence or recurrence of illness. This type of analysis may be conducted with a single case or a group of cases with a common factor. In the case of groups of cases, the drill down seeks to identify correlative factors. Statistical processes may be applied to determine the strength of relation between correlative factors.

Drug Court: A legal court, presided over by a judge, that includes an interdisciplinary team of probation officers, psychologists, social workers, and community members and handles individuals who have been arrested on offenses related to drug abuse and addiction problems.

Dual Relationships: When a professional has a relationship with one individual in two different contexts, and these contexts have different and potentially conflicting expectations and interests. A practitioner who also conducts research is said to have a dual relationship with a client when the client is involved in a therapeutic relationship and is also a participant in a study offered by the practitioner. The therapeutic relationship is focused on the needs and interests of the client and the research relationship is focused on scientific insights and discovery for the benefit of improved professional knowledge rather than the interests of the individual participant/client.

Dysthymic Disorder: The DSM-IVTR diagnosis for a person with a chronically depressed mood that occurs for most of the day, more days than not, for at least two years (APA, 2000). When depressed, the person experiences two or more of the following symptoms: poor appetite or overeating, insomnia or hypersomnia, low energy or fatigue, low self-esteem, poor concentration or difficulty making decisions, and feelings of hopelessness.

Ecological Perspective: A set of assumptions and concepts that focus on the reciprocal interactions between individuals and their environments across time to explain variations in the values, orientations, and behavior of individuals.

Ecological Survey: A survey based on aggregate data for a particular population as it exists at a specific point or points in time. The survey is conducted to study the relationship of exposure to an identified or presumed risk factor for a specified outcome.

EEG: Electroencephalogram

Effectiveness: Refers to a type of impact study where the focus is on the estimate of overall program impact, i.e., the difference between treatment and counterfactual conditions without adjustment for the fidelity of the treatment implementation. Effectiveness estimates are often referred to as lower bound estimates of treatment impact or impact that can be expected under actual practice conditions. Effectiveness studies refer to the ability of social interventions to produce desired outcomes in the lives of families and children. Also refers to the *clinical utility* of an intervention. The effectiveness of an intervention is related to the extent to which the effects of an intervention could generalize or extend to other settings, populations, etc.

Efficacy Studies: Often intervention outcomes are measured in highly controlled contexts to enhance internal validity. Such studies are often called efficacy trials and they are recommended prior to examining outcomes in realistic service contexts. If the outcomes of efficacy studies merit testing in realistic service contexts, effectiveness studies are carried out.

Efficacy: The *potency* of an intervention. The efficacy of an intervention is related to the extent to which changes in the individual are due to the active ingredients of the intervention. This is a type of impact study where the focus is on the estimate of maximum program impact, i.e., the difference between treatment and counterfactual conditions when treatment implementation proceeds as intended. Efficacy studies are often referred to as the upper bound estimates of treatment impact or impact that can be expected under ideal practice conditions.

Elder Abuse: The intentional or unintentional infliction of or threat of harm on an older adult over 60 years of age. Categories of elder abuse include physical, emotional, or financial harm, or neglect of a care-dependent older adult.

Elder Abuse Homicide: The murder of an older adult; an extreme form of physical abuse.

Elder Abuse Victim: An older person who experiences harm or threat of harm by another person.

Emotional Responsiveness: The degree to which an individual is emotionally available to another person and allows himself or herself to be empathically in touch with the inner experience of the other person.

Empirically Based Practice: Clinical services that demonstrate statistically significant effectiveness.

Empirically Supported Treatments (EST): Treatments whose efficacy or effectiveness has been supported through a program of research meeting certain scientifically established criteria.

Empirically Validated/Supported Treatments: Empirically validated/supported treatments are those that have met the rigorous criteria set forth by the American Psychological Association's Division 12 Task Force on Promotion and Dissemination of Psychological Procedures. The Task Force identified two primary categories for treatments—"well established" treatments and "probably efficacious" treatments.

Empowerment Evaluation: A collaborative evaluation process in the use of evaluation concepts, techniques, and findings to foster improvement and self-determination. This includes the evaluator, funder, program staff, and participants and community in data collection, analysis, and reporting. For example, as developed by the Kellogg Foundation empowerment evaluation utilizes ongoing communication about processes and continuous self-examination from all perspectives.

Environmental Strains: A combination of strains (i.e., ongoing stressors), which are caused by elements in an individual's social situation, over which the individual may have limited or no control (e.g., race, socioeconomic status, physical disability).

Epidemiology: The study of the distribution and determinants of various disorders in the population. *See also Incidence* and *Point Prevalence.*

Equal Probability Sampling: Any sampling method where every element in the sampling frame has an equal chance of selection. For example, a sample of households in a defined geographic area would be an equal probability sample if each household in that area had the same chance of inclusion in the sample.

Error (Type I): Error that concludes a particular cause when, in fact, this was not the cause.

Error (Type II): Acceptance of a hypothesis or statement as true when it is false.

Ethics: The branch of philosophy that deals with distinctions between right and wrong and with the moral consequences of human actions. Examples of ethical issues that arise in medical practice and research include informed consent, confidentiality, respect for human rights, and scientific integrity.

Ethnography: A qualitative research approach that involves the investigation of a culture or particular aspect of a culture, with reference to the meaning of certain behaviors or attributions for members of that culture. For example, a large group of convicted felons who are studied by members of the state parole board. A social scientific description of a people or group and the cultural basis of their identities, elicited from naturalistic, qualitative modes of inquiry (e.g., participant observation, semistructured interviews, focus groups).

Etiological Fraction: The proportion of people with a specific disease that can be attributed to a certain risk factor.

Evaluation: A systematic process of gathering and interpreting data to determine results generated by a specific set of procedures designed to meet specific goals. *See also outcome evaluation, outcome measures, process evaluation,* and *program monitoring.*

Evidence-Based Guidelines: Clinical recommendations to assist providers with managing and treating specific diseases that are based on research studies published in the scientific literature. Many consider clinical recommendations "evidence-based" if they are developed through a specific process that includes a systematic review and analyses of the scientific peer-reviewed journal literature. These professional practice guidelines are based on empirical studies preappraised for scientific validity and prescreened for clinical relevance.

Evidence-Based Health Care (EBH): The conscientious, explicit, and judicious use of current best practices and systematic reviews of evidence in making decisions about the care of individual patients. This involves all of the health professions, including health care information systems and management of health records.

Evidence-Based Medicine (EBM): The conscientious, explicit, and judicious use of current best evidence in making decisions about the care and medical treatment of individual patients. Best practices of EBM refers to integrating individual clinical expertise with the best available external clinical evidence from systematic research investigations.

Evidence-Based Practice (EBP): An approach to practice that requires the examination of research findings from systematic clinical research (e.g., randomized controlled clinical research) in making decisions about the care of a specific population with a specific problem. The process of critically identifying and employing treatment or practice approaches that have the strongest basis of empirical support for attaining desired outcomes. An evidence-based practice is considered any practice that has been established as effective through scientific research according to a set of explicit criteria. The term *evidence-based practice* is also used to describe a way of practicing in which the practitioner critically uses best evidence, expertise, and values to make practice decisions that matter to individual service recipients and patients about their care.

Evidence-based practice is the use of interventions that are based on rigorous research methods. Evidence-based practice includes the integration of different studies and establishing the combined probative value. An example of an EBP approach to supporting and serving families and children would be based on the likelihood that certain types of supports and services can be shown to be more effective than other interventions. See chapters 1 through 6 in this volume for specific definitions and discussion of the application of evidence-based practice in medicine, mental health, psychiatry, psychology, and social work settings.

Evidence-Based Practice Education: A lifelong problem-based learning approach to keep up-to-date on the scientific research and improve clinical practice and treatment outcomes. This process requires that the practitioner use theories and interventions based on empirical evidence of their effectiveness, apply approaches appropriate to the client and setting, and evaluate his/her own practice effectiveness.

Expected Nonconcordant Scores: The number of nonagreeing scores occurring by chance.

Experimental Design: A type of research design that uses random assignment of study participants to different treatment groups. Randomization provides some level of assurance that the groups are comparable in every way except for the treatment received. In general, a randomized experiment is regarded as the most rigorous and strongest research design to establish a cause-effect (treatment outcomes) relationship. These designs usually collect data before and after the program to assess the net effects of the program.

Experimental Study: One in which the independent variable is manipulated by the researcher in order to see its effect on the dependent variable(s). It is defined as a research study in which people are randomly assigned to different forms of the program or alternative treatments, including a control group and/or a placebo group.

Expert Consensus: Expert consensus is the synthesis of the evidence of treatment effectiveness using a panel of noted contributors of the field. The outcome of an expert consensus is often a treatment protocol or guideline.

Expert System: A computer program designed to draw inferences from data provided pertinent to some decision. Expert systems are developed through a process of data mining in which recognized experts in a specific knowledge domain are studied, such as through interviewing, to determine the type of information they use and the rules that they use to make decisions. Computer programs are then designed to request this information and to use the rules to draw inferences. This output is used by decision makers to support pertinent decision-making. An expert system is a form of artificial intelligence that is more sophisticated than a decision support system. An expert system is a computer software application that recommends a specific decision based on case information. Expert systems take several years to develop and typically include a knowledge base, an inference system, the facts of cases, and a question/answer system for the practitioner to interface with the expert system. Expert systems were intended to lend expert advice by capturing it in a software program that could then be accessed by staff that may not possess expert knowledge.

Exposure: A behavior therapy procedure used in the treatment of anxiety disorders to help the patient confront situations or stimuli they avoid yet which realistically pose acceptable risks of danger. During exposure, the patient gradually confronts situations in a prolonged and repeated fashion with the therapist's assistance and then on their own.

Externalizing Disorders: Also referred to as disruptive behavior disorders, this class of disorders is characterized by high rates of noncompliant, hostile, and defiant behaviors, including aggressiveness and hyperactivity. The *DSM-IV-TR* (APA, 2000) categorizes externalizing disorders into three headings: attention-deficit/hyperactivity disorder (ADHD), oppositional defiant disorder (ODD), and conduct disorder (CD).

Eye Movement Desensitization and Reprocessing: A theoretical approach developed in 1987 by Francine Shapiro to relieve posttraumatic stress symptoms. The EMDR model is based on the hypothesis that traumatization produces neural networking that interferes with successful processing of those memories, feelings, and experiences.

Factorial Analysis: The purpose of factor analysis is to examine the interrelationships of data such as scale items, to group items together, and make it possible to identify the underlying dimension or trait for a set of items. Data can be simplified by reducing the number of items from many to the most relevant items that best capture the construct of interest.

Family Caregiving: The use of immediate or extended family members to provide services for an ill, aging, or handicapped member. Family members might choose voluntarily to provide these services out of personal connection to the needy family member, or they may be obliged to provide these services in the absence of equivalent services being provided by social agencies.

Family Educational Interventions: Nonclinical intervention with the primary objective of meeting informational and practical needs of families with a relative who suffers from severe mental illness. There are a variety of models that are delivered by either professionals and/or peers (family members).

Family Etiology of Mental Illness: The belief (now discredited) that family interpersonal dynamics and communication problems (e.g., high "expressed emotion" or "communication deviance") were responsible for causing severe mental illness (i.e., schizophrenia or bipolar disorder). It is now believed that these are biologically based illnesses, which may be exacerbated by family communication dynamics.

Family Process: The way in which members of the family interact with each other.

Family Sense of Competence: The unique appraisal of family members about how well they are managing a particular problem as a group. This may be contrasted with "locus of control" (internal control/external control) appraisal, which tends to be an individual appraisal of global functioning.

Family Status: Refers to how the family position of an adult is characterized—single, married, engaged, divorced, widowed.

Family Structure: The composition of the family, such as grandmother, mother, father, and three children.

Father Hunger: The longing desire to have an emotionally close relationship with an admiring father.

Femicide: The killing of a woman.

First-Level Coding: The first step in the coding of qualitative data, where researchers identify conceptually distinct categories of information that reflect meaningful patterns and themes.

Fiscal: The financial elements of an organization such as the year, accounting and auditing procedures, and the organization budget. The fiscal year is the 12-month period in which the organization operates financially (often July 1 to June 30 in the United States; October 1 to September 30 for federal government agencies; or the calendar year, January 1 to December 31 in some cases).

Fish Bone Diagram: Also known as a Cause and Effect Analysis Diagram, used by a problem-solving team during brainstorming to logically list and display known and potential causes to a problem. Analysis of the listed causes is done to identify root causes.

Focus Group: A focus group interview consists of a small group of individuals who are gathered together in a permissive, nonthreatening environment to discuss a topic of interest to the researcher. Focus group studies are used to gain understanding of peoples' thoughts and behaviors, to pilot test ideas, or to evaluate programs, products, or services.

Follow-Up: Observation over a period of time of an individual, group, or initially defined population whose relevant characteristics have been assessed in order to observe changes in health status or health-related variables.

Formative Evaluation: Formative evaluation seeks to change and improve programs through ongoing data collection and interpretation about program activities, structures, and short-term results. While it may include data on long-term outcomes, formative evaluation emphasizes decision-making, process, and implementation variables that need to be improved in order to effect outcomes. It is similar in purpose and practice to action research and performance improvement. An evaluation, which has the primary goal of improving the program prior to full implementation.

Frequency Matching: A method of selecting controls for case-control studies in a manner such that the distribution of extraneous factors in controls is similar to that of cases. Frequency matching is often done for age and gender so that differences in these characteristics between cases and controls do not distort the relationship between case-control status and the factor under study.

Frisk: A "pat down" based on reasonable suspicion that a citizen has been involved in criminal behavior, or is about to commit a crime.

FTE: Total organization salary hours paid 2080; also refers to full-time college enrollments.

Functional Outcomes: Measures of programmatic effectiveness based on client ability to perform in day-to-day activities (e.g., stay in school, work, avoid conflict with the law, etc.).

Generalized Anxiety Disorder: An anxiety disorder resulting in a continuous state of anxiety or fear, lasting a month or more. Defining features include but are not limited to: signs of motor tension, autonomic hyperactivity (a pounding heart), constant apprehension, and difficulties in concentration. Persons who suffer from generalized anxiety disorders often describe a chronic, exaggerated, unprovoked state of worry and tension, often accompanied by physical symptoms (trembling, twitching, headaches, irritability, sweating, hot flashes, nausea, lump in throat). Anxiety disorders, if untreated, frequently lead to the emergence of a depressive disorder.

Geographic Information System (GIS): A computer system that allows the collection, storage, integration, analysis, and display of spatially referenced data.

Global Positioning System (GPS): L Satellites constellation that allows users equipped with a GPS receiver to determine in real time their location anywhere on Earth, with an accuracy ranging from a few millimetres to several meters.

Goal: A general aim, object, or end effect that one strives to achieve.

Government Performance and Results Act: The 1993 public law that established the requirement for all federal government agencies and their programs to gauge their success on results achieved instead of activities undertaken. Specific results or outcomes are to be used to justify funding rather than activity indicators or outputs.

Grant-making: A process or system of distributing and managing resources for program implementation.

Gray Murder: A homicide of an older victim that is disguised by the perpetrator to appear as a natural death. *See also Elder Abuse, Homicide, and Femicide.*

Grief and Bereavement Counseling: Therapy, often cognitive-behavioral in nature, utilized by a psychologist, social worker, or counselor to assist in understanding and adapting to grief related to the death of others.

Grief: A predictable series of feelings and psychological states occurring as a result of the loss, specifically death, of another.

Grounded Theory: An inductive research method in which a theory is developed from the data. The goal of grounded theory is to explain a phenomenon by drawing on data collected from the field and generating propositions from them.

Hawthorne Effect: People's behavior may change simply because they know they are in a study or being observed. The bias is introduced when this change is erroneously attributed to specific components of the study. *See also Placebo Effect* and *Blinding.*

Health Care: Services provided to individuals or communities by a health care system or by professionals to promote, maintain, monitor, or restore health. Health care contains a broad spectrum of services and activities delivered by a team of health personnel. This contrasts with medical care, which concentrates on diagnostic and therapeutic actions performed by or under the supervision of an individual physician.

Healthy Worker Bias: People who are selected for a study through their workplace are healthier than the population at large, because the population consists of people who are unable to work for health reasons.

Heterogeneity: This takes place when there is more variation between the results in systematic research reviews than would be expected to occur by chance alone.

High-Quality Data: Specific information, either numerical or nonnumerical, that is reliable, valid, and useful for decision-making. Said another way, high-quality data are data that allow the viewer to understand more clearly the underlying reality of the situation. In the case, for example, of program management, higher data quality allows you to understand more clearly what effects your program is having, and because you have a clearer picture of reality, you are able to make better decisions about your program.

Ill Member Level of Adaptation: The functional level of a person diagnosed with serious mental illness, living in the community. It is based on Likert-scale assessments of several areas of functioning by family members (but could also be completed by the person himself/herself, case managers, or other observers). It is intended to give a broader view of community functioning than can be gained from observing symptoms alone.

Illness-Related Strains: A combination of strains (i.e., ongoing stressors) that are the direct result of a person's illness history and which subsequently affect future capabilities (e.g., number of hospitalizations, limited functioning, substance abuse complications).

Impact: The marginal change in client functioning caused by a program or therapeutic intervention. This change is measured as the difference in outcomes for clients in the treatment and counterfactual conditions.

Impact Assessments: More formal research designs, which try to determine if it was the intervention and not other factors that created a program outcome. Impact assessments usually employ experimental and quasi-experimental designs.

Impact Evaluation: A study of what changed as a result of the intervention or program under investigation. Often inherent in the definition of an impact evaluation is the idea that a judgment will be placed on the whole; the program either works (shows results) or it does not (show results), and either it should be funded or should not be funded.

Implementation Strategy: While evidence may establish a specific practice as an evidence-based practice or a best practice, it has been found difficult to move these best practices into routine practice. Accordingly, systematic plans have been developed to disseminate and facilitate the use of best practices in service systems. Top-down or macro strategies disseminate best practices for use by frontline practitioners through agency directives, guidelines, manualized interventions, accreditation requirements, algorithms, toolkits, and so forth. Bottom-up or micro strategies focus directly on individual practitioners by engaging them in or teaching them the evidence-based practice process of critical decision-making. *See also Evidence-Based Practice* and *Evidence-Based Practice Guidelines.*

Incentives: To get people to attend a focus group interview, the recruiter offers an incentive. The incentive could be tangible, such as money, food, or gifts, or it could be intangible, such as a feeling of community service, helping a meaningful research effort, or contributing to society. Incentives are important because people need a compelling reason to give up their time to be involved in a focus group. *See also Focus Groups.*

Incidence: The proportion of new cases of a disorder in the population that appear within a specified time frame. The number of new cases in a given period divided by the number of people at risk for the disorder. To make results more understandable, incidence is sometimes expressed as cases per 1,000 or 10,000 people in the time period (or even per million per year for rare disorders).

Incidence-Prevalence (Neyman) Bias: A cross-sectional survey will tend to overlook people with less serious forms of a disorder (because they would have gotten better) and more serious forms (because they would have died).

Indicator: A measure of performance based on desired or expected outcome of a specific process or activity.

Indirect costs (IDC): A percentage of the budget (usually the overall total or sometimes the total excluding certain items) that is allocated to the grantee to cover overhead expenses, such as building space, administrative oversight and services, maintenance of facilities and equipment, insurance costs, etc. Usually a funder specifies an indirect cost rate that it allows, or negotiates with the grantee as to an acceptable IDC on a case-by-case basis.

Inferential Statistics: Estimates of population parameters based on probability sampling and theoretical distributions of sampling error. For example, an estimate of the mean GPA of the freshman class that is derived from a random sample of members of the freshman class would be classified as an inferential statistic.

Information exists when the significance of data is determined for a particular problem, patient, and practitioner (e.g., the physical examination is abnormal, laboratory test elevated, or treatment result successful). When data is displayed or analyzed in relationship to other data, it becomes information. Information becomes useful in asking the questions of why a particular organization achieves a certain result and another organization some other result. Data needs to be turned into information to become useful.

Information Management: A method used to organize information to avoid information overload and to keep information in a format that is efficient to retrieve whenever needed. Filing systems, cognitive maps, manuals, and electronic databases are examples of devices that can prove useful in information management. A network of consultants is an additional way to ensure that necessary information will be readily available.

Information-Rich: This is a term used to describe participants in a qualitative research study (including focus group interviewing) who possess the greatest information about the research topic. This concept assumes that certain people have more experience with the topic and therefore offer greater richness of insight for the purposes of the study. *See also Focus Groups.*

Informed Consent: Voluntary agreement based on information about foreseeable risks and benefits associated with the agreement. In the context of research, informed consent implies that participants have been informed about the nature of the research, the benefits and risks of participating, and what will happen with the information they share or is gathered about them during the research process.

Infrastructure: The hierarchical levels of management established to support a specific process or system.

Inner City: Geographic areas within large urban centers that are usually located in the older core of the city and characterized by high population density. Although there may be a wide range of socioeconomic status among inner-city residents, in many urban areas they are severely disadvantaged and prone to poor health.

Inner-city Health Research: Research focused on the health of disadvantaged urban populations, the social, economic, and health care factors that influence individual and population health in the inner city, and the evaluation of relevant interventions.

Inputs: Inputs are the resources needed to develop deliberate efforts intended to achieve desired outcomes. There are material and nonmaterial inputs. Material inputs include: funding, personnel, volunteers, equipment, and infrastructure. Nonmaterial inputs include leadership, vision, clearly formulated and measurable goals, strategies, strategic planning, a commitment to performance measurement, competence, realistic yet challenging performance targets, social capital, appropriate technology, interorganizational collaboration, stakeholder involvement, and so forth.

Inquiry: Involves activity that a private citizen would not be expected to make but where a police officer initiated what would be labeled non-offensive contact if it occurred between two ordinary citizens. These actions would not be considered a seizure, if questions were put in a conversational manner, demands by an officer were not made, orders were not issued, and if questions were not overbearing or harassing. It is an exchange of conversation between a police officer and a citizen that does not constitute a Fourth Amendment seizure.

Installation Phase: Fifth phase of EMDR that serves to close down the catalytic process and install more desired cognitive and affective responses. These positive, adaptive responses are elicited from the client; they illustrate how the client would prefer to think or feel about the trauma event or memory. Clients are asked to rank the validity of the new cognition as to how true it feels until it has been successfully installed. *See also Eye Movement Desensitization Reprocessing.*

Intake Interview: An initial set of in-person meetings between a clinician and a patient used to establish a working relationship and to make an assessment of client problems, symptoms, needs, strengths, and circumstances as relevant to services requested and available. The assessment can include the gathering and evaluation of biological, psychological, and social data pertaining to the patient. In mental health settings the assessment includes specification of differential psychiatric diagnoses.

Internal Consistency Reliability: Computing the internal consistency (Cronbach's alpha) of a measure allows one to estimate how consistently respondents performed across items of a measure. The internal consistency of a measure also lends support for evidence of its content validity.

Internal Consistency: The degree to which all of the items on a scale correlate with each other, indicating that they are all tapping the same attribute.

Interrater Reliability: The degree to which observations yield similar results from different judges.

Intrusiveness: The intensity of interference into a citizen's life. It can be perceived as a violation of rights if pushed too far by a police officer. However, in order to control crime and protect the public, an examination of a citizen under reasonable suspicion may be necessary.

The level of intensity of the encroachment and how imposing the interruption is determines the degree of interference.

Juvenile Delinquency: Delinquency is a legal designation that includes a range of behaviors that violate the law, such as robbery, drug use, and vandalism. Some acts are illegal for both adults and juveniles (referred to as index offenses) and cover serious offenses like homicide, aggravated assault, and rape. Other acts (referred to as status offenses) are illegal only for juveniles due to their age, such as underage drinking, truancy from school, and running away from home.

Key Information Needs: These are the data required for any program to measure effectiveness and are based on the logic model design. They include data, knowledge, etc., about program performance that is necessary to make judgments about the program and manage it for positive outcomes. The information necessary to measure a program's operations may also reflect needs of the program stakeholders (i.e., funders, board members).

Kinship care: An arrangement under which a relative or group of relatives serve on a temporary or permanent basis as substitute parent(s) for a child or sibling group whose biological parent(s) cannot ensure the safety and well-being of the child(ren).

Knowledge is abstracted from information when external evidence is used to anticipate how additional interventions could change the data (e.g., surgery will cure the physical finding, or a drug will normalize the laboratory test result and prevent disease).

Lay Health Advisor: A lay health advisor (LHA) is a person who is recognized as a natural helper and receives training to use her (or his) natural skills to raise health-related awareness and skills among her relatives, friends, and acquaintances. An LHA differs from a peer advisor or outreach work in that she does not seek to convey information to strangers. Moreover, unlike peer advisors and outreach workers, LHAs are often not employed by an agency. Rather, they share their knowledge and skills with people they know during the normal course of their lives.

Learning Factors: Interactions between the therapist and client or patient consisting of corrective emotional experiences, insight, and feedback processes.

Likelihood Ratio: This refers to the likelihood that a particular test finding would be expected in a patient with the target disorder when compared with the likelihood that this same test finding would be expected in a patient without the target disorder.

Likert Scale: Developed by Rensis Likert as a type of composite measure used to determine levels of measurement and the relative intensity of different items. For example, a bipolar scale with a neutral middle point (e.g., Strongly Agree / Agree / Neither Agree nor Disagree / Disagree / Strongly Disagree).

Line Item Budget: A fiscal plan that focuses on the monetary elements of the organization.

Literature: A written repository of knowledge pertaining to any given topic. It includes information sources such as refereed scientific journals, practice-oriented review journals, conference proceedings, trade journals, textbooks, product promotion materials, and Internet e-mail communications, literature sources vary widely in strength of evidence and can be weighted based on content and degree of rigor applied in the development of the literature.

Local Knowledge: Knowledge that is applicable to a given client or practice situation, and which derives from practitioner practice wisdom, experience, and characteristics of a practice setting. It is contrasted with knowledge that is generalized from research results.

Logic Model: An assessment/evaluation strategy used to determine the extent to which the intended outcomes of a program are consistent with the activities and resources of an agency. This is a single-page figure depicting the intended theory behind the program in terms of resources, activities, process, and outcomes. The process allows for an agency to determine the intermediate and long-term outcomes as they relate to program structure and operations.

Longitudinal Data: Involves the collection of data at different agreed-upon points in time, such as 1 month, 3 months, 6 months, and 12 months post-treatment completion. In the context of social interventions for families and children, a database that tracks the experience of families and children from their initial involvement with the formal service system through their continued involvement with that system, and which provides a valid and reliable basis for describing and assessing the experiences of families and children served by that system over time.

Longitudinal Survey: A research design in which the participants are followed at several different points in time, in comparison to a cross-sectional study, which examines participants at only one point in time.

Low-Quality Data: Information that is unreliable or invalid and does not reveal the underlying reality. These data are not useful for decision-making.

Macro: The level of results in which the organization itself is considered to be the primary beneficiary of organizational action.

Macro Results: The level of results in which the organization itself is considered to be the primary beneficiary of organizational action. Results at this level are called *outputs*, which specify the results internal to an organization that are accomplished (or not accomplished), that are *delivered* (or "put out") externally into society. A *product* becomes an *output* only when it is sold or otherwise matriculates to customers, consumers, or other external stakeholders.

Magnitude: The average absolute magnitude (as defined in microvolts) of a band over the entire epoch (1 second).

Maintenance Orientation: An approach to opioid agonist therapy that promotes long-term maintenance on an opioid agonist. Indefinite maintenance on an opioid agonist is considered a reasonable goal of treatment.

Marginalized Population: These are people in a community who do not sit in the seats of traditional power and who are often looked down upon by the people in those seats. A marginalized group is often a racial or ethnic minority but can also be the majority if the minority in power is effective in determining the social norms for the community.

Measurement: The quantification of some property or aspect of an object according to explicit rules of measurement. As an example, the mass of an object in a gravitational field is generally quantified in explicit measures of weight. The quantification of some property or aspect of an object measurement observed on each member of the reference population or measurements that are observed on each member of the reference population. In large populations, the specific values of parameters are often assumed or estimated rather than known.

Mega Results: The level of results in which external stakeholders and society are considered to be the primary beneficiaries of organizational action. Results at this level are called *outcomes*, which specify the *impact* on society of results that are accomplished (or not accomplished) by organizations, teams, and/or individuals. An output becomes an outcome when external stakeholders and society are impacted—positively or negatively, unintentionally or intentionally—by organizational actions.

Meta-Analysis: A study of studies, or collection and integration of experimental studies on a particular treatment or program where a statistical formula is used to measure the effect, size, and impact of the different treatment programs. Also known as a systematic literature review that utilizes quantitative methods to summarize the findings. For example, a formal synthesis of experimental research that seeks to understand how particular interventions affect specific outcomes for families and children.

Metacognition: Thinking about and documenting one's thought process; the monitoring of one's thinking for the critical thinking criteria as one acquires new information. Within the area of scientific thinking, this requires becoming aware of one's background knowledge, assumptions, and the rival hypotheses (how observing works) and assessing their validity as well.

Metric: A measure of performance.

Micro: The level of results in which individuals and teams within the organization are considered to be the primary beneficiaries of organizational action.

Micro Results: The level of results in which individuals and teams within the organization are considered to be the primary beneficiaries of organizational action. Results at this level are called *products*, which specify the results internal to organizations that are accomplished (or not accomplished) by individuals and/or teams that are produced for *other* individuals or teams *within* an organization.

Middle Range Theory: A theory that is between a total explanation of society and explaining discrete individual behavior.

Mission: The values and dreams of the group.

Mission-Based Research: Research projects whose inspiration is derived from political or social interests, in addition to purely scientific objectives.

Moderator: The term *moderator* is used to describe the individual leading a focus group interview. The moderator creates a nonthreatening environment where people feel comfortable talking, guides the discussion using predetermined questions, and keeps the discussion on track and on time.

Mortality Rate: The proportion of people at risk who die from a disorder within a specific time frame.

Mortality Rate: Number of deaths from a disorder in a time period divided by the number of people at risk. When the time period is one year, this number is called the *annual mortality rate*.

Need: A gap between "What Is" (current) and "What Should Be" (required) individual, small group, organizational and/or societal performance results (not perceived shortages of personnel, resources, finances, training or service provision). Used as a noun, not a verb, a need can be represented as a simple mathematical function: required results minus current results = need.

Needs Assessment: A formal process that identifies needs as gaps in results between "What Is" and "What Should Be," prioritizes those gaps on the basis of the costs and benefits of closing versus ignoring those needs, and selects the needs to be reduced or eliminated. Needs assessments serve to identify gaps between current and desired results that occur both within an organization (at the micro level of results) as well as outside (at the macro and mega levels of results) in order to provide useful information for decision-making.

Negative Verification: A pattern of communication typical of people with depression in which they make negative remarks posed as questions for their partners ("I look terrible, don't I?"). Either way—whether the partner agrees or disagrees—the individual will not feel better, and eventually the partner may feel frustrated by these demands.

Objective: An objective is a statement of what the proposed project aims to achieve. Objectives should specify a time period and be quantifiable. For example, "within 12 months, 75% of participants will have participated in job interviews and 50% will be employed in part-time or full-time stable jobs." Ideally, a proposed project should have a manageable number of objectives (e.g., 5 to 7).

Observational Study: One in which the researcher looks at the relationship among variables but does not alter the variables in any way.

Obsession: Intrusive thoughts, feelings, urges or images that trigger intense anxiety or discomfort associated with obsessive-compulsive disorder. Obsessions occur outside of the sufferer's control, and tend to increase with attempts to control, neutralize, or suppress them. Obsessions are not excessive worries about real problems. Several categories exist, including but not limited to contamination fears, violent or horrific obsessions, superstitious obsessions; scrupulous obsessions, obsessions related to fear of responsibility for harm coming to others, and a feeling that things need to be "just right." *See also Anxiety Disorder.*

Obsessions: A symptom of obsessive-compulsive disorder involving persistent unwanted intrusive thoughts, ideas, or images that seem senseless yet evoke high levels of anxiety or distress. Examples include unwanted ideas about violence, sex, or blasphemy; senseless fears of contamination from realistically safe situations; and exaggerated fears of making unlikely mistakes (e.g., discarding important papers).

Obsessive-Compulsive Disorder (OCD): A disorder characterized by recurrent obsessions and compulsions that take at least one hour per day or cause significant distress or impairment. In discerning the differential diagnosis, OCD must be distinguished from related disorders including Hypochondriasis, Body Dysmorphic Disorder, Generalized Anxiety Disorder, Delusional Disorders, Tic Disorders, and Obsessive-Compulsive Personality Disorder. *See also Anxiety Disorders or Comorbidity.*

Odds: A ratio of events to nonevents. If the event rate for a disease is 0.1 (10 per cent), its nonevent rate is 0.9 and therefore its odds are 1:9, or 0.111. Note that this is not the same expression as the inverse of event rate.

Odds Ratio: The odds of an experimental patient suffering an adverse event relative to a control patient.

Online Groups: Online groups are therapy or support groups that are conducted via the computer in real time through e-mail, bulletin boards, or chat rooms. Online groups can also be conducted without the real-time component through e-mails. Online groups may also be referred to as "e-therapy."

OpiATE Monitoring System (OMS): A toolkit designed to assist opioid agonist therapy clinics in assessing current practices and developing quality improvement goals. The OMS contains a quick and easy method for assessing current practices and comparing these practices to best-practice recommendations as well as educational materials on best practices and multiple tools to assist in successfully carrying out quality improvement projects.

Opioid Agonist Therapy: A form of treatment for opioid (mainly heroin) dependence in which counseling and other psychosocial services are coupled with provision of a daily dose of an opioid agonist medication (methadone, levo-acetyl methadol, or buprenorphine).

Opioid Agonist Therapy Effectiveness (OpiATE) Initiative: A Veterans Administration Health Services Research and Development funded project aiming to increase access to high quality opioid agonist therapy for veterans diagnosed with opioid dependence.

Oppositional Defiant Disorder: Defined by a pattern of negativity, noncompliant defiance to authority figures (e.g., parents, teachers, and other adults), and temperamental outbursts that impair a child's ability to function effectively in home, school, and peer environments. This maladaptive pattern of behavior must have endured for six months or longer for the diagnosis to be made accurately. The DSM-IV TR (APA, 2000) is careful to note that these behaviors must occur more often than in peers of comparable age and developmental level. *See also Comorbidity and Externalizing Disorders.*

Organization Development (OD): Organization development (OD) is a field of study founded on principles of humanizing and improving organizations by planned change initiatives focused on individual growth, group process, and organizational culture and structure. While based on the idea of data-based change, the practice of OD has placed less emphasis on empirical procedures and focused more on the process of intervention and change. Related fields and practices include human resource management, management consulting, and training. The field of program evaluation has much to offer OD in relation to methods and processes for gathering data about change interventions and their outcomes.

Organizational Learning: Organizational learning emphasizes structures and processes by which participants share, interpret, retain, and experiment with knowledge about their work. Some practitioners emphasize the individual skills necessary to create and share knowledge, while others focus on group, resource, policy and structural aspects of organizations that impede or facilitate knowledge sharing. Related concepts include knowledge organizations, sense making, and communities of practice.

Outcome: A change in a patient's current and future health status that can be attributed to antecedent health care.

Outcome-Based Accountability: A process by which providers of supports and services are held responsible for the effectiveness of their work in terms of improved outcomes rather than conformity to prescribed standards of practice that may, in fact, not affect those outcomes.

Outcome Evaluation: A determination of the extent to which the intervention produced the intended short-term or long-term goals. Usually, outcome evaluations involve comparisons with a preintervention state and/or with comparable, untreated (control) groups. In most cases, an outcome evaluation is not very useful unless preceded by a process evaluation, which helps interpret the results. Evaluations that focus on what happens to clients as a result of the program and the program's level of success. Outcome evaluations study goals such as changes in knowledge, attitude, behavior, or improvements in client conditions. A study conducted to determine the impact of the program on the intended target(s), sometimes called impact evaluation.

Outcomes: Conditions that interventions are intended to effect or change. Specifically defined, measurable and verifiable events, conditions, states, or changes. There are two kinds of outcomes in the OPM&M framework: community outcomes, which represent improvements that the entire community desires for its well-being and livability, and service-delivery outcomes, which refer to what the service-providing organization needs to do in order to express its social commitment to accountability, efficiency, and equity. Community outcomes encompass the community's entire population and/or its environmental conditions as indicated by measures of social justice, economic prosperity, health, education, safety, recreation, aesthetics, and so forth. Service-delivery outcomes include the organization's public intention to use resources wisely and to manage operations rigorously and transparently.

Outputs: Outputs in the OPM&M framework are narrower in scope and scale than are outcomes. They refer to specific impacts that service providers actually have on the clients/customers that are actually reached. In this sense, outputs are associated with a subset of the larger population to which outcomes are linked. The "performance" of service providers is gauged by examining their outputs, in terms of how efficiently and equitably (as judged by measures of effort) and how effectively (as judged by measures of effect) they are able to reach and satisfy their clients'/customers' needs and to what extent successes and gains along these lines can be associated with the attainment or at least the approximation of the overall desired outcomes of the community.

Panic Attack / Panic Disorders: A panic attack is a stress-related feeling of intense fear and impending doom or death, accompanied by intense physiological symptoms including but not limited to rapid breathing, rapid pulse, sweaty palms, smothering sensations, shortness of breath, choking sensations, and dizziness. Panic attacks can happen very frequently and leave the individual emotionally drained. Individuals with panic disorders frequently live in fear of having another panic attack and develop avoidance (phobic) behaviors. Sufferers often consult physicians, many times thinking they are having a heart attack or asthma attack.

Parameters: Statistical indices that are assumed to be derived from measurements that are observed on each member of the reference population. In large populations, the specific values of parameters are often assumed or estimated rather than known. One can speak of the average per capita income of the United States, but actually observing the annual income of each and every person residing in the U.S. has proved impossible—even for the I.R.S.!

Paraphilia: A group of disorders characterized by recurrent, intense sexually arousing urges and fantasies or behaviors involving nonhuman objects, the suffering or humiliation of self, partner, children, or other nonconsenting person(s).

Parasuicide: Intentional acute self-injury with or without suicide intent.

Participant Incentives: Payments, whether monetary or in-kind, made to study participants for the purpose of reimbursement of expenses, compensation for time and effort, and/or as an incentive for participation in the study.

Participant Observation: A research method in which researchers observe behavior in real-life settings in which they participate.

Partnership Model: An approach to helping people with serious mental illness that relies on a triangular partnership of patient, family members, and involved mental health professionals. The model assumes that all of the "partners" have equally valid ideas and information to contribute to successful community adaptation, and it represents an alternative to the "medical model," which sees illness as an internal individual biological process that does not require attention to social context.

Paternal Bond: The degree to which an adult offspring feels attached, emotionally close, and bonded to his/her father.

Paternal Deprivation: An often overlooked form of child maltreatment most often characterized by a lack of attachment between a father and his child, emotional abandonment, indifference, failure to claim paternity, abuse, or neglect.

Paternal Involvement: The ways in which fathers are involved with their children in one-on-one activities, the degree to which they are accessible, and their level of responsibility for the care and well-being of their children.

Paternal Roles: The ways in which men carry out their roles as fathers. Major roles include breadwinner, gender role model, moral father, nurturer, and supporter of the mother.

Perceptions: Views about characteristics, based on personal prejudices, feelings, reactions and judgments. They are usually determined by race, gender, religion, socio-economic status, and other demographic and situational factors.

Performance Indicator: A specification of how well something—typically an organization—is performing. This is normally expressed as a ratio: for example, the percent of service recipients who report a certain level of satisfaction. Ratios allow meaningful comparison of groups with different sizes. Data for calculating indicators are derived from *measures*.

Performance Management: Incorporating measures of performance into management decisions on a regular, ongoing basis. A hospital manager may examine data monthly and notice after three months that one ward has lower rates of secondary infections than the others. This manager may then go and talk to the staff on the ward, find out what they are doing, then require other wards to replicate the practices.

Performance Measure/Indicator: A quantitative standard to describe performance. Usually a percentage, where the numerator represents actual performance and the denominator represents the entire population. The methodology for deriving and calculating quantitative results that may be used in a *performance measure*. Some indicators are derived from administrative data. Others may be derived from an instrument: for example, a survey that has been developed to determine consumers' perceptions regarding the quality of services they received. A multiquestion survey measure may yield one or more scores, depending upon design, and may reflect one or more *dimensions*.

Performance: The results an individual or organization accomplishes in their progression toward measurable objectives of desired/required results at the societal (*see Mega*), organizational (*see Macro*), and individual/team (*see Micro*) levels. Performance is measured by the value that is added or subtracted by the results accomplished by individuals and organizations, regardless of preferred or mandated behaviors.

Performance-Measurement Literacy: Performance measurement literacy refers to the capacity of individuals and organizations to obtain, interpret, and understand performance measurement information and the competence to use such information to benefit clients, service delivery, and the entire community.

Period Prevalence: Number of people with a disorder during the interval divided by the number of people at risk during the interval. Prevalence is the *incidence* of the disorder multiplied by the *duration* of the event.

Perpetrator: An abuser who engages in a harmful act toward an older adult when the act meets the criteria for a crime as defined by a state penal code. An *alleged* perpetrator is a perpetrator who has not been convicted of a crime by a court of law.

Personalism: The practitioner's intentional observance of informality in open displays of warmth toward a client rather than adoption of a more formal presentation. It is used as a means of engaging clients who can only feel comfortable with an informal relationship. Latino persons, for example, often value personalism in their relationships with professionals.

Pharmacotherapy: A form of treatment for obsessive-compulsive disorder involving the use of psychotropic medications. For OCD, the most effective medications are the serotonin reuptake inhibitors (SRIs). Although less is known about the exact mechanisms by which SRIs reduce OCD symptoms, one possibility is that they work by changing the way that neurotransmitters, such as serotonin, function in the brain.

Phase: The time lag between two locations of a particular band as defined by how soon after the beginning of an epoch a particular waveform at location #1 is matched in location #2.

Phenomenology: The systematic study of particular, unique states, conditions, or events for the purpose of understanding.

Phenomenologically Based Treatment: Treatment designed to assist in achieving particular goals unique to an individual condition or event that had been systematically studied.

Process: Continuing dynamic interactions over time related to achieving a specific set of goals or conditions.

Phenomenology: The systematic study of particular, unique states, conditions, or events for the purpose of understanding.

Placebo Effect: Reacting to an inert substance or a deliberately ineffective treatment as if it were a real drug or an effective treatment. (*See Hawthorne Effect* and *Blinding*.)

Plan, Do, Check, Act (PDCA) Cycle of Improvement: (Also known as the *Plan, Do, Study, Act* cycle of improvement.) W. Edwards Deming, founder of the *Total Quality Management* movement, developed the cycle to assist organizations in making changes to improve their performances. First, an organization *plans* what it wants to improve and how to improve it. It tests the improvement in a pilot phase in the *Do* cycle. During the *Check* cycle, it analyzes performance data to determine if the change resulted in an improvement. If an improvement was made, then the organization implements the change fully in the *Act* cycle. The cycle is continuous until optimal performance is reached.

Planning for the Future: Establishing group goals and strategies (and agreeing on credible evidence to monitor change over time to determine if the strategies are working).

POEMS (Patient Oriented Evidence That Matters): Searchable databases from the Journal of Family Practice. POEMS are searchable summaries similar to journal club article summaries in methodology and format, targeted to family practitioners.

Point Prevalence: Number of people with a disorder at a time divided by the number at risk. As the name implies, the point prevalence describes how many people have a disorder at a single point in time, in contrast to incidence, which describes cases over a longer time period. Prevalence is the *incidence* of the disorder multiplied by the *duration* of the event.

Population-Based Case-Control Studies: A type of epidemiological study that identifies all newly diagnosed cases of a specified disease that occur during a specified time period in a defined population. Controls are identified in a manner such that they are representative of the population that gave rise to the cases. Data related to the study hypothesis are collected from as many cases and controls as possible using personal interviews, medical record reviews, and/or biologic samples. The presence and/or degree of the hypothesized factor in cases are compared to the presence and/or degree of the same factor in controls.

Positive Paternal Emotional Responsiveness: The degree to which a father is understanding, warm, empathic, and nurturing to his children.

PQRS Objectives: A simple mnemonic device for remembering that objective statements should specify the *p*erformer who is expected to achieve the desired result, relevant *q*ualifying criteria should be delineated (typically by indicating the time frame over which the result is to be accomplished), the *r*esults (ends) to be accomplished, and the *s*tandards or conditions under which the result or performance will be demonstrated. Performance objectives never include how a result will be achieved.

Practice Evidence: Practitioners typically consider evidence of all sorts, direct and indirect, circumstantial, and even hearsay evidence when making practice decisions. Most classifications of evidence stress the likely reliability and validity of sources of evidence. Evidence derived from controlled research conducted in realistic practice contexts is typically given the most weight. Replication of such studies by independent investigators adds to the weight of the evidence. *See also Evidence-Based Practice* and *Evidence-Based Practice Guidelines.*

Practice Guidelines for Intervention: A set of systematically compiled and organized knowledge statements designed to enable practitioners to find, select, and use interventions that are most effective and appropriate for a given client, situation, and desired outcome.

Practice Theory: Explains behavior and suggests interventions to maintain or change it.

Pragmatism: A philosophy based in social democratic values and which avoids absolutes. It does not propose a total explanation of society but says that social values are enduring but manifested differently as social conditions change.

Prevalence (Period): The proportion of the population that has the outcome of interest within a specified time frame.

Prevalence (Point): The proportion of the population that has the outcome of interest at a specific point in time.

Primary Prevention: Prevention steps that reduce disease incidence; primary prevention is directed to susceptible persons before they have developed a disease. (Examples: vaccination for a variety of communicable diseases; smoking prevention)

Prison Prelease: Actions undertaken to prepare an offender for release into the community so that the chances of recidivating are reduced. Usually a minimum security program 30–90 days prior to release where the offender is transitioning through a social education program and participation in work-release.

Problem-Solving Training: Instructing couples on strategies they can use for managing problems that everyday life brings. Problem-solving involves the following steps: defining the problem; brainstorming; examining possible options; deciding on an option; implementing an option; and evaluating the implementation.

Process Evaluation: A determination of whether the intervention was carried out as planned, in terms of timing, service type and amount, participant eligibility, staff expertise, and so on. Process evaluations should also include an assessment of the micro- and macro-environments in which the intervention was delivered to investigate their intended and unintended effects. A process evaluation asks questions such as whether the program is being implemented as intended and whether it is reaching its target audience. Program evaluation studies conducted early in the program's development and characterized by informal types of research designs and data collection procedures such as collecting qualitative data while the program is in operation, use of agency reports, small surveys, and direct observation of the program. The purpose is to identify program targets, determine if the program fits its plan or design, and examine issues in program implementation. Applied research, which examines a program for pragmatic reasons, such as determining whether it accomplished its objectives or whether it is more efficient than comparable programs. In a nutshell, a study of the activities involved in the implementation of a program.

Process Measure: A gauge used to track the accuracy and effectiveness of implementation of a series of steps designed to achieve a certain result.

Professional Consensus: When referring to how practice guidelines or best practices are established, the term *professional consensus* refers to agreement achieved through a critical review by an authoritative group of professional experts in the review area. Typically, the review process includes a consideration of scientific evidence, collective practice experience, potential risks and benefits, relevance, problem or condition prevalence and burden, cost, and values.

Program Activities: Specific interventions that are undertaken to achieve the designated program results. Activities are "owned" by the agency offering services. For example, a program activity might include a two-hour group meeting to present and discuss contraceptives or the assignment of a volunteer to work 4 days per week with a student on homework assignments.

Program Budget: A fiscal plan that focuses on the activities of the organization and the expenditures allocated to support them.

Program Effectiveness: The extent to which program objectives have been achieved.

Program Improvement Plan: A plan designed by the program stakeholders, which considers the needs of all constituents, key information needs, and resources available to the agency. It is a collaborative effort whereby key stakeholders are engaged in a process of designing, implementing, and evaluating a program innovation for its impact on program outcome.

Program Monitoring: Evaluation studies that focus on how the program is being implemented. Questions answered in monitoring studies include: Is the program reaching its intended audience? Who is being served? What changes have been made in the program? What are the program's initial effects? Monitoring studies frequently use management information system data, available data about the program, and informal surveys about the program.

Program Results: Shorter-term outcomes for program clients or participants that result from successful interventions. These results usually represent a change in knowledge, attitudes, or behavior in the client. For example, an agency program result could include an increase in awareness of contraceptives or a higher rate of homework completion among participants.

Program Stakeholders: The group of people who are responsible for or play an important role in the administration, implementation, or consumption of services. Depending upon program structure, this group could include administrators, board members, funders, social workers, community members, and clients. Ultimately, this group must include workers and clients.

Proportional Mortality Rate (PMR): The proportion of all deaths that are due to the disorder of interest.

Prospective Study: A study in which the data are collected after the start of the study and the participants are followed forward in time.

Protective Factors: Circumstances that moderate or mediate the effects of risks and enhance adaptation. Risk factors and protective processes exist and interact on a variety of levels with individual, familial, societal, or cultural manifestations.

Psychoanalysis: An old-fashioned approach to psychology that emphasizes unconscious motives and conflicts and is based on the works of Sigmund Freud. It encompasses both a theory of personality and a method of long-term psychotherapy.

Psychoanalytic Method: In psychoanalytic therapy, the effort to bring unconscious material into consciousness, often through dream recall and free association.

Psychodynamic Theory: Four major schools of thought are encompassed by psychodynamic theory: object relations, self-psychology, drive theory, and ego psychology. In psychodynamic therapy, the patient (as opposed to the client in other types of therapy) talks, during this process the therapist acts to facilitate the discovery process providing interpretations about the patient's words and behaviors. Psychodynamic therapy may include dream analysis as a function of the therapeutic process. As with other types of therapy, some psychodynamic therapists may utilize other methods of therapy such as cognitive-behavioral techniques for specific problems.

Psychoeducation: A model for combining education with therapeutic input when dealing with problems of emotional management of an illness. It was developed as a method of engaging participants who might not otherwise commit to psychotherapy. Generally facilitated by a mental health professional, it is usually provided on a time-limited basis, and frequently in a group or multifamily context, as a way of promoting group interaction or self-help support.

Psychometric Measurement Tool: A standard way of assessing a particular aspect of human behavior. Raw scores are converted into standard scores so that statements can be made about one score as compared to the mean score. Reliability and validity are critical concepts in the development of psychometric tools.

Psychometry: The science of testing and measuring mental and psychologic ability, efficiency potentials, and functioning, including psychopathy components.

Psychopharmacology: The management of psychiatric illness using medication such as antidepressants, antipsychotics, anti-anxiety medications and more.

Psychotherapy: The treatment of mental disorders, emotional problems, and personality difficulties through talking with a therapist. There are dozens of different approaches to psychotherapy; frequently therapists choose methods based upon individual responsiveness or strengths related to a particular approach.

Q fever: A zoonosis caused by the bacterium *Coxiella burnetii*. People become infected mainly by inhaling aerosols generated during parturition of contaminated animals. In French Guiana, an administrative French unit located between Suriname and Brazil, Q fever incidence has significantly increased since 1996. Presently, this original epidemic remains an enigma because the reservoir responsible for transmission has not yet been identified. Several facts make this epidemic different from the usual case: first, it occurs in the Cayenne region, the main urban area of the country, although Q fever is considered a rural disease. On the other hand, many facts strengthen the hypothesis of there being a wild reservoir whereas it is usually constituted by domestic ungulates.

Qualitative Data: Any information that is not numerical or quantitative in nature. Qualitative data are often obtained from in-depth interviews, direct observation of behavior, and examination of written documents.

Qualitative Research: A branch of research that is viewed as naturalistic and encompasses a range of methods that, broadly defined, describes and provides insights into naturally occurring phenomena and everyday experiences, and the meanings associated with those phenomena and experiences.

Quality Assurance (QA): A process or set of activities to maintain and improve the level of care provided to patients. (also known as quality improvement, or QI). These activities may include review, formal measurements, and corrective actions. The QA/QI function is a standard part of health insurance plans and all institutional health care providers. Managed care often demands that providers present QA/QI findings to the sponsoring plans, especially data on the outcome of care. In the era of managed care, it has become critical to demonstrate effective outcomes in measurable terms.

Quality Enhancement Research Initiative (QUERI): A large-scale initiative funded by the Veterans Administration Health Services Research and Development Service. QUERI's goal is to improve quality of care and outcomes for patients suffering from eight prevalent chronic illnesses, including substance use disorders, through the implementation of evidence-based practice guidelines.

Quality Improvement: Enhancement of products and/or services to obtain optimal levels of efficiency, effectiveness, and overall performance. Total quality management, an organization-wide approach geared to achieving better results by constantly making improvements in processes and performance.

Quantitative research: A type of research that tests well-specified hypotheses concerning predetermined variables. It gathers information in numeric form and produces findings by statistical procedures or other means of quantification. It aims to answer questions such as whether or how much. Examples include whether cancer mortality rates are higher in different immigrant populations; what proportion of older adults in the U.S. has chronic illnesses such as diabetes.

Quasi-experimental designs: Experimental designs in which people are not randomly assigned to different forms of the program. Quasi-experimental designs can compare different forms of the program that naturally occur or can use procedures such as matching or waiting lists to form quasi-control or comparison groups.

Questioning route: A questioning route is the set of questions developed for the focus groups. These questions are distinctive in that they are carefully sequenced or focused to lead the discussion into the areas of greatest importance to the researcher. In a two-hour focus group the questioning route might consist of about a dozen questions.

Quit rate (ratio): The proportion of smokers who quit smoking during a specified time period; many more smokers attempt to quit than actually achieve the goal of quitting.

Random Digit Dialing (RDD): A technique used to generate and call random telephone numbers. If properly executed, RDD can be used to identify a sample of households or individuals that is representative of all households/individuals with residential telephones in a designated geographic area.

Randomized Control Trials (RCT): A type of research design, also called experimental design, in which participants (subjects) are randomly assigned to a control (no treatment or treatment as usual) condition or to an experimental condition. The purpose of an RCT is to minimize biases, which may compromise, confound, or obscure the results of research contrasting the treatment with the control condition. The purpose of random assignment is to test the counter-factual—that is, what would the outcome be for the treatment group if they had not participated in the treatment?

Randomized Controlled Clinical Trial: A group of patients is randomized into an experimental group and a control group. These groups are followed up for the variables / outcomes of interest. *See also glossary of study designs.*

Randomized Controlled Study (RCT): A research design, also called an *experiment,* in which participants are randomly assigned to receive a specific intervention or to be in a control group.

Randomized Field Experiment: An explanatory research study conducted in a naturalistic setting in which subjects are randomly assigned

to intervention conditions. To enhance external validity, subjects are often randomly selected from a larger population. The experimental independent variable (e.g., an intervention) is actively manipulated by the researchers such as by randomly assigning active or placebo conditions to subjects. (Ideally subjects are not aware of which condition they are exposed to, e.g., an active treatment or a placebo, and information is gathered pertaining to the dependent variable in a manner that is blind to which condition the subject has experienced.)

Rapid Assessment Instruments (RAI): RAIs provide a brief standardized format for gathering information about clients. These instruments are scales, checklists, and questionnaires that are relatively brief, often less than 50 items, and easy to score and interpret. RAIs have established psychometrics and, thus, reliably and validly ascertain traits of an individual in terms of its frequency, intensity, or duration. Such instruments are useful for determining the nature and/or extent of specific behaviors, assessing the presence of psychiatric disorders, or monitoring client progress and evaluating treatment effectiveness.

Reassurance-Seeking: A pattern of negative communication typical of people with depression in which they request excessive reassurance from their partners, leading to rejection and dissatisfaction.

Receiver Operating Character Analysis (ROC): A nonparametric test that identifies the ability of a measure to determine presence or absence of a particular trait.

Recidivism: Recurrence of criminal activity in an offender. Recidivism rate refers to the general rate of re-offense in a particular group of offenders during a specified time period. For example, re-arrest, technical parole violation, or reconviction rate twelve months post-release from prison.

Regression toward the Mean: The phenomenon whereby people who are selected for a study because their score on some measure is significantly above (or below) the mean will, on retesting, have scores closer to the mean. This will occur simply because of the unreliability of the measure, and not because of the effectiveness of any treatment that may have been given between the two testing periods.

Relative Power: The relative magnitude of a band (absolute magnitude of the particular band divided by the total microvolt generated at a particular location by all bands).

Relative Risk Reduction (RRR): The percent reduction in events in the treated group event rate (EER) compared to the control group event rate (CER): RRR = (CER − EER) / CER * 100

Relaxation Training: A behavioral intervention in which the practitioner helps a client learn and master one or several exercises for physiological anxiety reduction. Common methods include deep breathing, progressive muscle relaxation, and imagery construction. All of these methods generally require practice by the client prior to mastery.

Reliability: The extent to which research/evaluation measures produce replicable and consistent results. Reliability is most commonly assessed between raters (inter-rater reliability), over time (test-retest reliability), or in terms of the internal consistency of a measure (e.g., split-half reliability, inter-item correlations, item-total correlations).

This concept relates to the consistency of a measure to yield the same results over multiple measures. It is assessed through test-retest reliability, alternate form reliability, split-half reliability, and internal consistency reliability. Reliability is especially important for tools used in making clinical assessments and practice decisions. When a scale is reliable, you get the same results every time. When using the term to describe a measure, it means the same thing. If the measure is a good measure, then each time you test it in the same way, you should get the same result. For example, let's say that you are a SCUBA diver. You take out your air gauge and measure that you've got 21% oxygen in your tank (that's good; it mirrors the percent of oxygen in the air we breathe). Then you immediately test the tank again with the same gauge and find that it reads 5% oxygen (that's a one-way track to brain damage). Do you go diving with the tank? Chances are you would opt to find a reliable gauge and measure again. An unreliable measure makes the data untrustworthy. In summary, reliability refers to the quality of an item, scale, or instrument that focuses on how consistently it collects information across time from the same respondents, or across raters. A commonly reported type of reliability is internal consistency reliability, which assesses the intercorrelations among the scale indicators used to measure a latent construct.

Reliability (Inter-Rater): The degree to which two people, observing the same behavior, give similar scores on a scale.

Reliability Test-Retest: The degree to which a scale, given at two times, yields similar results (assuming that the person has not changed in the interim).

Remote Sensing: Process of acquiring information about an object from a distance. This broad definition includes Earth observations using airborne and spaceborne sensors, which measure the electromagnetic radiation reflected or radiated from the Earth's surface and store the measurements in 2D images. There is a wide range of remote sensing sensors, which provide information about sea and land surfaces. Distinctions are usually made between passive (which responds to the natural radiation incident on the instrument) and active (which generates its own radiation and measures the reflected signal) sensors; between high spatial resolution (resolution <100 m) and low spatial resolution (resolution around 1 km) sensors; between imaging and non-imaging instruments. Remote sensing systems can also be categorized according to the range of wavelengths in which they are operating: visible and near-infrared sensors, thermal-infrared sensors, microwave sensors.

Research: Scientific inquiry using the scientific method or an organized quest for new knowledge and better understanding, such as of the natural world or determinants of health and disease. Research can take several forms: empiric (observational), analytic, experimental, theoretical, and applied.

Resilience: The capability of individuals to cope successfully in the face of significant change, adversity, or risk. This capability changes over time and is enhanced by protective factors in the individual and environment. Resilience is influenced by diversity. It is expressed and affected by multilevel attachments, both distal and proximal, including family, school, peers, neighborhood, community, and society. In addition, it is affected by the availability of environmental resources.

Resiliency: Factors that are present in the lives of families and children that may offset the risks facing those families and children and help produce better outcomes for them.

Response Bias: A specific type of selection bias. It occurs when relevant characteristics of respondents who participate in a study differ from those who do not participate. Response bias is more likely to introduce error into study results if the proportion of eligible persons who are included in the study is low.

Response Prevention: A behavior therapy technique in which the patient refrains from acting on urges to perform compulsive behaviors. Response prevention is typically used along with exposure in the treatment of obsessive-compulsive disorder.

Results-Based Accountability: Program oversight that includes resource and output monitoring but emphasizes performance measures to evaluate how well programs achieve desired outcomes and impacts.

Results Management: A planning and resource allocation strategy for achieving client or participant outcomes through designing and managing program operations with a clear focus toward achieving targeted results. Program results for clients are actively monitored and used to make adjustments in program interventions and to allocate program resources.

Retrospective Study: One in which the data exist before the start of the study, as in administrative or clinical databases.

Risk: A psychosocial adversity or event that would be considered a stressor to most people and that may hinder normal functioning. Risk is understood as a dynamic process rather than a causal mechanistic one. A confounding factor causally related to the outcome under study.

Risk Assessment: Methods of determining adverse factors or events that hinder normal functioning in a particular area, such as alcohol use. Quantitative methods are used to ascertain empirical factors and qualitative methods are valuable in gaining insight into the complexity and interrelationships of these factors.

Risk-Adjustment: The process of accounting for pertinent patient characteristics before making inferences about the effectiveness of care.

Risk Factor: An aspect of personal behavior or lifestyle, environmental exposure, or inborn or inherited characteristic, which on the basis of epidemiological evidence is known to be associated with an unfavorable health-related condition and considered important to prevent, if possible. It is used as an indication of increased probability of

a specified health outcome such as the occurrence of a disease but is not necessarily a causal factor. The term risk factor is further used to mean a determinant that can be modified by intervention, thereby reducing the probability of occurrence of disease or other specified outcomes.

Risk Ratio is the ratio of risk in the treated group (EER) to the risk in the control group (CER): RR = EER/CER. RR is used in randomized trials and cohort studies.

Root Cause: A factor that, if changed or removed, will permanently eliminate a nonconformance. Common to quality review process seeking to find the contributing factor to issues in service delivery.

Sample (Haphazard): A study group chosen simply on the basis of the availability of people (e.g., those who pass by a booth at a mall, or students in a class).

Sample (Random): A study group selected in such a way that everyone in the population has the same probability of being chosen.

Sample (Stratified): A study group chosen so that people are selected from different strata (e.g., by age, gender, social class). This is done either to ensure that there are a sufficient number of people in each stratum, or to ensure that the demographic characteristics of the final sample match that of the population.

Scenario: The presentation of case examples to reflect real life dilemmas of police decision-making. They allow an assessment of whether respondents are giving consistent answers by creating simulated situations and make it easier for respondents to understand the context of each encounter, so they can respond to the questions in the way they really believe they would if actually presented with the exact same encounter on the streets.

Scholar Practitioner: The term scholar practitioner expresses an ideal of professional excellence grounded in theory and research, informed by experiential knowledge and motivated by personal values, political commitments and ethical conduct. Scholar practitioners are committed to the well-being of clients and colleagues, to learning new ways of being effective, and to conceptualizing their work in relation to broader organizational, community, political, and cultural contexts. Scholar practitioners explicitly reflect upon and assess the impact of their work. Their professional activities and the knowledge they develop are based on collaborative and relational learning through active exchange within communities of practice and scholarship. Related concepts include reflective practice and wisdom.

Screens: People are selected and invited to a focus group interview because they have certain experiences or qualities in common. These criteria or qualifications are called screens. The screens could be social, demographic, geographic or the extent of exposure or use of a program or product. The screens ensure that those attending the focus groups have the characteristics or experiences that are of interest to the researcher. *See also Focus Groups.*

Secondary Data Analysis: This process involves the utilization of existing data, collected for the purposes of a prior study or quality improvement process in order to pursue a research interest that is distinct from that of the original work.

Secondary Prevention: Prevention steps used for early detection and treatment; secondary prevention is directed to asymptomatic persons who have developed biologic changes from a disease. Examples: mammography; Papanicoulaou (pap) tests

Second-Level Coding: The second step in the coding of qualitative data, where researchers identify conceptually distinct subcategories within larger conceptual categories that were identified in first-level coding. *See also Qualitative Research.*

Selection Bias: Occurs when the individuals (or units) included in a study are not representative of the population of interest. Selection bias is a result of flawed selection procedures and can threaten study validity.

Self-Efficacy: One's perceived capacity to meet some challenge or perform a particular response. An individual's beliefs that particular behaviors will produce the desired outcome and the confidence in his/her ability to perform the essential tasks involved in a particular behavior.

Self-Instruction Training: A cognitive intervention technique that is intended to increase the client's control over behavior by improving the quality of his or her internal, self-directed speech. The technique assumes that many behaviors are mediated by internal, self-directed speech, and negative cues or an absence of positive cues may characterize a client's self-

dialogue. The practitioner assesses the client's behavior and its relationship to deficits in sub-vocal dialogue, models more adaptive behavior, demonstrates how overt self-directed speech can be used to guide behavior, helps the client to rehearse new self-talk and behaviors, and helps the client make plans to risk more adaptive behavior while using covert self-directed speech.

Self Object: An individual's subjective psychological experience of an important relationship.

Self Object Functions: Empathic psychological responses that support the emerging sense of self in the child. They include mirroring, idealizing, and twinship.

Self-Psychology: A theory of how the self-structure of a person develops.

Self-Report Measure: A pen-and-pencil measurement tool designed to be completed by the client in order to measure his or her own attitudes, feelings, or behaviors.

Sense of Community: Feelings of connectedness to the physical characteristics and/or the social groups within the environment.

Sensitivity: A measure of the ability of any test to identify individuals with a selected trait. In other words, sensitivity gives us the proportion of cases picked out by the test, relative to all cases in which individuals actually have the disease. *Specificity* is the ability of the test to pick out individuals who do *not* have the selected trait. Results are reported in terms of an AUC.

Sentinel Events: Those events/incidents that the Joint Commission on Accreditation of Healthcare Organizations defines as reportable Sentinel Events (e.g., suicide, loss of limb or function, rape).

Sexual Predator: This is not a psychiatric term but rather has been defined by law. The Washington State law defines a sexual predator as anyone who seeks a relationship with another solely for the purposes of sexual assault.

Single-Subject Design: The structure for studying a single unit such as one person, one family, or one organization over time is called a single-subject design. Such designs typically require the researcher to clearly identify specific interventions to be studied, operational specification of measurable outcomes or dependent variables, and establishment of a baseline rate followed by measurement of rates following the intervention.

Situation Analysis: Any process of estimating how institutional policies and actions influence the state of the neighboring universe. Examination of the current reality of the organization utilizing statistical analysis rather than speculation to assess current status.

Short-Term Abuse: Victimization occurs one to three times during a relatively short time period of a day to several months. The abuse victim is usually in a dating relationship and breaks the relationship off permanently with the help of parents or older siblings after a few pushes, slaps, or punches.

Skill: The ability to perform a task well, usually gained by training or experience; a systematic and coordinated pattern of mental and/or physical activity.

Slot Zone: A specified area on the casino floor that contains one or more slot machines.

Snowball Sampling: This is a method to locate hidden groups such as drug abusers, incest survivors, and/or wealthy battered women who usually have no contacts with formal agencies and social institutions (e.g., hospital, police department, or prosecutor's office).

Social Environment: Collective processes in the neighborhoods, schools, families, and peer systems of children that organize, facilitate, and constrain their behavior over time.

Social Interventions: A blend of formal services and informal supports that is created with the intention of improving outcomes for a family, or the children in a family, and entails the combined efforts of professional service providers, paraprofessionals, friends, and family members.

Social Network: These are people who interact with each other on a regular basis. A social network is likely to include relatives, neighbors, coworkers, and members of one's church or faith organization. It is difficult to determine where a social network ends, particularly when considering network ties that are weak (i.e., remote acquaintances).

Social Phobia: Persistent anxiety surrounding social and/or performance situations. Symptoms are usually based in a fear of embarrassment. Social phobias often drive sufferers into self-imposed isolation resulting in dropping out of school, the tendency to avoid making friends, or job loss. Feelings induced by public speaking can provide insight into the types of issues faced by persons with social phobia when engaging in day-to-day functions such as meeting new people, going to parties, and going to school or work. *See also Anxiety Disorders.*

Social Policy: The statement of what is or should be in relation to meeting the needs of members of society.

Social Services: The help provided by the network of public and private agencies that serve the community's needs in relation to health and welfare.

Social Survey: Collection of data for the purpose of developing information to solve a specific problem. Technical criteria for collecting and handling data are the same as for hypothesis testing research.

Somatization: A process whereby psychological distress manifests as symptoms of physical illness. Specifically, it refers to complaints about or the manifestation of physical symptoms such as headaches, stomach aches, sleep problems, fatigue, and loss of concentration that have a psychological origin.

Soup Kitchen: A place where hungry people can obtain a free meal. Usually sponsored by religious organizations.

Space-Borne Remote Sensing: Process of acquiring information about the Earth by a space-borne sensor. Satellite remote sensing dates back to the early 70's, when images provided by space-borne sensors began to be used for environmental monitoring, either with wide field (e.g., NOAA AVHRR) or medium to high resolution (Landsat TM). Nowadays, wide field sensors, with resolution around 1 km have generally been designed for specific application, e.g. SeaWiFS or MeRIS for ocean colour, AATSR for sea surface temperature, or SPOT-Vegetation for biosphere monitoring. High-resolution sensors have reached performances comparable to those classically obtained with airborne sensors, i.e., resolution of 1–3 m (SPOT-5, IKONOS, QuickBird).

Special Cause Variation: A shift in output caused by a specific factor—for example, environmental conditions or process input parameters. It can be accounted for directly and potentially removed and is a measure of process control. Unlike common cause variability, special cause variation is based in known factors that result in a nonrandom distribution of output frequently referred to as "exceptional" or "assignable" variation.

Split-Half Reliability: The split-half method consists of administering one form of a scale to a group of subjects. Half of the items are used to compute one total score, and the other half to compute a second total score. To the extent that the two halves correlate, split-half reliability is established.

Stakeholder: People who will be affected by the project or can influence it but who are not directly involved with doing the project work. Examples are managers affected by the project, practitioners, who work with the process under study, and departments or businesses that support the process, e.g., suppliers, environmental management, and financial departments.

Standard: Refers to a model, example, or rule for the measure of quantity, weight, extent, value, or quality, established by authority, custom or general consent. It is also defined as a criterion, gauge, or yardstick by which judgments or decisions may be made. A meaningful standard should offer a realistic prospect of determining whether or not one actually meets it.

Standard Deviation: A statistical process to determine the expected range of responses for a particular set of collected data. Those responses that fall outside of the normal standard deviation become outliers and deserve particular attention.

Standardized Mortality Rate: Multiply the *Age-Specific Mortality Rate* by the proportion of people of a given age (compared to the rest of the general population across the United States, for example) and add up the results across the strata. The result is the mortality rate, standardized to the comparison group. This allows you to age-adjust mortality rates for a given disease and compare them to other, more general populations.

Statistical Significance: The observation of a statistical value that exceeds the explicitly stated limit of values that might occur by random chance. In most social science applications a statistical observation is considered statistically significant if its probability of occurrence simply by random chance is less than .05. The most straightforward example of this is a difference in means on a depression scale between two groups exposed to two different treatment conditions, where a difference in means is of sufficient magnitude to justify a conclusion that the observed difference is not due to random chance (i.e., random variation of the depression scale that is unrelated to the treatment conditions). Under such circumstances, it may be reasonable for the researcher to conclude that the difference in means is influenced by the difference in treatment conditions. It should be emphasized, however, that statistical significance is not proof but rather a statistical justification for the rejection of random chance as an explanation for the observed difference in means.

Strategic Planning: The process of determining an organization's long-term goals and then applying statistical analysis, review of best practice, and evidence-based approaches for identifying the best approach for achieving those goals.

Stress-Diathesis Theory: Based on the biopsychosocial model of understanding the functioning of the individual in a social context, this theory proposes that many people have a genetic or biological "weak link" or vulnerability (diathesis), which is the part of the organism that will break down first under stressful conditions. The theory advocates attention to those elements in the social context that put stress on that particular vulnerability.

Subjective Units of Disturbance (SUDS): Client self-report measure of the feelings and emotions associated with the trauma image on a scale from 0 to 7, with 7 being the most severe. The scale is done pre- and post-test for each counseling session to evaluate changes in those emotions and feelings.

Substance Abuse: Ingesting on a regular basis illegal chemical agents that alter perception, coordination, and mental and/or physical state and interfere with behaviors necessary for maintaining a healthy and prosocial lifestyle.

Suicidality: Refers to the degree and intensity of a person's desire to attempt to kill himself or herself. This includes suicidal ideas, thoughts, threats, and gestures and suicidal attempts. *See also Chronic Suicidality.*

Suicide Intent: The intensity and pervasiveness of one's wish to die.

Support Factors: Therapeutic interactions between therapist and client or patient, including therapeutic alliance, catharsis, and therapist warmth.

Surrogate End Point: A dependent variable that is measured rather than the outcome of interest (e.g., scores on a scale of proneness to suicide, rather than suicidal attempts themselves). This is usually done because the outcome of interest is either too difficult to measure directly or occurs too rarely.

Sustainable Execution: An extended period of time in which demonstration of sustained impact is documented with causation being assigned to the implementation of specific, well documented and defined strategic planning.

Symbolic Interaction: A social theory that says humans base their responses to what others do by taking account of their expectations and what they expect of themselves.

Systematic Critical Reviews: Reviews of research in a given area and/or on a given topic that are conducted according to an explicit, pre-established methodology, and which can be criticized and replicated.

Systematic Review: The process of searching for, recording, analyzing, and interpreting the evidence emanating from all valid research studies addressed to a specific question, using explicit criteria and methods, is called a systematic review. Sometimes systematic reviews use a quantitative method, meta-analysis, to analyze the data provided by the studies reviewed. Systematic reviews are often conducted by groups of researchers expert in the specific area examined. Also, the summary report of this process is called a systematic review. The process of retrieving and synthesizing empirical results in order to establish quantitative findings of the effects of an intervention.

Systems Theory: Evolved from the physical sciences as a method of analyzing complex interactions in closed systems. In family therapy, the behaviors of people cannot be understood without looking at the social system in which they live. The whole is greater than the individual parts.

Taking Stock: The prioritization of key activities a group will assess, the actual assessment of the activities on a 1 to 10 scale, and a dialogue about the ratings.

Target Results: These are longer-term outcomes toward which program activities and interventions are directed. These results are directly influenced by the interventions but are "owned" by the client or participant or community. Thus, the program cannot take full credit for their achievement or full blame if they

are not achieved. For example, a program may have a target result of lowering the dropout rate or teenage pregnancy rate in a community.

Tests of Significance: *See Statistical Significance.*

The Point-Counterpoint Technique: A cognitive intervention method for helping a client to challenge thinking patterns that are the source of his or her maladaptive emotional responses. The practitioner and client "argue" both sides of a client's arbitrary belief in a role-play. After a specified amount of time they switch roles and repeat the process. The client is thus forced to argue both sides of an issue, which is often helpful to his or her analyzing its validity and considering alternative thoughts.

Thanatology: The study of death and of actions and reactions associated with death.

Theory of Explanation: A theory that seeks to explain the cause of a problem.

Theory of Intervention: A theory that seeks to provide direction for intervening to solve a problem.

Theory: A proposition, perspective, or conceptual framework for interpreting data. A series of related hypotheses.

Therapeutic Alliance: According to L. Bickman, therapeutic alliance has generally been conceptualized as an agreement on tasks and goals between the client and the therapist, and a clients' affective bond with the therapist. Therapeutic alliance is recognized as one of the common factors related to therapeutic efficacy and effectiveness.

Theta: A frequency range in the EEG, defined as 4-8 Hertz per second.

Thought Stopping: A process of helping a client to eliminate an unwanted thought. The client is taught to concentrate on an unwanted thought and, after a short time, suddenly interrupt the thought with a vocal or subvocal command, some other loud noise, or some type of sensory jolt. The command serves as a punishment and thus inhibits the unwanted thinking behavior. The client can follow thought stopping with thought substitutions or reassuring, self-accepting statements.

Tolerance: A characteristic of substance dependence that may be shown by the need for markedly increased amounts of the substance to achieve intoxication or the desired effect, by markedly diminished effect with continued use of the same amount of the substance, or by adequate functioning despite doses or blood levels of the substance that would be expected to produce significant impairment in a casual user.

Toxicology: The branch of science concerned with the nature, effects, and detection of poisons and toxic substances.

Transportability: Transportability research examines the movement of efficacious interventions to usual direct care settings. This research examines not only the components of an intervention, but who is able to conduct the intervention and under what circumstances they can conduct it.

Trauma: This often be characterized by intrusive thoughts, bad dreams, nightmares, flashbacks, and psychological disequilibrium. Traumatic experiences involve the actual or threat of death, serious injury, or loss of physical integrity to which the person responds with fear, helplessness, or horror.

Treatment Effectiveness: Deals with issues of validity, specifically addressing whether a particular treatment works or not. Treatment effectiveness studies seek to increase understanding of the impact of a particular intervention assuring that said intervention is responsible for the identified impact.

Treatment Efficiency: Encompasses several aspects of accountability, effectiveness, efficiency, and effect. The focus is on more than a single intervention, asking the question Does more than one intervention provide an advantage for impact and change?

Treatment Manuals: Written instructions to practitioners on how to implement a particular treatment, specifying the components, dosage, and ordering of the practice approach.

Trend Lines: The establishment of the same information measured over a period of time with the intent to measure movement in a positive or negative direction over that period of time.

Type III error: First proposed in 1968 by statistician Howard Raiffa, type III error involves giving a precise answer to the wrong question, i.e., errors in question formulation or conceptualization of the problem, rather than statistical error.

Validity: The extent to which a measurement tool accurately measures a specified concept. There are four types of validity: content validity, criterion validity, construct validity, and factorial analysis. The type of validity that should be assessed depends on the measure being used and the measure's intended use. The extent to which data collection actually measures the construct of concern, also referred to as the accuracy of the measure. Measures may be reliable but not valid; however, reliability is a precondition of validity. Validity is assessed in numerous ways. All validation studies attempt to determine whether a measure reflects the "true" situation; for example, by examining correlations with expert opinions, established measures, current state, or eventual outcome. A scale or questionnaire is valid if you are measuring what you think you are measuring. For example, many of the intelligence tests done at Ellis Island on immigrants were not valid: they purported to measure intelligence when in fact they measured the ability to speak English. If you couldn't speak English, you did not pass. Validity is tricky because it is difficult to prove; how do we really know we are measuring what we want and nothing else? In summary, validity refers to a quality of an item, scale, or instrument that focuses on how well it measures the concept it is intended to measure.

Validity (Construct): Determining what a test is measuring through a process of hypothesis testing.

Validity (Content): Ensuring that all of the items in a scale pertain to the construct of interest (content relevance), and that all aspects of the construct are tapped by a sufficient number of items (content coverage).

Validity (Criterion): The degree to which one scale correlates with other measures of the same attribute. The other measures can be given at the same time (concurrent validity) or can be an outcome observable only at some time in the future (predictive validity).

Validity of Cognition (VOC): Client self-report measure of the validity of the cognition associated with the trauma, ranked on a scale 0–7, with 7 feeling the most true to the client. The scale is done pre- and post-test for each counseling session to evaluate changes in the cognition and during the installation phase to evaluate the desired cognition(s).

Variance: The variation in the values for a given variable.

Visual Analog Scale (VAS): A scale consisting of a 10 cm line, along which the respondent places a mark to indicate the amount of the attribute (e.g., pain) that he or she has.

Volunteer Bias: People who agree to be part of a study differ from those who refuse to participate. They are generally older, more likely to be married, working, and healthier.

Wisdom: Added to knowledge when internal data and external evidence is integrated with considerations of preference, values, and costs to determine whether and how the primary intervention should have been performed in the first place. Wisdom is also referred to as practice wisdom.

Woman Battering Continuum: A range of levels of the magnitude of woman battering based on the duration, severity, and frequency of battering incidents. Also taken into account is the psychosocial and demographic pattern of variables common to each of the levels. *See also Abuser, Domestic Violence Continuum, Elder Abuse, Short Term Abuse,* and *Chronic Battering.*

INDEX OF NAMES

SUBJECT INDEX